Supportive Oncology

Supportive Oncology

Mellar P. Davis MD, FCCP

Professor of Medicine
Cleveland Clinic Lerner School of Medicine
Case Western Reserve University
Clinical Fellowship Director
Palliative Medicine and Supportive Oncology Services
Division of Solid Tumor
Taussig Cancer Institute
Cleveland Clinic Foundation
Cleveland, Ohio

Petra Ch. Feyer MD, PhD

Professor of Radiation Oncology
Director, Clinic of Radiation Oncology
Vivantes Clinics Berlin Neukoelln
Berlin, Germany

Petra Ortner PharmD, PhD

German Supportive Care in Cancer Group (ASORS)
POMME-med Medical Communication
Munich, Germany

Camilla Zimmermann MD, PhD, FRCPC

Head, Palliative Care Program
Medical Director
Lederman Palliative Care Centre
Department of Psychosocial Oncology and Palliative Care
Princess Margaret Hospital
Associate Professor of Medicine
Division of Medical Oncology and Hematology
University of Toronto
Scientist, Campbell Family Cancer Research Institute
Ontario Cancer Institute
Toronto, Ontario, Canada

ELSEVIER
SAUNDERS

ELSEVIER
SAUNDERS

1600 John F. Kennedy Blvd.
Ste. 1800
Philadelphia, PA 19103-2899

SUPPORTIVE ONCOLOGY   ISBN: 978-1-4377-1015-1

Notices

Knowledge and best practice in this field are constantly changing. As new research and experience
broaden our understanding, changes in research methods, professional practices, or medical treatment may
become necessary.

Practitioners and researchers must always rely on their own experience and knowledge in evaluating
and using any information, methods, compounds, or experiments described herein. In using such
information or methods they should be mindful of their own safety and the safety of others, including
parties for whom they have a professional responsibility.

With respect to any drug or pharmaceutical products identified, readers are advised to check the most
current information provided (i) on procedures featured or (ii) by the manufacturer of each product to be
administered, to verify the recommended dose or formula, the method and duration of administration, and
contraindications. It is the responsibility of practitioners, relying on their own experience and knowledge
of their patients, to make diagnoses, to determine dosages and the best treatment for each individual
patient, and to take all appropriate safety precautions.

To the fullest extent of the law, neither the Publisher nor the authors, contributors, or editors, assume
any liability for any injury and/or damage to persons or property as a matter of products liability,
negligence or otherwise, or from any use or operation of any methods, products, instructions, or ideas
contained in the material herein.

International Standard Book Number

978-1-4377-1015-1

Acquisitions Editor: Pamela Hetherington
Publishing Services Manager: Patricia Tannian
Team Manager: Radhika Pallamparthy
Senior Project Manager: Claire Kramer
Project Manager: Jayavel Radhakrishnan
Designer: Louis Forgione

Working together to grow
libraries in developing countries

www.elsevier.com | www.bookaid.org | www.sabre.org

ELSEVIER   **BOOK AID**
International   Sabre Foundation

Printed in the United States of America

Last digit is the print number: 9   8   7   6   5   4   3   2   1

We dedicate this book to our families in gratitude for their love and support:

To my wife, Deborah, and my children Luke, Amanda, Meghan, Jessamyn, Emelin, and Lilian—Mellar Davis

To Otto Josef — Petra Feyer

To my daughter, Eva, and to my mother, Rose-Marie—Petra Ortner

To my husband, Richard, and my children, Erica, Hendrik, and Karl—Camilla Zimmermann

Contributors

Amy P. Abernethy, MD
Associate Professor of Medicine
Division of Medical Oncology
Department of Medicine
Duke University School of Medicine
Director
Duke Cancer Care Research Program
Duke University Medical Center
Durham, North Carolina

Douglas G. Adler, MD
Associate Professor of Medicine
Director of Therapeutic Endoscopy
Gastroenterology and Hepatology
University of Utah School of Medicine
Huntsman Cancer Center
Salt Lake City, Utah

Yesne Alici, MD
Attending Psychiatrist
Geriatric Services Unit
Central Regional Hospital
Butner, North Carolina

Eugene Balagula, MD
Clinical Research Fellow
Department of Dermatology
Memorial Sloan-Kettering Cancer Center
New York, New York

Ani Balmanoukian, MD
Johns Hopkins Hospital
Baltimore, Maryland

Nikhil Banerjee, MD
University of Utah
Salt Lake City, Utah

Gerhild Becker, MD, MSc
Palliative Care
King's College London
London, United Kingdom
Assistant Medical Director
Palliative Care Unit
University Medical Center Freiburg
Freiburg, Germany

Virginia Boquiren, MSc
Doctoral Fellow
Psychosocial Oncology and Palliative Care
Princess Margaret Hospital
University Health Network
Toronto, Ontario, Canada

Julie R. Brahmer, MD, MSc
Sidney Kimmel Comprehensive Cancer Center
  at Johns Hopkins
Baltimore, Maryland

William Breitbart, MD
Chief, Psychiatry Service
Vice Chairman
Department of Psychiatry and Behavioral
  Sciences
Memorial Sloan-Kettering Cancer Center
New York, New York

Michael T. Brennan, DDS, MHS
Associate Chairman
Department of Oral Medicine
Carolinas Medical Center
Charlotte, North Carolina

Eduardo Bruera, MD
F.T. McGraw Chair in the Treatment of Cancer
Medical Director
Department of Palliative Care and
  Rehabilitation Medicine
MD Anderson Cancer Center
Houston, Texas

Marianne Brydøy, MD
Department of Oncology
Haukeland University Hospital
Bergen, Norway

Robert Buckman, PhD, MB
Medical Oncologist
Princess Margaret Hospital
Professor
University of Toronto
Toronto, Ontario, Canada
Adjunct Professor
MD Anderson Cancer Center
University of Texas
Austin, Texas

Amanda Caissie, MD, PhD
Resident
Department of Radiation Oncology
University of Toronto
Princess Margaret Hospital
Toronto, Ontario, Canada

Joseph R. Carver, MD
Director
Cardiology Fellows Practice
Chief of Staff
Abramson Cancer Center
Clinical Professor
University of Pennsylvania
Philadelphia, Pennsylvania

Harvey M. Chochinov, MD, PhD
Distinguished Professor
Department of Psychiatry
University of Manitoba
Winnipeg, Manitoba, Canada

Edward Chow, PhD, MSc, MBBS
Professor
Department of Radiation Oncology
University of Toronto
Senior Scientist
Sunnybrook Research Institute
Chair of Rapid Response Radiotherapy Program
  and Bone Metastases Site Group
Odette Cancer Centre
Sunnybrook Health Sciences Centre
Toronto, Ontario, Canada

Ai-Ping Chua, MMED (Int Med), MBBS
Consultant
Assistant Professor
Division of Respiratory and Critical Care Medicine
Department of Medicine
National University Heathcare System
Singapore

Maureen E. Clark, MS
Associate Director
Center for Psycho-oncology and Palliative Care
  Research
Dana-Farber Cancer Institute
Boston, Massachusetts

Raimundo Correa, MD
Department of Oncology
Princess Margaret Hospital
University of Toronto
Toronto, Ontario, Canada

Kerry S. Courneya, PhD
Professor and Canada Research Chair
  in Physical Activity and Cancer
Faculty of Physical Education and Recreation
University of Alberta
Edmonton, Alberta, Canada

David C. Currow, MD
Professor
Palliative and Supportive Services
Flinders University
Chief Executive Officer
Cancer Australia
Adelaide, Australia

Shalini Dalal, MD
Assistant Professor
Department of Palliative Care and
  Rehabilitation Medicine
MD Anderson Cancer Center
Houston, Texas

Mellar P. Davis, MD, FCCP
Professor of Medicine
Cleveland Clinic Lerner School of
    Medicine
Case Western Reserve University
Clinical Fellowship Director
Palliative Medicine and Supportive
    Oncology Services
Division of Solid Tumor
Taussig Cancer Institute
Cleveland Clinic Foundation
Cleveland, Ohio

Maike de Wit, MD, PhD
Professor, Medical Oncology
Director, Clinic Hematology and Oncology
Vivantes Clinics Berlin Neukoelln
Berlin, Germany

Haryana Dhillon, PhD, MA(psych), BSc
Centre for Medical Psychology and Evidence-
    based Decision-making
Central Clinical School
Sydney Medical School and School of
    Psychology
Faculty of Science
University of Sydney
Sydney, Australia

Mario Dicato, MD
Department of Hematology-Oncology
Centre Hospitalier de Luxembourg
Luxembourg, Luxembourg

Ingo J. Diel, MD, PhD
Institute for Gynecological Oncology
Mannheim, Germany

Jason E. Dodge, MD, MEd
Gynecologic Oncologist
Assistant Professor
Department of OB/GYN
Division of Gynecologic Oncology
University of Toronto
Princess Margaret Hospital
University Health Network
Toronto, Ontario, Canada

Matthew Doolittle, MD
Fellow in Psychosomatic Medicine
Memorial Sloan-Kettering Cancer
    Center
New York, New York

Wolfgang Dörr, DVM, PhD
Department for Radiotherapy and Radiation
    Oncology
Medical Faculty Carl Gustav Carus
Technical University of Dresden
Dresden, Germany

Geoffrey P. Dunn, MD
Department of Surgery
Palliative Care Consultation Service
Hamot Medical Center
Erie, Pennsylvania

Alexandra M. Easson, MSc, MD
Assistant Professor
Department of Surgery
University of Toronto
General Surgery and Surgical Oncology
Mount Sinai Hospital
Princess Margaret Hospital
Toronto, Ontario, Canada

Edzard K. Ernst, MD, PhD
Department of Complementary Medicine
Peninsula Medical School
University of Exeter
Exeter, United Kingdom

Petra Ch. Feyer, MD, PhD
Professor of Radiation Oncology
Director, Clinic of Radiation Oncology
Vivantes Clinics Berlin Neukoelln
Berlin, Germany

David R. Fogelman, MD
Assistant Professor
Department of Gastrointestinal Medical
    Oncology
Division of Cancer Medicine
MD Anderson Cancer Center
Houston, Texas

Sophie D. Fosså, MD
National Resource Center for Late Effects
Department of Oncology
Oslo University
Hospital Montebello
Oslo, Norway

Orit Freedman, MD, MSc
Medical Oncologist
Durham Regional Cancer Centre
Toronto, Ontario, Canada

Debra L. Friedman, MD, MS
Associate Professor of Pediatrics
E. Bronson Ingram Chair in Pediatric Oncology
Department of Pediatrics
Vanderbilt University School of Medicine
Nashville, Tennessee

Surafel Gebreselassie, MD
Department of Nephrology and Hypertension
Cleveland Clinic
Cleveland, Ohio

Thomas R. Gildea, MD, MS
Head
Section of Bronchoscopy
Respiratory Institute
Department of Pulmonary
    Allergy and Critical Care Medicine and
    Transplant Center
Cleveland Clinic
Cleveland, Ohio

Marc Giovannini, MD, PhD
Department of Paediatrics
San Paolo Hospital
University of Milan
Milan, Italy

Paul A. Glare, MD
Chief, Pain and Palliative Care Service
Memorial Sloan-Kettering Cancer Center
New York, New York

Arin K. Greene, MD, MMSc
Department of Plastic and Oral Surgery
Co-Director Lymphedema Program
Children's Hospital Boston;
Assistant Professor of Surgery
Harvard Medical School
Boston, Massachusetts

Janet R. Hardy, BSc, MD
Director of Palliative and Supportive Care
Mater Health Services
Brisbane, Australia

Daniel B. Hinshaw, MD
Section of Geriatrics and Palliative Care Program
VA Ann Arbor Health Care System and
    Palliative Medicine Clinic
University of Michigan Geriatrics Center
    Professor of Surgery
University of Michigan Medical School
Ann Arbor, Michigan

Ulrike Hoeller, MD
Associate Professor, Radiation Oncology
Ambulatory Health Center of the Charité
Berlin, Germany

Juliet Hou, MD
Department of Physical Medicine and Rehabilitation
Cleveland Clinic
Cleveland, Ohio

Lynn Jedlicka, MD
Department of Physical Medicine and Rehabilitation
Cleveland Clinic
Cleveland, Ohio

Siri Beier Jensen, DDS, PhD
Department of Oral Medicine,
    Clinical Oral Physiology,
    Oral Pathology and Anatomy
Institute of Odontology
Faculty of Health Sciences
University of Copenhagen
Copenhagen, Denmark

Katherine T. Johnston, MD, MA, MSc
Instructor of Medicine
Harvard Medical School
Beth Israel Deaconess Medical Center
Breast Care Center and Women's Health
Boston, Massachusetts

Jason M. Jones, MD
Department of Oncology
Mayo Clinic
Rochester, Minnesota

Karin Jordan, MD, PhD
Associate Professor, University of Halle/Saale
Department of Oncology and Hematology
Halle, Germany

Karunakaravel Karuppasamy, MSc, MBBS
Department of Radiology
Cleveland Clinic
Cleveland, Ohio

Raghid Kikano, MD, MS
Fellow
Department of Neuroradiology
University of Chicago
Chicago, Illinois

Kenneth L. Kirsh, PhD
Assistant Professor in Pharmacy Practice and
   Science
University of Kentucky College of Pharmacy
Lexington, Kentucky

Cecilie Kiserud, MD
National Resource Center for Late Effects
Department of Oncology
Oslo University
Hospital Montebello
Oslo, Norway
Buskerud University College
Institute of Health
Drammen, Norway

David W. Kissane, MD, MPM
Jimmie C. Holland Chair of Psycho-oncology
Attending Psychiatrist and Chairman
Department of Psychiatry and Behavioral
   Sciences
Memorial Sloan-Kettering Cancer Center
Professor of Psychiatry
Weill Medical College of Cornell University
New York, New York

Małgorzata Krajnik, MD
Department and Chair of Palliative Medicine
Nicolaus Copernicus University in Torun
Collegium Medicum
Bydgoszcz, Poland

Christof Kramm, MD
University of Children's Hospital
Department of Pediatrics and Adolescent
   Medicine
Martin-Luther-University Halle-Wittenberg
Halle, Germany

Sheldon Kwok, MD
Odette Cancer Centre
Sunnybrook Health Sciences Centre
Toronto, Ontario, Canada

Mario E. Lacouture, MD
Dermatology Service
Department of Medicine
Memorial Sloan-Kettering Cancer Center
New York, New York

Abraham Levitin, MD
Staff, Interventional Radiology
Department of Radiology
Cleveland Clinic
Cleveland, Ohio

Madeline Li, MD, PhD
Psychiatrist
Psychosocial Oncology and Palliative Care
Princess Margaret Hospital
University Health Network
Assistant Professor
Department of Psychiatry
University of Toronto
Toronto, Ontario, Canada

S. Lawrence Librach, MD, CCFP
Director
Temmy Latner Centre for Palliative Care
Mount Sinai Hospital, Toronto
Professor and Head
Division of Palliative Care
Department of Family and Community
   Medicine
University of Toronto
Toronto, Ontario, Canada

Wendy G. Lichtenthal, PhD
Instructor
Department of Psychiatry and Behavioral
   Sciences
Memorial Sloan-Kettering Cancer Center
New York, New York

Isador Lieberman, MD
Professor of Surgery
Department of Orthopaedic Surgery
Cleveland Clinic Foundation
Cleveland, Ohio

Vernon W. H. Lin, MD
Department of Physical Medicine and
   Rehabilitation
Cleveland Clinic
Cleveland, Ohio

Hartmut Link, MD, PhD
Professor, Medical Oncology
Director, Department of Internal Medicine,
   Hematology
Oncology Westpfalz-Klinikum
Kaiserslautern, Germany

Christopher Lo, PhD
Assistant Professor of Psychiatry
University of Toronto
Psychologist
Department of Psychosocial Oncology and
   Palliative Care
Princess Margaret Hospital
University Health Network
Toronto, Ontario, Canada

César V. Lopes, MD, PhD
Santa Casa Hospital
Paoli-Calmettes Institute
Porto Alegre, Rio Grande do Sul, Brazil

Charles L. Loprinzi, MD
Regis Professor of Breast Cancer Research
Mayo Clinic
Rochester, Minnesota

Amy E. Lowery, PhD
Chief Postdoctoral Research Fellow
Department of Psychiatry and Behavioral
   Sciences
Memorial Sloan-Kettering Cancer Center
New York, New York

Robert Mader, MD
Division of Oncology
Department of Medicine
Medical University of Vienna
Vienna, Austria

Henriette Magelssen, MD
National Resource Center for Late Effects
Department of Oncology
Oslo University
Hospital Montebello
Oslo, Norway

Vincent Maida, MD, MSc, BSc
Assistant Professor
University of Toronto
Toronto, Ontario, Canada
Clinical Assistant Professor
McMaster University
Hamilton, Ontario, Canada
Division of Palliative Medicine
William Osler Health System
Toronto, Ontario, Canada

H. A. Marsman, MD
Department of Surgical Oncology
Erasmus University Medical Center
Daniel den Hoed Cancer Center
Rotterdam, The Netherlands

Susan E. McClement, RN, PhD
Associate Professor
Faculty of Nursing
University of Manitoba
Research Associate
Manitoba Palliative Care Research Unit
CancerCare Manitoba
Winnipeg, Manitoba, Canada

Erin L. McGowan, PhD, MSc, BSc
Post-Doctoral Fellow, Kinesiology
Canadian Cancer Society Research Institute
University of Alberta
Edmonton, Alberta, Canada

Daniel J. Moskovic, MD, MA, MBA
Scott Department of Urology
Baylor College of Medicine
Houston, Texas
Columbia University
New York, New York

Marissa Newman, MD
Department of Dermatology
Memorial Sloan-Kettering Cancer Center
New York, New York

Tanya Nikolova, MD
Chief Fellow
Pain and Palliative Care Service
Department of Medicine
Memorial Sloan-Kettering Cancer Center
New York, New York

Jan Oldenburg, MD, PhD
National Resource Center for Late Effects
Department of Oncology
Oslo University
Hospital Montebello
Oslo, Norway

Petra Ortner, PharmD, PhD
German Supportive Care in Cancer Group
   (ASORS)
POMME-med Medical Communication
Munich, Germany

Dierdre R. Pachman, MD
Department of Oncology
Mayo Clinic
Rochester, Minnesota

Jocelyn Pang, MD
Odette Cancer Centre
Sunnybrook Health Sciences Centre
Toronto, Ontario, Canada

Steven D. Passik, PhD
Associate Attending Psychologist
Memorial Sloan-Kettering Cancer Center
Associate Professor of Psychology
Weill College of Medicine
Cornell University Medical Center
New York, New York

Timothy M. Pawlik, MD, MPH, FACS
Associate Professor of Surgery and Oncology
Hepatobiliary Surgery Program Director
Director
Johns Hopkins Medicine Liver Tumor Center
   Multi-Disciplinary Clinic
Co-Director of Center for Surgical Trials and
   Outcomes Research
Johns Hopkins Hospital
Baltimore, Maryland

Júlio C. Pereira-Lima, MD, PhD
Serviço de Endoscopia Digestiva
Santa Casa de Caridade de Bagé
Bagé, Rio Grande do Sul, Brazil

Douglas E. Peterson, DMD, PhD
Professor
Oral Medicine
Department of Oral Health and Diagnostic
   Sciences School of Dental Medicine
Chair, Head and Neck Cancer and Oral
   Oncology
Neag Comprehensive Cancer Center
University of Connecticut Health Center
Farmington, Connecticut

Barbara F. Piper, DNSc, RN, AOCN
Professor and Chair of Nursing Research
Scottsdale Healthcare/University of Arizona
Scottsdale, Arizona

Laurent Plawny, MD
Department of Hematology-Oncology
Centre Hospitalier de Luxembourg
Luxembourg, Luxembourg

Kathy Pope, MBBS (Hons)
Consultant Radiation Oncologist
Division of Radiation Oncology
Peter MacCallum Cancer Centre
Melbourne, Victoria, Australia;
Clinical/Research Fellow
Palliative Radiation Oncology Program
University of Toronto Division of Radiation
   Oncology
Radiation Medicine Program
Princess Margaret Hospital
Toronto, Ontario, Canada

Jennifer Potter, MD
Director
Women's Health Center
Beth Israel Deaconess Medical Center
Women's Health Program
Fenway Health Associate Professor of Medicine
Harvard Medical School
Boston, Massachusetts

Holly G. Prigerson, PhD
Director
Center for Psycho-oncology and Palliative Care
   Research
Dana-Farber Cancer Institute
Associate Professor of Psychiatry
Brigham & Women's Hospital
Harvard Medical School
Boston, Massachusetts

Carla I. Ripamonti, MD
Head
Supportive Care in Cancer Unit
IRCCS Foundation
National Cancer Institute
Milano, Italy

Lizbeth Robles, MD
Resident
Department of Neurology
Cleveland Clinic
Cleveland, Ohio

Gary Rodin, MD
Professor of Psychiatry
University of Toronto
University Health Network/University of Toronto
Chair
Psychosocial Oncology and Palliative Care
Head
Department of Psychosocial Oncology and
   Palliative Care
Princess Margaret Hospital
Toronto, Ontario, Canada

Lisa Ruppert, MD
The Rehabilitation Medicine Service
Department of Neurology
Memorial Sloan-Kettering Cancer Center
New York, New York

Brenda M. Sabo, RN, BA, MA, PhD
Assistant Professor
Dalhousie University School of Nursing
Advance Practice Nurse
Psychosocial Oncology Team
Nova Scotia Cancer Centre
Capital District Health Authority
Halifax, Nova Scotia, Canada

Nadia Salvo, MD
Odette Cancer Centre
Sunnybrook Health Sciences Centre
Toronto, Ontario, Canada

Jose Fernando Santacruz, MD
Staff Physician
Pulmonary, Critical Care Medicine, and
   Interventional Pulmonology
Oncology Consultants
International Cancer Center
Houston, Texas

Josée Savard, PhD
Professor
School of Psychology
Université Laval
Laval University Cancer Research
   Center
Quebec City, Quebec, Canada

Carolyn C. Schook, BA
Harvard Medical School
Children's Hospital Boston
Boston, Massachusetts

Dale R. Shepard, MD, PhD
Associate Staff
Solid Tumor Oncology
Co-Director
Taussig Oncology Program for Seniors
   (TOPS)
Cleveland Clinic Taussig Cancer Institute
Assistant Professor of Medicine
Cleveland Clinic Lerner College of
   Medicine
Case Western Reserve University
Cleveland, Ohio

Heather L. Shepherd, PhD, BA (Hons)
NHMRC Public Health Postdoctoral Research
   Fellow
School of Public Health and Community
   Medicine
University of New South Wales, Australia
Centre for Medical Psychology and
   Evidence-based Decision-Making
   (CeMPED)
School of Public Health
University of Sydney
Sydney, Australia

Sumner A. Slavin, MD
Associate Clinical Professor
Plastic Surgery
Harvard Medical School
Beth Israel Deaconess Medical Center
Boston, Massachusetts

Martin L. Smith, STD
Director of Clinical Ethics
Department of Bioethics
Cleveland Clinic
Cleveland, Ohio

Fred K. L. Spijkervet, DDS, PhD
Department of Oral and Maxillofacial
    Surgery
University Hospital Groningen
Groningen, The Netherlands

Glen H. J. Stevens, DO, PhD
Section Head
Adult Neuro-Oncology
Brain Tumor and Neuro-Oncology Center
Neurologic Institute
Cleveland Clinic
Cleveland, Ohio

Michael D. Stubblefield, MD
Assistant Attending Physiatrist
Rehabilitation Medicine Service
Memorial Sloan-Kettering Cancer Center
Assistant Professor of Rehabilitation Medicine
Department of Physical Medicine and
    Rehabilitation
Weill Medical College of Cornell University
New York, New York

Nigel P. Sykes, MA
Consultant in Palliative Medicine
St. Christopher's Hospice
Honorary Senior Lecturer in Palliative Medicine
King's College
University of London
London, United Kingdom

Matthew Tam, MD
The Radiology Academy
Norfolk and Norwich University Hospital
Norwich, United Kingdom

Martin H. N. Tattersall, MD, MSc
Professor of Cancer Medicine
Sydney Medical School
University of Sydney
Clinical Academic
Sydney Cancer Centre
Royal Prince Alfred Hospital
Sydney, Australia

Mary L. S. Vachon, PhD, RN
Psychotherapist in Private Practice
Professor
Department of Psychiatry
Dalla Lana School of Public Health
University of Toronto
Clinical Consultant
Wellspring
Toronto, Ontario, Canada

A. E. van der Pool, MD
Department of Surgical Oncology
Erasmus University Medical Center
Daniel den Hoed Cancer Center
Rotterdam, The Netherlands

T. M. van Gulik, MD
Department of Surgery
Academic Medical Center
Amsterdam, The Netherlands

Janette Vardy, PhD, BMed (Hons)
Sydney Cancer Centre
University of Sydney
Sydney, Australia
Researcher-Clinician
Cancer Institute NSW
Eveleigh, Australia

Cornelis Verhoef, MD, PhD
Surgeon
Department of Surgical Oncology
Daniel den Hoed Cancer Center
Erasmus Medical Center
Rotterdam, The Netherlands

Arjan Vissink, DMD, MD, PhD
Department of Oral and Maxillofacial Surgery
University Medical Center Groningen
Groningen, The Netherlands

Hans-Heinrich Wolf, MD
Associate Professor, University Hospital
Department of Oncology, Hematology, and
    Hemostaseology
Halle, Germany

Rebecca K. S. Wong, MSc, MB, ChB
Professor
Department of Radiation Oncology
University of Toronto
Princess Margaret Hospital
Toronto, Ontario, Canada

Camilla Zimmermann, MD, PhD, FRCPC
Head
Palliative Care Program
Medical Director
Lederman Palliative Care Centre
Department of Psychosocial
    Oncology and Palliative Care
Princess Margaret Hospital
Associate Professor of Medicine
Division of Medical Oncology and Hematology
University of Toronto
Scientist
Campbell Family Cancer Research Institute
Ontario Cancer Institute
Toronto, Ontario, Canada

Zbigniew Zylicz, MD
Consultant in Palliative Medicine
Dove House Hospice
Hull, United Kingdom

Foreword

The new specialty of medical oncology emerged in the aftermath of World War II. Since then, it has expanded rapidly around the world as a vibrant and important area of specialist medicine. By definition, it often involves the care of people with cancer that recurred after definitive primary therapy or that presented de novo with metastatic disease. Because of advances in therapy and prevention, death from cancer in industrialized countries has declined, even as incidence has continued to increase. The latter is partly due to aging of the population; cancer is, in part, a disease of the aging process. In addition, lifestyle choices have a significant impact. Development of medical oncology was driven by the belief that cancer could be cured even when metastatic. Dramatic improvements in mortality (particularly pediatric oncology) have been obtained in some diseases. Over the same time frame, there have been dramatic improvements in medical technology with benefits in common structural complications of metastatic cancer. Examples include stenting techniques for gastrointestinal malignancies and sophisticated approaches to management of pleural effusions. Surgical oncology, oncology nursing, psychosocial oncology, and multidisciplinary care have also emerged as new allied areas of endeavor. It is still true that in most patients who are referred to a medical oncologist, death is a frequent (although not always explicitly recognized) outcome. Unfortunately, most common solid tumors remain incurable once they metastasize.

In medical oncology, an early commitment was made to structured investigation of new therapies. The vehicle for this this has been through clinical trials. This discipline has made a major impact on diseases such as breast cancer and multiple myeloma. There has been some debate that other advances in imaging and laboratory medicine have contributed to the apparent increased duration of survival (because of earlier diagnosis). Nevertheless, there seems little doubt that the systematic use of clinical trials has been of therapeutic benefit for many patients and has improved clinical care. An important part of clinical trial methodology is the assessment of therapeutic toxicity. This allows the medical oncologist to carefully balance the potential benefits of therapy against its adverse effects.

Therefore, we have come to realize that chemotherapy and radiation therapy are often blunt instruments. They can be associated with significant, sometimes life-threatening morbidity. Some of these effects are nonspecific, and others are particular to the therapeutic modality or specific drug used. Certain levels of morbidity have been considered acceptable (or inevitable) and part of the price for attempting to cure a catastrophic illness. Examples include the complications associated with certain high-dose chemotherapy regimens for breast cancer and those seen in patients after bone marrow transplant. The morbidity experienced during active treatment includes significant psychological and physical symptoms, emotional and financial distress, family dysfunction, and work and career disruption. In addition, such toxicities may be prolonged in nature beyond the treatment time frame and may be responsible for significant long-term morbidity or development of new diseases. Among those who survive cancer, there are significant effects on quality of life and residual issues, such as sexual dysfunction, that disrupt life long after cancer has been cured. In addition, the response rates to many common therapies are still disappointing, toxicity is notable, and nonresponders are often exposed to significant morbidity without any therapeutic benefit.

As the field of medical oncology progressed, certain common complications of cancer therapy, such as infections, were identified as requiring systematic attention. Later, the problems of nausea and vomiting associated with cis-platinum chemotherapy arose as another challenge. It was quickly realized that sophisticated management of these and the many other complications of therapeutic intervention was important in themselves as clinical challenges. Better management would also allow regimens to be administered most effectively. It also became apparent that the benefits to the patient were additive by improved quality of life, reduced hospitalization, and mitigated emotional and physical distress. In addition to the practical clinical benefits, a rigorous approach to the investigation and management of these common problems required significant academic endeavor. This field is now what is known as Supportive Oncology.

This major new book about supportive oncology is a timely recognition of the practical relevance, academic rigor, and increasing sophistication of the field. Supportive oncology is now recognized as an important part of practice in all areas of clinical oncology, with many benefits to the millions of people around the world in whom cancer is diagnosed every year. It can also rightly be seen as a sister specialty to another modern development, Palliative Medicine. Modern care of the cancer patient is a multidisciplinary endeavor, and everyone involved in the field will benefit from access to the wisdom and perspectives of this exciting new book.

T. Declan Walsh, MD

Preface

We are pleased to present this first edition of *Supportive Oncology*. The aim of supportive oncology is to minimize the physical, psychosocial, and spiritual suffering caused by cancer and the adverse effects of its treatment to ensure the highest possible quality of life for patients and their families. We believe that this book fulfills a unique need by providing a guide to supportive oncology throughout the cancer trajectory, from diagnosis to survivorship or bereavement. The book is based on an integrative model of care. We posit that supportive, rehabilitative, and palliative care measures should accompany patients throughout their course of disease and should be taken into account in the treatment goal in every situation, from diagnosis until cure or death. A well-defined integrative supportive care model should be included in every treatment protocol for cancer care. Supportive measures should be tailored to the special treatment or illness situation and must also reflect the wishes and needs of the patient.

This book is a collaborative venture including not only oncologists, but also palliative care physicians, nurses, pharmacists, psychologists, and psychiatrists. It is also an international collaboration, with editors from the United States, Canada, and Germany and contributors from across the globe. We are fortunate to have the contribution of many international experts in their respective fields and are grateful for their excellent contributions to this book.

This book is intended as a comprehensive resource for all oncology practitioners to assist in the management of physical and psychosocial symptoms and concerns throughout the illness trajectory. It is a useful resource for medical, radiation, and surgical oncologists; palliative medicine specialists; and oncology nurses. In addition, this book serves as a guide to supportive oncology for primary care practitioners and other health care workers seeking detailed, practical information on the supportive management of patients with cancer.

The fifty-nine chapters are organized into six sections: management of treatment-related adverse effects, management of tumor-related symptoms, management of complications in the palliative setting, rehabilitation and survivorship, communication and decision making, and psychosocial oncology. The organization of the book reflects the fact that supportive oncology encompasses symptoms and complications related to treatment, as well as those arising as a consequence of the malignancy. The section on rehabilitation and survivorship acknowledges the reality that cancer care continues after the cancer has been cured and addresses the important aspects of late effects of treatment, as well as ongoing recovery and rehabilitation The section on communication addresses decision making and supportive processes throughout the cancer trajectory. The psychosocial care not only of patients but also of professional caregivers is highlighted in the final section.

We wish to express our sincere gratitude to all the contributors to this book. We also extend our thanks to the editorial staff at Elsevier, particularly Pamela Hetherington, who guided us through this project with patience and perseverance.

Mellar P. Davis
Petra Ch. Feyer
Petra Ortner
Camilla Zimmermann

Contents

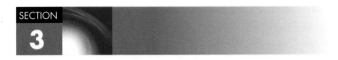

SECTION 3

MANAGEMENT OF COMPLICATIONS IN THE PALLIATIVE SETTING 257

SECTION 4

REHABILITATION AND SURVIVORSHIP 405

MANAGEMENT OF TREATMENT-RELATED ADVERSE EFFECTS

SECTION OUTLINE

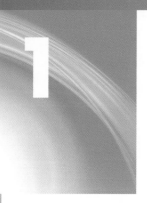

Chemotherapy extravasations (cutaneous and mucosal)

Maike de Wit and Robert Mader

Although intravenous drug administration is a basic requisite and daily routine for every physician, extravasation has been observed with a variety of agents, including electrolyte solutions, contrast media, blood products such as red blood cells, heparins, phenytoin, and cytotoxics.

The incidence and extent of injury are functions of localization, extravasating substance, absolute amount and concentration of the drug, and remedial action. Every physician should be aware of specific problems associated with different administration sites such as the back of the hand or foot and the inside of the elbow.

PREVALENCE AND PATHOPHYSIOLOGY

Accidental extravasation of cytotoxic agents is a relatively rare complication, with an incidence varying between 0%, 1%, and 5%.[1–3] In a recent survey of the MD Anderson Institute, 44 extravasations were observed in 40 to 60,000 chemotherapies during the same time period. Twelve extravasations included doxorubicin, and 10 of them needed surgical intervention.[4] Because of smaller vessels and more complicated venous access, extravasation is more common among children and is observed in up to 11%.[5] Obviously, only incidents identified by staff or patient are included.

DEFINITION

Extravasation is the process of unintentional instillation of a given infusion or injection, passing out of a vessel into surrounding tissue such as subcutaneous fat, underlying connective tissue, or muscle. Consequences depend on local drug effects and have been shown to be especially disastrous for some anticancer cytostatic agents, causing severe tissue damage within hours, days, or even months.

RISK FACTORS

The multiple risk factors can be divided in patient related, drug related, medical staff related (iatrogenic), or related to the intravenous access.

RISK FACTORS ASSOCIATED WITH THE INDIVIDUAL PATIENT

Frequency and extent of damage vary with different locations. Peripheral veins at the back of the hand, the dorsum of the foot, or the inside of an elbow are more vulnerable. If veins have been used several times already,[6] or if they are small and fragile[7] or are located near nerves, tendons, and arteries (e.g., of the hand), problems occur more frequently. Older patients and patients with sclerosis or smaller vessels suffer more damage from extravasations. The same is true for patients with higher venous pressure following thrombosis,[8] right cardiac insufficiency,[7] mediastinal tumors,[9] or a vena cava superior syndrome due to other reasons. Extremities with lymph edema following lymphadenectomy,[10] radiotherapy,[11] or problems like thrombophlebitis, venous spasms, or generalized vascular diseases like Raynaud's syndrome[7] hinder uncomplicated intravenous drug application. Patients with neurologic deficits like reduced sensitivity due to diabetes or chemotherapy-induced polyneuropathy[11] may report extravasation too late, and this results in more extensive tissue damage.

The probability of extravasation, attitudes that can help to avoid them, and signs and symptoms of early detection of an extravasation should be completely explained to the patient. Informed patients are more compliant, usually keep their arms immobilized to avoid extravasation, and inform nurses earlier, thus reducing the amount of extravasated drug. Restless patients with neurologic disorders or lack of understanding such as children,[12] psychotic patients, or patients with dementia suffer more problems related to intravenous access.

RISK FACTORS ASSOCIATED WITH THE DRUG

Tissue injury is caused by the drug itself (e.g., with anthracycline extravasation),[13,14] but sometimes it is caused by additives like solvents.[15] Cytotoxic agents are divided into three groups according to the damage potential of the respective drug: vesicant, irritant, or nontoxic (Table 1-1). For grading, only low-level evidence, mostly based on case reports and new drugs, has to be observed carefully.

Additional risk arises from osmolarity and pH value (e.g., undiluted 5-fluorouracil) as alkaline infusion (pH 9). Larger amounts of cytotoxic extravasation, longer exposure,[16] or hypersensitivity exponentiates tissue reaction.

RISK FACTORS ASSOCIATED WITH THE MEDICAL STAFF

Because intravenous devices are associated with a risk of extravasation, chemotherapy should be administered by experienced staff only. Insufficient puncture skills lead to higher rates of extravasation.[10] Overtired or too few personal[17] and time pressure[12,18] increase the risk of extravasation. The location of intravenous access has to be selected carefully and plays a major role in safety. Safety is highest with intravenous lines in the forearm and declines in this order from the back of the hand to the inside of the elbow.[19] Multiple punctures and veins punctured upstream within the last 48 hours should be avoided. High-pressure infusions to peripheral veins, large volumes, and longer duration of infusion are potential causes of extravasation. Extremities with lymphedema and neurologic problems like polyneuropathy should be avoided whenever possible.

Drugs with necrotizing potential should never be administered through steel cannulas but always with flexible intravenous devices.

Lack of experience and knowledge of medical staff,[11] as well as carelessness or underestimation of potential damage,[12] and lack of surveillance[5] such as disregard of patient complaints[20] delay diagnosis[21] and are reasons for greater damage. This risk is increased when the injection site is covered.[11]

Table 1-1 Graduation of necrotizing potential

High risk of ulceration (vesicans)	Irritating; rarely necrotizing (irritants)	Low/No risk of inflammation
Amsacrine	Bendamustine	Alemtuzumab
Carmustine[1]	Busulfan	Asparaginase
Cisplatin (concentration >0.4 mg/ml)	Carboplatin[1]	Azacytidine
	Cisplatin <0.4 mg/ml	Bevacizumab*
Dactinomycin	Dacarbazine*	Bleomycin
Daunorubicin	Etoposide	Bortezomib*
Docetaxel[1]	Fotemustine	Cladribine
Doxorubicin	Gemcitabine	Clofarabine
Epirubicin	Liposomal daunorubicin	Cyclophosphamide
Idarubicin	Liposomal doxorubicin*	Cytarabine
Mitomycin C	Melphalan	Decitabine
Mitoxantrone	Streptozocin	Etoposide-phosphate
Oxaliplatin[1]	Teniposide	Fludarabine
Paclitaxel[1]	Trabectedin*†	5-FU
Vinblastine	Treosulfan	Ifosfamide
Vincristine		Irinotecan
Vindesin		Methotrexate
Vinflunin*		Nelarabine
Vinorelbine		Nimustine
		Pegasparaginase
		Pemetrexed
		Pentostatin
		Raltitrexed
		Rituximab
		Thiotepa
		Topotecan
		Trastuzumab
		cytokines (interferon, interleukin)

[1]In the literature and according to experts, sometimes a lower necrotizing potential is estimated. Unknown: cetuximab, panitumumab, gemtuzumab-ozogamicin, arsenic trioxide, and estramustine.
*According to the manufacturer.
†Theman TA, Hartzell TL, Sinha I, et al. Recognition of a new chemotherapeutic vesicant: trabectedin (ecteinascidin-743) extravasation with skin and soft tissue damage. *J Clin Oncol.* 2009;27:e198–200. Epub 2009 Oct 5.

RISK CAUSED BY THE INTRAVENOUS ACCESS

The use of central venous catheters and intravenous port systems in patients with problematic veins minimizes the risk of extravasation. For a long time, central venous catheters in patients with difficult veins were considered a safe approach for complex therapeutic regimens with vesicant substances. However, clues suggest that even in central venous application, the incidence of extravasation is similar to that of peripheral application. Observations from the MD Anderson Institute included extravasation in one third of central venous devices.[4] Furthermore, delayed symptoms may mask the event, and extravasations may be noted only after necroses appear. In addition, extravasation most often involves a larger amount of cytotoxic agent, for which administration itself is complicated.

When a central venous device is used, the different endings of the line have to be kept in mind. If a triple-line catheter is displaced, the upper end may already be located outside the venous lumen, and use of it will cause extravasation.[22] Use of port systems is suggested in patients with difficult veins, but even then, extravasation to the thoracic wall,[23] mediastinum,[21] or pleura is possible. Some complications[24] involving the use of port systems result from malposition of the catheter tip. This is caused in part by primary misplacement and in part by misplacement due to movements of the head, coughing attacks, or flushing of the port. In spite of good positioning of the port system in 25% of patients, aspiration of blood is impossible after some time because of thrombosis of the port, the surrounding vein, or the complete system. Hypercoagulation in cancer patients, especially with mucinous adenocarcinomas, promotes thrombosis, as well as endothelial lesions caused by the catheter tip or precipitation of drugs. Fibrinolysis can be therapeutic, and low-dose anticoagulation may be prophylactic. Other possible complications of port systems include perforation of the vessel and pericardial tamponade. Attention has to be given to patients who describe pain in the neck or ear, or who cough continuously; these may be indicative of a dislocation.

Not only the tip but also the corpus of the port can be malpositioned or turned around 180 degrees[25] if absorbable surgical material is used.

The ligamentum costoclaviculare narrows the space between first rib and clavicula during shoulder movement and inhibits regular flow within the port (pinch-off phenomenon).[9,26–29]

Typical reasons for extravasation in port systems include malposition of the injection needle, use of a short needle, and displacement of the needle.[26] Less frequent causes are disconnection of the corpus from the catheter of the port, catheter dislocation, defective material, and incorrect handling.[30]

DIAGNOSIS

Extravasation is usually diagnosed with nonspecific symptoms such as pain, edema, and erythema; only rarely is a specific diagnosis possible (e.g., fluorescence microscopy in anthracycline extravasation). However, the extent of tissue damage is underestimated even after diagnosis of extravasation. When in doubt, magnetic resonance imaging (MRI) is a reasonable imaging method for visualizing extravasated fluids if difficult to assess otherwise.

Extravasation is rare, and differential diagnoses include the more common chemotherapy-induced thrombophlebitis and local hypersensitivity reactions. In clinical practice, distinguishing hypersensitivity reaction or phlebitis from extravasation may be difficult. This differential diagnosis rarely causes problems for experienced clinicians; this again emphasizes the need for training and education by experienced colleagues, as well as the need for specialization within hospitals and institutions that treat cancer patients.

DIFFERENTIAL DIAGNOSIS

Thrombophlebitis is the most common local complication of intravenous cytostatic drug infusion.[9,11] Local bacterial infection against cytotoxic agents, the carrier substance, or the diluent results in thrombophlebitis. Pain emerges immediately after injection, swelling after hours, and thrombosis and discoloration of the skin after days. Amsacrine leads to thrombophlebitis in up to 17%[31] and is better tolerated if it is more highly diluted and given with a longer infusion duration and with the use of heparin.[32] Bendamustine causes phlebitis in 35% as the result of low pH value in higher concentrations.

Local cutaneous hypersensitivity reaction is mediated immunologically and has to be distinguished from local toxicity. Gell and Coombs described four different hypersensitivity reaction types (types I through IV). Local type II has not been described in chemotherapeutic agents, but a systemic reaction is possible.[33] The most common type I reaction (immediate type) mediated by immunoglobulin (Ig)E-antibodies begins seconds to minutes after exposition, with a second reaction occurring 4 to 6 hours later. The vein hurts upstream of the injection site, inducing urticaria, erythema, and pruritus. Swelling is rare. Symptoms are reversible within hours and can be reduced by sufficiently rinsing the vein. This reaction is common with cisplatinum, bleomycin, and melphalan.[34]

Type III reactions (immune complex disease) begin 8 to 12 hours after infusion and are characterized by urticaria, erythema multiforme, vasculitis, and sometimes angioedema.

Type IV reaction is delayed, antibody independent, and cell mediated. The reaction begins even later—usually 12 to 72 hours after injection, as with allergic contact dermatitis.

Local allergy occurs rarely but mostly with anthracyclines. Hyperallergic reaction results in large necrotic areas. No acute reactions are noted, but days after infusion, pain develops at the injection site, and weeks later, redness and ulceration appear.

Local hypersensitivity reaction was described with asparaginase (types I and III) and taxanes.[35] Sometimes reactions are caused by additives (Cremophor, polysorbate 80) used to enhance solubility and stability.[36]

Local hypersensitivity allows continuation of chemotherapy[3] because it does not recur regularly.

Flare reaction

In 3% of doxorubicin applications, a flare reaction is reported, showing erythema, pruritus, and induration along the punctured vein; symptoms remain after cessation of infusion.[37]

Recall phenomenon

If a cutaneous reaction reemerges after previous chemotherapy or radiotherapy, this is called a *recall phenomenon*. Although chemotherapy may be given correctly, symptoms reappear at the site of previous extravasation.[38] Symptoms include hypersensibility, redness, swelling, inflammation, blistering, discoloration of the skin, and even necrosis. The recall phenomenon has been observed up to 15 years after radiotherapy,[39] but the probability of occurrence is lower if at least 10 days have passed since radiotherapy was given. Recall phenomenon is described for taxanes[40] and anthracyclines[41,42] and after radiotherapy with etoposide,[43] gemcitabine,[44] methotrexate,[45] and vinblastine.[46] The mechanism is unknown, and controversy is ongoing.[47,48]

Photosensitivity

Drugs may increase sensitivity against solar rays. Symptoms are identical to typical sunburn: erythema, edema, and blistering. Most published severe cases have occurred following administration of dacarbazine,[49] but bleomycin,[50] dactinomycin, 5-fluorouracil, methotrexate,[51,52] vinblastine, and taxanes[53] have caused similar damage. The only effective prophylaxis is avoiding direct exposure to sunlight.

Interventions

The most important measure against extravasation is primary prevention. This includes application of vesicants only by experienced staff and single puncture with flexible cannulas, preferably in the forearm. Applying central venous devices should be considered early.

Similar to all other adverse effects, the probability of an extravasation differs from patient to patient, requiring an individual risk-benefit balance for every subject scheduled for cytotoxic chemotherapy. Patients at risk need to be informed about possible side effects of treatment, to stimulate compliance and attention.

Patient information about possible extravasation must accentuate the need for minimizing movement of the extremity in question to diminish the probability of extravasation. Fully informed patients can stop the infusion themselves if they feel compromised; accordingly, they will call the nurse at once.

Before injection or infusion of vesicants, blood has to be aspirated from the catheter, and sodium chloride (NaCl) solution must be infused for 5 minutes. Rinsing should be repeated after the vesicant infusion. NaCl infusion is useful additionally for administration of cytotoxic drugs. The catheter and the infusion have to be fixed properly. Use of a port system is recommended in difficult veins, although extravasation to the thoracic wall, mediastinum, or pleura is possible.

Port systems are flushed and aspirated before infusion, as are all intravenous devices. If this is not possible, some maneuver such as movement of the head, the Valsalva maneuver, or supination or elevation of the shoulder and arm (pinch-off) may help to restore normal flow. These attempts are escalated with NaCl injection, use of ascorbic acid, or fibrinolysis.

GENERAL NONPHARMACOLOGIC MANAGEMENT

Extravasation calls for immediate action. Infusion or injection has to be stopped at once, even if extravasation remains doubtful. Before restart of the infusion, correct placement of the catheter must be assured.

In case of extravasation, use the extravasation kit, put on (sterile) gloves, and, after changing the infusion line or syringe, aspirate as much extravasated liquid as possible without applying pressure. Subsequently remove the cannula under aspiration. With blistering, aspirate liquid using a 1-ml syringe and a new cannula for every attempt. After finishing acute general measures, elevate and immobilize the extremity. Specific treatment starts thereafter. Primary findings are documented on an extravasation report form, which also can be used for follow-up. Photographic documentation with measuring tape and colored marker around the site of extravasation is recommended. Clinical findings are documented not only for clinical care, but for liability and law implications as well. In addition, the patient and his relatives are instructed and are called in for regular controls. Within 24 hours after extravasation with necrotizing potential, a (plastic) surgeon should be consulted, preferably one with expertise in handling extravasation. During this period, surgical interventions such as the flush-out technique or liposuction can be useful in severe cases of extravasation.

For tissue relief, early surgery and flushing with isotonic solution after extravasation of cytostatics and other toxic substances, such as potassium and high concentrated glucose (>10%), have been performed to overcome the painful feeling of tightness in the extremity. This approach is not recommended generally, but it can be useful in special cases, such as with extravasation of a highly vesicant compound at the dorsum of the hand or from a central venous device.

PHARMACOLOGIC MANAGEMENT

AMSACRINE, MITOMYCIN C, MITOXANTRONE, DACTINOMYCIN

Extravasation of these substances demands immediate dry local cooling for at least 1 hour and continuation for some days several times daily, 15 minutes each time. Topical use of dimethylsulfoxide (DMSO) 99% 4 to 6 times daily is recommended for at least 7 days. Experience with dexrazoxane has not been reported with these cytotoxic agents.

VINCA ALKALOIDS AND ETOPOSIDE

Perilesional hyaluronidase is injected subcutaneously or intradermally (1500 IU/ml in 10 ml NaCl), starting from the periphery and moving toward the center.[54] Specific measures include dry heat (no hot humidity!) for 1 hour the first time, then 4 times daily for 20 minutes each time.

CISPLATINUM

The toxicity of cisplatinum varies with concentration. Concentrations exceeding 0.4 mg/ml require specific management involving dry local cooling for at least 1 hour. This should be continued several (4 to 6) times daily for 15 minutes each time (e.g., DMSO 99% 4 to 6 times daily for at least 7 days).[55,56]

ANTHRACYCLINES

Anthracycline extravasation may lead to progressive destruction of tissues such as nerves, vessels, tendons, and muscles, causing pain for a long time and possible permanent functional defects. Sometimes chemotherapy has to be interrupted, and hospitalization is necessary.

Immediate pain, edema, and erythema are followed by vesication and induration with atrophic skin and ulceration 1 to 4 weeks later. The ulceration keeps growing for months, showing few tendencies toward spontaneous recovery but with the potential to destroy underlying structures. In addition, pain contractures, dystrophy, and functional loss of the extremity may follow.

Small extravasations are often observed, leading to slowly growing ulcerations and the possible need for more aggressive strategies. Overall, surgical intervention is necessary during follow-up in 35% to 40% of cases. On the other hand, surgical results are best for excisions made within 8 hours but not later than 1 week after extravasation. The need for wide margins free of anthracyclines can be verified by fluorescence microscopy, especially before skin transplantation.

Small uncontrolled series support conservative therapy but do not provide histologic verification. Although several therapeutic interventions have been tested in the past, the standard procedure so far consists of cooling in combination with topical DMSO 99%.

In 2006, dexrazoxane (Savene) was the first approved antidote for treatment of anthracycline extravasation. Approval of dexrazoxane (Savene) was based on two series that reported a 98% success rate (i.e., in 54 cases of anthracycline extravasation confirmed by fluorescence microscopy, one surgical intervention was necessary). Chemotherapy was not delayed. Dexrazoxane must be infused as soon as possible, but not later than 6 hours after extravasation, using a new intravenous access. Local cooling has to be stopped at least 15 minutes before the first infusion and should not be initiated again. Application of DMSO in combination with dexrazoxane has not been approved. For 3 consecutive days, dexrazoxane is infused daily: $1000 \, mg/m^2$ on days 1 and 2, and $500 \, mg/m^2$ on the third day, for a maximum overall dose of 2000 mg each day.[57,58]

Upon reviewing the data on more than 100 extravasations with anthracyclines, the authors determined that around 40% of extravasations are discovered only one or several days after the event itself. In these cases, the use of topical cooling combined with DMSO is still recommended.

SPECIFIC MEASURES

Immediate action is essential. Application of local warmth and cold is decided according to the cytotoxic agent. With most cytotoxic agents, low temperature slows diffusion and is beneficial, whereas with vinca alkaloids, cooling is never indicated because dry heat favors systemic resorption of vinca alkaloids.

Dry cold

- Use with anthracyclines (if not using dexrazoxane), cisplatinum, amsacrine, mitomycin C
- Initial duration of 1 hour, with topical cooling with cold packs

- Several times daily 15 minutes each time, with topical cooling for at least 1 week
- Including DMSO, with the exception of liposomal daunorubicin and liposomal doxorubicin
- Do not use DMSO when giving dexrazoxane.

Dry heat

- Vinca alkaloids
- Initial duration 1 hour with hot packs
- Several times daily at 15 minutes each for at least 1 week
- Do not use with DMSO.

ANTIDOTA
Dimethylsulfoxide (DMSO)

The 99% solution enhances permeability of the skin, leading to better systemic absorption (application over 8 days every 8 hours with stippling and air drying). DMSO is a solvent that is not approved for use as medicine in humans.

Hyaluronidase

The enzyme hyaluronidase loosens the structure of connective tissue. The exposed region is injected around the paravasate lesion with 10 ml of 1500 IU/ml hyaluronidase. The burning pain that results is alleviated with local anesthetics. Consideration of pain against benefit favors the treatment. With vinca alkaloids, hyaluronidase is combined with dry heat, but not with taxanes.

Dexrazoxane, the first approved antidote

The registration of dexrazoxane as a novel antidote to anthracyclines was a consequence of its effective performance in preclinical and clinical studies. Clinical data obtained in registration trials were convincing, with a single patient requiring surgical intervention, while 53 recruited patients with histologically verified extravasation recovered completely with conservative management only.[58] Nevertheless, several issues have not been addressed in these studies. First of all, it is not clear how the effectiveness of dexrazoxane compares with that of the highly established clinical use of DMSO/topical cooling, although the latter has not been approved for treatment of human patients. This reliable procedure has been tested in a prospective clinical trial under very similar circumstances (equal numbers of patients and very similar success rates), clearly proving that DMSO/topical cooling is an effective antidote for the management of anthracycline extravasation.[59] The serious flaw in the dexrazoxane study design indicates that we have lost an opportunity to directly compare the effectiveness of the two antidotes.

Other factors associated with the use of dexrazoxane include (1) that IV dexrazoxane is an invasive procedure requiring hospitalization over 3 days, and (2) that a higher rate of side effects is seen with dexrazoxane (elevation of liver enzymes and bilirubin) when compared with DMSO/cooling.

OTHER PHARMACEUTICAL INTERVENTIONS

Use of steroids is debatable; natrium thiosulfate and bicarbonate are no longer recommended.

Quality control and quality assurance

Although extravasation of cytotoxic agents is one of the rarer complications of chemotherapy, severe complications may result, particularly after extravasation of vesicants. Prevention and appropriate management are therefore essential to avoid sequelae. In this regard, quality control and quality assurance contribute to both prevention and extravasation management and should be implemented in all oncologic centers. The following issues related to quality of care are considered to be essential: information and education for patients, training for medical and nursing staff, an emergency number for consulting an experienced physician, interdisciplinary cooperation, implementation of guidelines, documentation of all extravasation events (even if only suspected), and knowledge management.

Regular training sessions help to raise sensitivity and awareness among medical and nursing staff. At the same time, they impart the knowledge necessary to promptly deliver an appropriate intervention in an emergency situation.

To support therapeutic staff members of the hospital, an experienced physician should be appointed as emergency consultant in case of extravasation. His responsibilities should include management of acute situations ("first aid") with information, communication, supervision of patient documentation, and coordination of the rescue procedure. The hospital pharmacy should provide an extravasation kit.

It is highly recommended that guidelines be established and regularly updated to provide scientifically based recommendations with a focus on clinical practice. Deviations from these guidelines require sound reasoning and appropriate documentation. Besides the usefulness of standardized procedures (SOPs) in emergency situations, it is increasingly important to be prepared for questions of legal liability. Guidelines should include a registry of relevant substances, risk factors, prophylaxis, symptoms, and general and special therapeutic measures, as well as components of an extravasation kit (Table 1-2) and an extravasation report form.

Standardized patient documentation is crucial for evaluating outcomes and should include the following: description of events, amount and concentration of extravasated substance, symptoms, measures taken, further developments/sequelae, aftercare, and outcomes (templates may be retrieved from <www.extravasation.at>). Because almost no prospective clinical studies on extravasation of cytotoxic drugs have been

conducted, our current knowledge is based primarily on low-level evidence. As long as this unsatisfactory situation persists, knowledge management is essential to gain experience and to share information.[60]

Open questions

In terms of extravasation, the focus should be on preventive measures proposed as a catalogue of the most important questions that should be asked before therapy is initiated. This checklist includes questions about the vascular condition of a patient, hyposensitivities or hypersensitivities, previous therapies, polyneuropathy or medications reducing perception, patient compliance, and others. Knowledge of these risk factors provides the basis for preventive measures and contributes to early detection, thus warranting our full attention.

The type of damage associated with novel cytotoxic agents usually requires an experienced clinician to determine its final classification. It may take years to obtain sufficient clinical information to properly assess cutaneous and tissue toxicity. Even after years of clinical use, some antineoplastic agents (e.g., busulfan, estramustine) are not conclusively classified. Although much pharmaceutical knowledge is available, it is not possible to extrapolate tissue toxicity on the basis of physical-chemical attributes. One possible approach would be to evaluate acute tissue toxicity, including vesicant potential, during the approval procedure of a novel substance, as has already been envisaged by the guidelines of the European Agency for the Evaluation of Medicinal Products (EMEA). From a clinical perspective, it would be helpful to explicitly define these requirements for extravasation by testing local and cutaneous tolerance. This information should be included in the summary of the product characteristics to inform physicians about the tissue toxicity of newly approved compounds, even before their first use.

Extravasations are not always noticed instantly. According to the literature, the delay is often longer than 5 days, thus raising the following question: How much time may lapse before antidotes are no longer effective? Antidotes have been tested immediately following the extravasation event, but animal studies have shown that the efficacy of dexrazoxane against anthracyclines persists for at least 3 hours after extravasation and is clearly reduced against daunorubicin after 6 hours. Even smaller time windows seem to apply to the antidote hyaluronidase. For this reason, informing patients, in addition to regular monitoring of the infusion, is of such crucial importance: Early detection is the key when time is critical.

Pathologic changes that occur in damaged tissue have not yet been sufficiently characterized. This lack of knowledge explains the ongoing discussion about the use of corticosteroids. Although we know that inflammation is not the prevailing process after extravasation, the literature still proposes the use of corticosteroids. The evidence needed can be achieved through cooperation with pathologists and examination of human tissue samples.

New therapeutic developments will change the pharmacologic landscape fundamentally over the next 15 years. In addition to antihormonal substances, which most often are given orally, molecular and targeted therapies will complement and substitute for traditional cytotoxic agents. These compounds hardly possess vesicant potential—most probably, not even irritant effects. Today's trend toward peroral formulations will increase (e.g., cytotoxic agents like vinorelbine or temozolomide;

Table 1-2　Table with overview for orientation

- Drugs and necrotizing risk (grades 1 to 3)
- General procedures
- Drug-specific procedures
  - Cold-hot packs (Cold/Hot 10 × 26)
    - At least two
  - Swabs, sterile, minimum two sets with four swabs each
  - DMSO (e.g., dimethylsulfoxide 99% [Merck Art. Nr. 16743])
  - Hyaluronidase (HYLASE 150 IE) 10 amp
  - Dexrazoxane 500 mg (10 vials) (Savene 10 vials with 500 mg and three bags Savene diluent) should be available on demand at the pharmacy or another central point within 4 hours to be administered within 6 hours.
  - Extravasation report form

oral tyrosine kinase inhibitors such as lapatinib, erlotinib, sorafenib, and others). Potentially toxic local taxanes such as paclitaxel will be used in polymer-bound form with reduced local toxicity, similar to the liposomal formulations of dauno-rubicin, doxorubicin, and vincristine. Monoclonal humanized antibodies are used increasingly often in oncology (e.g., rituximab, trastuzumab, bevacizumab, cetuximab). Thanks to these molecular therapeutic drugs, extravasation may become a less dreaded complication of chemotherapy. Notwithstanding, we should not forget that cytotoxic drugs will certainly remain the cornerstone of cancer therapy in less developed countries and will continue to do serve this purpose in our hospitals for the upcoming years.

SUMMARY FOR DAILY PRACTICE

Prophylaxis of extravasation is essential, as are instruction of patients, guidelines for physicians, and immediate action in cases of extravasation. If you have doubts or lack experience, do not lose time; get a specialist involved immediately. Appropriate and quick initiation of treatment is crucial.

REFERENCES

1. Laughlin RA, Landeen JM, Habal MB. The management of inadvertent subcutaneous Adriamycin infiltration. *Am J Surg.* 1979;137:408–412.
2. Cox K, Stuart-Harris R, Abdini G, et al. The management of cytotoxic-drug extravasation: guidelines drawn up by a working party for the Clinical Oncological Society of Australia. *Med J Aust.* 1988;148:185–189.
3. Barlock AL, Howser DM, Hubbard SM. Nursing management of Adriamycin extravasation. *Am J Nurs.* 1979;79:94–96.
4. Langstein HN, Duman H, Seelig D, et al. Retrospective study of the management of chemotherapeutic extravasation injury. *Ann Plast Surg.* 2002;49:369–374.
5. Brown AS, Hoelzer DJ, Piercy SA. Skin necrosis from extravasation of intravenous fluids in children. *Plast Reconstr Surg.* 1979;64:145–150.
6. Linder RM, Upton J. Prevention of extravasation injuries secondary to doxorubicin. *Postgrad Med.* 1985;77:105.
7. Ignoffo RJ, Friedman MA. Therapy of local toxicities caused by extravasation of cancer chemotherapeutic drugs. *Cancer Treat Rev.* 1980;7:17–27.
8. Larson DL. Treatment of tissue extravasation by antitumor agents. *Cancer.* 1982;49:1796–1799.
9. Jordan K, Grothe W, Schmoll HJ. Extravasation of chemotherapeutic agents: prevention and therapy. *Dtsche Med Wochenschr.* 2005;130:33–37.
10. Bowers DG, Lynch JB. Adriamycin extravasation. *Plast Reconstr Surg.* 1978;61:86–92.
11. Mullin S, Beckwith MC, Tyler LS. Prevention and management of antineoplastic extravasation injury. *Hosp Pharm.* 2000;35:57–76.
12. Upton J, Mulliken JB, Murray JE. Major intravenous extravasation injuries. *Am J Surg.* 1979;137:497–506.
13. Richardson DS, Johnson SA. Anthracyclines in haematology: preclinical studies, toxicity and delivery systems. *Blood Rev.* 1997;11:201–223.
14. Cox RF. Managing skin damage induced by doxorubicin hydrochloride and daunorubicin hydrochloride. *Am J Hosp Pharm.* 1984;41:2410–2414.
15. Larson DL. Treatment of tissue extravasation by anti-tumor agents. *Cancer.* 1982;49:1796–1799.
16. Reilly JJ, Neifeld JP, Rosenberg SA. Clinical course and management of accidental Adriamycin extravasation. *Cancer.* 1977;40:2053–2056.
17. Preuss P, Partoft S. Cytostatic extravasations. *Ann Plast Surg.* 1987;19:323–329.
18. Linder RM, Upton J, Osteen R. Management of extensive doxorubicin hydrochloride extravasation injuries. *J Hand Surg (Am).* 1983;8:32–38.

19. Lynch DJ, Key JC, White RR. Management and prevention of infiltration and extravasation injury. *Surg Clin North Am.* 1979;59:939–949.
20. MacCara ME. Extravasation: a hazard of intravenous therapy. *Drug Intell Clin Pharm.* 1983;17:713–717.
21. Anderson CM, Walters RS, Hortobagyi GN. Mediastinitis related to probable central vinblastine extravasation in a woman undergoing adjuvant chemotherapy for early breast cancer. *Am J Clin Oncol.* 1996;19:566–568.
22. Schummer W, Schummer C, Schelenz C. Case report: the malfunctioning implanted venous access device. *Br J Nurs.* 2003;12:210, 212–220.
23. Barutca S, Kadikoylu G, Bolaman Z, et al. Extravasation of paclitaxel into breast tissue from central catheter port. *Support Care Cancer.* 2002;10:563–565.
24. Ener RA, Meglathery SB, Styler M. Extravasation of systemic hemato-oncological therapies. *Ann Oncol.* 2004;15:858–862.
25. Gebarski SS, Gebarski KS. Chemotherapy port "Twiddler's syndrome." A need for preinjection radiography. *Cancer.* 1984;54:38–39.
26. Hofer S, Schnabel K, Vogelbach P, et al. The "pinch off" syndrome: a complication of implantable catheter systems in the subclavian vein. *Schweiz Med Wochenschr.* 1997;127:1247–1250.
27. Aitken DR, Minton JP. The "pinch-off sign": a warning of impending problems with permanent subclavian catheters. *Am J Surg.* 1984;148:633–636.
28. Hinke DH, Zandt-Stastny DA, Goodman LR, et al. Pinch-off syndrome: a complication of implantable subclavian venous access devices. *Radiology.* 1990;177:353–356.
29. D'Silva K, Dwivedi AJ, Shetty A, et al. Pinch-off syndrome: a rare complication of totally implantable venous devices. *Breast J.* 2005;11:83–84.
30. Biffi R, Orsi F, Grasso F, et al. Cenciarelli S, Andreoni B. Catheter rupture and distal embolisation: a rare complication of central venous ports. *J Vasc Access.* 2000;1:19–22.
31. Louie AC, Issell BF. Amsacrine (AMSA)—a clinical review. *J Clin Oncol.* 1985; 3:562–592.
32. Case Jr DC. Prevention of amsacrine-induced phlebitis with heparin. *Clin Pharm.* 1982; 1:490.
33. Weiss RB, Bruno S. Hypersensitivity reactions to cancer chemotherapeutic agents. *Ann Intern Med.* 1981;94:66–72.
34. Cornwell III GG, Pajak TF, McIntyre OR. Hypersensitivity reactions to IV melphalan during treatment of multiple myeloma: Cancer and Leukemia Group B experience. *Cancer Treat Rep.* 1979;63:399–403.

35. Haskell CM, Canellos GP, Leventhal BG, et al. Hansen HH. L-asparaginase toxicity. *Cancer Res.* 1969;29:974–975.
36. Markman M. Management of toxicities associated with the administration of taxanes. *Expert Opin Drug Saf.* 2003;2:141–146.
37. Vogelzang NJ. "Adriamycin flare": a skin reaction resembling extravasation. *Cancer Treat Rep.* 1979;63:2067–2069.
38. Koppel RA, Boh EE. Cutaneous reactions to chemotherapeutic agents. *Am J Med Sci.* 2001;321:327–335.
39. Burdon J, Bell R, Sullivan J, et al. Adriamycin-induced recall phenomenon 15 years after radiotherapy. *JAMA.* 1978;239:931.
40. Yeo W, Leung SF, Johnson PJ. Radiation-recall dermatitis with docetaxel: establishment of a requisite radiation threshold. *Eur J Cancer.* 1997;33:698–699.
41. Gabel C, Eifel PJ, Tornos C, et al. Radiation recall reaction to idarubicin resulting in vaginal necrosis. *Gynecol Oncol.* 1995;57:266–269.
42. McCarty MJ, Peake MF, Lillis P, et al. Paclitaxel-induced radiation recall dermatitis. *Med Pediatr Oncol.* 1996;27:185–186.
43. Fontana JA. Radiation recall associated with VP-16-213 therapy. *Cancer Treat Rep.* 1979;63:224–225.
44. Castellano D, Hitt R, Cortes-Funes H, et al. Side effects of chemotherapy. Case 2. Radiation recall reaction induced by gemcitabine. *J Clin Oncol.* 2000;18:695–696.
45. Camidge DR. Methotrexate-induced radiation recall. *Am J Clin Oncol.* 2001;24:211–213.
46. Nemecek PM, Corder MC. Radiation recall associated with vinblastine in a patient treated for Kaposi sarcoma related to acquired immune deficiency syndrome. *Cancer.* 1992;70:1605–1606.
47. Kitani H, Kosaka T, Fujihara T, et al. The "recall effect" in radiotherapy: is subeffective, reparable damage involved? *Int J Radiat Oncol Biol Phys.* 1990;18:689–695.
48. Camidge R, Price A. Characterizing the phenomenon of radiation recall dermatitis. *Radiother Oncol.* 2001;59:237–245.
49. Iwamoto T, Hiraku Y, Okuda M, et al. Mechanism of UVA-dependent DNA damage induced by an antitumor drug dacarbazine in relation to its photogenotoxicity. *Pharm Res.* 2008;25:598–604.
50. Douglas KT, Ratwatte HA, Thakrar N. Photoreactivity of bleomycin and its implications. *Bull Cancer.* 1983;70:372–380.
51. Goldfeder KL, Levin JM, Katz KA, et al. Ultraviolet recall reaction after total body irradiation, etoposide, and methotrexate therapy. *J Am Acad Dermatol.* 2007;56:494–499.

52. Pascu ML, Staicu A, Voicu L, et al. Methotrexate as a photosensitiser. *Anticancer Res.* 2004;24:2925–2930.

53. Ee HL, Yosipovitch G. Photo recall phenomenon: an adverse reaction to taxanes. *Dermatology.* 2003;207:196–198.

54. Bertelli G, Dini D, Forno GB, et al. Hyaluronidase as an antidote to extravasation of Vinca alkaloids: clinical results. *J Cancer Res Clin Oncol.* 1994;120: 505–506.

55. Dorr RT. Antidotes to vesicant chemotherapy extravasations. *Blood Rev.* 1990;4:41–60.

56. Louvet C, Bouleuc C, Droz JP. Tissue complications of cisplatin extravasation. *Presse Med.* 1989;18:725–726.

57. Jensen JN, Lock-Andersen J, Langer SW, et al. A promising antidote in the treatment of accidental extravasation of anthracyclines. *Scand J Plast Reconstr Surg Hand Surg.* 2003;37:174–175.

58. Mouridsen HT, Langer SW, Buter J, et al. Treatment of anthracycline extravasation with Savene (dexrazoxane): results from two prospective clinical multicentre studies. *Ann Oncol.* 2007;18:546–550.

59. Bertelli G, Gozza A, Forno GB, et al. Topical dimethylsulfoxide for the prevention of soft tissue injury after extravasation of vesicant cytotoxic drugs: a prospective clinical study. *J Clin Oncol.* 1995;13:2851–2855.

60. Mader I, Fürst-Weger PR, Mader RM, et al. *Extravasation of cytotoxic agents.* 2nd ed. New York: Springer; 2009.

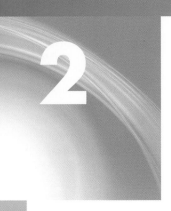

2

Allergic reactions to chemotherapy

Dale R. Shepard

Infusion reactions are relatively common during administration of chemotherapy. Unfortunately, too little attention is often paid to whether these reactions are simple hypersensitivity reactions or more serious immune-mediated allergic reactions. Patients with apparent allergic reactions to chemotherapy must be evaluated very carefully so the cause of the reaction can be determined. If these reactions are not evaluated appropriately, a patient with a true allergy may be harmed by inadequate treatment of the reaction or by reexposure to the allergen, or an active regimen may be discontinued in a patient with a simple hypersensitivity reaction.

Allergic reactions to chemotherapy can occur with both cytotoxic agents and monoclonal antibodies with systemic or cutaneous manifestations. Systemic allergic reactions to chemotherapy are more common than cutaneous reactions, are most important to differentiate from benign hypersensitivity reactions, and are most likely to influence further use of the causative agent. These systemic allergic reactions will be the focus of this chapter. This chapter will describe the types and mechanisms of allergic reactions, the chemotherapeutic agents that most commonly cause allergic reactions, and the clinical manifestations of allergic reactions. The diagnosis, prevention, and management of allergic reactions will be reviewed.

WHAT IS A SYSTEMIC ALLERGIC REACTION?

Reviewing the literature for trials, reviews, or guidelines pertaining to allergic reactions to chemotherapy is difficult because of the lack of standard terminology. Terms that occur frequently in the literature, although they usually are poorly defined, include *hypersensitivity reaction, infusion reaction, allergic reaction, pseudoallergic reaction, standard infusion reaction, severe infusion reaction, anaphylactic reaction,* and *anaphylactoid reaction.* Prevention, correct diagnosis, and management of allergic reactions to chemotherapy require an understanding of the distinctions between these terms and an ability to use them correctly when communicating with other clinicians. *Hypersensitivity reaction,* a term often used synonymously with *infusion reaction,* is a general term that is often used to describe an adverse reaction to a drug, which does not imply a mechanism. Infusion reactions can be characterized further as standard infusion reactions, severe infusion reactions, and anaphylactic or anaphylactoid reactions. Standard infusion reactions are not the result of an allergic mechanism, and anaphylactic reactions are immune mediated. Pseudoallergic reactions, also called *anaphylactoid reactions,* are not directly immune mediated, but may be severe. These reactions are due to indirect activation of the immune system by the drug or by an excipient. The National Cancer Institute (NCI) differentiates between infusion-related reactions, allergic reactions, and anaphylaxis in the Common Toxicity Criteria for Adverse Events (CTCAE), version 4 (Table 2-1).[1]

TYPES AND MECHANISMS OF ALLERGIC REACTIONS

Allergic reactions historically have been divided into categories on the basis of their immunologic mechanisms via a classification system initially described by Gell and Coombs

Table 2-1 Differences between hypersensitivity reactions and acute infusion reactions

Adverse event	Grade				
	1	2	3	4	5
Infusion-related reaction*	Mild transient reaction; infusion interruption not indicated; intervention not indicated	Therapy or infusion indicated but responds promptly to symptomatic treatment (e.g., antihistamines, NSAIDs, narcotics, IV fluids); prophylactic medications indicated for ≤24 hours	Prolonged (e.g., not rapidly responsive to symptomatic medication and/or brief interruption of infusion); recurrence of symptoms following initial improvement; hospitalization indicated for clinical sequelae	Life-threatening consequences; urgent intervention indicated	Death
Allergic reaction†	Transient flushing or rash, drug fever <38° C (<100.4° F); intervention not indicated	Intervention or infusion indicated; responds promptly to symptomatic treatment (e.g., antihistamines, NSAIDs, narcotics); prophylactic medications indicated for ≤24 hours	Prolonged (e.g., not rapidly responsive to symptomatic medication and/or brief interruption of infusion); recurrence of symptoms following initial improvement; hospitalization indicated for clinical sequelae (e.g., renal impairment, pulmonary infiltrates)	Life-threatening consequences; urgent intervention indicated	Death
Anaphylaxis‡			Symptomatic bronchospasm, with or without urticaria; parenteral intervention indicated; allergy-related edema/angioedema; hypotension	Life-threatening consequences; urgent intervention indicated	Death

Adapted from the classification for immune reactions first described by Gell and Coombs.[2]
NSAIDs, Nonsteroidal antiinflammatory drugs.
* A disorder characterized by an adverse reaction to the infusion of pharmacologic or biological substances.
CTCAE, October 15, 2009: General disorders and administration site conditions.
† A disorder characterized by an adverse local or general response from exposure to an antigen.
‡ A disorder characterized by an acute inflammatory reaction resulting from the release of histamine and histamine-like substances from mast cells, causing a hypersensitivity immune response. Clinically, it presents with breathing difficulty, dizziness, hypotension, cyanosis, and loss of consciousness and may lead to death.
CTCAE-4.02, October 15, 2009: Immune disorders.[1]

(Table 2-2).[2] Type I reactions are mediated by immunoglobulin (Ig)E, are usually immediate with onset less than 1 hour from the start of the infusion, and lead to release of vasoactive compounds through activation of basophils or mast cells. Type II reactions are slower in onset and are due to antibody-mediated cellular destruction. Type II reactions are usually due to IgG. Type III reactions are also delayed in onset compared with Type I reactions and are mediated by IgG antibodies. Type III reactions lead to deposition of IgG/drug immune complexes and activation of complement. Similar to Type I reactions, Type IV reactions are caused by activation of the immune system, but in contrast to Type I reactions, Type IV reactions are delayed in onset and are mediated by the activation of T cells. In addition to classification by pathogenesis, the World Allergy Organization (WAO) distinguishes between immediate reactions, reactions occurring within 1 hour, and delayed reactions, which occur after 1 hour.[3] Systemic anaphylactic reactions due to chemotherapeutic agents usually are always Type I reactions, in which IgE binds to FcεRI receptors on the surface of mast cells or basophils.[4] Activation of mast cells by binding of allergen-specific IgE to FcεRI receptors leads to the release of many mediators, including histamine, ser-

ine proteases, carboxypeptidase A, proteoglycans, tryptase, chymase, carboxypeptidase, prostaglandins, leukotrienes, tumor necrosis factor (TNF)-α, and interleukins.[5] Basophils are also activated by binding of IgE to FcεRI receptors but primarily release histamines, leukotrienes, interleukin-4, and interleukin-13.

AGENTS ASSOCIATED WITH SYSTEMIC ALLERGIC REACTIONS

CYTOTOXIC CHEMOTHERAPY

Although many cytotoxic chemotherapeutic agents can cause mild or moderate hypersensitivity reactions, fewer agents cause severe hypersensitivity reactions or systemic allergic reactions. Chemotherapy agents most frequently associated with hypersensitivity reactions include cisplatin, carboplatin, oxaliplatin, paclitaxel, docetaxel, l-asparaginase, and etoposide.[6-14] The platinum compounds are prototypic of classic IgE-mediated allergic reactions, with an increase in the incidence of infusion reactions with increased exposure to the

Table 2-2 Classification of allergic reactions

Type	Description	Mechanism	Clinical presentation
Type I	IgE-mediated immediate hypersensitivity	IgE-mediated activation of mast cells and basophils due to antigen exposure with release of vasoactive substances	Anaphylaxis, angioedema, bronchospasm, urticaria
Type II	Antibody-dependent cytotoxicity	Tissue or cell injury due to binding of an associated antigen or hapten to an antibody	Hemolytic anemia, thrombocytopenia, neutropenia
Type III	Immune complex disease	Damage to cells or tissues due to deposition of antigen-antibody complexes with resultant complement activation and/or recruitment of neutrophils	Serum sickness
Type IV	Cell-mediated/delayed hypersensitivity	Activation of T cells by antigen with resultant tissue damage	Contact dermatitis, Stevens Johnson syndrome, drug-induced hypertension

drug. For example, in one trial, 27% of patients who received seven or more cycles of carboplatin had an infusion reaction, compared with 1% for patients with fewer cycles.[13] By comparison, patients receiving the taxanes docetaxel and paclitaxel are most likely to have an infusion reaction with the first cycle of therapy, suggesting a nonimmune, anaphylactoid reaction.[15-17]

MONOCLONAL ANTIBODIES

Monoclonal antibodies are sometimes associated with systemic infusion reactions and may also cause cutaneous reactions, but this chapter focuses on systemic reactions and their management. In contrast to systemic allergic reactions, which often require acute management and discontinuation of therapy, cutaneous allergic reactions may be treated topically and may even indicate that the drug has efficacy.[18,19] The monoclonal antibodies that are most frequently associated with systemic allergic reactions are rituximab, cetuximab, and trastuzumab.[20-23]

The mechanism for systemic infusion reactions to monoclonal antibodies often is not IgE-mediated cytokine release, but rather cytokine release from antigen-antibody interactions.[24,25] Unlike traditional cytotoxic chemotherapy, which often requires pre-exposure to elicit an IgE-mediated reaction, systemic anaphylactic reactions to monoclonal antibodies often occur with the first or second infusion.[26,27] These allergic reactions to therapeutic monoclonal antibodies may be due to preexisting IgE to specific glycoproteins, which may be present on the therapeutic monoclonal antibody, causing an IgE-mediated anaphylactic reaction on initial exposure. The importance of a history of allergy or preformed antibodies for predicting the risk of an allergic reaction to monoclonal antibody therapy was shown in a review of data from patients receiving cetuximab in North Carolina and Tennessee—areas with a high incidence of infusion reactions to this therapy.[27] This hypothesis is supported by a higher incidence of bronchospasm and hypotension as symptoms of anaphylaxis to cetuximab in the southeastern United States, where a greater prevalence of an IgE specific for galactose-alpha-1,3-galactose, which is on the Fab heavy chain of cetuximab, has been noted.[23] Pretreatment antibodies against cetuximab were present in 21% of patients from Tennessee, but in only 0.6% of patients from Boston.

DIAGNOSIS OF SYSTEMIC ALLERGIC REACTIONS TO CHEMOTHERAPY

Correct identification of an allergic reaction to chemotherapy requires careful clinical evaluation, with laboratory testing to confirm the clinical diagnosis of anaphylaxis, as necessary. Clinical evaluation is critical for distinguishing between a standard infusion reaction, a severe infusion reaction, and an anaphylactic reaction, because this will determine the necessary management and risks associated with continued use of chemotherapy. The National Institute of Allergy and Infectious Disease and the Food Allergy and Anaphylaxis Network have developed diagnostic criteria for determining the likelihood that a patient is having an anaphylactic reaction (Table 2-3).

Patients who develop an infusion reaction to chemotherapy should be evaluated for fever, changes in heart rate or blood pressure, chest pain, back or abdominal pain, chills, nausea or vomiting, diarrhea, hypoxia, dyspnea or bronchospasm, and dizziness or syncope. The skin should always be carefully assessed for flushing, urticaria, hives, or rash because skin manifestations are very common.

Anaphylactic reactions are allergic reactions resulting from IgE-mediated release of histamine and many other vasoactive mediators. Symptoms of anaphylaxis include flushing; urticaria, often in the neck, trunk, abdomen, or axilla; angioedema, usually involving the face, lips, or eyelids; cough; shortness of breath; wheeze; chest pressure; laryngeal edema; and hypoxia. Patients with anaphylaxis may have tachycardia, hypotension, dizziness, tunnel vision, nausea, vomiting, and diarrhea.

Although anaphylaxis is a clinical diagnosis, the diagnosis of an allergic, IgE-mediated immediate reaction with activation of mast cells or basophils can be confirmed by a blood test to identify chemical mediators, in some cases. Anaphylactoid or pseudoallergic reactions in which mast cells and basophils are activated by indirect, nonimmune mechanisms may lead to positive skin or blood tests. Many chemical mediators, including tryptase, histamine, and leukotriene, are released from mast cells and basophils during

Table 2-3 National Institute of Allergy and Infectious Disease/Food Allergy and Anaphylaxis Network diagnostic criteria for anaphylaxis

Anaphylaxis is highly likely if a patient fulfills one of the following three criteria:

1. Acute illness within minutes to several hours with involvement of the skin, mucosal membranes, or both (e.g., hives, pruritus, flushing, swelling of the lips, tongue, or uvula)

AND AT LEAST ONE OF THE FOLLOWING:

   A. Respiratory compromise with dyspnea, wheeze, bronchospasm, stridor, hypoxemia, or decreased peak expiratory flow

   B. Reduced blood pressure or symptoms of end-organ dysfunction, such as syncope, collapse, or incontinence

2. Two or more of the following within minutes to several hours of exposure to a *likely* allergen:

   A. Involvement of the skin or mucosal membranes (e.g., hives, pruritus, flushing, swelling of the lips, tongue, or uvula)

   B. Respiratory compromise with dyspnea, wheeze, bronchospasm, stridor, hypoxemia, or decreased peak expiratory flow

   C. Reduced blood pressure or symptoms, such as syncope, collapse, or incontinence

   D. Persistent gastrointestinal symptoms, such as crampy abdominal pain or vomiting

3. Reduced blood pressure within minutes to several hours after exposure to a *known* allergen

   A. Infants and children: Low systolic blood pressure or a greater than 30% decrease in systolic blood pressure*

   B. Adults: Systolic blood pressure less than 90 mm Hg or a greater than 30% decrease from baseline

Adapted from Sampson HA, et al. Second symposium on the definition and management of anaphylaxis: summary report—Second National Institute of Allergy and Infectious Disease/Food Allergy and Anaphylaxis Network symposium. *J Allergy Clin Immunol.* 2006;117:391.

* Low blood pressure for children 1 month to 1 year: <70 mm Hg; 1 to 10 years: <(70 mm Hg + [2 × age]); 11 to 17 years: <90 mm Hg.

PREVENTION OF SYSTEMIC ALLERGIC REACTIONS TO CHEMOTHERAPY

SKIN TESTING

Although skin testing is a routine part of testing for many drugs to determine their ability to elicit a type I, IgE-mediated allergic reaction, this procedure is not as common for chemotherapy. Skin testing is used most frequently for platinum-based chemotherapy.[38-41] Unfortunately, these tests are not standardized and frequently are not sensitive or specific for predicting a patient's risk for an allergic reaction. The use of skin testing for other chemotherapeutic agents is limited by the irritative properties of most chemotherapy agents, or by the lack of an IgE-mediated allergic reaction. Other problems with skin testing that limit its use include false-negative tests due to allergy to the metabolite of the administered drug, negative tests due to hypogranulation of mast cells and basophils immediately following the allergic reaction, and decreasing allergic response caused by antihistamine use. Because of these limitations in testing to confirm a diagnosis or predict an anaphylactic reaction, systemic allergic reactions are diagnosed and treated on the basis of clinical criteria.

PREMEDICATIONS

It is important for clinicians to understand the role of premedications in preventing infusion or allergic reactions to chemotherapy. Although nonsteroidal antiinflammatory agents, antihistamines, and steroids are often used as premedications for many chemotherapy regimens, these agents do not prevent IgE-mediated allergic reactions to oxaliplatin, for example.[14,42] Premedications can prevent mild, nonimmune hypersensitivity or standard infusion reactions to paclitaxel or docetaxel, for example, and can limit the symptoms or severity of severe hypersensitivity reactions, but they do not prevent immune-mediated anaphylactic reactions.[43,44]

MANAGEMENT OF PATIENTS WITH ALLERGIC REACTIONS TO CHEMOTHERAPY

ACUTE MANAGEMENT

Systemic chemotherapy should be given to patients only by appropriately trained personnel in a setting equipped to provide emergent supportive medical care, because of the seriousness of anaphylaxis. The most important therapy for the acute management of an anaphylactic reaction to chemotherapy is to stop the infusion and the intramuscular administration of epinephrine.[45] The World Allergy Organization ad hoc Committee on Epinephrine in Anaphylaxis has determined that no absolute contraindications are known for administering epinephrine for suspected anaphylaxis, and this treatment can be administered every 5 to 15 minutes as needed for control of symptoms.[45] Epinephrine should be given promptly to patients with an anaphylactic reaction, because respiratory distress and hypotension can progress rapidly, and studies of patients with anaphylactic reactions to several allergens show that delays in treatment can be fatal.[46] In addition to receiving

an anaphylactic reaction, but the most reliable diagnostic test is serum tryptase.[28-30] Histamine is produced by both mast cells and basophils, but the half-life and plasma or serum and potential false elevations due to sample processing make confirming anaphylaxis with this marker difficult.[31,32] The levels of total tryptase and serum peak 3 hours after development of an anaphylactic reaction, remain stable in a refrigerated sample for 1 week, and constitute a frozen sample for 1 year.[30,31,33] A blood sample should be drawn between 15 minutes and 3 hours after development of the suspected anaphylactic reaction. Although other conditions, such as mastocytosis or myelodysplastic syndromes, may be associated with elevated serum total tryptase, this is a specific marker for anaphylaxis with no acute elevation in tryptase with other conditions that may be in the initial differential diagnosis for symptoms of anaphylaxis, such as vasovagal reactions or septic shock.[28,34-36] Serum total tryptase levels can be normal in a patient who has an anaphylactic reaction if the samples are drawn too early after the appearance of symptoms suggestive of anaphylaxis, or if the anaphylactic reaction is due to release of vasoactive mediators from basal cells relative to mast cells, given the significantly lower levels of tryptase in mast cells.[30,31,37]

epinephrine, patients should lie down with their lower extremities elevated, should be given supplemental oxygen because of the risk for respiratory compromise, and should be given IV fluids because of the risk for significant hypotension due to vasodilation. Patients having an anaphylactic reaction may benefit from albuterol to relieve bronchospasm and diphenhydramine for urticaria and pruritus; however, clinicians must recognize that beta-2 agonists and H$_1$-antihistamines are not substitutes for epinephrine for the acute management of anaphylaxis.[47-49] Patients with symptoms that are refractory to intramuscular epinephrine may require an infusion of epinephrine. Additionally, approximately 20% of patients with an anaphylactic reaction will have a biphasic response, with recurrence of symptoms of anaphylaxis up to 72 hours after the initial episode.[50-52] Unfortunately, no predictors indicate which patients will have a biphasic response, so all patients with anaphylaxis should be observed after confirmation of a systemic allergic reaction. An observation period of 24 hours has been recommended.[51,52]

FURTHER MANAGEMENT
Desensitization

Many chemotherapy options are often available for patients with cancer; however, some patients may benefit from a specific therapy because of the anticipated efficacy of, or intolerance to, other therapies. Unfortunately, patients can develop allergic reactions to chemotherapeutic agents, and this may limit their treatment options. Desensitization is a procedure for inducing tolerance to an agent by administering small amounts of the agent in incremental steps up to full therapeutic doses.[53] Many methods have been developed to desensitize patients to carboplatin, cisplatin, oxaliplatin, docetaxel, and paclitaxel—agents that cause systemic anaphylactic reactions directly by an IgE-mediated process or by indirect activation of mast cells.[54-60] Although traditional desensitization protocols for many allergens require exposure to increasing amounts of allergen over a prolonged time, many of the protocols for chemotherapeutic agents require rapid desensitization and are completed within hours. In one series, 98 patients underwent 412 desensitizations to carboplatin, cisplatin, oxaliplatin, paclitaxel, liposomal doxorubicin, or rituximab with a 12-step protocol.[54] Of 98 patients, 81 had severe hypersensivity reactions. The procedure took less than 6 hours, was well tolerated, and allowed all patients to subsequently receive full-dose therapy. This series showed successful desensitization to platinums, which cause systemic allergic reactions through traditional IgE-mediated mechanisms; taxanes, which cause systemic reactions via direct effects on mast cells; and a monoclonal antibody, which typically causes allergic reactions due to pre-formed antibodies. Desensitization may allow patients to safely receive the most appropriate therapy for their cancer.

CONCLUSION

Treating patients with cancer with cytotoxic chemotherapy or monoclonal antibodies can lead to serious systemic allergic reactions. Many of the frequently used oncology drugs cause mild or moderate, non–immune-mediated hypersensitivity or infusion reactions, which can be prevented with appropriate premedications, are easily managed, and do not hinder further use of the therapy. Rarely, patients will have an immune-mediated, systemic allergic reaction that, if not recognized promptly and treated appropriately, may be fatal. Anaphylaxis is a clinical diagnosis that may be properly recognized and differentiated from non–immune-mediated systemic reactions. Patients with unrecognized anaphylaxis or severe anaphylactoid reactions are at risk for serious adverse events with reexposure to the drug. For most tumors, treatment options known to be effective are limited. Incorrectly stopping treatment in a patient with a systemic reaction to therapy that is not immune mediated may have serious consequences for the effectiveness of treatment. It is imperative that all healthcare providers who treat patients with cancer chemotherapy recognize the signs of anaphylaxis and understand the acute management of this condition, so they can safely and effectively treat these patients.

REFERENCES

1. Institute, National Cancer. *Common terminology criteria for adverse events (CTCAE) and common toxicity criteria (CTC)*. Available at: http://ctep.cancer.gov/protocolDevelopment/electronic_applications/ctc.htm; 2009.
2. Gell PGH, Coombs R, eds. *Clinical aspects of immunology*. 1st ed. Oxford: Blackwell; 1963.
3. Johansson SG, Bieber T, Dahl R, et al. Revised nomenclature for allergy for global use: report of the Nomenclature Review Committee of the World Allergy Organization, October 2003. *J Allergy Clin Immunol*. 2004;113:832.
4. Simons FE. Anaphylaxis. *J Allergy Clin Immunol*. 2008;121(suppl 2):S402.
5. Prussin C, Metcalfe DD. IgE, mast cells, basophils, and eosinophils. *J Allergy Clin Immunol*. 2006;117(2 suppl mini-primer):S450.
6. Billett AL, Carls A, Gelber RD, et al. Allergic reactions to Erwinia asparaginase in children with acute lymphoblastic leukemia who had previous allergic reactions to *Escherichia coli* asparaginase. *Cancer*. 1992;70:201.
7. Kim BH, Bradley T, Tai J, et al. Hypersensitivity to oxaliplatin: an investigation of incidence and risk factors, and literature review. *Oncology*. 2009;76:231.
8. Koren C, Yerushalmi R, Katz A, et al. Hypersensitivity reaction to cisplatin during chemoradiation therapy for gynecologic malignancy. *Am J Clin Oncol*. 2002;25:625.
9. O'Dwyer PJ, Weiss RB. Hypersensitivity reactions induced by etoposide. *Cancer Treat Rep*. 1984;68:959.
10. Price KS, Castells MC. Taxol reactions. *Allergy Asthma Proc*. 2002;23:205.
11. Weiss RB, Donehower RC, Wiernik PH, et al. Hypersensitivity reactions from taxol. *J Clin Oncol*. 1990;8:1263.
12. Woo MH, Hak LJ, Storm MC, et al. Anti-asparaginase antibodies following *E. coli* asparaginase therapy in pediatric acute lymphoblastic leukemia. *Leukemia*. 1998;12:1527.
13. Markman M, Kennedy A, Webster K, et al. Clinical features of hypersensitivity reactions to carboplatin. *J Clin Oncol*. 1999;17:1141.
14. Thomas RR, Quinn MG, Schuler B, et al. Hypersensitivity and idiosyncratic reactions to oxaliplatin. *Cancer*. 2003;97:2301.
15. Ardavanis A, Tryfonopoulis D, Yiotis I, et al. Non-allergic nature of docetaxel-induced acute hypersensitivity reactions. *Anticancer Drugs*. 2004;15:581.
16. Robinson JB, Singh D, Bodurka-Bevers DC, et al. Hypersensitivity reactions and the utility of oral and intravenous desensitization in patients with gynecologic malignancies. *Gynecol Oncol*. 2001;82:550.
17. Syrigou E, Karapanagiotou EM, Alamara CV, et al. Hypersensitivity reactions to antineoplastic agents: an overview. *Anticancer Drugs*. 2009;20:1.
18. Perez-Soler R, Saltz L. Cutaneous adverse effects with HER1/EGFR-targeted agents: is there a silver lining? *J Clin Oncol*. 2005;23:5235.

19. Saltz L, Rubin MS, Hochster H. Acne-like rash predicts response in patients treated with cetuximab (IMC-C225) plus irinotecan (CPT-11) in CPT-11-refractory colorectal cancer (CRC) that expresses epidermal growth factor receptor (EGFR). *Clin Cancer Res.* 2001;7:3766. Abstract 559.

20. Brennan PJ, Rodriguez Bouza T, Hsu FL, et al. Hypersensitivity reactions to mAbs: 105 desensitizations in 23 patients, from evaluation to treatment. *J Allergy Clin Immunol.* 2009;124:1259.

21. Grillo-López AJ, White CA, Varns C, et al. Overview of the clinical development of rituximab: first monoclonal antibody approved for the treatment of lymphoma. *Semin Oncol.* 1999;26 (5 suppl 14):66.

22. Melamed J, Stahlman JE. Rapid desensitization and rush immunotherapy to trastuzumab (Herceptin). *J Allergy Clin Immunol.* 2002;110:813.

23. Chung CH, Mirakhur B, Chan E, et al. Cetuximab-induced anaphylaxis and IgE specific for galactose-alpha-1,3-galactose. *N Engl J Med.* 2008;358:1109.

24. Chung CH. Managing premedications and the risk for reactions to infusional monoclonal antibody therapy. *Oncologist.* 2008;13:725.

25. Dillman RO. Infusion reactions associated with the therapeutic use of monoclonal antibodies in the treatment of malignancy. *Cancer Metastasis Rev.* 1999;18:465.

26. McLaughlin P, Grillo-López AJ, Link BK, et al. Rituximab chimeric anti-CD20 monoclonal antibody therapy for relapsed indolent lymphoma: half of patients respond to a four-dose treatment program. *J Clin Oncol.* 1998;16:2825.

27. O'Neil BH, Allen R, Spigel DR, et al. High incidence of cetuximab-related infusion reactions in Tennessee and North Carolina and the association with atopic history. *J Clin Oncol.* 2007;25:3644.

28. Schwartz LB. Diagnostic value of tryptase in anaphylaxis and mastocytosis. *Immunol Allergy Clin North Am.* 2006;26:451.

29. Schwartz LB, Bradford TR, Rouse C, et al. Development of a new, more sensitive immunoassay for human tryptase: use in systemic anaphylaxis. *J Clin Immunol.* 1994;14:190.

30. Schwartz LB, Yunginger JW, Miller J, et al. Time course of appearance and disappearance of human mast cell tryptase in the circulation after anaphylaxis. *J Clin Invest.* 1989;83:1551.

31. Laroche D, Vergnaud MC, Sillard B, et al. Biochemical markers of anaphylactoid reactions to drugs: comparison of plasma histamine and tryptase. *Anesthesiology.* 1991;75:945.

32. Schwartz LB, Irani AM, Roller K, et al. Quantitation of histamine, tryptase, and chymase in

dispersed human T and TC mast cells. *J Immunol.* 1987;138:2611.

33. Schwartz LB, Metcalfe DD, Miller JS, et al. Tryptase levels as an indicator of mast-cell activation in systemic anaphylaxis and mastocytosis. *N Engl J Med.* 1987;316:1622.

34. Sperr WR, Jordan JH, Baghestanian M, et al. Expression of mast cell tryptase by myeloblasts in a group of patients with acute myeloid leukemia. *Blood.* 2001;98:2200.

35. Sperr WR, Stehberger B, Wimazal F, et al. Serum tryptase measurements in patients with myelodysplastic syndromes. *Leuk Lymphoma.* 2002;43:1097.

36. Valent P, Sperr WR, Schwartz LB, et al. Diagnosis and classification of mast cell proliferative disorders: delineation from immunologic diseases and non-mast cell hematopoietic neoplasms. *J Allergy Clin Immunol.* 2004;114:3.

37. Jogie-Brahim S, Min HK, Fukuoka Y, et al. Expression of alpha-tryptase and beta-tryptase by human basophils. *J Allergy Clin Immunol.* 2004;113:1086.

38. Leguy-Seguin V, Jolimoy G, Coudert B, et al. Diagnostic and predictive value of skin testing in platinum salt hypersensitivity. *J Allergy Clin Immunol.* 2007;119:726.

39. Pagani M, Bonadonna P, Senna GE, et al. Standardization of skin tests for diagnosis and prevention of hypersensitivity reactions to oxaliplatin. *Int Arch Allergy Immunol.* 2008;145:54.

40. Markman M, Zanotti K, Peterson G, et al. Expanded experience with an intradermal skin test to predict for the presence or absence of carboplatin hypersensitivity. *J Clin Oncol.* 2003;21:4611.

41. Garufi C, Cristaudo A, Vanni B, et al. Skin testing and hypersensitivity reactions to oxaliplatin. *Ann Oncol.* 2003;14:497.

42. Bhargava P, Gammon D, McCormick MJ. Hypersensitivity and idiosyncratic reactions to oxaliplatin. *Cancer.* 2004;100:211.

43. Eisenhauer EA, ten Bokkel Huinink WW, Swenerton KD, et al. European-Canadian randomized trial of paclitaxel in relapsed ovarian cancer: high-dose versus low-dose and long versus short infusion. *J Clin Oncol.* 1994;12:2654.

44. Trudeau ME, Eisenhauer EA, Higgins BP, et al. Docetaxel in patients with metastatic breast cancer: a phase II study of the National Cancer Institute of Canada-Clinical Trials Group. *J Clin Oncol.* 1996;14:422.

45. Kemp SF, Lockey RF, Simons FE. Epinephrine: the drug of choice for anaphylaxis. A statement of the World Allergy Organization. *Allergy* 1008;63:1061.

46. Greenberger PA, Rotskoff BD, Lifschultz B. Fatal anaphylaxis: postmortem findings and associated comorbid diseases. *Ann Allergy Asthma Immunol.* 2007;98:252.

47. Sheikh A, ten Broek V, Brown SG, et al. H1-antihistamines for the treatment of anaphylaxis with and without shock. *Cochrane Database Syst Rev.* 2007;(1): CD006160.

48. Simons FE. Advances in H1-antihistamines. *N Engl J Med.* 2004;351:2203.

49. Soar J, Pumphrey R, Cant A, et al. Emergency treatment of anaphylactic reactions—guidelines for healthcare providers. *Resuscitation.* 2008;77:157.

50. Ellis AK, Day JH. Incidence and characteristics of biphasic anaphylaxis: a prospective evaluation of 103 patients. *Ann Allergy Asthma Immunol.* 2007;98:64.

51. Kemp SF. The post-anaphylaxis dilemma: how long is long enough to observe a patient after resolution of symptoms? *Curr Allergy Asthma Rep.* 2008;8:45.

52. Lieberman P. Biphasic anaphylactic reactions. *Ann Allergy Asthma Immunol.* 2005;95:217.

53. Castells M. Rapid desensitization for hypersensitivity reactions to chemotherapy agents. *Curr Opin Allergy Clin Immunol.* 2006;6:271.

54. Castells MC, Tennant NM, Sloane DE, et al. Hypersensitivity reactions to chemotherapy: outcomes and safety of rapid desensitization in 413 cases. *J Allergy Clin Immunol.* 2008;122:574.

55. Choi J, Harnett P, Fulcher DA. Carboplatin desensitization. *Ann Allergy Asthma Immunol.* 2004;93:137.

56. Feldweg AM, Lee CW, Matulonis UA, et al. Rapid desensitization for hypersensitivity reactions to paclitaxel and docetaxel: a new standard protocol used in 77 successful treatments. *Gynecol Oncol.* 2005;96:824.

57. Goldberg A, Confino-Cohen R, Fishman A, et al. A modified, prolonged desensitization protocol in carboplatin allergy. *J Allergy Clin Immunol.* 1996;98:841.

58. Lee CW, Matulonis UA, Castells MC. Carboplatin hypersensitivity: a 6-h 12-step protocol effective in 35 desensitizations in patients with gynecological malignancies and mast cell/IgE-mediated reactions. *Gynecol Oncol.* 2004;95:370.

59. Lee CW, Matulonis UA, Castells MC. Rapid inpatient/outpatient desensitization for chemotherapy hypersensitivity: standard protocol effective in 57 patients for 255 courses. *Gynecol Oncol.* 2005;99:393.

60. Rosique-Robles D, Vicent Verge JM, Borrás-Blasco J, et al. Successful desensitization protocol for hypersensitivity reactions caused by oxaliplatin. *Int J Clin Pharmacol Ther.* 2007;45:606.

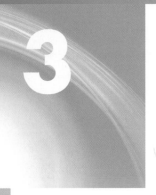

3

Prophylaxis and treatment of chemotherapy-induced nausea and vomiting

Karin Jordan, Petra Ch. Feyer, and Petra Ortner

The goal of antiemetic therapy is to completely prevent chemotherapy-induced nausea and vomiting (CINV). Few side effects of cancer treatment are more feared by the patient than nausea and vomiting.[1,2] Twenty years ago, these were inevitable adverse events of chemotherapy and forced up to 20% of patients to postpone or refuse potentially curative treatment.[3] Clinical and basic research over the past 25 years has lead to steady improvement in the control of CINV.

A main milestone in modern antiemetic therapy was the development of the 5-HT$_3$ receptor-antagonists (5-HT$_3$-RA) as antiemetics at the end of the 1980s. From the patient's view, this has been one of the most significant advances in the management of side effects of tumor therapy.[4]

Another group of antiemetics, the neurokinin-1 receptor antagonists (NK-1-RAs), were developed at the beginning of this century. The first drug in this class, aprepitant, was approved in 2003.[5] Studies have shown that in acute and delayed settings of highly and moderately emetogenic chemotherapy, patients benefit from the use of aprepitant in combination with standard antiemetic therapy. Old drugs also have a place in today's antiemetic strategies: The role of corticosteroids is often underestimated, even though they show good antiemetic efficacy in the prevention of acute and delayed emesis, respectively, especially when combined with other antiemetic agents.

However, although significant progress has been made with the development of a number of effective and well-tolerated antiemetic treatments, CINV remains an important adverse effect of tumor treatment.

PATHOPHYSIOLOGY AND CLASSIFICATION OF CHEMOTHERAPY-INDUCED NAUSEA AND VOMITING

The pathophysiology of CINV is not entirely understood; however, it is thought to have many contributing pathways.[6]

MECHANISMS OF CINV

Three key components involving areas of the hindbrain and the abdominal vagal afferents have been identified. Nowadays, it is thought that an anatomically discrete vomiting center is unlikely to exist.[6] The locations of neurons that coordinate bodily functions associated with emesis are spread throughout the medulla, supporting the notion that a central pattern generator coordinates the sequence of behaviors during emesis. The central pattern generator receives indirect input from both the area postrema (chemoreceptor trigger zone) and the abdominal vagus by means of the nucleus tractus solitarius.

Chemoreceptor trigger zone

The chemoreceptor trigger zone (CTZ) is located in the area postrema at the bottom end of the fourth ventricle. The CTZ is a circumventricular organ, which basically means that this structure lacks an effective blood-brain barrier and is able to detect emetic agents in both the systemic circulation and the cerebrospinal fluid. Studies in animal models have demonstrated that opioids and dopaminergic agonists can induce emesis when they bind to this site. The area postrema has afferent and efferent connections with underlying structures—the subnucleus gelatinosus and the nucleus tractus solitarius—receiving vagal afferent fibers from the gastrointestinal tract.

Abdominal vagal afferents

The abdominal vagal afferents appear to have the greatest relevance for chemotherapy-induced nausea and vomiting. A variety of receptors, including 5-hydroxytryptamine 3 (5-HT_3), neurokinin-1, and cholecystokinin-1, are located on the terminal ends of the vagal afferents. These receptors lie in close proximity to the enterochromaffin cells located in the gastrointestinal mucosa of the proximal small intestine, which contains a number of local mediators, such as 5-hydroxytryptamine (5-HT), substance P, and cholecystokinin.

Following exposure to radiation or cytotoxic drugs, serotonin (5-HT) is released from enterochromaffin cells in the small-intestinal mucosa, which are adjacent to the vagal afferent neurons on which 5-HT_3 receptors are located. Released serotonin activates vagal afferent neurons via the 5-HT_3 receptors, which leads ultimately to an emetic response mediated by the chemoreceptor trigger zone within the area postrema (Fig. 3-1). Although the vagal nerve relays information to the area postrema, most of the sensory information from the vagal nerve is relayed to the tractus solitarius, further interacting with the central pattern generator.

At present, this vagal-dependent pathway is considered the primary mechanism by which most chemotherapeutic agents initiate acute emesis. Delayed emesis is mainly centrally mediated, as is depicted in Fig. 3-2.

Neurotransmitters

Investigations over the past three decades have gradually elucidated the clinical significance of several neurotransmitters in the vomiting process. The neurotransmitters serotonin, substance P, and dopamine all appear to play important roles in this process.[6,7]

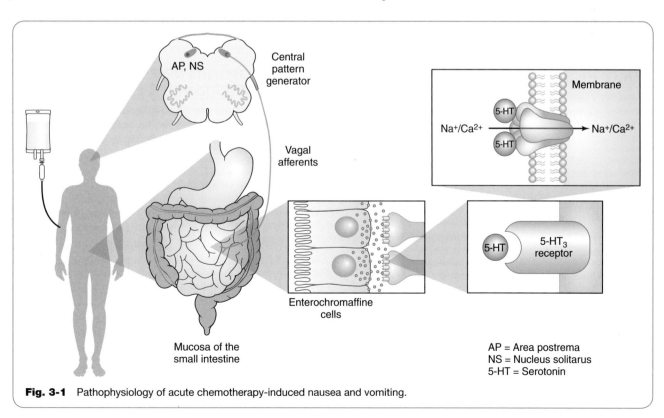

Fig. 3-1 Pathophysiology of acute chemotherapy-induced nausea and vomiting.

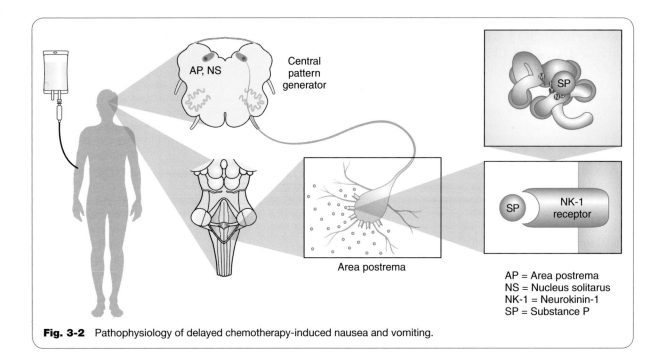

Fig. 3-2 Pathophysiology of delayed chemotherapy-induced nausea and vomiting.

CLASSIFICATION OF NAUSEA AND VOMITING

Chemotherapy-induced nausea and vomiting may be classified into three categories: acute onset, occurring within 24 hours of initial administration of chemotherapy; delayed onset, occurring 24 hours to several days after initial treatment; and anticipatory nausea and vomiting, observed in patients whose emetic episodes are triggered by taste, odor, sight, thoughts, or anxiety secondary to a history of poor response to antiemetic agents[8,9] (Table 3-1).

RISK FACTORS ASSOCIATED WITH NAUSEA AND VOMITING AFTER CHEMOTHERAPY

The severity and clinical presentation of CINV depend on several factors. The emetogenic potential of the che-

motherapeutic agents used is the main risk factor for the degree of CINV (Tables 3-2 and 3-3).[10-12] Individual patient characteristics, which may differ substantially from one patient to another, must also be taken into consideration (Table 3-4).

ANTIEMETIC DRUGS

Several classes of antiemetic drugs that antagonize the neurotransmitter receptors responsible for CINV are available.

5-HT$_3$ SEROTONIN RECEPTOR ANTAGONISTS (5-HT$_3$-RAs)

The 5-HT$_3$ serotonin receptor antagonists (5-HT$_3$-RAs) form the cornerstone of therapy for the control of acute emesis, along with chemotherapy agents with moderate to high emetogenic potential. However, some data suggest the potential value of these drugs, especially palonosetron for the treatment of delayed emesis associated with chemotherapy.[13]

Five 5-HT$_3$-RAs—dolasetron, granisetron, ondansetron, palonosetron, and tropisetron—are available. Guideline-based dose recommendations are shown in Table 3-5.

Palonosetron differs from the other four in having both a higher receptor binding affinity and a much longer half-life, and phase III trials in the setting of moderately emetogenic chemotherapy have suggested its possible superiority to older 5-HT$_3$ receptor antagonists.[14,15] In light of these results, the updated Multinational Association of Supportive Care in Cancer, European Society of Medical Oncology (MASCC/ESMO) 2009 guidelines recommend palonosetron as the preferred agent in patients receiving moderately emetogenic chemotherapy (MEC).[16]

When 5-HT$_3$-RAs are administered, several points should be taken into consideration[17-19]:

Table 3-1 Three categories of chemotherapy-induced nausea and vomiting

Acute nausea and vomiting

- Within the first 24 hours after chemotherapy
- Mainly by serotonin (5-HT) release from enterochromaffin cells

Delayed nausea and vomiting

- After 24 hours to 5 days after chemotherapy
- Various mechanisms: mainly substance P–mediated disruption of the blood-brain barrier and of gastrointestinal motility, adrenal hormones (9)

Anticipatory nausea and vomiting

- Occurrence is possible after one cycle of chemotherapy (8).
- Involves the element of classical conditioning

Adapted from (3).

Table 3-2 Emetogenic risk of intravenous chemotherapeutic agents

High (emesis risk >90% without antiemetics)	
Carmustine, BCNU	Lomustine
Cisplatin	Mechlorethamine
Cyclophosphamide (>1500 mg/m²)	Pentostatin
Dacarbazine, DTIC	Streptozotocin
Dactinomycin, Actinomycin D	

Moderate (emesis risk 30% to 90% without antiemetics)	
Alemtuzumab	Methotrexate (>100 mg/m²)
Altretamine	Idarubicin
Azacitidine	Ifosfamide
Bendamustine	Irinotecan
Carboplatin	Mitoxantrone (>12 mg/m²)
Clofarabine	Melphalan IV
Cyclophosphamide (<1500 mg/m²)	Oxaliplatin
Cytarabine (>1 g/m²)	Temozolomide
Doxorubicin	Trabectedin
Daunorubicin	Treosulfan
Epirubicin	

Low (emesis risk 10% to 30% without antiemetics)	
Asparaginase	Mitoxantrone (<12 mg/m²)

Bortezomib	Paclitaxel
Catumaxumab	Panitumumab
Cetuximab	Pegasparaginase
Cytarabine (<1 g/m²)	Pemetrexed
Docetaxel	Teniposide
Etoposide IV	Thiopeta
5-Fluorouracil	Topotecan
Gemcitabine	Trastuzumab
Ixabepilone	

Minimal (emesis risk <10% without antiemetics)	
Bevacizumab	Melphalan PO
Bleomycin	α-, β-, γ-Interferon
Busulfan	Mercaptopurine
Chlorambucil	Methotrexate (<100 mg/m²)
Cladribine	Thioguanine
Cytarabine (<100 mg/m²)	Vinblastine
Fludarabine	Vincristine
Hormone	Vinorelbine
Hydroxyurea	

Data from References 16, 33, 35, 38, 39.

- The lowest fully effective dose for each agent should be used; higher doses do not enhance any aspect of activity because of receptor saturation.
- Oral and intravenous routes are equally effective.
- No schedule is better than a single dose daily given before chemotherapy.

Side effects: The adverse effects of 5-HT₃-RAs are generally mild, with headache, constipation, diarrhea, and asthenia often described.[20] Small, transient, reversible changes in electrocardiographic parameters have been shown to occur with all available 5-HT₃-RAs. However, after more than 13 years of commercial use, clinically relevant cardiovascular effects have not been reported.[21]

STEROIDS

Steroids are an integral part of antiemetic therapy for acute and delayed CINV, although they are not approved as antiemetics.[22] When used in combination with other antiemetics, corticosteroids exert a booster effect, raising the emetic threshold. Besides the recently introduced neurokinin-1-receptor-antagonists, dexamethasone is the most important drug in preventing delayed CINV.

For prevention of acute CINV, 20 mg (12 mg when coadministered with aprepitant) in highly emetogenic chemother-

apy and a single dose of 8 mg dexamethasone in MEC should be the dose of choice (see Table 3-5)[23,24] and has been recommended by MASCC and ASCO guidelines.[12,16]

Side effects: Steroids are considered to be safe antiemetics. Side effects are usually dependent on dose and duration of therapy.

NEUROKININ-1-RECEPTOR ANTAGONISTS (NK-1-RAs)

Aprepitant, the first representative of this new group, blocks the NK-1 receptor in the brainstem (central pattern generator) and gastrointestinal tract.[5] Aprepitant is currently the only agent available in this class.

Aprepitant-containing regimens have been shown to significantly reduce acute and delayed emesis in patients receiving highly emetogenic chemotherapy (HEC)[25-27] and MEC, compared with regimens containing a 5-HT₃-RA plus dexamethasone only.[28,29]

A randomized study established the most favorable risk profile of aprepitant at doses of 125 mg PO on day 1 and 80 mg PO on days 2 and 3 (see Table 3-5).[30] A parenteral formulation of aprepitant (fosaprepitant, a water-soluble prodrug of aprepitant) has been available since 2008. The bioequivalent dose is 115 mg IV 30 minutes before chemotherapy on

Table 3-3   Emetic risk of oral chemotherapeutic agents

High (emesis risk >90% without antiemetics)	
Hexamethylmelamine	Procarbazine

Moderate (emesis risk 30% to 90% without antiemetics)	
Cyclophosphamide	Temozolomide
Imatinib	Vinorelbine

Low (emesis risk 10% to 30% without antiemetics)	
Capecitabine	Lapatinib
Etoposide	Lenalidomide,
Everolimus	Sunitinib
Fludarabine	Thalidomide

Minimal (emesis risk <10% without antiemetics)	
Chlorambucil	Melphalan
Erlotinib	Methotrexate
Gefitinib	Sorafenib
Hydroxyurea	6-Thioguanine
L-Phenylalanine mustard	

Data from Referecnes 16, 35, 38, 39.

Table 3-4   Patient characteristics influencing the occurrence of CINV

Risk factor	Raised (↑) or decreased risk (↓)
Experience of nausea and or vomiting during previous chemotherapy	↑
Age <50 years	↑
Female gender	↑
Pretreatment anxiety	↑
Pretreatment nausea	↑
Chemotherapy as an inpatient	↓
Chemotherapy as an outpatient	↑
Severe alcohol consumption	↓
Low intake of alcohol	↑
Impaired quality of life	↑
History of motion sickness	↑
Pain	↑
Hyperemesis gravidarum	↑
Fatigue	↑

Data from References 6, 40, 41.

day 1, followed by 80 mg of aprepitant orally on days 2 and 3. Recently it was determined that the fosaprepitant 150-mg single IV regimen is equally effective to the aprepitant 3-day oral regimen.[30a]

Side effects: In general, the incidence of adverse events reported with aprepitant plus 5-HT$_3$-RA and dexamethasone is similar to that with 5-HT$_3$-RA plus dexamethasone alone: headache, 8% versus 10%; anorexia, 12% versus 11%; asthenia/fatigue, 20% versus 17%; diarrhea, 11% versus 12%; and hiccups, 12% versus 9%.[31]

DOPAMINE RECEPTOR ANTAGONISTS

Before the introduction of 5-HT$_3$-RAs, dopamine-receptor antagonists formed the basis of antiemetic therapy.[3] These agents can be subdivided into phenothiazines, butyrophenones, and substituted benzamides.[3,32] The most frequently used benzamide is metoclopramide. Before the 5-HT$_3$-RAs were established in CINV prophylaxis, metoclopramide, usually at high doses and in combination with a corticosteroid, played a primary role in the management of acute CINV. However, in patients receiving cisplatin-based chemotherapy, the effects of conventional doses of metoclopramide are not significantly different from those of placebo. Consequently, current guidelines do not recommend metoclopramide for prevention of acute CINV.

OLANZAPINE

Olanzapine, an atypical antipsychotic drug, has potential antiemetic properties caused by its ability to antagonize several neurotransmitters involved in the CINV pathways. Adverse effects reported are typical of those seen with other antipsychotics and include sleepiness, dizziness, weight gain, and dry mouth but usually no extrapyramidal side effects.[32]

CANNABINOIDS

The combination of weak antiemetic efficacy with potentially beneficial side effects (sedation, euphoria) makes cannabinoids a useful adjunct to modern antiemetic therapy in selected patients. However, the associated side effects of dizziness and dysphoria should not be underestimated.[3] Cannabinoids are advised in patients intolerant of or refractory to 5-HT$_3$-RAs or steroids and aprepitant.[16,33]

BENZODIAZEPINES

Benzodiazepines can be a useful addition to the antiemetic regimen in certain circumstances. They are often used to treat anxiety and reduce the risk of anticipatory CINV. Benzodiazepines are also used in patients with refractory and breakthrough emesis.[3,32]

ANTIHISTAMINES

Antihistamines have been administered both as antiemetics and as adjunctive agents to prevent dystonic reactions with dopamine antagonists.[34] Studies with diphenhydramine or hydroxyzine in the prevention of CINV have not shown that these drugs have antiemetic activity.[18]

Table 3-5   Dose of antiemetics

5-HT$_3$-receptor antagonist	Route	Recommended dose (once daily)
Ondansetron	PO	24 mg (high) 16 mg* (moderate)
	IV	8 mg (0.15 mg/kg)
Granisetron	PO	2 mg
	IV	1 mg (0.01 mg/kg)
Tropisetron	PO	5 mg
	IV	
Dolasetron	PO	100 mg to 200 mg
	IV	100 mg (1.8 mg/kg)
Palonosetron	IV	0.25 mg
	PO	0.5 mg
Steroids		
Dexamethasone	PI/IV	12 mg (high emetogenic with aprepitant) to 20 mg w/o aprepitant 8 mg (moderate emetogenic), 8 mg (high/moderate) days 2 and 3
NK-1-Receptor Antagonist		
Aprepitant	PO	125 mg day 1, 80 mg days 2+3
Fosaprepitant	IV	115 mg day 1 (IV), 80 mg days 2+3 (orally) or 150 mg day 1 only

Adapted from (16, 33, 35, 39).
*8 mg twice daily is recommended.

ANTIEMETIC PROPHYLAXIS OF CINV

Before chemotherapy, it is crucial to clearly define the optimal prophylactic antiemetic therapy for acute and delayed nausea and vomiting and to implement it from the beginning, because symptom-oriented therapy at a later stage is ineffective in most cases. This is important especially for the prophylaxis of delayed emesis. First, the emetogenic potential of the planned chemotherapy regimen needs to be established. The cytostatic agent with the highest emetogenic potential determines the emetogenicity of the whole chemotherapy; no cumulative effect is caused by the addition of additional cytostatic agents with lower emetogenicity.[16,35]

For outpatients, it is important to establish a written treatment plan for the prophylaxis of delayed emesis. The lowest fully effective once-daily dose of each antiemetic agent should be used. At equivalent doses and bioavailabilities, PO and IV routes have similar efficacy and safety.[33,35,36]

Table 3-6 summarizes the antiemetic therapy schemes recommended for the prevention of acute and delayed nausea and vomiting, with consideration of the antiemetic potential of chemotherapies. These schemes are based on the recent 2009 MASCC/ESMO guidelines. Recommended daily doses of antiemetics for acute (day 1) and delayed (from day 2 onward) CINV are shown in Table 3-5.[16]

PREVENTION OF ACUTE NAUSEA AND EMESIS (WITHIN THE FIRST 24 HOURS FROM THE CHEMOTHERAPY TREATMENT)
Highly emetogenic chemotherapy

Patients should be treated with a combination of a 5-HT$_3$-RA, an NK-1-RA (aprepitant), and a corticosteroid.

Moderately emetogenic chemotherapy

1. Patients receiving a combination of anthracycline plus cyclophosphamide-based chemotherapy should be given a triple combination of a 5-HT$_3$-RA, an NK-1-RA (aprepitant), and a corticosteroid.
2. Patients undergoing other moderately emetogenic chemotherapy regimens should be given a combination of a 5-HT$_3$-RA (palonosetron is recommended as the preferred agent, owing to the convincing study situation) and a corticosteroid. On the basis of favorable results, it is expected that indications of the NK-1-RA (aprepitant) may be extended to the moderately emetogenic chemotherapy field. However, such a possible extension is not yet part of the updated MASCC/ESMO 2009 guidelines.

Low emetogenic chemotherapy

In patients receiving chemotherapy of low emetic risk, a single agent such as a low dose of a corticosteroid is effective. In principle, prophylaxis with a 5-HT$_3$-RA is not part of the prophylaxis. In this area, overtreatment has been observed in clinical practice, for example, a patient who is treated with paclitaxel does not routinely need a 5-HT$_3$-RA.

Minimally emetogenic chemotherapy

For patients treated with agents of minimal emetic risk, no antiemetic drug should be routinely administered before chemotherapy.

PREVENTION OF DELAYED NAUSEA AND EMESIS (DAYS 2 TO 5 AFTER CHEMOTHERAPY)
Highly emetogenic chemotherapy

Routinely, prophylaxis should be done with an NK-1-RA (aprepitant) and a corticosteroid. The addition of a further 5-HT$_3$-RA is not necessary.[27]

Moderately emetogenic chemotherapy

If an NK-1-RA (aprepitant) was part of the prophylaxis of acute nausea and vomiting, then NK-1-RA (aprepitant) is suggested for the prevention of delayed emesis for another 2 days.

In patients who do not receive an NK-1-RA (aprepitant) as part of the prophylaxis for acute emesis, dexamethasone is recommended. In case of contraindication for the use of a corticosteroid, it can be replaced by a 5-HT$_3$-RA.

Low and minimally emetogenic chemotherapy

No routinely prophylactic antiemetic treatment is planned for the delayed phase.

Table 3-6   Antiemetic prophylaxis of CINV according to MASCC/ESMO guidelines 2009 (16)

Emetogenicity of chemotherapy	Acute phase (up to 24 hr after chemotherapy)	Delayed phase (following the first 24 hours to 5 days after chemotherapy)
High	**5-HT$_3$-RA** Palonosetron: 0.25 mg IV Granisetron: 2 mg PO/1mg IV Ondansetron: 16-24 mg PO/8 mg IV Tropisetron: 5 mg PO/IV Dolasetron: 200 mg PO/100 mg IV + **Corticosteroid** Dexamethasone: 12 mg PO/IV + **NK-1-RA** Aprepitant: 125 mg PO or Fosaprepitant: 115 mg IV or Fosaprepitant: 150 mg on day 1 only	**Corticosteroid** Dexamethasone: 8 mg PO/IV days 2 to 4 + **NK-1-RA** Aprepitant: 80 mg PO on days 2 and 3
Moderate	*Anthracycline-/Cyclophosphamide (AC)-Based Chemotherapies* As for highly emetogenic chemotherapy *Other Chemotherapies* **5-HT$_3$-RA:** Palonosetron preferred + **Corticosteroid** Dexamethasone: 8 mg PO/IV	*Anthracycline-/Cyclophosphamide (AC)- Based Chemotherapies* **NK-1-RA** Aprepitant: 80 mg PO on days 2 and 3 + **(Corticosteroid)*** Dexamethasone: 8 mg PO/IV on days 2 and 3 *Other Chemotherapies* **Corticosteroid** Dexamethasone: 8 mg PO/IV on days 2 and 3 alternatively (not 1st choice) **5-HT$_3$-RA** (Dose s.a.)
Low	**Corticosteroid** Dexamethasone: 8 mg PO/IV	No routine prophylaxis
Minimal	No routine prophylaxis	No routine prophylaxis

*Administration of corticosteroids for delayed emesis with AC-based chemotherapies is not part of the MASCC/ESMO guidelines because of missing study information, but it is considered meaningful by the expert panel.

THERAPY AGAINST ANTICIPATORY NAUSEA AND VOMITING

The use of conventional antiemetics for anticipatory nausea and vomiting is mostly ineffective and has not been extensively tested. Treatment with low benzodiazepine doses has showed some efficacy, especially if it is given before chemotherapy. However, because anticipatory nausea and vomiting is a learned conditioned reflex, it should be managed by psychological techniques, although this may not represent an easy solution in daily practice. Possible interventions include muscle relaxation, systemic desensitization, hypnosis, and cognitive distraction.[8]

Multiple-day (cisplatin-containing) chemotherapy

For multiple-day cisplatin therapy, the use of a 5-HT$_3$-RA and a corticosteroid is recommended on the days when cisplatin is administered (acute phase). In addition, for prophylaxis of delayed CINV, a corticosteroid alone should be administered on days 2 and 3 after chemotherapy. The addition of an NK-1-RA can be considered.[16,35,37] If palonosetron is part of the prophylaxis, it has to be given only on days 1, 3, and 5 because of its higher receptor affinity and longer half-life.

High-dose chemotherapy

Studies in the high-dose chemotherapy setting are lacking. On days of high-dose chemotherapy (acute phase), use of a 5-HT$_3$-RA and a corticosteroid is recommended before chemotherapy is initiated. A corticosteroid alone should be given for the prevention of delayed CINV on days 2 and 3 after high-dose chemotherapy. Use of an NK-1-RA can be taken into consideration but is not explicitly recommended by recent guidelines.[16]

BRIEF SUMMARY: PRACTICAL TREATMENT APPROACH

- Establish the emetogenic potential of chemotherapy (see Tables 3-2 and 3-3). The chemotherapeutic agent with the highest emetogenic potential determines the emetogenic level of the whole therapy.
- A prophylactic antiemetic treatment is crucial! Important: The appearance of delayed emesis is often underestimated; consequently, prophylaxis for days 2 through 5 has to be well planned from the beginning.
- Antiemetic prophylaxis: See Table 3-6.
- For persistent CINV, it is necessary to consider possible differential diagnoses (e.g., brain metastases)

REFERENCES

1. Coates A, Abraham S, Kaye SB, et al. On the receiving end—patient perception of the side-effects of cancer chemotherapy. *Eur J Cancer Clin Oncol.* 1983;19:203–208.

2. Griffin AM, Butow PN, Coates AS, et al. On the receiving end. V: Patient perceptions of the side effects of cancer chemotherapy in 1993. *Ann Oncol.* 1996;7:189–195.

3. Jordan K, Schmoll HJ, Aapro MS. Comparative activity of antiemetic drugs. *Crit Rev Oncol Hematol.* 2007;61:162–175.

4. Aapro MS. Review of experience with ondansetron and granisetron. *Ann Oncol.* 1993;4(suppl 3):9–14.

5. Hesketh PJ, Grunberg SM, Gralla RJ, et al. The oral neurokinin-1 antagonist aprepitant for the prevention of chemotherapy-induced nausea and vomiting: a multinational, randomized, double-blind, placebo-controlled trial in patients receiving high-dose cisplatin—the Aprepitant Protocol 052 Study Group. *J Clin Oncol.* 2003;21:4112–4119.

6. Hesketh PJ. Chemotherapy-induced nausea and vomiting. *N Engl J Med.* 2008;358:2482–2494.

7. Gralla RJ. Current issues in the management of nausea and vomiting. *Ann Oncol.* 1993;4(suppl 3): 3–7.

8. Aapro MS, Molassiotis A, Olver I. Anticipatory nausea and vomiting. *Support Care Cancer.* 2005;13:117–121.

9. Roila F, Donati D, Tamberi S, et al. Delayed emesis: incidence, pattern, prognostic factors and optimal treatment. *Support Care Cancer.* 2002;10:88–95.

10. Grunberg SM, Osoba D, Hesketh PJ, et al. Evaluation of new antiemetic agents and definition of antineoplastic agent emetogenicity—an update. *Support Care Cancer.* 2005;13:80–84.

11. Hesketh PJ, Kris MG, Grunberg SM, et al. Proposal for classifying the acute emetogenicity of cancer chemotherapy. *J Clin Oncol.* 1997;15:103–109.

12. Kris MG, Hesketh PJ, Somerfield MR, et al. American Society of Clinical Oncology guideline for antiemetics in oncology: update 2006. *J Clin Oncol.* 2006;24:2932–2947.

13. Saito M, Aogi K, Sekine I, et al. Palonosetron plus dexamethasone versus granisetron plus dexamethasone for prevention of nausea and vomiting during chemotherapy: a double-blind, double-dummy, randomised, comparative phase III trial. *Lancet Oncol.* 2009;10:115–124.

14. Eisenberg P, Figueroa-Vadillo J, Zamora R, et al. Improved prevention of moderately emetogenic chemotherapy-induced nausea and vomiting with palonosetron, a pharmacologically novel 5-HT3 receptor antagonist: results of a phase III, single-dose trial versus dolasetron. *Cancer.* 2003;98:2473–2482.

15. Gralla R, Lichinitser M, Van Der Vegt S, et al. Palonosetron improves prevention of chemotherapy-induced nausea and vomiting following moderately emetogenic chemotherapy: results of a double-blind randomized phase III trial comparing single doses of palonosetron with ondansetron. *Ann Oncol.* 2003;14:1570–1577.

16. Roila F, Herrstedt J, Aapro M, et al. Guideline update for MASCC and ESMO in the prevention of chemotherapy- and radiotherapy-induced nausea and vomiting: results of the Perugia consensus conference. *Ann Oncol.* 2010;21:v232–v243.

17. Kris MG, Hesketh PJ, Herrstedt J, et al. Consensus proposals for the prevention of acute and delayed vomiting and nausea following high-emetic-risk chemotherapy. *Support Care Cancer.* 2005;13:85–96.

18. Gralla RJ, Osoba D, Kris MG, et al. Recommendations for the use of antiemetics: evidence-based, clinical practice guidelines. American Society of Clinical Oncology. *J Clin Oncol.* 1999;17:2971–2994.

19. Ettinger DS, Dwight D, Kris MG, eds. *National Comprehensive Cancer Network: antiemesis, clinical practice guidelines in oncology.* 1st ed. Jenkintown: NCCN; 2005.

20. Goodin S, Cunningham R. 5-HT(3)-receptor antagonists for the treatment of nausea and vomiting: a reappraisal of their side-effect profile. *Oncologist.* 2002;7:424–436.

21. Navari RM, Koeller JM. Electrocardiographic and cardiovascular effects of the 5-hydroxytryptamine3 receptor antagonists. *Ann Pharmacother.* 2003;37:1276–1286.

22. Grunberg SM. Antiemetic activity of corticosteroids in patients receiving cancer chemotherapy: dosing, efficacy, and tolerability analysis. *Ann Oncol.* 2007;18:233–240.

23. Double-blind, dose-finding study of four intravenous doses of dexamethasone in the prevention of cisplatin-induced acute emesis. Italian Group for Antiemetic Research. *J Clin Oncol.* 1998;16:2937–2942.

24. Italian Group for Antiemtic Research. Randomized, double-blind, dose-finding study of dexamethasone in preventing acute emesis induced by anthracyclines, carboplatin, or cyclophosphamide. *J Clin Oncol.* 2004;22:725–729.

25. Hesketh P, Grunberg S, Gralla R, et al. The oral neurokinin-1 antagonist aprepitant for the prevention of chemotherapy-induced nausea and vomiting: a multinational, randomized, double-blind, placebo-controlled trial in patients receiving high-dose cisplatin—the Aprepitant Protocol 052 Study Group. *J Clin Oncol.* 2003;21:4112–4119.

26. Poli-Bigelli S, Rodrigues-Pereira J, Carides AD, et al. Addition of the neurokinin 1 receptor antagonist aprepitant to standard antiemetic therapy improves control of chemotherapy-induced nausea and vomiting: results from a randomized, double-blind, placebo-controlled trial in Latin America. *Cancer.* 2003;97:3090–3098.

27. Schmoll HJ, Aapro MS, Poli-Bigelli S, et al. Comparison of an aprepitant regimen with a multiple-day ondansetron regimen, both with dexamethasone, for antiemetic efficacy in high-dose cisplatin treatment. *Ann Oncol.* 2006;17:1000–1006.

28. Warr D, Grunberg SM, Gralla RJ, et al. The oral NK(1) antagonist aprepitant for the prevention of acute and delayed chemotherapy-induced nausea and vomiting: pooled data from 2 randomised, double-blind, placebo controlled trials. *Eur J Cancer.* 2005;41:1278–1285.

29. Rapoport B, Jordan K, Boice J, et al. Aprepitant for the prevention of chemotherapy-induced nausea and vomiting associated with a broad range of moderately emetogenic chemotherapies and tumor types: a randomized, double-blind study. *Support Care Cancer.* 2010;18:423–431.

30. Chawla SP, Grunberg SM, Gralla RJ, et al. Establishing the dose of the oral NK1 antagonist aprepitant for the prevention of chemotherapy-induced nausea and vomiting. *Cancer.* 2003;97:2290–2300.

30a. Grunberg S, Chua DT, Roila F, Herrstedt J. Phase III randomized double-blind study of single-dose fosaprepitant for prevention of cisplatin-induced nausea and vomiting (CINV). *J Clin Oncol.* 2010;28:Abstr 9021.

31. Depre M, Van Hecken A, Oeyen M, et al. Effect of aprepitant on the pharmacokinetics and pharmacodynamics of warfarin. *Eur J Clin Pharmacol.* 2005;61:341–346.

32. Lohr L. Chemotherapy-induced nausea and vomiting. *Cancer J.* 2008;14:85–93.

33. Kris MG, Hesketh PJ, Somerfield MR, et al. American Society of Clinical Oncology guideline for antiemetics in oncology: update 2006. *J Clin Oncol.* 2006;24:2932–2947.

34. Kris MG, Gralla RJ, Clark RA, et al. Antiemetic control and prevention of side effects of anti-cancer therapy with lorazepam or diphenhydramine when used in combination with metoclopramide plus dexamethasone: a double-blind, randomized trial. *Cancer.* 1987;60:2816–2822.

35. Roila F, Hesketh PJ, Herrstedt J. Prevention of chemotherapy- and radiotherapy-induced emesis: results of the 2004 Perugia International Antiemetic Consensus Conference. *Ann Oncol.* 2006;17:20–28.

36. Jordan K, Bokemeyer C, Langenbrake C, et al. Antiemetische prophylaxe und therapie gemäß den MASCC und ASCO guidelines. In: *Kurzgefasste interdisziplinäre Leitlinien 2008.* München: Zuckschwerdt Verlag; 2008:348–354.

37. Jordan K, Kinitz I, Voigt W, et al. Schmoll HJ. Safety and efficacy of a triple antiemetic combination with the NK-1 antagonist aprepitant in highly and moderately emetogenic multiple-day chemotherapy. *Eur J Cancer.* 2009;45:1184–1187.

38. National Comprehensive Cancer Network. *Antiemesis, clinical practice guidelines in oncology.* 1st ed. Jenkintown: NCCN; 2007.

39. Jordan K, Sippel C, Schmoll HJ. Guidelines for antiemetic treatment of chemotherapy-induced nausea and vomiting: past, present, and future recommendations. *Oncologist.* 2007;12:1143–1150.

40. Morrow GR, Roscoe JA, Hickok JT, et al. Nausea and emesis: evidence for a biobehavioral perspective. *Support Care Cancer.* 2002;10:96–105.

41. Jordan K, Grothey A, Pelz T, et al. Impact of quality of life parameters and coping strategies on postchemotherapy nausea and vomiting (PCNV). *Eur J Cancer Care.* 2010;19:603–609.

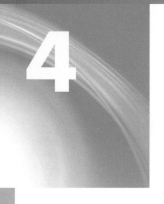

4

Antimicrobial therapy of unexplained fever and infection in neutropenic cancer patients

Hartmut Link

Neutropenia is a common complication in patients undergoing cytostatic chemotherapy and one of the most important risk factors for infection. Additional factors that contribute markedly to increased susceptibility to infection include damage to the skin and to the mucous membranes of the oral pharynx and gastrointestinal tract, which can be due to toxic effects of chemotherapy or radiotherapy, or to the neutropenia itself. Fever is often the only indication of infection in neutropenic patients.

Although 50% of febrile neutropenic patients have a documented infection initially, infection cannot be localized in the other patients. Even if the infection site cannot be identified, antibiotic therapy must be started immediately to prevent progression to a life-threatening infection. This means that therapy usually will be empirical, based on the results of therapeutic trials and local experience.

Prognostic parameters for infection progression are mainly neutropenia as a surrogate marker and such factors as mucosal damage, severe comorbidity, and antibody deficiency.

DEFINITIONS

Neutropenia is defined as a neutrophil count <500/µl (i.e., segments and bands) or <1000/µl with predicted decline to 500/µl over the next 2 days.

Fever is defined as temperature taken orally or at the tympanum with no signs of noninfectious causes, a temperature of ≥38.3° C once or a temperature of ≥38.0° C twice, lasting for at least 1 hour or measured twice within 12 hours.

Note: Simultaneous infection can be expected in up to 5% of all patients who experience a febrile reaction receiving blood transfusions.

RISK GROUPS

Risk of progression to a life-threatening infection depends on the overall duration of neutropenia (Table 4-1). For general aspects of classification into risk groups, see Table 4-2.

Numerous study groups have tried to incorporate further risk-adapted concepts into the decision-making process of empirical therapy. In the case of the so-called low-risk group, two different concepts apply: outpatient management and therapy with oral antibiotics. So far, the definitions are not satisfactory, but they can be used for orientation. Apart from general criteria, the low-risk definitions that have been used so far include criteria for oral therapy and for outpatient management (Table 4-3). In nonselected patients, approximately 30% to 40% of all febrile neutropenic episodes can be classified as low risk. The initial classification can be changed during the course of the infection. The state of a patient who initially fails to meet low risk criteria might have stabilized

Table 4-1   Risk groups

Low risk

Duration of neutropenia ≤5 days, in the absence of any high risk factor as listed in Table 4-2.

Intermediate risk

Duration of neutropenia 6 to 9 days

High risk

Duration of neutropenia ≥10 days

Neutropenia

Neutrophil count <500/μl (i.e., segments and bands) or <1000/ml with predicted decline to 500/μl within the next 2 days

after 12 to 24 hours of therapy; hence outpatient management and oral therapy might be feasible after reclassification. Some investigators never include patients with hematologic neoplasia in the low-risk group.

The Multinational Association for Supportive Care in Cancer (MASCC) has established a risk index by evaluating nonselected consecutive patients with febrile neutropenia, according to which low risk patients were defined as defervescing during antibiotic therapy without developing any of the complications listed in Table 4-2.[1]

IDENTIFICATION OF TRUE PATHOGENS

In approximately one third of all patients, the causative pathogen can be identified during the initial infection phase. In approximately 20% to 30% of cases, pathogenic evidence can be found at a later stage. The species listed in Table 4-4 represent 90% of all proven microorganisms, although fungal infections initially may play a more significant role in pulmonary infiltrates. If pathogens are identified after more than 5 days, fungi can be identified in approximately 30% to 40% of all microbiologically documented infections.

INFECTIONS

Infections in febrile neutropenia can be classified in accordance with the recommendations of the consensus conference of the International Immunocompromised Host Society and the Infectious Diseases Society of America as follows diagnostics (see Box 4-1):

Unexplained fever

Unexplained fever or fever of unknown origin (FUO) is defined as a new fever not accompanied by clinical or microbiological evidence of infection: single incident of fever (oral) without evident cause, temperature ≥38.3° C or ≥38.0° C lasting for at least 1 hour, or measured twice within 12 hours.

Table 4-2   Criteria of the low-risk group*

Hypotension: systolic blood pressure less than 90 mm Hg or need for pressor support to maintain blood pressure

Respiratory failure: arterial oxygen pressure less than 60 mm Hg while breathing room air, or need for mechanical ventilation

Admission to intensive care

Disseminated intravascular coagulation

Confusion or altered mental state

Congestive heart failure seen on chest x-ray and requiring treatment

Bleeding severe enough to require transfusion

Arrhythmia or ECG changes requiring treatment

Renal failure requiring investigation and/or treatment with IV fluids, dialysis, or any other intervention

Other complications judged serious and clinically significant

Microbiologically documented primary viral or microbial infection during the febrile episode, without any described complication and resolving under therapy, was considered a part of the infectious process and was not considered a serious complication.

A multivariate analysis including many different factors yielded the following risk factors that were weighted in a scoring system that allocates a high number of points to low risk:

Scoring system (characteristic weight)

- Burden of illness: no or mild symptoms 5
- No hypotension 5
- No chronic obstructive pulmonary disease 4
- Solid tumor or no previous fungal infection 4
- No dehydration 3
- Burden of illness: morate symptoms 3
- Outpatient status 3
- Age, <60 years 2

Note: Points attributed to the variable "burden of illness" are not cumulative, and the maximum theoretical score is therefore 26. Patients with 21 or more points on this MASCC index can be classified easily into the low-risk group. Positive predictive value was 91%, specificity was 68%, and sensitivity was 71%. The commonly used risk criterion "remaining duration of neutropenia" did not correlate well with the actual duration of neutropenia in the present concept and therefore could not be considered.

*Medical complications considered serious, and risk classification according to the Multinational Association of Supportive Care in Cancer (MASCC) (1).

Table 4-3   Low risk criteria for therapy and management

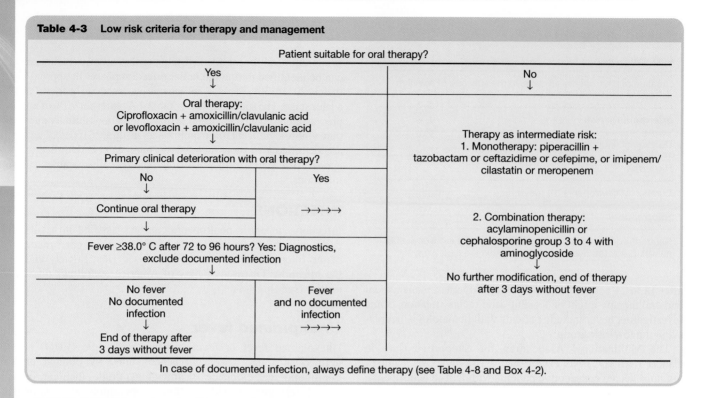

In case of documented infection, always define therapy (see Table 4-8 and Box 4-2).

Table 4-4   Probable initial pathogenic spectrum upon diagnosis

Frequent	Less frequent
Gram-positive bacteria	
Coagulase-negative staphylococci	
Staphylococcus aureus	
Streptococcus spp.	
Enterococcus faecalis/faecium	
Corynebacterium spp.	
Gram-negative bacteria	
Escherichia coli	*Enterobacter* spp.
Klebsiella	*Proteus* spp.
Pseudomonas aeruginosa	*Salmonella* spp.
	Haemophilus influenzae
	Acinetobacter species
	Stenotrophomonas
	maltophilia
	Citrobacter species
Anaerobic	
Clostridium difficile	*Bacteroides* species
	Clostridium species
	Fusobacterium species
	Propionibacterium species
Fungi	
Candida spp.	*Mucor* species
Aspergillus spp.	

Pathogens not relevant lung infiltrates, but possibly for simultaneous other infections

Enterococci from blood cultures, coagulase-negative staphylococci, or *Coryneiform* bacilli spp. from all materials.
Candida spp., swabs, saliva, sputum, tracheal secretions or bronchoalveolar lavage, surveillance cultures from stools or urine.
Other analyses (e.g., *Staphylococcus aureus* or *Legionella* from respiratory secretions should be assessed critically for relevance, before the decision is made to modify antimicrobial therapy accordingly).

Clinically documented/defined infection

Clinically documented infection (CDI) is defined as fever accompanied by unambiguous, clinically localized evidence (e.g., in the case of pneumonia or skin/tissue infection) when pathogens cannot be identified or examined microbiologically.

Microbiologically documented/defined infection with/without bacteremia

A microbiologically documented infection (MDI) is present if infection has been localized and microbiologically plausible evidence, which is also plausible with regard to timing, has been found, or if an infectious agent can be demonstrated in a blood culture even if a localized infection site has not been identified. Coagulase-negative staphylococci and corynebacteria must be demonstrated at least twice in separate blood cultures. A single isolation of these potential pathogens is viewed as contamination. In the case of pulmonary infiltrates, pathogen isolation from blood or a bronchoalveolar lavage specimen is regarded as a reliable source. Throat swabs, sputum, saliva, or a mouth rinse can be viewed as reliable only if a true pathogen is found in timely correlation with the development of pulmonary infiltrates. If symptoms of abdominal infection are present, evidence of *Clostridium difficile* toxin from stool culture is acceptable, whereas other potentially pathogenic agents must be found in at least two consecutive stool cultures. In catheter-associated infections, positive blood culture in conjunction with evidence of the same pathogen from the sampled catheter material or a swab taken from the infected entry site is required. For urinary tract infections, a significant pathogen count is necessary; for wound infections, swab or puncture material is acceptable (Box 4-1).

If microorganisms are detected in any culture, a further sample should be taken, even if the treatment is successful, so that a surveillance culture can be established to ensure microbiological

---

BOX 4-1   Initial diagnostics

1. Initial clinical diagnostic procedures when febrile neutropenia is identified
   a. Before initiation of antimicrobial therapy
      i. Thorough clinical examination, performed every day as long as fever persists: alterations of skin and mucosa
         - Exit sites of central and peripheral venous access routes, puncture sites
         - Upper and lower respiratory tract
         - Urogenital tract
         - Abdomen and perianal region
         - Monitoring of blood pressure, pulse rate, and respiratory frequency
   b. Further imaging and other diagnostics according to clinical symptoms or risk situation
      - Chest x-ray, two views, or high-resolution CT scan of the chest
      - Other images as indicated in the presence of specific symptoms (e.g., paranasal sinuses by computed tomography or magnetic resonance tomography)
      - Abdominal ultrasound, echocardiography, retinal examination, etc.
2. Initial microbiological diagnosis:
   - At least two separate pairs of peripheral venous blood samples for culture (aerobic/anaerobic) taken immediately after rise in temperature (i.e., immediately before initiation of antibiotic therapy). If a venous catheter is in place, two blood cultures should also be taken from the catheter.
3. Microbiological diagnosis (only if indicated on the basis of infection symptoms)
   - *Aspergillus galactomannan:* antigen in serum
   - Urine culture
   - Stool culture, including demonstration of *Clostridium difficile* enterotoxin in case of diarrhea, suspected enteritis, or enterocolitis; if applicable, viral diagnostics: Rota-, Noro-virus
   - If necessary:
      - Wound swab (nasal pharynx, anal region)
      - Liquor: Culture for bacteria, fungi, eventually PCR for HSV
      - Puncture material (histology and culture)
   - In the case of positive chest radiography findings, bronchoscopy with bronchoalveolar lavage (BAL): culture and microscopy; if suspected: cytomegalovirus (CMV), herpes simplex virus (HSV), respiratory syncytial virus (RSV), mycobacteria, *Legionella, Pneumocystis jiroveci,* other fungi.
   - If a catheter-associated induction is suspected: After removal of the venous catheter: Perform a microbiological examination of the catheter tip using a standard technique.
   - Check diagnostics with specialist.

effectiveness. Susceptibility testing for medication in use is required for all cultures of potentially pathogenic agents.

CLINICAL-CHEMICAL DIAGNOSIS

These minimal diagnostic requirements should be tested twice a week before and during therapy: leukocytes and differential blood count, hemoglobin, platelets, serum glutamic oxaloacetic transaminase (SGOT), serum glutamic pyruvic transaminase (SGPT), lactate dehydrogenase (LDH), alkaline phosphatase, gamma-glutamyl transpeptidase (GT), bilirubin, uric acid, creatinine, sodium, potassium, Quick's test, partial thromboplastin time, D-dimers, and C-reactive protein (CRP); repeated lactate examination if signs of sepsis are noted; and procalcitonin.

For patients receiving aminoglycosides, it is recommended that plasma trough levels be determined at least twice a week or more often if indicated. For patients with renal failure, particularly those simultaneously receiving other potentially nephrotoxic substances, the intervals for plasma level determination should be shortened if aminoglycosides cannot be avoided. It is recommended that creatinine clearance be determined at the outset to guide dosage decisions and evaluate potential nephrotoxicity.

DIAGNOSTIC MEASURES AFTER 72 TO 96 HOURS OF THERAPY WITHOUT RESPONSE

The diagnostic procedures described above should be repeated if radiography of the lungs is still negative and neutropenia persists, and there is obligatory high resolution CT-scan of the chest.

WHEN TO START ANTIMICROBIAL THERAPY

Prompt initiation of antimicrobial therapy is indicated in cases of the following diagnostics (see Box 4-1):

1. Fever and neutropenia $<500/\mu l$ or $<1000/\mu l$ if decline to $<500/\mu l$ is expected
   Type of fever: Single (oral) temperature $\geq 38.3°$ C or $\geq 38.0°$ C lasting for at least 1 hour or measured twice within 12 hours with no evident cause. *Exception:* Fever that is known to be due to noninfectious causes.
   or, in addition (see separate protocols [Table 4-8]):
   - Microbiologically documented infection
   or, in addition
   - Clinically or radiologically documented infection

   or

2. Signs of infection in afebrile neutropenia
   - Symptoms or evidence of an infection

   or

   - Clinical diagnosis of septic syndrome or septic shock

Therapy is empirical or calculated; proof of an infection by a microbial organism cannot be awaited.

Treatment must begin within 2 hours; diagnosis should not delay its initiation.

THERAPEUTIC CONCEPTS

Essentially, combination therapies or monotherapy is possible. Antibiotics chosen should have been investigated adequately and must be effective against Enterobacteriaceae, *Pseudomonas aeruginosa, Staphylococcus aureus,* and streptococci. Monotherapies should be administered only by an experienced team. Patients must be examined regularly and monitored closely for early detection of treatment failure, additional infections, side effects, and resistant pathogens.

Hospital- and ward-specific susceptibility patterns of pathogens have to be considered when an antibiotic regimen is chosen. For several years, 60% to 70% of all documented infections have been caused by gram-positive pathogens, primarily coagulase-negative staphylococci and *Corynebacterium jeikeum*. The prognosis for these infections is favorable, even if initial therapy was not directed against them, compared with life-threatening infections by the gram-negative microorganisms *Staphylococcus aureaus*, viridans streptococci, and pneumococci.

CLASSIFICATION INTO RISK GROUPS

Classification follows the criteria described in Table 4-1.

- Low risk
- Intermediate risk
- High risk

Treatment of low-risk patients

For low-risk patients (see Tables 4-2 and 4-3) eligible for oral antibiotic therapy, we recommend the combination of ciprofloxacin plus amoxicillin/clavulanic acid. This combination is also suitable for sequential therapy (possibly only after initial intravenous pretreatment and stabilization). A high rate of attributable gastrointestinal adverse effects should be taken into account.

Monotherapy with ciprofloxacin, ofloxacin, or levofloxacin has not been investigated sufficiently. In the case of penicillin allergy, amoxicillin/clavulanic acid can possibly be replaced by clindamycin or cefalexin (little experience) or cefuroxim-axetil. For patients with questionable compliance or contraindications for oral therapy, the parenteral medication recommended for intermediate- and high-risk patients should be used. See Table 4-5 for dosages.

Treatment of intermediate- and high-risk patients

Note: Effectiveness against *Pseudomonas aeruginosa* and streptococci must be guaranteed. (See Box 4-2, Tables 4-6 and 4-7.[3-5])

> **BOX 4-2 Strategy for patients with pulmonary infiltrate and possible fungal infection**
>
> Antibiotic therapy: piperacillin-tazobactam or ceftazidime or cefepime or imipenem/cilastatin or meropenem combined with antimycotic therapy: liposomal amphotericin B or caspofungin or voriconazole

Table 4-5 Part 1: Anti-infective drugs, alphabetic sorting; antibiotics (dosage in normal renal function)

Substance	Group*	Dose per day	Route	Notes
Amikacin	AG*	15 mg/kg (maximum 1.5 g daily, maximum 10 days)	IV	Control of serum levels, see below
Amoxicillin/Clavulanic acid	Aminopenicillin/BLI	2 × 1 g	PO	
Cefalexin	Ceph gr 1	2 × 1 g	PO	
Cefepime	Ceph gr 4	2 to 3 × 2 g	IV	
Cefixime	Ceph gr 3	1 × 400 mg or 2 × 200 mg	PO	
Cefotaxime	Ceph gr 3a	3 × 2 g	IV	
Ceftazidime	Ceph gr 3b	3 × 2 g	IV	
Ceftriaxone	Ceph gr 3a	1 × 2 g	IV	
Cefuroxime-Axetil	Ceph gr 2	2 × 250 to 2 × 500 mg	PO	
Ciprofloxacin	Chinolon	2 × 0.4 g	IV	
		2 × 0.75 g	PO	In low-risk patients
Clindamycin	Lincosamide	Moderately severe infections: 1200 to 1800 mg; severe infections: 2400 to 2700 mg in 2 to 4 equal doses	IV	
		3 × 600 mg	PO	After IV therapy
Cotrimoxazole (sulfamethoxazole / trimethoprim, fixed combination)	Sulfonamide/ Diaminopyrimidine	Sulfamethoxazole 100 mg/kg; trimethoprim 20 mg/kg; in 3 to 4 IV doses, 2 to 3 weeks	IV	In *Pneumocystis* pneumonia (PcP)
		2× (sulfamethoxazole 800 mg; trimethoprim 160 mg) until 2× (sulfamethoxazole 1200 mg; trimethoprim 240 mg)	PO IV	Normal dosing

Table 4-5 Part 1: Anti-infective drugs, alphabetic sorting; antibiotics (dosage in normal renal function)—cont'd

Substance	Group*	Dose per day	Route	Notes
Flucloxacillin	Isoxazolyl- penicillin	3 to 4 × 2 g	IV	
Gentamicin	AG*	3 to 6 mg/kg	IV	Serum level controls, see below
Imipenem/Cilastatin	Carbapenem	3 × 1 g or 4 × 0.5 g	IV	
Levofloxacin	Chinolon	1 × 0.5 g	IV PO	
Linezolid	Oxazolidinone	2 × 0.6 g	IV PO	
Meropenem	Carbapenem	3 × 1 g	IV	
Metronidazole	Nitroimidazole	3 × 500 mg	IV	
		3 × 400 mg	PO	
Mezlocillin	Acylam	3 × 4 to 5 g or 2 × 10 g	IV	
Netilmicin	AG*	4 to 7.5 mg/kg	IV	Serum level controls, see below
Piperacillin	Acylam	3 to 4 × 4 g	IV	
Piperacillin/ Tazobactam	Acylam/BLI	3 to 4 × 4.5 g	IV	
Teicoplanin	Glycopeptide	1 × 400 mg, day 2 × 400 mg	IV	
Tobramycin	AG*	3 to 5 mg/kg	IV	Serum level controls, see below
Vancomycin	Glycopeptide	2 × 1000 mg	IV	Serum level controls, see below
Vancomycin	Glycopeptide	4 × 125 mg	PO	In case of *C. diffficile* colitis

Refer to Summary of Product Characteristics (SmPC) and to labeling for different countries.
*Groups of substances: *acylam*, Acylaminopenicillin; *AG*, aminoglycoside; *BLI*, β-lactamase inhibitor; *ceph*, cephalosporin and group.

ASSESSMENT AND DURATION OF THERAPY

- Initial response at 72 to 96 hours after initiation of antimicrobial therapy
- Final response at the end of antimicrobial therapy
- After an adequate follow-up period (e.g., 7 days)

Assessment criteria should be based on the recommendations of the consensus conference of the International Immunocompromised Host Society and the Infectious Diseases Society of America.[2]

SUCCESSFUL TREATMENT: CONTINUATION AND FOLLOW-UP

If success criteria are met within 72 hours of antimicrobial treatment and the neutrophil granulocyte count is stable at <1000/μl, the regimen should be continued until the patient is afebrile for 7 consecutive days. If, however, the neutrophil granulocyte count has risen to >1000/μl, two consecutive afebrile days are sufficient. Treatment should not be shorter than 7 days. After completion of antimicrobial therapy, a follow-up period of 7 days is necessary to detect a relapse or a secondary infection. Some infections become apparent only after an increase in neutrophil count is noted. Patients with an adequate neutrophil count whose clinical state is improving thus also require follow-up (e.g., on an outpatient basis).

ADDITIONAL TREATMENT OPTIONS

Granulocyte-colony stimulating factor (G-CSF) for stimulation of granulopoiesis in persistent neutropenia is indicated in cases of severe or progressive infection, pneumonia, or fungal infection.

In severe hypogammaglobulinemia, 7S-polyvalent intravenous immunoglobulins should be substituted.

See Table 4-8.

Table 4-5 Part 2: Target serum concentrations of aminoglycosides and vancomycin

1. First determination: days 5 to 7 of therapy, then twice per week, together with creatinine serum level. Earlier determinations might be reasonable if renal function changes and the dosing must be adapted, especially trough levels and 8-hour levels correlate with nephrotoxicity

2. Time points: trough levels just before the next application, 8h-level. 8h after the beginning of infusion.

3. Dose adaptation: for aminoglycosides: dose reduction by ⅓ or ½ if treatment intervals are identical; or prolonging treatment intervals to 36 or 48 hours

Substance	Peak level, mg/l	8h-level, mg/l	Trough level, mg/l
Amikacin (single dose)	45-75	2–15	<5
Amikacin q8h	20-30	–	5-10
Gentamicin (single dose)	4-10	1.5-6	<1
Gentamicin q8h	4-10	–	<2
Netilmicin (single dose)	15-25	1-5	<1
Netilmicin q8h	6-10	–	<2
Vancomycin	30-40	–	5-15
Tobramycin (single dose)	4-10	1.5-6	<1
Tobramycin q8h	4-10	–	<2

Table 4-5 Part 3: Antimycotics, alphabetical sorting; dosage in normal renal function

Substance	Group*	Dose per day	Route	Notes
Amphotericin B lipid complex	Polyen, lipid complex	5 mg/kg	IV	
Amphotericin B, liposomal	Polyen, liposomes	Start with 3 mg/kg; then dose according to disease, clinical stage, and age of the patient; 1 mg to 3 mg/kg; 3 mg/kg in lung infiltrates; at least 5 mg/kg in zygomycoses	IV	
Caspofungin	Echinocandin	70 mg; in patients <80 kg 50 mg from day 2 onward	IV	
Fluconazole	Triazole	400 to 800 mg	IV	
Itraconazole	Triazole	2 × 200 mg day 1 and 2 IV, followed by 1 × 200 mg until at least day 5; then oral therapy with suspension 2 × 200 mg possible	IV PO	Oral therapy: trough plasma levels day 5; target value: >500 ng/ml
Posaconazole	Triazole	2 × 400 mg or 4 × 200 mg	PO	
Voriconazole	Triazole	IV: Day 2 × 6 mg/kg, dann 2 × 4 mg/kg; PO: Day 2 × 400 mg/d, then 2 × 200 mg	IV PO	
Virustatics				
Acyclovir	Nucleoside-analogue	5 to 14 days, depending on indication	IV	
Ganciclovir	Nucleoside-analogue	2 × 5 mg/kg, duration according to clinical response	IV	

Refer to Summary of Product Characteristics (SmPC) and to labeling for different countries.

Table 4-6   Intermediate-risk criteria for therapy and management*

1. Monotherapy: Piperacillin + Tazobactam or Ceftazidime or Cefepime, or Imipenem/cilastatin or Meropenem
2. Combination therapy: Acylaminopenicillin or Cephalosporine group 3 to 4 with Aminoglycoside

Primary clinical deterioration?	
No ↓	Yes ↓
Fever after 72-96 hours? Yes: → Diagnostics, exclude documented infection ↓	After 1: additional aminoglycoside After 2: imipenem/cilastatin or meropenem After initial imipenem/cilastatin or meropenem also: quinolone and vancomycin or teicoplanin ↓ ↓ ↓

No fever No documented infection ↓ ↓	Fever ≥38.0° C No documented infection ↓	
	Clinically stable ↓	Clinically unstable →

No modification if clinically stable Total therapy: 7 days without fever After increase in neutrophils >1000/μl, 2 days without fever	Fever after 72 to 96 hours? → Diagnostics ↓	
	Yes, and no documented infection ↓	No ↓
	Additional fluconazole: after 72 hours of fever Change to: liposomal amphotericin B or caspofungin or itraconazole or voriconazole	End of therapy after 3 days without fever; total therapy at least 10 days

In case of documented infection, always defined therapy (see Table 4-8 and Box 4-2).

*In modifications of therapy, no period without antibiotics for diagnostics during neutropenia.
Note for fluconazole: Only if no prophylaxis with azole and no risk of infection with filamentous fungi.

Table 4-7   High-risk criteria for treatment and management*

1. Monotherapy: Piperacillin + Tazobactam or Ceftazidime or Cefepime, or Imipenem/cilastatin or Meropenem
2. Combination therapy: Acylaminopenicillin or Cephalosporine group 3 to 4 with Aminoglycoside

Primary clinical deterioration?	
No ↓	Yes ↓
Fever after 72 to 96 hours? → Diagnostics, exclude documented infection ↓	Imipenem/cilastatin or meropenem, after initial imipenem/cilastatin or meropenem: quinolone and vancomycin or teicoplanin In all treatments, additional: Fluconazole or liposomal amphotericin B or caspofungin or itraconazole or voriconazole

No fever No documented infection ↓ ↓	Yes, fever ≥38.0° C No documented infection ↓	
	Clinically stable ↓	Clinically unstable →→

No modification if clinically stable Total therapy: 7 days without fever; After increase in neutrophils >1000/μl, 2 days without fever	If fluconazole, after 72 hours of fever, change to: liposomal amphotericin B or caspofungin or itraconazole or voriconazole

In case of documented infection, always defined therapy (see Table 4-8 and Box 4-2).

*In modifications of therapy, no period without antibiotics for diagnostics during neutropenia.
Note for fluconazole: Only if no prophylaxis with azole and no risk of infection with filamentous fungi (2–5).

Table 4-8 **Diagnostic and therapeutic strategies**

Finding or symptom	Modification of strategy*
Persistent or renewed fever at regeneration of neutrophils or increase in cholestasis	Suspicion of hepatolienal candidiasis: in negative abdominal ultrasound; abdominal CT scan or MRI, and decide if antifungal therapy is indicated (see Candidemia)
Positive blood culture **Bevor therapy**	
Gram-positive bacteria, MSSA, MRSA	Flucloxacillin according susceptibility; if necessary, vancomycin, teicoplanin; linezolid (antibiogram)
Coagulase-negative staphylococci; (relevance see Diagnostics, Table 4-4)	Vancomycin, teicoplanin
Gram-negative bacteria	Continue with therapy, if patient stable and pathogen sensitive; if not, therapy according to antibiogram
Candida spp.	See below
Pathogen isolated during antibiotic therapy	
Gram-positive bacteria	According to antibiogram
Gram-negative bacteria	According to antibiogram
Candida spp.	Depending from prophylaxis/previous therapy/pathogen/antibiogram (not awaiting result of MHC determination)
1. fluconazole-sensible + clinically stable + no previous azole-therapy 2. All other cases, especially if C. krusei or C. glabrata	Fluconazole Caspofungin or liposomal amphotericin B or ampho B-lipid-complex; In response and regeneration of neutrophils change to fluconazole or voriconazole orally, if reasonable by antibiogram, caspofungin or voriconazol, if not given initially
Sepsis, septic shock	
	See also Tables 4-6 and 4-7; or therapy by antibiogram; according to usual treatment guidelines of sepsis
Respiratory tract	See also Box 4-2
Lung infiltrate during recovery of neutrophils	Close monitoring, possible inflammatory reaction in neutrophil recovery (n.b. ARDS) Directed bronchoalveolar lavage, if not performed yet
Interstitial pneumonia	Diagnostics: if induced sputum or bronchoalveolar lavage not possible: suspicion of Pneumocystis pneumonia: consider therapy with high-dose trimethoprim-sulfamethoxazole or pentamidine; consider infection by herpes-viruses (herpes simplex, cytomegalovirus) and Legionella

Finding or symptom	Modification of strategy*
Invasive aspergillosis	
	Dependent from previous prophylaxis or therapy Initial therapy: voriconazole (preferred in CNS infections) Alternatively: liposomal amphotericin B Secondary: caspofungin or liposomal amphotericin B or amphotericin B-lipid-complex or posaconazole or voriconazole
Head, eyes, ears, throat	
Necrotizing or borderline gingivitis, periodontitis, necrotizing gingivitis	Additional drugs active against anaerobic pathogenszusätzlich (clindamycin, metronidazole, imipenem/cilastatin, or meropenem)
Vesicles or ulcer	Suspicion of herpes simplex infection; where appropriate, viral cultures; additional empirical acyclovir therapy
Infiltration of paranasal sinuses or nasal ulcer	Suspicion of fungal infection by Aspergillus spp. or Zygomyces, biopsy needed! Therapy of aspergillosis (see above) Treatment of zygomycosis: high-dose liposomal amphotericin B or amphotericin B lipid complex; 5 to 10 mg/kg/day or posaconazole (if amphotericin B not possible); local surgery when indicated
Gastrointestinal tract	
Retrosternal pain	Suspicion of Candida and/or herpes simplex infection; bacterial esophagitis possible: consider endoscopy by 48 hours at the latest
	Primary therapy against Candida: additional antimycotics: possibly fluconazole, itraconazole, or voriconazole
	If not successful: suspicion of herpes virus infection and therapy with acyclovir
Acute abdominal pain	Suspicion of typhlitis, appendicitis: additional substances active against anaerobic bacteria: metronidazole, clindamycin, imipenem/cilastatin, or meropenem; close monitoring, possible indication for surgery (!) in case of acute abdomen!
Diarrhea	Suspicion of colitis by Clostridium difficile: analysis of toxin in stools, metronidazole orally (in case of need IV); in ineffectiveness: oral vancomycin

Table 4-8 Diagnostic and therapeutic strategies—cont'd

Finding or symptom	Modification of strategy*
Perianal pain	Additional substances active against anaerobic bacteria (see above), frequent and close monitoring, because of possible surgery, especially during regeneration of neutrophils; herpes simplex virus infection possible as well
Central venous catheter	
Positive culture for pathogens except for aerobe spore-forming (*Bacillus* spp.) or *Candida* spp.	Attempt of IV treatment with antibiotics; application via changing of lumen in case of multiple-lumina catheter
Staphylococcus aureus (methicillin/oxacillin-sensitive)	Catheter removal, isoxazolylpenicillin (penicillinase-resistant penicillin) (e.g., flucloxacillin), at least 2 weeks
Staphylococcus aureus (methicillin/oxacillin-resistant)	Catheter removal, therapy according to antibiogram, at least 2 weeks intravenously
Coagulase-negative staphylococci	According to antibiogram; vancomycin or teicoplanin only in methicillin/oxacillin resistance; duration 5 to 7 days
Enterococci	Aminopenicillin plus aminoglycoside; in ampicillin-resistance: vancomycin or teicoplanin plus aminoglycoside; in vancomycin resistance: linezolid; duration of 5 to 7 days

Finding or symptom	Modification of strategy*
Coryneform bacteria	According to antibiogram; vancomycin or teicoplanin only in resistance against other antibiotics
Positive culture with *Bacillus* spp.	Catheter removal, directed therapy
Escherichia coli, *Klebsiella* spp. or other Enterobacteriaceae	According to antibiogram with effective antibiotic: cephalosporin group 3, acylaminopenicillin, imipenem/cilastatin or meropenem, quinolone antibiotics
Pseudomonas aeruginosa	Combination of β-lactam antibiotic with activity against *Pseudomonas* plus aminoglycoside, at least 2 weeks
Acinetobacter baumannii	According to antibiogram
Stenotrophomonas maltophilia	According to antibiogram (cotrimoxazole!)
Candidemia	Replace catheter, therapy (see above)
Clinical infection at exit site	Vancomycin or teicoplanin
Infection of tunnel or pouch	Replace catheter; vancomycin or teicoplanin

*Modification or amendment according to symptoms or clinical or microbiological finding in patients with neutropenia and fever.

REFERENCES

1. Klastersky J, Paesmans M, Rubenstein EB, et al. The Multinational Association for Supportive Care in Cancer risk index: a multinational scoring system for identifying low-risk febrile neutropenic cancer patients. *J Clin Oncol*. 2000;18:3038–3051.
2. Hughes WT, Armstrong D, Bodey GP, et al. 2002 guidelines for the use of antimicrobial agents in neutropenic patients with cancer. *Clin Infect Dis*. 2002;34:730–751.
3. Böhme A, Ruhnke M, Buchheidt D, et al. Treatment of invasive fungal infections in cancer patients "Recommendations of the Infectious Diseases Working Party (AGIHO) of the German Society of Hematology and Oncology (DGHO). *Ann Hematol*. 2009;88:97–110.
4. Link H, Bohme A, Cornely OA, et al. Antimicrobial therapy of unexplained fever in neutropenic patients—guidelines of the Infectious Diseases Working Party (AGIHO) of the German Society of Hematology and Oncology (DGHO), Study Group Interventional Therapy of Unexplained Fever, Arbeitsgemeinschaft Supportivmassnahmen in der Onkologie (ASO) of the Deutsche Krebsgesellschaft (DKG-German Cancer Society). *Ann Hematol*. 2003;82(suppl 2):S105–S117.
5. Maschmeyer G, Thomas B, Dieter B, et al. Diagnosis and antimicrobial therapy of lung infiltrates in febrile neutropenic patients: guidelines of the infectious diseases working party of the German Society of Haematology and Oncology. *Eur J Cancer*. 2009;14:2462.

5 Radiotherapy-induced adverse events

Ulrike Hoeller

Radiation is a very efficient treatment option for many tumors. However, radiation toxicity can be dose-limiting. The dose-response relationship for tumor control is well defined, as it is for adverse effects. Therefore, from the beginning of radiotherapy on, the aim of any irradiation technique has been to increase the dose to the target tumor and reduce the incidental dose in surrounding normal tissues. Modern radiation techniques and advances in diagnostic imaging have greatly improved the risk-benefit ratio, so that effective radiotherapy can be given with usually mild, sometimes moderate, and rarely severe radiation-induced toxicity.

The nature and symptoms of the adverse effects are determined by the organ/normal tissue included in the radiation volume. General symptoms such as nausea and fatigue may occur during radiation of the upper abdomen and/or large irradiation volumes.

Generally, adverse effects are defined by the time of onset as acute or late effects. The time was set arbitrarily as less than or greater than 90 days after radiotherapy. Acute effects are usually reversible; late effects occur after months to many years and are mostly irreversible. The risk of late effects is lifelong.[1]

This review will focus on adverse effects encountered in the daily routine that are amenable to therapy and/or prevention. Oral mucositis, osteoradionecrosis, and xerostomia are discussed in detail in other chapters.

PATHOPHYSIOLOGY AND PREVALENCE OF ADVERSE EFFECTS

ACUTE EFFECTS

Acute effects are caused by direct cytotoxicity to rapidly proliferating tissues with continuous cell turnover (e.g., bone marrow, mucosa, intestine). Radiation results in cell depletion. Epithelial barrier functions are impaired and infections may be enhanced by radiation toxicity. Usually, accompanying inflammation is noted. Proinflammatory cytokines and tumor necrosis factor are expressed, and inducible nitric oxide synthase[2] is activated. Lesions are repaired ad integrum by proliferation from stem cells that survived within or migrated into the volume. If tissues relevant for late effects (vasculature, soft tissue) are affected, consequential late effects may occur.

LATE EFFECTS

Late effects are expressed after a latency period of months to years. The mechanisms of late effects are much more complex and are not fully understood. Radiation induces damage to the vasculature, fibrosis, atrophy, neural damage, and a variety of endocrine and growth-related effects, and affects the nonspecific immune system. Two mechanisms were thought to be essential: (1) depletion of target cells, slowly proliferating stem cells, or functional subunits in parenchymal organs, resulting in functional changes, and (2) endothelial damage leading to fibrosis and tissue breakdown. During the past decade, radiobiological research could demonstrate that radiation activates a cytokine cascade and induces functional changes during the latency period.[3,4] An increasing number

of signaling pathways, cell cross-talk, and other mechanisms are being discovered. The role of transforming growth factor (TGF)-β in radiation-induced fibrosis is well known. Fibrosis is understood as a nonhealing wound.[3]

RISK FACTORS FOR ADVERSE EFFECTS

RADIATION TECHNIQUE AND DOSE

The severity of adverse effects is related to the radiation dose, the specific radiation tolerance of the tissue, and the volume of irradiated tissue.

Generally, the total dose is fractionated, conventionally 5 times weekly by 1.8 to 2 Gy, up to total doses of 30 to 50 to 80 Gy, and in palliative symptomatic settings by 3 to 5 Gy, with total doses of 20 to 30 Gy. The shorter the overall time for application of a given total dose, the more severe is the acute reaction; the higher the dose per fraction of a given total dose, the more severe is the late reaction. Modern radiotherapy techniques are targeted at reducing incidental irradiation of normal tissue surrounding the tumor because small-volume irradiation is tolerated better in most organs (e.g., lung, gut, kidneys).

Radiation tolerance is also modified by patient-specific factors such as age, gender, and comorbidities. Children are much more vulnerable than adults, and radiation before the age of 3 is avoided whenever possible. Elderly patients are not at higher risk of adverse effects. The role of gender is not clear; females carry a higher risk of radiation-induced malignancy and cataract formation.[5,6] Comorbidities may reduce tolerance to radiation through impaired organ capacity (chronic obstructive pulmonary disease [COPD], renal insufficiency) or through additive pathologic effects (e.g., arteriosclerosis, radiation-induced endothelial lesions), resulting in myocardial infarction.

DRUGS

Chemotherapy frequently enhances radiation cytotoxic effects on tumors, as well as radiation toxicity, especially when applied concurrently; for example, erlotinib combined with radiation has evoked severe skin toxicity.[2] Drugs and herbs (usually considered harmless by patients and doctors) that enhance photosensitivity should be avoided during radiotherapy.

INDIVIDUAL RADIOSENSITIVITY

It is well known that patients who undergo comparable treatment protocols differ widely in the extent of adverse radiation effects.[7] This is attributed to individual radiosensitivity as determined by genetic factors.[8] If the individual patient's radiosensitivity were known, radiotherapy could be tailored to the patient. Dose could be escalated in fairly radioresistant patients. It was calculated that such individualization of radiotherapy might improve the overall success rate by up to 20%. Various predictive assays were evaluated (survival of skin fibroblasts, chromosomal aberrations in lymphocytes, single nucleotide polymorphisms in selected genes). Results are controversial, and large-scale prospective studies with robust clinical endpoints are needed (review[9]).

Prevention

Adverse effects are prevented best by reducing the radiation dose in normal tissue. Modern radiotherapy techniques use image fusion (microbeam radiation therapy [MRT] and positron emission tomography [PET]) for optimal target definition (tumor localization), computer-assisted three-dimensional (3D) and 4D (including target movement over time) planning for highly specific dose distribution (conformal radiotherapy), patient immobilization to reduce safety margins, and image-guided radiotherapy that allows optimal dose delivery to the target in the breathing and moving patient.

Hopefully, the evolving knowledge of radiation-induced processes will allow medical modification of these processes and prevention of radiation-induced adverse effects with specific drugs. To date, there are few examples: amifostine may reduce xerostomia and mucositis (controversial results), keratinocyte growth factors may reduce mucositis and bladder inflammation, captopril alleviates renal dysfunction. Radioprotectors should act selectively on normal tissue. Studies to exclude radioprotection of the tumor by the mentioned drugs have yet to be performed.

SKIN

PATHOPHYSIOLOGY

Acute skin reactions are the result of an inflammatory response and depletion of actively proliferating cells. Late effects include fibrosis, atrophy, and reduction of cell and vessel density.

SYMPTOMS AND MANAGEMENT

Acute skin reactions include erythema, edema, pigmentation, dry/moist desquamation, alopecia, and, in severe cases, ulcer. Only one or any combination of these symptoms may occur in the individual patient.

Skin care for erythema/dry desquamation is identical to preventive measures (see below). For treatment of moist desquamation or ulcer, general principles of wound management are applied; no specific treatment has been found superior. Alginate dressing and black tea compress for moist desquamation and silver-coal dressing for areas of superinfection have been useful.

Late skin reactions include photosensitivity, xerosis (dry skin), hypo-/hyperpigmentation, atrophy, fibrosis, teleangiectasia, and, rarely, skin breakdown/necrosis.

Dry skin should be treated with cream. Fibrosis is understood as a complex wound with development of excess fibrosis.[3,4] It is an ongoing process throughout years. Pentoxifylline and tocopherol have been shown to reverse subcutaneous fibrosis. However, results of clinical studies are controversial.[10,11]

In the rare case of radiation-induced skin ulcer, advice on wound management should be sought. Intense systemic and topical antibiotic treatment followed by cautious debridement is advocated. Before surgery, the extent of necrosis should be defined by MRT. Experimental and case studies have shown that hyperbaric oxygen stimulates angiogenesis and increases cell density so that ulcers heal.

RADIATION RECALL DERMATITIS

Radiation recall dermatitis is a rare phenomenon. It "represents the 'recalling' of an effect similar in appearance to that of an acute radiation reaction in a previously irradiated field."[12] Recall is triggered by a drug months to years after radiation. The cause is not known, but it may be caused by a local drug hypersensitivity reaction. Skin reactions settle within days after the drug is stopped. Rechallenge is possible and usually is associated with mild symptoms only; steroids can be helpful. Triggering drugs are frequently cytotoxic agents but may include a great number of other drugs (refer to review[12]).

PREVENTION

General recommendations for skin care during and after radiotherapy are endorsed by most institutions. A wide variety of creams, lotions, and agents have been advocated for prevention of acute skin reaction. However, few scientifically sound studies have been conducted, and even fewer substances have been shown to mitigate the acute skin reaction. In contrast to old beliefs, double-blind randomized studies have shown that patients should be encouraged to wash.[13] No evidence was found in a prospective noninferiority trial to suggest that the use of deodorants without aluminium should be restricted.[14] Topical potent steroids have been shown to reduce and delay skin inflammation,[15] but most institutions do not use them for fear of skin atrophy.

General recommendations include the following: Shower or bathe with warm water, avoid harsh soaps, do not use deodorant or perfume, avoid tight-fitting clothing and irritating fabrics, do not expose skin to the sun, use hydrophilic cream (e.g., urea 3% cream, linimentum aquosum), do not use tape or adhesive bandages in the radiation field, and do not apply topical agents with greater than 2 mm thickness before radiotherapy. Bright erythema and discomfort/itching can be alleviated with steroid cream.

BRAIN

Radiation-induced brain injuries include edema, subacute delayed reaction with fatigue or somnolence syndrome, neurocognitive dysfunction, and necrosis of white matter.

PATHOPHYSIOLOGY

The acute reaction is characterized by disruption of the blood-brain barrier that induces vasogenic edema in the intercellular space of white matter. Subacute delayed reaction is associated with transient demyelination of oligodendroglial cells. Late effects are predominantly abnormalities of small vessels and demyelination and eventually necrosis. Long-lasting controversy continues regarding whether reduction in clonogenic cells of parenchymal (oligodendrocytes) or vascular structures (endothelial) is the predominant mechanism. Currently, brain injury is understood as a complex and orchestrated interaction of several cell types.[16] Astrocytes, microglia, neurons, and neuronal stem cells are involved. The hippocampus is the major site of postnatal neurogenesis. Radiation to this area has been shown to decrease cell proliferation and stem cell differentiation into neurons.[17]

Risk factors for brain injury include high dose per fraction, large radiation volumes, concurrent or previous neurotoxic agents (e.g., methotrexate), young age of the patient, and pre-existing vascular disease caused by diabetes mellitus and arterial hypertension.

SYMPTOMS AND MANAGEMENT
Edema

The predominant acute adverse reaction is edema. Headache, vomiting without nausea in the morning, singultus, and psychic abnormalities like aspontaneity should lead to initiation of steroid treatment. Dexamethasone 4 to 8 mg in the morning is indicated; in severe cases, dexamethasone 50 to 100 mg IV initially is followed by 24 to 32 mg daily; more than 40 mg of medication daily is ineffective. Mannitol or glycerol (IV 10%, 125 ml short infusion 4 times a day, or liquid PO 50%, 50 ml 4 times a day) is proposed for refractory edema. However, the effect does not last long, so that additional diuretics are frequently necessary. The increased thromboembolic risk of brain tumor patients should be taken into account.

ACUTE DELAYED REACTION/SOMNOLENCE SYNDROME

Six to eight weeks after radiotherapy, lethargy, fatigue, and loss of appetite may occur and will resolve spontaneously after some time. Steroids may help. Methylphenidate has proved ineffective with therapeutic and preventive intent in double-blind studies.[18,19]

NEUROCOGNITIVE FUNCTION

Very few prospective studies of adequate size and method have focused on the severity and incidence of radiation-induced impairment of neurocognitive functioning in adult patients. It should be kept in mind that uncontrolled tumor is the most important cause of neurocognitive deterioration, and a high baseline deficit can be found even in patients without brain tumor or metastases.[20,21]

During and shortly after radiotherapy, visual and verbal memory and learning function are affected.[22,23] Years after high-dose radiotherapy, attention, impaired memory, and executive function affect daily functioning, and quality of life is affected in a subgroup of patients.[24] The younger the patient, the more severe is the impairment.[25]

No standard therapy is yet available. A variety of substances are being studied in the preclinical and phase I/II study setting. Donepezil, also used for Alzheimer's disease, is promising.[26]

NECROSIS

Necrosis usually develops at or near the site of the brain tumor (i.e., the site of high dose). Focal symptoms depend on the location of the necrosis. Radiation-induced necrosis becomes apparent months to many years after radiation. It is an ongoing, dynamic process. Necrosis can resolve spontaneously, remain stable, or enlarge.

Differential diagnosis of radiation-induced necrosis and tumor relapse is crucial and extremely difficult. Standard computed tomography and magnetic resonance imaging (MRI) cannot distinguish between necrosis and tumor regrowth. Recently it was suggested that a ratio of specific aspects of the lesion in standard MRI can distinguish tumor enlargement from necrosis.[27] Dynamic susceptibility contrast-enhanced MRI and methionine PET are currently being evaluated.[28] O-2-18F-fluoroethyl-L-tyrosine (FET)-PET with tyrosine is a very promising tool for improving MRI diagnosis.[29] The phenomenon of pseudoprogression, that is, enhanced contrast enhancement on the first posttreatment MRI scan, was described for patients with glioblastoma treated with radiation and temozolamide.[30]

Dexamethasone should be initiated as soon as marked reactive edema is noted. Animal studies have shown that dexamethasone can modify vascular and inflammatory changes and reduce subsequent necrosis. Dexamethasone therapy can mitigate symptoms of early necrosis but is often ineffective once cystic liquefaction has developed.[31] Reduction of necrosis by hyperbaric oxygen treatment has been reported, especially in children.[32,33] Debulking surgery is warranted in cases of intractable symptoms.

SYMPTOMATIC EPILEPSY

Edema and necrosis can induce symptomatic epilepsy (e.g., necrosis of temporal lobe after treatment of nasopharyngeal carcinoma). Simple seizures or complex seizures associated with impaired consciousness may occur. Grand mal seizures include tonic-clonic spasms, loss of consciousness, frequent tongue bites and incontinence, and sometimes bone fractures (e.g., impression fractures of vertebrae). Status epilepticus is described as a series of seizures in which the individual does not regain consciousness between seizures. If it is not interrupted within hours, lethal brain edema may develop.

The course of a single seizure is self-limiting. Intravenous injections during the seizure are difficult and should not be attempted. Barbiturates shortly after the seizure are not recommended because of the risk of ischemic brain injury. Symptomatic epilepsy should be treated because of the high risk of repetition and transition into status epilepticus. Monotherapy with carbamazepine or phenytoin is preferred. Continued therapy until 3 years after the last seizure has been recommended. However, the side effects of carbamazepine are indistinguishable from and add to the clinical symptoms of radiation toxicity.[34] The frequency of preexisting seizures may increase during radiotherapy and is reduced with low/moderate doses of dexamethasone. Patients with status epilepticus are immediately transferred to a critical care unit.

HYPOPITUITARISM

Neuroendocrine dysfunction of anterior pituitary hormone secretion is common after radiation of the anterior hypothalamic-pituitary axis. Severity and time of onset depend on radiation dose, interval to radiotherapy, and age and sex of the patient.

The somatotropic axis is the most vulnerable, and growth hormone deficiency is the most frequent disorder. In adults, compensatory stimulation of the partially damaged somatotropic axis maintains normal spontaneous growth hormone secretion. In children, the increased demand for growth hormone during growth and puberty may not be met, and development may be insufficient. High-dose radiation induces gonadotropin, adrenocorticotropic hormone (ACTH), and thyroid-stimulating hormone (TSH) deficiency, resulting in the respective clinical disorders. Children are at risk of precocious puberty. Regular testing throughout the lifetime and substitution are mandatory to prevent serious disturbances of growth, body image, sexual function, and quality of life.

Prevention

Volume sparing treatment planning is suggested.

Medical prevention of cerebral or myelin injury has not yet been established. A variety of substances are being studied in preclinical and phase I/II study settings: thiazolidinedione pioglitazone,[35] an insulin sensitizer, inhibitors of the angiotensin-converting enzyme, and linoleic (omega-6) acid[36] are promising. Sparing the dentate gyrus of the hippocampus and the subventricular zone of the lateral ventricles, where neural stem cells are probably located, has been suggested to enable repopulation of damaged areas.[37]

LUNG

The lungs are very sensitive to radiation. The acute reaction is radiation pneumonitis or pneumopathy; the late reaction is lung fibrosis. Depending on the affected lung volume, both conditions may produce more radiologic findings or may lead to symptoms and morbidity. Fibrosis frequently evolves from pneumonitis but may occur without obvious preceding pneumonitis, or, vice versa, mild pneumonitis may resolve completely.

PATHOPHYSIOLOGY

Radiation pneumonitis resembles interstitial pneumonitis. An acute inflammatory reaction, an alveolar component, and vascular lesions are observed. Vascular endothelial cells and type II pneumocytes are postulated as the major target cells. The latter line the alveolar walls, produce surfactant factor, and are stem cells of type I pneumocytes. Radiation reduces type I pneumocytes and inhibits the proliferation of type II pneumocytes, resulting in cell depletion, loss of surfactant, and loss of alveolar membrane barrier function. The endothelial cells become vacuolated, endothelial gaps form, capillary permeability is increased, and intraalveolar exudation is enhanced. Inflammatory cells, predominantly macrophages, lymphocytes, and mononuclear cells are found in the interstitial spaces and in the alveoli.

Gradually, as the acute reaction is resolved, perivascular fibrosis becomes apparent and capillary density is reduced. Collagen is deposited in the alveolar wall and in the alveolar space. The process of lung fibrosis is not fully understood. However, TGF-β, along with other cytokines, plays a major role.

SYMPTOMS AND MANAGEMENT

Four weeks to six months after radiotherapy, pneumonitis sets in with nonproductive cough and, in more severe cases, shortness of breath and low-grade fever. The white blood count is normal, and carbon monoxide (CO)-diffusion capacity is reduced. High-resolution computed tomography confirms the diagnosis and helps to differentiate pneumonitis from infectious pneumonia, progressive tumor, and pulmonary embolism. Severe pneumonitis will result in adult respiratory distress syndrome.

Therapy for pneumonitis is symptomatic only. Steroids reduce alveolitis and symptoms but do not prevent fibrosis.[38] Mild to moderate, clinically apparent pneumonitis is treated with an initial adequate dose of prednisone (50 to 60 mg/day) that is reduced after 1 week to 30 mg/day and to 12 mg daily after 2 weeks, and is tapered, depending on the clinical course, after 4 to 6 weeks. The treatment should not be stopped too early because rebound effects may occur. Superinfections are treated with antibiotics. Prophylactic antibiotic treatment is controversial and should be considered for patients at risk for superinfection (i.e., those with stenotic lung cancer or immunosuppression). If bronchial lavage is not performed, antibiotics are chosen according to the guidelines for community-acquired pneumonia (i.e., aminopenicillin and beta-lactamase inhibitor [amoxilline + clavulan acid or sultamicilline]) or fluochinolon against pneumococces (moxifloxacin), because lung cancer is frequently associated with COPD. When long-lasting symptoms do not respond to treatment, bronchial lavage is indicated.

Severe pneumonitis is treated with oxygen, prophylaxis of right heart failure, and assisted respiration.

Lung fibrosis develops within 0.5 to 1 year after radiotherapy. The formation of lung fibrosis is an ongoing process that cannot yet be modified. Depending on the affected fibrotic lung volume and the pretreatment lung function, dyspnea, pulmonary hypertension, and cor pulmonale will develop and should be treated accordingly.

PREVENTION

Amifostine, a radical scavenger, has been shown to reduce pneumonitis after combined chemoradiotherapy in some but not all studies.[39-43] Amifostine has not been established in the clinical routine because of drug toxicity and the lack of studies on possible tumor protection. Experimental studies with captopril[44] or modifiers of TGF-β expression[45] promise modulation of pneumopathy.

ESOPHAGUS

PATHOPHYSIOLOGY

The esophagus reacts acutely through inflammation of the mucosa, in rare instances leading to ulcer and perforation. Late reactions include chronic inflammation of the lamina propria and fibrosis of the submucosa and muscularis. Stenosis can result. In rare cases, chronic ulcers and fistulas may form.

SYMPTOMS AND MANAGEMENT

Acute esophagitis occurs in week 3 to 4 of conventionally fractionated radiotherapy—2 weeks earlier in cases of additional chemotherapy. Patients experience dysphagia, odynophagia, and heart burn similar to gastroesophageal reflux, and will develop weight loss and dehydration if not treated early.

The purposes of therapy are to reduce pain and to maintain a good nutritional status. Literature is scarce, so institutional protocols have been proposed. Mild esophagitis is treated effectively with a suspension of aluminium hydroxide, magnesium hydroxide, and oxetacain. A mouthwash consisting of Maalox (4 oz), benadryl elixir (4 oz), viscous lidocaine

(100 ml), and mycostatin oral suspension (1 oz), 5 to 10 ml swallowed every 2 to 3 hours, was suggested.[46] More severe symptoms necessitate analgesic drugs, frequently including morphine. Proton pump inhibitors can alleviate heartburn symptoms. Spasms can be treated with calcium antagonists. Candidiasis should be looked for and treated with oral nystatin or fluconazole. If dehydration occurs despite intensive pain management, it should be corrected. Nutrition via percutaneous gastrostomy tube or parenteral nutrition should be considered early to improve quality of life, to reduce adverse radiation effects and the risk of superinfection, and to minimize the rate of treatment interruptions. Intervention is recommended for patients who are expected to receive <500 kcal/day over 7 days, or <60% to 80% of calculated need over 14 days, in case of initial undernourishment earlier.[47]

PREVENTION

General recommendations are to reduce additional mucosal irritation by avoiding alcohol, smoking, and spicy or acidic or hot food. An effective medical way to prevent esophagitis is not known. The effect of amifostine is controversial for chemoradiotherapy and has not been studied for radiotherapy as a single treatment modality.[39–42] Sucralfate[48] or immunoglobulin did not prevent esophagitis.

STOMACH

SYMPTOMS AND MANAGEMENT

Patients complain of nausea, vomiting, abdominal pain, and dyspepsia. Late effects consist of chronic dyspepsia and, rarely, ulcers. Treatment is symptomatic, employing antacids, sucralfate, H_2-receptor inhibitors, and proton pump inhibitors.

Prophylactic antiemetic therapy is strongly recommended for radiation of the upper abdomen.

ENTEROPATHY

The small bowel is highly radiosensitive. Because it is included in typical radiation fields for tumors in the upper and lower abdomen and in the pelvis, small-bowel toxicity is dose-limiting (e.g., for gastric, pancreatic, cervical, or rectal tumors).

PATHOPHYSIOLOGY

The crypts of Langerhans are the most sensitive structures. Radiation damages the rapidly proliferating cells, so that cells cannot be replaced fast enough. The epithelial barrier breaks down, and mucosal inflammation results. Villi are shortened and the absorption surface is decreased, leading to malabsorption.

Late effects include vascular sclerosis and intestinal wall fibrosis, leading to abnormal motility, malabsorption, strictures, fistulas, or perforation. It may be the result of a plethora of pathophysiologic processes, including inflammation, epithelial regeneration, tissue remodeling, collagen deposition, and activation of the coagulation system. The reaction is orchestrated and sustained by a number of cell types and interacting molecular signals, cytokines, growth factors, and endothelial cell surface molecules.[4,49–51]

SYMPTOMS AND MANAGEMENT

During and 2 to 6 weeks after radiotherapy, patients complain of diarrhea, abdominal pain and cramps, bloating, and anorexia. Delayed enteropathy is characterized by recurrence of these symptoms, in mild cases triggered by indigestible food, and in severe cases occurring with a high frequency of diarrhea and malabsorption, bleeding, and short bowel syndrome. Malnutrition, anemia, and hypoalbuminemia may result. Strictures, fistulas, and perforation may occur.

Chronic diarrhea can have several causes, such as small bowel bacterial overgrowth, bile salt malabsorption, carbohydrate malabsorption, motility changes, strictures, and even nonradiogenic onset of primary inflammatory bowel disease. Gastroenterologic workup is recommended in cases of severe chronic enteropathy. A low-fat, glutamine-rich, low-fiber diet is recommended. Avoidance of lactose may be useful and should be tested. Antidiarrheals (loperamide, tincture of opium), spasmolytics, and anticholinergics are indicated. Bowel motility is frequently abnormal; propulsion may be indicated, and octreotide has some effect. Bile acid malabsorption is treated with cholestyramine. Malnutrition should be corrected by parenteral substitution. Parenteral nutrition alleviates severe chronic enteropathy.[52]

Strictures, fistulas, and perforation are treated surgically if necessary. It should be kept in mind that the complication rate is very high because these patients are nutritionally depleted, and usually several regions of the bowel are affected (review[53]).

PREVENTION

Several agents were tested; however, the results have been disappointing. Prophylactic 5-aminosalicylic acid (ASA) (mesalazine and olsalazine) increased the incidence and severity of diarrhea and are contraindicated.[54,55] In contrast, sulfasalazine, which has a different formulation, decreased acute enteropathy symptoms in a double-blind placebo-controlled study.[56] Oral sucralfate,[57,58] octreotide,[59] and smectite[60] are ineffective. Amifostine was studied in a single, open-label study with inconclusive results.[61]

PROCTITIS

SYMPTOMS AND MANAGEMENT

Symptoms of acute proctitis include urgency, tenesmus, winds, anorectal pain, bleeding, and loose bowel movements.

The main symptoms of delayed proctopathy include urgency, tenesmus, and fecal incontinency, mainly caused by fibrosis of the sphincter and bleeding due to telangiectases and/or friable rectal mucosa. Symptoms peak at 18 to 24 months after treatment. It is very important to discuss the symptoms in detail with the patient. The complaint of loose bowels may mean diarrhea, a minor change in bowel habits, frequent defecation, or tenesmus. Of all gastrointestinal symptoms, urgency causes the greatest distress, but it is the most difficult symptom for patients to discuss.[62] In cases of bleeding, complete colposcopy should always be performed to exclude other sources (e.g., tumors). In 25% to 60% of patients, bleeding is not radiotherapy induced. Proctitis-induced bleeding subsides spontaneously in up to half of patients.[63]

Therapy for acute proctitis is topical. Urgency and anorectal irritation are ameliorated by topical lidocaine 1%, steroid foam, and butyrate. Tenesmus and loose bowels are reduced by loperamide. Butyrate acts as an antiinflammatory and was effective in a small study.[64] Acute proctitis rarely causes severe bleeding; usually treatment is not required.

In contrast to acute proctitis, sucralfate enema (2 g at 30 to 50 ml) reduces proctopathy and is superior to 5-ASA and steroids.[65] Sucralfate forms a complex with mucosal proteins, binds to epidermal growth factor, stimulates angiogenesis, and protects the mucosa. Short fatty acids, butyrate enema, and metronidazole per os have had effect. However, studies were small and only partially double-blind controlled.[66] It is important to use only one intervention at a time and to maintain the medication over at least 3 to 6 months. Bleeding does not require intervention unless it causes anemia or impairs quality of life. Well-defined bleeding sources can be treated with laser, argon plasma coagulation, or formalin. However, all interventions carry a risk. In a recent placebo-controlled crossover study, hyperbaric oxygen therapy improved healing responses and symptoms of therapy-refractory proctopathy.[67] Incontinence is difficult to treat. Antidiarrheal drugs (loperamide), stool-bulking agents (e.g., sterculia), toileting exercises, biofeedback, mechanical devices (e.g., anal tampons), and phenylephrine gel are helpful.

PREVENTION

Prevention or amelioration of acute proctitis is sought because acute effects predict late radiation proctitis.[68] In double-blind prevention studies, oral sucralfate and topical mesalazine increased acute bleeding,[69,70] and intrarectal sucralfate and hydrocortisone enema did not reduce the incidence and severity of symptoms.[70,71] Data on topical intrarectal application of amifostine for prevention of late radiation rectal injury are preliminary.[72]

BLADDER

PATHOPHYSIOLOGY

The bladder is covered by urothelium consisting of several layers of transitional epithelial cells that are replenished by very slowly differentiating basal cells. The surface is covered by a monomolecular film of sulfonated polysaccharides or glycosaminoglycan that plays a role in maintaining internal impermeability of the bladder. Acute reactions of the bladder are predominantly functional disorders and infrequently hematuria caused by hyperemia.

Late radiation effects are a consequence of loss of impermeability and of vascular changes. Chronic inflammation, reactive tumor-like epithelial proliferation with hemorrhage, fibrin deposits, fibrinoid vascular changes and multinucleated stromal cells, thinning of transitional epithelium, formation of telangiectases, and bladder contracture due to muscle fibrosis occur over the course of years.

SYMPTOMS AND MANAGEMENT

Acute reactions include frequency, urgency, dysuria, spasms, and incontinence. Symptoms are relieved by antispasmodics (e.g., oxybutynin), by phenazopyridine hydrochloride, which has an analgesic effect on the bladder mucosa, and by analgesics. Bladder outlet resistance is increased by ephedrine hydrochloride, pseudoephedrine hydrochloride, and phenylpropanolamine.

Late effects include persistent dysuria and/or urgency, and in severe cases severe pain, bladder contraction, and hematuria. Ulcers and vesicovaginal/vesicorectal fistulas are rare events.

Treatment is symptomatic, as was described earlier. Hematuria is treated primarily with irrigation. Intravesical application of formalin is effective but is associated with a substantial risk of renal papillary necrosis and bladder rupture. Instillation of silver nitrate and prostaglandin-F2α and systemic application of estrogen have been reported in select cases. (Super)selective vascular embolization[73] and fibrin sealant[74] have been employed for severe hemorrhage. Radiation-induced cystitis was treated like interstitial cystitis of other origin. Topical hyaluronic acid, a protective barrier of the urothelium (40 mg every week for 4 to 6 weeks),[75] or pentosanpolysulfate (initial 100 mg 3 times daily, maintenance dose 100 mg per day).[76] Hyperbaric oxygen was effective in approximately 80% of patients with refractory hemorrhagic cystitis.[77] However, controlled studies for any of the aforementioned regimens are not available, and efficacy is not proven. If the symptoms are severe and do not respond to treatment, cystectomy is performed.

Incontinence is treated according to established urologic recommendations.

PREVENTION

Effective prevention is not known. Superoxide dismutase, a radical scavenger, is not recommended because of questionable radioprotective effects and a high rate of allergic reactions.[78,79]

SEXUAL FUNCTION

FEMALE SEXUAL FUNCTION

Radiation of the pelvis has a moderate to severe impact on the sexual life of 50% to 80% of patients.[80,81] Vaginal shortening and stenosis, dyspareunia, insufficient lubrication, and bleeding or concerns of bleeding are well-known sequelae that compromise intercourse and cause considerable distress. However, vaginal changes and an unsatisfying sexual life do not correlate well. The frequency and pleasure of orgasm are not influenced by radiation.[82] Other causes of low or absent sexual interest and of dissatisfaction are important (e.g., emotional stress caused by cancer diagnosis, fear of relapse, injury, transmitting cancer, etc). Because patients frequently hesitate to address sexual issues, these should be discussed and counseling offered to the patient and her partner, as well as to the elderly patient.

Little information is available on the treatment of vaginal changes.[83] Vaginal stenosis is decreased by vaginal dilatation. Careful instructions on the use of vaginal dilators and on potential sexual difficulties, as well as suggestions of alternate sexual practices, improve compliance with vaginal dilatation and reduce sexual fears.[84] Topical estrogens decrease vaginal irritation and increase lubrication but are contraindicated for patients with hormone-sensitive tumors.

MALE SEXUAL FUNCTION

Up to 60% of patients report dissatisfaction with sex life and decreased libido and sexual desire. Erectile dysfunction develops after high-dose radiotherapy of the prostate, penile bulb, and floor of the pelvis. Lack of ejaculation after brachytherapy of the prostate, hematospermia, and pain at orgasm are reported. The likelihood of dysfunction correlates with pretreatment potency and the patient's age and comorbidities, especially diabetes mellitus. Sildenafil citrate improves function in two thirds of patients. Vacuum pumps and a penile prosthesis can help. Counseling of the patient and his partner provided by psychotherapists who specialize in sexual medicine is strongly recommended.

BONE MARROW

LEUKOPENIA

Leukopenia after myelotoxic therapy is a known, potentially dangerous adverse effect. Myelotoxicity can be dose limiting and life threatening. Clinically important are bacterial, viral, or fungal infections. Mucositis and leukopenia in head and neck carcinoma patients in the course of simultaneous radiochemotherapy carry a high risk of sepsis. Septicemia with gram-negative bacteria has a high lethality if calculated antibiosis is not started within 24 hours. Therapy should be started immediately after the first febrile episode. Choice of antibiosis follows general guidelines.

Prevention of leukopenia with growth factors in radio-oncologic settings was not studied and is not recommended.

ANEMIA

Anemia occurs after approximately 2 to 3 months, in line with the 120-day lifetime of erythrocytes.

Symptomatic anemia is treated with transfusions or erythropoietin[85]; hemoglobin level of 12 ng/dl is the goal. Erythropoietin has a longer durable effect and no infection risk; however the effect is delayed and growth induction of tumors via erythropoietin (EPO) receptors is possible. Improved local control has been proposed but not yet proven.[86–90] Therefore use of EPO is not recommended outside of clinical studies. See also guidelines on the use of growth factors.

NAUSEA AND EMESIS

Radiotherapy also induces acute, delayed, and anticipatory nausea and emesis. The risk is predominantly determined by the site and volume of radiation (Table 5-1). High dose per fraction, concomitant chemotherapy, and patient characteristics—female sex, young age, little in contrast to high alcohol consumption, previous emesis of any cause—increase the emetogenic risk. Prophylaxis is indicated for patients at moderate to high risk, and rescue is an option for patients at minimal to low risk. The NK-1 receptor antagonist enhances the $5-HT_3$ receptor antagonist effect on acute emesis and is useful in delayed emesis (see Table 5-1).

Table 5-1 Treatment of radiation-induced emesis

Emetogen risk	Typical radiation	Medication
High	Total body irradiation	$5-HT_3$ receptor antagonist prophylaxis + dexamethasone
Moderate	Upper abdomen	$5-HT_3$ receptor antagonist prophylaxis + dexamethasone as needed
Low	Lower thorax, pelvis, brain, craniospinal axis, head, and neck	$5-HT_3$ receptor antagonist prophylaxis or rescue
Minimal	Extremities, breast	Rescue with dopamine receptor or $5-HT_3$ receptor antagonist

REFERENCES

1. Jung H, Beck-Bornholdt HP, Svoboda V, et al. Quantification of late complications after radiation therapy. *Radiother Oncol.* 2001;61:233–246.
2. Bolke E, Gerber PA, Lammering G, et al. Development and management of severe cutaneous side effects in head-and-neck cancer patients during concurrent radiotherapy and cetuximab. *Strahlenther Onkol.* 2008;184:105–110.
3. Denham JW, Hauer-Jensen M. The radiotherapeutic injury—a complex 'wound. *Radiother Oncol.* 2002;63:129–145.
4. Bentzen SM. Preventing or reducing late side effects of radiation therapy: radiobiology meets molecular pathology. *Nat Rev Cancer.* 2006;6:702–713.
5. Constine LS, Tarbell N, Hudson MM, et al. Subsequent malignancies in children treated for Hodgkin's disease: associations with gender and radiation dose. *Int J Radiat Oncol Biol Phys.* 2008;72:24–33.

6. Ainsbury EA, Bouffler SD, Dorr W, et al. Radiation cataractogenesis: a review of recent studies. *Radiat Res.* 2009;172:1–9.
7. Safwat A, Bentzen SM, Turesson I, et al. Deterministic rather than stochastic factors explain most of the variation in the expression of skin telangiectasia after radiotherapy. *Int J Radiat Oncol Biol Phys.* 2002;52:198–204.
8. Borgmann K, Haeberle D, Doerk T, et al. Genetic determination of chromosomal radiosensitivities in G0- and G2-phase human lymphocytes. *Radiother Oncol.* 2007;83:196–202.
9. Andreassen CN, Alsner J, Overgaard J. Does variability in normal tissue reactions after radiotherapy have a genetic basis—where and how to look for it? *Radiother Oncol.* 2002;64:131–140.
10. Delanian S, Porcher R, Balla-Mekias S, et al. Randomized, placebo-controlled trial of combined pentoxifylline and tocopherol for regression of

superficial radiation-induced fibrosis. *J Clin Oncol.* 2003;21:2545–2550.
11. Gothard L, Cornes P, Earl J, et al. Double-blind placebo-controlled randomised trial of vitamin E and pentoxifylline in patients with chronic arm lymphoedema and fibrosis after surgery and radiotherapy for breast cancer. *Radiother Oncol.* 2004;73:133–139.
12. Camidge R, Price A. Characterizing the phenomenon of radiation recall dermatitis. *Radiother Oncol.* 2001;59:237–245.
13. Roy I, Fortin A, Larochelle M. The impact of skin washing with water and soap during breast irradiation: a randomized study. *Radiother Oncol.* 2001;58:333–339.
14. Theberge V, Harel F, Dagnault A. Use of axillary deodorant and effect on acute skin toxicity during radiotherapy for breast cancer: a prospective randomized noninferiority trial. *Int J Radiat Oncol Biol Phys.* 2009;75:1048–1052.

15. Shukla PN, Gairola M, Mohanti BK, et al. Prophylactic beclomethasone spray to the skin during postoperative radiotherapy of carcinoma breast: a prospective randomized study. *Indian J Cancer*. 2006;43:180–184.

16. Tofilon PJ, Fike JR. The radioresponse of the central nervous system: a dynamic process. *Radiat Res*. 2000;153:357–370.

17. Mizumatsu S, Monje ML, Morhardt DR, et al. Extreme sensitivity of adult neurogenesis to low doses of X-irradiation. *Cancer Res*. 2003;63:4021–4027.

18. Bruera E, Valero V, Driver L, et al. Patient-controlled methylphenidate for cancer fatigue: a double-blind, randomized, placebo-controlled trial. *J Clin Oncol*. 2006;24:2073–2078.

19. Butler Jr JM, Case LD, Atkins J, et al. A phase III, double-blind, placebo-controlled prospective randomized clinical trial of d-threo-methylphenidate HCl in brain tumor patients receiving radiation therapy. *Int J Radiat Oncol Biol Phys*. 2007;69:1496–1501.

20. Aoyama H, Tago M, Kato N, et al. Neurocognitive function of patients with brain metastasis who received either whole brain radiotherapy plus stereotactic radiosurgery or radiosurgery alone. *Int J Radiat Oncol Biol Phys*. 2007;68:1388–1395.

21. Komaki R, Meyers CA, Shin DM, et al. Evaluation of cognitive function in patients with limited small cell lung cancer prior to and shortly following prophylactic cranial irradiation. *Int J Radiat Oncol Biol Phys*. 1995;33:179–182.

22. Chang EL, Wefel JS, Hess KR, et al. Neurocognition in patients with brain metastases treated with radiosurgery or radiosurgery plus whole-brain irradiation: a randomised controlled trial. *Lancet Oncol*. 2009;10:1037–1044.

23. Welzel G, Fleckenstein K, Mai SK, et al. Acute neurocognitive impairment during cranial radiation therapy in patients with intracranial tumors. *Strahlenther Onkol*. 2008;184:647–654.

24. Klein M, Heimans JJ, Aaronson NK, et al. Effect of radiotherapy and other treatment-related factors on mid-term to long-term cognitive sequelae in low-grade gliomas: a comparative study. *Lancet*. 2002;360:1361–1368.

25. Merchant TE, Conklin HM, Wu S, et al. Late effects of conformal radiation therapy for pediatric patients with low-grade glioma: prospective evaluation of cognitive, endocrine, and hearing deficits. *J Clin Oncol*. 2009;27:3691–3697.

26. Shaw EG, Rosdhal R, D'Agostino Jr RB, et al. Phase II study of donepezil in irradiated brain tumor patients: effect on cognitive function, mood, and quality of life. *J Clin Oncol*. 2006;24:1415–1420.

27. Dequesada IM, Quisling RG, Yachnis A, et al. Can standard magnetic resonance imaging reliably distinguish recurrent tumor from radiation necrosis after radiosurgery for brain metastases? A radiographic-pathological study. *Neurosurgery*. 2008;63:898–903 discussion 904.

28. Alexiou GA, Tsiouris S, Kyritsis AP, et al. Glioma recurrence versus radiation necrosis: accuracy of current imaging modalities. *J Neurooncol*. 2009;95:1–11.

29. Rachinger W, Goetz C, Pöpperl G, et al. Positron emission tomography with O-(2-[18F] fluoroethyl)-L-thyrosine versus magnetic resonance imaging in the diagnosis of recurrent gliomas. *Neurosurgery*. 2005;57:505–511.

30. Gerstner ER, McNamara MB, Norden AD, et al. Effect of adding temozolomide to radiation therapy on the incidence of pseudo-progression. *J Neurooncol*. 2009;94:97–101.

31. Lee AW, Ng SH, Ho JH, et al. Clinical diagnosis of late temporal lobe necrosis following radiation therapy for nasopharyngeal carcinoma. *Cancer*. 1988;61:1535–1542.

32. Wanebo JE, Kidd GA, King MC, et al. Hyperbaric oxygen therapy for treatment of adverse radiation effects after stereotactic radiosurgery of arteriovenous malformations: case report and review of literature. *Surg Neurol*. 2009;72:162–167; discussion 167–8.

33. Chuba PJ, Aronin P, Bhambhani K, et al. Hyperbaric oxygen therapy for radiation-induced brain injury in children. *Cancer*. 1997;80:2005–2012.

34. Nieder C, Leicht A, Motaref B, et al. Late radiation toxicity after whole brain radiotherapy: the influence of antiepileptic drugs. *Am J Clin Oncol*. 1999;22:573–579.

35. Zhao W, Payne V, Tommasi E, et al. Administration of the peroxisomal proliferator-activated receptor gamma agonist pioglitazone during fractionated brain irradiation prevents radiation-induced cognitive impairment. *Int J Radiat Oncol Biol Phys*. 2007;67:6–9.

36. Sims EC, Plowman PN. Stereotactic radiosurgery. XII. Large AVM and the failure of the radiation response modifier gamma linolenic acid to improve the therapeutic ratio. *Br J Neurosurg*. 2001;15:28–34.

37. Barani IJ, Cuttino LW, Benedict SH, et al. Neural stem cell-preserving external-beam radiotherapy of central nervous system malignancies. *Int J Radiat Oncol Biol Phys*. 2007;68:978–985.

38. Inoue A, Kunitoh H, Sekine I, et al. Radiation pneumonitis in lung cancer patients: a retrospective study of risk factors and the long-term prognosis. *Int J Radiat Oncol Biol Phys*. 2001;49:649–655.

39. Antonadou D, Coliarakis N, Synodinou M, et al. Randomized phase III trial of radiation treatment ± amifostine in patients with advanced-stage lung cancer. *Int J Radiat Oncol Biol Phys*. 2001;51:915–922.

40. Komaki R, Lee J, Kaplan B, et al. Randomized phase III study of chemoradiation with or without amifostine for patients with favorable performance status inoperable stage II-III non-small cell lung cancer: preliminary results. *Semin Radiat Oncol*. 2002;12:46–49.

41. Sasse AD, Clark LG, Sasse EC, et al. Amifostine reduces side effects and improves complete response rate during radiotherapy: results of a meta-analysis. *Int J Radiat Oncol Biol Phys*. 2006;64:784–791.

42. Leong S, Tan E, Fong K, et al. Randomized double-blind trial of combined modality treatment with or without amifostine in unresectable stage III non-small-cell lung cancer. *J Clin Oncol*. 2003;21:1767–1774.

43. Brizel DM, Wasserman TH, Henke M, et al. Phase III randomized trial of amifostine as a radioprotector in head and neck cancer. *J Clin Oncol*. 2000;18:3339–3345.

44. Ghosh SN, Zhang R, Fish BL, et al. Renin-angiotensin system suppression mitigates experimental radiation pneumonitis. *Int J Radiat Oncol Biol Phys*. 2009;75:1528–1536.

45. Haiping Z, Takayama K, Uchino J, et al. Prevention of radiation-induced pneumonitis by recombinant adenovirus-mediated transferring of soluble TGF-beta type II receptor gene. *Cancer Gene Ther*. 2006;13:864–872.

46. Bradley J, Movsas B. Radiation pneumonitis and esophagitis in thoracic irradiation. In: *Radiation toxicity: a practical guide*. New York: Springer Berlin; 2008.

47. Arends J, Bodoky G, Bozzetti F, et al. ESPEN guidelines on enteral nutrition: non-surgical oncology. *Clin Nutr*. 2006;25:245–259.

48. McGinnis WL, Loprinzi CL, Buskirk SJ, et al. Placebo-controlled trial of sucralfate for inhibiting radiation-induced esophagitis. *J Clin Oncol*. 1997;15:1239–1243.

49. Wang J, Boerma M, Fu Q, et al. Significance of endothelial dysfunction in the pathogenesis of early and delayed radiation enteropathy. *World J Gastroenterol*. 2007;13:3047–3055.

50. Haydont V, Vozenin-Brotons MC. Maintenance of radiation-induced intestinal fibrosis: cellular and molecular features. *World J Gastroenterol*. 2007;13:2675–2683.

51. Richter KK, Langberg CW, Sung CC, et al. Increased transforming growth factor beta (TGF-beta) immunoreactivity is independently associated with chronic injury in both consequential and primary radiation enteropathy. *Int J Radiat Oncol Biol Phys*. 1997;39:187–195.

52. Andreyev J. Gastrointestinal symptoms after pelvic radiotherapy: a new understanding to improve management of symptomatic patients. *Lancet Oncol*. 2007;8:1007–1017.

53. Hauer-Jensen M, Wang J, Denham JW. Bowel injury: current and evolving management strategies. *Semin Radiat Oncol*. 2003;13:357–371.

54. Martenson JA, Hyland G, Moertel CG, et al. Olsalazine is contraindicated during pelvic radiation therapy: results of a double-blind, randomized clinical trial. *Int J Radiat Oncol Biol Phys*. 1996;35:299–303.

55. Resbeut M, Marteau P, Cowen D, et al. A randomized double blind placebo controlled multicenter study of mesalazine for the prevention of acute radiation enteritis. *Radiother Oncol*. 1997;44:59–63.

56. Kilic D, Egehan I, Ozenirler S, et al. Double-blinded, randomized, placebo-controlled study to evaluate the effectiveness of sulphasalazine in preventing acute gastrointestinal complications due to radiotherapy. *Radiother Oncol*. 2000;57:125–129.

57. Martenson JA, Bollinger JW, Sloan JA, et al. Sucralfate in the prevention of treatment-induced diarrhea in patients receiving pelvic radiation therapy: a North Central Cancer Treatment Group phase III double-blind placebo-controlled trial. *J Clin Oncol*. 2000;18:1239–1245.

58. Stellamans K, Lievens Y, Lambin P, et al. Does sucralfate reduce early side effects of pelvic radiation? A double-blind randomized trial. *Radiother Oncol*. 2002;65:105–108.

59. Martenson JA, Halyard MY, Sloan JA, et al. Phase III, double-blind study of depot octreotide versus placebo in the prevention of acute diarrhea in patients receiving pelvic radiation therapy: results of North Central Cancer Treatment Group N00CA. *J Clin Oncol*. 2008;26:5248–5253.

60. Hombrink J, Frohlich D, Glatzel M, et al. Prevention of radiation-induced diarrhea by smectite: results of a double-blind randomized, placebo-controlled multicenter study. *Strahlenther Onkol*. 2000;176:173–179.

61. Athanassiou H, Antonadou D, Coliarakis N, et al. Protective effect of amifostine during fractionated radiotherapy in patients with pelvic carcinomas: results of a randomized trial. *Int J Radiat Oncol Biol Phys*. 2003;56:1154–1160.

62. Andreyev J. Gastrointestinal complications of pelvic radiotherapy: are they of any importance? *Gut*. 2005;54:1051–1054.

63. O'Brien PC, Hamilton CS, Denham JW, et al. Spontaneous improvement in late rectal mucosal changes after radiotherapy for prostate cancer. *Int J Radiat Oncol Biol Phys*. 2004;58:75–80.

64. Vernia P, Fracasso PL, Casale V, et al. Topical butyrate for acute radiation proctitis: randomised, crossover trial. *Lancet*. 2000;356:1232–1235.

65. Denton A, Forbes A, Andreyev J, et al. Nonsurgical interventions for late radiation proctitis in patients who have received radical radiotherapy to the pelvis. *Cochrane Database Syst Rev*. 2002; CD003455.

66. Venkitaraman R, Price A, Coffey J, et al. Pentoxifylline to treat radiation proctitis: a small and inconclusive randomised trial. *Clin Oncol (R Coll Radiol)*. 2008;20:288–292.

67. Clarke RE, Tenorio LM, Hussey JR, et al. Hyperbaric oxygen treatment of chronic refractory radiation proctitis: a randomized and controlled double-blind crossover trial with long-term follow-up. *Int J Radiat Oncol Biol Phys*. 2008;72:134.

68. O'Brien PC, Franklin CI, Poulsen MG, et al. Acute symptoms, not rectally administered sucralfate, predict for late radiation proctitis: longer term follow-up of a phase III trial—Trans-Tasman Radiation Oncology Group. *Int J Radiat Oncol Biol Phys*. 2002;54:442–449.

69. Kneebone A, Mameghan H, Bolin T, et al. The effect of oral sucralfate on the acute proctitis associated with prostate radiotherapy: a double-blind, randomized trial. *Int J Radiat Oncol Biol Phys*. 2001;51:628–635.

70. Sanguineti G, Franzone P, Marcenaro M, et al. Sucralfate versus mesalazine versus hydrocortisone in the prevention of acute radiation proctitis during conformal radiotherapy for prostate carcinoma: a randomized study. *Strahlenther Onkol*. 2003;179:464–470.

71. O'Brien PC, Franklin CI, Dear KB, et al. A phase III double-blind randomised study of rectal sucralfate suspension in the prevention of acute radiation proctitis. *Radiother Oncol*. 1997;45:117–123.

72. Ben-Josef E, Han S, Tobi M, et al. A pilot study of topical intrarectal application of amifostine for prevention of late radiation rectal injury. *Int J Radiat Oncol Biol Phys*. 2002;53:1160–1164.

73. De Berardinis E, Vicini P, Salvatori F, et al. Superselective embolization of bladder arteries in the treatment of intractable bladder haemorrhage. *Int J Urol*. 2005;12:503–505.

74. Ouwenga MK, Langston MD, Campbell SC. Use of fibrin sealant in recalcitrant hemorrhagic cystitis. *J Urol*. 2004;172:1348.

75. Iavazzo C, Athanasiou S, Pitsouni E, et al. Hyaluronic acid: an effective alternative treatment of interstitial cystitis, recurrent urinary tract infections, and hemorrhagic cystitis? *Eur Urol*. 2007;51:1534–1540 discussion 1540–51.

76. Sandhu SS, Goldstraw M, Woodhouse CR. The management of haemorrhagic cystitis with sodium pentosan polysulphate. *BJU Int*. 2004;94:845–847.

77. Corman JM, McClure D, Pritchett R, et al. Treatment of radiation induced hemorrhagic cystitis with hyperbaric oxygen. *J Urol*. 2003;169:2200–2202.

78. Sanchiz F, Milla A, Artola N, et al. Prevention of radioinduced cystitis by orgotein: a randomized study. *Anticancer Res*. 1996;16:2025–2028.

79. Nielsen OS, Overgaard J, Overgaard M, et al. Orgotein in radiation treatment of bladder cancer: a report on allergic reactions and lack of radioprotective effect. *Acta Oncol*. 1987;26:101–104.

80. Jensen PT, Groenvold M, Klee MC, et al. Longitudinal study of sexual function and vaginal changes after radiotherapy for cervical cancer. *Int J Radiat Oncol Biol Phys*. 2003;56:937–949.

81. Davidson SE, Burns MP, Routledge JA, et al. The impact of radiotherapy for carcinoma of the cervix on sexual function assessed using the LENT SOMA scales. *Radiother Oncol*. 2003;68:241–247.

82. Bergmark K, Avall-Lundqvist E, Dickman PW, et al. Vaginal changes and sexuality in women with a history of cervical cancer. *N Engl J Med*. 1999;340:1383–1389.

83. Denton AS, Maher EJ. Interventions for the physical aspects of sexual dysfunction in women following pelvic radiotherapy. *Cochrane Database Syst Rev*. 2003;CD00378.

84. Robinson JW, Faris PD, Scott CB. Psychoeducational group increases vaginal dilation for younger women and reduces sexual fears for women of all ages with gynecological carcinoma treated with radiotherapy. *Int J Radiat Oncol Biol Phys*. 1999;44:497–506.

85. Adepoju LJ, Symmans WF, Babiera GV, et al. Impact of concurrent proliferative high-risk lesions on the risk of ipsilateral breast carcinoma recurrence and contralateral breast carcinoma development in patients with ductal carcinoma in situ treated with breast-conserving therapy. *Cancer*. 2006;106:42–50.

86. Lambin P, Ramaekers BL, van Mastrigt GA, et al. Erythropoietin as an adjuvant treatment with (chemo) radiation therapy for head and neck cancer. *Cochrane Database Syst Rev*. 2009;CD001658.

87. Machtay M, Pajak TF, Suntharalingam M, et al. Radiotherapy with or without erythropoietin for anemic patients with head and neck cancer: a randomized trial of the Radiation Therapy Oncology Group (RTOG 99-03). *Int J Radiat Oncol Biol Phys*. 2007;69:1008–1017.

88. Strauss HG, Haensgen G, Dunst J, et al. Effects of anemia correction with epoetin beta in patients receiving radiochemotherapy for advanced cervical cancer. *Int J Gynecol Cancer*. 2008;18:515–524.

89. Henke M, Laszig R, Rube C, et al. Erythropoietin to treat head and neck cancer patients with anaemia undergoing radiotherapy: randomised, double-blind, placebo-controlled trial. *Lancet*. 2003;362:1255–1260.

90. Shasha D, George MJ, Harrison LB. Once-weekly dosing of epoetin-alpha increases hemoglobin and improves quality of life in anemic cancer patients receiving radiation therapy either concomitantly or sequentially with chemotherapy. *Cancer*. 2003;98:1072–1079.

6

Chemotherapy toxicities of the kidney

Surafel Gebreselassie

Patients with malignancy can present with acute kidney injury from prerenal, renal (acute tubular necrosis in tumor lysis), obstructive nephropathy (cast nephropathy) or direct neoplastic infiltration (renal involvement with lymphoma). Such patients can have features of (1) tubular (Fanconi's syndrome from multiple myeloma) or (2) glomerular injury presenting with combinations of a decrease in glomerular filtration rate or a rise in creatinine and proteinuria (podocytopathies such as minimal change disease in lymphoproliferative malignancies, membranous nephropathy in patients with adenocarcinoma, or nodular glomerulosclerosis such as amyloidosis or light/heavy chain deposition disease in patients with multiple myeloma), or (3) vascular involvement such as renal vein thrombosis and glomerular thrombotic microangiopathy. Aside from this, currently used chemotherapeutic agents can cause both glomerular and tubular damage manifesting as acute or chronic kidney injury, hypertension, thrombotic microangiopathy, tubulopathies or electrolyte abnormalities such as hypomagnesemia, and hypokalemia contributing to significant morbidity and mortality. This chapter focuses on the nephrotoxicity of commonly used therapeutic agents and emerging targeted therapies, and their molecular mechanism of action and toxicity.

CISPLATIN NEPHROTOXICITY (Fig. 6-1)

DIAGNOSTIC FEATURES
- Acute kidney injury (can lead to chronic kidney disease)
- Renal magnesium wasting
- Hypokalemia
- Urinary concentrating defect

MECHANISM OF RENAL INJURY
Cisplatin (*cis*-diamminedichloroplatinum [II]) and other platinum-based compounds are commonly used in testicular, ovarian, head and neck, and other solid tumors. The antineoplastic activity of cisplatin is a result of DNA cross-links and adducts and generation of superoxide radicals. Cisplatin requires activation by an aquatic reaction involving exchange of the two chlorides, leaving groups with water or hydroxyl ligands facilitated by low intracellular concentrations of chloride.[1-3] It is neutral in chloride-rich medium such as isotonic saline.

Cisplatin is highly protein bound and is excreted by the kidney. The primary elimination mechanism is through proximal tubular secretion. Up to one third of patients treated or exposed to cisplatin develop renal dysfunction starting within days to weeks in a dose-dependent manner. Electrolyte abnormalities such as hypokalemia, hypomagnesemia, and urinary concentrating defect can persist for weeks to months after cessation of therapy. Cisplatin uptake involves at least two distinct transporters in the proximal tubule. A high-affinity copper transporter (Ctr1), which is abundantly expressed in the proximal tubule, has been shown to mediate cisplatin uptake in yeast cells. Furthermore, mouse cells lacking the *CTR1* gene that encodes Ctr1 protein exhibited cisplatin resistance. Likewise, increased concentrations of copper decreased uptake of cisplatin in wild-type yeast cells compared with Crt1 lacking mutants.[4] Organic cation transporters, particularly human organic cation transporter 2 (OCT2) isoform, have also been demonstrated to mediate cisplatin

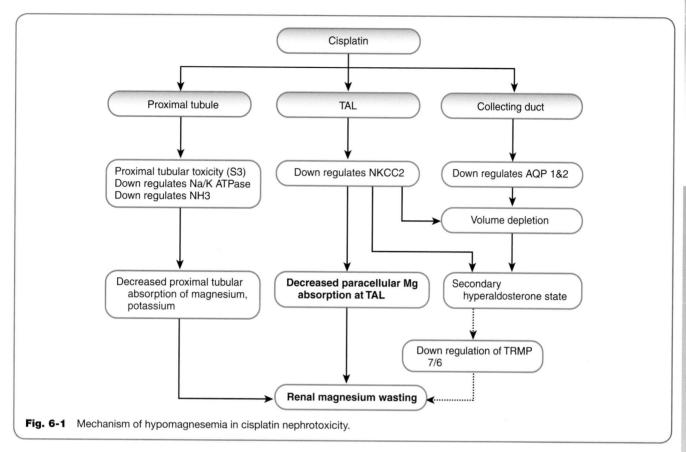

Fig. 6-1 Mechanism of hypomagnesemia in cisplatin nephrotoxicity.

nephrotoxicity in human embryonic kidney cortex cells (HEK293-cells).[5,15] OCT2-mediated uptake of cisplatin was competitively reduced in the presence of other cations transported by the same protein—cimetidine and corticosterone. Furthermore, cumulative excretion of cisplatin was reduced in organic cation 1 and 2 knockout mice compared with wild type.[6,7] Gamma-glutamyl transpeptidase (GGT) knockout mice and pharmacologic inhibition of GGT also demonstrated inhibition of cisplatin nephrotoxicity.

Once cisplatin is taken up by the proximal tubular cell, in particular the corticomedullary S3 segment of the proximal tubule, which is highly susceptible to toxic injury,[8] it undergoes an aqueous reaction, substituting the chloride groups with water or hydroxyl ligands that bind sites in the DNA, particularly at the high nucleophilic N-7 site, forming DNA adducts and cross-links that inhibit DNA replication and induce apoptosis. It has been shown to induce tubular apoptosis in a caspase-dependent and -independent manner. Furthermore, activation of proinflammatory markers such as tumor necrosis factor (TNF)-α leads to robust inflammation that contributes to acute tubular injury. The balance between activation of cytoprotective molecules such as P21, death, and inflammation promoters such as cdk2, MAPK, P53, and ROS[8,9] and the tubular abundance of free radical scavenger gluthathione (GSH) determines the likelihood of developing cisplatin nephrotoxicity in a dose-dependent manner. The progressive decrease in GSH synthesis along segments of the proximal tubule partially explains the susceptibility of the S3 segment to cisplatin toxicity.[10,16]

Patients with cisplatin toxicity often present with hypomagnesemia, hypokalemia, and distal urinary concentrating defects weeks to months after cessation of therapy. Magnesium is freely filtered but primarily reabsorbed through a paracellular route in the thick ascending loop of Henle. Only about 5% of the filtered magnesium is actively regulated in the distal tubule through the cationic channel TRPM6. Although the proximal tubule is primarily affected in cisplatin-induced tubular injury, cisplatin can also affect tubular transport in the distal tubular segments, such as the sodium potassium two-chloride cotransporter (NKCC2) in the thick ascending limb of the loop of Henle and the collecting duct. In experimental studies, NKCC2 expression was significantly reduced in rats exposed to cisplatin. Furthermore, expression of Na/K ATPase, NH3, and AQP1 and 2 was significantly reduced by cisplatin. It is interesting to note that low magnesium alone in these experimental models reduced both NKCC2 and AQP1 and 2 expressions even in the absence of cisplatin, but the effect was magnified in the presence of both cisplatin and low magnesium.[11,18] The mechanisms of hypokalemia, including impaired absorption in the proximal tubule, excessive distal sodium delivery as a result of impaired NKCC2, and secondary hyperaldosteronism, are likely multifactorial. Hypomagnesemia impairs renal potassium conservation through its permissive role in an inward-rectifying K+ channel responsible for basal K+ secretion; ROMK[12] in the distal tubule and the principal cell of the collecting duct and direct inhibitory effects on Na/K ATPase contribute to renal potassium wasting. The magnesuric effect of aldosterone is perhaps mediated through downregulation of transient receptor potential melastatin cation channel 7 (TRPM7), an important player in cellular Mg^{2+} homeostasis, along with TRPM6.[13] Whether cisplatin induced secondary hyperaldosteronism as a result of polyuria and tubular inhibition of transporters (Na/K ATPase, NH3, NKCC2, AQP1, and AQP2) plays a major role in cisplatin-induced renal magnesium wasting needs to be further elucidated.

PREVENTIVE AND TREATMENT STRATEGIES

Intravenous hydration and magnesium supplementation along with avoidance of concomitant Mg wasting medications (such as HCTZ, aminoglycosides, and amphotericin) are commonly employed as treatment and prophylactic measures in cisplatin exposure. Amifostine (Ethyol), an inorganic thiophosphate, is a selective broad-spectrum cytoprotector of normal tissues that provides cytoprotection against ionizing radiation and chemotherapeutic agents; it is FDA approved and may be considered for the prevention of nephrotoxicity in patients receiving cisplatin-based chemotherapy.[14,37] It is metabolized by alkaline phosphatase bound to cell membranes to the active form WR-1065, which scavenges free radicals. Its use is limited by side effects such as nausea, vomiting, flushing, transient hypotension, and, rarely, Stevens-Johnson syndrome. Antioxidants such as N-acetylcysteine, vitamin C, and sodium thiosulfate can be used, but their efficacy has not been established. Medications such as rosiglitazone, carvedilol, inhibitors of cisplatin metabolism (acivicin, amino-oxaloacetic acid), fibrate, erythropoietin, p53 inhibitors, MAPK inhibitors, and alpha-lipoic acid are all experimental at this time.[20]

Vascular endothelial growth factor inhibition and other targeted therapies

DIAGNOSTIC FEATURES

- Proteinuria
- Hypertension (new onset or worsening of existing hypertension)
- Thrombotic microangiopathy

Vascular endothelial growth factor (VEGF) plays a central role in angiogenesis, hence inhibitors of VEGF target tumor angiogenesis. It has been shown that VEGF expression is highest in structures with fenestrated capillaries such as the glomerulus. VEGF receptors are present in endothelial cells, mesangial cells, and podocytes, along with other molecules that mediate angiogenesis such as platelet-derived growth factors (PDGFs).[21,22]

BEVACIZUMAB (AVASTIN)

Bevacizumab is an anti-VEGF165 humanized monoclonal antibody that has been approved by the FDA for use for metastatic renal carcinoma and in combination for treatment of other malignancies. It is a potent inhibitor of angiogenesis, leading to endothelial cell apoptosis, but it is often associated with proteinuria, hypertension, and thrombotic microangiopathy. In a meta-analysis by Zhu et al[23] involving 1850 patients from seven clinical trials, 21% to 63% of patients developed some degree of proteinuria. In all, 1.8% of patients who received high doses of bevacizumab developed nephrotic range proteinuria, although two patients had focal segmental sclerosis and cryoglobulinemic glomerulonephritis, which was believed to be unrelated to bevacizumab, on subsequent renal biopsy; hence it is difficult to ascertain the true incidence of nephrotic range proteinuria in patients receiving VEGF inhibitors. Eremina et al[24] described six patients with proteinuria and renal pathologic features of thrombotic microangiopathy after bevacizumab therapy. They were able to show thrombotic microangiopathy in a murine model with genetic deletion of VEGF. On the other hand, the incidence of hypertension ranged from 3% to 36% in a dose-dependent

manner,[23] with few patients developing hypertensive crisis, including hypertensive encephalopathy. It has been reported that sunitinib, a small molecule inhibiting tyrosine kinase receptors, can induce similar renal side effects, including features of thrombotic microangiopathy, hypertension, and proteinuria, suggesting a class effect.[25,26] The mechanism appears to be similar to what happens in preeclampsia/eclampsia, in which VEGF starvation plays a major role.

Electrolyte abnormalities such as hypocalcemia (sorafenib) and hypomagnesemia (cetuximab) have been reported with other inhibitors of angiogenesis.

TREATMENT STRATEGIES

Evidence is lacking regarding the choice of antihypertensive agents in patients who develop hypertension. The role of angiotensin receptor blockers and angiotensin-converting enzyme inhibitors in the management of proteinuria and hypertension associated with VEGF inhibitors is not well defined. It is recommended that patients who develop hypertensive crisis or nephrotic range proteinuria be taken off permanently. Patients with severe hypertension and those with proteinuria greater than 2 g/day would benefit from temporary cessation of therapy and reassessment as to whether or not these abnormalities persist.

Alkylating agents (ifosfamide)

DIAGNOSTIC FEATURES

- Acute kidney injury
- Proximal tubulopathy such as phosphaturia with hypophosphatemic rickets in children, glucosuria, proteinuria, and elevated urinary β_2-microglobulin
- Renal tubular acidosis
- Hemorrhagic cystitis

Ifosfamide is widely used to treat malignancies in children such as rhabdomyosarcoma. Acrolein and chloroacetaldehyde are metabolites of ifosfamide responsible for urotoxicity and nephrotoxicity, respectively. The urotoxic effects of acrolein have been well mitigated by sodium 2-mercaptoethanesulfonate (MESNA) given concurrently. It binds acrolein and prevents its direct contact with uroepithelium. In isolated perfused rat kidney, Zamlauski-Tucker et al have shown that the ifosfamide metabolite chloroacetaldehyde can cause a clinical condition resembling Fanconi's syndrome with markedly decreased renal para-aminohippurate (PAH) clearance.[27,28] Ifosfamide can induce acute kidney injury in both children and adults in a dose-dependent manner. Survivors can have long-term tubulopathy manifesting as renal tubular acidosis, glucosuria, or phosphaturia. Cyclophosphamide, another commonly used alkylating agent in both benign and malignant conditions, can cause hemorrhagic cystitis. Its metabolism produces much less chloroacetaldehyde compared with ifosfamide, hence proximal tubulopathy is rarely observed; however electrolyte abnormalities such as hyponatremia have been reported with cyclophosphamide.

TREATMENT STRATEGIES

Various strategies, including limiting the cumulative dose of ifosfamide, discontinuing the medication when nephrotoxicity (low glomerular filtration rate [GFR] or tubular toxicity) occurs, avoiding other potential nephrotoxic drugs, and close monitoring of renal function during and after completion of therapy, have been employed.[27-29] New ifosfamide analogues with less chloracetaldehyde formation are currently investigational.[30]

Antimetabolites: Gemcitabine
DIAGNOSTIC FEATURES

- Acute kidney injury
- Hypertension
- Thrombotic microangiopathy

Gemcitabine is an antimetabolite used in various advanced malignancies. Reports of thrombotic microangiopathy have been associated with its use. In a report of 29 cases from a single institution, the median cumulative dose of gemcitabine was 22 g/m^2 and 19 patients had partial or complete recovery of renal function after cessation of therapy, but a significant proportion of patients (7 of 29) progressed to end-stage kidney disease[31]; concomitant use of mitomycin was reported to result in more severe renal injury. The mechanism of gemcitabine-induced thrombotic microangiopathy is not clear.

TREATMENT STRATEGIES

- High index of suspicion
- Cessation of therapy when evidence indicates thrombotic microangiopathy

Methotrexate nephrotoxicity
DIAGNOSTIC FEATURES

- Acute kidney injury
- Crystalluria

Methotrexate (MTX) is an antifolate that blocks dihydrofolate reductase and acts to disrupt protein and DNA synthesis. It has been used in both benign and malignant conditions. It is excreted primarily by the kidneys. MTX is poorly soluble at acidic pH and can precipitate, leading to intratubular obstruction, particularly in high-risk patients with concomitant volume depletion, and use of nonsteroidal antiinflammatory drugs and other nephrotoxic agents. The risk of acute renal failure after high-dose methotrexate administration can be as high as 10%. An increase in urine pH from 6.0 to 7.0 results in five- to eightfold greater solubility of MTX and its metabolites.[32,33]

TREATMENT STRATEGIES

- Leucovorin rescue
- Carboxypeptidase G2 hydrolyzes MTX to inactive metabolites.
- Intravenous hydration and urine alkalinization are mainstays of treatment, along with avoidance of other nephrotoxic agents.

Immune Modulators (Interleukin-2, Interferon)
DIAGNOSTIC FEATURES

- Capillary leak and intravascular volume depletion
- Various glomerulopathies

Interleukin-2 has been used in metastatic renal cancer and can cause a capillary leak with marked intravascular volume depletion. The renal complication is often dose related and can manifest within 24 to 48 hours. Patients with concomitant comorbidities such as coronary heart disease are at higher risk and may not tolerate the massive fluid resuscitation that such patients may require. Reports have described return of renal function to baseline in 95% of patients after discontinuation within 30 days.

Interferons can cause mild reversible proteinuria in 15% to 20% of patients. In addition, associated reports have described renal histologic changes consistent with membranous, membranoproliferative, focal segmental glomerulosclerosis, minimal change, acute tubular necrosis, and thrombotic microangiopathy following use of interferon.[35,36]

TREATMENT STRATEGIES

- Safe administration of high dose IL-2[34]
- Fluid resuscitation and cessation of therapy when appropriate

Nitrosoureas (Streptozocin, Carmustine)
DIAGNOSTIC FEATURES

- Acute kidney injury
- Proximal tubular dysfunction

Streptozocin-based regimens are used in pancreatic neuroendocrine tumors.[38] It is highly nephrotoxic, and several reports have described associated proximal tubular dysfunction. It is often used to induce diabetes in experimental conditions.

TREATMENT STRATEGIES

Discontinuation of therapy usually improves renal function, but progression to chronic kidney disease can occur in certain cases.

Antitumor antibiotics (mitomycin C)
DIAGNOSTIC FEATURES

- Thrombotic microangiopathy
- Noncardiogenic pulmonary edema

Mitomycin C is associated with thrombotic microangiopathy when used alone or in combination with antimetabolites and platinum compounds.[39] Reports have described high mortality among patients who developed thrombotic microangiopathy, along with noncardiogenic pulmonary edema, and hypertension in patients treated with mitomycin C.

TREATMENT STRATEGIES

- Cessation of therapy when appropriate
- Symptomatic treatment

Lenalidomide

Acute renal failure requiring renal replacement therapy after use of lenalidomide has been reported rarely in patients with plasma dyscrasia, although it is a very effective and well-tolerated agent used in multiple myeloma. Dose reduction is recommended in patients with low GFR.[40]

REFERENCES

1. Barabas K, Milner R, Lurie D, et al. Cisplatin: a review of toxicity and therapeutic applications. *Vet Comp Oncol.* 2008;6:1–18.
2. Hanigan MH, Devarajan P. Cisplatin nephrotoxicity: molecular mechanisms. *Cancer Ther.* 2003;1:47–61.
3. Sahni V, Choudhury D, Ahmed Z. Chemotherapy-associated renal dysfunction. *Nature Rev Nephrol.* 2009;5:450–462.
4. Ishida S, Lee J, Thiele DJ, et al. Uptake of the anticancer drug cisplatin mediated by the copper transporter Ctr1 yeast and mammals. *Proc Natl Acad Sci U S A.* 2002;99:14298–14302.
5. Ciarimboli G, Ludwig T, Lang D, et al. Cisplatin nephrotoxicity is critically mediated via the human organic cation transporter 2. *Am J Pathol.* 2005;167:1477–1484.
6. Ciarimboli G. Organic cation transporters. *Xenobiotica.* 2008;38:936–971.
7. Choi M-K, Song I-S. Organic cation transporters and their pharmacokinetic and pharmacodynamic consequences. *Drug Metab Pharmacokinet.* 2008;23:243–253.
8. Pabla N, Dong Z. Cisplatin nephrotoxicity: mechanisms and renoprotective strategies. *Kidney Int.* 2008;73:994–1007.
9. Cristofori P, Zanetti E, Fregona D, et al. Renal proximal tubule segment-specific nephrotoxicity: an overview on biomarkers and histopathology. *Toxicol Pathol.* 2007;35:270–275.
10. Parks LD, Zalups R, Barfuss DW. Heterogeneity of glutathione synthesis and secretion in the proximal tubule of the rabbit. *Am J Physiol.* 1998;274:F924–F931.
11. Lajer H, Kristensen M, Hansen HH, et al. Magnesium depletion enhances cisplatin-induced nephrotoxicity. *Cancer Chemother Pharmacol.* 2005;56:535–542.
12. Huang CL, Kuo E. Mechanism of hypokalemia in magnesium deficiency. *J Am Soc Nephrol.* 2007;18:2649–2652.
13. Sontia B, Montezano AC, Paravicini T, et al. Downregulation of renal TRPM7 and increased inflammation and fibrosis in aldosterone-infused mice: effects of magnesium. *Hypertension.* 2008;51:915–921.
14. Koukourakis MI. Amifostine in clinical oncology: current use and future applications. *Anticancer Drugs.* 2002;13:181–209.
15. Yonezawa A, Masuda S, Nishihara K, et al. Association between tubular toxicity of cisplatin and expression of organic cation transporter rOCT2 (Slc22a2) in the rat. *Biochem Pharmacol.* 2005;70:1823–1831.
16. Kuhlmann MK, Burkhardt G, Köhler H. Insights into potential cellular mechanisms of cisplatin nephrotoxicity and their clinical application. *Nephrol Dial Transplant.* 1997;12:2478–2480.
17. Kishore BK, Rane CM, Iulio DD, et al. Expression of renal aquaporins 1, 2 and 3 in a rat model of cisplatin-induced polyuria. *Kidney Int.* 2000;58:701–711.
18. Price PM, Safirstein RL, Megyesi J, et al. Protection of renal cells from cisplatin toxicity by cell cycle inhibitors. *Am J Physiol Renal Physiol.* 2004;286:F378–F384.
19. Portilla D, Li S, Nagothu KK, et al. Metabolomic study of cisplatin-induced nephrotoxicity. *Kidney Int.* 2006;69:2194–2204.
20. Bae EH, Lee J, Ma SK, et al. Alpha-lipoic acid prevents cisplatin-induced acute kidney injury in rats. *Nephrol Dial Transplant.* 2009;24:2692–2700.
21. Kelly RJ, Billemont B, Rixe O. Renal toxicity of targeted therapies. *Targeted Oncol.* 2009;4:121–133.
22. Ivy SP, Wick JY, Kaufman BM. An overview of small-molecule inhibitors of VEGFR signaling. *Nat Rev Clin Oncol.* 2009;6:569–579.
23. Zhu X, Wu S, Dahut WL, et al. Risks of proteinuria and hypertension with bevacizumab, an antibody against vascular endothelial growth factor: systemic review and meta-analysis. *Am J Kidney Dis.* 2007;49:186–193.
24. Eremina V, Jefferson JA, Kowalewska J, et al. VEGF inhibition and renal thrombotic microangiopathy. *N Engl J Med.* 2008;358:1129–1136.
25. Bollée G, Patey N, Cazajous G, et al. Thrombotic microangiopathy secondary to VEGF pathway inhibition by sunitinib. *Nephrol Dial Transplant.* 2009;24:682–685.
26. Launay-Vacher V, Deray G. Hypertension and proteinuria: a class-effect of antiangiogenic therapies. *Anticancer Drugs.* 2009;20:81–82.
27. Hanley L, Chen N, Rieder M, et al. Ifosfamide nephrotoxicity in children: a mechanistic base for pharmacological prevention. *Expert Opin Drug Saf.* 2009;8:155–168.
28. Zamlauski-Tucker MJ, Morris ME, Springate J. Ifosfamide metabolite chloracetaldehyde causes Fanconi syndrome in the perfused rat kidney. *Toxicol Appl Pharmacol.* 1994;129:170–175.
29. Oberlin O, Fawaz O, Rey A, et al. Long-term evaluation of ifosfamide-related nephrotoxicity in children. *J Clin Oncol.* 2009;27:5350–5355.
30. Storme T, Deroussent A, Mercier L. New ifosfamide analogs designed for lower associated neurotoxicity and nephrotoxicity with modified alkylating kinetics leading to enhanced in vitro anticancer activity. *J Pharmacol Exp Ther.* 2009;328:598–609.
31. Glezerman I, Kris MG, Miller V, et al. Gemcitabine nephrotoxicity and hemolytic uremic syndrome: report of 29 cases from a single institution. *Clin Nephrol.* 2009;71:130–139.
32. Widemann BC, Adamson P. Understanding and managing methotrexate nephrotoxicity. *Oncologist.* 2006;11:694–703.
33. Green MR, Chamberlain MC. Renal dysfunction during and after high-dose methotrexate. *Cancer Chemother Pharmacol.* 2009;63:599–604.
34. Schwartzentruber DJ. Guidelines for the safe administration of high-dose interleukin-2. *J Immunother.* 2001;24:287–293.
35. Shah M, Jenis EH, Mookerjee BK, et al. Interferon-alpha-associated focal segmental glomerulosclerosis with massive proteinuria in patients with chronic myeloid leukemia following high dose chemotherapy. *Cancer.* 1998;83:1938–1946.
36. Stokes MB, Foster K, Markowitz GS, et al. Development of glomerulonephritis during anti-TNF-alpha therapy for rheumatoid arthritis. *Nephrol Dial Transplant.* 2005;20:1400–1406.
37. Hensley ML, Hagerty KL, Kewalramani T, et al. American Society of Clinical Oncology 2008 clinical practice guideline update: use of chemotherapy and radiation therapy protectants. *J Clin Oncol.* 2009;27:127–145.
38. Chan JA, Kulke MH. Emerging therapies for the treatment of patients with advanced neuroendocrine tumors. *Expert Opin Emerg Drugs.* 2007;12:253–270.
39. Verweij J, van der Burg ME, Pinedo HM. Mitomycine C-induced hemolytic uremic syndrome: six case reports and review of the literature on renal, pulmonary and cardiac side effects of the drug. *Radiother Oncol.* 1987;8:33–41.
40. Batts ED, Sanchorawala V, Hegerfeld Y, et al. Azotemia associated with use of lenalidomide in plasma cell dyscrasias. *Leuk Lymphoma.* 2008;49:1108–1115.

Hepatic toxicity as a result of chemotherapy in the treatment of colorectal liver metastases

A. E. van der Pool, H. A. Marsman, T. M. van Gulik, and Cornelis Verhoef

COLORECTAL LIVER METASTASES

Colorectal cancer is a leading cause of cancer death. The liver is the most common site of metastases, with 25% of patients presenting with liver metastases at diagnosis; an additional 25% to 35% develop liver metastases during follow-up. Surgical resection is still the gold standard in the curative treatment of colorectal liver metastases (CLMs), with 5-year survival rates reported to be 30% to 50%.[1,2] Unfortunately, most patients (80%) are unresectable at presentation because of extrahepatic disease involvement or insufficient future liver remnant. In addition, 60% to 80% of patients who underwent hepatic surgery develop disease recurrence.

New effective systemic chemotherapeutics and the introduction of advanced surgical and anesthesiologic techniques have increased the percentage of patients with initially unresectable CLM who become candidates for curative hepatic resection.[3] In patients with normal liver, the future liver remnant should be at least 20%.[4] The question nowadays has shifted from "What can be resected?" to "What can be left?"

CHEMOTHERAPY

Over the past decade, as a result of improved chemotherapy regimens for colorectal liver metastases, a rising number of patients with unresectable and resectable disease are treated with systemic chemotherapy (CTx) before undergoing a potentially curative liver resection. Theoretical advantages include the treatment of undetectable distant micrometastases, both in the future remnant liver and at extrahepatic sites, thereby reducing the risk of disease recurrence after resection. It may also be useful to determine chemo-responsiveness of the tumor to select the optimal adjuvant therapy and to identify patients with progressive intrahepatic or extrahepatic disease under chemotherapy in whom surgery would be inappropriate. Furthermore, preoperative CTx is being used increasingly to downsize colorectal liver metastases; it appears to be able to convert 10% to 20% of initially deemed unresectable disease to resectable disease.[5,6] Neoadjuvant chemotherapy may also allow for a smaller resection (the potential to preserve hepatic parenchyma) and may increase the probability of achieving a margin-negative resection. It must be stressed that up to now, no randomized trial has proven that the use of neoadjuvant CTx after hepatic colorectal metastases prolongs survival. The European Organisation for Research and Treatment of Cancer (EORTC) 40983-trial[22] showed that perioperative chemotherapy did not influence overall survival but could result in longer disease-free survival compared with surgery only. In a consensus meeting, the panel's recommendation was that most patients with colorectal carcinoma (CRC) liver metastases should be treated up front with chemotherapy, irrespective of the initial resectability status of their metastases.[7]

CHEMOTHERAPY REGIMENS

In the late 1950s, 5-fluorouracil (5-FU) was developed, and for many years it was the CTx of choice, delivered in various bolus schedules. In the 1980s, many studies demonstrated superior response rates for 5-FU combined with leucovorin (LV), as compared with 5-FU alone, and this combination has response rates up to 20%. Since 2000, the introduction of new chemotherapy regimens has dramatically improved the outcome of CLM by combining fluoropyrimidines with irinotecan (FOLFIRI [folinic acid, fluorouracil, irinotecan]) or oxaliplatin (FOLFOX [fluorouracil, leucovorin, and oxaliplatin]). The addition of irinotecan, a topoisomerase I inhibitor, and oxaliplatin, a platinum derivative, to 5-FU and LV has yielded clinical response rates up to 55%, with a median survival of 22 months, in patients with stage IV colorectal cancer.[8,9] In addition to these novel cytotoxic agents, new molecular targeted therapies have been developed. Both bevacizumab, a monoclonal antibody to vascular endothelial growth factor (VEGF), and cetuximab, a monoclonal antibody against epidermal growth factor receptor (EGFR), have produced clinical response rates approaching 70% when combined with cytotoxic agents.[10] The possible advantage of combining different chemotherapy regimens is shortening the length of chemotherapy while receiving the same (or even better) tumor response.

RESPONSE TO CHEMOTHERAPY

Several studies indicated the response to chemotherapy before resection as a powerful predictor of outcome following resection of CLM.[11–13] When disease is stable, outcome following resection is good, and when disease responds to chemotherapy, outcome is even better. In addition, several studies showed that a "relative contraindication" exists for liver surgery if disease progression occurs under chemotherapy; Adam et al[11] reported in patients with multiple (≥4) colorectal metastases not only that response to preoperative chemotherapy was a prognostic indicator for survival, but that progressive disease under chemotherapy could represent a contraindication to surgery. Allen et al[12] showed that administration of CTx did not statistically influence survival, but that patients on CTx showing clinical response or stable disease had significantly improved survival compared with patients with progressive disease (87% vs. 38%, 5-year specific survival; $P = .03$). In contrast, Gallagher et al[14] found in their study that response to neoadjuvant chemotherapy was not related to survival after hepatic resection in patients with resectable synchronous CLM.

Complete response

A concern of effective neoadjuvant chemotherapeutics may be the complete disappearance of lesions after several lines of chemotherapy and the complexity of identifying these lesions during surgery. The question arises as to what should be resected in such clinically complete responders. Several studies demonstrated that a complete clinical response to chemotherapy with a complete pathologic response remains elusive. Adam et al[5] found that only 0.3% (2/767) of patients showed a radiographic complete response after treatment with preoperative chemotherapy, and 4% (29/767) of patients were found to have a pathologic complete response. Moreover, none of the patients with a complete radiologic response had a complete pathologic response, and vice versa. Benoist et al[15] support the need for surgical resection of CLMs despite the radiologic disappearance of the lesions after computed tomography (CT): 83% of tumors that disappeared on CT recurred upon follow-up or contained viable tumor cells at pathologic examination after liver resection. Tan et al[16] showed that 81% of patients whose tumors disappeared on fluorodeoxyglucose–positron emission tomography (FDG-PET) were not pathologic com-

plete responders. For these reasons, we recommend an evaluation scan after two or three cycles in our center, and in cases of partial response, to stop the chemotherapy and perform a partial liver resection if the disease is still resectable. Although it has been demonstrated that a pathologic response predicts survival after preoperative chemotherapy and resection of CLM,[17,18] and that complete pathologic response is associated with high survival rates,[13] concern has arisen regarding the "loss of opportunity to resect" due to progressive disease under preoperative chemotherapy. This was of significant relevance in the study by Nordlinger et al,[19] who demonstrated comparable percentages of patients who were resected in the chemotherapy group (83%) as in the group randomized to surgery directly (84%). In this study, only 7% progressed on chemotherapy. Furthermore, the nontherapeutic laparotomy rate in this prospective study was lower in the chemotherapy group (only 5% of patients in the chemotherapy group underwent a laparotomy but no resection vs. 11% of patients in the surgery-only group). This higher rate of unnecessary laparotomy in the surgery-only group may suggest that patients were better selected for surgery after using chemotherapy.

The rising use of chemotherapy combinations for CLM raises concerns about the potential hepatotoxicities induced by systemic drugs and the effects of these drugs on perioperative and postoperative outcomes. The hypothesis that systemic chemotherapy before hepatic surgery can adversely affect the liver parenchyma is strongly suggested by the increased fragility of the liver parenchyma as observed in some patients during hepatic surgery. The phenotype of hepatic injury after preoperative chemotherapy is regimen specific.[20] In the following paragraphs, this aspect will be further elucidated.

5-Fluorouracil/Leucovorin

The combination of 5-fluorouracil and leucovorin (LV) has been in clinical use for several decades. Metabolically, 5-FU acts by blocking the enzyme thymidylate synthase and inhibiting both RNA and DNA synthesis. Like most chemotherapeutic agents, 5-FU induces marked apoptosis in sensitive cells through excessive production of reactive mitochondria-derived oxygen species (ROS). Paradoxically, ROS can promote normal cellular proliferation and carcinogenesis, and can also induce apoptosis of tumor cells. Primarily, 5-FU affects the tumor itself, which leads to tumor necrosis and tumor fibrosis.

Hepatoxicity of 5-FU is mediated by excessive production of ROS, which results in accumulation of lipid vesicles in hepatocytes with the histomorphologic correlate of steatosis. The association of 5-FU with liver steatosis has been shown in several studies:

- Zeiss et al[21] reported steatosis in parts of the liver parenchyma that were overperfused with floxuridine via hepatic artery infusion.
- Peppercorn et al[22] reported CT findings of steatosis associated with 5-FU and folinic acid administration. Furthermore, high body mass index (BMI) and administration of 5-FU resulted in marked steatosis.[23]
- More recently, it has been demonstrated that all chemotherapeutic agents used in colorectal cancer may cause steatosis.[24]

Several case series observed that moderate to severe steatosis is associated with greater postoperative morbidity.[25,26] Patients with severe steatosis are at higher risk of developing postoperative liver dysfunction and infectious complications and of longer intensive care unit stay. However, no differences in mortality rates have been described.[23,27] Although 5-FU–based chemotherapy may cause profound changes in liver parenchyma, it can be safely applied.

Oxaliplatin

Oxaliplatin is a diaminocyclohexane platinum compound that acts as an alkylating cytotoxic agent, inhibiting DNA replication by forming adducts between two adjacent guanines or guanine plus adenine. Most cancer cell lines are sensitive to oxaliplatin, and it has synergistic activity with 5-FU. The EORTC 40983 trial[19] showed an absolute increase in rate of progression-free survival at 3 years of 7% in patients who received preoperative oxaliplatin-based CTx, but no difference in overall survival was found.

Various studies have demonstrated that oxaliplatin's liver injury appears to be directed against the endothelial cells lining the sinusoids.[20,24,28,29] Oxaliplatin leads to depletion of glutathione and impairs mitochondrial oxidation, which results in the production of reactive oxygen species that may induce this injury.[30] Damage to the endothelial cells will lead to circulatory compromise of centrilobular hepatocytes with fibrosis and obstruction of liver blood flow—the sinusoidal obstruction syndrome. These histopathologic alterations result in a characteristic discoloration of the liver with associated edema and spongiform consistency, referred to as "blue liver syndrome" (Figs. 7-1 and 7-2). In severe cases, sinusoidal obstruction can lead to portal hypertension, ascites, and jaundice. One of the histologic features of the sinusoidal obstruction syndrome is sinusoidal dilatation (Fig. 7-3A compared with Fig. 7-3B). Oxaliplatin is also associated with other parenchymal hepatic injuries, such as nodular regenerative hyperplasia, peliosis, and centrilobular vein fibrosis. Rubbia-Brandt et al[28] showed that 51% of post–oxaliplatin-based chemotherapy liver resection specimens had sinusoidal dilatation. Other studies have confirmed this observation, with an incidence of 10% to 52% in patients receiving preoperative oxaliplatin.[20,24,29]

No study to date has demonstrated increased mortality after hepatic resection in patients who have received preoperative oxaliplatin-based CTx, but several studies have revealed that

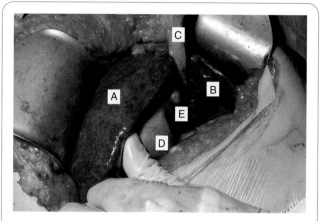

Fig. 7-2 D, Gallbladder. **E,** Necrotic colorectal metastases after oxaliplatin.

postoperative complications could be associated with the use of preoperative oxaliplatin-based CTx.[20,31,32] Nordlinger et al[19] showed that the use of oxaliplatin-based chemotherapy appeared to be associated with some increased and reversible morbidity (25% vs. 16%; $P = .04$). This may be related to the short interval between cessation of chemotherapy and performance of surgery (the protocol initially mandated surgery within 3 weeks of chemotherapy but was later amended). The duration of time off chemotherapy before surgery may have an impact on complications. Karoui et al[33] found prolonged CTx (≥6 cycles of oxaliplatin) to be a risk factor for postoperative complications after major liver resection. Therefore, in patients undergoing an extended liver resection after a high number of CTx cycles (>6), additional risk factors, such as a high degree of steatosis, should be ruled out. Vauthey et al[24] found that grade 2 to 3 sinusoidal dilatation was associated with oxaliplatin-based CTx (19% vs. 2%; $P < .001$) but found no increase in postoperative morbidity or mortality. Aloia et al[32] noted that patients with liver injury due to oxaliplatin-based chemotherapy required more perioperative blood transfusions than patients who received 5-FU. Perioperative blood transfusion has been shown to be a risk factor for poor outcomes following hepatic resection.[34] Another study found that sinusoidal injury was associated with higher morbidity and longer hospital stay in patients undergoing major hepatectomy, and that it resulted in an impaired liver functional reserve before hepatectomy.[35] The association between postoperative morbidity and sinusoidal injury might be attributable to the intensive chemotherapy given in this study: 90 patients received an average of nine cycles, and 27% (24/90) received two different lines of chemotherapy. The link between sinusoidal injury and morbidity is still under debate.

Irinotecan

Irinotecan is a semisynthetic analog of the natural alkaloid camptothecin and is commonly used in combination with 5-fluorouracil and leucovorin. After administration, it is hydrolyzed into SN-38, a topoisomerase inhibitor, which prevents DNA replication and transcription. It is mainly used in patients with metastatic colorectal cancer and has shown increased response rates (>50%) and improved survival.

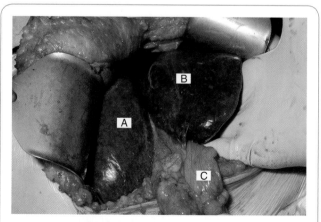

Fig. 7-1 A, Right liver lobe. **B,** Left liver lobe. **C,** Ligamentum teres.

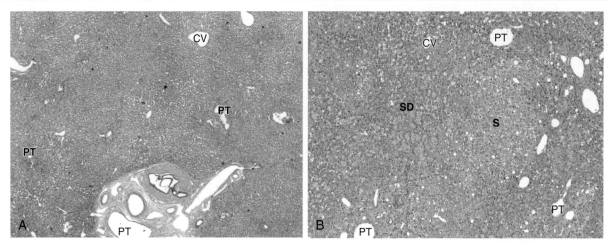

Fig. 7-3 **A,** Normal liver parenchyma with portal tract (PT) and central vein (CV). No significant steatosis or sinusoidal dilatation of fibrosis is seen.**B,** Liver parenchyma after treatment with XELOX (capecitabine plus oxaliplatin); areas with sinusoidal dilatation (SD) are seen together with foci of steatosis (S).

However, an important downside of the use of irinotecan is the induction of chemotherapy-associated steatohepatitis (CASH). CASH is characterized by increased accumulation of hepatic fat in combination with hepatic inflammation following chemotherapy treatment. It is closely related to the upcoming Western disease known as nonalcoholic fatty liver disease (NAFLD), a condition inextricably associated with the current obesity epidemic. In NAFLD, simple steatosis can progress over time into nonalcoholic steatohepatitis. Although the exact mechanism is still under debate, a theory put forth to explain disease progression in NAFLD refers to the "two-hit" mechanism. The first hit is the unbridled hepatic fatty acid accumulation caused by a high caloric intake and insulin resistance. The second hit consists of increased oxidative stress response caused mainly by mitochondrial dysfunction through excessive microsomal and peroxisomal ω- and β-oxidation of fatty acids. This leads to activation of Kuppfer cells and a consequent inflammatory cascade. As was mentioned in a previous section, 5-FU, with or without LV, is the foundation to which other chemotherapy regimens are added. This regimen alone is already associated with steatosis induction caused by impaired mitochondrial function. In the FOLFIRI regimen, irinotecan is added to 5-FU and LV. In a small study by Fernandez et al,[36] 28% (4/14) of patients developed steatohepatitis following the FOLFIRI regimen. Lower rates of steatohepatitis were detected after FOLFIRI by Pawlik et al[20]: 2 of 55 (4%) patients. In a larger study, Vauthey et al[24] showed that irinotecan treatment was associated with steatohepatitis in 20% (19/94) of patients. Furthermore, this study showed that a higher degree of steatohepatitis development occurred in obese (BMI > 25 kg/m²) patients (25%;15/61) as opposed to patients with a normal BMI (<25 kg/m²) (12%; 4/33). A similar association between obesity and increased steatohepatitis induction following irinotecan treatment was noted by Pawlik et al[20] and by Fernandez et al.[36] Mechanistic studies shedding light on increased induction of steatohepatitis are lacking. It can be postulated that 5-FU treatment serves as the "first hit," leading to hepatic fatty acid accumulation (i.e., simple steatosis). Subsequently, the addition of irinotecan can be considered the "second hit," finally resulting in an inflammatory cascade and consequent steatohepatitis.

Additionally, obese patients already suffer from steatosis before undergoing chemotherapy, and when exposed to irinotecan are at higher risk for development of steatohepatitis.

The largest study investigating liver resection outcomes following irinotecan treatment was performed by Vauthey et al.[24] Investigators found that 90-day mortality was significantly higher in patients with steatohepatitis, as compared with patients without steatohepatitis (14.7% vs. 1.6%; $P = .001$). An almost sixfold higher incidence of liver failure was observed as a cause of death in patients with steatohepatitis, as compared with chemo-naïve patients. It was suggested that because of limited regenerative capacity, progressive liver failure occurs in the remnant liver affected by steatohepatitis. In contrast to findings of the latter study, Pawlik et al[20] reported a lower incidence of steatohepatitis induction and consequently no difference in morbidity and mortality following liver resection. Ideally, patients should be evaluated for the presence of steatohepatitis before, during, and after irinotecan treatment before liver resection. However, a liver biopsy is an invasive procedure that can be associated with serious complications. Instead, noninvasive tests could be employed for the possible detection of steatohepatitis. For instance, a combination of elevated transaminases and increased hepatic fat content on radiologic studies could serve as an indication to perform a biopsy preoperatively. For noninvasive detection of hepatic fat, several modalities are available, such as ultrasound, CT scan, and magnetic resonance imaging (MRI), with the latter considered the most reliable. When steatohepatitis is detected, a limited liver resection should be performed to prevent postoperative liver failure of the remnant liver. In general, a remnant liver volume in a healthy liver can be as low as 20%. However, in the setting of steatosis or steatohepatitis, a safer margin of 40% is recommended.[37] This, on the other hand, could be a negative influence on the radicality of a liver resection.

Bevacizumab

VEGF mediates liver growth through hepatocyte and sinusoidal endothelial cell proliferation and is essential for wound healing.[38,39] Activation of the VEGFR-1 receptor results in secretion of paracrine cytokines (including hepatocyte growth factor and interleukin-6), which stimulate hepatocyte division; binding of VEGF to VEGFR-2 receptors induces proliferation of the sinusoidal endothelium. Several studies have demonstrated that VEGF prevents hepatocyte injury, reduces the severity of acute liver injury, and initiates hepatic regeneration after CCL4, D-galactosamine, and lipopolysaccharide-mediated liver damage.[40] Bevacizumab is a recombinant humanized version of a murine monoclonal antibody with angiogenesis-inhibiting effects. It binds to VEGF, preventing activation of the corresponding receptor kinases VEGFR-1 and VEGFR-2. It neutralizes free VEGF and thus inhibits VEGF-mediated endothelial cell proliferation, survival, and migration in vitro. On the other hand, bevacizumab induces apoptosis in hypoxia-susceptible tumor cell lines.

Prospective, randomized trials have shown that bevacizumab added to oxaliplatin-based CTx regimens in patients with stage IV colorectal cancer improves overall survival, progression-free survival, and response rate.[41,42] As a result, it might allow a higher proportion of patients with unresectable disease to become resectable. It would also be likely that bevacizumab has an effect on dormant micrometastases, promoting tumor shrinkage and inhibition of angiogenesis. The antiangiogenic effect and the long half-life of bevacizumab have raised concerns about wound healing and liver regeneration.[43,44] The addition of bevacizumab in the TREE-2 (Three Regimens of Eloxatin in Advanced Colorectal Cancer) study caused more grade 3 or 4 hypertension, impaired wound healing, and bowel perforation.[45] On the other hand, Kesmodel et al[46] showed that neither the use of bevacizumab nor the timing of its administration was associated with an increase in complication rates in patients treated with different types of CTx regimens. Other studies[40,47] have shown that bevacizumab can be given before hepatectomy without affecting postoperative morbidity, if the interval between discontinuation of bevacizumab and hepatic resection is at least 8 weeks. The results from a study by Gruenberger and colleagues[48] suggest that this interval could be shortened to 5 weeks without an increase in perioperative complications. Bevacizumab is associated with gastrointestinal perforation and poor wound healing across clinical trials, but reported incidences are rare.[49] Moreover, bevacizumab does not impair liver regeneration, even in response to portal vein embolization (PVE).[50]

Evidence suggests that bevacizumab might decrease the incidence of sinusoidal injury. Ribero et al[51] showed that bevacizumab reduces the occurrence of sinusoidal injury related to oxaliplatin when therapy is relatively short. Sinusoidal dilatation of any grade was reduced in patients who received oxaliplatin plus bevacizumab (27% vs. 54% without bevacizumab), and severe (grade 2-3) sinusoidal obstruction was reduced significantly by the addition of bevacizumab to oxaliplatin (8% vs. 28%; $P = .006$). Ribero et al[51] also showed an improved pathologic response. Klinger et al[29] found no improved clinical tumor response with the addition of bevacizumab but demonstrated that when given in five cycles, bevacizumab protects against the sinusoidal obstruction syndrome. The exact mechanism responsible for this is still unknown, but it is possible that the VEGF blockade acts by downregulating metalloproteinases, thereby decreasing the rate of apoptosis in endothelial cells.

Cetuximab

One of the new members of the family of biological agents for treatment of colorectal cancer is cetuximab. This mouse/human chimeric monoclonal antibody has inhibiting effects on epidermal growth factor receptor (EGFR). Several studies have shown an increased response rate when added to the FOLFIRI regimen.[10,52–54] In particular, patients with KRAS wild-type metastatic colorectal cancer may greatly benefit from this regimen. In a recent study, response rates up to 70% were reported.[10] Also, increased resection rates following metastatic disease irresponsive to traditional regimens have been reported, of which the largest study (CRYSTAL [Cetuximab Combined With Irinotecan in First-Line Therapy for Metastatic Colorectal cancer]) was performed by Van Cutsem et al.[53] In this study, 1198 unresectable patients were randomized to FOLFIRI or FOLFIRI + cetuximab chemotherapy. The addition of cetuximab resulted in a significantly increased resection rate (7.0% vs. 3.7%) and an increase in R0 resections (4.8% vs. 1.7%). Similarly, in the OPUS (Oxaliplatin and Cetuximab in First-Line Treatment of mCRC) trial,[52] the addition of cetuximab to FOLFOX and R0 resulted also in an increased resection rate (91% vs. 81%).

Reported side effects of cetuximab included skin reactions and in select cases infusion reactions and hypomagnesemia.[52] Unfortunately, no histologic analysis of liver tissue was performed in either study. As far as we know, the only study performing histologic analysis of liver tissue following cetuximab treatment was conducted by Adam et al.[54] Twenty-seven of 151 patients were downsized after irresponsiveness to traditional regimens. Hepatic lesions were found in 37% of patients; they were not attributable to cetuximab but were related to traditional chemotherapy regimes. No clinical studies to date have investigated whether cetuximab impairs regenerative capacity. In this respect, experimental reports are contradictory. Natarajan et al[55] indicated that EGFR is a key regulator of liver regeneration. However, van Buren et al[44] showed that inhibition of EGFR by cetuximab, as opposed to bevacizumab, does not impair liver regenerative capacity in a murine model. Additional clinical studies will have to be employed to investigate whether cetuximab can be used safely before liver resection is performed.

Because it is one of the newest biological agents available, only a few studies have been performed on perioperative outcomes after liver resection following cetuximab treatment. Adam et al[54] showed encouraging operative results in a modest series of 27 patients. One of 27 patients (3.7%) died as a consequence of liver failure after a second partial liver resection was performed. The overall complication rate was 50%. It must be noted that in this study, patients had received several different combinations of chemotherapy treatment before undergoing liver resection, thus making it difficult to point out the exact influence of cetuximab on outcomes of liver resection alone. With respect to measures for the safe preoperative use of cetuximab, too few studies have been completed to allow any recommendations to be put forth regarding safe use of this type of chemotherapy.

In summary, increased use of preoperative chemotherapy in initially resectable patients or in those converted to a resectable status offers several theoretical benefits, but outcomes have enhanced awareness of the adverse effects of chemotherapy on the liver parenchyma. Concerns regarding chemotherapy-associated liver injury may prevent clinicians from offering potentially curative therapy, and such treatment may increase morbidity in some patients. Prolonged use of preoperative chemotherapy should be avoided, and choice of therapy should be individualized on the basis of resectability status, extent of hepatic resection required, and associated comorbid conditions.

REFERENCES

1. Abdalla EK, Vauthey JN, Ellis LM, et al. Recurrence and outcomes following hepatic resection, radiofrequency ablation, and combined resection/ablation for colorectal liver metastases. *Ann Surg.* 2004;239:818–825; discussion 825-7.

2. Choti MA, Sitzmann JV, Tiburi MF, et al. Trends in long-term survival following liver resection for hepatic colorectal metastases. *Ann Surg.* 2002;235:759–766.

3. Jarnagin WR, Gonen M, Fong Y, et al. Improvement in perioperative outcome after hepatic resection: analysis of 1,803 consecutive cases over the past decade. *Ann Surg.* 2002;236:397–406; discussion 406-7.

4. Charnsangavej C, Clary B, Fong Y. Selection of patients for resection of hepatic colorectal metastases: expert consensus statement. *Ann Surg Oncol.* 2006;13:1261–1268.

5. Adam R, Delvart V, Pascal G, et al. Rescue surgery for unresectable colorectal liver metastasis downstaged by chemotherapy: a model to predict long-term survival. *Ann Surg.* 2004;240:644–657; discussion 657-8.

6. Adam R, Wicherts DA, de Haas RJ, et al. Patients with initially unresectable colorectal liver metastases: is there a possibility of cure? *J Clin Oncol.* 2009;27:1829–1835.

7. Nordlinger B, Van Cutsem E, Gruenberger T, et al; European Colorectal Metastases Treatment Group. Sixth International Colorectal Liver Metastases Workshop. Combination of surgery and chemotherapy and the role of targeted agents in the treatment of patients with colorectal liver metastases: recommendations from an expert panel. *Ann Oncol.* 2009;20:985–992.

8. de Gramont A, Figer A, Seymour M, et al. Leucovorin and fluorouracil with or without oxaliplatin as first-line treatment in advanced colorectal cancer. *J Clin Oncol.* 2000;18:2938–2947.

9. Tournigand C, Andre T, Achille E, et al. FOLFIRI followed by FOLFOX6 or the reverse sequence in advanced colorectal cancer: a randomized GERCOR study. *J Clin Oncol.* 2004;22:229–237.

10. Folprecht G, Gruenberger T, Bechstein WO, et al. Tumour response and secondary resectability of colorectal liver metastases following neoadjuvant chemotherapy with cetuximab: the CELIM randomised phase 2 trial. *Lancet Oncol.* 2010;11:38–47.

11. Adam R, Pascal G, Castaing D, et al. Tumor progression while on chemotherapy: a contraindication to liver resection for multiple colorectal metastases? *Ann Surg.* 2004;240:1052–1061; discussion 1061-4.

12. Allen PJ, Kemeny N, Jarnagin W, et al. Importance of response to neoadjuvant chemotherapy in patients undergoing resection of synchronous colorectal liver metastases. *J Gastrointest Surg.* 2003;7:109–115; discussion 116-7.

13. Adam R, de Haas RJ, Wicherts DA, et al. Is hepatic resection justified after chemotherapy in patients with colorectal liver metastases and lymph node involvement? *J Clin Oncol.* 2008;26:3672–3680.

14. Gallagher DJ, Zheng J, Capanu M, et al. Response to neoadjuvant chemotherapy does not predict overall survival for patients with synchronous colorectal hepatic metastases. *Ann Surg Oncol.* 2009;16:1844–1851.

15. Benoist S, Brouquet A, Penna C, et al. Complete response of colorectal liver metastases after chemotherapy: does it mean cure? *J Clin Oncol.* 2006;24:3939–3945.

16. Tan MC, Linehan DC, Hawkins WG, et al. Chemotherapy-induced normalization of FDG uptake by colorectal liver metastases does not usually indicate complete pathologic response. *J Gastrointest Surg.* 2007;11:1112–1119.

17. Blazer DG, Kishi Y, Maru DM, et al. Pathologic response to preoperative chemotherapy: a new outcome end point after resection of hepatic colorectal metastases. *J Clin Oncol.* 2008;26:5344–5351.

18. Rubbia-Brandt L, Giostra E, Brezault C, et al. Importance of histological tumor response assessment in predicting the outcome in patients with colorectal liver metastases treated with neoadjuvant chemotherapy followed by liver surgery. *Ann Oncol.* 2007;18:299–304.

19. Nordlinger B, Sorbye H, Glimelius B, et al. Perioperative chemotherapy with FOLFOX4 and surgery versus surgery alone for resectable liver metastases from colorectal cancer (EORTC Intergroup trial 40983): a randomised controlled trial. *Lancet.* 2008;371:1007–1016.

20. Pawlik TM, Olino K, Gleisner AL, et al. Preoperative chemotherapy for colorectal liver metastasis: impact on hepatic histology and postoperative outcome. *J Gastrointest Surg.* 2007;11:860–868.

21. Zeiss J, Merrick HW, Savolaine ER, et al. Fatty liver change as a result of hepatic artery infusion chemotherapy. *Am J Clin Oncol.* 1990;13:156–160.

22. Peppercorn PD, Reznek RH, Wilson P, et al. Demonstration of hepatic steatosis by computerized tomography in patients receiving 5-fluorouracil-based therapy for advanced colorectal cancer. *Br J Cancer.* 1998;77:2008–2011.

23. Kooby DA, Fong Y, Suriawinata A, et al. Impact of steatosis on perioperative outcome following hepatic resection. *J Gastrointest Surg.* 2003;7:1034–1044.

24. Vauthey JN, Pawlik TM, Ribero D, et al. Chemotherapy regimen predicts steatohepatitis and an increase in 90-day mortality after surgery for hepatic colorectal metastases. *J Clin Oncol.* 2006;24:2065–2072.

25. Belghiti J, Hiramatsu K, Benoist S, et al. Seven hundred forty-seven hepatectomies in the 1990s: an update to evaluate the actual risk of liver resection. *J Am Coll Surg.* 2000;191:38–46.

26. McCormack L, Petrowsky H, Jochum W, et al. Hepatic steatosis is a risk factor for postoperative complications after major hepatectomy: a matched case-control study. *Ann Surg.* 2007;245:923–930.

27. Gomez D, Malik HZ, Bonney GK, et al. Steatosis predicts postoperative morbidity following hepatic resection for colorectal metastasis. *Br J Surg.* 2007;94:1395–1402.

28. Rubbia-Brandt L, Audard V, Sartoretti P, et al. Severe hepatic sinusoidal obstruction associated with oxaliplatin-based chemotherapy in patients with metastatic colorectal cancer. *Ann Oncol.* 2004;15:460–466.

29. Klinger M, Eipeldauer S, Hacker S, et al. Bevacizumab protects against sinusoidal obstruction syndrome and does not increase response rate in neoadjuvant XELOX/FOLFOX therapy of colorectal cancer liver metastases. *Eur J Surg Oncol.* 2009;35:515–520.

30. Chun YS, Laurent A, Maru D, et al. Management of chemotherapy-associated hepatotoxicity in colorectal liver metastases. *Lancet Oncol.* 2009;10:278–286.

31. Welsh FK, Tilney HS, Tekkis PP, et al. Safe liver resection following chemotherapy for colorectal metastases is a matter of timing. *Br J Cancer.* 2007;96:1037–1042.

32. Aloia T, Sebagh M, Plasse M, et al. Liver histology and surgical outcomes after preoperative chemotherapy with fluorouracil plus oxaliplatin in colorectal cancer liver metastases. *J Clin Oncol.* 2006;24:4983–4990.

33. Karoui M, Penna C, Amin-Hashem M, et al. Influence of preoperative chemotherapy on the risk of major hepatectomy for colorectal liver metastases. *Ann Surg.* 2006;243:1–7.

34. Kooby DA, Stockman J, Ben-Porat L, et al. Influence of transfusions on perioperative and long-term outcome in patients following hepatic resection for colorectal metastases. *Ann Surg.* 2003;237:860–869; discussion 869-70.

35. Nakano H, Oussoultzoglou E, Rosso E, et al. Sinusoidal injury increases morbidity after major hepatectomy in patients with colorectal liver metastases receiving preoperative chemotherapy. *Ann Surg.* 2008;247:118–124.

36. Fernandez FG, Ritter J, Goodwin JW, et al. Effect of steatohepatitis associated with irinotecan or oxaliplatin pretreatment on resectability of hepatic colorectal metastases. *J Am Coll Surg.* 2005;200:845–853.

37. Vetelainen R, van Vliet A, Gouma DJ, et al. Steatosis as a risk factor in liver surgery. *Ann Surg.* 2007;245:20–30.

38. Donahower B, McCullough SS, Kurten R, et al. Vascular endothelial growth factor and hepatocyte regeneration in acetaminophen toxicity. *Am J Physiol Gastrointest Liver Physiol.* 2006;291:G102–G109.

39. Redaelli CA, Semela D, Carrick FE, et al. Effect of vascular endothelial growth factor on functional recovery after hepatectomy in lean and obese mice. *J Hepatol.* 2004;40:305–312.

40. Reddy SK, Morse MA, Hurwitz HI, et al. Addition of bevacizumab to irinotecan- and oxaliplatin-based preoperative chemotherapy regimens

does not increase morbidity after resection of colorectal liver metastases. *J Am Coll Surg.* 2008;206:96–106.

41. Hurwitz H, Fehrenbacher L, Novotny W, et al. Bevacizumab plus irinotecan, fluorouracil, and leucovorin for metastatic colorectal cancer. *N Engl J Med.* 2004;350:2335–2342.

42. Saltz LB, Clarke S, Diaz-Rubio E, et al. Bevacizumab in combination with oxaliplatin-based chemotherapy as first-line therapy in metastatic colorectal cancer: a randomized phase III study. *J Clin Oncol.* 2008;26:2013–2019.

43. Scappaticci FA, Fehrenbacher L, Cartwright T, et al. Surgical wound healing complications in metastatic colorectal cancer patients treated with bevacizumab. *J Surg Oncol.* 2005;91:173–180.

44. Van Buren G, Yang AD, Dallas NA, et al. Effect of molecular therapeutics on liver regeneration in a murine model. *J Clin Oncol.* 2008;26:1836–1842.

45. Hochster HS, Hart LL, Ramanathan RK, et al. Safety and efficacy of oxaliplatin and fluoropyrimidine regimens with or without bevacizumab as first-line treatment of metastatic

colorectal cancer: results of the TREE study. *J Clin Oncol.* 2008;26:3523–3529.

46. Kesmodel SB, Ellis LM, Lin E, et al. Preoperative bevacizumab does not significantly increase postoperative complication rates in patients undergoing hepatic surgery for colorectal cancer liver metastases. *J Clin Oncol.* 2008;26:5254–5260.

47. D'Angelica M, Kornprat P, Gonen M, et al. Lack of evidence for increased operative morbidity after hepatectomy with perioperative use of bevacizumab: a matched case-control study. *Ann Surg Oncol.* 2007;14:759–765.

48. Gruenberger B, Tamandl D, Schueller J, et al. Bevacizumab, capecitabine, and oxaliplatin as neoadjuvant therapy for patients with potentially curable metastatic colorectal cancer. *J Clin Oncol.* 2008;26:1830–1835.

49. Saif MW, Elfiky A, Salem RR. Gastrointestinal perforation due to bevacizumab in colorectal cancer. *Ann Surg Oncol.* 2007;14:1860–1869.

50. Zorzi D, Chun YS, Madoff DC, et al. Chemotherapy with bevacizumab does not affect liver regeneration after portal vein embolization

in the treatment of colorectal liver metastases. *Ann Surg Oncol.* 2008;15:2765–2772.

51. Ribero D, Wang H, Donadon M, et al. Bevacizumab improves pathologic response and protects against hepatic injury in patients treated with oxaliplatin-based chemotherapy for colorectal liver metastases. *Cancer.* 2007;110:2761–2767.

52. Bokemeyer C, Bondarenko I, Makhson A, et al. Fluorouracil, leucovorin, and oxaliplatin with and without cetuximab in the first-line treatment of metastatic colorectal cancer. *J Clin Oncol.* 2009;27:663–671.

53. Van Cutsem E, Kohne CH, Hitre E, et al. Cetuximab and chemotherapy as initial treatment for metastatic colorectal cancer. *N Engl J Med.* 2009;360:1408–1417.

54. Adam R, Aloia T, Levi F, et al. Hepatic resection after rescue cetuximab treatment for colorectal liver metastases previously refractory to conventional systemic therapy. *J Clin Oncol.* 2007;25:4593–4602.

55. Natarajan A, Wagner B, Sibilia M, et al. The EGF receptor is required for efficient liver regeneration. *Proc Natl Acad Sci U S A.* 2007;104:17081–17086.

8

Acute neurotoxicity induced by common chemotherapies

Daniel J. Moskovic and David R. Fogelman

CHEMOTHERAPIES KNOWN TO INDUCE TOXICITY

OVERVIEW

Chemotherapy-induced neurotoxicity occurs in up to 40% of patients receiving treatment.[1] It is important to note that the neurotoxic effects of the therapy—both central and peripheral—can be the dose-limiting event in treatment of a variety of cancers. This may adversely affect prognosis, quality of life, and survival. Most notably, many of the central and peripheral neurotoxic effects of chemotherapy may be prevented or reversed if identified early and managed properly.[2] Thus, the astute clinician must be aware of common neurologic manifestations of toxicity and the appropriate diagnostic and management approach. This chapter provides a basic overview of common neurotoxicities associated with specific therapies. It is crucial to appreciate that few chemotherapies are administered alone. Therefore, many of the descriptions involve combination treatment. Additionally, the most severe neurotoxicities are reported in case series rather than in large clinical trials because of low incidence. These are mentioned here to provide a comprehensive reference for those involved in managing the patient on chemotherapy.

In general, the diagnosis of neurotoxicity is determined through a comprehensive history and physical examination. In certain cases, imaging and diagnostic tests may help confirm the diagnosis. Additionally, prevention and treatment strategies represent a growing body of research. Little is known about the pathogenesis of neurotoxicity in some cases. The literature has focused on prevention strategies, although treatment options remain sparse.

PLATINUM COMPOUNDS

The platinum compounds (i.e., cisplatin, carboplatin, oxaliplatin) act by cross-linking DNA strands. By inducing intrastrand and interstrand cross-links, platinum compounds damage the integrity of cells and induce necrosis. Widely utilized in chemotherapy, these compounds are often limited by their acute and chronic neurotoxicities. More recently, the genetic basis for susceptibility of patients to the neurotoxic effects of these drugs has been explored and described.[3]

CISPLATIN

Highly utilized in head and neck, gastrointestinal, urologic, and gynecologic cancers, cisplatin can cause both central and peripheral nervous system toxicity. Although blood-brain barrier penetration of cisplatin is limited, its use in intra-arterial therapy can lead to dose-limiting central neurotoxicity soon after treatment.[4] Up to 6% of patients will experience headache, encephalopathy, seizures, or focal neurologic deficits. Previous brain radiation is also associated with an increased risk of neurotoxicity. It is unknown whether cisplatin leads directly to neurotoxicity, or whether electrolyte disturbances secondary to therapy cause central toxicity, but in any case, withdrawal of therapy often leads to resolution of symptoms.

The peripheral effects of cisplatin, although widely known, occur most often in the setting of continual therapy, usually when total dose exceeds $400 \, mg/m^2$.[5] In addition, peripheral neuropathy can occur up to several months after completion of therapy.[6] For patients treated with intra-arterial therapy, the risk of acute, reversible radiculopathy is due to toxic levels of the drug at the administration site.[7] Pathologic investigation of cisplatin toxicity reveals chronic axonal changes (Fig. 8-1), thus precluding recognition of these changes in the acute setting.[8] Most commonly, patients will develop transient muscle cramps in the acute setting, but it is not known if this is a predictor of subsequent neurotoxicity. Occasionally, patients report Lhermitte's sign during or shortly after administration of high-dose cisplatin.[9]

CARBOPLATIN

Carboplatin is a platinum analog that is associated with fewer overall neurologic complications as compared with cisplatin but is known to have slightly increased central nervous system penetration. This finding does not appear to be of much clinical significance. Peripheral administration has not been linked to acute central neurotoxicity; however, intra-arterial therapy has been shown to cause acute retinopathy and, less often, focal neurologic deficits.[10]

Peripheral toxicity is similar to cisplatin but requires greater exposure because of the less potent neurotoxic effects of carboplatin. Specifically, toxicity typically manifests only after several cycles of therapy.[11]

OXALIPLATIN

Oxaliplatin is a newer compound that is used most commonly in colorectal cancer. Central neurologic side effects are not common with oxaliplatin, but peripheral toxicity can be the dose-limiting side effect. These peripheral effects are grouped into acute and chronic toxicities. Acute toxicities include muscle fasciculations, cold-induced paresthesias, and contractures. These develop within hours of treatment in most patients.[12–14] Nearly 25% of patients will develop perioral or laryngeal dysesthesias during infusion, although only a small fraction will develop laryngospasm with difficulty breathing.[12] Continued administration will lead to chronic toxicities such as paresthesias and loss of deep tendon reflexes (DTRs); thus careful consideration of subsequent therapy is necessary.[13]

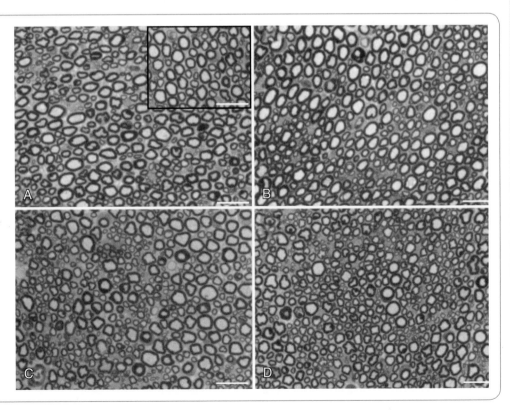

Fig. 8-1 **Panel A** represents mouse sciatic nerve light photomicrographs from specimens obtained after treatment, showing mild axonopathy. A = cisplatin 4 mg/kg *(the inset in the upper right corner is a control photo)*. B = paclitaxel 10 mg/kg; C = paclitaxel 10 mg/kg + cisplatin 4 mg/kg; D = cisplatin 4 mg/kg + paclitaxel 10 mg/kg. *(Reprinted from Carozzi V, et al. Effect of the chronic combined administration of cisplatin and paclitaxel in a rat model of peripheral neurotoxicity. Eur J Cancer 2009;45:656-65.)*

VINCA ALKALOIDS

The vinca alkaloids represent a class of compounds that block microtubule formation during mitosis, thus arresting cell division. These chemotherapies are most useful in hematologic malignancies and are occasionally used as immunosuppressants because of their ability to inhibit rapidly dividing cells. It is not surprising that the main side effects of therapy involve bone marrow suppression. It is important to note that vinblastine, commonly used in lung cancers, is not strongly associated with significant neurotoxicity.

VINCRISTINE

Central neuropathies due to vincristine are rare but serious. When administered intrathecally, even small doses of this drug can cause a devastating and fatal myeloencephalopathy that begins within hours of treatment.[14] A potentially reversible encephalopathy can develop while on vincristine therapy (dose >4 mg), although this is very uncommon.[15]

The acute peripheral neurotoxicity of vincristine is most likely related to inhibition of the axonal microtubule infrastructure (Fig. 8-2). Symptoms of toxicity include paresthesias of the distal extremities, numbness, and loss of ankle DTRs.[16] These symptoms occur in a large majority (up to 70%) of patients treated with vincristine and present in a dose-dependent fashion. Once cumulative doses exceed the toxic threshold, symptoms appear soon after treatment. Cessation of treatment resolves the neuropathy in most cases; however, about 25% of patients experience worsening of symptoms when off therapy. A more worrisome peripheral complication is a collection of polyradicular findings similar to the Guillain-Barré syndrome. Although it occurs only on rare occasions, this complication can pose a diagnostic challenge to clinicians.[17] The Guillain Barré–like syndrome has been shown to present progressively after cumulative doses of at least 4 mg of vincristine and is not regarded with the spectrum of acute or subacute toxicity. Vocal cord paralysis can present as an emergency requiring ventilatory support, although this rare complication has been reported in only a little more than 1% of children receiving vincristine therapy.[18] An extremely rare multiple cranial and peripheral neuropathy within a few days of treatment can be fatal.[19]

SEMISYNTHETIC VINCA ALKALOIDS

The semisynthetic vinca alkaloids, including vindesine and vinorelbine, are used in hematologic malignancies, as well as in breast and lung cancers. Vinorelbine holds a far lower risk of neurotoxicity as compared with vincristine.[20] Peripheral neuropathy manifested by sensory changes and paresthesias will occur in 20% of patients, although significant symptoms appear in less than 1%. Additionally, constipation is frequently encountered and is believed to represent autonomic neuropathy. Both peripheral and autonomic neuropathies are readily reversible upon discontinuation of therapy. Similarly, vindesine can cause reversible peripheral and autonomic neuropathies at rates similar to vincristine neuropathies.[21] In addition, vindesine has been found to induce a reversible Guillain Barré–like syndrome.[22]

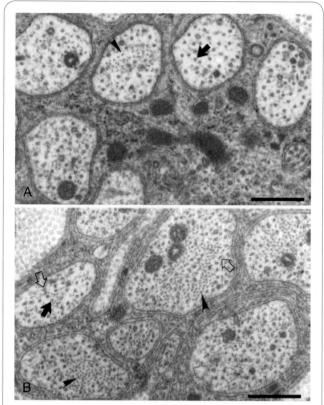

Fig. 8-2 Cross sections of mictotubules in control **(A)** and vincristine-treated **(B)** rat nerves. Whereas neurofilaments were distributed throughout the axoplasmin control axons, there appeared to be more neurofilaments in many vincristine-treated axons. Neurofilaments in vincristine-treated axons also appeared to be abnormally clustered in the central portion of the axoplasm. In addition, many vincristine-treated unmyelinated axons were larger and more irregularly shaped compared with controls. *(From Tanner KD, Levine JD, Topp KS. Microtubule disorientation and axonal swelling in unmyelinated sensory axons during vincristine-induced painful neuropathy in rat. J Comp Neurol 1998;395:481-2. Permission from www.copyright.com, academic subscription.)*

ANTIMETABOLITES

The antimetabolite class of chemotherapy includes agents that inhibit cellular metabolism at various points throughout the metabolic processes that are ongoing in the dividing cell. These drugs primarily interfere with processes involved in the synthesis and replication of DNA.

METHOTREXATE

Methotrexate is a dihydrofolate reductase inhibitor that is used very commonly in hematologic and breast cancers. It is also used at high doses for central nervous system (CNS) lymphomas and intrathecally for acute lymphocytic leukemias. Debate has arisen over the pathogenesis of methotrexate-induced neurotoxicity, and it is unknown whether magnetic resonance imaging (MRI) changes precede symptoms or serve as evidence of irreversible damage. Intrathecal methotrexate administration has been associated with the development of aseptic meningitis, and a recent case description of methotrexate-induced meningitis following intramuscular administration has been described.[23] The symptoms present within a few hours of treatment and resolve within 72 hours. Other common complaints following intrathecal therapy include back pain, weakness, and sensory changes. These are precursory to the development of a rare but reversible transverse myelopathy.[24] High doses of systemic methotrexate have been associated with subacute, reversible mental status changes and focal neurologic deficits in up to 15% of patients.[25] Some of the damage induced by methotrexate therapy is irreversible, and more than 25% of patients show long-term cognitive and functional changes. Thus early recognition of toxicity is crucial in maintaining quality of life for these patients. A partially reversible lumbosacral radiculopathy has been reported on rare occasions.[26] Symptoms of radiculopathy are progressive and often do not present immediately after treatment.

5-FLUOROURACIL

5-Fluorouracil (5-FU) is an inhibitor of thymidylate synthase that prevents nucleotide synthesis and arrests cell division. This therapy is widely utilized for the treatment of gastrointestinal and head and neck tumors. Although rarely implicated in neurotoxicity, 5-FU has been associated with acute onset of encephalopathy, a cerebellar syndrome, seizures, or isolated cranial nerve deficits.[27] Cerebellar (ataxia, slurred speech, nystagmus) or encephalopathic (cognition, confusion, sensation) changes manifest themselves within hours of chemotherapy and are reversible within days upon cessation of treatment. Either of these syndromes will present in fewer than 10% of patients, and rarely will a patient develop both conditions simultaneously. Although the mechanism of neurotoxicity is not entirely characterized, it is thought to be related to metabolic interference by 5-FU. Less acutely, a multifocal leukoencephalopathy has been described several days after therapy.

Recent evidence indicates that susceptibility to 5-FU neurotoxicity may be related to genetic factors, although this concept is new and requires further development.[28] It is known that patients with dihydropyrimidine dehydrogenase deficiency are at increased risk of developing 5-FU neurotoxicity, in addition to other 5-FU–mediated adverse events.

Peripheral toxicity due to 5-FU is very rare, presenting with mild sensorimotor deficits that are reversible with cessation of therapy.[29]

CYTOSINE ARABINOSIDE (CYTARABINE, ARA-C)

Cytarabine is a pyrimidine analog that inhibits DNA polymerase and is used primarily in hematologic cancers. Several case studies have documented aseptic meningitis after intrathecal cytarabine administration.[30] This complication is largely reversible but can last for several weeks after therapy. Symptoms develop after a cumulative dose of about 20 mg. Seizures can also present in up to 20% of patients receiving intrathecal therapy. About 10% of patients will develop cerebellar dysfunction with high-dose cytarabine following cumulative doses of 36 mg/m^2.[31] Symptoms are largely reversible with cessation of therapy but occasionally (in <1% of patients) can be permanent.

Peripheral polyneuropathy occurs in 1.5% to 2% of patients receiving high-dose cytarabine.[32] Symptoms can present up to

20 days after therapy and result in a devastating demyelinating sensorimotor course. Patients may require mechanical ventilatory support, and the course can be fatal. More commonly, reversible sensory neuropathy (with or without neuropathic pain) will develop as the result of inhibition; this is followed by rebound overexpression of a specific capsaicin receptor on peripheral nerves.[33]

IFOSFAMIDE

Ifosfamide is a nitrogen mustard alkylating agent used in the treatment of hematologic, gynecologic, urologic, and bone cancers. Transient central neurotoxicity has been observed in about 5% of children and presents as partial and generalized seizures.[34] Reversible encephalopathy has been found to develop in the elderly, with men older than age 65 presenting with encephalopathic symptoms at a rate of up to 30%.[35]

TAXANES

The taxane class of chemotherapeutic agents disrupts the mitotic cycle by stabilizing microtubule formation after the S phase. Thus, their neurotoxicity is purported to be related to dysfunctional axonal transport of neurotransmitters and neuronal constituents (Fig. 8-3). Neurotoxicity in the setting of these agents is very common and can often be the dose-limiting side effect.

PACLITAXEL

Paclitaxel is commonly used in ovarian, breast, and lung cancers, and is being applied to pancreatic cancer as well. Central neurotoxicity of this agent is very limited, although high doses (>600 mg/m^2) have been associated with a reversible encephalopathy (<5%) and an altered visual sensorium.[36] Peripheral toxicity is dose dependent and usually requires at least a cumulative dose of 100 mg/m^2.[37,38] Typical signs and symptoms of peripheral neuropathy develop first in almost all patients and include numbness, proximal and distal muscle weakness, myalgias, arthralgias, and paresthesias. These can be severe enough to interfere with activities of daily living and can be intensified when paclitaxel is administered in combination with cisplatin.[39] At higher cumulative doses, loss of reflexes and vibratory sensation will occur in some patients.[40] Pathologically, axonal atrophy and absence of axonal sprouting are hallmarks of late paclitaxel-induced neurotoxicity.[40]

Abraxane is an albumin-bound paclitaxel that is now being used in breast cancer and is under investigation in other cancer types. Early studies of abraxane have found that sensory neurotoxicity and fatigue are the most commonly reported side effects (in up to 65% of patients), although severe neurotoxicity is far less common (5%–10% of patients).[41] Neurotoxicity was more common with abraxane than with paclitaxel alone. Additionally, initial experience with this drug reveals that reversal of symptoms is more rapid once the medication is discontinued. Further studies are needed to evaluate the neurotoxic potential of this new chemotherapeutic agent.

DOCETAXEL

Similar to paclitaxel, docetaxel is used commonly in gynecologic and lung malignancies. Side effects are similar to paclitaxel, although mild symptoms appear in only about 10%

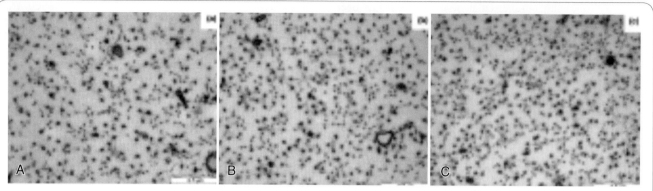

Fig. 8-3 Electron micrograph of small myelinated axons in **(A)** control animal, **(B)** paclitaxel 10 mg/kg, and **(C)** docetaxel 10 mg/kg. Increased density of microtubules is induced by docetaxel treatment. *(With permission from Persohn E, Canta A, Schopefer S, et al. Morphological and morphometric analysis of paclitaxel and docetaxel-induced peripheral neuropathy in rats. Eur J Cancer 2005;41:1460-6.)*

of patients, and more severe symptoms tend to present only after cumulative doses of 400 mg/m^2.[41,42] In addition to general peripheral toxicities, 5% of patients receiving docetaxel may experience Lhermitte's sign.[43] Nerve biopsy of patients with docetaxel-induced peripheral neuropathy demonstrates pathologic findings similar to patients with paclitaxel-induced neuropathy.

NITROSOUREAS

These compounds are a class alkylating agents whose mechanism of action is not well understood. They readily cross the blood-brain barrier and are often used to treat neurologic malignancies. Although neurotoxicity with this class of chemotherapy is uncommon in the systemic setting, intra-arterial carmustine (200 mg/m^2)–induced encephalopathy and focal neurologic deficits are common (15%) within hours of treatment. Computed tomographic (CT) changes are evident within days in a large number of patients, although no specific pattern is diagnostic.[44] About 15% of patients treated with lomustine in combination with methotrexate and vincristine for malignant glioma developed cognitive deficits, seizures, and focal neurologic deficits.[45]

DIAGNOSIS OF NEUROTOXICITY

Careful history and physical examination remain the mainstay of diagnosis of neurotoxicity. History should specifically elicit recent chemotherapies, previous responses, and any history of past neurotoxicity. Additionally, medications, medical problems, predisposing conditions, and preexisting neurologic injuries should be identified. For example, it has been suggested that pretreatment nerve conduction velocity (NCV) studies and family history of neuropathy may be predictors of vincristine-induced neurotoxicity, although no prospective data are available to test this hypothesis. Additionally, patients with hereditary motor and sensory neuropathy (Charcot-Marie-Tooth type I) have been found to be at higher risk for severe acute and chronic neurotoxicity when treated with vincristine.[46]

To aid history taking, various neuropathy scales have been designed and validated in the setting of chemotherapy-induced neurotoxicity. The comprehensive and reduced Total Neuropathy Scale[50] has been shown to correlate with clinical symptoms of peripheral neuropathy. Additionally, a comprehensive survey used to characterize oxaliplatin-induced neurotoxicity may be useful to clinicians because it includes a comprehensive list of central and peripheral symptoms of neurotoxicity.[47]

Physical examination should be comprehensive and should test motor, sensory, and cerebellar functions. Concerns regarding central toxicity should prompt further examination. Various domains of sensory function (e.g., vibration, pain, two-point discrimination) should be tested, as different peripheral nerve subtypes are affected by various chemotherapies.

Diagnostic tests can be useful but should be given only when needed. Electromyelogram and NCV studies were abnormal within hours of oxaliplatin therapy and indicated nerve hyper-excitability. However, patients reported symptoms and demonstrated signs consistent with hyperexcitability. Cerebrospinal fluid (CSF) pleocytosis with the absence of bacterial culture is the typical finding for patients who develop methotrexate meningitis.[26] Sural nerve NCV studies demonstrated slow action potentials in paclitaxel-induced neurotoxicity.[43] Additional history of conditions that predispose patients to develop neuropathy (e.g., diabetes) should be elicited.[48] Patients treated with lomustine, methotrexate, and vincristine who develop cognitive deficits and central neurotoxicity typically show slowing of electroencephalographic output.[48]

IDENTIFICATION OF HIGH-RISK PATIENTS

Emerging data demonstrate that patients bearing individual or combinations of unfavorable polymorphisms may be at higher risk for neuropathy. This is particularly true for oxaliplatin, for which extensive pharmacogenomic studies have been performed. Although not now in routine use, increasing knowledge of such polymorphisms may soon provide a rationale for routine a priori testing of patients' genetic makeup before treatment is initiated. Several of these polymorphisms are listed in Table 8-1.

Table 8-1 Unfavorable polymorphisms

Genetic Predisposition for Neuropathy

Chemotherapy	Genes associated with neuropathy
Oxaliplatin	AGXT
	GSTP1-I105V
Cisplatin	GSTM1
Docetaxel	ABCB1
	GSTP1
Paclitaxel	ABCB1

For instance, Gamelin and others demonstrated that a minor haplotype of glyoxylate aminotransferase (AGXT) was found to predict both acute and chronic neurotoxicity from oxaliplatin.[49] In this study, glutathione-S-transferase P1 polymorphisms did not predict oxaliplatin sensitivity, although a later study found that the I105V polymorphism in this gene was associated with increased neurotoxicity.[50] Two other studies—one French, one Italian—found a similar association between the I105V polymorphism and neuropathy among patients treated with oxaliplatin, thereby validating this finding.[51,52] A study of polymorphisms among voltage-gated sodium channel genes themselves failed to find a relationship between the SCN2A R19K polymorphism and oxaliplatin use.[53]

As with oxaliplatin, polymorphisms may predict cisplatin and taxane toxicity. A polymorphism in the glutathione-S-transferase *M1* gene, for instance, may predispose patients to cisplatin neurotoxicity.[54] Likewise, patients with a polymorphism in the P-glycoprotein *(ABCB1)* gene may benefit from a longer time to development of neuropathy during treatment with paclitaxel[55] and docetaxel alone or in combination with thalidomide.[56] Additionally, the GST I105V allele described above may predispose patients toward docetaxel-induced peripheral neuropathy.[57]

As we further our knowledge of the relationship between genotype and predilection toward neuropathy and other side effects, the benefit of testing will increase. And as we develop alternative chemotherapies and medications capable of preventing neuropathy, we will ultimately be able to steer high-risk patients toward less toxic outcomes.

PREVENTION AND TREATMENT OF NEUROPATHY

Several agents have been tested for prevention of neuropathy and for treatment of existing neuropathy as caused by neurotoxic agents. In this section, we review a number of these strategies; many of the larger studies are listed in Table 8-2.

CALCIUM AND MAGNESIUM

Oxaliplatin-induced neuropathy can alter a patient's quality of life, and this is a frequent reason for discontinuation of the drug. Infusion of calcium and magnesium may reduce the incidence of neuropathy. Interest in this treatment is based on

the mechanism of action of oxaliplatin itself. Oxaliplatin is broken down in cells to oxalate, which chelates intracellular calcium. The absence of intracellular calcium then potentiates calcium-dependent sodium channels, leading to hyperexcitability of the nerve (the acute neuropathy), and later to a more chronic neuropathy. Hypothetically, increasing the amount of extracellular calcium and magnesium might decrease oxaliplatin-induced hyperexcitability of peripheral neurons.[58]

Replacing lost calcium and magnesium has been tested as a means of preventing the hyperexcitability of peripheral nerves. The French Neuroxa study retrospectively examined colorectal cancer patients treated with FOLFOX (fluorouracil, leucovorin, and oxaliplatin) with or without electrolyte replacement.[59] In this review, 95 patients were treated with calcium and magnesium infusion before and after treatment, and 65 patients were treated without these electrolytes. Less toxicity was seen in the treatment group, along with fewer grade 3 paresthesias (7% vs. 26%), less paresthesia, and less neuropathy at the end of treatment (20% vs. 45%). Efficacy was similar between the two groups.

This strategy was then tested in a randomized, placebo-controlled, double-blind phase III study among patients receiving oxaliplatin (as FOLFOX) as adjuvant chemotherapy for colon cancer.[60,61] Neuropathy was assessed through conventional common toxicity criteria (CTC), as well as with a patient-reported outcome scale specific for oxaliplatin. The primary endpoint of this study was grade 2 or greater chronic peripheral neuropathy. Time to onset of neuropathy, percentage of patients with acute neuropathy, and percentage of patients discontinuing treatment were secondary endpoints. Although the study was designed to include 300 patients, accrual was halted and the study was closed when an interim analysis of the CONcePT study (Comparison of Oxaliplatin vs. Conventional Methods With Calcium/Magnesium in First-Line Metastatic Colorectal Cancer; later) suggested that the two salts reduced the efficacy of treatment. At that point, 50 patients had received FOLFOX with the salts, and 52 had received FOLFOX without them.

Differences in acute and chronic toxicity were reported. Some acute toxicity, specifically muscle cramps, was decreased in the Ca/Mg group (23% vs. 6%; $P = .002$), although sensitivity to cold and discomfort when swallowing were similar between the two groups. A reduction in chronic neurotoxicity occurred as well, with less grade 2 or worse neuropathy in the Ca/Mg group (22% vs. 41%; $P = .038$), less numbness and tingling in the fingers and toes, and less inability to button shirts. The time to neuropathy was significantly prolonged in the Ca/Mg group. No difference in non-neurologic toxicities was noted between the groups.

The CONcePT trial[62] simultaneously tested two strategies for prevention of oxaplatin-induced neuropathy. Patients with metastatic colorectal cancer were randomized to arms with or without calcium and magnesium salts, as well as to arms with continuous treatment or a "stop-and-go" strategy, whereby oxaliplatin was discontinued after 8 cycles of treatment; it was reintroduced after an additional 8 cycles of chemotherapy. The study evaluated time to treatment failure as its primary endpoint. After 270 patients were enrolled, randomization to Ca/mg was halted, and all patients received these salts. This study was halted early because an unplanned interim analysis suggested a higher response rate in the arm without calcium and magnesium. However, a subsequent review of imaging

Table 8-2   Agents tested for prevention of neuropathy and for the treatment of existing neuropathy as caused by neurotoxic agents

Intermittent Oxaliplatin Strategy	Pts.		Study findings	Comments
Optimox-1	2006	620	Grade 3 sensory neuropathy in 18% of continuously and 13% of intermittently treated patients; $P = .12$	
Grothey (CONcePT)	2008	139	Decreased neuropathy (24% vs. 10%), improved TTF (5.6 vs. 4.2 months) in the intermittent arm	
Glutathione				
Cascinu	1995	50	Decreased neuropathy in GSH-treated patients as compared with placebo	Small, prospective, randomized study; no change in platinum activity
Smyth	1997	151	Decreased neurosensory toxicity but not significant (49% vs. 39%; $P = .22$).	Prospective trial of ovarian cancer patients randomized to GSH or placebo
Cascinu	2002	52	Decreased grade 2-4 neurotoxicity in the GSH arm (11 vs. 2; $P = .003$)	Small, prospective, randomized study; no change in platinum activity
Glutamine/Glutamate				
Wang	2007	86	Significant decrease in grade 3-4 neuropathy in oxaliplatin-treated patients	Small, prospective, randomized trial
Stublefield	2005	46	Less weakness and loss of vibration in patients treated with high-dose paclitaxel	
Vitamin E				
NCCTG	2009	189	No difference in grade 2+ neurotoxicity	Patients received multiple chemo regimens. Numbers are too small to assess for each chemotherapy

showed no difference in response rates based on the use of these salts. In total, 140 patients were randomized to the 2×2 protocol. Response rate and time to treatment failure were similar between the two groups. Calcium and magnesium did not show an effect on the incidence of neurotoxicity. Because it consisted of small numbers of patients, it is difficult to draw conclusions from this study.

In all, trials that evaluated calcium and magnesium in preventing oxaliplatin toxicity do not show a significant deleterious effect of these electrolytes and suggest that they may provide benefit in reducing neuropathy. However, the numbers of patients evaluated remain small, making it difficult to draw definitive conclusions on the efficacy of this treatment.

STOP-AND-GO STRATEGIES

One means of preventing the development of oxaliplatin-related neuropathy is reducing the patient's exposure to the drug. The first study to assess this approach was the Optimox-1 study,[63] in which oxaliplatin was given continuously as FOLFOX4 or was omitted after six cycles of FOLFOX7 and reintroduced after 12 cycles. In this study, 623 patients were randomized to either arm. Grade 3 sensory neuropathy was seen in 18% in the continuous treatment arm and in only 13% in the intermittent treatment arm, but this did not reach statistical significance. Response rate, progression-free survival, and overall survival were similar.

Patients in the CONcePT trial were randomized to discontinuing oxaliplatin after eight cycles of chemotherapy or continuing oxaliplatin until the occurrence of disease progression or unacceptable toxicity. Patients in the early discontinuation

arm resumed oxaliplatin treatment after an additional eight cycles of 5-FU and leucovorin alone, or earlier if the disease progressed. Time to treatment failure was prolonged in those patients undergoing the intermittent infusion schedule of oxaliplatin: 5.6 vs. 4.2 months, with $P = .0025$. Progression-free survival was also prolonged in the intermittent treatment group (12 vs. 7.3 months; hazard ratio [HR] = .53; $P = .048$). Less grade 3-4 neurotoxicity was reported (10% vs. 24%), along with fewer dose delays or reductions (22% vs. 8%) and fewer discontinuations (22% vs. 10%) in the intermittent treatment arm.

GLUTATHIONE

Glutathione (GSH) is a tripeptide originally developed to protect against the nephrotoxicity of cisplatin; it was later found to have a neuroprotective effect. Its efficacy might be attributed to its ability to form cisplatin-GSH complexes, and evidence suggests that it reduces platinum concentrations in dorsal root ganglia.[64] Alternatively, exogenous GSH may act by scavenging free radicals induced by platinum, by repleting intracellular GSH, or by affecting renal clearance of cisplatin.

Cascinu and others evaluated the ability of GSH to prevent glutathione-induced neurotoxicity. In a study of 50 patients, those with gastric cancer undergoing cisplatin treatment were randomized to $1.5 \, g/m^2$ GSH or to placebo given before cisplatin, with IM injections given on days 2 to 5. Clinical evaluation and electrophysiologic (EP) studies were used to assess toxicity. After 9 weeks, no patients in the GSH arm demonstrated neuropathy, and 16 of 25 in the placebo arm had some degree of neuropathy; 4 of these were grade 2-3.

At week 15, 4 of 24 in the GSH arm had neuropathy, all of which were grade 1-2. Conversely, in the placebo arm, 16 of 18 had some neuropathy, 3 of which were grade 3-4. One of the placebo patients and none of the GSH patients discontinued for neuropathy. Responses and survival were at least similar and possibly better in the GSH arm. Glutathione also demonstrated efficacy in a larger study of 151 ovarian cancer patients receiving cisplatin chemotherapy.[65] Patients receiving GSH demonstrated better quality-of-life scores with improved neurotoxicity scores and remained more functional than placebo-controlled patients. A trend toward better outcomes was observed in the GSH group, but this was not statistically significant. Likewise, GSH patients received more cisplatin (median 440 mg/m^2 vs. 401 mg/m^2), although this was not statistically significant.

GSH has also been tested in colorectal cancer patients receiving oxaliplatin in the form of FOLFOX chemotherapy.[66] Fifty-two patients were randomized to GSH or placebo. As in the earlier study, significantly fewer patients experienced grade 2-4 neurotoxicity in the GSH than the placebo arm. Response rates and progression-free survival were similar in the two arms. Other forms of toxicity were similar between the two arms.

Taken as a whole, these studies of glutathione offer promise in their ability to reduce neurotoxic effects of chemotherapy. However, larger studies are needed to validate these findings before their routine use can be recommended.

GLUTAMINE/GLUTAMATE

The precise mechanism by which glutamine acts as a neuroprotectant remains unknown. It may be that this agent stimulates nerve growth factor release. Wang and others[67] conducted a pilot trial evaluating oral glutamine in patients receiving oxaliplatin-based chemotherapy for colorectal cancer. Patients receiving 15 g twice daily had less grade 3-4 neuropathy after four cycles (18.2% vs. 4.8%; $P = .05$) and six cycles (31.8% vs. 11.9%; $P = .04$) of chemotherapy. Glutamine also reduced neuropathy in patients receiving paclitaxel in preparation for stem cell transplants. In a study of 46 patients, the treatment group showed less weakness and less loss of vibratory sensation.[68]

A small, recent study of glutamate in 43 patients receiving paclitaxel failed to show a significant benefit.[69] However, this was a small study that used a lower dose of glutamate than either of the previous studies. As a whole, these studies may warrant a larger clinical trial.

N-ACETYLCYSTEINE

N-acetylcysteine (NAC) is used as an antioxidant in various types of poisoning and in prevention of contrast-induced nephrotoxicity. Laboratory work demonstrated its ability to prevent nerve cell apoptosis from cisplatin exposure, suggesting a possible clinical role.[70] Additionally, NAC may increase circulating glutathione. Lin and colleagues[71] found that one of five colon cancer patients receiving FOLFOX chemotherapy with NAC demonstrated neurotoxicity after 12 cycles, and 8 of 12 patients on placebo had such toxicity. These numbers remain too small to be conclusive, however.

VITAMIN E

Investigators have studied antioxidants such as vitamin E as a means of reducing free-radical damage to neurons posed by chemotherapies such as cisplatin. Indeed, pathologic features of cisplatin-damaged cells appeared similar to those damaged by vitamin E deficiency, both of which occur in the dorsal root ganglia.

This interest led to early but small clinical studies of vitamin E supplementation. Pace and others[72] assigned 47 patients receiving cisplatin to vitamin E (300 mg/day) before cisplatin and for 3 months after treatment, or to cisplatin alone. The incidence of neurotoxicity was significantly lower in the vitamin E group (30.7% vs. 85.7%; $P < .01$). Furthermore, the severity of neurotoxicity was significantly less. Limitations of this study included its small size: Only 27 patients were assessable for neurotoxicity. Also, the impact of vitamin E on treatment efficacy was not recorded.

This open-label study has prompted a larger, double-blind study by the same group.[73] As of their latest analysis, published in 2007, 81 patients receiving cisplatin chemotherapy were randomized in a double-blind fashion to vitamin E (400 mg/day) or placebo. Patients were followed by neurologic and neurophysiologic examinations during treatment. At interim analysis of 25 evaluable patients, a significant improvement in median neurotoxicity scores favoring the vitamin E group was noted.

Perhaps the largest study of vitamin E was that conducted by the North Central Cancer Treatment Group.[74] This was a phase III, double-blind, placebo-controlled study wherein patients were treated with vitamin E, 400 mg twice daily, or placebo. Eligible patients were those receiving adjuvant neurotoxic chemotherapy with curative intent. Head and neck cancer patients were excluded from this study. The primary endpoint was grade 2 or higher sensory neuropathy. Most patients received taxanes (109), but those receiving cisplatin (8), carboplatin (2), oxaliplatin (50), or combinations thereof (20) were also included. In total, 189 patients were evaluable. Disappointing findings revealed no difference in the incidence of grade 2+ neurotoxicity in the vitamin E group as opposed to the placebo group (34% vs. 29%; $P = .043$). Also, no differences in time to neuropathy onset, in the number of dose reductions or omissions due to neuropathy, or in overall patient-reported symptoms were noted.

Because this study included a minority of patients receiving platinum therapies, it is unclear whether vitamin E is simply ineffective, or if damage from taxanes in particular is not prevented by the vitamin. It is noteworthy that taxane-treated patients do not show the same dorsal root ganglia changes that platinum-treated patients experience. In this case, the number of platin-treated patients may not be large enough to make a judgment on this question.

A small, early study by Argyriou and others[75] evaluated vitamin E in patients receiving both taxanes and platins. This randomized but open-label study assessed the vitamin's effect on neurotoxicity. This study is notable in that 21 of 40 patients received paclitaxel. They were split 11/10 among the vitamin E and control groups; the remaining patients received cisplatin (15) or the combination (4). Less neuropathy was seen among patients on the vitamin E arm (25% vs. 73.3%; $P = .023$).

However, the authors do not give specific data on outcomes in taxane- and platin-treated patients. Thus, questions remain as to whether the vitamin has efficacy, and whether this role might be unique for platinum agents.

One of the controversies of vitamin E focuses on whether it has an impact on the efficacy of treatment. Animal studies had suggested that the drug does not interfere with anti-tumor efficacy in cell lines and mouse models.[76] However, a study of vitamin E[77] and β-carotene as a protectant suggested a detriment to local recurrence rates with the use of these vitamins. Patients receiving the combination had a hazard ratio of recurrence of 1.37, although this was not statistically significant (0.93–2.02). Quality of life was not improved by the supplementation. A second placebo-controlled study[78] evaluating a vitamin E mouthwash in preventing mucositis during radiation showed somewhat inferior survival rates for the treatment group; however, the difference was not statistically significant, and the treatment group had more stage III and IV patients than the placebo group.

Contradicting these studies, a study of chemotherapy with or without vitamin supplementation, including vitamin E, ascorbic acid, and β–carotene, found no difference in response rates.[79] Survival was not statistically different, but a trend favored the vitamin group. Given the small size of these studies and the discordant results, we feel that it is too early to draw conclusions on the role of vitamin E in treatment.

ANTIDEPRESSANTS AND ANTIEPILEPTICS

Interest in tricyclic antidepressants stems from their role in treating neuropathic pain associated with diabetes mellitus. Unfortunately, trials of amitriptyline[80] and nortriptyline[81] failed to demonstrate significant benefit. These trials were fairly small, with 44 and 51 patients, respectively, and revealed only modest changes in neuropathy.

Gabapentin and pregabalin are antiepileptics that have had some use in treating diabetic neuropathy. Thus, they have been considered worthy of testing in chemotherapy-induced peripheral neuropathy (CIPN). A randomized trial of 115 patients assigned to gabapentin or placebo failed to demonstrate any benefit associated with using this agent in the treatment of CIPN.[82] A nonrandomized trial of 23 patients receiving pregabalin showed improvement by one grade level in 8 patients.[83] These results await confirmation in a larger, randomized trial.

CONCLUSION

A significant number of chemotherapeutic agents are capable of causing peripheral neuropathy. These agents have different mechanisms of action, although the resulting neuropathy is often clinically similar. Therefore, it is conceivable that the different mechanisms of action of the various neurotoxic chemotherapy agents may confound clinical trials aimed at preventing the development of or reducing existing neuropathy. Future clinical trials may be more likely to succeed if they focus on specific chemotherapy agents. Furthermore, improving our ability to identify individuals at high risk of neuropathy may allow us to better target these patients for intervention, and to better select study candidates, thereby assisting in the development of preventive and therapeutic agents.

Of the clinical trials performed to date, the most compelling data are related to avoidance of neurotoxic agents when possible (e.g., Optimox-1 for colon cancer) and the use of calcium and magnesium in the specific case of oxaliplatin. Unfortunately, most other agents have failed to demonstrate a clear strategy for avoiding neuropathy. At the moment, antiepileptics represent the best available treatment for neuropathy, but further research is necessary before patients can be provided with neuroprotective agents that do not impair the antitumor efficacy of the causative agents.

REFERENCES

1. Wolf S, Barton D, Kottschade L, et al. Chemotherapy-induced peripheral neuropathy: prevention and treatment strategies. *Eur J Cancer.* 2008;44:1507–1515.
2. Quasthoff S, Hartung HP. Chemotherapy-induced peripheral neuropathy. *J Neurol.* 2002;249:9–17.
3. McWhinney SR, Goldberg RM, McLeod HL. Platinum neurotoxicity pharmacogenetics. *Mol Cancer Ther.* 2009;8:10–16.
4. Tfayli A, Hentschel P, Madajewicz S, et al. Toxicities related to intraarterial infusion of cisplatin and etoposide in patients with brain tumors. *J Neurooncol.* 1999;42:73–77.
5. Boogerd W, ten Bokkel Huinink WW, Dalesio O, et al. Cisplatin induced neuropathy: central, peripheral and autonomic nerve involvement. *J Neurooncol.* 1990;9:255–263.
6. Siegal T, Haim N. Cisplatin-induced peripheral neuropathy: frequent off-therapy deterioration, demyelinating syndromes, and muscle cramps. *Cancer.* 1990;66:1117–1123.
7. Nishimura T, Sanada J, Furukawa M. Cervical radiculopathy due to intra-arterial infusion of cisplatin. *J Laryngol Otol.* 2005;119:649–650.

8. Gregg RW, Molepo JM, Monpetit VJ, et al. Cisplatin neurotoxicity: the relationship between dosage, time, and platinum concentration in neurologic tissues, and morphologic evidence of toxicity. *J Clin Oncol.* 1992;10:795–803.
9. Walther PJ, Rossitch Jr E, Bullard DE. The development of Lhermitte's sign during cisplatin chemotherapy: possible drug-induced toxicity causing spinal cord demyelination. *Cancer.* 1987;60:2170–2172.
10. Watanabe W, Kuwabara R, Nakahara T, et al. Severe ocular and orbital toxicity after intracarotid injection of carboplatin for recurrent glioblastomas. *Graefes Arch Clin Exp Ophthalmol.* 2002;240:1033–1035.
11. Markman M, Kennedy A, Webster K, et al. Neurotoxicity associated with a regimen of carboplatin (AUC 5-6) and paclitaxel (175 mg/m2 over 3 h) employed in the treatment of gynecologic malignancies. *J Cancer Res Clin Oncol.* 2001;127:55–58.
12. de Gramont A, Figer A, Seymour M, et al. Leucovorin and fluorouracil with or without oxaliplatin as first-line treatment in

advanced colorectal cancer. *J Clin Oncol.* 2000;18:2938–2947.
13. Cassidy J, Misset JL. Oxaliplatin-related side effects: characteristics and management. *Semin Oncol.* 2002;29:11–20.
14. Bain PG, Lantos PL, Djurovic V, et al. Intrathecal vincristine: a fatal chemotherapeutic error with devastating central nervous system effects. *J Neurol.* 1991;238:230–234.
15. Whittaker JA, Parry DH, Bunch C, et al. Coma associated with vincristine therapy. *Br Med J.* 1973;4:335–337.
16. Verstappen CC, Koeppen S, Heimans JJ, et al. Dose-related vincristine-induced peripheral neuropathy with unexpected off-therapy worsening. *Neurology.* 2005;64:1076–1077.
17. Gonzalez Perez P, Serrano-Pozo A, Franco-Macias E, et al. Vincristine-induced acute neurotoxicity versus Guillain-Barre syndrome: a diagnostic dilemma. *Eur J Neurol.* 2007;14:826–828.
18. Kuruvilla G, Perry S, Wilson B, et al. The natural history of vincristine-induced laryngeal paralysis in children. *Arch Otolaryngol Head Neck Surg.* 2009;135:101–105.

19. Tarlaci S. Vincristine-induced fatal neuropathy in non-Hodgkin's lymphoma. *Neurotoxicology.* 2008;29:748–749.

20. Hohneker JA. A summary of vinorelbine (Navelbine) safety data from North American clinical trials. *Semin Oncol.* 1994;21:42–46; discussion 46–7.

21. Vats T, Buchanan G, Mehta P, et al. A study of toxicity and comparative therapeutic efficacy of vindesine-prednisone vs. vincristine-prednisone in children with acute lymphoblastic leukemia in relapse. A Pediatric Oncology Group study. *Invest New Drugs.* 1992;10:231–234.

22. Liu L, Shi B, Ye L, et al. Vindesine-induced neuropathy mimicking Guillain-Barre syndrome. *Leuk Res.* 2009;33:e232–e233.

23. Hawboldt J, Bader M. Intramuscular methotrexate-induced aseptic meningitis. *Ann Pharmacother.* 2007;41:1906–1911.

24. Teh HS, Fadilah SA, Leong CF. Transverse myelopathy following intrathecal administration of chemotherapy. *Singapore Med J.* 2007;48:e46–e49.

25. Jaffe N, Takaue Y, Anzai T, et al. Transient neurologic disturbances induced by high-dose methotrexate treatment. *Cancer.* 1985;56:1356–1360.

26. Koh S, Nelson Jr MD, Kovanlikaya A, et al. Anterior lumbosacral radiculopathy after intrathecal methotrexate treatment. *Pediatr Neurol.* 1999;21:576–578.

27. Pirzada NA, Ali II, Dafer RM. Fluorouracil-induced neurotoxicity. *Ann Pharmacother.* 2000;34:35–38.

28. Ruzzo A, Graziano F, Loupakis F, et al. Pharmacogenetic profiling in patients with advanced colorectal cancer treated with first-line FOLFOX-4 chemotherapy. *J Clin Oncol.* 2007;25:1247–1254.

29. van Laarhoven HW, Verstappen CC, Beex LV, et al. 5-FU-induced peripheral neuropathy: a rare complication of a well-known drug. *Anticancer Res.* 2003;23:647–648.

30. van den Berg H, van der Flier M, van de Wetering MD. Cytarabine-induced aseptic meningitis. *Leukemia.* 2001;15:697–699.

31. Herzig RH, Hines JD, Herzig GP, et al. Cerebellar toxicity with high-dose cytosine arabinoside. *J Clin Oncol.* 1987;5:927–932.

32. Openshaw H, Slatkin NE, Stein AS, et al. Acute polyneuropathy after high dose cytosine arabinoside in patients with leukemia. *Cancer.* 1996;78:1899–1905.

33. Anand U, Otto WR, Bountra C, et al. Cytosine arabinoside affects the heat and capsaicin receptor TRPV1 localisation and sensitivity in human sensory neurons. *J Neurooncol.* 2008;89:1–7.

34. Di Cataldo A, Astuto M, Rizzo G, et al. Neurotoxicity during ifosfamide treatment in children. *Med Sci Monit.* 2009;15:CS22–CS25.

35. Brunello A, Basso U, Rossi E, et al. Ifosfamide-related encephalopathy in elderly patients : report of five cases and review of the literature. *Drugs Aging.* 2007;24:967–973.

36. Nieto Y, Cagnoni PJ, Bearman SI, et al. Acute encephalopathy: a new toxicity associated with high-dose paclitaxel. *Clin Cancer Res.* 1999;5:501–506.

37. Postma TJ, Vermorken JB, Liefting AJ, et al. Paclitaxel-induced neuropathy. *Ann Oncol.* 1995;6:489–494.

38. Freilich RJ, Balmaceda C, Seidman AD, et al. Motor neuropathy due to docetaxel and paclitaxel. *Neurology.* 1996;47:115–118.

39. Chaudhry V, Rowinsky EK, Sartorius SE, et al. Peripheral neuropathy from taxol and cisplatin combination chemotherapy: clinical and electrophysiological studies. *Ann Neurol.* 1994;35:304–311.

40. Sahenk Z, Barohn R, New P, et al. Taxol neuropathy: electrodiagnostic and sural nerve biopsy findings. *Arch Neurol.* 1994;51:726–729.

41. Green MR, Manikhas GM, Orlov S, et al. Abraxane, a novel Cremophor-free, albumin-bound particle form of paclitaxel for the treatment of advanced non-small-cell lung cancer. *Ann Oncol.* 2006;17:1263–1268.

42. New PZ, Jackson CE, Rinaldi D, et al. Peripheral neuropathy secondary to docetaxel (Taxotere). *Neurology.* 1996;46:108–111.

43. van den Bent MJ, Hilkens PH, Sillevis Smitt PA, et al. Lhermitte's sign following chemotherapy with docetaxel. *Neurology.* 1998;50:563–564.

44. Mahaley Jr MS, Whaley RA, Blue M, et al. Central neurotoxicity following intracarotid BCNU chemotherapy for malignant gliomas. *J Neurooncol.* 1986;3:297–314.

45. Postma TJ, van Groeningen CJ, Witjes RJ, et al. Neurotoxicity of combination chemotherapy with procarbazine, CCNU and vincristine (PCV) for recurrent glioma. *J Neurooncol.* 1998;38:69–75.

46. Naumann R, Mohm J, Reuner U, et al. Early recognition of hereditary motor and sensory neuropathy type 1 can avoid life-threatening vincristine neurotoxicity. *Br J Haematol.* 2001;115:323–325.

47. Leonard GD, Wright MA, Quinn MG, et al. Survey of oxaliplatin-associated neurotoxicity using an interview-based questionnaire in patients with metastatic colorectal cancer. *BMC Cancer.* 2005;5:116.

48. Chaudhry V, Chaudhry M, Crawford TO, et al. Toxic neuropathy in patients with pre-existing neuropathy. *Neurology.* 2003;60:337–340.

49. Gamelin L, Capitain O, Morel A, et al. Predictive factors of oxaliplatin neurotoxicity: the involvement of the oxalate outcome pathway. *Clin Cancer Res.* 2007;13:6359–6368.

50. Chen YC, Tzeng CH, Chen PM, et al. Influence of GSTP1 I105V polymorphism on cumulative neuropathy and outcome of FOLFOX-4 treatment in Asian patients with colorectal carcinoma. *Cancer Sci.* 2010;101:530–535.

51. Lecomte T, Landi B, Beaune P, et al. Glutathione S-transferase P1 polymorphism (Ile105Val) predicts cumulative neuropathy in patients receiving oxaliplatin-based chemotherapy. *Clin Cancer Res.* 2006;12:3050–3056.

52. Ruzzo A, Graziano F, Loupakis F, et al. Pharmacogenetic profiling in patients with advanced colorectal cancer treated with first-line FOLFOX-4 chemotherapy. *J Clin Oncol.* 2007;25:1247–1254.

53. Argyriou AA, Antonacopoulou AG, Scopa CD, et al. Liability of the voltage-gated sodium channel gene SCN2A R19K polymorphism to oxaliplatin-induced peripheral neuropathy. *Oncology.* 2009;77:254–256.

54. Khrunin AV, Moisseev A, Gorbunova V, et al. Genetic polymorphisms and the efficacy and toxicity of cisplatin-based chemotherapy in ovarian cancer patients. *Pharmacogenomics.* 2010;10:54–61.

55. Sissung TM, Mross K, Steinberg SM, et al. Association of ABCB1 genotypes with paclitaxel-mediated peripheral neuropathy and neutropenia. *Eur J Cancer.* 2006;42:2893–2896.

56. Sissung TM, Baum CE, Deeken J, et al. ABCB1 genetic variation influences the toxicity and clinical outcome of patients with androgen-independent prostate cancer treated with docetaxel. *Clin Cancer Res.* 2008;14:4543–4549.

57. Mir O, Alexandre J, Tran A, et al. Relationship between GSTP1 ILE(105)Val polymorphism and docetaxel-induced peripheral neuropathy: clinical evidence of a role of oxidative stress in taxane toxicity. *Ann Oncol.* 2009;20:736–740.

58. Armstrong CM, Cota G. Calcium block of Na+ channels and its effect on closing rate. *Proc Natl Acad Sci U S A.* 1999;96:4154–4157.

59. Gamelin L, Boisdron-Celle M, Delva R, et al. Prevention of oxaliplatin-related neurotoxicity by calcium and magnesium infusions: a retrospective study of 161 patients receiving oxaliplatin combined with 5-fluorouracil and leucovorin for advanced colorectal cancer. *Clin Cancer Res.* 2004;10:4055–4061.

60. Nikcevich DA, Grothey A, Sloan JA, et al. Intravenous calcium and magnesium prevents oxaliplatin-induced sensory neurotoxicity in adjuvant colon cancer: results of a phase III placebo-controlled, double-blind trial (N04C7). *J Clin Oncol.* 2008;26:Abstr 4009.

61. Grothey A, Nikcevich DA, Sloan JA, et al. Evaluation of the effect of intravenous calcium and magnesium (CaMg) on chronic and acute neurotoxicity associated with oxaliplatin: results from a placebo-controlled phase III trial. *J Clin Oncol.* 2009;27:Abstr 4025.

62. Grothey A, Hart L, Rowland K, et al. Intermittent oxaliplatin administration improves time-to-treatment failure in metastatic colorectal cancer: final results of the phase III CONcePT trial. *J Clin Oncol.* 2008;26:Abstr 4010.

63. Tournigand C, Cervantes A, Figer A, et al. Optimox1: a randomized study of FOLFOX4 or FOLFOX7 with oxaliplatin in a stop-and-go fashion in advanced colorectal cancer—a GERCOR study. *J Clin Oncol.* 2006;24:137–400.

64. Hamers FP, Brakkee JH, Cavalletti E, et al. Reduced glutathione protects against cisplatin-induced neurotoxicity in rats. *Cancer Res.* 1993;53:544–549.

65. Smyth JF, Bowman A, Perren T, et al. Glutathione reduces the toxicity and improves quality of life of women diagnosed with ovarian cancer treated with cisplatin: results of a double-blind, randomized trial. *Ann Oncol.* 2007;8:569–573.

66. Cascinu S, Catalano V, Cordella L, et al. Neuroprotective effect of reduced glutathione on oxaliplatin-based chemotherapy in advanced colorectal cancer: a randomized, double-blind, placebo-controlled trial. *J Clin Oncol.* 2002;20:3478–3483.

67. Wang WS, Lin JK, Lin TC, et al. Oral glutamine is effective for preventing oxaliplatin-induced neuropathy in colorectal cancer patients. *Oncologist.* 2007;12:312–319.

68. Stubblefield MD, Vahdat LT, Balmaceda CM, et al. Glutamine as a neuroprotective agent in high-dose paclitaxel-induced peripheral neuropathy: a clinical and electrophysiologic study. *Clin Oncol (R Coll Radiol).* 2005;17:271–276.

69. Loven D, Levavi H, Sabach G, et al. Long-term glutamate supplementation failed to protect against peripheral neuropathy of paclitaxel. *Eur J Cancer Care.* 2009;18:78–83.

70. Park SA, Choi KS, Bang JH, et al. Cisplatin-induced apoptotic cell death in mouse hybrid neurons is blocked by antioxidants through suppression of cisplatin-mediated accumulation of p53 but not of Fas/Fas ligand. *J Neurochem.* 2000;75:946–953.

71. Lin PC, Lee MY, Wang WS, et al. N-acetylcysteine has neuroprotective effects against oxaliplatin-based adjuvant chemotherapy in colon cancer patients: preliminary data. *Support Care Cancer.* 2006;14:484–487.

72. Pace A, Savarese A, Picardo M, et al. Neuroprotective effect of vitamin E supplementation in patients treated with cisplatin chemotherapy. *J Clin Oncol.* 2003;21:927–931.

73. Pace A, Carpano S, Galie E, et al. Vitamin E in the neuroprotection of cisplatin induced peripheral neurotoxicity and ototoxicity. *J Clin Oncol.* 2007;25:Abstr 9114.

74. Kottschade LA. Oral presentation, ASCO Annual Meeting 2009, Orlando, Florida. *J Clin Oncol.* 2009;27:Abstr 9532.

75. Argyriou AA, Chroni E, Koutras A, et al. Vitamin E for prophylaxis against chemotherapy-induced neuropathy. *Neurology.* 2005;64:26–31.

76. Leonetti C, Biroccio A, Gabellini C, et al. α-Tocopherol protects against cisplatin-induced toxicity without interfering with antitumor efficacy. *Int J Cancer.* 2003;104:243–250.

77. Bairati I, Meyer F, Gelinas M, et al. Randomized trial of antioxidant vitamins to prevent acute adverse effects of radiation therapy in head and neck cancer patients. *J Clin Oncol.* 2005;23:5805–5813.

78. Ferreira PR, Fleck JF, Diehl A, et al. Protective effect of alpha-tocopherol in head and neck cancer radiation-induced mucositis: a double-blind randomized trial. *Head Neck.* 2004;26:313–321.

79. Pathak AK, Bhutani M, Guleria R, et al. Chemotherapy alone vs. chemotherapy plus high dose multiple antioxidants in patients with advanced non small cell lung cancer. *J Am Coll Nutr.* 2005;24:16–21.

80. Kautio AL, Haanpaa M, Saarto T, et al. Amitriptyline in the treatment of chemotherapy-induced neuropathic symptoms. *J Pain Symptom Manage.* 2008;35:31–39.

81. Hammack JE, Michalak JC, Loprinzi CL, et al. Phase III evaluation of nortriptyline for alleviation of symptoms of cisplatinum-induced peripheral neuropathy. *Pain.* 2002;98:195–203.

82. Rao RD, Michalak JC, Sloan JA, et al. Efficacy of gabapentin in the management of chemotherapy-induced peripheral neuropathy. *Cancer.* 2007;110:2110–2118.

83. Isufi I, James E, Keley K, et al. Pregabalin (PGB) in treatment of oxaliplatin-induced neuropathy. *J Clin Oncol.* 2009;27:AbstrE15045.

Management of cardiac and pulmonary treatment–related side effects

Joseph R. Carver

MANAGEMENT OF CARDIAC AND PULMONARY TREATMENT–RELATED SIDE EFFECTS

Significant advances have occurred in chemotherapy and radiation therapy over the past decades, leading to improved outcomes in patients with cancer. Cardiotoxicity (CT) and pulmonary toxicity (PT) are well known and potentially catastrophic complications of these therapies.

In this chapter, a broad overview of common treatment-related side effects will be described. For each subject, diagnostic and therapeutic recommendations will be presented. Toxicity that is rare and mild (<1% and grade I/II) or known because of isolated case reports will not be included.

INCIDENCE

The incidence of CT and PT continues to be controversial, with wide ranges in published numbers. Multiple factors confound our understanding of the true incidence; these are listed in Table 9-1. In the past, an attempt to standardize the reporting of drug adverse events was seen in the grading system proposed by the World Health Organization,[1] and the National Cancer Institute Common Terminology Criteria for Adverse Events were put forth to define symptomatic CT.[2] The latter document has been updated recently, and version 4.0 is now in the public domain.

SUPPORTIVE ONCOLOGY CARE

Care of the cancer patient in the 21st century is multidisciplinary, consisting of a diverse team of professionals that includes experts in cancer rehabilitation, cancer nutrition, and cancer psychosocial counseling. In addition to the traditional pharmacologic approach to the treatment of chemotherapy-induced CT and PT, the complimentary contribution of nonpharmacologic interventions (complementary and alternative medicine [CAM] or integrative medicine)

Table 9-1 Factors that influence the reported incidence of treatment-related cardiotoxicity and pulmonary toxicity

Definitions	Multiple grading systems
Reporting thresholds	Grade vs. % incidence, absolute vs. relative change in measured parameter
Patient characteristics	Demographic cutoff (age, sex), exclusions due to comorbidity
Treatment regimens	Initial treatment vs. retreatment, multiagent therapy, multimodality therapy

Table 9-2 Complementary and integrative interventions

Modality	Intervention
Physical therapy and cancer rehabilitation	Prevention /restoration of functional loss, strength training, endurance training
Nutritional counseling	Weight maintenance during treatment and weight loss after therapy. Specific diets: salt restriction, lipid lowering
Psychosocial counseling	Cognitive-behavioral therapy, pharmacologic interventions
Pain management	Acupuncture, nerve blocks, analgesic pharmacology
Nonpharmacologic interventions	Acupuncture, massage, exercise, meditation

will be highlighted when appropriate. Modalities and potential interventions are listed in Table 9-2.

CHEMOTHERAPY-RELATED CARDIOTOXICITY

Chemotherapy may affect the myocardium and may cause cardiomyopathy with or without overt heart failure (HF). Treatment may affect the vascular endothelium with resultant ischemia due to vasospasm or to direct coronary vessel injury; in other vascular beds, treatment may have profound effects on blood pressure, resulting in hypotension or hypertension. Treatment may lead to pericardial inflammation with acute pericarditis and/or tamponade, and in the long term the development of constrictive pericarditis. Treatment can cause virtually every known electrocardiographic abnormality and/or a full range of arrhythmias from asymptomatic single, isolated atrial/ventricular premature depolarizations to sustained tachycardia (reentrant supraventricular tachycardia, atrial fibrillation/flutter, or ventricular tachycardia), bradyarrhythmias (sinus or junctional bradycardia, all degrees of heart block, and QT prolongation), left ventricular and valvular dysfunction, and alterations of atherosclerotic risk factors. Table 9-3 offers an overview of chemotherapy-related CT by drug class.

Key point: CT may involve all parts of the heart from the pericardium to the endocardium.

HEART FAILURE

The anthracyclines (doxorubicin [Adriamycin], daunorubicin [Cerubidine], idarubicin[Zavedose], epirubicin [Ellence]) and mitoxantrone (Novantrone) have been the anchor drugs of cancer chemotherapy for longer than 60 years and continue to be critical components of the modern treatment of breast cancer and lymphomas (Table 9-4). CT associated with their use has been the most extensively studied nonhematologic complication of chemotherapy and is the most widely recognized cardiac complication of cancer therapy by clinicians. Anthracycline CT may present at three distinct times defined from the onset of treatment initiation.

Acute CT is a broadly defined syndrome that occurs during or immediately after treatment initiation. The manifestations can be electrophysiologic with transient electrocardiogram (ECG) changes (nonspecific ST and T wave changes, low voltage, QT prolongation), arrhythmias (sinus tachycardia, atrial/ventricular premature depolarizations or tachycardia, atrioventricular block), and overt myopericarditis.[3–5] Isolated cases of sudden death have been reported that may be due to sustained ventricular arrhythmias, hypersensitivity, or hypotension.[6,7] Preexisting ECG abnormalities do not influence the incidence or predict the occurrence of CT.[8]

This manifestation of CT is not dose related, and withdrawal of the anthracycline usually results in recovery. The development of acute CT does not increase the risk or affect the incidence of late CT. The mechanism is most likely due to drug-induced myocardial damage and/or an associated catecholamine or histamine surge.

Key point: Most instances of acute anthracycline cardiotoxicity consist of minor electrocardiographic changes.

Subacute CT presents in the first year in approximately 3% of patients. *Late CT* occurs after the first year. Both have been characterized by various degrees of HF historically defined by a symptomatic decrease in left ventricular ejection fraction (LVEF). It has become increasingly clear that this decrease in systolic function may be preceded by a decrease in diastolic function[9] and/or may exist without clinical manifestations (i.e., an asymptomatic latent period). Late CT can occur decades after treatment completion. Several factors increase the risk and include extremes of age (young and elderly), female sex, cumulative anthracycline dose, mediastinal radiation, and preexisting cardiovascular disease and risk factors. The clinical presentation is indistinguishable from other types of nonischemic cardiomyopathy.

The classic relationship for the risk of developing CT was described by Von Hoff, who showed an association with the total cumulative dose of anthracycline.[10] We have subsequently learned that the "real-world" risk, although generally proportional to the total accumulated dose, actually can occur in a less linear fashion and may be more time dependent.[11] It is increasingly recognized that asymptomatic abnormalities in noninvasive studies can be found in greater frequency and at a lower cumulative anthracycline dose than was previously reported.[12] A case for ongoing monitoring and for the need for a systematic study of late survivors has been made.[13,14]

Key point: Late asymptomatic cardiomyopathy can have a latent period of up to 30 years from treatment completion and may occur at any anthracycline dose, so there probably is no safe dose of medication that is 100% protective.

Table 9-3 Summary of chemotherapeutic toxicity

Chemotherapeutic agent by class	Cardiac toxicity
Anthracyclines	
Doxorubicin Mitoxantrone Daunorubicin Idarubicin Epirubicin Liposomal preparations	Acute CT: arrhythmias, myocarditis, pericarditis, sudden cardiac death Subacute and late CT: asymptomatic and symptomatic reductions in LVEF
Monoclonal antibodies	
Rituximab	Infusion-related hypotension, atrial and ventricular arrhythmias, heart block, chest pain, and acute myocardial infarction
Cetuximab	Possible hypomagnesemia-induced arrhythmia, atrial fibrillation
Alemtuzumab	First dose infusion-related hypotension
Trastuzumab	Asymptomatic and symptomatic decrease in LVEF
Lapatinib	Asymptomatic decrease in LVEF
Bevacizumab	Hypertension, venous and arterial thromboembolism
Antimetabolites	
Gemcitabine	Rare radiation recall
Cytarabine	Pericarditis, asymptomatic bradycardia
Fluorouracil	Chest pain with or without ST segment elevation, arrhythmia, heart failure, sudden cardiac death
Capecitabine	Chest pain due to coronary vasospasm with ST elevations ± arrhythmias ± HF
Histone deacetylase (HDAC) inhibitors	QT prolongation, supraventricular and ventricular premature depolarizations, supraventricular and ventricular tachycardia, decreased LVEF, sudden death
Alkylating agents	
Cyclophosphamide (high doses)	Myopericarditis
Ifosfamide (high doses)	Asymptomatic decrease in LVEF, myopericarditis
Microtubule-targeting agents	
Vinca alkaloids	Myocardial infarction or ischemia
Vinflunine	Angina
Taxanes	
Paclitaxel	Asymptomatic sinus bradycardia, premature ventricular depolarizations, ventricular tachycardia, and atrioventricular block
Docetaxel	None
Epilithones	
Ixabepilone	Symptomatic palpitation, atrial flutter, myocardial infarction

Chemotherapeutic agent by class	Cardiac toxicity
Immunomodulating agents	
Thalidomide	Venous thromboembolism, sinus bradycardia
Lenalidomide	Venous thromboembolism
Pomalidomide	Venous thromboembolism
Tyrosine kinase inhibitors (TKIs)	
Imatinib	Heart failure in patients with risk factors or preexisting CV disease
Sunitinib	Hypertension, myocardial infarction, heart failure, cardiovascular death
Sorafenib	Hypertension
Epidermal growth factor TKI	
Erlotinib	None reported
Gefitinib	None reported
Retinoids	
Bexarotene	Hypertriglyceridemia, hypercholesterolemia
Proteasome inhibitors	
Bortezomib	Heart failure, QT prolongation, angina, atrioventricular block, atrial fibrillation
Platinum agents	
Cisplatin	Acute: small- and large-vessel vasospasm Long-term: hypercholesterolemia, hypertension, increased incidence of CV events
Oxaliplatin	Chest pain
Folate antagonists	
Methotrexate	Sinus bradycardia, ventricular tachycardia, chest pain
Pemtrexed	None reported
Cytokines	
Interferon	Arrhythmia, dilated cardiomyopathy, myocardial ischemia, myocardial infarction
Interleukins	Infusion-related hypotension, myocardial ischemia, arrhythmias
Radioimmunotherapy	
Tositumomab	None reported
Ibritumomab tiuxetan	Hypertension
Gemtuzumab ozogamicin	Nonspecific arrhythmias, hypotension, hypertension
Arsenic trioxide	QT prolongation, atrioventricular block
Tamoxifen	Stroke, venous thromboembolism

CT, Cardiotoxicity; *CV,* cardiovascular; *HF,* heart failure; *LVEF,* left ventricular ejection fraction; *TKI,* tyrosine kinase inhibitor.

Table 9-4 Nonanthracycline chemotherapy drugs associated with heart failure

Drug	Dose relationship	Incidence	Reversibility
Cyclophosphamide	Yes	7%–28%	Yes
Trastuzumab	No	<16% asymptomatic <4% symptomatic	Yes
Lapatinib	No	<1%	Yes
TKIs			
Imatinib Sorafenib Sunitinib	No	1%–10%	Yes
Bevicizumab	?	1%–3%	Yes

Although less studied than doxorubicin, the incidence of CT with daunorubicin, idarubicin, mitoxantrone, and epirubicin (a semisynthetic derivative) is similar with equivalent dosing regimens.[15]

In an effort to preserve or increase antitumor efficacy while reducing CT, pegylation or liposomal encapsulation of anthracyclines was developed. It appears that encapsulated doxorubicin/daunorubicin (Doxil or Caelix, Lipodox, DaunoXome) probably has a decreased incidence of CT compared with conventional anthracycline administration.[16,17]

Key point: Liposomal anthracyclines have a lower risk of CT, but their use is limited by their increased cost and limited evidence base.

The human epidermal growth factor receptor 2 (HER2) is a transmembrane tyrosine kinase receptor that is involved in many cellular processes, including regulation of cell growth and cellular survival in normal healthy tissue. In 20% to 25% of new cases of breast cancer, the *HER2* gene is amplified or the HER2 protein is overexpressed, and these patients have a relatively poor prognosis.[18]

Trastuzumab (Herceptin) is a humanized monoclonal antibody designed to target HER2 on the surface of HER2-overexpressing tumor cells. Trastuzumab is approved for the treatment of HER2-positive breast cancer in both metastatic and adjuvant settings. Trastuzumab is generally well tolerated and is not associated with the side effects common to cytotoxic chemotherapy, but it has been associated with an increased incidence of CT. This can manifest as an asymptomatic decline in LVEF (1%–28%) or as symptomatic HF that occurs less frequently (0.9%–3.2%). Unlike CT associated with the anthracyclines, in most patients, cardiac dysfunction is reversible without direct myocardial damage with the potential for posttreatment recovery of cardiac function.

Consistently identified risk factors for development of CT are related to the age of the patient (elderly), pretreatment with anthracyclines, a lower pretreatment LVEF, and possibly the co-association of hypertension.[19–35] Although less intensely studied, it appears that the potential for CT with lapatinib, a dual kinase antagonist, is less than with trastuzumab and is probably no more than 1%.[36,37]

Key point: The incidence of reversible asymptomatic and symptomatic cardiomyopathy with trastuzumab use is <16% and <4%, respectively, and <1% with lapatinib.

CYCLOPHOSPHAMIDE

CT has been associated with high-dose chemotherapy (120–180 mg/kg/day over a standard 7-day delivery regimen) with an incidence of 22% and a fatality rate of 11%. Gottdiener and colleagues[38] described their experience in 32 patients with hematologic malignancies treated with 180 mg/kg/day for 4 days and reported a 28% incidence of HF and a 33% incidence of pericardial effusion. In their series, six patients (19%) died and six patients (19%) had pericardial tamponade.

More recently, with the advent of multifractionated schedules of administration, the incidence of overt HF has declined, and subclinical myocardial dysfunction has been recognized. Zver and his group studied 23 consecutive patients with multiple myeloma and found evidence of consistent neurohormonal activation with elevation of biomarker levels after treatment compared to baseline, with echocardiographic evidence of diastolic dysfunction.[39]

Unlike the chronic CT associated with anthracyclines that is related to cumulative dosing, the CT associated with cyclophosphamide is related to the magnitude of single dosing, is more often reversible without permanent structural myocardial damage, and lacks the latency for development, with all cases occurring within a week to 10 days of treatment.

Key point: The cardiotoxicity of cyclophosphamide is not related to cumulative dose.

IFOSFAMIDE

Ifosfamide (Mitoxana) is an oxazaphosphorine nitrogen mustard compound that is structurally similar to cyclophosphamide, with indications and side effects that are virtually identical.[40]

IMATINIB

Imatinib mesylate (Gleevec) is a tyrosine kinase inhibitor (TKI) that targets BCR-ABL, platelet-derived growth factor receptor, and stem cell receptor *c*-Kit. Imatinib is used for the treatment of chronic myeloid leukemia, Philadelphia chromosome–positive acute lymphoblastic leukemia, gastrointestinal stromal tumor (GIST), and other diseases.

Fluid retention and edema occur in up to 66% of patients (4%–5% grade 3–4) and dyspnea in up to 16% of patients (4%–5% grade 3–4).[41]

In patients with risk factors and/or preexisting cardiovascular (CV) disease, the incidence of CT manifested by HF with imatinib is in the range of 1% to 2%.[41–46] Noncardiac edema is common, and asymptomatic increases in biomarker levels with unknown clinical significance may be detected. In most reported studies, rechallenge with a lower dose of imatanib has been tolerated after resolution of acute HF.

Key point: Imatinib use is associated with edema and fluid retention and a low incidence of HF.

TRANSMEMBRANE RECEPTOR INHIBITORS: SMALL MOLECULE EPIDERMAL GROWTH FACTOR RECEPTOR (EGFR)/TYROSINE KINASE INHIBITOR (TKI)

Transmembrane receptors are involved in a complex set of essential biological processes. Dysregulation is associated with altered tumor development, growth, metastasis, and survival. Inhibition of tumor-specific receptors produces antitumor effects.

Sunitinib

Sunitinib maleate (Sutent) is a multitarget receptor TKI with activity against vascular endothelial growth factor (VEGF) receptors 1 through 3, platelet-derived growth factor receptors α and β, c-KIT, FLT3 kinase, colony-stimulating factor 1 receptor, and RET kinase.[47] Sunitinib is approved for the treatment of advanced renal cell carcinoma (RCC) and imatinib-resistant GISTs, or in patients with GISTs who do not tolerate imatinib.

The first indication of LV dysfunction and HF was seen when sunitinib was compared with interferon in patients with metastatic RCC. Sunitinib was associated with decreases in LVEF that were uniformly twice as frequent as with interferon.[48]

The incidence of myocardial infarction (MI), HF, or cardiovascular death has been observed to be as high as 11% in sunitinib-treated patients with imatinib-resistant GIST.[48,49]

In a recent study by Telli and associates, in a more "real-world" population of patients, 15% of patients developed symptomatic decreases in LVEF,[50] while a retrospective review from M.D. Anderson showed a 2.7% (6/224) incidence of grade 3–4 CT in a population with underlying hypertension and a mean age of 65 years.[51]

The cause of CT is not fully understood. An animal model suggested a potential correlation between mitochondrial dysfunction, cardiomyocyte apoptosis, and underlying hypertension.[52]

Sorafenib

Sorafenib (Nexavar) is another oral multikinase inhibitor (Raf-1, A-Raf, and B-Raf), as are VEGF receptor (VEGFR)2/3, FLT3, c-Kit, and platelet-derived growth factor receptors (PDGFRs). Sorafenib is approved for the treatment of metastatic RCC as a second-line agent and for hepatocellular carcinomas.[53]

In summary, both sunitinib and sorafenib are associated with varying degrees of LV dysfunction. The reported incidence is blurred by varying definitions of CT, the lack of distinction in most studies between asymptomatic decreases in LVEF and overt HF, and the high incidence at baseline of cardiac risk factors and underlying cardiovascular disease in treated patients. Similar to CT defined by trastuzumab, it appears that CT associated with sunitinib and sorafenib is not associated with permanent myocardial damage and is largely reversible when the offending drugs are discontinued. Rechallenge with lower doses of medication has been successful in treatment continuation.

Key point: Sunitinib and sorafenib are associated with hypertension and a reversible cardiomyopathy

DIAGNOSIS

Detection of CT requires a defined monitoring scheme that begins with baseline pretreatment assessment, follows treatment serially, and continues for some time post treatment completion. On the basis of risk factors, multiple strategies have been proposed for the early detection of chemotherapy-related cardiomyopathy.

These include serial endocardial biopsy, exercise testing, serial biomarker measurements (B-type natriuretic peptide [BNP] and troponin), and serial measurements of LVEF by radionucleotide multigated acquisition (MUGA) scan or echocardiogram.[54] Currently, none of these strategies has reached guideline status.

Echocardiography is the most widely used noninvasive tool to evaluate cardiac function. Routine studies include measurements of chamber size, pericardial integrity and function, and associated valvular disease. The echocardiogram is particularly sensitive for measuring diastolic function, and the addition of tissue Doppler studies provides more accurate evaluation of diastolic function; measurement of regional myocardial wall motion velocity may be important in the early detection of local abnormalities before global function change is apparent.[55,56]

With recognition and acceptance that HF can occur with a normal LVEF (i.e., diastolic HF), coupled with the fact that a decrease in the LVEF represents more advanced disease, often with irreversible structural changes, there is a renewed interest in biomarkers with indications that an increase in troponin after chemotherapy is a strong predictor of CT; the highest risk is observed in patients with a >1 month elevation.[57,58] An increased risk of HF has been reported with measurement of serial BNP levels.[59]

Key point: Regardless of the test used, serial studies should be done with the same testing modality at the same institution to avoid intertest and interfacility nonclinical variation.

TREATMENT

Currently, no guidelines are specifically related to the treatment of chemotherapy-induced HF. Because the clinical manifestations and behavior are similar to those of other forms of dilated cardiomyopathy, it is logical that the guidelines published for those cardiomyopathies should be applicable to the management of this patient population.[60] Similar to most forms of cardiomyopathy, treatment is palliative and is rarely curative.

Treatment starts by withdrawal of the offending chemotherapeutic agent, along with patient and family education about the disease and the effects of diet on its natural history (salt and fluid restriction, achieving ideal weight, alcohol use); it includes risk factor modification (treatment of hypertension, lipid level reduction, smoking cessation, alcohol abstinence or moderation). Pharmacologic interventions begin with initiation of an angiotensin-converting enzyme (ACE) inhibitor[61] or an angiotensin II receptor blocker (ARB)[62] or a beta blocker (BB)[63,64] as initial therapy with slow titration to achieve maximally tolerated doses of an ACE/ARB and a BB. Exclusion of an ischemic cause of cardiomyopathy should be part of the assessment, especially in patients with risk factors and/or who present at an age when ischemic heart disease becomes prevalent. Loop diuretics should be reserved and used only when fluid overload is evident.

The addition of digoxin or spironolactone[65] and the use of implantable devices (biventricular pacemaker, implantable cardioverter defibrillator [ICD]) should be considered after titration of medical treatment in patients with more advanced disease. Use of a nitrate/hydralazine combination has been effective in the African American population with heart failure,[66] and when renal function precludes the use of an ACE/ARB.

Because the HF associated with trastuzumab does not produce structural changes in the myocardium and may be reversible, initial management of this condition consists of the removal of trastuzumab from therapy. In many cases, the drug can be reintroduced with or without standard HF therapies, driven by the oncologic need for that medication.[67] When trastuzumab-induced HF occurs in patients who previously were treated with anthracyclines, lifelong treatment with HF medication may be indicated, because withdrawal in these patients has resulted in HF-related morbidity and mortality.[68]

Key point: Treatment of chemotherapy-induced heart failure after withdrawal of the offending medication is similar to standard treatment of dilated cardiomyopathy.

PREVENTION

Attempts to prevent the myocardial toxicity of chemotherapeutic agents focused on drug formulation and delivery and chemoprotective agents.

Semisynthetic formulations of the anthracyclines (e.g., epirubicin) promised to maintain efficacy with reduced CT. As was noted earlier, in equivalent doses for efficacy, CT remains virtually identical to the original preparations. Liposomal pegylation may offer reduced CT in exchange for increased acquisition costs of the medication.[69] Varying the administration duration from bolus to prolonged infusion has had limited acceptance and has not been widely adopted.[70] More toxic sequencing schedules (e.g., concurrent taxane and anthracycline combination with myocardial toxicity up to 27%) have been abandoned for sequential delivery with reduced toxicity.[71]

Chemoprotective agents have also been controversial. Dexrazoxane, an iron chelator, was originally reported as the first drug to reduce CT from anthracyclines.[72] Subsequently, reports of decreased chemotherapeutic efficacy tempered its use, and currently, it is recommended only for high-risk patients who have received a cumulative dose of more than 300 mg/m^2 of doxorubicin.[73]

Recently, the use of standard heart failure therapy in a chemopreventive mode has been reported in a number of small adult patient populations. These include valsartan, an ARB[74]; carvedilol, a BB[75]; and enalapril, an ACE.[76]

In summary, general recommendations to minimize the myocardial CT of chemotherapy are presented in Table 9-5.

SUPPORTIVE ONCOLOGY

Depression has a major impact on HF, and awareness of the high incidence of this coexistent disorder is important, along with an approach to provide psychosocial support.

Patients with heart failure receive an average of 6.8 medications per day; this presents logistical, drug-interaction, financial, and potential side-effect ramifications. In the current economic climate, an awareness of cost considerations is important in initial prescribing and follow-up of maintenance therapy.

Table 9-5 Minimizing chemotherapy/radiation-induced cardiotoxicity

Baseline assessment and individualization of therapy
- Provide appropriate treatment of hypertension.
- Diagnose and treat correctable disease (e.g., CAD, anemia, tachycardia).
- Follow published guidelines for cardiac risk reduction.

Modification of chemotherapy regimen based on cardiovascular risk
- Use nonanthracycline regimen in high-risk patient.
- Use cardioprotective drugs: **dexrazoxane**, ACE inhibitors/ARBs + beta blocker.

Modification of monitoring
- Total awareness of cumulative drug and radiation dosing
- Cardiology input and comanagement
- Biomarkers with each dose
- More frequent assessment of LVEF
- Long-term follow-up and treatment of asymptomatic decreases in LVEF

ACE, Angiotensin-converting enzyme; *ARBs,* angiotensin II receptor blocker; *CAD,* coronary artery disease; *LVEF,* left ventricular ejection fraction.

Heart failure disease management programs have been successful in reducing hospitalizations and providing proactive care.

Family education and support to maintain dietary and medication compliance is essential in successfully treating the patient with heart failure.

Key point: Management of patients with HF requires a team approach.

ISCHEMIA AND CHEST PAIN

Chest pain in patients with cancer undergoing chemotherapy may be due to a variety of causes. These include local effects of the tumor, referred pain from the gastrointestinal (GI) tract or musculoskeletal system, associated pleuritis, and associated pericarditis or coronary ischemia. The latter may be caused by increased demand (immunomodulating medicine medications, interleukin interferon) or may result from hypersensitivity or coronary vasospasm.

FLUOROURACIL (5-FU)

Fluorouracil (5-FU; Efudex) has been used for longer than five decades as first-line therapy for GI cancer, head and neck cancers, and breast cancer.

CT has been manifested by chest pain without ECG changes, ST changes without chest pain and with ST elevation suggestive of acute ST segment elevation myocardial infarction (STEMI), arrhythmias, HF, and sudden death. Coronary vasospasm has been implicated in the pathophysiology of ischemia. In the literature, the incidence of chest pain ranges from less than 1% to 1.8%, with an associated mortality rate of 2.2% to 13%.[77,78]

CT manifested by acute nonischemic HF has been described by case report with an incidence of less than 1%. In one case, myocardial biopsy showed proliferation of the sarcoplasmic reticulum with marked vacuolization.[79,80]

A large body of literature attempts to predict 5-FU CT. This includes patient profiles (hereditary dihydropyrimidine dehydrogenase [DPD] deficiency, underlying ischemia, older age, female sex, elevated creatinine) and delivery method (infusion, bolus vs. continuous, cycle >1) and screening studies (for single-nucleotide polymorphisms [SNPs], DPD deficiency, and individual response to the drug by giving test doses, measuring blood levels).[81] Currently, no reliable markers for predicting 5-FU toxicity have been validated to permit their use as a standard of care. CT is not satisfactorily explained by age, sex, hepatic or renal function, method of administration, comorbidity, or comedication.[82]

Key point: Chest pain with and without electrocardiographic changes occurs in 1% to 2% of patients treated with fluorouracil.

CAPECITABINE

Capecitabine (Xeloda), an oral fluoropyrimidine, is a 5-FU prodrug drug used in the treatment of female breast cancer and colorectal cancer (CRC). Capecitabine is metabolized to 5-FU via a complex enzymatic pathway. More than 50 case reports to date have described capecitabine-induced chest pain. The most frequent description implicates coronary spasm suggested by ST segment elevation with or without arrhythmias,[83] global left ventricular dysfunction, or overt HF.[84,85]

A meta-analysis of 53 patients from the literature found 38 (71%) cases with angina, 6 (11.3%) with arrhythmias, and 6 (11.3%) with myocardial infarction. Rechallenge in 16 patients led to symptoms in 10.[86]

Typically, ECG changes and symptoms are transient and respond to drug withdrawal, nitrates, and/or calcium channel blockers. Coronary arteriography[87] or CT angiography[88] has typically demonstrated no obstructive epicardial lesions in the coronary arteries.

Chest pain without ECG changes has been infrequently seen to occur at rest or with activity only during treatment weeks and responds to cessation of therapy or the addition of oral calcium channel blockers.[89]

Key point: The spectrum and incidence of chest pain with and without electrocardiographic changes associated with capecitabine are similar to fluorouracil.

VINCA ALKALOIDS

The vinca alkaloids are microtubule-targeting drugs derived from the pink periwinkle plant; they are part of the backbone of regimens for hematologic and solid malignancies. Four drugs in this class vary by minor structural differences with different spectrums of clinical efficacy: vincristine (Oncovin), vinblastine (Velban), vindesine (Eldisine), and the semisynthetic vinorelbine (Navelbine).

The most commonly reported CT is the development of myocardial ischemia and infarction. The mechanism for CT is speculative and includes drug-induced vasoconstriction and hypertension, a direct effect on cellular microtubules with impairment of myocardial metabolism, and coronary spasm.[90–92]

Key point: Chest pain occurs in approximately 1.5% of patients receiving vinca alkaloids.

CISPLATIN

Heightened vascular reactivity and/or arterial thrombosis have been described with short-term administration of cisplatin. When the coronary arteries are the "target," manifestations may include angina, acute coronary syndrome (ACS), or MI.[93] A 1% incidence of chest pain is reported in the approval summary for oxaliplatin.[94]

Mechanisms postulated include direct endothelial damage leading to vasospasm, increased thrombogenicity with increased platelet aggregation, an increase in von Willebrand factor (vWF), and hypomagnesemia.[95] A higher incidence may be seen in patients with preexisting high levels of vWF.[96] The incidence of arterial thrombosis may be 1% to 3%, and venous thromboembolism as high as 10% to 15%, when cisplatin is combined with a vinca alkaloid and bleomycin.[97]

Key point: Short-term cardiotoxicity of platinum-containing chemotherapy consists of small and large vessel arterial spasm with a 1% incidence of chest pain.

SYSTEMIC FIRST DOSE INFUSION REACTIONS
Cytokines

Cytokines are signaling polypeptides that are critical for the immune response. They have anticancer effects when used alone or in combination chemotherapy.

Interferons

The interferons are a family of glycoproteins that include interferon-alpha (from leukocytes), --beta (from fibroblasts), and -gamma (from T lymphocytes). Interferon was the first cytokine to show activity in patients with metastatic RCC. All three interferons cause a flu-like syndrome whose hemodynamic burden may increase the myocardial oxygen demand beyond the limits of coronary blood flow and/or ventricular function in patients with underlying cardiac disease. Sonnenblick and Rosin reviewed the literature and found 15 reports on 44 patients with interferon-induced CT. In their review, CT was not related to type of interferon nor to the daily or cumulative dose. CT was manifested by arrhythmia, dilated cardiomyopathy, and ischemia, including MI.[98] Because of the relationship to febrile illness, symptoms usually occur within the first 2 to 8 hours of treatment.

With modern awareness of the potential for CT and with the major risk factor being underlying cardiac disease, screening, especially for coronary artery disease, is the standard before interferon use. Patients with unrevascularized coronary artery disease virtually never receive this drug; therefore the currently reported incidence of CT is extremely low, and it occurs in patients with pretreatment unrecognized cardiac disease.

Interleukin

Since the 1980s, interlukin-2 has been utilized as a cancer therapy, with improved survival in RCC and metastatic melanoma. It is a glycoprotein produced by activated lymphocytes that induces T-cell proliferation. Toxicity is secondary to a capillary leak syndrome with resultant tachycardia, decreased peripheral vascular resistance (PVR), hypotension, and increased cardiac output—a picture similar to septic shock that is probably related to the release of tumor necrosis factor. Early studies

QE Hospital Library
Tel: 0121 371 2485

Items that you have returned

Title: Oncology.
ID: UH00003098

Title: Understanding prostate disorders :
ID: UH00003380

Title: Washington and Leaver's
principles and practice of radiation
therapy
ID: UH00010660

Total items: 3
15/02/2021 14:21

You should retain this receipt

Email: qelibrary@uhb.nhs.uk

showed grade 3–4 CT that included a 3% incidence of ischemia and an 81% incidence of hypotension. The decrease in PVR may last for days following infusion. Postulates regarding mechanisms include direct CT and demand ischemia.[99,100]

Key point: Cytokines (interferons and interleukins) cause a febrile reaction that increases cardiac demand and may lead to ischemia and/or ventricular dysfunction in susceptible patients.

Monoclonal antibodies

The monoclonal antibodies rituximab, cetuximab and alemtuzumab are all associated with first dose reactions that increase myocardial demand and may precipitate chest pain in patients with underlying coronary artery disease (CAD).

Rituxumab infusion is associated with some combination of fever, chills, nausea, vomiting, urticaria, hypotension, and bronchospasm in more than 80% of patients. This occurs most often during the first treatment and is a result of cytokine release. Symptoms can be attenuated by preparatory regimens and adjustment of the infusion rate. Moderate to severe reactions occur in about 15% of patients.[101,102]

The incidence of first dose infusion–related hypotension is real, and isolated cases of non–life-threatening arrhythmias, cardiac ischemia, and reversible LV dysfunction may occur in patients with underlying cardiovascular disease.

DIAGNOSIS

Diagnosis is based on clinical suspicion coupled with a detailed history and review of the electrocardiogram, especially when recorded during symptoms combined with serial monitoring of appropriate biomarkers (troponins and creatine phosphokinase [CPK]). A role for echocardiography is likely in defining the extent of ischemia and/or infarction and its effect on left ventricular and valvular function.

Noninvasive stress testing to exclude underlying CAD is appropriate in the stable patient, and results of that study dictate the need for coronary angiography.

TREATMENT

Treatment is based on making a correct diagnosis. Patients may present with an acute syndrome or subacutely with typical chest pain unassociated with hemodynamic sequelae.

For patients who present with typical exertional angina without ECG changes or elevation of biomarkers, the offending drug should be withheld and treatment instituted for CAD according to the current American Heart Association (AHA)/American College of Cardiology (ACC) guidelines for angina.[103] For patients with ECG changes and/or elevation of biomarkers, treatment should proceed according to the AHA/ACC guidelines for ACS/non–ST segment MI (NSTEMI)[104] and STEMI or myocardial infarction.[105] Medical therapy includes beta blockers and ACE inhibitors with reduction of all cardiac risk factors to normalize blood pressure, as well as aggressive treatment of lipids. Once stabilized, the decision to continue with the culprit drug is based on the oncologic benefit of treatment. For drugs that induce ischemia via vasospasm, first-line treatment includes calcium blockers and nitrates. We have been able to restart or continue the continuous infusion of 5-FU and oral capecitabine when oncologically indicated.

At some point after stabilization, we exclude the presence of major obstructive coronary disease with stress testing. If nuclear perfusion is normal, we ascribe the symptoms to the culprit drug, and when abnormal, we have proceeded with coronary arteriography to define the coronary anatomy and to attempt percutaneous revascularization.

Acute coronary syndromes are managed according to current AHA/ACC treatment guidelines, which include prompt pain relief, hemodynamic stabilization, antiplatelet agents, and selective coronary arteriography.

For patients who develop chest pain without evidence of myocardial infarction and who are taking oral capecitabine or continuous infusion of 5-FU, the first step is initiation of medical therapy and stabilization. Rechallenge with the offending drug at the same or a lower dose may be successful. Recurrence of chest pain after rechallenge is a signal for drug discontinuation.[106]

SUPPORTIVE ONCOLOGY

A proactive approach to these patients is important. When drugs that can cause first dose systemic reactions and/or known coronary vasospasm are contemplated, it is beneficial to have a pretreatment evaluation by a cardiologist who is familiar with these drugs to assess the risk of CT, to develop a plan for pretreatment testing and monitoring during therapy, and to initiate therapy to minimize risk.

HYPERTENSION

Hypertension is one of the most frequent comorbid conditions in patients with cancer[107] and is a major side effect of several of the new chemotherapeutic agents.

BEVACIZUMAB

Bevacizumab (Avastin) is a recombinant humanized monoclonal antibody with activity against vascular endothelial growth factor (VEGF) that disrupts tumor angiogenesis. It has been studied in various malignancies, including CRC, non–small cell lung carcinoma (NSCLC), RCC, and breast cancer, when used alone or as part of combination chemotherapy.

Because of the physiologic role of VEGF in regulating arterial tone and promoting vasodilatation, it is not surprising that the most common adverse effect of bevacizumab therapy is hypertension, which has been recognized consistently from the first phase I trial.[108] Hypertension may be newly diagnosed, or existing hypertension may be exacerbated.

The publication from the pivotal phase III trial of bevacizumab, fluorouracil, and leucovorin in metastatic CRC reported a 22.4% incidence of any grade of hypertension in the bevacizumab treatment arm, of which 11% of patients had grade 3 hypertension.[109]

Bevacizumab-induced hypertension is reversible, may occur early or late in treatment, and may be dose related. In a meta-analysis of 1850 patients in 10 trials treated with bevacizumab, the incidence of hypertension ranged between 2.7% and 32% and between 17.6% and 36% in low- and high-dose treatment.[110]

Overall, the incidence of hypertension may be >60% and grade 3–4 hypertension has been reported in 8% to 19% with initial or subsequent doses.[111]

Key point: Bevacizumab causes dose-related hypertension.

TRANSMEMBRANE RECEPTOR INHIBITORS: SMALL MOLECULE EGFR/ TYROSINE KINASE INHIBITORS

Sunitinib

Hypertension (defined as ≥150/100 mmHg) is the most common manifestation of CT, with an incidence of 30% according to the package insert.[112]

Sorafenib

Similar to other VEGFR inhibitors, hypertension is the most frequent treatment-related serious adverse effect.

In a meta-analysis of nine studies that included 4599 patients with various solid tumors, the overall incidence of hypertension was 23.4% (95% confidence interval [CI], 16.0%–32.9%), and grade 3–4 incidence was 5.7% (95% CI, 2.5%–12.6%).[113]

An observational study of sorafenib and sunitinib reported the incidence of cardiac events to be higher than reported in clinical trials. Use of TKIs led to mild asymptomatic to severe symptomatic cardiac events in 33.8% of patients, and the incidence may be higher in sunitinib- than in sorafenib-treated patients (5% vs. 14%).[114]

In summary, both sunitinib and sorafenib are associated with CT manifested by hypertension.

Key point: Sunitinib and sorafinib are associated with hypertension.

DIAGNOSIS

Diagnosis is based on three factors. The first occurs in the pretreatment evaluation and recognition of preexisting hypertension. The second involves recognition of potential hypertension associated with the contemplated regimen. The third is actual measurement of blood pressure regularly during treatment.

Hypertension during treatment may be new, or preexisting hypertension may be aggravated. In most cases, a standard approach to hypertension and hypertension management enables continuation of chemotherapy.

TREATMENT

The treatment of hypertension always begins with an assessment to exclude secondary causes of high blood pressure. In most cases, hypertension is primary.

Initial treatment maneuvers are based on lifestyle modification that includes dietary approaches limiting total calories and sodium and weight loss. Avoidance of alcohol may also be helpful. Withdrawing nonchemotherapy drugs that elevate blood pressure (e.g., nonsteroidal antiinflammatory drugs) may also be beneficial.

The choice of antihypertensive agent should be based on guidelines put forth by the Seventh Report of the Joint National Committee on Prevention, Detection, Evaluation, and Treatment of High Blood Pressure (JNC 7).[115] With coexisting LV dysfunction, ACE inhibitors and beta blockers should be the therapy of choice. With coexistent CAD, beta blockers, ACE inhibitors, and calcium blockers provide dual benefits.

Early experience suggests that hypertension related to the TKIs is due to vasoconstriction. Therefore, drugs whose mechanism of action is vasodilatation may be excellent first choices to mange hypertension. We have had success using calcium channel blockers and ACE inhibitors in this population and have avoided using beta blockers as first-line antihypertensive agents.

Special caution should be exercised when adding drugs metabolized by the CYP 4A pathway, because sorafinib is metabolized by this pathway; drug-drug interactions, especially with the calcium channel blockers diltiazem and verapamil, may increase sorafenib levels. The dihydropyridine calcium blockers do not interact with this pathway, and they are safe to use with this medication. Similarly, no interaction with ACE inhibitors or beta blockers is noted, except with carvedilol.[114]

SUPPORTIVE ONCOLOGY

Using the CT associated with chemotherapy as a trigger for nonpharmacologic counseling and vigorous long-term follow-up has enhanced value.

After treatment completion, proactive nutritional counseling for weight maintenance and/or reduction and for education regarding sodium, calorie, and saturated fat restriction may be more beneficial in this population than in the general population.

Cancer patients who have self-limited CT manifested by an increase in cardiac risk factors (e.g., hypertension) require long-term monitoring. This is exemplified by the late effects of platinum-based chemotherapy (PBCT) on atherosclerotic risk factors and future cardiac risk. Survivors of PBCT have an excess of cardiac risk factors (hypertension, dyslipidemia, obesity, and insulin resistance [metabolic syndrome]) and an increased risk of premature atherosclerosis that appears to become evident 10 or more years after treatment completion.[116,117]

Meinardi et al[118] studied 87 patients treated with cisplatin-containing chemotherapy who were in remission for at least 10 years, and whose ages were ≤50 years at the time of analysis. Patients were evaluated for the occurrence of cardiovascular events. Sixty-two of 87 patients were additionally evaluated for cardiac damage and cardiovascular risk factors. Their cardiovascular risk profile was compared with that of 40 patients with comparable age and follow-up treated with orchidectomy only for stage I disease: 79% had hypercholesterolemia, 39% had hypertension, and 25% experienced Raynaud's phenomenon. Major vascular events were noted in 6.9% of patients (6/87) who were 30 to 42 years old at the time of study and 9 to 16 years post chemotherapy: two with MI, three with angina pectoris with proven myocardial ischemia, and one CVA. An increased observed-to-expected ratio of 7.1 (95% CI, 1.9–18.3) for coronary artery disease, as compared with the general male Dutch population, was reported.[118]

Key point: Long-term follow-up by a cardiologist with input from a nutritionist in patients who have had cardiotoxicity during chemotherapy and/or have received PBCT is beneficial.

ARTERIAL AND VENOUS THROMBOEMBOLISM

In addition to increasing risk of thrombosis associated with cancer and its nonpharmacologic treatment (indwelling catheters; immobilization from fatigue, sepsis, surgery), several chemotherapeutic agents are associated with arterial and/or venous thromboembolism.

BEVICIZUMAB

Early studies in patients with metastatic CRC and NSCLC treated with bevacizumab suggested that these patients are at increased risk for venous thromboembolic (VTE) and/or arterial thromboembolic events (ATE). Arterial events can occur in any arterial bed, but are reported most commonly in the coronary and cerebral circulations, manifested by transient ischemic attack (TIA)/cerebrovascular accident (CVA) and ACS.

The mechanism for increased thrombosis is multifactorial and includes decreased production of endothelial nitric oxide with a decrease in vasodilatation, an increase in platelet aggregation, and enhanced thrombin formation. Current analyses suggest that bevacizumab doubles the risk for ATE.

In a pooled analysis from five randomized, controlled trials that included a total of 1745 patients with metastatic CRC, breast cancer, or NSCLC, published by Scappiticci and associates, the risk of arterial or venous thromboembolism was assessed when bevacizumab was combined with chemotherapy versus when chemotherapy alone was used. Among patients treated with both, 3.8% experienced ATE events, compared with 1.7 % of patients on chemotherapy alone. Death from ATE was 0.62% compared with 0.26%, respectively. No statistically significant difference in the incidence of VTE was noted. Risk factors for blood clots in both arteries and veins included a prior history of thrombosis and age >65 years.[119]

A similar incidence of ATE was found in a study of 1401 patients who were randomly assigned in a 2×2 factorial design to oxaliplatin-based chemotherapy with or without bevacizumab. The incidence of grade 3–4 ATE was 1% and 2%, respectively, in the bevacizumab treatment groups.[120]

The risk of ATE is not related to dose or duration of bevacizumab therapy. In a preliminary report of the BRITE (Bevacizumab Regimens: Investigation of Treatment Effects and Safety) study of 1953 patients, the incidence of ATE was 2.1% in the first year and 0.7% beyond 12 months.[121] The incidence of hypertension and ATE is increased in the elderly and in patients who have had prior arterial embolic events.[122,123]

Although no statistical difference for VTE was reported in the Scappiticci pooled analysis, an increased risk of venous thrombosis in addition to the risk associated with malignancy has been reported with incidences that range from 3% to 19.4% across phase II and phase III trials. In a recent meta-analysis, a total of 7956 patients with a variety of advanced solid tumors from 15 randomized controlled trials were identified. Among patients receiving bevacizumab, the summary incidences of all-grade and high-grade VTE were 11.9% (95% CI, 6.8%–19.9%) and 6.3% (95% CI, 4.8%–8.3%), respectively, compared with controls.

Tumor type and the bevacizumab dose may influence the risk of thromboembolism. Patients with metastatic CRC were found to have an incidence of all-grade VTE of 19.1% (95% CI, 16.1%–22.6%), NSCLC 14.9% (95% CI, 8.2%–25.5%), breast cancer 7.3% (95% CI, 4.6%–11.5%), and renal cell carcinoma 3.0% (95% CI, 1.6%–5.5%).[124]

Key point: The use of bevacizumab is associated with an increased incidence of arterial and venous thrombosis.

IMMUNOMODULATING AGENTS

Immunomodulating compounds are novel small molecule, orally available compounds that affect the immune system and other biologically important targets through multiple mechanisms of action, including angiogenesis inhibition, modulation of the levels of key proinflammatory and regulatory cytokines, and immune cell co-stimulation.

Thalidomide

The immunomodulatory drug thalidomide inhibits angiogenesis and induces apoptosis of established neovasculature in experimental models. Thalidomide is an oral cancer drug that has been used to treat multiple myeloma and some non-Hodgkin's lymphoma (NHL). The known toxicities of thalidomide include peripheral neuropathy, constipation, fatigue, and sedation. Therapy for myeloma has revealed a new and previously unrecognized toxicity of thalidomide: deep venous thrombosis with a 2% incidence when used as a single agent.[125]

The incidence of DVT increases substantially when thalidomide is administered with other cytotoxic agents. In a group of 100 patients who received induction chemotherapy including four cycles of continuous infusion of combinations of dexamethasone, vincristine, doxorubicin, cyclophosphamide, etoposide, and cisplatin, VTE developed in 14 of 50 patients (28%) randomly assigned to receive thalidomide, but in only 2 of 50 patients (4%) not given the agent ($P = .002$). All episodes of DVT occurred during the first three cycles of induction. Administration of thalidomide was resumed safely in 75% of patients after receiving anticoagulation therapy.[126] A similar increased incidence of VTE has been seen when thalidomide is combined with doxorubicin, fluorouracil, or gemcitabine.[127–130]

Lenalidomide

Lenalidomide (Revlimid) is structurally similar to thalidomide and was developed to enhance its efficacy while reducing its neurotoxicity. It is used in patients with multiple myeloma and chronic lymphocytic leukemia (CLL). The major CT, similar to thalidomide, is the development of VTE. The overall incidence of VTE is increased in patients with multiple myeloma and with concurrent steroid use. Overall, the incidence of grade 3–4 VTE in myeloma patients is 13% when lenalidomide and dexamethasone are used compared with 4% with dexamethasone alone.

The relationship of VTE to steroid use is dose-related: An incidence of 6.3% was noted with low-dose versus 18% with high-dose dexamethasone.[131] In a study with patients with relapsed and refractory multiple myeloma, a 2% incidence of VTE was noted, and events occurred only when dexamethasone was added to the treatment regimen.[132]

Pomalidomide

Pomalidomide (Actimid) is structurally similar to thalidomide with similar immunomodulating effects and is under investigation. Early results show a similar incidence of VTE.[133]

Cisplatin

An increased rate of arterial thrombosis is seen with acute administration of cisplatin. The incidence of stroke has been reported as 1 in 2000.[134,135]

VEGF

Chemotherapeutic drugs that target VEGF and TK are associated with an increased risk of arterial embolic events that are more common in patients over the age of 65 years and/or who have pretreatment cardiac risk factors or prior arterial disease. The relationship to age is highlighted by the 2.2% incidence of thrombosis/embolism described in a recent study of young women with carcinoma of the cervix (median age, 46 years, with a range of 29–62 years) treated with bevacizumab.[136]

DIAGNOSIS AND TREATMENT
VTE diagnosis

Venous thromboembolism commonly occurs in patients with cancer; an increased incidence during chemotherapy has been reported.[137] Diagnosis is based on clinical suspicion and vigilance in assessing symptoms and performing a thorough physical examination.

Only 30% of patients presenting with symptoms suggestive of VTE actually have a confirmed diagnosis. The most common presenting symptoms associated with VTE are leg edema (80%), pain (75%), and erythema (26%).[138]

Clinical prediction algorithms that combine clinical presentation, imaging, and d-dimer testing have been developed to help make the diagnosis.[139] Clinical characteristics of a high-risk population are listed in Table 9-6. d-Dimer is a marker of endogenous fibrinolysis and should be detectable in patients with VTE. It has a high negative predictive value and is a sensitive but nonspecific marker of VTE.

When VTE is suspected, venous ultrasound is the primary diagnostic imaging modality. It has a sensitivity and specificity of 97% and 94%, respectively, for clot in the proximal leg veins. Sensitivity decreases to 73% for the calf veins, and more distally, sensitivity drops to 53%. For suspected VTE proximal to the inguinal ligament, contrast-enhanced computed tomography or magnetic resonance venography should be considered. For upper extremity disease, duplex ultrasound is a useful imaging modality with a sensitivity of 82% and a specificity of 82%.

Untreated DVT can result acutely in pulmonary embolism (PE) or chronic venous insufficiency. Making the diagnosis early to institute treatment and to avoid these complications is critical. The most common presenting symptoms of PE are dyspnea (85%), chest pain (40%), tachypnea (30%), and tachycardia (23%). Hemoptysis is rare in the absence of pulmonary infarction. Clinical presentation, hypoxemia, hypocapnia, and the ECG and echocardiogram have low sensitivity and specificity for the diagnosis. Computed tomography angiography is the primary imaging modality for the diagnosis of PE.

Ventilation /perfusion scanning is less sensitive and should be reserved for patients who have an allergy to contrast dye or who have compromised renal function. An alternative in these patients is magnetic resonance angiography.

Predisposing factors and diagnostic algorithms for suspected pulmonary embolism and treatment recommendations have been reviewed recently.[140,141]

Cancer patients with VTE have a higher incidence of recurrent thrombosis, as well as an increase in bleeding during anticoagulation therapy.[142]

In patients with confirmed VTE, full anticoagulation with heparin or low-molecular-weight heparin (LMWH) transitioned to oral warfarin therapy is the standard of care.

The risk of VTE is increased in patients with multiple myeloma beyond that associated with cancer. This risk is especially magnified in patients treated with thalidomide and lenalidomide. Palumbo and a panel of experts recently reviewed VTE risk and prevention in detail. Their model defines risk for VTE according to patient (age, prior VTE, central venous catheter in place, infection, diabetes, cardiovascular disease, immobilization, surgery, inherited thrombophilia), disease (diagnosis of myeloma and hyperviscosity), and treatment (high-dose dexamethasone, doxorubicin, multiagent chemotherapy) characteristics. They recommended aspirin for patients with less than one risk factor, LMWH equivalent to enoxaparin 40 mg/day for those with two or more risk factors, and LMWH for all concurrently being treated with high-dose dexamethasone or doxorubicin. Full-dose warfarin (international normalized ratio [INR], 2–3) is an alternative to LMWH.[143]

VTE prevention

Several studies have looked at VTE prophylaxis with oral warfarin or LMWH. In spite of trends toward a reduction in VTE incidence, the concept of VTE prophylaxis with systemic anticoagulation has not been widely adopted.[144,145]

Current practice is driven by guidelines developed by the American Society of Clinical Oncology that include the following: (1) All hospitalized cancer patients should be considered for VTE prophylaxis with anticoagulants in the absence of bleeding or other contraindications; (2) routine prophylaxis of ambulatory cancer patients with anticoagulation is not recommended, with the exception of patients receiving thalidomide or lenalidomide; (3) patients undergoing major surgery for malignant disease should be considered for pharmacologic thromboprophylaxis; (4) LWMH represents the preferred agent for both initial and continuing treatment of cancer patients with established VTE; and (5) the impact of anticoagulants on cancer patient survival requires additional study, and their use cannot be recommended.[146]

Table 9-6   High-risk factors for DVT/PE

Factor	DVT	PE
Active cancer	√	√
Immobilization	√	√
Recent surgery	√	√
Physical signs	Leg swelling edema, collateral veins	DVT, tachycardia, hemoptysis
Prior documented	DVT √	PE √
Alternative less likely diagnosis	√	√

Adopted from Wells PS, Owen C, Doucette S, et al. Does this patient have deep vein thrombosis? *JAMA.* 2006;259:199–207; van Belle A, Büller HR, Huisman MV, et al. Effectiveness of managing suspected pulmonary embolism using an algorithm combining clinical probability. D-dimer testing and computed tomography. *JAMA.* 2006;295:172–179.
DVT, Deep vein thrombosis; *PE,* pulmonary embolism.

VTE treatment

Most evidence supports the use of LMWH with efficacy and safety that are comparable to unfractionated heparin and oral warfarin. LMWH is the recommended first-line approach to diagnosed VTE. Treatment duration should be individualized according to the stage of cancer, risk of bleeding, and chemotherapy treatment regimen.[147–150]

Evidence for the use of inferior vena cava (IVC) filters is limited, and their use should be reserved for patients who cannot receive systemic anticoagulation.[151]

Key point: The safety and efficacy of LMWH are established in cancer patients. For patients with PE and cancer, LMWH should be considered for the first 3 to 6 months, followed by oral warfarin or LMWH indefinitely, or until the cancer is considered cured.

ARTERIAL THROMBOEMBOLISM

Prophylaxis for arterial embolic issues revolves around reducing comorbidity before treatment. The keystone of this is treating hypertension and avoiding hypotension associated with treatment. The potential for the latter occurs because of weight loss, dehydration, and sepsis. Clinicians need to be vigilant and must closely monitor blood pressure with regular reassessment of dosing schedules and overall regimens with up or down titration as treatment proceeds.

When an acute arterial embolic event occurs, it is reasonable to interrupt chemotherapy until full anticoagulation is achieved.

Key point: The treatment goal for arterial and venous thromboembolism is first to relieve the hemodynamic burden, then to relieve symptoms, and then to prevent recurrence.

LIPIDS
Tamoxifen and aromatase inhibitors

Tamoxifen treatment has been associated with a protective effect against atherosclerotic cardiovascular events because of its favorable effects on cholesterol: reducing low-density lipoprotein (LDL) and raising high-density lipoprotein (HDL) levels.[152,153]

The aromatase inhibitors (AIs) consisting of anastrozole (Arimidex), letrozole (Femara), and exemestane (Aromasin) have a neutral effect on lipids. As a result of early trials, researchers thought that the AIs may have a negative effect on lipids; changes in lipid levels were observed when women were treated sequentially with tamoxifen followed by an AI. Letrozole was found to increase total cholesterol and LDL over 16 weeks in a small study of 20 patients with advanced breast cancer. Patients switched to anastrozole from tamoxifen in the Italian Tamoxifen Arimidex (ITA) trial showed a higher incidence of lipid abnormalities (9.3%) than those in the tamoxifen alone arm (4.0%; $P = .04$). The difference was thought to be due to the discontinuation of tamoxifen (favorable effect) and the addition of anastrozole (neutral effect).[154–156]

Key point: Tamoxifen lowers LDL cholesterol and raises HDL cholesterol, and the aromatase inhibitors have a neutral effect on lipids.

RETINOIDS

Retinoids are a class of compounds structurally related to vitamin A that have anticancer effects.

Bexarotene

Bexarotene (Targretin) is a synthetic retinoid that selectively binds to retinoid X receptors. It is approved for the treatment of recurring or refractory cutaneous T-cell lymphoma.

Treatment may be limited by reversible drug-related adverse effects that include hypothyroidism in up to 30% of patients.[157]

Major CT is manifested by a mixed hyperlipidemia, primarily hypertriglyceridemia in more than 80% and hypercholesterolemia in more than 30% of patients. Hyperlipidemia is dose related and begins 1 to 2 weeks after initiation of therapy. Triglyceride levels left untreated can lead to acute pancreatitis. Prophylactic and therapeutic use of lipid-lowering agents can temper the degree of lipid elevation.[158]

Key point: Bexarotene causes marked hypertriglyceridemia in more than 80% of patients.

ARRHYTHMIAS

ECG changes and arrhythmias are probably the most common manifestations of cardiotoxicity related to chemotherapy. Every electrophysiologic abnormality known has been described. Most are incidental and have no hemodynamic or clinical significance. The subject was recently reviewed by Guglin and colleagues.[159] Table 9-7 lists the electrophysiologic abnormalities associated with commonly used chemotherapeutic drugs. Detailed highlights of some common electrophysiologic effects ascribed to specific drugs are described in the following sections.

ANTIMETABOLITES

Antimetabolites are chemically similar to substances required in normal biochemical pathways. These "decoys" interfere with normal function preferentially in cancer cells, leading to abnormalities in cell division and replication.

Gemcitabine

Gemcitabine (Gemzar) is an antimetabolite that is effective as monotherapy or in combination with other drugs in a variety of solid tumors. Toxicity related to the cardiovascular system is rare. Preclinical and phase I data from 1997 described incidences of ventricular tachycardia in 1.4%, 0.7%, 0.2%, and 0%.[160]

Three case reports have described atrial fibrillation within 18 to 24 hours of gemcitabine infusion with recurrence following second and/or third subsequent infusions. One patient had paroxysmal atrial fibrillation before treatment, and two patients had advanced lung cancer.[161–163]

HISTONE DEACETYLASE INHIBITORS (HDACS)

Epigenetic modification is an important mechanism in tumor cell biology. Drugs that target epigenetic silencing mechanisms are under development. Depsipeptide is one such drug.

Table 9-7 Chemotherapy-induced rhythm and conduction abnormalities

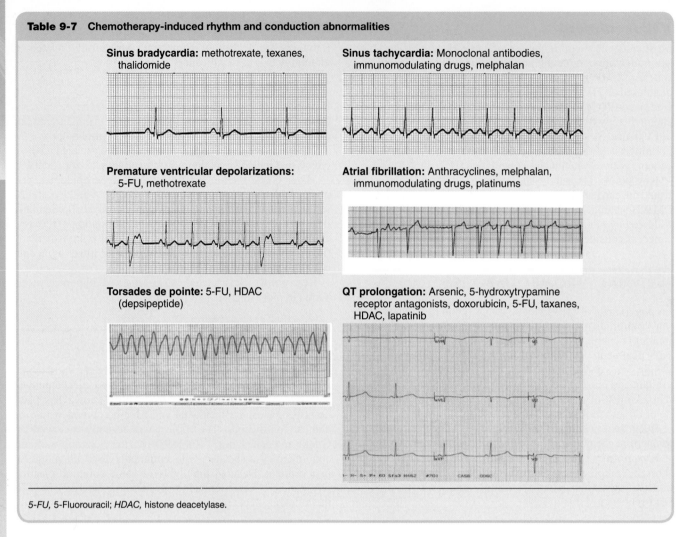

Sinus bradycardia: methotrexate, texanes, thalidomide

Sinus tachycardia: Monoclonal antibodies, immunomodulating drugs, melphalan

Premature ventricular depolarizations: 5-FU, methotrexate

Atrial fibrillation: Anthracyclines, melphalan, immunomodulating drugs, platinums

Torsades de pointe: 5-FU, HDAC (depsipeptide)

QT prolongation: Arsenic, 5-hydroxytrypamine receptor antagonists, doxorubicin, 5-FU, taxanes, HDAC, lapatinib

5-FU, 5-Fluorouracil; *HDAC,* histone deacetylase.

A phase I preclinical trial of 15 patients with metastatic neuroendocrine tumors was stopped prematurely because of serious CT that included one case of sudden death, two cases of grade 2 ventricular tachycardia, and three cases of grade 2 QT prolongation.[164] Toxicity of depsipeptide may be mediated through histone deacetylase (HDAC) inhibition.

To date, more than 500 patients have been treated with depsipeptide. In one eloquently documented study, more than 50% of patients had nonspecific ST-T wave changes, 65% and 38% had isolated supraventricular and ventricular premature depolorizations, respectively, and 38%/14% had unsustained supraventricular tachycardia/ventricular tachycardia. Decreases in LVEF or liberation of cardiac biomarkers (creatine phosphokinase [CPK]-MB or troponin) has been reported.[165]

The drug is arrhythmogenic, and the issue of associated potential QT prolongation modulates the severity of drug-induced arrhythmias. The true incidence of QT prolongation remains speculative, but probably real, and less than that seen in preclinical studies. This warrants electrocardiographic (ECG) monitoring and QT measurement with treatment.

TAXANES

The taxanes (paclitaxel [Taxol], docetaxel [Taxotere]) are derived from the bark of the Yew tree and have demonstrated clinical efficacy in a variety of solid tumors since the early 1990s. Their antitumor activity is caused by inhibition of microtubular function. Paclitaxel, but not docetaxel, is formulated in a Cremophor EL vehicle that enhances drug solubility.

Paclitaxel infusion has been associated with asymptomatic sinus bradycardia in up to 29% of patients, with a 5% incidence of other cardiac arrhythmias (premature ventricular depolarizations, ventricular tachycardia, and atrioventricular block).[166] It is speculated that these arrhythmias are a result of histamine release triggered by Cremophor EL.

MISCELLANEOUS DRUGS
Arsenic trioxide

Arsenic trioxide has efficacy in the treatment of acute promyelocytic leukemia, pancreatic carcinoma, and metastatic melanoma.

QTc prolongation may occur in up to 63% of treated patients, with <1% incidence of torsade de pointes and case reports of sudden death. QT prolongation is due to dose-dependent inhibition of the potassium ion channel by arsenic. Less QT prolongation is seen with oral versus intravenous dosing.[167–169]

Other less frequent electrophysiologic adverse events include high-grade atrioventricular block that occasionally requires pacemaker implantation.[170]

5-Hydroxytryptamine₃ receptor antagonists

Three 5-hydroxytryptamine₃ receptor antagonists are available in the United States for the prevention and treatment of chemotherapy-induced and postoperative nausea and vomiting: dolasetron (Anzemet), granisetron (Kytril), and ondansetron (Zofran).

These agents are generally well tolerated. Studies in healthy subjects showed ECG changes (prolongation of PR, QRS, and QT intervals) with the use of all three drugs. In less than 10%, an asymptomatic and transient intraventricular conduction delay may be seen on the ECG, as well as minor (<15 msec) prolongation of the QT interval that returns to baseline within 6 to 8 hours after infusion. These changes are more prominent with dolasetron. Proarrhythmia is rare, and clinical consequences of these cardiovascular changes have not been reported in practice.[171–174]

Key point: Caution should be used in patients with preexisting conduction delay and underlying heart disease and chemotherapy that can cause QT prolongation, because most of the experience described in the literature is based on events in healthy subjects.

TUMOR LYSIS SYNDROME

Tumor lysis syndrome is a complication of cancer therapy with a constellation of metabolic abnormalities (hyperkalemia, hyperphosphatemia, and hypocalcemia) that result from treatment-related tumor necrosis. These metabolic abnormalities can lead to a wide range of cardiac arrhythmias and typical ECG changes (e.g., hyperkalemia can lead to tall peaked T waves and life-threatening cardiac arrhythmia and conduction delay, and hypocalcaemia can lead to QT interval lengthening).

Key diagnostic and subsequent management issues regarding tumor lysis syndrome involve the identification of high-risk patients, proactive monitoring, and initiation of prophylactic therapy with rapid correction of metabolic abnormalities.

DIAGNOSIS

Routine electrocardiographic monitoring is not required during the administration of chemotherapy. Routine measurement of vital signs (pulse rate) and remeasurement in response to patient symptoms or in detection of asymptomatic or symptomatic changes in heart rate or regularity may prompt the recording of an ECG to help make the diagnosis. Rarely, patients complain of postchemotherapy palpitations, which may trigger short-term (24- to 48-hour Holter monitor) or long-term ambulatory electrocardiographic monitoring (outpatient telemetry or cardiac event monitoring) to make a diagnosis and to exclude a life-threatening arrhythmia.

For patients with known preexisting heart disease or prior documented arrhythmias, more intense ECG monitoring during chemotherapy administration may be indicated.

SUPPORTIVE ONCOLOGY

Stressing that patients should continue their antiarrhythmic medication during chemotherapy, and especially on chemotherapy administration days, is crucial, and members of the oncology team may need to reinforce this principle frequently. For patients who are anticoagulated with warfarin, more frequent monitoring from baseline may be indicated as medications are added and discontinued during treatment with resultant changes in INR.

TREATMENT

A major tenet in proactive treatment of significant and potentially life-threatening arrhythmias is to avoid chemotherapy-induced ischemia, fluid overload, and heart failure, while providing vigilant monitoring of potential shifts in serum electrolytes, especially in levels of magnesium and potassium.

In patients with documented arrhythmias, we recommend cardiology consultation for appropriate decisions regarding antiarrhythmic medications.

No special decisions or treatment modifications are necessary for patients with implanted devices (i.e., pacemakers and internal defibrillators).

SUMMARY

CT is a frequent complication in the treatment of both solid and hematologic malignancies. Large variation is seen in quantitating the incidence, but the potential for chemotherapy-related CT is real. Clinicians should be vigilant and should approach chemotherapy in the context of both a high-risk patient and a high-risk chemotherapy regimen with the knowledge that as much individual variation is seen in CT incidence as in regimen efficacy.

RADIATION-INDUCED CARDIOTOXICITY

Mediastinal radiation (MR) is effective for the treatment of many cancers, especially Hodgkin's lymphoma. In addition, craniospinal radiation contributes to cardiotoxicity. For this discussion, everything attributed to mediastinal radiation also applies to the risks and cardiotoxicity of craniospinal radiation.

It has been established that MR may cause cardiotoxicity. MR-induced cardiotoxicity can be subclinical and asymptomatic or symptomatic with overt disease.[175]

All parts of the heart are potentially at risk, from the pericardium to the endocardium, including the coronary vasculature. Manifestations include acute and chronic pericarditis, asymptomatic decreases in LVEF to overt congestive heart failure (CHF), valvular stenosis and insufficiency, arrhythmias and conduction disease, and accelerated CAD causing angina, myocardial infarction, or sudden death. Radiation probably increases the incidence of anthracycline-induced CT. Several recent comprehensive reviews describe details of incidence, pathophysiology, and testing recommendations.[176–179]

A spectrum of structural abnormalities is presented in Table 9-8.

Similar to anthracyclines, several factors increase the risk of cardiotoxicity after MR. These are reviewed in Table 9-9. When the incidence of radiation-induced CT is considered, it is important to separate patients who were treated before 1985 from those treated subsequently in the "modern era," when more conformational techniques such as image-guided therapy, linear accelerator source, daily fraction size to <2 Gy, equal

Table 9-8 Spectrum of radiation-induced cardiotoxicity

Site	Manifestation
Pericardium	Late pericarditis; late constriction
Myocardium	Diastolic dysfunction, systolic dysfunction: Both can be asymptomatic or be associated with heart failure
Coronary vessels	Proximal anterior vessel CAD- LM, LAD, and RCA
Cardiac valves	Aortic regurgitation/stenosis, mitral regurgitation manifested 10 to 20 years after therapy completion
Conduction system	Conduction delay (right bundle branch block most common): All forms of AV block, including complete heart block

AV, atrioventricular; CAD, coronary artery disease; LAD, left anterior descending coronary artery, LM, left main coronary artery; RCA, right coronary artery.

Table 9-9 Risk factors for chemotherapy-induced pulmonary toxicity

Patient related	Treatment related
Preexisting lung disease	Dose of chemotherapy
Current smoking	(Bleomycin)
Abnormal baseline imaging study	History of MR
Chronic kidney disease	
Prior pneumonectomy	

MR, Mediastinal radiation.

weighting between anterior and posterior portals, minimizing heart exposure with subcarinal blocking, and a shrinking field technique have reduced the potential for cardiotoxicity.

Similar to anthracycline therapy, the risk of radiation-induced cardiotoxicity can be immediate (acute) or late with long latency periods up to several decades post treatment completion.

Almost always, when late radiation-induced cardiotoxicity occurs, more than one cardiac structure is involved, for example, restrictive heart disease often accompanies chronic pericardial disease, and heart block frequently occurs coincidentally with aortic valvular stenosis.

The aggregate incidence of radiation-induced cardiotoxicity is estimated at between 10% and 30% up to 10 years post treatment completion, and more than 70% of patients have asymptomatic abnormalities in various cardiac structures. These data may overestimate the current risk following contemporary treatment.

Heidenreich et al[175] studied 294 asymptomatic patients (mean age, 42 ± 9 years) who had received MR for Hodgkin's lymphoma (average radiation dose, 43 ± 0.3 Gy). Valvular disease was common and increased over time following treatment completion; patients treated for longer than 20 years before evaluation had significantly more valvular disease than those evaluated 10 years post treatment completion. Thirty-six percent of this cohort had abnormal systolic function marked by decreased fractional shortening that was statistically

significantly less than that seen in a "matched" Framingham population who did not receive MR.

This population was also observed for ischemic heart disease; 63 (21.4%) had abnormal resting images during stress, 42 (14%) developed perfusion defects or abnormal wall motion or both, and 40 had coronary arteriography based on noninvasive testing, with stenosis >50% in 22 patients (55%) and less than 50% in 9 patients (22.5%), and with no stenosis in 9 patients.[180,181]

Key point: MR can improve outcomes in malignant disease, but the trade-off is increased risk of late cardiotoxicity.

HEART FAILURE

Acute radiation-induced cardiotoxicity can cause perimyocarditis, ranging from asymptomatic decreases in measured LVEF to full-blown CHF with or without manifestations of pericarditis. In a study from 2003 that was previously referenced, Heidenreich and associates looked at myocardial disease in long-term Hodgkin's lymphoma (HL) survivors. They prospectively performed echocardiogram screening in 294 asymptomatic patients with a mean age of 42 ± 9 years who received a mean radiation dose of 43.3 Gy and were studied from 2 to 23 years (mean, 15 years) after treatment completion. Investigators found frequent abnormalities in left ventricular mass and systolic function. The prevalence of these abnormalities was greater than expected for a generally closely matched population. The incidence of all abnormalities increased as time from treatment completion elapsed.

Radiation-induced myocardial disease differs from the predominantly systolic dysfunction associated with chemotherapy, with preponderance in late-onset disease for diastolic dysfunction and restrictive hemodynamics. Moderate techniques have reduced the risk of systolic dysfunction but have not changed the course of restrictive disease. In a group of 21 asymptomatic survivors treated with 20 to 70 cGy (mean, 35.9 Gy) before 1983, 57% had an abnormal LVEF by RNA 20 years after treatment completion (mean, 14.1 years) compared with the modern technique group, which evaluated 50 Hodgkin's lymphoma survivors (mean age, 35.1 years) 1 to 30 years after treatment (mean, 14.1 years); 4% had an abnormal LVEF by RNA, but 60% had RNA evidence of diastolic systolic dysfunction. Of Heidenrich's 294 patients, 26 (9%) had mild and 14 (5%) had moderate diastolic dysfunction.[182]

The use of modern techniques has led to a lower expected incidence of CT.

Glanzmann et al reported their experience with 352 patients with the use of modern techniques; the incidence of acute pericarditis decreased from 20% to 2.5%. Giordano et al reviewed the risk of cardiac death after adjuvant radiotherapy for breast cancer and found a progressive decrease over time with the use of contemporary radiation delivery techniques.[183–185]

Key point: Radiation-induced myocardial disease is unusual with exposure less than 30 Gy, is increased with any anthracycline exposure, and has a predilection for diastolic dysfunction.

CORONARY ARTERY DISEASE

Laboratory and clinical evidence supports the fact that MR can accelerate the development of coronary artery disease. Manifestations of CAD are unusual before 5 years from treatment completion. Hancock and associates at Stanford

University reviewed the records of 635 patients younger than 21 years of age treated for Hodgkin's lymphoma between 1961 and 1991. After a mean follow-up of 10.3 years, 12 patients died of cardiac disease (relative risk [RR], 29.6; 95% confidence interval [CI], 16.0–49.3), including seven from acute myocardial infarction (AMI; RR, 41.5; 95% CI, 18.1–82.1), three from valvular heart disease, and two from radiation pericarditis/pancarditis. Death occurred 3 to 22 years after patients received 42 to 45 Gy to the mediastinum.[186]

The development of CAD differs from the development of atherosclerotic CAD in the lack of conventional risk factors for atherosclerosis seen in patients who have received MR.

The clinical presentation of radiation-induced CAD is similar to that of CAD in the general population: It may be silent or may present with angina, ACS, myocardial infarction, or sudden death. The distribution of disease, however, is different and somewhat characteristic. It more commonly affects the ostial or proximal right coronary artery, the left anterior descending coronary artery, and the left main coronary artery, with relative sparing of the left circumflex system.[187]

The relative risk of right versus left chest radiation in females with breast cancer is controversial. Data from the early literature that was focused on women who were treated after mastectomy with adjuvant radiation suggested that those with left-sided breast cancer had an increased incidence of fatal cardiovascular disease compared with those with right-sided breast cancer.[188–190]

These studies, published before 1990, reflect pre-modern and modern radiation techniques. A preponderance of studies published after the institution of modern radiotherapy techniques show no increase in ischemic heart disease and no increased risk when treatment to the left versus the right breast is compared,[191–195] and no difference in any other cardiac disease (valvular conduction or heart failure) with adjuvant radiotherapy for local stage I or II breast cancer after breast conservation surgery performed up to 15 years post treatment completion.[192]

Key point: Radiation-induced CAD may double the risk of death from CAD compared with the nonradiated population.

PERICARDITIS

Pericardial disease is the most common manifestation of radiation-induced cardiotoxicity.

During the delivery of radiation therapy, the pericardium can become inflamed and presents like typical acute pericarditis. Acute pericarditis that occurs during active radiation or within weeks of treatment completion is rare; incidence is probably less than 2%. Positional pleuritic chest pain is the hallmark feature of acute pericarditis that is often associated with dyspnea. Fever and other constitutional symptoms are less common. Cardiac auscultation reveals a typical three-component pericardial friction rub. Varying degrees of pericardial fluid may be present from asymptomatic effusions to acute pericardial tamponade.

The ECG shows diffuse ST elevation with or without PR interval depression in acute pericarditis and may be completely normal other than sinus tachycardia. An echocardiogram confirms the presence or absence of pericardial fluid and measures systolic and diastolic left ventricular function.

Similarly, radiation-induced late pericardial disease (within the first year post treatment completion) may be silent with the incidental discovery of an asymptomatic pericardial effusion, or it may present with hemodynamic compromise secondary to reduction in ventricular filling and cardiac output. The latter can be due to pericardial fluid and can present as tamponade, may be purely constrictive without pericardial fluid, or may be caused by a combination of both—effusive constrictive pericarditis. All of the latter presentations are symptomatic with typical signs and symptoms. No evidence suggests that interventions can alter the course of hemodynamically inconsequential and clinically silent effusions.

The literature reflecting pre-modern MR suggests that approximately 20% to 25% of those with late pericarditis progress to develop constrictive disease or acute tamponade 5 to 10 years after therapy. With modern techniques, the incidence of chronic pericardial disease is lower, with pericarditis occurring in less than 2% and chronic pericarditis in less than 5% of treated patients.

Key point: The most frequent manifestation of radiation-induced pericardial disease is late-onset chronic pericarditis.

VALVULAR DISEASE

The same process that can cause myocardial fibrosis is responsible for thickening and fibrosis that may occur on the cardiac valves. In the Heidenreich study, which used echocardiographic screening, the most common valvular abnormality was aortic regurgitation, with less frequent involvement of the mitral and tricuspid valves. Sixty percent of patients followed for 20 years or longer had at least mild aortic insufficiency. Of interest, only 5% of these patients were recognized to have an aortic insufficiency murmur on physical examination performed by an experienced cardiologist.

Most patients present with asymptomatic murmurs without any hemodynamic consequence.

Key point: Radiation-induced valvular disease is unusual before 10 years after treatment completion.

ARRHYTHMIAS

The spectrum from simple isolated premature depolarizations to life-threatening arrhythmias and all forms of conduction disease may occur during treatment or years after treatment completion. A wide spectrum of abnormalities includes the development of sick sinus syndrome, all forms of atrioventricular block, and bundle branch block. Right bundle branch block is more commonly seen because of its anterior location in the heart.

The frequency of serious conduction abnormalities in long-term asymptomatic survivors following MR is not known and is probably overstated in the literature, making causality a difficult assumption. A few prospective studies are reporting the incidence.

Key point: Right bundle branch block is the most frequent conduction abnormality caused by MR.

DIAGNOSIS

Diagnosis is based on clinical suspicion. At every encounter, questions about symptoms of cardiac disease and assessment of functional capacity are critical components. For the most part, until late in the progression of most cardiac disease related to radiation, physical findings are minimal. Although not generally used by cardiologists, assessment of functional capacity using the Karnofsky score or performance status is valuable.

Typical physical findings of heart failure are uncommon; even edema is rare in the early stages of radiation-induced heart failure.

In appropriate patients with risk factors for CAD, we exclude ischemia as the cause of heart failure by a stress echocardiogram or an exercise nuclear perfusion study.

Even though the incidence of CAD is increased in patients with prior MR, no evidence indicates that treatment of asymptomatic lesions favorably influences survival. We do not routinely screen patients for CAD in the absence of a change in functional capacity or with development of exercise-induced symptoms. We do, however, take an aggressive approach to risk factor management and target all patients who have had MR secondary prevention lipid values (i.e., an LDL <70 and an HDL >45). For most, statin therapy is employed because it is difficult to get to those target values by diet alone. Additional counseling regarding diet, weight, exercise, smoking, and substance abuse should be part of every evaluation of long-term survivors of MR.

As a late complication of MR, constrictive pericarditis is suspected with a constellation of symptoms that include dyspnea, fatigue, and edema. Physical examination may show an inspiratory increase in jugular venous pressure (Kussmaul's sign) and a characteristic pericardial knock in diastole. The ECG may show low voltage and/or electrical alternans (beat-to-beat variation in total voltage). We confirm the diagnosis by echocardiography (showing characteristic pericardial thickening and restriction of filling with pronounced respiratory variation) and cardiac MRI with pericardial tagging. This combination of testing has been most valuable in defining anatomy for the surgeon if pericardiectomy is considered. All of these patients undergo right and left heart catheterization to confirm the diagnosis and exclude associated CAD that may need revascularization during open heart surgery.

Of interest, because of the high incidence of hypothyroidism following MR, we check thyroid function in all patients who present with pericardial effusions.

When a murmur suspected of arising from valvular disease is appreciated, we follow with a baseline echocardiogram to quantitate the degree of valvular stenosis/insufficiency and measure associated LV function.

Symptoms of palpitation and dizziness are evaluated by ECG and longer-term ambulatory cardiac monitoring.

Because the incidence of all CT tends to increase over time, we have been doing serial echocardiograms routinely at 5-year intervals even in asymptomatic patients. The latter is a recommendation and not an official guideline at this time.

The American College of Radiology[46] has developed appropriateness criteria for routine follow-up of asymptomatic patients who received MR.[196]

Key point: Hallmarks of radiation-induced CT include pericarditis, ostial or proximal CAD, aortic valve stenosis and insufficiency, and right bundle branch block

TREATMENT

The general approach to the patient with radiation-induced heart disease is similar to that used for patients with cardiac disease that is unrelated to radiation. The medical management of pericardial disease, heart failure, arrhythmias, and coronary artery disease is virtually identical, regardless of the cause. When invasive procedures or surgery is contemplated, decisions may be tempered by the presence of scarring from prior surgery and/or radiation and coagulopathy related to the cancer and/or its treatment. For all, risk factor modification and reduction and the management of noncardiac comorbidity are essential starting points.

The following represents some unique features related to radiation-induced cardiac disease by syndrome.

Pericardial disease

When pericardial symptoms occur during treatment, the cause is more likely directly related to the tumor rather than to the treatment. Treatment in the absence of hemodynamic compromise is symptomatic with aspirin and/or NSAIDs. We try to avoid systemic steroids whenever possible because the latter tend to ultimately extend the course of the illness. As in acute idiopathic pericarditis, we use colchicine 0.6 mg twice daily for 6 to 12 weeks to help prevent recurrent pericarditis and the development of constrictive pericarditis. More common is the development of delayed pericarditis manifested by acute symptoms or asymptomatic pericardial effusions. In the absence of pericardial tamponade, symptomatic treatment is warranted, with careful monitoring of symptoms and physical examination to recognize the development of hemodynamically significant pericardial tamponade.

In the presence of hemodynamic compromise, if an anterior window with clearance allows for safe percutaneous drainage, we first attempt pericardiocentesis in the Cath Lab to relieve the hemodynamic burden. Patients with recurrent effusions after drainage may require a pericardial window or a pericardiectomy.

If no window for drainage is provided and if hemodynamic compromise occurs, we proceed with the surgical creation of a pericardial window.

In the absence of significant restrictive cardiomyopathy, the treatment for documented constriction is surgical pericardiectomy. The presence of restrictive cardiac disease increases operative mortality to >50%, and long-term survival is limited by restrictive cardiomyopathy.

Heart failure

We follow current guidelines for the treatment of heart failure in both asymptomatic and symptomatic patients. Because radiation-induced myocardial disease is more often manifested as diastolic dysfunction (impaired relaxation) or restrictive hemodynamics, medical management is more difficult than for purely garden-variety systolic heart failure. We use a combination of ACE inhibitors or ARBs and beta blockers, depending on the patient's major clinical presentation. Strict management of fluid status is critical with a narrow window of effectiveness: Over-diuresis leads to hypotension and renal insufficiency, and under-dieresis leads to symptoms of congestion. The therapeutic window between these two points is often extremely narrow. For many patients, just managing fluid, blood pressure, and associated coronary disease and diabetes provides adequate treatment for heart failure.

When ischemia is reversible and a component of ischemic cardiomyopathy is present, a role for revascularization may be identified.

Small series case reports of cardiac transplantation for end-stage CHF due to MR describe outcomes that are comparable with those of non–MR-induced disease.[197]

Valvular disease

When radiation-induced valvular disease progresses to consideration of surgical correction, the decision process is not much different from that seen in "ordinary" valve disease.

Additional consideration of altered chest anatomy caused by mediastinal disease, prior surgery, and radiation has an impact on the risks of the operation. In the absence of constrictive pericarditis or restrictive heart disease, risks and outcomes comparable to those seen without prior MR can be expected for mechanical valve replacement.

Surgical repair of regurgitant valves has been reported to have technical feasibility but limited durability, with a percentage of patients requiring reoperation 3 to 5 years down the line.[198,199]

Coronary artery disease

Medical management consisting of risk factor reduction, combined with a pharmacologic armamentarium that includes various combinations of nitrates, beta blockers, ACE inhibitors/ARBs, calcium blockers, and ranolazine, is the standard of care for radiation-induced CAD. More often than not, patients present with acute coronary syndromes that require revascularization. Percutaneous and operative revascularization can be done safely and effectively in this population. Specific risks regarding malignancy status, enhanced risk of thrombosis, and ability to institute and maintain long-term dual antiplatelet therapy may dictate the type of revascularization to be used, from balloon angioplasty to the choice between bare metal and drug-eluting stents to operative bypass surgery. In spite of prior exposure to radiation, the internal thoracic artery can be safely utilized for grafting.[200,201]

Early results of coronary artery bypass grafting for the treatment of MR-induced CAD are good. Late survival, however, is limited by malignancy (recurrent or second) and the development of heart failure. Many patients require concomitant or a later second valvular operation. Careful assessment of any valvular lesion is important during the initial coronary artery bypass grafting, as is careful follow-up.[202]

Key point: Radiation-induced CAD is marked by an ostial or proximal location of stenoses and sparing of the left circumflex coronary artery.

The surgical approach to radiation-induced heart disease is complicated by fibrosis of mediastinal structures and association of multiple cardiac abnormalities that may need repair or may have an impact on ventricular function; early mortality is similar to that of a matched general population, with a higher rate of reexploration for postoperative bleeding, a greater number of sternal wound infections, and a higher rate of sternal dehiscence. Late results differ by the more rapid development of new valve disease and the lack of long-term durability of valve repair. In general, to a greater extent than in the general population, more rigid individualized decision making is critical.[203,204]

Arrhythmias

The treatment of arrhythmias for radiation-induced disease is identical to the standard approach to conduction disease and rhythm disturbances for non–radiation-induced disease.

CAROTID DISEASE AND STROKE

Carotid artery stenosis is a recognized complication of radiation treatment for head and neck tumors, with an increased incidence of carotid and/or subclavian artery atherosclerosis compared with the nonradiated population and an increased actuarial stroke rate.

TIA/CVA may be asymptomatic or minimally symptomatic, and carotid bruits may be absent on examination. We recommend carotid duplex imaging at 5 years post treatment completion to establish a baseline. Subsequent monitoring interval and treatment options are driven by the imaging results. For all, we attempt to achieve secondary prevention levels for lipids because we consider MR another risk factor for atherosclerosis.

For patients with any demonstrable disease, we recommend the addition of aspirin and a more intense serial monitoring schedule.[205,206]

SUPPORTIVE ONCOLOGY

The presence of extracardiac abnormalities due to MR can complicate diagnosis and treatment. They include skeletal abnormalities and muscle wasting that can lead to hypoventilation, hypothyroidism whose lack of treatment or treatment has major cardiac effects, and pulmonary fibrosis with restrictive lung disease that can contribute to exertional breathlessness.

In summary, many of the features of radiation-induced cardiotoxicity mimic the natural history timelines and dose relationships of chemotherapy-induced cardiotoxicity. Radiation-induced disease differs by having a preponderance of diastolic as opposed to systolic dysfunction, development of valvular disease, late pericardial inflammation/fibrosis, conduction system disease, and coronary artery atherosclerosis.

RADIATION-INDUCED PULMONARY TOXICITY (PT)

MR can cause acute pneumonitis and chronic fibrosis as manifestations of pulmonary toxicity. The cause of radiation-induced lung damage is multifactorial. Radiation can injure both capillary endothelial cells and type I cells, triggering the release of transcription factors (e.g., nuclear factor [NF]-κ B), cytokines, and growth factors that lead to localized or general inflammation and consolidation.

The incidence and severity of radiation-induced PT are related to the volume of lung tissue radiated (minimal exposure of least 10% of the lung is required for the development of pneumonitis), the total dose of radiation, and the delivery technique used. Radiation pneumonitis is unusual when total exposure does not exceed 20 Gy, and its incidence increases progressively with higher doses; when 70 Gy is exceeded, the incidence is almost 100%. Delivering the total dose over more fractions also reduces the risk. The underlying disease that is being treated also plays a role: With all other factors being equal, the risk for pneumonitis is lower when Hodgkin's lymphoma or breast cancer is treated, rather than primary lung cancer. With modern techniques, the incidence of subacute pneumonitis is less than 3% in lymphoma and less than 1% for breast cancer compared with 5% to 20% for lung cancer. A higher percentage of patients have asymptomatic changes in pulmonary function testing, and as more sophisticated imaging and testing are employed, the incidence of asymptomatic disease rises. Thus the true incidence of pulmonary toxicity is dependent on definition and diagnostic criteria: The more sensitive the technique, the higher the incidence that is reported.[207–210]

Other high-risk factors include any exposure to anthracycline chemotherapy, previous lung radiation, and steroid withdrawal. Increased age and/or underlying chronic obstructive lung disease does not increase risk, but disease may be more severe in the elderly and in patients with underlying parenchymal lung disease.[211]

Risk factors for MR-induced PT are listed in Table 9-10.

Most patients who develop radiation pneumonitis have a self-limited course without long-term late consequences. The severity of illness is somewhat proportional to the time of onset, with early-appearing disease associated with a more aggressive course.[212]

Key point: The major manifestation of radiation-induced pulmonary toxicity is acute pneumonitis.

Dyspnea, the most frequent presenting symptom, may be associated with cough and/or fever. These symptoms may be insidious and typically occur within months of treatment completion. Aside from hypersensitivity reactions, it is usual to find symptoms in the first month or beyond 8 months.

Physical examination may be unremarkable or minimally abnormal with moist crackles, a pleural friction rub, or evidence of a pleural effusion.

Most patients with acute pneumonitis have complete resolution of the process, become asymptomatic, and return to their baseline level; some develop a degree of fibrosis. In some cases, patients may present with late-onset progressive dyspnea due to radiation fibrosis, even in the absence of a history of an acute event. When fibrosis occurs, it generally evolves over several months and almost always stabilizes by 2 years. Similar to patients with acute pneumonitis, patients with fibrosis can be asymptomatic or may have varying degrees of dyspnea. At the worst end of the spectrum, patients may develop cor pulmonale and respiratory failure.[213]

Additional pulmonary complications of high-dose radiation, including bronchial stenosis, mediastinal fibrosis, and injury to the pulmonary veins, lymphatic system, and recurrent laryngeal nerve, have been reported.[214]

Diagnosis is based on clinical history and is confirmed by radiographic imaging. The chest x-ray may be normal or may present with nonspecific and nondiagnostic reticulonodular opacities to alveolar infiltrates. Fibrosis is recognized by linear streaks, often with volume loss with or without a shift in mediastinal structures. One of the most characteristic features is that the area of fibrosis generally conforms to the field of radiation. Rarely, changes are seen in the contralateral lung. The latter may represent a hypersensitivity reaction to radiation. Computed tomography scans with and without contrast and positron emission tomography (PET) imaging may be more sensitive than a plain chest X-ray in making a diagnosis.

Key point: The chest X-ray may be normal or may have nonspecific changes that limit its utility as a diagnostic tool for radiation-induced lung injury.

Pulmonary function tests (PFTs) may show a decrease in lung volumes, diffusing capacity of carbon monoxide (DLCO), and arterial hypoxemia. In general, some recovery occurs in the first year after treatment completion.[215]

The role of plasma transforming growth factor (TGF)-β_1 in predicting radiation-induced pulmonary toxicity has recently been reviewed.[216]

Key point: The hallmark symptom of radiation-induced pulmonary toxicity is dyspnea.

Radiation-induced bronchiolitis obliterans with organized pneumonia (BOOP) has been reported. Similar to pneumonitis, dyspnea is the major symptom, and temperature elevation is common. The radiographic picture shows infiltrates that always extend beyond the radiation field, with an incidence up to 40% of contralateral lung involvement. This disease almost universally responds to steroids, and recurrence is often seen when steroids are tapered rapidly or are discontinued. This subject has recently been extensively reviewed.[217]

With interstitial pneumonitis, the differential diagnosis is between recurrent malignancy, lymphangitic spread of tumor, alveolar hemorrhage, and infection. In some cases, lung biopsy is needed to sort this out. Some researchers thought that biomarkers, including intercellular adhesion molecule-1 or TGF-β, may indicate a slightly higher risk of developing pulmonary toxicity.

Corticosteroids (e.g., prednisone 1 mg/kg) are the cornerstone of treatment, although no controlled clinical trials have proved their benefit. Prophylactic steroids are not prophylactic and do not prevent the development of PT. Use of steroids for the treatment of radiation fibrosis is not indicated.

Use of the protective agent amifostine to prevent lung injury has been controversial, with inconsistent results reported in major trials during radiation treatment.[218] Guidelines have been generated for the use of amifostine during the course of radiation treatment.[219]

SUPPORTIVE ONCOLOGY

Proactive recognition and treatment are provided for potential extrapulmonary complications of radiation, including esophagitis and aspiration pneumonia.

Because esophageal injury frequently accompanies the pulmonary complications of radiation treatment, vigilance to the maintenance of caloric intake and constant reassessment of the ability to take oral medications are essential, especially for patients with comorbid conditions that require continuation of maintenance medication.

For patients who have had head and neck radiation and are susceptible to recurrent bouts of aspiration pneumonia, aspiration should always be included in the differential diagnosis of a clinical picture that includes a pulmonary infiltrate, especially in a debilitated population.

Table 9-10 Risk factors for radiation-induced pulmonary toxicity

Patient related	Treatment related
Anthracycline exposure	Total volume of lung at risk
Preexisting lung disease	Radiation dose >2 Gy
Current smoking	Fractionization
Oxygen use	Radiation quality
Cancer diagnosis (Lung cancer>breast cancer> HL)	Hilum/mediastinal structures included in field
Steroid withdrawal	

HL, Hodgkin's lymphoma.

CHEMOTHERAPY-ASSOCIATED PULMONARY TOXICITY

Chemotherapy-induced pulmonary toxicity was first reported in the 1960s with busulfan, with subsequent recognition that lung injury is common to a wide variety of chemotherapy agents, with an incidence of up to 10%. Patients may present with **acute or early lung injury** during or soon after treatment or **late** after treatment completion. Diagnosis is often complicated and difficult because of the underlying cancer, the associated immunosuppression, similar presentation of infiltrates due to multiple causes, use of multimodality and multiagent chemotherapy, and lack of specific diagnostic criteria.[220–224]

Key point: Manifestations of chemotherapy-induced pulmonary toxicity involve the parenchyma (alveolar or interstitial disease), the airways (bronchospasm), the pleura (effusions), and the pulmonary circulation (hemorrhage or embolism) with asymptomatic changes on pulmonary function testing.

A summary of chemotherapeutic agents that can cause PT is presented in Tables 9-11 and 9-12.

ACUTE LUNG INJURY

Acute chemotherapy-induced PT is more common than late disease, and acute interstitial pneumonitis is the most common presentation. No universal mechanism of lung injury is known. It may be related to hypersensitivity, the generation of toxic metabolites, the induction of free radicals and/or genetic factors (gefitinib toxicity in the Japanese), and/or the presence of pretreatment pulmonary comorbidity.[224–226]

Similar to the anthracyclines and their associated cardiac toxicity, bleomycin (Blenoxane) is the "poster-child" and the best known and studied cause of chemotherapy-induced pulmonary toxicity. Bleomycin is an antineoplastic antibiotic effective in germ cell tumors, lymphomas, sarcomas, and carcinomas of the head and neck and esophagus. Its use is limited by its potential PT, which is fatal in 2% to 3% of treated patients.[227–231]

A specific entity, bleomycin-induced pneumonitis (BIP), is recognized. However, a wide range of pulmonary toxicity similar to chemotherapy-induced cardiotoxicity is associated with the pharmacologic treatment of cancer.

The most important criteria for diagnosis include recognition of exposure and exclusion of progression of cancer, pulmonary infection, diffuse alveolar hemorrhage, pulmonary embolism, and nonpulmonary causes of interstitial edema that may occur with cardiac or renal failure.

Progressive dyspnea is the most common presenting symptom, occurring in >90% of patients. Clinical presentation is similar to that seen in radiation-induced disease. Patients present with some combination of cough (50%), dyspnea, fever, and varying degrees of arterial hypoxemia. Pleural effusions may be associated, and patients may progress to respiratory failure and acute respiratory distress syndrome (ARDS) requiring mechanical ventilation.

Timing of disease onset is unpredictable, and symptoms may occur with first dosing to anytime during treatment; similar to radiation-induced disease, prophylactic treatment with steroids may not prevent the development of toxicity.

Key point: The major manifestation of chemotherapy-induced pulmonary toxicity is acute interstitial pneumonitis.

Table 9-11 Chemotherapy-induced pulmonary toxicity by drug

Type	Example
Parenchymal	
Interstitial pneumonitis	ARA-C, Bleomycin*, busulfan, chlorambucil, cyclophosphamide, doxorubicin, erlotinib, etoposide, fludarabine, FOLFIRI, FOLFOX, gefitinib, gemcitabine, ifosfamide, imatinib, irinotecan*, melphalan, methotrexate, mitomycin, oxaliplatin, procarbazine, rituximab, taxanes, vincristine/vinblastine
Pneumonitis with fibrosis	BCNU (carmustine), CCNU (lomustine)
Airways	
Bronchospasm	Gemcitabine, methotrexate monoclonal antibodies, taxanes, trastuzumab, vinblastine
Pleura	
Effusion	Gemcitabine, docetaxel, fludarabine, imatinib, mitocycin, thalidomide
Circulation	
Noncardiac pulmonary edema	ARA-C, all trans-retinoic acid, cytoxan, gemcitabine, imatinib, immunomodulating drugs, monoclonal antibodies
Alveolar hemorrhage	Etoposide, gefitinib, gemcitabine
Veno-occlusive disease	Gemcitabine
Hemoptysis	Bevacizumab
Thromboembolic events	Thalidomide

*Dose dependent.

Table 9-12 Chemotherapy-induced pulmonary toxicity by timing of onset

Time	Example
Early or Acute	
Immediate or days	Etoposide, methotrexate, procarbazine, rituximab, taxanes, vincristine/vinblastine
Subacute	
1 month to 8 years	ARA-C, bleomycin, chlorambucil, gemcitabine, melphalan
Late	
10 or more years	BCNU, busulfan, cyclophosphamide,

For simplicity, lung injury related to chemotherapy can be classified according to five syndromes defined by clinical presentation.

Interstitial lung disease

The parenchymal manifestation of pulmonary toxicity is pneumonitis. This can be nonspecific, and may be due to hypersensitivity or allergy or alveolar hemorrhage. An illustrative example is the diffuse alveolar damage that occurs most commonly with bleomycin. The radiographic picture is not dissimilar from that seen with ARDS. It may also present with patchy/ground glass opacities. When bronchoalveolar lavage (BAL) yields a preponderance of eosinophils, and/or peripheral eosinophilia occurs, this interstitial pneumonitis is classified as eosinophilic pneumonia.

Risk factors for BIP include the cumulative dose of bleomycin, the patient's age and smoking history, the presence of renal dysfunction, and concomitant use of supplemental oxygen. Prior MR also increases the risk. The reported incidence has varied from zero to 46% depending on the population studied and the criteria to make the diagnosis. BIP generally starts insidiously during treatment but can also develop up to 2 years after treatment completion. Most patients recover with discontinuation of bleomycin and/or steroid treatment. A minority of patients progress and develop pulmonary fibrosis.

Another variation seen with methotrexate, cyclophosphamide, busulfan, and bleomycin is what used to be called organized pneumonia (BOOP). Currently, this entity is recognized as drug-induced organizing pneumonia. Its hallmark is the radiographic appearance of migratory opacities, often nodular and perilobular/perihilar, that change on serial imaging over weeks to months, often interspersed with a normal chest X-ray.

Radiation recall pneumonitis is seen in patients who received prior chest radiation and following radiation develop symptoms of pneumonitis associated with radiographic infiltrates corresponding to the fields of prior radiation. This has been reported with gemcitabine, doxorubicin, carmustine, etoposide, paclitaxel, and trastuzumab.

HYPERSENSITIVITY PNEUMONITIS

When symptoms occur during drug infusion or immediately after its completion and/or are accompanied by some combination of rash, urticaria, angioedema, changes in blood pressure, or bronchospasm, a hypersensitivity reaction should be suspected. This is often associated with diffuse interstitial edema or infiltrates. The taxanes are the most frequent culprits for this hypersensitivity reaction; this has been reported recently with the use of temozolomide.[232]

Muller and colleagues published a comprehensive review of chemotherapy-induced interstitial lung disease.[233]

Isolated bronchospasm

Less common is isolated bronchospasm with evidence of airflow obstruction characterized by wheezing and prolonged expiration. This has been reported with gemcitabine, the taxanes, methotrexate, vinblastine, the immunomodulating drugs (interleukins and interferons), and most monoclonal antibodies.

Treatment includes withdrawal of the offending agent and use of bronchodilators.

Pulmonary edema

This all-encompassing category is based on the development of interstitial edema that can be primarily cardiac or noncardiac (without elevation of left heart filling pressures). Noncardiogenic pulmonary edema occurs in a time frame that is closely related to administration; it is often preceded by self-limited dyspnea that may have occurred during previous exposure to the drug (previous cycles). Noncardiogenic pulmonary edema is due to an increase in capillary permeability. It is frequently associated with cytosine arabinoside (ARA-C)[234] and with the use of all trans-retinoic acid (especially with a large number of circulating blasts).

Early recognition and withdrawal of the offending drug or drugs are suggested as the most important steps toward successful management. Intravenous corticosteroids, diuretic therapy, and respiratory support with or without mechanical ventilation have been successfully employed.[235]

Pleural effusions

The development of pleural fluid is most often a manifestation of metastatic disease. However, a primary pleural toxicity has been associated with several chemotherapy drugs (gemcitabine, docetaxel).

Patients present with dyspnea that may be accompanied by pleuritic chest pain. Examination reveals marked dullness to percussion and decreased breath sounds and absent fremitus over the affected lung. A plain chest X-ray is often sufficient to make a diagnosis. Treatment consists of removing fluid to alleviate symptoms; a variety of longer-term solutions are available for recurrent accumulation of fluid, including chemical pleurodesis and the insertion of long-term indwelling drainage catheters.[236]

Asymptomatic decrease in pulmonary function testing

Similar to that described with radiation, asymptomatic decreases in lung volumes and DLCO may occur. The incidence is unknown because of its clinically insignificant standing and the lack of a standardized and rigorous pursuit of this in patients without clinical symptoms.[237]

Diagnosis

Chemotherapy-induced PT is almost always a diagnosis of exclusion. Physical examination may be unremarkable, crackles may be diffuse or localized, and pleural fluid may be evident. Clubbing almost never occurs even with profound hypoxemia. No specific radiologic pattern is known for parenchymal disease induced by chemotherapy. In fact, in the early stages, plain chest X-rays may be normal, and high-resolution computed tomography scanning may provide the first diagnostic clue. The benefit of computed tomography scanning is its virtual absence of risk compared with lung biopsy. However, because clinical presentations and radiographic patterns are often similar and nondiagnostic, bronchoscopy with BAL and/or open lung biopsy may be necessary to make a definitive diagnosis.

Key point: Clinical presentation and plain chest radiography most often do not distinguish between drug-induced and other causes of pneumonitis.

An echocardiogram may help to exclude a cardiac cause, especially when pulmonary edema is present; serologically, the measurements of BNP may also be useful.

Key point: A normal BNP and a normal echocardiogram virtually exclude any cardiac causes.

Treatment

Treatment is dictated by the diagnosis. The first step is when drug-induced pulmonary toxicity is suspected to stop the most likely offending drug. Assessment of hypoxemia dictates the use of supplemental oxygen or mechanical ventilation.

Until a definitive diagnosis is made, empirical use of broad-spectrum antibiotics until cultures are returned is the usual standard of care.

In the absence of sepsis that dictates appropriate antibiotic use, a trial of high-dose steroids may be beneficial.

Supportive oncology

It is essential to be overcautious and avoid iatrogenic fluid overload, especially when the patient presents with initial hypotension that may be initially managed with a fluid challenge. During the acute phase of chemotherapy-induced pulmonary injury, renal function may be temporarily compromised, which may contribute to fluid retention and higher drug levels. In addition to strict measurements of fluid intake and output, we recommend strict adherence to a policy of daily weights to help follow fluid status.

CHRONIC LUNG INJURY

Less common than acute pneumonitis is the development of pulmonary fibrosis resulting in restrictive lung disease. The latter is defined by reductions in lung volumes, especially total lung capacity, with accompanying reductions in diffusing capacity (DLCO).

Symptoms consist of varying degrees of dyspnea that may occur insidiously and may progress over time, with or without a nonproductive cough. Physical examination may be unremarkable, or dry rales may be appreciated on lung auscultation. Imaging studies may show areas of fibrosis and/or a decrease in lung volume with a shift of mediastinal structures. PFTs typically show a restrictive pattern. The pathogenesis is most likely initial lung injury followed by ongoing inflammation with immune activation and the liberation of inflammatory cytokines, ultimately leading to fibrosis.

Key point: Chronic chemotherapy-induced pulmonary fibrosis is less common than acute interstitial pneumonitis.

Because this ends up being mainly a mechanical problem (i.e., a reduction in lung volume), supportive therapy and supplemental oxygen when indicated are limited management options. The value of long-term immunosuppression with steroids has not been proved. Infections should be aggressively treated in the early phases to avoid respiratory decompensation.[238–240]

Supportive oncology

Pulmonary rehabilitation has a role in this population to maintain or improve functional capacity and to provide psychosocial support.

LUNG INJURY AFTER BONE MARROW TRANSPLANTATION

The range of pulmonary toxicity after bone marrow transplant is similar to that described for chemotherapy in general. In addition, consideration of graft-versus-host disease (GVHD) is always a possibility. In-depth reviews of this subject have been published.[241,242]

CLINICAL PEARLS

- Chemotherapy- and radiation therapy–induced pulmonary injury may be insidious or may present with severe and rapidly fatal pulmonary decompensation.
- The presentation of various possible syndromes is generally similar in spite of multiple pathophysiologic entities, and the diagnosis is almost always one of exclusion.
- Because most of these patients are immunocompromised, opportunistic infections are always in the background.

SUMMARY

Current treatment of cancer with multimodality therapies that include chemotherapy and radiation has been effective in curing many cancers and has converted others to chronic diseases. This has created a group of long-term survivors that numbers hundreds of thousands, whose ranks continue to swell. The downside of this miraculous increase in cure and survival is the potential for acute and chronic cardiac and pulmonary toxicity. As treatments continue to be more effective, the potential risk for late toxicity increases in proportions that make diagnostic and management knowledge essential for most caregivers in the future. Successful management of this population requires a team approach that includes physicians of many specialties, as well as nursing and support personnel.

REFERENCES

1. Miller AB, Hoogstraten B, Staquet M, et al. Reporting results of cancer treatment. *Cancer.* 1981;47:207–214.
2. National Cancer Institute. *Cancer treatment evaluation program: common terminology criteria for adverse events, v 3.0 (CTCAE).* Available at: http://ctep.cancer.gov/protocol Development/ electronic_applications/docs/ctcaev3.pdf; August 9, 2006. Accessed 20.01.09.
3. Von Hoff DD, Rozencweig M, Picart M. The cardiotoxicity of anticancer drugs. *Semin Oncol.* 1982;9:23–33.
4. Shan K, Lincoff AM, Young JB. Anthracycline-induced cardiotoxicity. *Ann Intern Med.* 1996;125:47–58.
5. Killckap S, Akgul E, Aksoy S, et al. Doxorubicin-induced second degree and complete heart block. *Europace.* 2005;7:227–230.
6. Wortman JE, Lucas VS, Schuster E, et al. Sudden death during doxorubicin administration. *Cancer.* 1979;44:1588–1591.
7. O'Brian RM, Luce JK, Talley RW, et al. Phase II evaluation of adriamycin in human neoplasm. *Cancer.* 1973;32:1–8.
8. Steinberg J, Cohen AJ, Wasserman AG, et al. Acute arrhythmogenicity of doxorubicin administration. *Cancer.* 1987;60:1213–1218.

9. Lipshultz SE, Colan SD, Gelber RD, et al. Late cardiac effects of doxorubicin therapy for acute lymphoblastic leukemia in childhood. *N Engl J Med.* 1991;324:808–815.

10. Von Hoff DD, Layard MW, Basa P, et al. Risk factors for doxorubicin induced congestive heart failure. *Ann Intern Med.* 1979;91:710–717.

11. Steinherz LJ, Steinherz PG, Tan CTC, Heller G, Murphy ML. Cardiac toxicity 4 to 20 years after completing anthracycline therapy. *JAMA.* 1991;266:1672–1677.

12. Hequet O, Le QH, Moulliet I, et al. Subclinical late cardiomyopathy after doxorubicin therapy for lymphoma in adults. *J Clin Oncol.* 2004;22:1864–1871.

13. Carver JR, Shapiro CL, Ng A, et al. American Society of Clinical Oncology clinical evidence review on the ongoing care of adult cancer survivors: cardiac and pulmonary late effects. *J Clin Oncol.* 2007;25:3991–4008.

14. Carver JR, Ng A, Meadows AT, et al. Cardiovascular late effects and the ongoing care of adult cancer survivors. *Dis Manag.* 2008;11:1–6.

15. Von Dalen EC, Michiels EM, Caron HM, et al. Different anthracycline derivatives for reducing cardiotoxicity in cancer patients. *Cochrane Database Syst Rev.* 2006;(4) CD005006.

16. Batist G, Ramakrishan G, Rao CS, et al. Reduced cardiotoxicity and preserved antitumor efficacy of liposome-encapsulated doxorubicin and cyclophosphamide compared to conventional doxorubicin and cyclophosphamide in a randomized, multicenter trial of metastatic breast cancer. *J Clin Oncol.* 2001;19:1444–1454.

17. O'Brien MER, Wigler N, Inbar M, et al. Reduced cardiotoxicity and comparable efficacy in a phase III trial of pegylated liposomal doxorubicin-HCL for the first line treatment of metastatic breast cancer. *Ann Oncol.* 2004;15:440–449.

18. Slamon DJ, Clark GM, Wong SG, et al. Human breast cancer: correlation of relapse and survival with amplification of the HER-2/neu oncogene. *Science.* 1987;235:177–182.

19. Slamon DJ, Leyland-Jones B, Shak S, et al. Use of chemotherapy plus a monoclonal antibody against HER2 for metastatic breast cancer that overexpresses HER2. *N Engl J Med.* 2001;344:783–792.

20. Seidman A, Hudis C, Pierri MK, et al. Cardiac dysfunction in the trastuzumab clinical trials experience. *J Clin Oncol.* 2002;20:1215–1221.

21. Seidman AD, Berry D, Cirrincione C, et al. Randomized phase III trial of weekly compared with every-3-weeks paclitaxel for metastatic breast cancer, with trastuzumab for all HER-2 overexpressors and random assignment to trastuzumab or not in HER-2 nonoverexpressors: final results of Cancer and Leukemia Group B protocol 9840. *J Clin Oncol.* 2008;26:1642–1649.

22. Marty M, Cognetti F, Maraninchi D, et al. Efficacy and safety of trastuzumab combined with docetaxel in patients with human epidermal growth factor receptor 2-positive metastatic breast cancer administered as first-line treatment: results of a randomized phase II trial by the M77001 Study Group. *J Clin Oncol.* 2005;23:4265–4274.

23. Robert N, Leyland-Jones B, Asmar L, et al. Randomized phase III study of trastuzumab, paclitaxel, and carboplatin compared with trastuzumab and paclitaxel in women with HER-2-overexpressing metastatic breast cancer. *J Clin Oncol.* 2006;24:2786–2792.

24. Pegram M, Forbes J, Pienkowski T, et al. BCIRG 007: first overall survival analysis of randomized phase III

trial of trastuzumab plus docetaxel with or without carboplatin as first line therapy in HER2 amplified metastatic breast cancer (MBC). *J Clin Oncol.* 2007;25:18S Abstract 1008.

25. Burstein H, Lyndsay N, Harris P, et al. Trastuzumab and vinorelbine as first-line therapy for HER2-overexpressing metastatic breast cancer: multicenter phase II trial with clinical outcomes, analysis of serum tumor markers as predictive factors, and cardiac surveillance algorithm. *J Clin Oncol.* 2003;21:2889–2895.

26. O'Shaughnessy J, Vukelja SJ, Marsland T, et al. Phase II trial of gemcitabine plus trastuzumab in metastatic breast cancer patients previously treated with chemotherapy: preliminary results. *Clin Breast Cancer.* 2002;3(suppl 1):17–20.

27. Wardley A, Anton-Torres A, Pivot X, et al. Evaluation of trastuzumab, docetaxel and capecitabine as first line therapy for HER2-positive locally advanced or metastatic breast cancer. *Breast Cancer Res Treat.* 2007;106(suppl 1):S33 Abstract 309.

28. Guarneri V, Lenihan DJ, Valese V, et al. Long-term cardiac tolerability of trastuzumab in metastatic breast cancer: the M.D. Anderson Cancer Center experience. *J Clin Oncol.* 2006;24:4107–4115.

29. Untch M, Eidtmann H, du Bois A, et al. Cardiac safety of trastuzumab in combination with epirubicin and cyclophosphamide in women with metastatic breast cancer: results of a phase I trial. *Eur J Cancer.* 2004;40:988–997.

30. Tan-Chiu E, Yothers G, Romond E, et al. Assessment of cardiac dysfunction in a randomized trial comparing doxorubicin and cyclophosphamide followed by paclitaxel, with or without trastuzumab as adjuvant therapy in node-positive, human epidermal growth factor receptor 2-overexpressing breast cancer: NSABP B-31. *J Clin Oncol.* 2005;23:7811–7819.

31. Perez E, Suman V, Davidson N, et al. Cardiac safety analysis of doxorubicin and cyclophosphamide followed by paclitaxel with or without trastuzumab in the North Central Cancer Treatment Group N9831 adjuvant breast cancer trial. *J Clin Oncol.* 2008;26:1231–1238.

32. Slamon D, Eiermann W, Robert N, et al. *BCIRG 006: 2nd interim analysis phase III randomized trial comparing doxorubicin and cyclophosphamide followed by docetaxel (ACT) with doxorubicin and cyclophosphamide followed by docetaxel and trastuzumab ACTH) with docetaxel, carboplatin and trastuzumab (TCH) in HER2neu positive early breast cancer patients.* Presented at: 29th Annual San Antonio Breast Cancer Symposium, San Antonio, TX: December 14–17; 2006. Abstract 52.

33. Joensuu H, Kellokumpu-Lehtinen PL, Bono P, et al. Adjuvant docetaxel or vinorelbine with or without trastuzumab for breast cancer. *N Engl J Med.* 2006;354:809–820.

34. Suter TM, Procter M, van Veldhuisen DJ, et al. Trastuzumab-associated cardiac adverse effects in the Herceptin adjuvant trial. *J Clin Oncol.* 2007;25:3859–3865.

35. Rayson D, Richel D, Chia S, et al. Anthracycline-trastuzumab regimens for HER2/neu-overexpressing breast cancer: current experience and future strategies. *Ann Oncol.* 2008;19:1530–1539.

36. Gomez HL, Doval DC, Chavez MA, et al. Efficacy and safety of lapatinib as first-line therapy for ERB2-amplified locally advanced or metastatic breast cancer. *J Clin Oncol.* 2008;26:2999–3005.

37. Perez EA, Koehler M, Byrne J, et al. Cardiac safety of lapatinib: pooled analysis of 3689 patients enrolled in clinical trials. *Mayo Clin Proc.* 2008;83:679–686.

38. Gottdiener JS, Appelbaum FR, Ferrnac VJ, et al. Cardiotoxicity associated with high dose cyclophosphamide therapy. *Arch Intern Med.* 1981;141:758–763.

39. Zver S, Zadnik V, Bunc M, et al. Cardiac toxicity of high dose cyclophosphamide in patients with multiple myeloma undergoing autologous hematopoietic stem cell transplantation. *Int J Hemat.* 2007;85:408–414.

40. Klastersky J. Side effects of ifosfamide. *Oncology.* 2003;65(suppl 2):7–10.

41. Cohen MH, Williams G, Johnson JR, et al. Approval summary for imatinib mesylate capsules in the treatment of chronic myelogenous leukemia. *Clin Cancer Res.* 2002;8:935–942.

42. Beccia M, Cannella L, Frustaci A, et al. Cardiac events in imatinib mesylate-treated chronic myeloid leukemia patients: a single institution experience. *Leuk Res.* 2008;32:835–836.

43. Park YH, Park HJ, Kim BS, et al. BNP as a marker of the heart failure in the treatment of imatinib mesylate. *Cancer Lett.* 2006;243:16–22.

44. Atallah E, Durand JB, Kantarjian H, et al. Congestive heart failure is a rare event in patients receiving imatinib therapy. *Blood.* 2007;110:1233–1237.

45. Lloyd-Jones DM, Larson MG, Leip EP, et al. Life-time risk for developing congestive heart failure: the Framingham heart study. *Circulation.* 2002;106:3068–3072.

46. Ribeiro AL, Soriano-Marcolino M, Bittencourt HNS, et al. An evaluation of the cardiotoxicity of imatinib mesylate. *Leuk Res.* 2008;32:1809–1814.

47. Motzer RJ, Rini BI, Bukowski RM, et al. Sunitinib in patients with metastatic renal cell carcinoma. *JAMA.* 2006;295:2516–2524.

48. Motzer RJ, Hutson TE, Tomczak P, et al. Sunitinib versus interferon alpha in metastatic renal cell carcinoma. *N Engl J Med.* 2007;356:115–124.

49. Chu TF, Rupnick MA, Kerkela R, et al. Cardiotoxicity associated with the tyrosine kinase inhibitor sunitinib. *Lancet.* 2007;370:2011–2019.

50. Telli ML, Witteles RM, Fisher GA, et al. Cardiotoxicity associated with the cancer therapeutic agent sunitinib malate. *Ann Oncol.* 2008;19:1613–1618.

51. Khakoo AY, Kassiotis CM, Tannir N, et al. Heart failure associated with sunitinib malate: a multitargeted receptor tyrosine kinase inhibitor. *Cancer.* 2008;112:2500–2508.

52. Chen MH, Kerkela R, Force T. Mechanisms of cardiac dysfunction associated with tyrosine kinase inhibitor cancer therapeutics. *Circulation.* 2008;117:84–95.

53. Escudier B, Eisen T, Stadler WM, et al. Sorafenib in advanced clear-cell renal-cell carcinoma. *N Engl J Med.* 2007;356:125–134.

54. Ganz WI, Sridhar KS, Ganz SS, et al. Review of tests for monitoring doxorubicin-induced cardiomyopathy. *Oncology.* 1996;53:461–470.

55. Kapusta L, Thijssen JM, Groot-Loonen J, et al. Discriminative ability of conventional echocardiography and tissue Doppler imaging techniques for the detection of subclinical cardiotoxic effects of treatment with anthracyclines. *Ultrasound Med Biol.* 2001;27:1605–1614.

56. Kapusta L, Thijssen JM, Groot-Loonen J, et al. Tissue Doppler imaging in detection of myocardial dysfunction in survivors of childhood cancer treated with anthracyclines. *Ultrasound Med Biol.* 2000;26:1099–1108.

57. Cardinale D, Sandri MT, Martinoni A, et al. Left ventricular dysfunction predicted by early troponin I release after high-dose chemotherapy. *J Am Coll Cardiol.* 2000;36:517–522.

58. Cardinale D, Sandri MT, Colombo A, et al. Prognostic value of troponin I in cardiac risk stratification of cancer patients undergoing high-dose chemotherapy. *Circulation.* 2004;109:2749–2754.

59. Lenihan DJ, Massey MR, Baysinger K, et al. Early detection of cardiotoxicity during chemotherapy using biomarkers. *J Clin Oncol.* 2007;25:19525.

60. Adams KF, Lindenfeld J, Arnold JMO, et al. Executive summary: HFSA 2006. Comprehensive heart failure practice guideline. *J Cardiac Failure.* 2006;12:10–38.

61. The SOLVD Investigators. Effect of enalapril on survival in patients with reduced left ventricular ejection fractions and congestive heart failure. *N Engl J Med.* 1991;325:293–302.

62. Pfeffer MA, Swedberg K, Granger CB, et al. Effects of candesartan on mortality and morbidity in patients with chronic heart failure: the CHARM-overall programme. *Lancet.* 2003;362:759–766.

63. Giesler G, Lenihan DJ, Durand JB. The update on the rationale, use and selection of [beta]-blockers in heart failure. *Curr Opin Cardiol.* 2004;19:250–253.

64. Bristow MR, Gilbert EM, Abraham WT, et al. Carvedilol produces dose-related improvements in left ventricular function and survival in subjects with chronic heart failure. *Circulation.* 1996;94:2807–2816.

65. Pitt B, Zannad F, Remme WJ, et al. The effect of spironolactone on morbidity and mortality in patients with severe heart failure. *N Engl J Med.* 1999;341:709–717.

66. Taylor AL, Ziesche S, Yancy C, et al. Combination of isosorbide dinitrate and hydralazine in blacks with heart failure. *N Engl J Med.* 2004;351:2049–2057.

67. Ewer MS, Vooltich MT, Durand JB, et al. Reversibility of trastuzumab-related cardiotoxicity: new insights based on clinical course and response to medical treatment. *J Clin Oncol.* 2005;23:7820–7826.

68. Lenihan DJ, Tong AT, Woods M, et al. Withdrawal of ACE-inhibitors and beta-blockers in chemotherapy induced heart failure leads to severe adverse cardiovascular events. *Circulation.* 2003;108(suppl IV):IV–665.

69. Gianni L, Munzone E, Capri G, et al. Paclitaxel by 3-hour infusion in combination with bolus doxorubicin in women with untreated metastatic breast cancer: high antitumor efficacy and cardiac effects in a dose-finding and sequence-finding study. *J Clin Oncol.* 1995;13:2688–2699.

70. Legha SS, Benjamin RS, Mackay B, et al. Reduction of doxorubicin cardiotoxicity by prolonged continuous intravenous infusion. *Ann Intern Med.* 1982;96:133–139.

71. Swain SS, Whaley FS, Gerber S, et al. Cardioprotection with dexrazoxane for doxorubicin-containing therapy in advanced breast cancer. *J Clin Oncol.* 1997;15:1315–1332.

72. Tebbi CK, London WB, Friedman D, et al. Dexrazoxane-associated risk for acute myeloid leukemia/myelodysplastic syndrome and other secondary malignancies in pediatric Hodgkin's disease. *J Clin Oncol.* 2007;25:493–500.

73. Hensley ML, Hagerty KL, Kewalramani T, et al. American Society of Clinical Oncology 2008 clinical practice guideline update: use of chemotherapy and radiation therapy protectants. *J Clin Oncol.* 2009;27:127–145.

74. Nakamae H, Tsumura K, Terada Y, et al. Notable effects of angiotensin II receptor blocker, valsartan, on acute cardiotoxic changes after standard chemotherapy with cyclophosphamide, doxorubicin, vincristine and prednisone. *Cancer.* 2005;104:2492–2498.

75. Kalay N, Basar E, Ozdogru I, et al. Protective effects of carvedilol against anthracycline-induced cardiomyopathy. *J Am Coll Cardiol.* 2006;48:2258–2262.

76. Cardinale D, Colombo A, Sandri MT, et al. Prevention of high-dose chemotherapy-induced cardiotoxicity in high-risk patients by angiotensin-converting enzyme inhibition. *Circulation.* 2006;114:2474–2481.

77. Labianca R, Beretta G, Glenici M, et al. Cardiac toxicity of 5-fluorouracil: a study of 1,083 patients. *Tumori.* 1982;68:505–510.

78. Keefe DL, Roistacher N, Pierri MK. Clinical cardiotoxicity of 5-fluorouracil. *J Clin Pharmacol.* 1993;33:1060–1070.

79. Kuropkat C, Griem K, Clark J, et al. Severe cardiotoxicity during 5-fluorouracil chemotherapy: a case and literature report. *Am J Clin Oncol.* 1999;22:466.

80. Sasson Z, Morgan CD, Wang B, et al. 5-fluorouracil related toxic myocarditis: case reports and pathological confirmation. *Can J Cardiol.* 1994;10:861–864.

81. Bertino J, Gameli E. Milano G. 5-Fluorouracil drug management: pharmacokinetics and pharmacogenomics meeting summary. *Clin Colorectal Cancer.* 2007;6:407–422.

82. Ezzeldin HH, Diasio RB. Predicting fluorouracil toxicity: can we finally do it? *J Clin Oncol.* 2008;26:2080–2082.

83. Papadopulos CA, Wilson H. Capecitabine-associated coronary vasospasm: a case report. *Emerg Med.* 2008;25:307–309.

84. To AC, Looi KL, Danmianovich D, et al. A case of cardiogenic shock caused by capecitabine treatment. *Nat Clin Pract Cardiovasc Med.* 2008;5:725–729.

85. Dalzell JR, Samuel LM. The spectrum of 5-fluorouracil cardiotoxicity. *Anticancer Drugs.* 2009;20:79–80.

86. Manojiovic N, Babic D, Stojanovic S, et al. Capecitabine cardiotoxicity—case reports and literature review. *Hepatogastroenterology.* 2006;55:1249–1256.

87. Scott PA, Ferchow L, Hobson A, et al. Coronary spasm induced by capecitabine mimics ST elevation myocardial infarction. *Emerg Med J.* 2008;25:699–700.

88. Goldsmith YB, Roistacher N, Baum MS. Capecitabine-induced coronary vasospasm. *J Clin Oncol.* 2008;26:3802–3804.

89. Personnel data on file

90. Mandel E, Lewinski U, Djaldetti M. Vincristine-induced myocardial infarction. *Cancer.* 1975;36:1979–1982.

91. Lejonc JL, Vernant JP, Macquin J, et al. Myocardial infarction following vinblastine treatment. *Lancet.* 1980;2:692.

92. Yancey RS, Talpaz M. Vindesine associated angina and ECG changes. *Cancer Treat Rep.* 1982;66:587–589.

93. Hansen SW, Olsen N, Rossing N, et al. Vascular toxicity and the mechanism underlying Raynaud's phenomenon in patients treated with cisplatin, vinblastine and bleomycin. *Ann Oncol.* 1990;1:289–292.

94. Ibrahim A, Hirschfeld S, Cohen MH, et al. FDA drug approval summaries: oxaliplatin. *Oncologist.* 2004;9:8–12.

95. Icli F, Karaoguz H, Dincol D, et al. Severe vascular toxicity associated with cisplatin-based chemotherapy. *Cancer.* 1993;72:587–593.

96. Vogelzang NH, Torkelson JL, Kennedy BJ. Hypomagnesemia, renal dysfunction, and Raynaud's phenomenon in patients treated with cisplatin, vinblastine, and bleomycin. *Cancer.* 1985;56:2765–2770.

97. Sonnenblick M, Rosin A. Cardiotoxicity of interferon: a review of 44 cases. *Chest.* 1991;99:667–671.

98. Vial T, Descotes J. Immune-mediated side-effects of cytokines in humans. *Toxicology.* 1995;105:2002–2008.

99. Nora R, Abrmas JS, Tait NS, et al. Myocardial effects during recombinant interleukin-2 therapy. *J Natl Cancer Inst.* 1989;81:59–63.

100. Chesson BD, Leonard JP. Monoclonal antibody therapy for B-cell non-Hodgkin's lymphoma. *N Engl J Med.* 2008;359:613–626.

101. Siano M, Lerch E, Negretti L, et al. A phase I-II study to determine the maximum tolerated infusion rate of rituximab with special emphasis on monitoring the effect of rituximab on cardiac function. *Clin Cancer Res.* 2008;14:7935–7939.

102. Fraker Jr TD, Fihn SD, writing on behalf of the 2002 Chronic Stable Angina Writing Committee. 2007 chronic angina focused update of the ACC/AHA 2002 guidelines for the management of patients with chronic stable angina: a report of the American College of Cardiology/American Heart Association task force on practice guidelines writing group to develop the focused update of the 2002 guidelines for the management of patients with chronic stable angina. *Circulation.* 2007;116:2762–2772.

103. Anderson JL, Adams CD, Antman EM, et al. ACC/AHA 2007 guidelines for the management of patients with unstable angina/non–ST-elevation myocardial infarction: executive summary: a report of the American College of Cardiology/American Heart Association task force on practice guidelines (Writing Committee to Revise the 2002 Guidelines for the Management of Patients With Unstable Angina/Non–ST-Elevation Myocardial Infarction). *Circulation.* 2007;116:803–877.

104. Kushner FG, Hand M, Smith Jr SC, et al. 2009 focused updates: ACC/AHA guidelines for the management of patients with ST-elevation myocardial infarction (updating the 2004 guideline and 2007 focused update) and ACC/AHA/SCAI guidelines on percutaneous coronary intervention (updating the 2005 guideline and 2007 focused update): a report of the American College of Cardiology Foundation/American Heart Association task force on practice guidelines. *Circulation.* 2009;120:2271–2306.

105. Saif MW, Tomita M, Ledbetter L, et al. Capecitabine-related cardiotoxicity: recognition and management. *Support Oncol.* 2008;6:41–48.

106. Jain M, Townsend RR. Chemotherapy agents and hypertension: a focus on angiogenesis blockade. *Curr Hypertens Rep.* 2007;9:320–328.

107. Arriaga Y, Becerra CR. Adverse effects of bevacizumab and their management in solid tumors. *Support Cancer Ther.* 2006;3:247–250.

108. Genentech Inc. *Avastin (bevacizumab) prescribing information.* San Francisco, CA: Genentech Inc; 2008 Last Accessed 22.02.09.

109. Zhu X, Wu S, Dahut W, et al. Risks of proteinuria and hypertension with bevacizumab, an antibody against vascular endothelial growth factor: systematic review and meta-analysis. *Am J Kidney Dis.* 2007;49:186–193.

110. Kabbinavar F, Hurwitz H, Fehrenbacher L, et al. Phase II randomized trial comparing bevacizumab plus fluorouracil (FU)/leucovorin (LV) with FU/LV alone in patients with metastatic colorectal cancer. *J Clin Oncol.* 2003;21:60–65.

111. Hurwitz H, Fehrenbacher L, Novotny W, et al. Bevacizumab plus irinotecan, fluorouracil and leucovorin for metastatic colorectal cancer. *N Engl J Med.* 2004;350:2335–2342.

112. Pfizer. *Sutent (sunitinib malate) prescribing information*. New York, NY: Pfizer; 2008 Last Accessed 21.02.09.

113. Wu S, Chen JJ, Kudelka A, et al. Incidence and risk of hypertension with sorafenib in patients with cancer: a systematic review and meta-analysis. *Lancet Oncol*. 2008;9:117–123.

114. Schmidinger M, Zielinski CC, Vogl UM, et al. Cardiac toxicity of sunitinib and sorafenib in patients with metastatic renal cell carcinoma. *J Clin Oncol*. 2008;26:5204–5212.

115. Chobanian AV, Bakris GL, Black HR, et al. Seventh report of the Joint National Committee on Prevention, Detection, Evaluation, and Treatment of High Blood Pressure. *Hypertension*. 2003;42:1206–1252.

116. Huddart RA, Norman A, Shahidi M, et al. Cardiovascular disease as a long-term complication of treatment for testicular cancer. *J Clin Oncol*. 2003;21:1513–1523.

117. Raghavan D, Cox K, Childs A, et al. Hypercholesterolemia after chemotherapy for testis cancer. *J Clin Oncol*. 1992;10:1386–1389.

118. Meinardi MT, Gietema JA, van der Graaf WT, et al. Cardiovascular morbidity in long-term survivors of metastatic testicular cancer. *J Clin Oncol*. 2000;18:1725–1732.

119. Scappaticci FA, Skillings JR, Holden SN, et al. Arterial thromboembolic events in patients with metastatic carcinoma treated with chemotherapy and bevacizumab. *J Natl Cancer Inst*. 2007;99:1232–1239.

120. Saltz LB, Clarke S, Diaz-Rubio E, et al. Bevacizumab in combination with oxaliplatin-based chemotherapy as first-line therapy in metastatic colorectal cancer: a randomized phase III study. *J Clin Oncol*. 2008;26:2013–2019.

121. Purdie DM, Berlin JD, Flynn PJ, et al. The safety of long-term bevacizumab use: results from the BRITE observational cohort study. *J Clin Oncol*. 2008;26:4103 Abstract.

122. Richardson S, Dickler M, Dang C, et al. Tolerance of bevacizumab in an older patient population: the Memorial Sloan-Kettering Cancer Center experience. *J Clin Oncol*. 2008;26: Abstract 519.

123. Sereno M, Brunello A, Chiappori A, et al. Cardiac toxicity: old and new issues in anticancer drugs. *Clin Transl Oncol*. 2008;10:35–46.

124. Nalluri SR, Chu D, Kereszetes R, et al. Risk of venous thromboembolism with the angiogenesis inhibitor bevacizumab in cancer patients: a meta-analysis. *JAMA*. 2008;300:2277–2285.

125. Barlogie B, Desikan R, Eddlemon P, et al. Extended survival in advanced and refractory multiple myeloma after single agent thalidomide: identification of prognostic factors in a phase II study of 169 patients. *Blood*. 2001;98:492–494.

126. Zangari M, Analssie E, Barlogie B, et al. Increased risk of deep-vein thrombosis in patients with multiple myeloma receiving thalidomide and chemotherapy. *Blood*. 2001;98:1614–1615.

127. Zangari M, Siegel E, Barlogie B, et al. Thrombogenic activity of doxorubicin in myeloma patients receiving thalidomide: implications for therapy. *Blood*. 2002;100:1168–1171.

128. Osman K, Comenzo R, Rajkumar SV. Deep vein thrombosis and thalidomide therapy for multiple myeloma. *N Engl J Med*. 2001;344:1951–1952.

129. Urbauer E, Kaufmann H, Nosslinger T, et al. Thromboembolic events during treatment with thalidomide. *Blood*. 2002;99:4247–4248.

130. Desai AA, Vogelzang NJ, Rini B, et al. A phase II trial of weekly intravenous gemcitabine (G) with prolonged continuous infusion 5-fluorouracil (F) and oral thalidomide (T) in patients with metastatic renal cell cancer. *J Clin Oncol*. 2008;20:2448 Abstract.

131. Richardson RG, Blood E, Mitsiades CS, et al. A randomized phase 2 study of lenalidomide therapy for patients with relapsed and refractory multiple myeloma. *Blood*. 2006;108:3458–3464.

132. Chanan-Khan AA, Cheson BD. Lenalidomide for the treatment of B-cell malignancies. *J Clin Oncol*. 2008;26:1544–1552.

133. Schey SA, Fields P, Bartlett JB, et al. Phase I study of an immunomodulatory thalidomide analog, CC-4047, in relapsed or refractory multiple myeloma. *J Clin Oncol*. 2004;22:3269–3276.

134. Pretner-Oblak J, Zaletel M, Jagodic M, et al. Thrombosis of internal carotid artery after cisplatin-based chemotherapy. *Eur Neurol*. 2007;57:109–110.

135. King M, Fernando I. Vascular toxicity associated with cisplatin. *Clin Oncol*. 2003;13:36–37.

136. Monk BJ, Sill MW, Burger RA, et al. Phase II trial of bevacizumab in the treatment of persistent or recurrent squamous cell carcinoma of the cervix: a gynecologic oncology group study. *J Clin Oncol*. 2009;27:1069–1074.

137. Rivkin SE, Green S, Metch B, et al. Adjuvant CMFVP versus tamoxifen versus concurrent CMFVP and tamoxifen for postmenopausal, node-positive, and estrogen receptor-positive breast cancer patients: a Southwest Oncology Group study. *J Clin Oncol*. 1994;12:2078–2085.

138. Agnelli G, Verso M, Ageno W, et al. The MASTER registry of venous thromboembolism: description of the study cohort. *Thromb Res*. 2008;121:605–610.

139. Wells PS, Owen C, Doucette S, et al. Does this patient have deep vein thrombosis? *JAMA*. 2006;295:199–207.

140. Torbicki A, Perrier A, Konstantinides SV, et al. Guidelines on the diagnosis and management of acute pulmonary embolism: the Task Force for the Diagnosis and Management of Acute Pulmonary Embolism of the European Society of Cardiology (ESC). *Eur Heart J*. 2008;29:2276–2315.

141. Konstantinides S. Acute pulmonary embolism. *N Engl J Med*. 2008;359:2804–2813.

142. Hutten BA, Prins MH, Gent M, et al. Incidence of recurrent thromboembolic and bleeding complications among patients with venous thromboembolism in relation to both malignancy and achieved international normalized ratio: a retrospective analysis. *J Clin Oncol*. 2000;18:3078–3083.

143. Palumbo A, Rajkumar SV, Dimopoulos MA, et al. Prevention of thalidomide- and lenalidomide-associated thrombosis in myeloma. *Leukemia*. 2008;22:414–423.

144. Alikhan R, Cohen AT, Combe S, et al. Prevention of venous thromboembolism in medical patients with enoxaparin: a subgroup analysis of the MEDOXOX study. *Blood Coagul Fibrinolysis*. 2003;12:341–346.

145. Levine M, Hirsh J, Gent M, et al. Double-blind randomized trial of a very low-dose warfarin for prevention of venous thromboembolism in stage IV breast cancer. *Lancet*. 1994;343:886–889.

146. Lyman GH, Khormana AA, Falanga A, et al. American Society of Clinical Oncology guideline: recommendations for venous thromboembolism prophylaxis and treatment in patients with cancer. *J Clin Oncol*. 2007;25:5490–5505.

147. Lee AYY, Rickles FR, Julian JA, et al. Randomized comparison of low molecular-weight heparin and coumarin derivatives on the survival of patients with cancer and venous thromboembolism. *J Clin Oncol*. 2005;23:2123–2129.

148. Kakkar AK, Levine MN, Kadziola Z, et al. Low molecular weight heparin, therapy with dalteparin, and survival in advanced cancer: the Fragmin Advanced Malignancy Outcome Study (FAMOUS). *J Clin Oncol*. 2004;22:1944–1948.

149. Klerk CPW, Smorenburg SM, Otten J.M.M.B., et al. *Malignancy and low-molecular-weight heparin therapy: the MALT trial*. Presented at: International Society of Thrombosis and Haemostasis XIX International Congress; Birmingham, UK: July 12–18; 2003.

150. Lee AYY, Levine MN, Baker RI, et al. Low-molecular-weight heparin versus a coumarin for the prevention of recurrent venous thromboembolism in patients with cancer. *N Engl J Med*. 2003;349:146–153.

151. Carrier M, Lee AYY. Prophylactic and therapeutic anticoagulation for thrombosis—major issues in oncology. *Nat Clin Pract Oncol*. 2009;6:74–84.

152. Early Breast Cancer Trialists' Collaborative Group (EBCTCG). Effects of chemotherapy and hormonal therapy for early breast cancer on recurrence and 15-year survival: an overview of the randomized trials. *Lancet*. 2005;365:1687–1717.

153. Mouridsen H, Keshaviah A, Coates AS, et al. Cardiovascular adverse events during adjuvant endocrine therapy for early breast cancer using letrozole or tamoxifen safety analysis of BIG 1–98 trial. *J Clin Oncol*. 2007;25:5715–5722.

154. Boccardo F, Rubagotti A, Puntoni M, et al. Switching to anastrozole vs. continued tamoxifen treatment of early breast cancer: preliminary results of the Italian Tamoxifen Anastrozole Trial. *J Clin Oncol*. 2005;23:5138–5147.

155. Elisaf MS, Bairaktari ET, Nicolaides C, et al. Effect of letrozole on the lipid profile in postmenopausal women with breast cancer. *Eur J Cancer*. 2001;37:1510–1513.

156. Kataja V, Hietanen P, Joensuu H, et al. The effects of adjuvant anastrozole, exemestane, tamoxifen, and toremifene on serum lipid in postmenopausal breast cancer patientsa preliminary study. *Eur J Cancer*. 2004; (suppl 2):143.

157. Duvic M, Martin AG, Kim Y, et al. Phase 2 and 3 clinical trial of oral bexarotene (Targretin capsules) for the treatment of refractory or persistent early-stage cutaneous t-cell lymphoma. *Arch Dermatol*. 2001;137:581–593.

158. Straus DJ, Duvic M, Kuzel T, et al. Results of a phase II trial of oral bexarotene (Targretin) combined with interferon alfa-2b (Intron-A) for patients with cutaneous T-cell lymphoma. *Cancer*. 2007;109:1799–1803.

159. Guglin M, Aljayah M, Salyad S, et al. Introducing a new entity: chemotherapy-induced arrhythmia. *Europace*. 2009;11:1579–1586.

160. Storniolo AM, Allerheiligen SR, Pearce HL. Preclinical, pharmacologic and phase I studies of gemcitabine. *Semin Oncol*. 1997;24(suppl 2): S72–S77.

161. Santini D, Tonini G, Abbate A, et al. Gemcitabine-induced atrial fibrillation: a hitherto unreported manifestation of drug toxicity. *Ann Oncol*. 2000;11:479–481.

162. Ferrari D, Carbone C, Codeca C, et al. Gemcitabine and atrial fibrillation: a rare manifestation of chemotherapy toxicity. *Anticancer Drugs*. 2006;17:359–361.

163. Tavil Y, Arslan K, Sen N, et al. Atrial fibrillation induced by gemcitabine treatment in a 65 year old man. *Onkologie*. 2007;30:253–255.

164. Shah M, Binkley P, Chan K, et al. Cardiotoxicity of histone deacetylase inhibitor depsipeptide in patients with metastatic neuroendocrine tumors. *Clin Cancer Res.* 2006;12:3997–4003.

165. Pierkarrz RL, Frye R, Wright JJ, et al. Cardiac studies in patients treated with depsipeptide, FK228, in a phase II trial for T-cell lymphoma. *Clin Cancer Res.* 2006;80:3762–3772.

166. Rowinsky EK, McGuire WP, Guaerlieri T, et al. Cardiac disturbances during the administration of paclitaxel. *J Clin Oncol.* 2000;22:1029–1033.

167. Ohnishi K, Yoshida H, Shigeno K, et al. Prolongation of the QT interval and ventricular tachycardia in patients treated with arsenic trioxide for acute promyelocytic leukemia. *Ann Intern Med.* 2000;133:881–886.

168. Wesrrevelt P, Brown RA, Adkins DR, et al. Sudden death among patients with acute promyelocytic leukemia treated with arsenic trioxide. *Blood.* 2001;98:266–271.

169. Barbey J, Pezzulllo J, Soignet S. Effect of arsenic trioxide on QT interval in patients with advanced malignancies. *J Clin Oncol.* 2003;21:3609–3615.

170. Huang CH, Chen WJ, Wu CC, et al. Complete atrioventricular block after arsenic trioxide treatment in an acute promyelocytic leukemia patient. *Pacing Clin Electrophysiol.* 1999;22:965–967.

171. Keefe DL. The cardiotoxic potential of the 5-HT$_3$ receptor antagonist antiemetics: is there cause for concern? *Oncologist.* 2002;7:65–72.

172. Navari RM, Koeller JM. Electrocardiographic and cardiovascular effects of the 5-hydroxytryptamine$_3$ receptor antagonists. *Ann Pharmacother.* 2003;37:1276–1286.

173. De Ponti F, Poluzzi E, Cavalli A, et al. Safety of non-antiarrhythmic drugs that prolong the QT interval or induce torsade de pointes. *Drugs.* 2002;21:263–286.

174. Frothingham R. Rates of torsade de pointes associated with ciprofloxacin, ofloxacin, levofloxacin, gatifloxacin, and moxifloxacin. *Pharmacotherapy.* 2001;21:1468–1472.

175. Heidenreich PA, Hancock SL, Lee BK, et al. Asymptomatic cardiac disease following mediastinal irradiation. *J Am Coll Cardiol.* 2003;42:743–749.

176. Adams MJ, Hardenbergh PH, Constine LS, et al. Radiation-associated cardiovascular disease. *Crit Rev Oncol Hematol.* 2003;45:55–75.

177. Glanzmann C, Kaufmann P, Jenni R, et al. Cardiac risk after mediastinal irradiation for Hodgkin's disease. *Radiother Oncol.* 1998;46:51–62.

178. Prosnitz RG, Chen YH, Marks LB. Cardiac toxicity following thoracic radiation. *Semin Oncol.* 2005;32:S71–S80.

179. Hull MC, Morris CG, Pepine CJ, et al. Valvular dysfunction and carotid, subclavian, and coronary artery disease in survivors of Hodgkin lymphoma treated with radiation therapy. *JAMA.* 2003;290:2831–2837.

180. Heidenreich PA, Schnittger I, Strauss HW, et al. Screening for coronary artery disease after mediastinal irradiation for Hodgkin's disease. *J Clin Oncol.* 2007;25:43–49.

181. Hull MC, Morris CG, Pepine CJ, et al. Valvular dysfunction and carotid, subclavian, and coronary artery disease in survivors of Hodgkin's lymphoma treated with radiation therapy. *JAMA.* 2003;290:2831–2837.

182. Heidenreich PA, Hancock SL, Vagelos RH, et al. Diastolic dysfunction following mediastinal irradiation. *Am Heart J.* 2005;150:977–982.

183. Boivin J-F, Hutchison G, Lubin J, et al. Coronary artery disease mortality in patients treated for Hodgkin's disease. *Cancer.* 1992;69:1241–1247.

184. Glanzmann C, Kaufmann P, Jenni R, et al. Cardiac risk after mediastinal irradiation for Hodgkin's disease. *Radiother Oncol.* 1998;46:51–62.

185. Giordano SH, Kuo YF, Freeman JL, et al. Risk of cardiac death after adjuvant radiotherapy for breast cancer. *J Natl Cancer Inst.* 2005;97:419–424.

186. Hancock SL, Donaldson SS, Hoppe RT. Cardiac disease following treatment of Hodgkin's disease in children and adolescents. *J Clin Oncol.* 1993;11:1208–1215.

187. Heidenreich PA, Kapoor JR. Radiation induced heart disease. *Heart.* 2009;95:252–258.

188. Cuzick J, Stewart H, Rutqvist L, et al. Cause-specific mortality in long-term survivors of breast cancer who participated in trials of radiotherapy. *J Clin Oncol.* 1994;12:447–453.

189. Jones JM, Ribeiro GG. Mortality patterns over 34 years of breast cancer patients in a clinical trial of post-operative radiotherapy. *Clin Radiol.* 1989;40:204–208.

190. Paszat LF, Mackillop WJ, Groome PA, et al. Mortality from myocardial infarction after adjuvant radiotherapy for breast cancer in the surveillance, epidemiology, and end-results cancer registries. *J Clin Oncol.* 1998;16:2625–2631.

191. Nixon AJ, Manola J, Gelman R, et al. No long-term increase in cardiac-related mortality after breast-conserving surgery and radiation therapy using modern techniques. *J Clin Oncol.* 1998;16:1374–1379.

192. Patt DA, Goodwin JS, Kuo YF, et al. Cardiac morbidity of adjuvant radiotherapy for breast cancer. *J Clin Oncol.* 2005;23:7475–7482.

193. Vallis KA, Pintilie M, Chong N, et al. Assessment of coronary heart disease morbidity and mortality after radiation therapy for early breast cancer. *J Clin Oncol.* 2002;20:1036–1042.

194. Harris EE, Correa C, Hwang WT, et al. Late cardiac mortality and morbidity in early-stage breast cancer patients after breast-conservation treatment. *J Clin Oncol.* 2006;24:4100–4106.

195. Correa CR, Litt HI, Hwang WT, et al. Coronary artery findings after left-sided compared to right-sided radiation treatment for early stage breast cancer. *J Clin Oncol.* 2007;25:3031–3037.

196. Ng AK, Constine LS, Deming RL, et al. *American College of Radiology appropriateness criteria: follow-up of Hodgkin's disease.* Reston, VA: Department of Quality and Safety, ACH; 2005. Available at: http:www.acr.org/SecondaryMainMenuCategories/quality_safety/app_criteria/pdf/rtPanelonRadiationOncologyHodgkinsWorkGroup/FollowUpofHodgkinsDiseaseDoc2.asp.

197. Handa N, McGregor CGA, Daly RC, et al. Heart transplantation for radiation-associated end stage heart failure. *Trans Int.* 2000;13:162–165.

198. Romano MA, Patel HJ, Pagoni FD, et al. Anterior leaflet repair with patch augmentation for mitral regurgitation. *Ann Thorac Surg.* 2005;79:1500–1504.

199. Crestanenello JA, McGregor CGA, Danielson GK, et al. Mitral and tricuspid valve repair in patients with previous mediastinal radiation therapy. *Ann Thorac Surg.* 2004;78:826–831.

200. Veeragandham RS, Goldin MD. Surgical management of radiation-induced heart disease. *Ann Thorac Surg.* 1998;65:1014–1019.

201. Gansera B, Schmidtler F, Angelis I, et al. Quality of the internal thoracic artery grafts after mediastinal radiation. *Ann Thorac Surg.* 2007;34:1479–1484.

202. Handa N, McGregor CGA, Danielson GK, et al. Coronary artery bypass grafting in patients with previous mediastinal radiation therapy. *J Thorac Cardiovasc Surg.* 1999;117:1136–1143.

203. Tamura A, Takahara Y, Mogi K, et al. Radiation-induced valvular disease is the logical consequence of irradiation. *Gen Thorac Cardiovasc Surg.* 2007;55:53–56.

204. Chang ASY, Smedira NG, Chang CL, et al. Cardiac surgery after mediastinal radiation: extent of exposure influences outcome. *J Thorac Cardiovasc Surg.* 2007;133:404–413.

205. De Bruin ML, Dorresteijn LD, van't Veer MB, et al. Increased risk of stroke and transient ischemic attack in 5-year survivors of Hodgkin lymphoma. *J Natl Cancer Inst.* 2009;101:928–937.

206. Morris B, Partap S, Yeom K, et al. Cerebrovascular disease in childhood cancer survivors. A Children's Oncology Group Report. *Neurology.* 2009;73:1906–1913.

207. Yorke ED, Jackson A, Rosenszweig KE, et al. Dose-volume factors contributing to the incidence of radiation pneumonitis in no small cell cancer patients treated with three-dimensional conformal radiation therapy. *Int J Radiat Oncol Phys.* 2002;54:329–339.

208. Abratt RP, Ong FT, Morgan GW, et al. Pulmonary complications of radiation therapy. *Clin Chest Med.* 2004;25:167–177.

209. Brady LW, Germon PA, Cander L. The effects of radiation therapy on pulmonary function in carcinoma of the lung. *Radiology.* 1965;85:130–134.

210. Marks LB. The pulmonary effects of thoracic irradiation. *Oncology.* 1994;8:89–100.

211. McDonald S, Rubin P, Phillips TL, et al. Injury to the lung from cancer therapy: clinical syndromes, measurable endpoints, and potential scoring systems. *Int J Radiat Oncol Biol Phys.* 1995;31:1187–1203.

212. Garipagalou M, Munley MT, Hollis D, et al. The effect of patient specific factors on radiation induced lung injury. *Int J Radiat Oncol Biol Phys.* 1999;45:3331–3338.

213. Roach M, Grandara DR, You HS, et al. Radiation pneumonitis following combined modality therapy for lung cancer: analysis of prognostic factors. *J Clin Oncol.* 1995;13:2606–2612.

214. Dechambre S, Dorzee J, Fastrez J, et al. Bronchial stenosis and sclerosing mediastinitis: an uncommon complication of external thoracic radiotherapy. *Eur Respir J.* 1998;11:1188–1190.

215. Hirsch A, Vander els N, Strauss DJ, et al. Effect of ABVD chemotherapy with and without mantle or mediastinal radiation on pulmonary function in early stage Hodgkin's disease. *J Clin Oncol.* 1996;14:1297–1305.

216. Zhao L, Sheldon K, Chen M, et al. The predictive role of plasma TGF-β1 during radiation therapy for radiation-induced lung toxicity deserves further study in patients with non-small cell lung cancer. *Lung Cancer.* 2008;59:232–239.

217. Yahalon J, Portlock CS. Long-term cardiac and pulmonary complications of cancer therapy. *Hematol Oncol Clin North Am.* 2008;22:305–318.

218. Mao J, Oluwatoyosi A, Fatunase, et al. Cytoprotection for radiation-associated normal tissue injury. *Radiat Oncol Adv.* 2008;139:302–322.

219. Hensley ML, Hagerty KL, Kewalramani T, et al. American Society of Clinical Oncology 2008 clinical practice guideline update: use of chemotherapy and radiation therapy protectants. *J Clin Oncol.* 2009;27:127–145.

220. Limper AH. Chemotherapy-induced lung disease. *Clin Chest Med.* 2004;25:53–64.

221. Vahid B, Marik PE. Pulmonary complications of novel antineoplastic agents for solid tumors. *Chest*. 2008;133:528–538.

222. Dimopoulou I, Bamias A, Lyberpoulos P, et al. Pulmonary toxicity from novel antineoplastic agents. *Ann Oncol*. 2005;17:373–379.

223. Shimura T, Kuse N, Yoshinto T, et al. Clinical features of interstitial lung disease induced by standard chemotherapy (FOLFOX or FOLFARI) for colo-rectal cancer. *Ann Oncol*. 2010; March.

224. Liu V, White DA, Zakowski MF, et al. Pulmonary toxicity associated with erlotinib. *Chest*. 2009;132:1042–1044.

225. Camus P, Fanton A, Bonniaud P, et al. Interstitial lung disease induced by drugs and radiation. *Respiration*. 2004;71:301–326.

226. Takano T, Ohe Y, Kusumoto M, et al. Risk factors for interstitial lung disease and predictive factors for tumor response in patients with advanced non-small cell lung cancer treated with gefitinib. *Lung Cancer*. 2004;45:93–104.

227. Kudoh S, Kato H, Nishiwaki Y, et al. Interstitial ling disease in Japanese patients with lung cancer: a cohort and nested case-control study. *Am J Respir Crit Care Med*. 2008;177:1348–1357.

228. White DA, Stover DE. Severe bleomycin-induced pneumonitis: clinical features and response to corticosteroids. *Chest*. 1984;86:723–728.

229. Maher J, Daly PA. Severe bleomycin lung toxicity: reversal with high dose corticosteroids. *Thorax*. 1993;48:92–94.

230. Sleijfer S. Bleomycin-induced pneumonitis. *Chest*. 2001;120:617–624.

231. Simpson AB, Paul J, Graham J, et al. Fatal bleomycin pulmonary toxicity in the west of Scotland 1991–95: a review of patients with germ cell tumours. *Br J Cancer*. 1998;78:1061–1066.

232. Koschel D, Handzhiev S, Leucht V, et al. Hypersensitivity pneumonitis associated with the use of temzolomide. *Eur Respir J*. 2009;33:931–934.

233. Muller NL, White DA, Gemma A. Diagnosis and management of drug-associated interstitial lung disease. *Brit J Cancer*. 2004;91(suppl 2):524–530.

234. Hupt HM, Hutchins GM, Moore GW. Ara-C lung: noncardiogenic pulmonary edema complicating cytosine arabinoside therapy of leukemia. *Am J Med*. 1981;70:256–261.

235. Briasoulis E, Pavlidis N. Noncardiogenic pulmonary edema: an unusual and serious complication of anticancer therapy. *Oncologist*. 2001;6:153–161.

236. Antony VB, Loddenkemper R, Astoul P, et al. Management of malignant pleural effusions. *Eur Respir J*. 2001;18:402–419.

237. Dimopoulou I, Galani H, Dafni U, et al. A prospective study of pulmonary function in patients treated with paclitaxel and carboplatin. *Cancer*. 2002;94:452–458.

238. O'Driscoll BR, Hasleton PS, Taylor PM, et al. Active lung fibrosis up to 17 years after chemotherapy with carmustine (BCNU) in childhood. *N Engl J Med*. 1990;323:378–382.

239. Alvarado CS, Boat TF, Newman AJ. Late-onset pulmonary fibrosis and chest deformity in two children treated with cyclophosphamide. *J Pediatr*. 1978;92:443–446.

240. Codling BW, Chakera TM. Pulmonary fibrosis following therapy with melphalan for multiple myeloma. *J Clin Pathol*. 1972;25:668–673.

241. Chan CK, Hayland RH, Hutcheon MA. Pulmonary complications following bone marrow transplantation. *Clin Chest Med*. 1990;11:323–332.

242. Wah TM, Moss HA, Robertson RJ, et al. Pulmonary complications following bone marrow transplantation. *Br J Radiol*. 2003;76:373–379.

Gonadal function after cancer treatment

10

Jan Oldenburg, Cecilie Kiserud, Henriette Magelssen, Marianne Brydøy, and Sophie D. Fosså

Human gonads (i.e., testicles and ovaries) are endocrine organs containing our germ cells. Cancer and its treatment may compromise both endocrine function and chances to generate and foster healthy offspring. In general, cancer is more common in elderly patients for whom fertility preservation might no longer be an issue, whereas younger patients might base their preferred treatment option on in-depth counseling about the risk of infertility.[1]

Gonadotoxicity is an unintended complication of cancer treatment, but in cases of hormone-driven cancers (e.g., those of the breast or of the prostate), complete disruption of endocrine function may be unavoidable. Principally, reduced endocrine gonadal function may be caused by insufficiency of the gonad (i.e., primary hypogonadism) or by insufficient hormonal stimulation (i.e., secondary hypogonadism). In this chapter, we provide an overview of different aspects of gonadal toxicity in cancer treatment.

NORMAL GONADAL FUNCTION

MALES

The two main functions of the testicles are production of sperm and production of testosterone (i.e., endocrine and exocrine). Gonadotropin-releasing hormone (GnRH) is produced in the hypothalamus, and its oscillating levels stimulate the production of luteinizing hormone (LH) and follicle-stimulating hormone (FSH) in the anterior pituitary gland and their release to the bloodstream.

Sperm cells (spermatozoa) are continuously produced by the testicular germinal epithelium, and maturation of spermatogonias to mature sperm cells takes approximately 70 days. New cycles of spermatogenesis are initiated at regular time intervals (every 2–3 weeks) before the previous ones are completed. FSH and testosterone stimulate the Sertoli cells to provide hormonal and nutritional support for spermatogenesis.[2,3] Sertoli cells, regulated by FSH and spermatogenic status, secrete inhibin B, which limits FSH secretion through a negative feedback mechanism.[4] In the adult, serum inhibin B levels correlate with total sperm count and testicular volume. Therefore, both FSH and inhibin B are considered useful markers of spermatogenesis. Spermatogenesis is usually evaluated by semen analyses, but in some cases, a testicular biopsy may be required.

Testosterone production, the principal testicular endocrine function, is prone to an age-related decrease. Testosterone is mostly bound to circulating plasma proteins: 40% to 50% is loosely bound to albumin, 50% to 60% is bound tightly to sexual hormone–binding globulin (SHBG), and only 1% to 2% represents free testosterone. The latter and the albumin-bound testosterone fraction form the effective pool determining the biological activity of testosterone. Because the amount of SHBG increases by age, the decrease in free serum testosterone is more pronounced than the total testosterone concentration.[5]

FEMALES

Female germ cells, as opposed to their male counterparts, do not proliferate post partum. At birth, the ovaries contain 1 to 2 million primordial follicles, most of which are destined to regression by a process called *follicular atresia*. From menarche to menopause, only 400 to 500 of the remaining 400,000 follicles are progressively released, whereas roughly 1000 per month are lost by apoptosis. By the age of 50, about 1000 remain; thus chances of natural conception are markedly reduced already, some years before menopause.

Each oocyte remains in meiotic division from birth to ovulation. Interplay of a follicular two-cell system regulates the generation of steroidal hormones and follicular growth. LH and FSH stimulate cells of the theca and granulosa to produce and secrete estrogen, whereas initiation of follicular maturation is promoted by paracrine growth factors. A growth-stimulated follicle develops over a 3-month period until the time of degeneration or ovulation.

Reduced numbers of follicles increase the risk of premature ovarian failure (POF), defined as menopause before 40 years of age in combination with low estrogen levels. A low oocyte reserve may decrease the chance of subsequent conception, despite a normal menstrual cycle.[6] The number of remaining oocytes determines the tolerance of the ovaries toward an injury, ranging from continuously normal function to immediate loss of function.

Even before the occurrence of POF, periods of transient amenorrhea may alternate with periods of apparently normal function. Menopause (i.e., the end of menstruation) defines the end of reproductive capability, but female fertility begins to decline already by the age of 30 years. The trend in the Western world to postpone pregnancy to the 30s contributes to the increasing demand for assisted reproduction techniques. For many women, the time required for diagnosis and treatment of their malignancy and subsequent recovery can reduce the chances of motherhood, because already by the age of 40 years, natural and artificial conception may be hampered by decreasing follicle numbers and oocyte quality. Simultaneously with lower chances of pregnancy, the risks of aneuploidy and abortion are increased.

GONADAL FUNCTION AND CANCER

Cancer itself, and sometimes susceptibility to develop a malignancy, may impair gonadal function. Occult ovarian dysfunction may be associated with *BRCA* mutations.[7] Thus, women with *BRCA*-associated breast cancer may experience a higher infertility risk already, before undergoing cancer treatment.[7] Men requiring artificial reproduction techniques are estimated to have an almost 20 times higher incidence of testicular cancer as compared with men without infertility problems.[8] For men with testicular cancer and Hodgkin's lymphoma, reduced spermatogenesis as compared with the general population before the time of diagnosis has been reported.[9,10]

In testicular cancer patients, Skakkebaek et al hypothesize a testicular dysgenesis syndrome, comprising low sperm count, hypospadias, and cryptorchidism.[11] The association between decreased male fertility and testicular cancer is well documented,[12] and about half of patients diagnosed with testicular cancer have reduced spermatogenesis after orchiectomy before receiving additional treatment.[13] Furthermore, biopsies have revealed that 24% of patients with unilateral testicular cancer probably have irreversibly impaired spermatogenesis in the contralateral testicle.[14]

POSTTREATMENT GONADAL FUNCTION

Cancer treatment is changing over time, and evaluation of its gonadotoxic effects, particularly on the parenthood rate, requires sufficiently long follow-up. Therefore, published observations related to these topics often pertain to yesterday's treatment and do not take into account risk-adapted treatment options attempted today, particularly in the youngest patients.

MALES
Chemotherapy

Gonadotoxic effects of cytostatic drugs hinge on several factors, among them the type of chemotherapy, the cumulative doses, the time since treatment, and the pretreatment fertility of the patient.[6] Alkylating agents (cyclophosphamide, ifosfamide, chlorambucil, nitrosoureas, melphalan, busulfan, and procarbazine) are the most gonadotoxic cytostatic drugs (Table 10-1).

The so-called "blood–testis barrier" refers to an intratubular nutritional germ cell compartment formed by Sertoli cells. However, blood vessels at that site are permeable, and cytostatic drugs reach intratubular cells (i.e., Leydig and Sertoli

Table 10-1 Expected gonadotoxicity of chemotherapy regimens

High	Medium	Low	Unknown
procarbazine	cisplatin	methotrexate	trastuzumab
cyclophosphamide	carboplatin	Adriamycin	(herceptin)
nitrogen mustard	oxaliplatin	prednisolone	docetaxel
chlorambucil	BEP	doxorubicin	(taxaner)
mechlorethamine	CHOP	vincristine	monoclonal
ifosfamide		vinblastine	antibodies
busulfan		5-FU	
MOPP		bleomycin	
MVPP		ABVD	
ChIVPP			
MOPP/ABVD			
COPP/ABVD			
COPP			
HDT			

ABVD, Doxorubicin, bleomycin, vinblastine, dacarbazine; *BEP*, bleomycin, etoposide, cisplatin; *ChIVPP*, chlorambucil, vinblastine, prednisolone, procarbazine; *CHOP*, cyclophosphamide, doxorubicin, vincristine, prednisolone; *CMF*, cyclophosphamide, methotrexate, 5-FU; *COPP*, cyclophosphamide, vincristine, procarbazine, prednisolone; *FEC*, cyclophosphamide, epirubicin, 5-FU; *5-FU*, 5-fluorouracil; *HDT*, high-dose chemotherapy with autologous stem cell support; *MOPP*, nitrogen mustard, vincristine, procarbazine, prednisolone; *MVPP*, mustine, vinblastine, procarbazine, prednisolone.

cells) and may affect spermatogonia. Consequently, sperm production is reduced after many types of chemotherapy. However, because late-stage germ cells are less sensitive to cytotoxic treatment than early-stage germ cells, it may take weeks until an effect on spermatogenesis is observable by sperm counts. Recovery of spermatogenesis relies on the ability of spermatogonial stem cells to survive drug toxicity and to retain the potential to differentiate to spermatocytes.

In unilaterally orchiectomized long-term survivors of testicular cancer, the prevalence of primary hypogonadism, as defined by LH levels > 12 IU/l and/or testosterone < 8 nmol/l, increases with treatment intensity.[15] Hypogonadism was observed in 19% and 27% of testicular cancer (TC) survivors after ≤ 850 mg and > 850 mg cisplatin, respectively, as compared with 9% of those who underwent surgery only (Fig. 10-1). Almost one third of male lymphoma survivors are hypogonadal, with risk increasing by age >50 years, with treatment with alkylating agents, and with high-dose chemotherapy with autologous stem cell support.[16]

Sperm production recovers in approximately 80% of TC patients after cisplatin-based chemotherapy within 2 years after treatment.[17] Among TC survivors attempting fatherhood, the likelihood of succeeding correlates with treatment intensity: Those requiring chemotherapy have inferior fatherhood rates compared with those who were cured by surveillance, retroperitoneal lymph node dissection, or radiotherapy only (Fig. 10-2).[18]

Elevated FSH was reported in roughly one third of males treated for early-stage Hodgkin's lymphoma (HL).[19] The probability of elevated FSH increased after treatment with alkylating agents, with age over 50 years at treatment, and with stage II versus stage I disease. After treatment with CHOP (cyclophosphamide, hydroxydaunorubicin, Oncovin [vincristine], and prednisone/prednisolone)-like chemotherapy

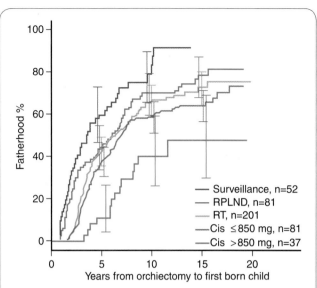

Fig. 10-2 Actuarial posttreatment fatherhood rates for testicular cancer survivors attempting conception by natural means according to treatment groups (*P* < .001, two-sided log-rank test). *cis,* Cisplatin; *RPLND,* retroperitoneal lymph node dissection; *RT,* radiotherapy. Vertical bars indicate 95% confidence intervals. *(Redrawn from Brydoy M, Fossa SD, Klepp O, Bremnes RM, Wist EA, Wentzel-Larsen T, et al. Paternity following treatment for testicular cancer. J Natl Cancer Inst 2005;97:1580–1588.)*

for non-Hodgkin's lymphoma, spermatogenesis is reported to recover in about two thirds of patients,[20] whereas approximately 80% of TC patients will have sperm production after cisplatin-based chemotherapy within 2 years after treatment.[17]

High-dose chemotherapy with stem cell support will render most patients infertile.[21]

Radiotherapy

The gonadotoxic effect of radiation therapy depends on dose, fractionation, and site of radiotherapy. Cranial radiation in doses of 40 to 70 Gy (e.g., for brain tumor) may cause hypogonadotropic hypogonadism (secondary hypogonadism) and is seen in up to 61% of patients.[21a,21b] Sperm cells are highly radiosensitive and may be damaged by direct or scattered radiation to the testicles. The latter effect is observed, for example, in radiotherapy for prostate, bladder, or rectal cancer, with irradiation given in doses of 0.4% to 18.7% of the target dose during treatment.[22–24]

The testicles, as opposed to most other organs, appear to tolerate single doses of radiation better than fractionated radiotherapy. The lowest sperm counts after radiotherapy are usually observed 4 to 6 months after treatment. Duration of oligozoospermia depends on the applied dose, and recovery of spermatogenesis can be expected 9 to 18 months after unfractionated radiation doses of 1 Gy or less to the testicles, 30 months after doses of 2 to 3 Gy, and 5 years or longer after doses of 4 Gy and above, whereas radiation doses of 4 Gy and above may result in permanent azoospermia.[25,26] However, recovery of spermatogenesis is reported in 15% of patients receiving single doses of 8 Gy as total body irradiation before

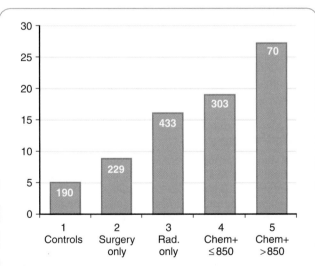

Fig. 10-1 Percentage of testicular cancer survivors (TCSs) with hypogonadism as defined by serum testosterone <8 nmol/l and/or LH >12 IU/l. Controls, Age-matched males from the normal population; Surgery only, TCSs treated by surgery only; Rad. only, TCSs treated by radiotherapy only; Chem+ ≤850 mg/>850 mg, TCSs treated by chemotherapy with a cumulative cisplatin dose ≤850 mg/>850 mg. *(Data from Nord et al [2003],[15] with permission by the authors.)*

bone marrow transplantation,[27] and recovery from azoospermia has been observed as long as 9 years after treatment.[27]

Pelvic radiotherapy with 46 to 50 Gy for rectal cancer results in testicular doses between 3.7 and 13.7 Gy and causes a 100% increase in serum FSH, a 70% increase in LH, and a 25% reduction in testosterone levels among men with a median age of 65 years.[28] Thus, irradiation of the prostate is more often associated with hypogonadism than with radical prostatectomy.[29] External beam radiotherapy with 70 Gy, as opposed to surgery, led to a decline of total and free testosterone levels by 27.3% and 31.6%, respectively, and LH and FSH increased by roughly 50% and 100%, respectively. The effect on gonadotropin levels was most significant in men older than 70 years. Scatter radiation is increased when inguinal lymph nodes are included in the radiation field for prostate cancer; the resulting decreased testosterone values may actually unfold a therapeutic effect.[30]

Radiotherapy for prostate, bladder, or rectal cancer may result in scattered irradiation in doses of 0.4% to 18.7 % of the target dose during treatment.[22–24] However, most men in their middle and late 60s do not attempt to achieve fatherhood, and impaired spermatogenesis is usually not considered a problem for most of these patients.

Some gonadotoxic effects of radiotherapy cannot be assessed by sperm count or hormone levels. DNA integrity of sperm may be compromised after irradiation: Ståhl et al[31] demonstrated DNA damage in 38% of normospermic testicular cancer patients 1 to 2 years after irradiation of infradiaphragmatic para-aortic and ipsilateral iliac lymph nodes (i.e., so-called hockey stick field) as compared with 7% in healthy controls. The radiotherapy dose of 25.2 Gy was applied in 14 fractions, and the contralateral testicle, shielded by lead, probably did not receive more than 0.5 Gy (i.e., <2% of target dose). It is intriguing that the proportion of spermatogonia with damaged DNA decreased approximately 2 years after radiation.

Surgery

Bilateral orchiectomy, which sometimes is performed as treatment for metastatic prostate cancer, is probably the most dramatic surgery with regard to gonadotoxicity. Its many consequences illustrate the importance of endocrine testicular functioning.

Unilateral orchiectomy, the first step in treatment of testicular cancer, usually does not necessitate hormone replacement therapy nor assisted reproduction techniques, but may be indicated in men with insufficient function of the remaining contralateral testicle. Contralateral testicular cancer, which occurs in 2% to 5% of patients, may be cured by organ sparing surgery and postoperative radiation.[32]

Hormonal Cancer Treatment

Typically, hormonal treatment aims at abolishing or at least minimizing stimulatory effects on the cancer by testosterone. This is principally achieved by interaction with the hypothalamic-pituitary-gonadal axis or by blocking of peripheral testosterone receptors. Gonadotropin-releasing hormone (GnRH) agonists, also known as luteinizing hormone–releasing hormone (LHRH) agonists (e.g., leuprolide, goserelin), by abolishing the oscillating binding of its natural analog, reduce testosterone to castrate levels. However, this effect requires

1 to 2 weeks, during which a surge of LH and FSH initially increases testosterone levels. GnRH antagonists should not release gonadotropins and therefore are probably better tolerated by prostate cancer patients. Chemical castration reduces sexual desire and erectile function and leads to testicular atrophy, which may become irreversible over the long term.

Oral nonsteroidal antiandrogens (i.e., substances like flutamide, bicalutamide, cyproterone acetate, or nilutamide) block androgen receptors, causing a rise in FSH and LH and thereby also in serum testosterone.[33] These drugs are applied to patients with prostate cancer, either as monotherapy or concomitant with LHRH. When given as monotherapy, impotence and loss of libido are significantly lower as compared with LHRH agonists, and sexual activity and morning erections may be preserved in 1 of 5 patients.[34]

FEMALES
Chemotherapy

In females, chemotherapy may cause loss of germ cells, probably through induction of apoptosis, leading to a reduction in the number of primordial follicles to fewer than the minimum required for cyclic menstruations. Permanent amenorrhea is observed by the patient and often is used to document gonadotoxicity. In cancer patients, however, hypothalamic activity and estrogen metabolism altered by malnutrition, weight loss, or stress may also mimic gonadotoxicity-related amenorrhea. Detailed data on the risk of POF or compromised fertility due to decreased ovarian reserve are sparse. Permanent amenorrhea was observed in 20% of women after ABVD (doxorubicin, bleomycin, vinblastine, dacarbazine) or four to six cycles of CHOP.[6] The impact of age on the risk of permanent amenorrhea can be observed in breast cancer survivors who received six cycles of FEC (5-fluorouracil, epirubicin, and cyclophosphamide) as adjuvant treatment: high (>80%) risk at age > 40 years, medium risk for women in their 30s, and low risk (<20%) at <30 years.[6] Approximately 37% of female survivors of Hodgkin's lymphoma experienced POF within 10 years of follow-up; a clear association was noted between POF and use of alkylating agents.[35] High-dose chemotherapy with stem cell support will render most patients infertile.[21] The combination of infradiaphragmatic radiotherapy with chemotherapy does aggravate gonadotoxicity.

Radiotherapy

The gonadotoxic effect of radiation therapy hinges mainly on the patient's age and on the dose, fractionation, and site of radiotherapy. As opposed to the testicles, the ovaries suffer less damage when radiation dose is given fractionated rather than as a single nonfractionated dose.

The high number of follicles in prepubertal girls and adolescents renders their ovaries relatively resistant to radiation-induced damage. Generally, oocytes are less radiosensitive than sperm cells but may be damaged by direct or scattered irradiation. If the ovaries are within the radiation field, a dose of 2 Gy may be enough to destroy half of the follicles.[36] The impact of the patient's age on vulnerability toward radiation is indicated by the doses required to irreversibly damage the ovaries: Whereas 6 Gy may be sufficient in women older than 40 years, 10 to 20 Gy is required in children or adolescents.[37] Total body irradiation usually leads to permanent amenorrhea. Some women, however, particularly the younger ones, may recover ovarian function.[38]

Surgery

Cancer of the genital organs (e.g., ovaries, uterine cervix) may affect women during their reproductive age, and infertility in most cases is inevitable as the genital organs are removed. In women with early-stage cervical cancers, however, laser conization or trachelectomy may preserve fertility.[39] Unilateral salpingo-ophorectomy may be pursued in women with borderline tumors of the ovary.

Hormonal Cancer Treatment

Typically, hormonal treatment aims at abolishing or at least minimizing stimulatory effects on cancer by estrogen. This may be achieved principally by interaction with the hypothalamic-pituitary-gonadal axis, blocking of peripheral estrogen receptors, or inhibition of enzymatic conversion of steroids to estrogen in postmenopausal women.

Gonadotropin-releasing hormone (GnRH) agonists, also known as luteinizing hormone–releasing hormone (LHRH) agonists (e.g., leuprolide, goserelin), produce castrate levels of estrogens by abolishing the oscillating binding of the natural ligand. GnRH agonists may induce several side effects (e.g., an increased rate of sexual dysfunction), but the symptoms usually are reversible on discontinuation of therapy.[40]

Selective estrogen receptor ligands such as tamoxifen are commonly used in the adjuvant setting. Estrogenic effects of amoxifen in the bone help to prevent osteoporosis, whereas its antiestrogenic effects in breast tissue unfold an antitumor effect.

Blocking of estrogen receptors in the hypothalamus causes release of LH and FSH in premenopausal women and results in hyperestrogenemia, whereas in postmenopausal women, already increased FSH and LH gonadotropin levels are reduced by tamoxifen. Aromatase inhibitors decrease estrogen synthesis outside the ovaries and today are considered the standard of hormonal therapy for postmenopausal women with breast cancer.[41]

EFFECTS OF GONADOTOXICITY ON THE OFFSPRING

To the best of the authors' knowledge, an association between cancer treatment–related gonadotoxicity and impaired health of children of parents treated for cancer has not been established. Elucidation of these potential effects is challenging in that the cancer itself, as well as impairment of organs other than the gonads, might account for observable deviations. In women treated by pelvic or spinal radiotherapy, preterm birth and low birthweight were probably due to reduced function of the uterus and other pelvic structures.[42]

However, one of several studies assessing the health of children fathered by cancer survivors reported a slightly increased risk of mild congenital malformations.[43] These findings, however, require corroboration by other studies, as the results are based on only 487 male cancer survivors, among whom 27 children were found to have a congenital anomaly.

PREVENTION OF GONADAL DYSFUNCTION

Even if many cancer patients have restored fertility after treatment, it is not possible to predict recovery in the individual patient. Fertility preservation starts with counseling before treatment about treatment options and their related risks of compromised fertility.[44] Depending on the patient's circumstances, the partner or parents should be included in these discussions. Information about the possibility of a cure and about inherent risks of infertility can be provided by a knowledgeable consulting physician.

MALES

The consequences of orchiectomy for testicular cancer can be reduced by tumor enucleation, if the following conditions are fulfilled: small tumor (i.e., <20 mm), cold ischemia, multiple biopsies of the tumor bed, adjuvant local irradiation postoperatively to avoid local recurrence, close follow-up, and high expected compliance.[32] Postponement of planned testicular radiotherapy can be considered in patients with carcinoma in situ in the remaining testis, to allow repeated sperm cryopreservation and/or natural conception.

So far, pharmacologic methods to protect spermatogenesis during chemotherapy or radiotherapy have not been established. Application of GnRH analogs has been promising in rodents but lacks efficacy in the clinical situation.[45] Testicular shielding, as well as more precise dose application to organs in the vicinity of the testicles, may prevent radiotherapy-induced gonadotoxicity to some degree. Radiotherapy in TC patients has become less common, and reduced radiation doses and target field size should limit damage to the contralateral testicle.[46] Cryopreservation should be offered to all patients who consider future fatherhood before treatment is started.

The diagnostic workup of patients following cancer treatment starts with history taking, including asking the patient about erectile dysfunction (ED) or "dry" ejaculation, followed by a physical examination.[44] The patient should be followed up on a regular basis for a long time, and serum FSH, LH, testosterone levels, and levels of inhibin B should be determined to reveal any signs of primary or secondary hypogonadism. A semen sample is mandatory, provided that patients are able to provide one. In patients with "dry" ejaculation, the postmasturbation urine should be investigated for the presence of sperm cells.

Men with secondary hypogonadism (e.g., after cranial radiotherapy) may recover spermatogenesis after gonadotropin injections, which might be required over up to 2 years.[47] Upon restored sperm production or achieved pregnancy, gonadotropin treatment is discontinued and substitution treatment with testosterone can be started.

Refinements in surgery and pharmacologic interventions developed during recent years to prevent and relieve ejaculatory problems and ED will certainly contribute to fertility preservation.

FEMALES

Preservation of ovarian function by suppression of ovarian activity by GnRH analogs before chemotherapy did not confer any benefit according to two randomized trials, such that this approach is not indicated.[48] Gonadotoxic effects of different cytostatica regimens may, however, vary hugely, such that incorporation of the estimated risks is important for selection of the optimal chemotherapy for younger patients. Transposition of the ovaries outside the planned area of radiation by oophoropexy may help to preserve fertility.[49] The current 5-year survival rate of pediatric malignancy is 70% to 90%, rendering infertility treatment increasingly important. To ensure fertility, oophorectomy or cryopreservation of the ovarian cortex may be performed before cancer treatment is provided.[50]

Before in vitro fertilization, the probability of pregnancy and live birth following treatment should be estimated. The follicle cohort size may be assessed by transvaginal ultrasound. Further, ovarian reserve correlates with levels of FSH, inhibin B, and, probably most reliably, anti-Müllerian hormone.

Hormonal stimulation, required for cryopreservation of fertilized oocytes or embryos, may postpone cancer treatment by 2 to 6 weeks because it has to be started at the beginning of the menstrual cycle.[6] Therefore, these approaches may not be an option for women with highly aggressive and/or hormone-responsive tumors. Concomitant tamoxifen or aromatase inhibitors with gonadotropins may, however, limit especially estrogen's stimulatory effect on the cancer, as indicated by satisfactory fertilization results and uncompromised survival.[51] Cryopreservation damages unfertilized oocytes and ovarian cortical strips; although this procedure is well tolerated by embryos,[52] the advantage may be offset by obviation of hormonal stimulation with freezing of ovarian tissue (cortical strips or biopsies). Resumption of endocrine function and live birth has been described after transplantation of frozen-banked ovarian tissue.[52]

CONCLUSIONS

Cancer survivors may experience gonadal dysfunction after treatment and should be informed about treatment-related toxicities and possible alternatives to circumvent or limit these before initiation of cancer therapy. Patients wishing to become parents should be offered appropriate support, for example, by cryopreservation of their germ cells.

REFERENCES

1. Brydoy M, Fossa SD, Dahl O, et al. Gonadal dysfunction and fertility problems in cancer survivors. *Acta Oncol.* 2007;46:480–489.
2. Dohle GR, Smit M, Weber RF. Androgens and male fertility. *World J Urol.* 2003;21:341–345.
3. Islam, Trainer. The hormonal assessment of the infertile male. *BJU Int.* 1998;82:69–75. Available at: http://www.blackwell-synergy.com/doi/abs/10.1046/j.1464-410x.1998.00692.x.
4. Meachem SJ, Nieschlag E, Simoni M. Inhibin B in male reproduction: pathophysiology and clinical relevance. *Eur J Endocrinol.* 2001;145:561–571.
5. Perheentupa A, Huhtaniemi I. Aging of the human ovary and testis. *Mol Cell Endocrinol.* 2009;299:2–13.
6. Lee SJ, Schover LR, Partridge AH, et al. American Society of Clinical Oncology recommendations on fertility preservation in cancer patients. *J Clin Oncol.* 2006;24:2917–2931.
7. Oktay K, Kim JY, Barad D, et al. Association of BRCA1 mutations with occult primary ovarian insufficiency: a possible explanation for the link between infertility and breast/ovarian cancer risks. *J Clin Oncol.* 2010;28:240–244.
8. Raman JD, Nobert CF, Goldstein M. Increased incidence of testicular cancer in men presenting with infertility and abnormal semen analysis. *J Urol.* 2005;174:1819–1822.
9. Fitoussi EH, Tchen N, Berjon JP, et al. Semen analysis and cryoconservation before treatment in Hodgkin's disease. *Ann Oncol.* 2000;11:679–684.
10. Joensen UN, Jorgensen N, Rajpert-De ME, et al. Testicular dysgenesis syndrome and Leydig cell function. *Basic Clin Pharmacol.Toxicol.* 2008;102:155–161.
11. Skakkebaek NE, Rajpert-De Meyts E, Main KM. Testicular dysgenesis syndrome: an increasingly common developmental disorder with environmental aspects. *Human Reprod.* 2001;16:972–978.
12. Berthelsen JG. Testicular cancer and fertility. *Int J Androl.* 1987;10:371–380.
13. Fossa SD, Abyholm T, Aakvaag A. Spermatogenesis and hormonal status after orchiectomy for cancer and before supplementary treatment. *Eur Urol.* 1984;10:173–177.

14. Berthelsen JG, Skakkebaek NE. Gonadal function in men with testis cancer. *Fertil Steril.* 1983;39:68–75.
15. Nord C, Bjoro T, Ellingsen D, et al. Gonadal hormones in long-term survivors 10 years after treatment for unilateral testicular cancer. *Eur Urol.* 2003;44:322–328. Available at: http://www.sciencedirect.com/science/article/B6X10-48V6XPD-1/2/d7bb0694cca7039dabc8fc3951d3e26e.
16. Kiserud CE, Fossa A, Holte H, et al. Post-treatment parenthood in Hodgkin's lymphoma survivors. *Br J Cancer.* 2007;96:1442–1449.
17. Huddart RA, Norman A, Moynihan C, et al. Fertility, gonadal and sexual function in survivors of testicular cancer. *Br J Cancer.* 2005;93:200–207.
18. Brydoy M, Fossa SD, Klepp O, et al. Paternity following treatment for testicular cancer. *J Natl Cancer Inst.* 2005;97:1580–1588.
19. van der Kaaij MAE, Heutte N, Le Stang N, et al. Gonadal function in males after chemotherapy for early-stage Hodgkin's lymphoma treated in four subsequent trials by the European Organisation for Research and Treatment of Cancer: EORTC Lymphoma Group and the Groupe d'Etude des Lymphomes de l'Adulte. *J Clin Oncol.* 2007;25:2825–2832. Available at: http://jco.ascopubs.org/cgi/content/abstract/25/19/2825.
20. Pryzant RM, Meistrich ML, Wilson G, et al. Long-term reduction in sperm count after chemotherapy with and without radiation therapy for non-Hodgkin's lymphomas. *J Clin Oncol.* 1993;11:239–247.
21. Hammond C, Abrams JR, Syrjala KL. Fertility and risk factors for elevated infertility concern in 10-year hematopoietic cell transplant survivors and case-matched controls. *J Clin Oncol.* 2007;25:3511–3517. Available at: http://jco.ascopubs.org/cgi/content/abstract/25/23/3511.
21a. Constine LS, Woolf PD, Cann D, et al. Hypothalamic-pituitary dysfunction after radiation for brain tumors. *N Engl J Med.* 1993;328:87–94.
21b. Yeung SCJ, Chiu AC, Vassilopoulou-Sellin R, et al. The endocrine effects of nonhormonal antineoplastic therapy. *Endocr Rev.* 1998;19:144–172.

22. Budgell GJ, Cowan RA, Hounsell AR. Prediction of scattered dose to the testes in ominopelvic radiotherapy. *Clin Oncol.* 2001;13:120–125. Available at: http://www.sciencedirect.com/science/article/B6WXW-45WYK3K-3Y/2/d9c9b14844f11a8097b23a0709d6008d.
23. Dueland S, Gronlie Guren M, Rune Olsen D, et al. Radiation therapy induced changes in male sex hormone levels in rectal cancer patients. *Radiother Oncol.* 2003;68:249–253. Available at: http://www.sciencedirect.com/science/article/B6TBY-49CRJ7P-1/2/8da6410f89d94d621311bf7bcb875c33.
24. Hermann RM, Henkel K, Christiansen H, et al. Testicular dose and hormonal changes after radiotherapy of rectal cancer. *Radiother Oncol.* 2005;75:83–88. Available at: http://www.sciencedirect.com/science/article/B6TBY-4FV9MC0-1/2/69100a574572f8aa1c7106c26452b624.
25. Howell SJ, Shalet SM. Effect of cancer therapy on pituitary-testicular axis. *Int J Androl.* 2002;25:269–276.
26. Rowley MJ, Leach DR, Warner GA, et al. Effect of graded doses of ionizing radiation on the human testis. *Radiat Res.* 1974;59:665–678.
27. Anserini P, Chiodi S, Spinelli S, et al. Semen analysis following allogeneic bone marrow transplantation: additional data for evidence-based counselling. *Bone Marrow Transplant.* 2002;30:447–451.
28. Dueland S, Guren MG, Olsen DR, et al. Radiation therapy induced changes in male sex hormone levels in rectal cancer patients. *Radiother Oncol.* 2003a;68:249–253.
29. Daniell HW, Clark JC, Pereira SE, et al. Hypogonadism following prostate-bed radiation therapy for prostate carcinoma. *Cancer.* 2001;91:1889–1895.
30. King CR, Kapp DS. To treat pelvic nodes or not: could the greater testicular scatter dose from whole pelvic fields confound results of prostate cancer trials? *J Clin Oncol.* 2009;27:6076–6078. Available at: http://jco.ascopubs.org.
31. Stahl O, Eberhard J, Jepson K, et al. Sperm DNA integrity in testicular cancer patients. *Hum Reprod.*

2006;21:3199–3205. Available at: http://humrep. oxfordjournals.org/cgi/content/abstract/21/12/3199.

32. Heidenreich A, Weissbach L, Holtl W, et al. Organ sparing surgery for malignant germ cell tumor of the testis. *J Urol*. 2001;166:2161–2165.

33. Vis AN, Schroder FH. Key targets of hormonal treatment of prostate cancer. Part 1: The androgen receptor and steroidogenic pathways. *BJU Int*. 2009;104:438–448.

34. Schroder FH, Collette L, de Reijke TM, et al. Prostate cancer treated by anti-androgens: is sexual function preserved? EORTC Genitourinary Group. *Br J Cancer*. 2000;82:283–290.

35. Haukvik UK, Dieset I, Bjoro T, et al. Treatment-related premature ovarian failure as a long-term complication after Hodgkin's lymphoma. *Ann Oncol*. 2006;17:1428–1433.

36. Wallace WH, Thomson AB, Kelsey TW. The radiosensitivity of the human oocyte. *Hum Reprod*. 2003;18:117–122.

37. Sklar C. Maintenance of ovarian function and risk of premature menopause related to cancer treatment. *J Natl Cancer Inst Monogr*. 2005;34:25–27.

38. Sanders JE, Buckner CD, Amos D, et al. Ovarian function following marrow transplantation for aplastic anemia or leukemia. *J Clin Oncol*. 1988;6:813–818.

39. Cibula D, Slama J, Svarovsky J, et al. Abdominal radical trachelectomy in fertility-sparing treatment of early-stage cervical cancer. *Int J Gynecol Cancer*. 2009;19:1407–1411.

40. Berglund G, Nystedt M, Bolund C, et al. Effect of endocrine treatment on sexuality in premenopausal breast cancer patients: a prospective randomized study. *J Clin Oncol*. 2001;19:2788–2796.

41. Gibson L, Lawrence D, Dawson C, et al. Aromatase inhibitors for treatment of advanced breast cancer in postmenopausal women. *Cochrane Database Syst Rev*. 2009;(4): CD003370.

42. Critchley HO, Wallace WH. Impact of cancer treatment on uterine function. *J Natl Cancer Inst Monogr*. 2005;(34):64–68.

43. Magelssen H, Melve KK, Skjaerven R, et al. Parenthood probability and pregnancy outcome in patients with a cancer diagnosis during adolescence and young adulthood. *Hum Reprod*. 2008;23:178–186.

44. Magelssen H, Brydoy M, Fossa SD. The effects of cancer and cancer treatments on male reproductive function. *Nat Clin Pract Urol*. 2006;3:312–322.

45. Shetty G, Meistrich ML. Hormonal approaches to preservation and restoration of male fertility after cancer treatment. *J Natl Cancer Inst Monogr*. 2005;(34):36–39.

46. Fossa SD, Horwich A, Russell JM, et al. Optimal planning target volume for stage I testicular seminoma: a Medical Research Council randomized trial. Medical Research Council Testicular Tumor Working Group. *J Clin Oncol*. 1999;17:1146.

47. Oldereid NB, Tanbo T. [Induction of spermatogenesis in hypogonadotrophic hypogonadism]. *Tidsskr Nor Laegeforen*. 2008;128:327–329.

48. Oktay K, Oktem O. Fertility preservation medicine: a new field in the care of young cancer survivors. *Pediatr Blood Cancer*. 2009;53:267–273.

49. Terenziani M, Piva L, Meazza C, et al. Oophoropexy: a relevant role in preservation of ovarian function after pelvic irradiation. *Fertil Steril*. 2009;91:935–936.

50. Nisker J, Baylis F, McLeod C. Choice in fertility preservation in girls and adolescent women with cancer. *Cancer*. 2006;107:1686–1689.

51. Azim AA, Costantini-Ferrando M, Oktay K. Safety of fertility preservation by ovarian stimulation with letrozole and gonadotropins in patients with breast cancer: a prospective controlled study. *J Clin Oncol*. 2008;26:2630–2635.

52. von Wolff M, Donnez J, Hovatta O, et al. Cryopreservation and autotransplantation of human ovarian tissue prior to cytotoxic therapy—a technique in its infancy but already successful in fertility preservation. *Eur J Cancer*. 2009;45:1547–1553.

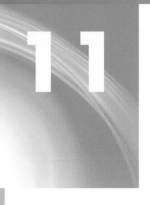

Oral and gastrointestinal mucosal adverse effects

Douglas E. Peterson

Alimentary tract mucosal injury caused by cancer therapies has long been an adverse event in the oncology setting.[1–3] Once viewed as an inevitable consequence of cancer treatment, the pathobiologic and clinical paradigm has fundamentally shifted over the past decade such that new insights for prevention and treatment have been delineated. The evolution of the study of mucositis has paralleled that of prior development of antiemetic interventions in the oncology setting. The stage is now set for achievement of new advances relative to understanding of mucositis causation, prediction of individual patient risk for severity and duration, and use of molecularly targeted treatments as they emerge from the drug pipeline in the future.

This chapter is directed to clinicians involved in management of the cancer patient at risk or currently experiencing oral and/or gastrointestinal mucositis. Evidence-based guidelines will be highlighted. The chapter will also identify current research directions that may in turn lead to strategic new advances in the prevention and treatment of the toxicity.

CLINICAL AND ECONOMIC IMPACT

Oral mucositis (Fig. 11-1) and gastrointestinal mucositis (Figs. 11-2 and 11-3) can have a clinically and economically significant impact on the overall course of the cancer patient.[4–6] An example of this impact from oral mucositis is illustrated in Figure 11-4. Clinical sequelae, when occurring in combination with other toxicities, can lead to a constellation of toxicities that collectively in the patient can be highly significant[3,5] (Fig. 11-5).

For example, patients with oral mucositis are significantly more likely to experience severe pain and weight loss of ≥5%.[5] Severity of oral mucositis has been correlated with decreased swallowing and the need for feeding via a gastrostomy tube.[7,8] The pain can be sufficiently severe as to require hospitalization with supportive care, including opioid narcotics and/or total parenteral nutrition. Associated hospitalization and additional medications in turn result in increased cost of care. For example, in one study of patients receiving chemotherapy for solid tumors or lymphoma, estimated hospitalization cost was $3893 per chemotherapy cycle without mucositis, $6277 per cycle with oral mucositis, and $9132 per cycle with both oral and gastrointestinal (GI) mucositis.[5] Costs of managing the sequelae of oral mucositis in hematopoietic stem cell patients can be substantial as well[9] and have been estimated at up to $42,000 per patient.[4] Oral mucositis has been significantly associated with increased rates of infection during cancer treatment.[5]

Mucositis can also contribute to interruption or dose reduction of cancer therapy, with potential impact on tumor response and long-term patient survival. For example, up to 11% of patients receiving radiation therapy for head and neck cancer had unplanned breaks in radiation therapy caused by severe mucositis.[7] Patients on multicycle chemotherapy regimens may reduce chemotherapy dose reductions in subsequent cycles because of the pain.[5,7] Multicycle dose modifications

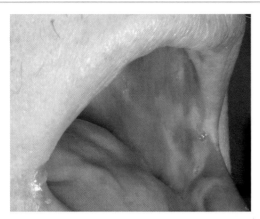

Fig. 11-1 Oral mucositis in a patient being treated for squamous cell carcinoma of the lateral tongue. The patient was receiving high-dose head and neck radiation and concomitant chemotherapy *(Photo courtesy of Ms. Linda Choquette, RDH, MSHS, CCRP).*

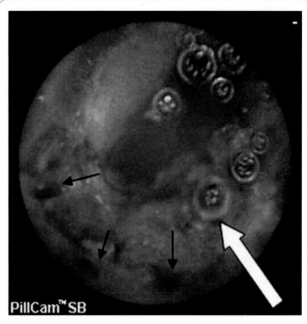

Fig. 11-3 Video-capsule endoscopy: ulceration and bleeding. Black arrows identify hemorrhage. White arrow identifies confluent ulceration. *(From Triantafyllou K, Dervenoulas J, Tsirigotis P, Ladas SD. The nature of small intestinal mucositis: a video-capsule endoscopy study. Support Care Cancer 2008;16:1173–1178.)*

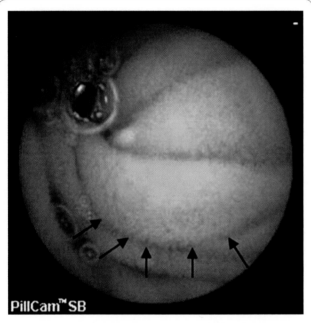

Fig. 11-2 Video-capsule endoscopy: normal jejunal mucosa. Black arrows indetify normal villi. *(From Triantafyllou K, Dervenoulas J, Tsirigotis P, Ladas SD. The nature of small intestinal mucositis: a video-capsule endoscopy study. Support Care Cancer 2008;16:1173–1178.)*

have been associated with increased cancer recurrence and decreased survival rates.[10]

In addition to these clinical and economic issues, the subjective experience for patients can be important. For example, patients developing oral mucositis secondary to intensive conditioning regimens before hematopoietic cell transplantation have reported oral mucositis as the single most distressing complication of the transplant experience.[11,12]

Despite these important adverse outcomes, clinical management of oral and gastrointestinal mucositis continues to be primarily palliative and empiric because of limitations in drug and device technology. For example, only one U.S. Food &

Drug Administration–approved molecularly targeted drug is currently approved for oral mucositis prevention; it is directed to patients with hematologic malignancies who are undergoing high-dose chemotherapy with or without total body irradiation, followed by hematopoietic cell rescue.[13] Several additional oral mucositis drugs are in clinical development, and selected devices are currently available as well. These opportunities may well enhance the ability of clinicians in the future to customize delivery of molecularly targeted drugs to prevent and treat the toxicity.

DEFINITION, INCIDENCE, AND RISK OF DEVELOPMENT

DEFINITION

Mucositis is defined as inflammation of the oral and gastrointestinal mucosa secondary to cancer therapies. Alimentary tract mucositis involves both oral and gastrointestinal mucosal injury, ranging from the oral to the anal mucosa.

Inflammatory changes associated with oral mucositis are typically characterized by erythema, ulceration, and pain.[14] Pain is the major symptom that leads to the need for increased supportive care, as described in greater detail later (see "Treatment"). By comparison, gastrointestinal mucositis is characterized by ulceration and/or loss of villi structure and function, with symptoms manifesting as cramping and/or diarrhea.[15]

In the neutropenic cancer patient, ulceration of the oral and/or gastrointestinal mucosa can represent a portal of entry for systemic infection that, in a subset of patients, can lead to sepsis and death.[16]

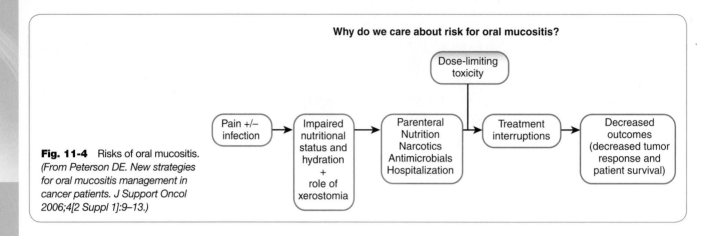

Fig. 11-4 Risks of oral mucositis. *(From Peterson DE. New strategies for oral mucositis management in cancer patients. J Support Oncol 2006;4[2 Suppl 1]:9–13.)*

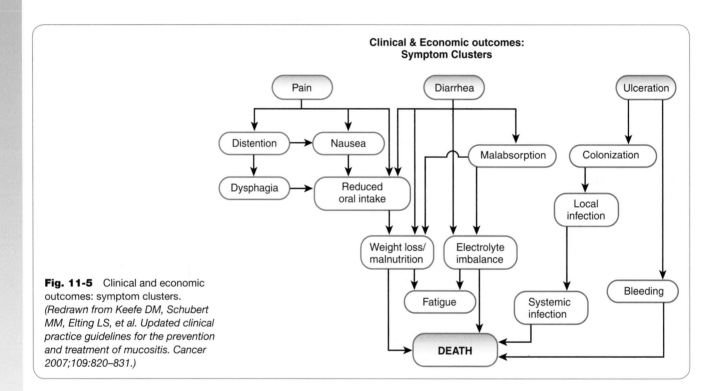

Fig. 11-5 Clinical and economic outcomes: symptom clusters. *(Redrawn from Keefe DM, Schubert MM, Elting LS, et al. Updated clinical practice guidelines for the prevention and treatment of mucositis. Cancer 2007;109:820–831.)*

INCIDENCE OF MUCOSITIS

The intensity of the cancer treatment regimen is a prime but not exclusive risk factor for oral and gastrointestinal mucositis (Fig. 11-6). Risk of mucositis has classically been directly associated with modality, intensity, and route of delivery of the cancer therapy. However, and as described later (see "Pathobiology"), fundamental mechanistic causes of the lesion along the continuum of the alimentary tract represent a multifactorial and complex interplay of multiple patient-based and treatment-based variables.

Patient cohorts classically associated with mucositis consist of (1) patients treated with radiation, including high-dose head and neck radiotherapy for head and neck cancer; (2) hematopoietic cell transplant patients; and (3) patients receiving single or multiple cycles of chemotherapy for solid tumors[2,3,17]

(Table 11-1). Although most patients in the first two cohorts develop clinically significant mucositis as summarized below, the incidence of World Health Organization (WHO) grade 3-4 oral mucositis and/or diarrhea caused by chemotherapy is considerably less frequent, as is cited in Table 11-2.[18]

Incidence of oral and oropharyngeal mucositis in patients receiving head and neck radiation with or without concurrent chemotherapy

WHO grade 3 or 4 oral and/or oropharyngeal mucositis occurs in approximately 85% of patients receiving head and neck radiation for primary tumors of the oral cavity, oropharynx, or nasopharynx.[14] Severity of the lesion is principally governed

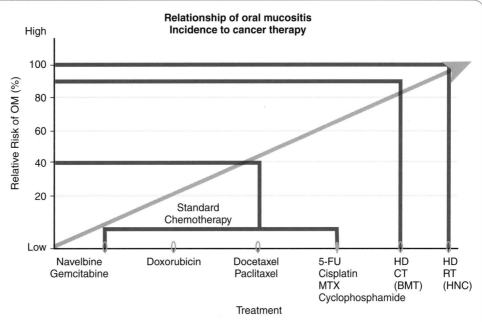

Fig. 11-6 Relationship of oral mucositis incidence to cancer therapy. *(From Peterson DE. New strategies for oral mucositis management in cancer patients, J Support Oncol 2006;4[2 Suppl 1]: 9–13.)*

If patients develop OM during the first chemotherapy cycle, the risk of OM is increased in subsequent cycles.

by the radiation dosimetry to mucosal tissue, with greater than 2500 cGy considered to be a risk factor for the development of clinically significant toxicity. The most severe lesions are observed in those patients receiving at least 5000 cGy; hyperfractionation further increases the risk.[6,19] Severity of the lesion can be escalated in patients receiving concurrent chemoradiotherapy.

Incidence of oral and gastrointestinal mucositis in patients undergoing hematopoietic cell transplantation (HCT)

Up to 75% of patients undergoing HCT can develop WHO grade 3 or 4 oral and/or gastrointestinal mucositis.[14] Intensity of the conditioning regimen is a principal but not exclusive

Table 11-1   Incidence of oral mucositis

1.3 million patients* receive cytotoxic therapy annually and at least 400,000 will develop some degree of oral mucositis.

Cancer therapy	Incidence, %	Grade 3-4, %
Solid tumor with myelosuppression	5–40	5–15
Stem cell transplantation	75–100	25–60
Radiotherapy for head and neck cancer	85–100	25–45

*U.S. statistics.
Adapted from Trotti A et al. *Radiother Oncol.* 2003;66:253–262.

Table 11-2   Risk of grade 3-4 oral mucositis and diarrhea by chemotherapy regimen*

Regimen	No. of studies	No. of patients	Risk of grade 3-4 oral mucositis		Risk of grade 3-4 diarrhea	
			%	95% CI	%	95% CI
NHL ALL	19	1444	6.55	5.54, 8.00	1.23	1.15, 2.12
NHL-15: non-Hodgkin's lymphoma regimen 15	1	100	3.00	0.50, 7.00	0.50	0.50, 2.00
CHOP-14: cyclophosphamide + Adriamycin + vincristine + prednisone	9	623	4.82	3.53, 6.78	1.04	0.95, 2.15
CHOP-DI-14: cyclophosphamide + Adriamycin + vincristine + prednisone, dose-intensified	4	231	7.85	5.28, 11.32	2.36	1.32, 4.65

Table 11-2   Risk of grade 3-4 oral mucositis and diarrhea by chemotherapy regimen*—cont'd

Regimen	No. of studies	No. of patients	Risk of grade 3-4 oral mucositis		Risk of grade 3-4 diarrhea	
			%	95% CI	%	95% CI
CHOEP-14: cyclophosphamide + Adriamycin + vincristine + etoposide + prednisone	2	346	10.40	7.23, 13.44	0.29	0.29, 1.01
CEOP/IMVP-Dexa: cyclophosphamide + etoposide + vincristine + prednisone/ifosfamide + methotrexate + dexamethasone	3	144	4.17	1.74, 7.99	2.78	1.39, 5.90
Breast ALL	21	2766	4.08	3.44, 4.85	3.41	2.86, 4.224
A→T→C Adriamycin, taxane, cyclophosphamide administered sequentially	4	594	2.29	1.30, 3.46	2.53	1.36, 3.92
AC→T Adriamycin + cyclophosphamide, taxane administered sequentially	2	515	2.80	1.40, 4.20	1.07	0.27, 2.07
A→CT Adriamycin + cyclophosphamide + taxane administered sequentially	1	19	5.26	2.63, 15.79	5.26	2.63, 15.79
A→T Adriamycin, taxane administered sequentially	2	60	4.17	1.67, 10.00	9.17	4.17, 15.83
AT Adriamycin + taxane	1	36	8.33	1.39, 19.44	1.39	1.39, 5.56
FAC (weekly): 5-FU + Adriamycin + cyclophosphamide	1	30	3.33	1.67, 10.00	1.67	1.67, 6.67
AC (weekly): Adriamycin + cyclophosphamide	1	22	13.64	2.27, 27.27	2.27	2.27, 9.09
Taxol (paclitaxel) (weekly)	2	87	2.87	1.15, 6.90	1.15	1.15, 4.02
TAC docetaxel + Adriamycin + cyclophosphamide	7	1403	4.92	3.83, 6.07	4.38	3.27, 5.54
Lung ALL (No XRT)	49	4750	0.79	0.88, 1.33	1.38	1.30, 1.99
Platinum + paclitaxel	16	2009	0.49	0.52, 1.06	1.59	1.08, 2.44
Platinum + paclitaxel (low dose)	1	49	1.02	1.02, 4.08	1.02	1.02, 4.08
Platinum + docetaxel	1	38	1.32	1.32, 5.26	1.32	1.32, 5.26
Platinum + paclitaxel + other	7	451	1.47	1.20, 3.07	2.80	2.17, 4.54
Platinum + docetaxel + other	1	83	0.60	0.60, 2.41	0.60	0.60, 2.41
Gemcitabine + platinum	18	1476	1.08	0.09, 1.91	1.08	0.99, 1.89
Gemcitabine + paclitaxel	2	109	1.84	1.02, 5.33	3.69	2.05, 6.97
Gemcitabine + vinorelbine	1	67	0.75	0.75, 2.99	2.99	0.75, 7.46
Vinorelbine + paclitaxel	1	175	0.29	0.29, 1.14	0.29	0.29, 1.14
Vinorelbine + platinum	1	203	0.25	0.25, 0.99	0.25	0.25, 0.99
Colon ALL	10	898	1.67	1.17, 2.67	15.42	13.14, 17.82
FOLFOX: 5-fluorouracil + leucovorin + oxaliplatin	5	482	1.35	0.73, 2.59	10.06	7.52, 12.97
FOLFIRI: 5-fluorouracil + leucovorin + irinotecan	2	79	4.43	1.90, 9.49	10.13	4.43, 16.46
IROX: irinotecan + oxaliplatin	3	337	1.48	0.59, 2.97	24.33	19.59, 29.08

From Keefe DM, Schubert MM, Elting LS, et al. Updated clinical practice guidelines for the prevention and treatment of mucositis. *Cancer.* 2007;109:820–831.
*Taxane is paclitaxel or docetaxel.

risk factor. In addition, prophylactic use of methotrexate to prevent graft-versus-host disease can increase this risk.

Incidence of mucositis associated with standard multicycle chemotherapy, with or without radiotherapy

Incidence of 1% to 14% WHO grade 3 or 4 mucositis has been reported in selected cohorts, including non-Hodgkin's lymphoma and breast, lung, and colorectal cancers (18). Single agents that have been classically associated with oral mucositis include methotrexate, doxorubicin, 5-fluorouracil (5-FU), busulfan, and bleomycin.[17] Combination therapy can escalate the risk of clinically significant mucosal injury. For example, anthracycline-based regimens in general are associated with an estimated 10% risk of clinically significant oral mucositis. However, 5-FU given in combination with docetaxel is associated with a considerably higher risk of clinically significant oral mucositis (e.g., 58%–74%).[16] Novel, molecularly targeted agents such as the mammalian targets of rapamycin (mTORs)[20] are now reported to contribute to the mucositis profile.[21] The mechanisms, clinical appearance, and possible preventive or therapeutic interventions require further investigation.

PATHOBIOLOGY

Historically, the primary if not exclusive cause of oral mucositis was viewed to be the direct effect of cytotoxic cancer treatments regimens on the basal cell compartment of the oral epithelium. However, this modeling has evolved over the past 10 years such that the pathobiology is now viewed as a complex interplay among epithelial and connective tissue components, as well as cancer-treatment–related variables[3,24] (Box 11-1). The current pathobiologic model is conceptualized into five phases. Injury associated with these phases, while occurring sequentially over time, can also occur concurrently. The combined effect is one of an escalating cascade of inflammation biology that peaks and eventually resolves several weeks after cessation of cancer therapy. In addition, proinflammatory cytokines may influence pain levels in patients with oral mucositis. For example, levels of tumor necrosis factor-alpha (TNF-α) RNA content based on buccal epithelial cell specimens have been significantly associated with worst intensity of oral pain with swallowing in patients undergoing hematopoietic stem cell transplantation.[22]

BOX 11-1 Risk Factors for Oral Mucositis: Patient-Related Variables (examples)

- Oral microflora and oral hygiene
- Inflammation
- Salivary function
- Genetic polymorphisms
- Age and gender (possible risk factor; further research needed)
- Nutritional status (possible risk factor; further research needed)

Data from Peterson D, et al[24]; Barasch A, Peterson D.[25]

Linkage of this pathobiologic model for oral mucositis with that of gastrointestinal mucositis is also relevant and includes potentially common pathways. For example, TNF-α, nuclear factor (NF)-κB, interleukin (IL)-1β, and IL-6 immunohistochemistry levels in oral mucosa, jejunum, and colon have been demonstrated to be elevated following administration of irinotecan in a rat model.[23] These research findings suggest a potentially common mechanistic basis for injury across the alimentary tract mucosa (Fig. 11-7).

Other variables, in addition to inflammation biology, may be operative as well. Several groups have studied the association of mucositis incidence with nongenetic factors such as age, gender, and race[2,24] (Boxes 11-2 and 11-3). No consistent trend across these variables has emerged following an analysis published in 2003.[25] For example, it has been reported that women experience significantly more mucositis than men when receiving specific treatment regimens.[26,27]

Dose delivery may be relevant as well. Some studies report that administration of 5-FU (bolus vs. continuous infusion) is not correlated with incidence of mucositis[27,28]; others have found bolus administration to be more toxic.[26]

In addition, mucosal defense systems may contribute to the risk for and clinical expression of mucosal injury. Regarding oral mucositis, the level of epidermal growth factor (EGF) in saliva, as well as xerostomia and/or baseline neutrophil counts, may be relevant. For example, reduced mucositis has been reported in patients with higher levels of salivary EGF.[29] Saliva also appears to protect oral tissues from mucositis; patients with xerostomia preceding or during 5-FU administration are significantly more likely to develop oral mucositis than those with normal levels of saliva.[28] Oral mucositis incidence may increase in patients with reduced neutrophil counts[28]; whether a causative role exists is unclear. The role of the colonizing microflora in relation to mucositis causation and progression is not fully delineated. Although historically the microflora has not been viewed as a key contributor, a recent study has identified new oral microbial profiles that provide an important basis for future investigation.[30]

In addition, variation in genetic polymorphisms across patients may account for variability in expression. For example, more than 29 genes are involved in the 5-fluorouracil metabolic pathway; genetic variations in any of these genes could have an impact on toxicity expression associated with 5-FU.[31] Differences across individuals relative to drug metabolism systemically may influence plasma drug levels. For example, targeted adjusted dosing resulted in longer survival and less toxicity[32]; implications relative to severity and duration of mucositis warrant further study.

The extent to which these variables contribute to the specific, variable expression of oral and/or gastrointestinal mucositis in solid tumor regimens[2] is an important consideration that requires new research. Mechanisms in this modeling for variable risk of oral and gastrointestinal mucositis appear to include proinflammatory cytokines[33,34] tissue-based genetic risk, and drug resistance mechanisms.[35–37] In addition, a mucosal epithelium biological threshold for clinical oral mucositis may occur secondary to mechanisms of apoptosis or decreasing proliferation.[38]

Despite these advances in understanding, however, key gaps in knowledge remain across the molecular, tissue, and clinical continuum relative to strategically advancing this multidimensional modeling. Closing these research gaps in

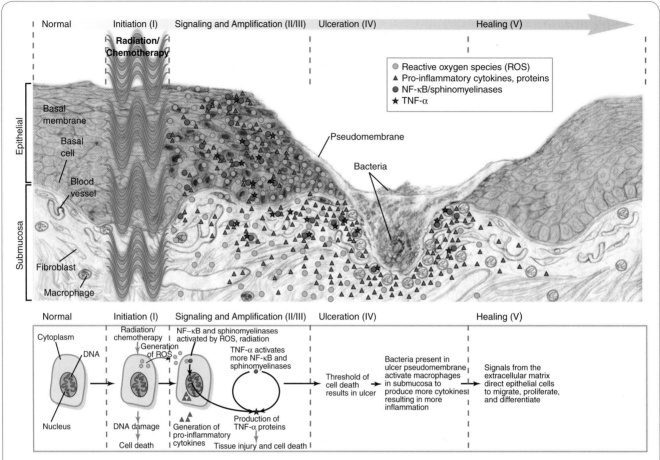

Fig. 11-7 Multistage model of mucosal injury secondary to cancer therapy. *(Redrawn from Sonis ST. Oral Oncol 2009;45:1015–1020.)*

BOX 11-2   Risk Factors for Oral Mucositis: Treatment-Related Variables (examples)

1. Modality, intensity, and route of administration
2. Combination therapy, including:
   - Chemoradiotherapy
   - Oxaliplatin and 5-fluorouracil (5-FU)
   - Bolus versus infusion

Data from Peterson D, et al.[24]; Barasch A, Peterson D.[25]

BOX 11-3   Oral Mucositis Assessment Scale (OMAS)

Ulceration/Pseudomembrane
   0= no lesion
   1= <1 cm²
   2= 1 cm²–3 cm²
   3= >3 cm²
Erythema
   0= none
   1= not severe
   2= severe

---

turn can lead to identification of specific targeting of hubs that, when perturbed by drugs or devices, could produce significant resolution in severity and duration of the lesion. The concept of targeting centrally important pathway hubs that are fragile yet pivotally important to the generation of downstream effects has been well established in the literature[39] (Fig. 11-8). Application of this modeling to mucosal injury caused by cancer therapies represents an exciting frontier for development of combination interventions in the future that could significantly obviate the trajectory of injury. In addition, mucosal injury can contribute to overall symptom burden[40,41]; the potentially beneficial effect of reducing the overall symptom complex profile in these patients by reducing severity of mucosal injury is therefore also of high importance.

Understanding the origin of oral mucositis is the first step toward development of targeted drug therapies for prevention or treatment. Until 2004, therapies were palliative but not preventive in nature. In 2004, the U.S. Food and Drug Administration (FDA) approved palifermin for the prevention and treatment of mucositis in hematopoietic stem cell transplant patients. Palifermin has been associated with significant reductions in incidence of oral mucositis, soreness of the oral cavity, and use of opioid analgesics.[13] Palifermin has also been associated with reducing hospital costs by an estimated $3595 per patient.[42] Amifostine, epithelial-specific growth factors, and hematopoietic growth factors have also been studied as potential mucositis therapies with mixed

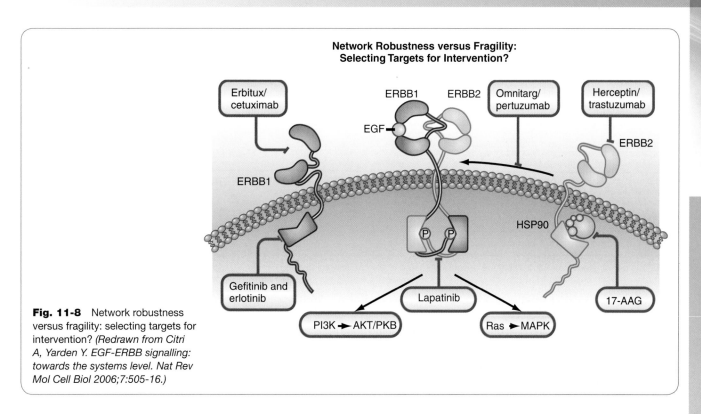

Fig. 11-8 Network robustness versus fragility: selecting targets for intervention? *(Redrawn from Citri A, Yarden Y. EGF-ERBB signalling: towards the systems level. Nat Rev Mol Cell Biol 2006;7:505-16.)*

results.[10,43] Developing new understandings relative to causation of mucosal injury in cancer patients is clearly needed, so as to identify opportune molecular targets for prevention and/or treatment of the toxicity.

Improving knowledge of the mechanism of oral mucositis in these patients can predictably lead to improved quality of life for cancer patients and reduced cost of treatment. The ability to predict risk or severity of oral mucositis for a given patient could allow clinicians to select and adjust cancer treatments for optimal results.

> **BOX 11-4   World Health Organization (WHO) Scale**
>
> Grade 0 = no oral mucositis
> Grade 1 = erythema and soreness
> Grade 2 = ulcers, able to eat solids
> Grade 3 = ulcers, requires liquid diet (owing to mucositis)
> Grade 4 = ulcers, alimentation not possible (owing to mucositis)

ASSESSMENT OF MUCOSITIS

Assessment of oral mucositis has the advantage of allowing direct examination of the oral mucosa. Multiple scales are available for use in the clinical research or clinical care setting. Research-based tools typically include objective measures of tissue injury (e.g., erythema and/or ulceration), in addition to symptom and functional assessment. One example of a research-based scale is the Oral Mucositis Assessment Scale (OMAS)[14] (see Box 11-3). This scale, developed via a multicenter study, demonstrates high reproducibility across examiners, as well as a strong correlation with more global scales such as the National Cancer Institute (NCI) Common Toxicity Criteria (CTC) instrument.

Most clinical care instruments are global in extent and incorporate general assessment of symptoms (e.g., pain), signs (e.g., erythema and/or ulceration), and functional disturbances (e.g., not able to eat solid foods). For example, the WHO scale[14] (Box 11-4) is a validated scale that can be readily incorporated into clinical care of patients and thus is suitable for ongoing use in clinical practice.

TREATMENT OF MUCOSITIS

Current management of mucositis is based, to a large extent, on supportive care approaches designed to (1) reduce oral pain via standardized pain management ladders, (2) reduce gastro-intestinally based symptoms such as diarrhea, and (3) enhance mucosal infection prevention or treatment. Additional interventions including providing nutritional support can be utilized as clinically indicated. As noted earlier, only one molecularly targeted oral mucositis agent, palifermin, is approved by the FDA. The label for this product is directed to patients with hematologic malignancies undergoing high-dose chemotherapy with or without radiation, followed by hematopoietic cell transplant. With the exception of this specific cohort, therefore, there is no definitive preventive strategy.

Current day mucositis management is thus supportive in nature and can be challenging for both the clinician and the patient. Despite these limitations, however, it is essential to practice a comprehensive approach to minimize the impact of oral and/or gastrointestinal mucositis on the overall clinical course of the patient. If successful, such approaches can have a direct, positive impact on a number of parameters, including improving patient quality of life, reducing risk for bacteremia/septicemia in the neutropenic setting, and permitting optimal dosing of cancer therapy over time.

The Mucositis Study Group of the Multinational Association for Supportive Care in Cancer and the International Society of Oral Oncology (MASCC/ISOO) recognized the need for an evidence-based review of the literature to produce guidelines for mucositis management (Table 11-3). The original guidelines were published in 2002[44] and were updated in 2007.[18] The review process, including weighing the quality of the literature, was been as based on criteria as reported by the American Society of Clinical Oncology and summarized in the 2004 and 2007 publications.

Table 11-3   Summary of evidence-based clinical practice guidelines for care of patients with oral and gastrointestinal mucositis (2005 update)

I. Oral mucositis

Basic oral care and good clinical practices

1. The panel suggests multidisciplinary development and evaluation of oral care protocols, as well as patient and staff education on the use of such protocols to reduce the severity of oral mucositis from chemotherapy and/or radiation therapy. As part of the protocols, the panel suggests the use of a soft toothbrush that is replaced on a regular basis. Elements of good clinical practice should include the use of validated tools to regularly assess oral pain and oral cavity health. Inclusion of dental professionals is vital throughout the treatment and follow-up phases.
2. The panel recommends patient-controlled analgesia with morphine as the treatment of choice for oral mucositis pain in patients undergoing hematopoietic stem cell transplantation (HSCT). Regular oral pain assessment using validated instruments for self-reporting is essential.

Radiotherapy: prevention

3. The panel recommends the use of midline radiation blocks and three-dimensional radiation treatment to reduce mucosal injury.
4. The panel recommends benzydamine for prevention of radiation-induced mucositis in patients with head and neck cancer receiving moderate-dose radiation therapy.
5. The panel recommends that chlorhexidine not be used to prevent oral mucositis in patients with solid tumors of the head and neck who are undergoing radiotherapy.
6. The panel recommends that sucralfate not be used for the prevention of radiation-induced oral mucositis.
7. The panel recommends that antimicrobial lozenges not be used for the prevention of radiation-induced oral mucositis.

Standard-dose chemotherapy: prevention

8. The panel recommends that patients receiving bolus 5-fluorouracil (5-FU) chemotherapy undergo 30 minutes of oral cryotherapy to prevent oral mucositis.
9. The panel suggests the use of 20 to 30 minutes of oral cryotherapy to decrease mucositis in patients treated with bolus doses of edatrexate.
10. The panel recommends that acyclovir and its analogs not be used routinely to prevent mucositis.

Standard-dose chemotherapy: treatment

11. The panel recommends that chlorhexidine not be used to treat established oral mucositis.

High-dose chemotherapy with or without total body irradiation plus hematopoietic cell transplantation: prevention

12. In patients with hematologic malignancies receiving high-dose chemotherapy and total body irradiation with autologous stem cell transplant, the panel recommends the use of keratinocyte growth factor-1 (palifermin) at a dose of 60 μg/kg/day for 3 days before conditioning treatment and for 3 days post transplant for the prevention of oral mucositis.
13. The panel suggests the use of cryotherapy to prevent oral mucositis in patients receiving high-dose melphalan.
14. The panel *does not recommend* the use of pentoxifylline to prevent mucositis in patients undergoing HSCT.
15. The panel suggests that granulocyte-macrophage colony-stimulating factor (GM-CSF) mouthwashes *not be used* for the prevention of oral mucositis in patients undergoing HSCT.
16. The panel suggests the use of low-level laser therapy (LLLT) to reduce the incidence of oral mucositis and its associated pain in patients receiving high-dose chemotherapy or chemoradiotherapy before HSCT, if the treatment center is able to support the necessary technology and training, as LLLT requires expensive equipment and specialized training. Because of interoperator variability, clinical trials are difficult to conduct and their results are difficult to compare; nevertheless, the panel is encouraged by accumulating evidence in support of LLLT.

II. Gastrointestinal mucositis

Basic bowel care and good clinical practices

17. The panel suggests that basic bowel care should include the maintenance of adequate hydration, and that consideration should be given to the potential for transient lactose intolerance, and the presence of bacterial pathogens.

Table 11-3 Summary of evidence-based clinical practice guidelines for care of patients with oral and gastrointestinal mucositis (2005 update)—cont'd

Radiotherapy: prevention

18. The panel suggests the use of 500 mg sulfasalazine orally twice daily to help reduce the incidence and severity of radiation-induced enteropathy in patients receiving external beam radiotherapy to the pelvis.

19. The panel suggests that amifostine at a dose of at least 340 mg/kg may prevent radiation proctitis in those receiving standard-dose radiotherapy for rectal cancer.

20. The panel recommends that oral sucralfate not be used to reduce related side effects of radiotherapy; it does not prevent acute diarrhea in patients with pelvic malignancies undergoing external beam radiotherapy, and compared with placebo, it is associated with more gastrointestinal side effects, including rectal bleeding.

21. The panel recommends that 5-aminosalicylic acid and its related compounds mesalazine and olsalazine not be used to prevent GI mucositis.

Radiotherapy: treatment

22. The panel suggests the use of sucralfate enemas to help manage chronic radiation-induced proctitis in patients who have rectal bleeding.

Standard-dose and high-dose chemotherapy: prevention

23. The panel recommends ranitidine or omeprazole for the prevention of epigastric pain following treatment with cyclophosphamide, methotrexate, and 5-FU or treatment with 5-FU with or without folinic acid chemotherapy.

24. The panel recommends that systemic glutamine not be used for the prevention of GI mucositis.

Standard-dose and high-dose chemotherapy: treatment

25. When loperamide fails to control diarrhea induced by standard-dose or high-dose chemotherapy associated with HSCT, the panel recommends octreotide at a dose of at least 100 µg subcutaneously, twice daily.

Combined chemotherapy and radiotherapy: prevention

26. The panel suggests the use of amifostine to reduce esophagitis induced by concomitant chemotherapy and radiotherapy in patients with non–small-cell lung cancer.

From Keefe DM, Schubert MM, Elting LS, et al. Updated clinical practice guidelines for the prevention and treatment of mucositis. *Cancer.* 2007;109:820–831.
5-FU, 5-Fluorouracil; *HSCT,* hematopoietic stem cell transplant; *LLLT,* low-level laser therapy.

Despite the utility of such systematic reviews for clinical guidelines, the recommendations and suggestions are by definition limited by the quality and scope of the literature. The more rigorous the review criteria, the fewer definitive statements can be produced. The clinician thus needs to consider both the guidelines themselves and the value of empiric approaches relative to both safety and efficacy. Examples of empirically based interventions that have been utilized by many clinicians for many years are listed in Table 11-4.[45]

The principal clinically significant outcomes associated with oral mucositis are (1) pain and (2) infection of oral mucosal origin during myelosuppression. In addition to providing specific pharmacologically directed interventions, the MASCC/ISOO mucositis guidelines address the importance of foundational mouth care, including the use of nonmedicated rinses to maximize effective oral mucosal hygiene throughout the phase of cancer therapy. Effective oral hygiene can play an important role in the management of oral mucositis. This care, often easily administered in the clinical setting, can reduce the oral microbial burden and provide important lubrication and cleansing of the oral mucosa. A basic mouth care protocol should thus be incorporated into management strategies for the patient at risk for or who has developed oral mucositis. The MASCC/ISOO guidelines recommend utilization of a standardized oral care protocol, including brushing with a soft toothbrush, flossing, and using nonmedicated rinses (e.g., saline, sodium bicarbonate rinse).

In addition to oral mucosal cleansing, a topical analgesic/anesthetic approach can be considered (see Table 11-4). If using topical agents that reduce the sensory component (e.g., topical local anesthetic), patients should be cautioned to be careful to not traumatize the oral mucosa when speaking or chewing.[17] It is usually safest if patients apply the local anesthetic agent directly to the painful lesion. Swishing and gargling may lead to risk for aspiration of food.

It is common practice in many institutions to utilize topical oral rinses that combine the properties of adherence to mucosa, local anesthesia, and soothing secondary to antihistaminic effects. The following considerations are useful before advising the patient to use these products[17]:

1. Will the patient gain benefit from the combination of agents?
2. Will the patient be able to tolerate the rinse, including considerations of taste and texture?
3. Will the combination rinse contribute added clinical benefit, versus single-agent therapy?

Table 11-4 Supportive care approaches for management of oral mucositis

Efficacy, patient tolerability, and dosing are important factors when a supportive care approach to the management of oral mucositis is considered. A step-wise strategy can be considered, in which progression from one level to the next occurs, based on the following sequence:

Bland rinses
- 0.9% saline solution
- Sodium bicarbonate solution
- 0.9% saline/sodium bicarbonate solution

Topical anesthetics
- Lidocaine: viscous, ointments, sprays
- Benzocaine: sprays, gels
- 0.5% or 1.0% dyclonine hydrochloride (HCl)
- Diphenhydramine solution

Mucosal coating agents (e.g., antacid solutions, kaolin solutions)
- Amphojel
- Kaopectate
- Hydroxypropyl methylcellulose film-forming agents (e.g., Zilactin)
- Cyanoacrylate mucoadherent film
- Gelclair (approved by the FDA as a device). This gel soothes oral mucositis pain by forming a protective coating that shields exposed and overstimulated nerve endings.

Analgesics
- Benzydamine HCl topical rinse (not approved in the United States)
- Opioid drugs: oral, intravenous (e.g., bolus, continuous infusion, patient-controlled analgesia [PCA]), patches, transmucosal

Adapted from NCI Supportive Care (PDQ website). Oral complications of chemotherapy and head/neck radiation. Available at: http://www.cancer.gov/cancertopics/pdq/supportivecare/oralcomplications/healthprofessional.

4. Is the rinse cost-effective, that is, does the combination therapy have cost superiority versus the cost of a single agent (e.g., topical viscous lidocaine) in relation to benefit/risk?

Depending on the intensity and duration of the oral mucositis, topical oral approaches may or may not be sufficient to control oral pain. As noted previously, achieving adequate to excellent oral pain control is very important in having the patient complete the optimal cancer therapy regimen, without dose reduction or treatment interruption.

Morphine-based medications, including patient-controlled analgesia,[17] are frequently utilized in these settings. Hydromorphone, meperidine, and timed-release oral or intravenous morphine and fentanyl (intravenous, transdermal patches, and oral transmucosal) are opiate drugs that can also be considered for use.

The MASCC/ISOO guidelines address empiric and evidence-based approaches for management of the patient with gastrointestinal mucositis (see Table 11-3). As with the oral mucositis guidelines, the combination of evidence-based general bowel care recommendations and specific, pharmacologically based approaches is delineated.

NUTRITIONAL SUPPORT

Oral mucositis and gastrointestinal disturbances associated with mucositis can impair enteral nutrition administration. This complication can be further compounded by the dysgeusia that occurs secondary to mucosal injury of the dorsal tongue, including the taste buds. Maintaining body weight can be critically important throughout the cancer treatment phase, as can maximizing compliance with outpatient visits and optimizing tumor cell response to head and neck radiation.

It is thus essential that nutritional intake and weight status be assessed and managed as needed by a nutritional specialist, when risk for compromise of these parameters is evident. Diets can be tailored to continue enteral administration via a soft or liquid diet. If clinically indicated, a gastrostomy for outpatient management or total parenteral nutrition for inpatient care may be necessary to preserve nutrition and body mass.

Strategies for the patient include the following[17]:

1. Utilize a bland, soft diet, thus avoiding spiced, acidic, or salted foods.
2. Avoid foods that are excessively hot or cold.
3. Utilize liquid nutritional supplements.
4. Chew sugar-free gum or sugar-free hard candy to stimulate saliva if salivary hypofunction is present secondary to head and neck radiation.
5. Implement the use of nasogastric or nasoduodenal tube feedings, or total parenteral nutrition if necessary.
6. If indicated in the patient with gastrointestinal mucositis, use antiemetics to reduce the discomfort associated with enteral intake.

FUTURE DIRECTIONS FOR MUCOSITIS RESEARCH AND CLINICAL TRANSLATION

Exciting new frontiers are being delineated relative to mucositis caused by cancer therapy, including pathobiology, clinical intervention, impact of alimentary tract mucositis on overall symptom burden, and risk prediction. These advances are being fostered by the novel use of biological, imaging, and computational strategies and by comprehensive, multidisciplinary research collaborations that embrace the biological, clinical, mathematical, and physical sciences.

Examples of new research directions include the following:

- Comprehensive coordination of future mucositis guideline development across the several guidelines that currently exist. As noted previously, the Mucositis Study Group of MASCC/ISOO produced the initial set of guidelines in 2002, followed by an updated version published in 2007. Since the time of publication of the original guidelines, other organizations including the National Comprehensive Cancer Network and the Oncology Nursing Society have produced mucositis guidelines. It will be important that guideline management be coordinated in the future to ensure clear, usable recommendations for clinicians.
- New drugs in development that, if successful, could permit new approaches for prevention and/or treatment of mucositis on a molecularly targeted basis
- Increased recognition of the contributions that oral and gastrointestinal mucositis play relative to the overall

symptom toxicity expression secondary to cancer therapy. In this model, even grade 2 toxicities, when they occur in combination with other ≥grade 2 toxicities, can cause clinically significant adverse outcomes.

- Enhanced understanding of the genetic and epigenetic basis for a given patient's response to cancer therapy, including the side effect profile. The ability to predict the severity and duration of oral and gastrointestinal mucositis in advance of cancer treatment could permit clinicians to customize ("personalize") single-agent or multiagent approaches to mucositis management.
- Novel biochemical and imaging strategies to assess severity of gastrointestinal mucositis
- Increasing recognition of the importance of conducting high-quality clinical trials relative to products that have

been approved as devices for the management of mucosal injury. These new studies may well serve to validate commercial claims that currently exist and may permit identification of which patient cohorts are likely to benefit most from use of the devices.

While these advances are occurring, new molecularly targeted cancer therapies are being tested and utilized in the clinical setting with increasing frequency. These novel agents in some cases are redefining the side effect toxicity profile that cancer patients are experiencing, including oral and gastrointestinal mucositis. Thus, comprehensive reporting of the trajectory of mucositis caused by these new drugs will be important in establishing risk, severity, and duration for the given cohorts.

REFERENCES

1. Peterson DE, et al. Oral mucositis: the new paradigms. *Curr Opin Oncol*. 2010;22:318–322.
2. Raber-Durlacher JE, Elad S, Barasch A. Oral mucositis. *Oral Oncol*. 2010;.
3. Sonis ST. Regimen-related gastrointestinal toxicities in cancer patients. *Curr Opin Support Palliat Care*. 2009;4:26–30.
4. Sonis ST, et al. Oral mucositis and the clinical and economic outcomes of hematopoietic stem-cell transplantation. *J Clin Oncol*. 2001;19:2201–2205.
5. Elting LS, et al. The burdens of cancer therapy: clinical and economic outcomes of chemotherapy-induced mucositis. *Cancer*. 2003;98:1531–1539.
6. Elting LS, et al. Risk, outcomes, and costs of radiation-induced oral mucositis among patients with head-and-neck malignancies. *Int J Radiat Oncol Biol Phys*. 2007;68:1110–1120.
7. Trotti A, et al. Mucositis incidence, severity and associated outcomes in patients with head and neck cancer receiving radiotherapy with or without chemotherapy: a systematic literature review. *Radiother Oncol*. 2003;66:253–262.
8. Murphy BA. Clinical and economic consequences of mucositis induced by chemotherapy and/or radiation therapy. *J Support Oncol*. 2007;5(9 suppl 4):13–21.
9. Jones JA, et al. In-hospital complications of autologous hematopoietic stem cell transplantation for lymphoid malignancies: clinical and economic outcomes from the Nationwide Inpatient Sample. *Cancer*. 2008;112:1096–1105.
10. Rosenthal DI. Consequences of mucositis-induced treatment breaks and dose reductions on head and neck cancer treatment outcomes. *J Support Oncol*. 2007;5(9 suppl 4):23–31.
11. Bellm LA, et al. Patient reports of complications of bone marrow transplantation. *Support Care Cancer*. 2000;8:33–39.
12. Stiff P. Mucositis associated with stem cell transplantation: current status and innovative approaches to management. *Bone Marrow Transplant*. 2001;27(suppl 2):S3–S11.
13. Spielberger R, et al. Palifermin for oral mucositis after intensive therapy for hematologic cancers. *N Engl J Med*. 2004;351:2590–2598.
14. Lalla RV, Sonis ST, Peterson DE. Management of oral mucositis in patients who have cancer. *Dent Clin North Am*. 2008;52:61–77.

15. Keefe DM. Gastrointestinal mucositis: a new biological model. *Support Care Cancer*. 2004;12:6–9.
16. Sonis ST, et al. Perspectives on cancer therapy-induced mucosal injury: pathogenesis, measurement, epidemiology, and consequences for patients. *Cancer*. 2004;100(suppl 9):1995–2025.
17. Peterson DE, et al. Mucositis in patients receiving high-dose cancer therapy. In: Lyman C, ed. *Cancer supportive care*. London/New York: Elsevier; 2008:187–205.
18. Keefe DM, et al. Updated clinical practice guidelines for the prevention and treatment of mucositis. *Cancer*. 2007;109:820–831.
19. Elting LS, et al. Patient-reported measurements of oral mucositis in head and neck cancer patients treated with radiotherapy with or without chemotherapy: demonstration of increased frequency, severity, resistance to palliation, and impact on quality of life. *Cancer*. 2008;113:2704–2713.
20. Easton JB, Houghton PJ. mTOR and cancer therapy. *Oncogene*. 2006;25:6436–6446.
21. Sonis S, et al. Preliminary characterization of oral lesions associated with inhibitors of mammalian target of rapamycin in cancer patients. *Cancer*. 2009;116:210–215.
22. Fall-Dickson JM, et al. Oral mucositis-related oropharyngeal pain and correlative tumor necrosis factor-alpha expression in adult oncology patients undergoing hematopoietic stem cell transplantation. *Clin Ther*. 2007;29(suppl):2547–2561.
23. Logan RM, et al. Characterisation of mucosal changes in the alimentary tract following administration of irinotecan: implications for the pathobiology of mucositis. *Cancer Chemother Pharmacol*. 2008;62:33–41.
24. Peterson DE, Bensadoun R-J, Roila F, on behalf of the ESMO Guidelines Working Group. Management of oral and gastrointestinal mucositis: ESMO Clinical Recommendations. *Ann Oncol*. 2010;21(suppl 5):v257–v261.
25. Barasch A, Peterson DE. Risk factors for ulcerative oral mucositis in cancer patients: unanswered questions. *Oral Oncol*. 2003;39:91–100.
26. Schwab M, et al. Role of genetic and nongenetic factors for fluorouracil treatment-related severe toxicity: a prospective clinical trial by the German 5-FU toxicity study group. *J Clin Oncol*. 2008;26:2131–2138.

27. Chansky K, Benedetti J, Macdonald JS. Differences in toxicity between men and women treated with 5-fluorouracil therapy for colorectal carcinoma. *Cancer*. 2005;103:1165–1171.
28. McCarthy GM, et al. Risk factors associated with mucositis in cancer patients receiving 5-fluorouracil. *Oral Oncol*. 1998;34:484–490.
29. Epstein JB, et al. The correlation between epidermal growth factor levels in saliva and the severity of oral mucositis during oropharyngeal radiation therapy. *Cancer*. 2000;89:2258–2265.
30. Napenas JJ, et al. Molecular methodology to assess the impact of cancer chemotherapy on the oral bacterial flora: a pilot study. *Oral Surg Oral Med Oral Pathol Oral Radiol Endod*. 2010;109:554–560.
31. Marsh S, McLeod HL. Cancer pharmacogenetics. *Br J Cancer*. 2004;90:8–11.
32. Gamelin E, et al. Individual fluorouracil dose adjustment based on pharmacokinetic follow-up compared with conventional dosage: results of a multicenter randomized trial of patients with metastatic colorectal cancer. *J Clin Oncol*. 2008;26:2099–2105.
33. Lalla RV, et al. Anti-inflammatory agents in the management of alimentary mucositis. *Support Care Cancer*. 2006;14:558–565.
34. Sonis S, et al. Gene expression changes in peripheral blood cells provide insight into the biological mechanisms associated with regimen-related toxicities in patients being treated for head and neck cancers. *Oral Oncol*. 2007;43:289–300.
35. Duan S, et al. Mapping genes that contribute to daunorubicin-induced cytotoxicity. *Cancer Res*. 2007;67:5425–5433.
36. Boerma M, et al. Local administration of interleukin-11 ameliorates intestinal radiation injury in rats. *Cancer Res*. 2007;67:9501–9506.
37. Belinsky MG, et al. Multidrug resistance protein 4 protects bone marrow, thymus, spleen, and intestine from nucleotide analogue-induced damage. *Cancer Res*. 2007;67:262–268.
38. Anthony L, et al. New thoughts on the pathobiology of regimen-related mucosal injury. *Support Care Cancer*. 2006;14:516–518.
39. Citri A, Yarden Y. EGF-ERBB signalling: towards the systems level. *Nat Rev Mol Cell Biol*. 2006;7:505–516.

40. Aprile G, et al. Application of distance matrices to define associations between acute toxicities in colorectal cancer patients receiving chemotherapy. *Cancer*. 2008;112:284–292.

41. Campagnaro E, et al. Symptom burden after autologous stem cell transplantation for multiple myeloma. *Cancer*. 2008;112: 1617–1624.

42. Elting LS, et al. Economic impact of palifermin on the costs of hospitalization for autologous hematopoietic stem-cell transplant: analysis of phase 3 trial results. *Biol Blood Marrow Transplant*. 2007;13:806–813.

43. Posner MR, Haddad RI. Novel agents for the treatment of mucositis. *J Support Oncol*. 2007; 5(9 suppl 4):33–39.

44. Rubenstein EB, et al. Clinical practice guidelines for the prevention and treatment of cancer therapy-induced oral and gastrointestinal mucositis. *Cancer*. 2004;100(9 suppl):2026–2046.

45. *Oral complications of chemotherapy and head/neck radiation*. 2010. Available at: http://www.cancer.gov/cancertopics/pdq/supportivecare/oralcomplications/healthprofessional.

Management of treatment-related dermatologic adverse effects

12

Marissa Newman, Eugene Balagula, and Mario E. Lacouture

Targeted chemotherapeutics developed over the past decade have revolutionized cancer treatment, but have brought with them a new set of challenges, particularly cutaneous toxicities. Because chemotherapy is most effective in destroying rapidly dividing cells, organs such as the skin, mucous membranes, hair, and nails are most susceptible to damage because of their rapid proliferation and turnover. This chapter will familiarize the practitioner with the pathophysiology, grading scale, incidence, characteristic patterns, and management of these dermatologic manifestations.

GRADING OF DERMATOLOGIC TOXICITY

Uniform grading of cutaneous toxicity is essential for choosing an initial treatment, assessing response to treatment, and giving practitioners a standardized scale for research purposes.[1] In 2009, the U.S. Department of Health and Human Services published the Common Terminology Criteria for Adverse Events (CTCAE), version 4.0, which is commonly used to classify toxicities in both clinical practice and research trials (Table 12-1). This updated scale takes into account body surface area of the rash, the variety of nail disorders, and the degree to which dermatologic toxicities have an impact on quality of life and activities of daily living (ADLs).

PATHOPHYSIOLOGY

The characteristics of each rash are tightly connected to the target molecule or receptor of a particular chemotherapeutic. For example, epidermal growth factor receptors (EGFRs) are essential in skin structure and function in that they regulate keratinocyte proliferation, differentiation, and longevity.[2] Epidermal growth factor receptor inhibitors (EGFRIs) include small molecules such as erlotinib and gefitinib, as well as monoclonal antibodies such as cetuximab and panitumumab. Inhibiting the EGFR causes keratinocyte dysregulation, which manifests in skin rash, as well as in hair and nail changes. When epithelial cells are exposed to EGFRIs, an increase is seen in the synthesis of chemokines, which recruit inflammatory cells such as leukocytes and neutrophils.[2] This inflammatory reaction and subsequent histologic derangement can be observed clinically in the erythematous papular and pustular rash.

PAPULOPUSTULAR (ACNEIFORM) RASH

The classic papulopustular rash is the most common cutaneous manifestation of EGFRIs and is observed in 75% to 90% of patients receiving traditional EGFRI therapy (Fig. 12-1). The dual EGFRI and human epidermal growth factor receptor 2 (HER2) inhibitor lapatinib has a lower incidence of the acneiform rash. Additionally, multikinase inhibitors (MKIs) such as sorafenib and sunitinib can produce the papulopustular rash, although with lower frequency. Forty percent of patients on sorafenib and 20% of patients on sunitinib develop this eruption.

The papulopustular or acneiform rash is characterized by papules and pustules often on the face and scalp, in a seborrheic distribution. Of note, comedones are not observed with this rash as they are in true acne because the histopathology differs.[3] This rash is associated with pruritus and pain and most frequently starts 2 weeks after therapy is initiated.[2] The rash typically peaks at weeks 4 to 6 of treatment and then gradually improves despite further EGFRI therapy.[2] Most important, the

Table 12-1   Common terminology criteria for adverse events (CTCAE), version 4.0

Skin and subcutaneous tissue disorders

Adverse events	Grade				
	1	*2*	*3*	*4*	*5*
Dry skin	Covering <10% BSA with no associated erythema or pruritus	Covering 10%–30% BSA and associated with erythema or pruritus; limiting instrumental ADLs	Covering >30% BSA and associated with pruritus; limiting self-care ADLs	–	–

Definition: A disorder characterized by flaky and dull skin; the pores are generally fine, and the texture is paper thin.

Nail discoloration	Asymptomatic; clinical or diagnostic observations only; intervention not indicated	–	–	–	–

Definition: A disorder characterized by change in the color of the nail plate.

Nail loss	Asymptomatic separation of the nail bed from the nail plate or nail loss	Symptomatic separation of the nail bed from the nail plate or nail loss; limiting instrumental ADLs	–	–	–

Definition: A disorder characterized by loss of all or a portion of the nail.

Nail ridging	Asymptomatic; clinical or diagnostic observations only; intervention not indicated	–	–	–	–

Definition: A disorder characterized by vertical or horizontal ridges on the nails.

Palmar-plantar erythrodysesthesia syndrome	Minimal skin changes or dermatitis (e.g., erythema, edema, hyperkeratosis) without pain	Skin changes (e.g., peeling, blisters, bleeding, edema, hyperkeratosis) with pain; limiting instrumental ADLs	Severe skin changes (e.g., peeling, blisters, bleeding, edema, hyperkeratosis) with pain; limiting self-care ADLs	–	–

Definition: A disorder characterized by redness, marked discomfort, swelling, and tingling in the palms of the hands or the soles of the feet.

Photosensitivity	Painless erythema and erythema covering <10% BSA	Tender erythema covering 10%–30% BSA	Erythema covering >30% BSA and erythema with blistering; photosensitivity; oral corticosteroid therapy indicated; pain control indicated (e.g., narcotics, NSAIDs)	Life-threatening consequences; urgent intervention indicated	Death

Definition: A disorder characterized by an increase in sensitivity of the skin to light.

Pruritus	Mild or localized; topical intervention indicated	Intense or widespread; intermittent; skin changes from scratching (e.g. edema, papulation, excoriations, lichenification, oozing/crusts); oral intervention indicated; limiting instrumental ADLs	Intense or widespread; constant; limiting self-care ADLs or sleep; oral corticosteroid or immunosuppressive therapy indicated	–	–

Definition: A disorder characterized by an intense itching sensation.

Rash acneiform	Papules and/or pustules covering <10% BSA, which may or may not be associated with symptoms of pruritus or tenderness	Papules and/or pustules covering 10%–30% BSA, which may or may not be associated with symptoms of pruritus or tenderness; associated with psychosocial impact; limiting instrumental ADLs	Papules and/or pustules covering >30% BSA, which may or may not be associated with symptoms of pruritus or tenderness; limiting self-care ADLs; associated with local superinfection with oral antibiotics indicated	Papules and/or pustules covering any % BSA, which may or may not be associated with symptoms of pruritus or tenderness and which are associated with extensive superinfection with IV antibiotics indicated; life-threatening consequences	Death

Table 12-1   Common terminology criteria for adverse events (CTCAE), version 4.0—cont'd

			Skin and subcutaneous tissue disorders		
			Grade		
Adverse events	**1**	**2**	**3**	**4**	**5**
Definition: A disorder characterized by an eruption of papules and pustules, typically appearing on face, scalp, upper chest, and back.					
Rash maculopapular	Macules/papules covering <10% BSA with or without symptoms (e.g., pruritus, burning, tightness)	Macules/papules covering 10%–30% BSA with or without symptoms (e.g., pruritus, burning, tightness); limiting instrumental ADLs	Macules/papules covering >30% BSA with or without associated symptoms; limiting self-care ADLs	–	–
Definition: A disorder characterized by the presence of macules (flat) and papules (elevated). Also known as morbilliform rash, it is one of the most common cutaneous adverse events, frequently affecting the upper trunk, spreading centripetally, and associated with pruritus.					

Source: Available at: http://ctep.cancer.gov/protocoldevelopment/electronic_applications/docs/ctcaev4.pdf. Accessed June 20, 2010.

ADLs, Activities of daily living; *BSA,* body surface area; *NSAID,* nonsteroidal antiinflammatory drug.

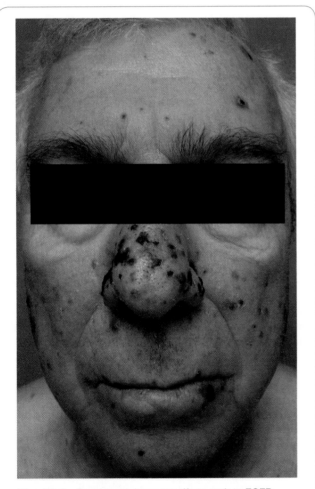

Fig. 12-1   Papulopustular or acneiform rash to EGFR inhibitors.

presence and severity of rash positively correlate with tumor response to chemotherapy and survival.[1] Thus, it is crucial for clinicians to be able to treat this rash, so patients have fewer interruptions or dose reductions in their chemotherapy.

Although most cases are mild to moderate, up to 32% of providers discontinue, and up to 76% temporarily stop, therapy. This dose interruption may negatively affect morbidity and mortality.[4] Therefore, it is essential for providers to educate patients of this potential toxicity and to act preemptively. Patients should be counseled to minimize the frequency and duration of bathing, limiting showers or baths to a maximum of once daily and for less than 10 minutes in tepid water.[2] Immediately after bathing, non–alcohol-based emollients should be applied liberally. Patients should avoid sun by wearing sunscreen and protective clothing such as a hat, sunglasses, and long sleeves. In the randomized controlled trial Skin Toxicity Evaluation Protocol With Panitumumab (STEPP), patients used moisturizer, sunscreen, 1% hydrocortisone cream, and doxycycline 100 mg twice daily prophylactically as compared with patients who were treated after the development of toxicity as determined by their physician.[5] Preemptive therapy decreased the development of a grade 2 rash by 50% and delayed the onset of grades 2 and 3 skin toxicity. Treatment mainstays for the acneiform rash include topical steroids, antibacterial washes, and, in more severe cases, antibiotics and/or oral steroids. Although the EGFR rash is not thought to be due to a true bacterial infection, the antiinflammatory properties of antibiotics have been shown to be beneficial.[4] One study demonstrated efficacy in decreasing facial lesions and pruritus with the use of prophylactic oral minocycline as compared with placebo in patients with metastatic colon cancer before cetuximab therapy.[4] In up to 38% of cases, bacterial superinfection can occur, most commonly *Staphylococcus aureus,* which may be methicillin resistant.[4] Any change in the appearance of the rash, yellow fluid oozing, or crusting should prompt the provider to culture the fluid to identify the causative organism so treatment can be tailored.

HAND FOOT SYNDROME

Hand foot syndrome (HFS), or palmar-plantar erythrodys-esthesia, most commonly occurs with cytotoxic agents, including 5-fluorouracil, **capecitabine**, cytarabine, methotrexate, docetaxel, and doxorubicin (Fig. 12-2). These drugs are believed to be transported by eccrine sweat glands to the stratum corneum, where they extravasate and accumulate, thereby causing cutaneous toxicity.[6,7] The skin reaction is characterized initially by paresthesias, followed by diffuse erythema and edema of the palms and soles.[8,9] Without treatment, the skin lesions may blister, desquamate, and progress to epidermal necrosis. Although variable, onset can occur from 3 days until 10 months after the first dose of chemotherapy.[7] The reaction is dose dependent and is associated with the means of delivery of the drug. For example, one meta-analysis found that 34% of patients administered a continuous infusion of 5-fluorouracil developed HFS, whereas only 13% of patients who received the same drug in bolus form developed the rash.[7]

Several lifestyle modifications have been suggested to decrease the incidence and progression of HFS. Such suggestions include tepid to cool bathing water so as to limit vasodilation and extravasation of the drug to the outer skin layers, loose clothing that does not cause friction with the skin, elevating the lower extremities when possible, and avoiding vigorous activity such as running[7] (Table 12-2). It is interesting to note that topical emollients, aloe vera, and petrolatum ointments, which have demonstrated efficacy against the papulopustular rash, have not shown benefit in randomized trials.[6]

MORBILIFORM ERUPTION (MACULOPAPULAR RASH)

A morbiliform eruption is marked by uniform erythematous macules and papules that blanch under pressure. This is one of the most common skin reactions to chemotherapy agents such as cytarabine, docetaxel, cladribine, gemcitabine,

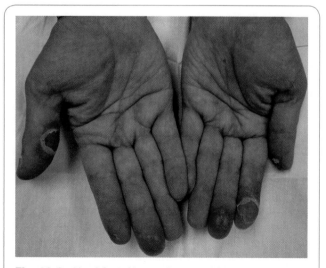

Fig. 12-2 Hand-foot skin reaction to multikinase inhibitors (sorafenib, sunitinib).

Table 12-2 Preemptive strategies for HFS[8]

- Full-body examination to look for hyperkeratotic regions on palms and soles and removal of calluses
- Avoidance of hot water when taking shower, bathing, or dish washing
- Avoidance of trauma and friction during the first 2 to 4 weeks
- Avoidance of vigorous exercise, especially during the first month of therapy
- Avoidance of tight-fitting shoes and evaluation by orthotist if necessary
- Avoiding excessive pressure when applying lotions
- Using moisturizing creams (before and during therapy) that contain keratolytics, such as ammonium lactate or urea
- Wearing thick cotton gloves and/or socks and slippers

Source: Lacouture M, Wu S, Robert C, et al. Evolving strategies for the management of hand-foot skin reaction associated with the multitargeted kinase inhibitors sorafenib and sunitinib. *Oncologist.* 2008;13:1001–1011.

premetrexed, liposomal doxorubicin, topotecan, imatinib, and dasatinib.[10] However, because patients with cancer often have an extensive drug regimen, other culprit drugs may include antibiotics, antipsychotics, and anticonvulsants. The rash most often starts on the trunk and may spread centrifugally to the extremities. Treatment consists of topical or oral steroids and antihistamines. Before chemotherapy is given, patients may be pretreated with steroids and antihistamines to minimize this eruption.[11] It is important to differentiate this rash from the more severe Stevens Johnson syndrome.

STEVENS JOHNSON SYNDROME AND TOXIC EPIDERMAL NECROLYSIS

Stevens Johnson syndrome (SJS) and toxic epidermal necrolysis (TEN), which are part of the same spectrum and disease mechanism, can be severe and even fatal mucocutaneous disorders.[12] These entities are distinguished on the basis of total body surface area (BSA) involved.[13] Less than 10% of BSA involved is referred to as SJS, and greater than 30% BSA involvement is termed TEN. Thus, an overlap of SJS and TEN occurs when 11% to 29% of BSA is involved. Often, the triggers for SJS are drugs, followed by infections, vaccinations, and graft-versus-host disease. Most TEN cases are presumed to be drug related. The most common drug culprits for both SJS and TEN include allopurinol, sulfonamide antibiotics, nonsteroidal antiinflammatories, and anticonvulsants. Chemotherapeutics that have been implicated in these disorders include monoclonal antibodies, antimetabolites, and alkylating agents.[14]

The incidence of SJS and TEN is 1.2 to 6 and 0.4 to 1.2 per million people, respectively. Mortality, which is dependent on the extent of epidermal detachment, ranges from 1% to 5% in SJS and up to 35% in TEN.[15] The pathophysiology underlying this reaction is believed to be an immune-mediated response involving cytotoxic T cells and macrophages. The keratinocyte necrosis is thought to be a direct result of increased activity of the Fas ligand, perforin, and granzyme B pathway.[12]

The classic lesion of SJS or TEN is the target lesion or purpuric macules with a necrotic center.[15] When the epidermis detaches from the underlying dermis, flaccid blisters are produced.

The overlying skin may slough off, causing erosions. The mucosa of the eye, oropharynx, and pulmonary and gastrointestinal tracts, as well as the genitalia, may be involved. The clinical diagnosis may be confirmed by biopsy, which shows diffuse keratinocyte apoptosis and full-thickness epidermal necrosis.[12]

Treatment of SJS and TEN relies upon identifying and stopping the offending agent.[16] Providing excellent wound care and maintaining euvolemia are essential. Intravenous immune globulin (IVIG) has been shown to decrease mortality in these patients when the total dose is greater than 2 g/kg over 3 to 5 days.[15,17] Corticosteroid use is controversial and has been associated with increased risk of infection.

XEROSIS AND PRURITUS

Many chemotherapeutics cause xerosis (dryness) and pruritus of the skin (Fig. 12-3). Up to 35% of patients treated with EGFRIs gradually develop scaly skin, xerosis, and pruritus over the course of their treatment. Of note, patients with a history of eczema experience the dry skin and itchiness more prominently.[18] In this patient population, risk of progression to chronic xerotic dermatitis is associated with secondary *S. aureus* or *Herpes simplex* infection. Xerosis that occurs on the palms of the hands and soles of the feet may lead to painful deep fissures on the tips of the fingers or toes (Fig. 12-4). These carry a similar risk of becoming infected.[19] To prophylax against these skin changes, patients should be instructed to use tepid water, keep showers short and only once daily, and use gentle cleansers. Oral antihistamines and gamma-aminobutyric acid analogs such as gabapentin and pregabalin are useful for calming intense pruritus.

NAIL TOXICITY

Several chemotherapy agents have been linked to nail toxicity, but none are more common than the taxanes.[20] When such drugs affect nail development, they can do so in several ways. They may damage the nail bed, causing onycholysis or subungual hemorrhage. Damage to the nail plate causes grooves, brittleness, and pigment changes. Nail fold damage is considered a paronychia.

PARONYCHIA

Paronychia or periungual inflammation is observed in up to 15% of patients on EGFRIs and occurs after 1 to 2 month of

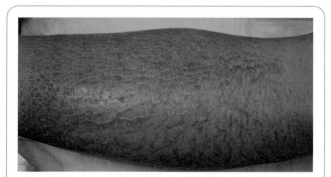

Fig. 12-3 EGFR inhibitor-induced xerosis in an arm.

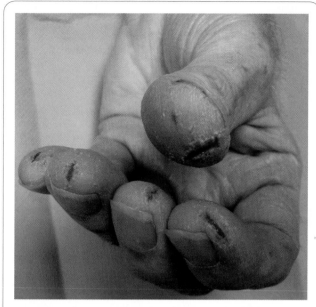

Fig. 12-4 EGFR inhibitor-induced xerosis, manifesting as fissures in the fingertips.

therapy.[18] Initially, the paronychia presents as erythema and edema of the lateral nail fold, which may progress into a tender pyogenic lesion, as with capecitabine, or abscess with the taxanes. This can mimic an ingrown nail. Secondary infection with *S. aureus* may occur and may be treated with oral cephalosporins pending culture and sensitivity results.

ONYCHOLYSIS

Onycholysis, or painful separation of the nail plate from the underlying nail bed, is a direct result of toxicity to the nail bed epithelium from chemotherapy (Fig. 12-5). The most frequently implicated drugs in onycholysis include paclitaxel and docetaxel, followed by capecitabine, doxorubicin, and 5-fluorouracil.[20] Prevention and treatment include trimming

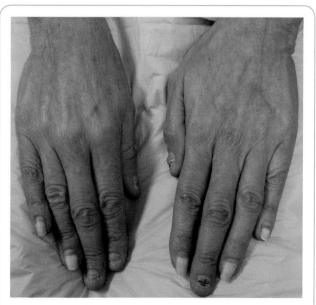

Fig. 12-5 Onycholysis secondary to taxanes (paclitaxel, docetaxel).

the nails short, applying topical antimicrobials, and minimizing exposure to chemical irritants. Frozen gloves and slippers worn 15 minutes before, during, and after the docetaxel infusion have been shown to reduce nail toxicity.[21]

SUMMARY

A wide variety of dermatologic manifestations resulting from anticancer therapies range from skin toxicity to hair and nail changes. These adverse events may cause significant discomfort and decreased quality of life, causing the oncologist to interrupt, terminate, or reduce the dose of therapy. Such changes in the chemotherapy regimen can adversely affect the treatment outcome. The guidelines provided in this chapter are intended to help prevent or mitigate these dermatologic toxicities, so that chemotherapy can be given as seamlessly as possible. Even before therapy is initiated, the patient should be educated on the most common cutaneous adverse events of chemotherapy, methods to prevent these eruptions, and when to seek specialized assistance. Patients must be carefully monitored and examined at each visit so these common dermatologic toxicities from chemotherapy are recognized. This will facilitate early intervention, minimize treatment interruption, and provide the highest quality of life for patients on chemotherapy.

REFERENCES

1. Lynch Jr TJ, Kim ES, Eaby B, et al. Epidermal growth factor receptor inhibitor-associated cutaneous toxicities: an evolving paradigm in clinical management. *Oncologist.* 2007;12:610–621.
2. Li T, Perez-Soler R. Skin toxicities associated with epidermal growth factor receptor inhibitors. *Target Oncol.* 2009;4:107–119.
3. Perez-Soler R, Delord JP, Halpern A, et al. HER1/EGFR inhibitor-associated rash: future directions for management and investigation outcomes from the HER1/EGFR inhibitor rash management forum. *Oncologist.* 2005;10:345–356.
4. Melosky B, Burkes R, Rayson D, et al. Management of skin rash during EGFR-targeted monoclonal antibody treatment for gastrointestinal malignancies: Canadian recommendations. *Curr Oncol.* 2009;16:16–26.
5. Mitchell EP, Lacouture ME, Shearer H, et al. A phase II, open-label trial of skin toxicity (ST) evaluation (STEPP) in metastatic colorectal cancer (mCRC) patients (pts) receiving panitumumab (pmab) + FOLFIRI or irinotecan-only chemotherapy (CT as 2nd-line treatment (tx): interim analysis. *J Clin Oncol.* 2008;644s: Abstract 15007.
6. Lorusso D, Di Stefano A, Carone V, et al. Pegylated liposomal doxorubicin-related palmar-plantar erythrodysesthesia ('hand-foot' syndrome). *Ann Oncol.* 2007;18:1159–1164.
7. von Moos R, Thuerlimann BJ, Aapro M, et al. Pegylated liposomal doxorubicin-associated hand-foot syndrome: recommendations of an international panel of experts. *Eur J Cancer.* 2008;44:781–790.
8. Lacouture ME, Wu S, Robert C, et al. Evolving strategies for the management of hand-foot skin reaction associated with the multitargeted kinase inhibitors sorafenib and sunitinib. *Oncologist.* 2008;13:1001–1011.
9. Lacouture ME, Reilly LM, Gerami P, et al. Hand foot skin reaction in cancer patients treated with the multikinase inhibitors sorafenib and sunitinib. *Ann Oncol.* 2008;19:1955–1961.
10. Heidary N, Naik H, Burgin S. Chemotherapeutic agents and the skin: an update. *J Am Acad Dermatol.* 2008;58:545–570.
11. Agha R, Kinahan K, Bennett CL, et al. Dermatologic challenges in cancer patients and survivors. *Oncology (Williston Park).* 2007;21:1462–1472 discussion 1473, 1476, 1481 passim.
12. Borchers AT, Lee JL, Naguwa SM, et al. Stevens-Johnson syndrome and toxic epidermal necrolysis. *Autoimmun Rev.* 2008;7:598–605.
13. Bastuji-Garin S, Rzany B, Stern RS, et al. Clinical classification of cases of toxic epidermal necrolysis, Stevens-Johnson syndrome, and erythema multiforme. *Arch Dermatol.* 1993;129:92–96.
14. Sorrell J, West DP, Bennett CL, et al. Life-threatening dermatologic toxicities to cancer drug therapy: an assessment of the published peer-reviewed literature. *J Clin Oncol.* 2009;27(suppl): Abstract 20592.
15. French LE. Toxic epidermal necrolysis and Stevens Johnson syndrome: our current understanding. *Allergol Int.* 2006;55:9–16.
16. Hazin R, Ibrahimi OA, Hazin MI, et al. Stevens-Johnson syndrome: pathogenesis, diagnosis, and management. *Ann Med.* 2008;40:129–138.
17. Enk A. Guidelines on the use of high-dose intravenous immunoglobulin in dermatology. *Eur J Dermatol.* 2009;19:90–98.
18. Lacouture ME, Boerner SA, Lorusso PM. Non-rash skin toxicities associated with novel targeted therapies. *Clin Lung Cancer.* 2006;8(suppl 1): S36–S42.
19. Segaert S, Van Cutsem E. Clinical signs, pathophysiology and management of skin toxicity during therapy with epidermal growth factor receptor inhibitors. *Ann Oncol.* 2005;16:1425–1433.
20. Gilbar P, Hain A, Peereboom VM. Nail toxicity induced by cancer chemotherapy. *J Oncol Pharm Pract.* 2009;15:143–155.
21. Scotte F, Tourani JM, Banu E, et al. Multicenter study of a frozen glove to prevent docetaxel-induced onycholysis and cutaneous toxicity of the hand. *J Clin Oncol.* 2005;23:4424–4429.

MANAGEMENT OF TUMOR-RELATED SYMPTOMS

SECTION OUTLINE

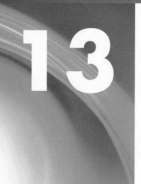

13 Cancer pain

Mellar P. Davis

Pain is one of the most common, feared, and distressing cancer symptoms.[1-3] It occurs as a presenting symptom in a significant minority; most (60%–80%) have significant pain with advanced cancer.[2] Most have moderate to severe pain, and more than 60% experience transient flares of pain.

An international survey characterized cancer pain and pain syndromes in more than 1000 individuals: 70% had metastatic disease, and 75% had a Karnofsky performance score of ≤70. One in four had more than one type of pain, and 20% had pain caused by treatment.[4] Sixty-six percent had severe pain (numeric rating of ≥7 on an 11-point scale). The same percentage had transient flares of pain, in addition to chronic pain. Radiographic procedures were helpful in detecting the cause in 82%. Cancer pain syndromes evolved from bone and joint lesions in 41%; visceral lesions in 28%; soft tissue metastases in 28%; and peripheral nerve injury in 28%. Individuals experiencing pain frequently had more than one distinct pain syndrome. Twenty-two common pain syndromes could be identified in cancer-related clusters.[4] Pain mechanisms were nociceptive in 72% (visceral nociceptive in 58%) and neuropathic in 40% (usually mixed neuropathic-nociceptive). Factors associated with the highest pain intensity included (1) transient flares of pain, (2) somatic and neuropathic pain, (3) age <60 years, and (4) reduced performance status.[4]

Neuropathic pain has several positive symptoms (burning, electric "shock," paroxysm, dysesthesia, and allodynia) in areas of sensory or motor deficits.[5] Post-herpetic neuralgia (a frequent complication in individuals with cancer) has a high prevalence of burning pain and allodynia, whereas amputation-related neuropathic pain and plexopathies have a high prevalence of paroxysmal electric shock–like pain.[5] Besides these associations, no correlations have been noted between neuropathic symptoms and origin, type, or location of the lesion causing pain. Major medications used to treat neuropathic pain (tricyclic antidepressants, gabapentins, pregabalin, and opioids) do not discriminate as to specific mechanisms responsible for pain. Drug choices therefore are based on severity, and not on pain characteristics.[5]

CANCER PAIN ANATOMY

Two main sensory fibers (C, unmyelinated; A-delta, lightly myelinated) enter the spinal cord through the dorsal root ganglion to synapse in the superficial (I-II) and deep (IV-V) dorsal horn laminae. These two fiber types are often silent and respond only to noxious stimuli[6,7] (Fig. 13-1). These sensory neurons have neurokinin receptors (NK-1) and contain substance P (SP) and glutamate.

Several receptors and channels are found in primary afferents. Acid-sensing ion channels (ASICs) are proton-gated nociceptors that are upregulated by inflammation. These receptors are activated in acidic environments such as occur in hypoxic tumors and within osteolytic lesions from osteoclast activation.[7–10] Sodium channels (particularly Na 1.3, Na 1.7, Na 1.8, and Na 1.9) are altered by neuropathic pain. These channels are located at the nerve endings and within the nodes of Ranvier. Sodium channels will be expressed in areas of demyelination within neuromas or within nerve sprouts. Activation causes depolarization. These channels become more active when phosphorylated, which occurs in pathologic pain.[8] Certain medications (lidocaine, mexiletine, phenytoin, carbamazepine, oxcarbazepine, lamotrigine, and tricyclic antidepressants) block sodium channels. These medications will reduce mechanical allodynia and thermal hyperalgesia.[8]

Voltage-gated calcium channels are classified into three subtypes. L-type channels found on postsynaptic membranes are blocked by verapamil and diltiazem. N-type channels on presynaptic membranes are blocked by gabapentinoids and ziconotide. N-type channels contain alpha-2/delta-1 subunits, which are bound by gabapentin and pregabalin, and block release of substance P and glutamate from sensory afferents.[8]

Transient receptor potential vanilloid receptor-1 (TRPV-1) channel cations respond to thermal injury and capsaicin. Inflammation activates kinases, which phosphorylate and activate these channels.[7]

PROSTAGLANDINS

Prostaglandins are not stored in vesicles (unlike substance P, monoamines, and glutamates) but are synthesized from membrane arachidonic acid by prostaglandin synthase and cyclooxygenase (Fig. 13-2). Arachidonate is mobilized from membranes by phospholipases. Cyclooxygenases cyclize arachidonic acid, which are oxidized at two separate sites. Two cyclooxygenases (COX-1 and COX-2) are constitutively expressed in neurons and glia.[11] Peripheral inflammation upregulates cyclooxygenase in the spinal cord, which leads to central sensitization and extension of the area of hypersensitivity around the site of injury. Cyclooxygenase is also found in the brainstem (periaqueductal gray), which facilitates somatosensory processing.[11,12] Prostaglandin (PG)E_2 decreases sodium channel thresholds, increases TRPV-1 cation channels, and inhibits voltage-gated K^+ channels (which repolarizes neurons). PGE_2 binds to presynaptic and postsynaptic prostaglandin receptors (EP_1, EP_2, EP_3, EP_4), amplifies pain (via activation of presynaptic neurons), and facilitates neurotransmission (by activating postsynaptic neurons).[11,12] Inflammation, inflammatory cytokines, and neuron activation (by SP and glutamate) upregulate cyclooxygenases. Salicylates irreversibly and nonsteroidal antiinflammatory drugs (NSAIDs) reversibly inhibit cyclooxygenases. Differences in the antiinflammatory potency and analgesic benefits of NSAIDs have been noted. The two properties of NSAIDs do not correlate. Central pain mechanisms are more responsive to NSAIDs than are peripheral mechanisms.[11] NSAIDs enter the central nervous system (CNS) by passive diffusion. Certain NSAIDs (ketoprofen, ibuprofen, and indomethacin) can be measurable in the CNS 15 to 30 minutes after dosing; levels in the CNS will exceed plasma levels.[11] NSAIDs also interfere with transcription factors (nuclear factor [NF]-κB, AP_1, and peroxisome proliferator–activated receptor [PPAR]) responsible for inflammation and pain independent of cyclooxygenase inhibition.[11] This may explain in part the dissociation between cyclooxygenase inhibitor activity and analgesia.

N-METHYL-D-ASPARTATE RECEPTORS

Glutamate is released from primary afferents in the dorsal horn and binds to and activates secondary afferent and wide dynamic range (WDR) neurons. Three receptors are activated by glutamate: N-methyl-D-aspartate (NMDA) receptors, alpha amino-3-hydroxy-5-methyl-4-isoxazelopropionic (AMPA) receptors, and G protein–coupled metabotropic receptors.[7] Repetitive and high-frequency C-fiber stimulation amplifies and prolongs nociceptive transmission through activation

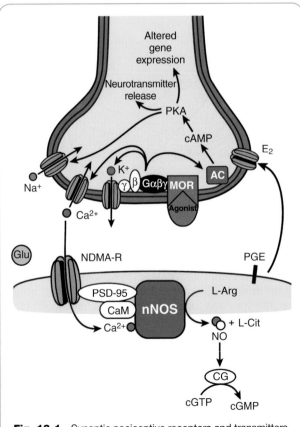

Fig. 13-1 Synaptic nociceptive receptors and transmitters.

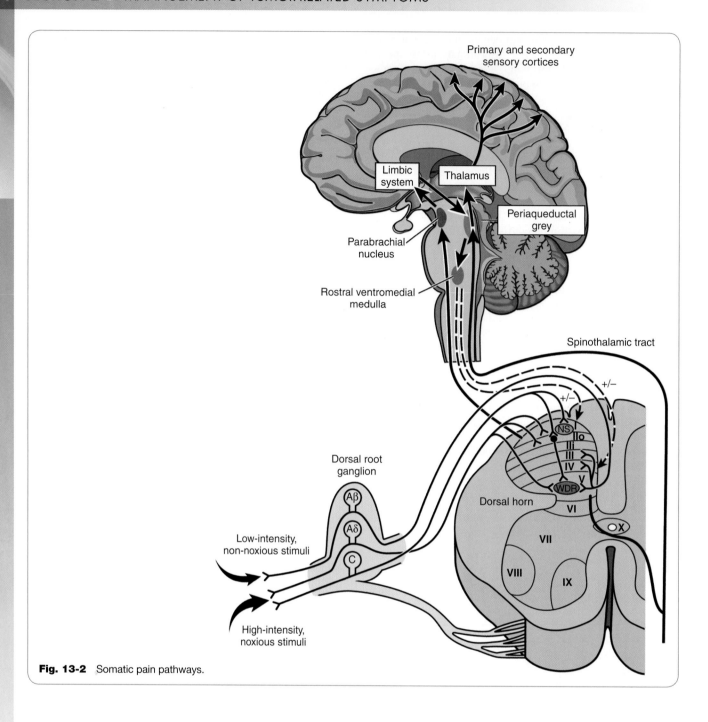

Fig. 13-2 Somatic pain pathways.

of NMDA receptors on WDR neurons. Presynaptic release of glutamate and SP and the presence of glycine unhinge the magnesium plug at the center of the NMDA channel and allow calcium to enter the neuron. Activated NMDA receptors not only increase calcium flux, they also increase nitric oxide synthase and intracellular kinase activity, leading to phosphorylation of other channels and opioid receptors. This results in long-term potentiation of afferent input and allodynia. Ketamine, a noncompetitive NMDA receptor antagonist, reduces pain at subanesthetic doses. Three opioids inhibit NMDA receptors: dextromethorphan, levorphanol, and methadone. Coactivation of WDR neurons with SP and a second neurotransmitter, calcitonin gene-related protein, causes WDR neurons to become resistant to ketamine inhibition.[7]

OPIOIDS

Morphine receptors were first described in 1973, and endogenous opioids were characterized 2 years later.[13] Three major receptors (mu, kappa, and delta) are derived from separate genes; subtypes are formed from mRNA splicing.[13] Opioid receptors are found presynaptically on C and A-delta fibers and on postsynaptic secondary afferents in the brainstem, thalamus, cingulated gyrus, insular and prefrontal cortex, ventral tegmentum amygdale, and nucleus tractus solitares.[14] Activation prevents depolarization through inhibition of calcium channels and adenylyl cyclase and activation of inward rectifying potassium (K^+) channels.[14] This prevents release of SP and glutamate. Activation of opioid receptors in the mesolimbic cortex increases dopamine and rewarding effects to opioids. Activation of opioid receptors on enteric neurons causes increased segmentation and reduced peristalsis, resulting in constipation.[14] Opioids reduce pituitary hypogonadotropin release, resulting in sexual dysfunction. Within the nucleus tractus solitarius, activation of opioid receptors causes nausea and vomiting.[14]

Three classes of opioids are used clinically: phenanthrenes (morphine derivatives), phenylpiperidines (fentanyl and other lipophilic opioids), and diphenylheptanes (methadone). Tramadol resembles venlafaxine in structure but is metabolized through cytochrome CYP2D6 to O-desmethyltramadol, which binds and activates opioid receptors. Partial agonists (morphine) need to bind more receptors to produce the same degree of analgesia.[15] Certain partial agonists such as buprenorphine have a high affinity for new receptors but poorly activate receptors.[15] This will cause a "ceiling" to analgesia at high doses and will change the equianalgesic ratio between opioids at high doses (as occurs between morphine and methadone, a full agonist).[14]

The genetics of the opioid receptor splice variants, dimer formation, G-protein interactions, and subcellular proteins (such as RGS proteins and beta-arrestin) determine analgesic responses to a greater extent than differences in opioid metabolism and clearance.[14,15] As a result, no universal or standard opioid doses or serum levels correlate with pain response. Each individual has a "minimally effective opioid concentration." Analgesic responses are log linear with dose, hence the practice of using percentage dose adjustments during titration for pain control. No "ceiling doses" are recommended, which is unlike most adjuvant analgesics and nonopioid analgesics. Doses are limited by side effectives (cognitive deficits, sedation, myochronus, hallucinations, nausea, and vomiting[15]).

BONE PAIN

Bone pain has a particular "signature" within the spinal cord. Superficial WDR neurons become increasingly activated and increasingly responsive to mechanical and thermal stimuli.[16] This clinically causes hypersensitivity in the area around the painful bone metastases. Trabecular sensory afferents are destroyed by cancer, and the remaining afferents are activated by the acidic environment caused by bone lyses and osteoclast activation.[16] Cytokines promote prostaglandin production, which increases pain and promotes tumor growth.[16] Within the spinal cord, glia are activated and increase in number. Gabapentinoids reduce the neuropathic component of and reduce bone pain,[17] and may be important in the treatment of breakthrough pain. Bisphosphonates inhibit osteoclasts, while NSAIDs and corticosteroids inhibit prostaglandin production within bone metastases; acutely radiation downregulations algesic mediators and subacutely reduces tumor mass. Calcitonin blocks parathyroid hormone (PTH)-related protein stimulation of bone resorption.[16]

VISCERAL PAIN

Visceral pain is poorly localized because of underrepresentation within the lateral (S_1) cortex.[18–20] Visceral primary sensory afferents converge on dorsal horn somatic sensory pathways, and this leads to somatic referral to somatic sites (to the back, shoulder, or abdomen as seen with pancreatic cancer, or to the ear as seen with lung cancer). Only types of visceral damage

are sensed. Tissue cutting, certain crushing, or burning is not painful, whereas ischemia, inflammation, and obstruction are painful.[18] Primary afferents travel with visceral sympathetic fibers in chest and abdomen and with parasympathetic fibers in the pelvis. Afferents converge on the celiac plexus and the paravertebral sympathetic ganglion in the chest. A celiac and hypogastric block relieves visceral pain, and a thoracic sympathetic neurolytic block relieves pain arising from the esophagus.[18]

Visceral afferents synapse within laminae I and V in the ventral horn. Second order neurons send projections to the brainstem and cortex through the ipsilateral dorsal funiculus (whereas somatic sensory afferents send projections through the contralateral anterolateral spinal cord). Visceral pain is relieved by midline myelotomy at the cervical cord level, where dorsal funiculus visceral afferents cross over to the contralateral side, whereas somatic pain is relieved by lateral cordotomy (without producing motor deficits)[7,18] (see Figs. 13-1, 13-2, and 13-3).

NEUROPATHIC PAIN

Two main mechanisms generate neuropathic pain: (1) sensitization of primary afferents, and (2) central sensitization due to increased or decreased peripheral input or CNS damage. Normally, there is a balance between inhibition and facilitation at different synaptic relay sites; with neurologic damage, this balance is lost.[18–20] The end result consists of spontaneous pain, continuous burning (C-fiber) pain, pain with innocuous stimuli (allodynia), or exaggerated pain with noxious stimuli

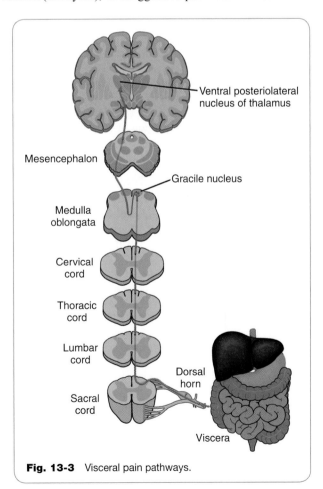

Fig. 13-3 Visceral pain pathways.

(hyperpathia) in areas (usually dermatomal) of sensory or motor deficits.

Neuropathic injury causes release of algesic mediators (bradykinin, histamine, serotonin, glutamate, nerve growth factor, prostaglandins) and cytokines (tumor necrosis factor-alpha [TNF-α], interleukin-1), which depolarizes surviving neurons and/or stimulates immunocyte infiltration and glia proliferation (centrally). Certain sodium channels (Na 1.8) are upregulated in surviving neurons, while other channels (Na 1.3) are upregulated in injured neurons. Both are slowly inactivated.[18–20] Opioid receptors are downregulated,[19] and alpha-2 delta calcium channel subunits are upregulated.[18] Expression of TRPV1 channels, SP, and calcitonin gene-related protein is maintained within areas of nerve damage by nerve growth factor.[19]

Long-lasting peripheral nerve discharges modify neuron phenotype and function (neuroplasticity). Spinal cord inhibitory interneurons undergo degeneration, NMDA receptors are upregulated, and rectifying potassium channels (which repolarize neurons) are lost.[19] Descending inhibition from brainstem structures (periaqueductal gray and rostral ventromedial medulla) to the dorsal horn becomes facilitatory. Spinal cord glia are activated through release of cytokines, which increases production of PGE_2 and downregulates glutamate transporters (increasing glutamate levels in synaptic clefts).[18] Loss of descending inhibition occurs because of downregulation of alpha-2 adrenergic receptors in the dorsal horn. Spinal cord serotonin enhances spinal excitability through serotonin ($5\text{-}HT_3$) receptors, which are upregulated.[7]

Clinically, neuropathic pain is less responsive to opioids. Adjuvants such as calcium channel blockers (gabapentin, pregabalin), sodium channel blockers (lidocaine, mexiletine, carbamazepine, lamotrigine, and phenytoin), NMDA receptors blockers (ketamine), monoamine reuptake inhibitors (tricyclic antidepressants, selective norepinephrine serotonin reuptake inhibitors), and alpha-2 adrenergic receptor agonists (clonidine) are needed to reduce pain.[19] Combinations of adjuvants with different mechanisms of action of opioids may improve pain control better than single-drug therapy.[20]

SECOND ORDER NEURONS AND CEREBRAL PAIN MATRIX

Second order neurons from lamina I of the dorsal horn contain NK-1 receptors and bind SP. These projections travel by way of the contralateral spinothalamic to the brainstem parabrachial area and periaqueductal gray (PAG). PAG, along with the rostral ventromedial medulla (RVM), modulates incoming nociceptive dorsal horn traffic through a spinobulbospinal loop. Brainstem projections to the dorsal horn inhibit or facilitate pain. Serotonin, when bound to $5\text{-}HT_3$ receptors, facilitates pain, and through $5\text{-}HT_{1A}$ receptors inhibits pain.[7] Norepinephrine from the locus coeruleus (brainstem) binds to dorsal horn alpha-2 adrenergic receptors to dampen nociceptive activity. Serotonin and norepinephrine brainstem projections travel via the dorsal funiculus to reach the spinal cord, norepinephrine is predominantly inhibitory, and serotonin inhibits or facilitates pain. Antidepressants, which inhibit norepinephrine transport, are better analgesics than antidepressants, which inhibit only serotonin transport.[7,8,19,20] Mu receptor agonists reduce pain by preventing brainstem pain facilitation.

Spinothalamics project to the ventral posterolateral thalamus and lateral (S_1) sensory cortex, which involves sensory discrimination and location. Projections through the medial thalamus synapse within the prefrontal, cingulate, and insular cortex and are responsible for motivation and affective pain experiences.[18] Prefrontal, cingulated, and insular cortex, in turn, projects back to the PAG, and RVM and will influence pain modulation within the dorsal horn (see Fig. 13-2).

PAIN ASSESSMENT

Pain has several characteristics: severity, quality, location, aversiveness, meaning, frequency, and interference with activities, social life, and role within the family. Pain intensity guides analgesic choices as outlined by the World Health Organization (WHO) in a three-step analgesic ladder. Pain intensity is assessed reliably by categorical scales (none, mild, moderate, severe), numeric scales (0 = no pain, 10 = severe pain), and visual analog scales (10-cm lines with anchors of "no pain" and "severe pain").[21] Visual analog scales (VAS) are more independent of language than categorical scales and hence more adaptable across translations, but they are more difficult to understand and are more dependent on instructions for completion. Numeric rating scales (NRS) are easier for patients to complete than VAS, and for those who are cognitively impaired, categorical scales should be used.[21]

Multidimensional scales assess intensity and the influence of pain on function, emotions, social life, meaning and spirituality, pain relief, quality, location, variations and intensity, flares, and temporal pattern.[21–23] Multidimensional tools most often assess pain intensity, relief, and location, but rarely reveal a temporal pattern.[22] Most multidimensional tools will not help in sculpting an analgesic dosing strategy because treatment strategies are mainly dependent on the temporal pattern. Pain tools with a large number of items and VAS will have a poor completion rate in advanced cancer.[22,23] Certain multidimensional tools are short (Brief Pain Inventory–Short Form) and can be easily completed by those without cognitive deficits.[20] Instruments must be sensitive to change over time if they are to be used to measure outcomes and responses. Many instruments have not been tested for sensitivity to change in pain intensity over time, whereas VAS, NRS, and categorical scales are sensitive to changes in pain.[21–23] A summary of expert opinion regarding assessment tools is provided in Table 13-1.

Analgesic trials use summed pain intensity differences (SPID) and total pain relief over time (TOTPAR) as primary outcomes. Secondary outcomes are patient-rated global efficacy and analgesic toxicity.[24] A 33% to 50% reduction in pain intensity is clinically meaningful to patients and has been used to define response.[25–27] The number of responders is compared with the number treated to generate the numbers needed to treat (NNT). In general, the NNT for neuropathic pain is 3, which means three individuals need to be treated to reduce pain in a single individual by 50%.[24–26] Analgesic trials use two different methods for outcomes: (1) changes in mean differences between groups, and (2) anchor methods, which compare percentages of responders. Trials that use changes in mean intensity are difficult to interpret as to clinical relevance. Pain intensity differences between analgesics may reflect significant pain reduction in only a few individuals, whereas most do not respond or most experience small reductions in

Table 13-1 Expert opinion of pain assessment[21,22]

- Pain intensity is the most important characteristic.
- Worst pain and average pain intensity over 24 hours correlate with impaired function.
- NRS is preferred to VAS and categorical scales in cognitively intact individuals.
- Temporal pattern, interference, and physical function are additional features that need to be assessed for optimum therapy.
- Palliative factors (position, activity, self-administered therapies) should be obtained during assessment.
- The number of flares of pain (breakthrough pain) during the day is critical in pain assessment because most individuals experience episodic pain.
- Treatment-related relief scales are important ancillary scales for analgesic trials.
- Computerized body mapping of worse pain is important (if available).

pain.[28] The anchor method uses responders between groups; these values have greater clinical relevance.[26,28] If interference with daily activities and mood were secondary outcomes to be measured during treatment, an independent meaningful clinical difference would have to be established for the scale. One could not assume a 33% to 50% reduction in interference, or improvement in mood or function would define response, as it does for pain intensity.[28]

IMAGING

SKELETAL METASTASES

Bone is a more frequent site of metastases than anticipated on the basis of cardiac output and perfusion. The most common cancers to spread to bone are prostate, breast, and lung, and are seen as multiple myeloma. Metastases are almost exclusively limited to red marrow, hence are most commonly found in the vertebra and axial skeleton and less frequently in appendages, and rarely in distant long bones.[29] Hematogenous metastases enter trabecular areas via interosseous vessels. Interactions with stromal cells and tumor cells stimulate osteoclasts and osteoblasts, which leads to bone destruction sclerosis and tumor growth.

Plain bone radiographs do not reveal osteolysis until >50% of the cortex is destroyed. Pathologic fracture is anticipated if >75% of the cortex is lost.[29] Surgeons who are considering surgical repair screen painful bone lesions with plain radiographs for this reason.

Bone scans have high sensitivity but low specificity for bone metastases. Positivity is dependent on reactive bone around metastases. Bone scans do not reveal pure osteolytic lesions (as occur with multiple myeloma).[29] Only one third of bone metastases imaged by bone scans are painful. The distribution using technetium 99 is as follows: 39% vertebral; 38% rib and sternum; 12% pelvis, and 10% skull and long bones. Osteolytic lesions appear as "cold spots."[29] Scans are positive for nonmalignant reasons in 23% to 30% of individuals with metastatic cancer. Super scans reveal red marrow extension to juxta-articular areas. The super scans appear "normal," except there is an absence of kidney shadows and diffuse juxta-articular uptake is noted.[29] Bone scans can appear to worsen with response to chemotherapy (called "flare") in prostate and breast cancer, which can persist for 6 months. Treating oncologists can be misled by bone scans during this time. Screening of asymptomatic individuals with early-stage cancer with bone scans has a low yield (<10%). Single areas of positivity are as likely to be benign as malignant, even in those with advanced cancer.[29] The yield in those with persistent musculoskeletal complaints, aged >50 years and without a history of cancer, is 9%.[30] In this situation, it is better to obtain plain radiographs followed by computed tomography (CT) scans or magnetic resonance imaging (MRI). Bone scans can be positive 3 to 18 months before metastases are visualized on plain radiographs.[31]

CT SCANS

Computed tomography imaging is guided by symptoms and plain radiographs.[31] CT scanning is more cumbersome, is not portable, and gives only limited views of the bone. CT scans clarify bone scan–positive lesions in individuals unable to undergo MRI, or who are intolerant of MRI procedures because of claustrophobia. CT scans are combined with myelography to image spinal cord compression.[31,32] CT scans will differentiate vertebral hemangiomas from metastases and will detect bone marrow metastases independent of bone destruction (differences of >20 Hounsfield units compared to normal fatty marrow).[31,32]

MRI

Magnetic resonance imaging detects skeletal metastases with greater sensitivity and specificity than bone scans but provides limited views of the bone. Bone scans detect only one third to two thirds of lesions found on MRI.[31,32] Skeletal metastases have low signal on T_1-weighted images (marrow has high signal on T_1 images) and high signal on T_2-weighted images caused by water content found in metastases.[31,32] A rim of bright T_2 signal may be found around metastases (halo sign). Fat suppression T_1-weighted images differentiate localized fatty deposits in bone and bone marrow from metastases.[31,32] MRI differentiates bone edema, degeneration, and inflammation from metastases and visualizes bone marrow metastases.[31,32] Gadolinium-enhanced MRI is important when imaging spinal soft tissues, epidural space, and spinal canal, but is not needed for bone images.[31,32] Short-tau inversion recovery (STIR) sequences and coronal and axial views help clarify the locations and extent of metastases. MRI is the image modality of choice for vertebral metastases.[29] MRI, like bone scans, is subject to super scan artifact from diffuse bone marrow and bone metastases.[31] Malignant fractures in contrast to osteoporotic fractures have diminished T_1 sequences and are associated with pedicle and posterior vertebral body involvement and epidural or paraspinal masses.[29]

LIVER METASTASES

Each imaging modality has size limitations; lesions <1 cm are difficult to image. Edge definition is key to imaging liver metastases. For each metastasis detected, one to four liver metastases are missed because of size and indistinct edge definitions.[33] Ultrasounds are limited by acoustic windows, obesity, and intervening bowel gas. High-frequency transducers and operator experience increase detection rates.[33] Doppler ultrasound detects metastases because of increased hepatic arterial blood flow to metastases.

Iodine contrast is needed to detect metastases by CT scans. Images should be obtained during the arterial (early) and portal (late) phases of contrast injection.[33] Renal and breast cancers, melanomas, and sarcomas enhance early because of the hypervascular characteristics of metastases. Hypovascular tumors are seen in the portal phase of imaging.[33] CT portography, which involves contrast injection into splenic or superior mesenteric arteries, bypasses the hepatic artery. Liver is enhanced (because most of the blood flow to the liver is portal) and metastases are unenhanced (because most of the blood flow to metastases is from the hepatic artery).[33]

Metastases enhance on T_2-weighted MRI images. Gadolinium does not improve MRI images of liver metastases. However, specific agents that collect in hepatocytes and/or reticuloendothelial cells (MnDPDP, Gd-BoPTA) do improve detection.[33]

LUNG IMAGING

Initial assessment involves anteroposterior and lateral plain chest radiographs. CT scans detect more lung metastases and better define lesions seen on plain radiographs. Contrast-enhanced CT scans should extend through the liver and adrenals to screen for common sites of extrathoracic metastases.[34] Bone lesions and axillary nodal metastases may also be seen on thoracic CT scans. CT scans have a sensitivity of 61% and a specificity of 79% in detecting mediastinal nodal involvement.[34] Positron emission tomography (PET) scans use deoxyfluoroglucose to image metastases. Metastases have increased glucose transporters, which take up the deoxyfluoroglucose. PET scans are combined with CT scans to better characterize small lesions.[35] Increased enhancement is characteristic of metastases and lung cancer. Whole body PET scans detect distant metastases and may be substituted for bone scans with certain cancers. PET scans do not image the brain well; this requires contrast-enhanced CT scans or MRIs. Quantitative expression of standardized uptake values (SUVs) on PET scan images not only clarifies whether a particular lesion is benign or malignant but is also prognostic.[36]

CANCER PAIN MANAGEMENT

Most cancer patients obtain significant relief from pain using a combination of antitumor treatment, systemic analgesics, and nonpharmacologic modalities (surgery, radiation, and psychological and interventional therapies).[37] The WHO analgesic ladder involves a step-wise approach to analgesic drug choices based on pain intensity.[38] NSAIDs or acetaminophen plus adjuvant analgesics are used for mild pain; weak opioids (codeine, tramadol, and dihydrocodeine) plus adjuvants are used for moderate pain; and potent opioids (morphine, methadone, hydromorphone, oxycodone, and fentanyl) are used for severe pain. Five principles guide the use of the WHO analgesic ladder: (1) Oral administration is preferred; (2) around the clock (ATC) dosing should be done for chronic pain; (3) drug choices should be based on pain severity; (4) treatment should be individualized because of variability in analgesic responses among individuals; and (5) constant attention should be paid to details of treatment and assessment.[37–39] Opioid dosing

strategies are based on pain intensity and changes in temporal pain pattern. Adjuvant analgesics are based on the type of pain and are initiated early in those experiencing pain that is poorly responsive to opioids.

Normal-release morphine (or oxycodone or hydromorphone) by mouth is started at 5 mg every 4 hours (oxycodone 5 mg, hydromorphone 1 mg) ATC in the opioid naïve.[40] Individuals with moderate to severe pain on weak opioids are started on 10 mg of immediate-release morphine every 4 hours.[40] Alternatively, sustained-release morphine at 15 mg every 12 hours is substituted for immediate-release morphine for the opioid naïve.[38,39] Steady state is achieved in 24 hours with immediate-release morphine and in 48 hours with sustained-release morphine.[38] The ATC dose should not be adjusted until steady state is reached. The final ATC dose can range from 5 mg to >250 mg every 4 hours.[41]

Transient flares of pain on ATC opioids are managed by "rescue" doses of the same potent opioid if at all possible. Several recommendations have been made for rescue: (1) the 4-hourly dose as the rescue dose every 1 to 2 hours as needed[38]; (2) 10% to 20% of the daily morphine dose (or equivalent)[39]; or (3) 50% of the 4-hourly dose given every 2 hours.[42] Pain flares are volitional incident, nonvolitional incident, spontaneous, or end-of-dose failure. End-of-dose failure is managed by increasing the ATC opioid dose.[43] Some consider end-of-dose failure to be an indicator of suboptimal ATC doses, and not of breakthrough pain.

Transdermal fentanyl is increasingly being used for cancer pain. The initial dose is 12 μ per hour, which is equivalent to 30 mg of oral morphine per day.[44] Transdermal fentanyl generic patches are commercially available as matrix and reservoir patches. Systematic experimental and clinical evidence of bioequivalence between the different patches is not established. Single case reports have described respiratory depression when matrix patches using the same dose are switched for reservoir patches.[44] Time to maximum concentration after placement of a transdermal patch ranges between 12 and 40 hours. Patches should not be changed more frequently than every 48 hours during titration. Oral morphine and transmucosal or transbuccal fentanyl is used for rescue.[45] Alternatively, intravenous or subcutaneous fentanyl is titrated to pain response and the effective dose converted to transdermal fentanyl using a 1:1 ratio. Dermal absorption is highly variable between individuals, so doses will need to be adjusted after conversion.[45]

Pain flares often peak within 2 to 5 minutes of onset and resolve within 30 to 60 minutes. Half of pain flares are spontaneous.[46,47] Volitional incident and procedural pain may be treated preemptively. Onset and offset of most pain flares do not match the onset of oral opioid analgesia (≥30 minutes). The opioid dose needed to relieve pain flares poorly corresponds to the effective ATC dose, particularly when transmucosal or transbuccal fentanyl is used.[48–50] Particular opioid formulations have been developed that bypass hepatic clearance, have a rapid onset and offset of action, and are relatively easy to administer, with high patient acceptance (Tables 13-2 and 13-3).[43]

OPIOID TITRATION

If pain is uncontrolled with ATC opioid doses and breakthrough (rescue) doses, ATC and rescue doses over the last 24 hours are summed and increased by 30% to 50%. For example, an individual on sustained-released morphine 60 mg

Table 13-2* Opioid formulations for pain flares[48]

Transmucosal fentanyl
 ACTIQ (Cephalon Inc., Frazer, PA, USA)
Transbuccal fentanyl
 Fentora (Cephalon Inc., Frazer, PA, USA)
 Abstral (Prostakan, Galashiels, UK)
Intranasal fentanyl
 Instranyl (Nycomed, Zurich, Switzerland)
 Nasalfent (Archimedes Pharma, Reading UK)

*Rescue doses are titrated to response after chronic pain is under control.[49]

Table 13-3 Recommendations for managing cancer-related breakthrough pain[47,49,50]

Assess for presence and severity of pain flares.
Consider treating the underlying mechanism.
 • Single-fraction radiation, bisphosphonates, and radioisotopes for bone pain
 • Kyphoplasty for vertebral fractures
Use avoidance treatment of precipitating factors.
Preemptively treat volitional incident pain and procedural pain.
Use nonopioid analgesics.
 • NSAIDs for bone pain
 • Gabapentin, pregabalin for neuropathic spontaneous pain
 • Ketamine rescue for spinal analgesia
 • Anticholinergics for colic from bowel obstruction
Maximize ATC opioid dose, particularly for end-of-dose failure.
Use interventional techniques.
 • Neurolytic blocks
 • Regional anesthesia
Use behavioral modalities, imagery, and mind/body techniques with analgesics.
Assess breakthrough pain response with each change in analgesics.

every 12 hours and 20 mg of immediate-release morphine every 4 hours who has taken four rescue doses over 24 hours has a baseline pain >7 (NRS), and the summed dose is 120 mg + 80 mg, or 200 mg. The dose is increased by 30%, or 260 mg. The adjusted dose should then be sustained-release morphine 130 mg every 12 hours with rescue dose adjusted to 30 mg to 45 mg every 1 to 2 hours as needed.[43]

If pain is controlled but more than four rescue doses are needed to control chronic pain, the rescue doses are added to the ATC dose unless the pain is predominantly incident pain.

If chronic pain is controlled but pain flares remain severe, the rescue dose is increased incrementally (by 30%–50%) for pain control. Alternatively, transmucosal, transbuccal, or intranasal fentanyl is used and titrated to response.[48]

ACUTE PAIN DOSING STRATEGY

Severe and rapidly changing pain is not to be treated the same way that chronic pain is treated. Morphine is given at a dose of 1 mg to 2 mg intravenously every 1 to 2 minutes until significant pain reduction is achieved.[51] Responses are generally seen within 30 to 60 minutes. Alternatively, 1.5 mg is given every 10 minutes, or 10 mg to 15 mg every 15 minutes. This should be done by a physician at the bedside. Naloxone should be available for potential overdose.[51] Pain assessment is done frequently; significant pain response, but not total analgesia, is the goal. Alternative opioids include hydromorphone 0.2 mg or fentanyl 20 μ every 1 to 2 minutes in place of morphine.[51] Maintenance doses after titration are one third to one fourth of the effective dose given as an hourly continuous dose. Alternatively, the effective dose is converted to oral equivalent morphine equivalents (by multiplying by 3) and is given every 4 hours ATC. The chronic opioid dose before titration in opioid-tolerant individuals will have to be added to the effective dose to avoid a relapse of pain.

Naloxone hydrochloride reverses opioid-induced respiratory depression at small doses (40 μ–100 μ) and should be given intravenously until the level of consciousness improves and spontaneous respirations are >10 per minute.[52–55] Naloxone can be given subcutaneously and intranasally to reverse opioid toxicity. Continuous infusion may be needed in those on sustained-release morphine, transdermal fentanyl, or methadone.[52–55]

OPIOID POORLY RESPONSIVE PAIN

Unrelieved chronic pain and concurrent dose-limiting side effects (delirium, hallucinations, myoclonus, nausea, or vomiting) are managed in three different ways: (1) opioid switch, (2) opioid route conversion, or (3) the addition of an adjuvant analgesic and opioid reduction (30%–50%).[56–59] Several factors predict for opioid responsiveness. Neuropathic pain, breakthrough pain, opioid tolerance, and young age predict for less opioid responsiveness.[59]

OPIOID ROTATION

Opioid switches or rotations reduce pain and opioid side effects in part because of lack of cross-tolerance between opioids.[56] Disadvantages or pitfalls to rotation are that opioid conversion tables are largely based on single-dose studies, availability of certain opioid formulations is limited, potential drug interactions may occur with the second opioid, and treatment expenses are increased.[58] Wide variability in equivalence is seen between individuals, and therefore wide confidence intervals with ratios[56] (Tables 13-4 and 13-5).

OPIOID ROUTE CONVERSION

Route conversions for uncontrolled pain and side effects are usually epidural or intrathecal.[60-64] Conversions from oral to parenteral morphine may improve pain control and reduce side effects, but the usual reason is mucositis, dysphagia, nausea, vomiting, enteric fistula, or bowel obstruction due to the number of tablets or the need for rapid opioid titration.[65] Epidural opioids are usually initiated when opioid rotation and adjuvants have failed to reduce pain or are limited by side effects.[65] Epidural opioid analgesia should not be selected solely because systemic opioids have failed to relieve pain. Low doses of opioid will reduce pain via the epidural route in those experiencing intractable opioid side effects with

Table 13-4 Equianalgesic table[60,61]

Opioid	Oral	Parenteral
Morphine	30	10
Hydromorphone	6	2–3
Fentanyl	1:70–100	
Oxycodone	20–30	
Methadone	4:1 (morphine <90 mg/day) 8:1 (morphine >90 mg<300 mg/day) 12:1 (morphine >300 mg–<1000 mg/day) 15–20:1 (morphine >1000 mg/day)	

Equivalents have a clinical context such as organ function, medication, and individual genetic constitution, which governs opioid metabolism and opioid receptor activation.[56,62,63] Equianalgesic ratios are not bidirectional equivalents. Rotations are usually "stop-start," in which the first opioid is stopped while the second is started.

Table 13-5 Guidelines for Opioid Rotation[56,62,63]

- Be sure the patient was compliant with the ATC and rescue doses.
- Be sure there is no other cause for symptoms that mimic opioid toxicity (hypercalcemia, brain metastases).
- Consider route conversion or the addition of adjuvant analgesic as an alternative to opioid rotation.
- Assess the clinical context of the patient (organ function, age, comedications, reasons for rotation, previous opioid response, comorbidities).
- When rotating for opioid toxicity, a 30% to 50% dose reduction in the opioid equivalent should be the initial dose.
- When rotating predominantly for pain, the initial opioid dose is the equivalent.
- Individuals who are frail, elderly, or on high opioid doses and who are experiencing toxicity should have opioid rotations at a 50% reduction of equivalence.
- Rotations to methadone should be performed with extreme care by using an experienced prescriber and a linear equivalent ratio (see Table 14-4) or 10% of the total daily oral morphine dose, up to 30 mg at the single maximum dose, every 3 hours orally as needed.

Table 13-6 Indications for Epidural Analgesia[65]

- Short life expectancy (usually ≤1 month)
- Pain scores >6 (NRS) after opioid titration, rotation, and systemic adjuvants with limited side effects or intolerance
- Neuropathic and somatic pain
- Continuous plus intermittent or intermittent pain
- Patient acceptance
- Adequate community resources and support systems to maintain epidural analgesia at home

Table 13-7 Contraindications to Epidural Analgesia[65]

- Patient refusal
- Lack of community support system or adequate informal caregivers
- Platelet counts <20,000
- Systemic coagulopathy or inherited bleeding disorder
- Oral anticoagulation
- Chemotherapy with expected myelosuppression
- Radiation to the vertebral site of epidural catheter insertion
- Occlusion of epidural site with tumor
- Uncontrolled infection
- Delirium and cognitive failure, which precludes consent or safe maintenance of epidural catheters
- Psychosis, suicide risk

systemic opioids.[65] Ranking order for responsive pains with epidural analgesia is as follows: somatic continuous pain, visceral continuous pain, somatic intermittent, neuropathic intermittent or continuous, and cutanous (cancer or fistula).[65] Epidural opioids are used for individuals who have 1 month or less to survive.[65] Indications and contraindications for epidural analgesia are outlined in Tables 13-6 and 13-7.

Individuals who undergo spinal analgesia are opioid tolerant, thus combinations of opioids and local anesthetics are frequently needed to improve pain control.[65–68] Metastatic vertebral metastases account for one of the most severe pain syndromes. Vertebral body metastases involve the posterior spinous process and lamina and will not affect the usual route of catheter placement (at the dermatome where the pain is experienced).[66] MRIs or CT scans are necessary before catheter placement to ensure that the epidural space is not involved with cancer. Patient-controlled epidural analgesia allows patients to bolus themselves before activities or at the onset of severe pain. Temporary catheters can be safely placed at the bedside tunneled to avoid infection and provide catheter stability.[65] Bupivacaine concentrations range from 0.1% to 0.25%, and clonidine dosage should start at 10 μ to 15 μ/ml. Both clonidine and bupivacaine are effective in neuropathic pain.[66–68] The opioid can be rotated from morphine to preservative-free hydromorphone or fentanyl in those poorly responding to morphine.[68]

Intrathecal opioid dose requirements are approximately 100 times lower than those for systemic opioids for analgesic. Forty-percent of individuals who are started on intrathecal opioids will require the addition of intrathecal adjuvants[66] (Table 13-8). Indications and contraindications are similar to those for epidural analgesia; however, fewer long-term complications occur with intrathecal catheters and internal pump placement than with epidural catheters and external pump placement. Individuals anticipated to live longer than 3 to 6 months are considered for intrathecal analgesia with implantable pump. Most individuals have significant reductions in pain severity and improved pain relief (60%–80% reduction in VAS, 60% improvement by relief scales).[66] Opioid side effects are fewer but still can be present (Table 13-9). Both systemic and spinal opioids are associated with an unusual side effect: hypogonadotropic hypogonadism.[69,70]

Table 13-8   Spinal Adjuvant Analgesic[66-68]

Local anesthetics	
• Bupivacaine	10 mg–30 mg/day
• Ropivacaine	10 mg–30 mg/day
Alpha-2 adrenergic drugst	
• Clonidine	50 μ–200 μ/day
Calcium channel blocker	
• Ziconotide	0.01–0.05 mcg/hr up to 19.4 mcg/day
Gamma-aminobutyric acid agonists	
• Baclofen	Up to 2 mg/day
• Midazolam	1 mg–2.5 mg/day

Table 13-9   Opioid Side Effects

- Constipation
- Urinary retention
- Nausea
- Vomiting
- Sweating
- Impotence
- Pruritus
- Sedation
- Nightmares
- Visual hallucinations
- Fatigue
- Xerostomia
- Myoclonus
- Peripheral edema
- Hyperalgesia
- Respiratory depression

The most common side effect noted with spinal opioid is pruritus. Inhibition of micturition reflex is more common with spinal opioids than with systemic opioids. Both spinal and systemic opioids cause hypogonadotropic hypogonadism, resulting in hot flashes, sweats, loss of libido, and menopausal symptoms that are reversible.[69,70]

NSAIDs

NSAIDs are not adjuvants but analgesics; however, NSAIDs have been combined with opioids, similar to adjuvant analgesics. In a meta-analysis of NSAID and opioid combinations for postoperative pain, nausea, vomiting, and sedation were lessened with the combination, and analgesia was better than opioids alone. NSAIDs have a 30% opioid sparing effect on opioid consumption.[71] Less evidence related to benefit is seen with NSAIDs plus opioid given for cancer pain. Trials are heterogeneous in design and population, a fact that precludes meta-analysis.[72] NSAIDs are better than placebo, and a dose-response effect is seen in multiple trials with NSAIDs alone. Not one particular NSAID is more effective than another. Nine of 14 trials demonstrated a slight but statistically significant benefit with the combination of NSAIDs and opioids for cancer pain.[72] Responses may be dependent on the particular NSAID and opioid used in combination.[73] Rotating NSAIDs or opioids within a combination could theoretically improve pain relief.[73]

CORTICOSTEROIDS

Corticosteroids have opioid sparing effects.[74] Corticosteroids reduce headache from brain metastases and back pain from spinal cord compression. Injections into or around bone metastases (ribs and sacroiliac joints) and epidural space may significantly reduce localized pain, which is not responsive to opioid titration.[74–76] Half of individuals in palliative and hospice programs will be placed on corticosteroids some time during the course of their illness to treat not only pain but anorexia and fatigue, and to improve a sense of well-being.[75,76] Treatment benefits are limited.[74,77,78] To avoid long-term complications, doses should be tapered to the lowest effective dose after response. If no response is seen within 1 week, corticosteroids should be discontinued.

ADJUVANT ANALGESICS

Adjuvant analgesics rebalance the opioid/analgesia side effect ratio in favor of widening the therapeutic index. Adjuvants improve pain relief, are opioid dose sparing, and thus reduce opioid side effects.[79] Adjuvants have primary indications other than pain but are analgesic with certain pains and may be used before opioids for pain (in this case, the term "adjuvant" is a misnomer).[79] Choices depend on the type of pain. Certain adjuvants are effective for several pains. Gabapentin, for instance, is effective in relieving neuropathic pain and bone pain.[17] Adjuvants are listed in Tables 13-8, 13-10, and 13-11.

Corticosteroids relieve bone pain and improve appetite in individuals suffering from anorexia. Anticonvulsants treat neuropathic pain and reduce seizures associated with brain metastases.[79] Concurrent syndromes may help in the selection

Table 13-10   Adjuvants[80,84,86]

Drug	Mechanism	NNT	Dose per Day
Carbamazepine	Sodium channel blocker	2.5	400 mg–800 mg
Phenytoin	Presynaptic glutamine, inhibits presynaptic release, sodium channels	2.1	300 mg–450 mg
Gabapentin	Voltage-gated calcium channel blocker	2.9–4.3	900 mg–3600 mg
Pregabalin	Voltage-gated calcium channel blocker	4.2	150 mg–600 mg
Amitriptyline	Monoamine reuptake inhibitor	3.6	50 mg–150 mg
Venlafaxine	Selective norepinephrine/serotonin reuptake inhibitor	3.1	75 mg–225 mg
Duloxetine	Selective norepinephrine/serotonin reuptake inhibitor	–	60 mg–120 mg
Transdermal lidocaine	Sodium channel blocker	3.6–4.4	1 to 3, 5% plasters

Table 13-11 Miscellaneous adjuvants[80,84,86]

Drug	Mechanism	Dose per Day
Bupropion	Dopamine reuptake inhibitor	100 mg–300 mg
Dexamethasone	Corticosteroid	1 mg–60 mg
Lamotrigine	Sodium channel blocker, prevents glutamate release	200 mg–400 mg
Oxcarbazepine	Sodium channel blocker	300 mg–1600 mg
Levetiracetam	Calcium channel blocker, antagonizes negative GABA/glycine modulators	1000 mg–3000 mg
Baclofen	Gamma-aminobutyric acid receptor beta blocker	20 mg–200 mg
Ketamine	NMDA receptor blocker	100 mg–500 mg PO or 0.8 mg/kg IV
Clonazepam	Gamma-aminobutyric acid	2 mg–4 mg
Mexiletine	Local anesthetic sodium channel blocker	100 mg–300 mg

of adjuvant medications. The NNT suggests that only one of three individuals experienced significant relief with the addition of a single adjuvant for neuropathic pain.[80] Few studies have focused on cancer, and most drug selections are based on the experience of treating nonmalignant pain. Combinations of gabapentin plus morphine and pregabalin plus oxycodone improve neuropathic pain to a greater extent and at lower doses of both drugs than single-drug therapy.[81–83] Adding an antidepressant to a gabapentinoid plus opioid combination theoretically could improve pain relief; however, published experience with two adjuvant combinations is limited.[80]

Tricyclic antidepressants, although effective, have multiple adverse effects, including cardiac toxicity, orthostatic hypotension, urinary retention, drowsiness, and confusion. Secondary amine tricyclic antidepressants have fewer anticholinergic side effects .Venlafaxine, duloxetine, mirtazapine, and bupropion are better tolerated.[80,84,85]

Oxcarbazepine can be substituted for carbamazepine to avoid drug interactions and myelosuppression.[86] Phenytoin should be avoided because of potential drug interactions. Pregabalin and gabapentin reduce not only pain intensity, but the affective component of pain, and also improve sleep. Both produce dizziness, somnolence, asthenia, and headache in a minority of patients. Pregabalin is reported to produce peripheral edema.[86] Few drug interactions have been reported with either of these anticonvulsants. Pregabalin is a more potent calcium channel blocker; it has dose linear pharmacokinetics and hence provides an advantage. Gabapentin absorption is dependent on L-amino acid transporters, which become saturated at high doses. Gabapentin must be given at least

3 times a day because it has a short half-life; pregabalin is dosed twice daily.[86] The type of pain (allodynia, spontaneous shooting pain, or burning pain) does not predict response to either agent. However, the genetic constitution of an individual could possibly determine pain response.[87]

Systemic administration of local anesthetics is reported to reduce pain.[88] Intravenous lidocaine or oral mexiletine is most frequently reported. Both are as effective as carbamazepine, amantadine, gabapentin, and morphine.[86,88] Local anesthetics are usually third-line adjuvants because of the risk of cardiac toxicity.

NMDA receptor antagonists reduce central sensitization and wind-up. The NMDA receptor antagonist (ketamine) is a receptor state–dependent antagonist and a noncompetitive blocker. Ketamine may also inhibit monoamine reuptake.[89] Oral bioavailability is 20%; however, the metabolite norketamine is an active NMDA receptor blocker. Ketamine may cause hypertension and tachyarrhythmia. Cognitive complications occur in a minority at low doses. The use of lorazepam or haloperidol reduces side effects.[89] Cognitive complications are more frequent in those with a psychiatric history or personality disorder. Ketamine should be avoided by those who are delirious.[89]

MISCELLANEOUS ADJUVANT MEDICATIONS AND INTERVENTIONS

BISPHOSPHONATES

Thirty randomized trials using bisphosphonates to relieve bone pain have been reported. The NNT at 4 weeks is 11, and at 12 weeks is 7. The number needed to harm (NNH) is 16.[90] Bisphosphonates in general do not work quickly. Pamidronate 60 mg to 90 mg or zolendronate 4 mg is usually given monthly. Side effects include fever and achiness after treatment. Doses are adjusted to renal function. Jaw osteonecrosis is a long-term adverse effect associated with bisphosphonates. This complication occurs particularly in individuals undergoing dental extractions while receiving bisphosphonates. Bisphosphonates are recommended early with the onset of bone metastases to prevent fractures and other bone complications; they can be considered as "add-on" therapy when analgesics or radiation therapy is inadequate.[90] Another bisphosphonate, ibandronate, has been used with loading doses; this rapidly relieves bone pain. A 4 to 6-day IV loading dose (4 mg–6 mg/day) does not produce renal toxicity and reduces pain within 7 days.[91]

Small, prospective, nonrandomized and randomized trials have demonstrated bone pain relief with salmon calcitonin.[92–96] Doses of 100 μ to 400 μ are given subcutaneously daily. Side effects are minimal. Calcitonin can be used in those with renal failure in lieu of NSAIDs. One study found that calcitonin causes increases in beta endorphin blood levels associated with gradual pain relief.[94]

RADIOISOTOPES

Three isotopes—phosphorous-32, strontium-89, and samarium-153—have affinity for bone.[97,98] They accumulate in areas of bone remodeling around metastatic sites. These isotopes are beta emitters and do not pose risk of radiation exposure to relatives.[97] Radioisotopes may relieve pain over a 1 to 6-month period. Adverse effects are leukopenia and thrombocytopenia.[97]

IMAGE-GUIDED THERAPIES

INTERVENTIONAL APPROACHES

Percutaneous ethanol injections cause dehydration and coagulation necrosis of tumor. Pain relief from bone metastases can occur within 24 to 48 hours. The best results are seen with small metastases (3 cm–6 cm).[98] Pain relief is experienced in 74% within 4 to 10 weeks. Twenty-three percent (23%) will have pain again as tumor progresses. This may occur over 2 to 4 months after the procedure. Ethanol injections do not improve mechanical stability of bone; incident pain due to mechanical instability is not likely to respond. Ethanol can diffuse into vital structures or within joints, resulting in pain, disability, or neurologic deficits.[98]

Radiofrequency ablation uses shielded needle electrodes and alternating currents to produce coagulation necrosis of tumor. Friction heat generated through the alternating current produces tumor damage. Tumors should measure <4 cm to use this modality. Several ablations are usually needed in multiple sessions. Nearly 60% experience pain relief within 4 weeks, 95% within 12 weeks.[98] Complication rates are low. Adverse effects are skin burns from grounding pads and delayed fractures. Contraindications are tumors near vital structures, large lesions (≥10 cm), and blastic lesions. Radiofrequency ablation does not provide stability to bone, and so fractures can occur post procedure.[98]

Percutaneous vertebroplasty and kyphoplasty are used to treat painful and mechanically unstable vertebral metastases. A recent randomized trial of vertebroplasty versus sham vertebroplasty in osteoporotic fractures failed to demonstrate a benefit for vertebroplasty.[99] Kyphoplasty uses balloon tamponade to reestablish vertebral height before filling the vertebral body with bone cement (polymethyl methacrylate) and thus differs from vertebroplasty. Kyphoplasty produces pain relief and improves functional outcomes.[100] Asymptomatic cement extravasation and new vertebral fractures occur in <10%. Kyphosis is corrected in 90%, with a mean correction of 7.6 degrees.[100]

Arterial embolization using polyvinyl alcohol particles reduces pain and bleeding from hypervascular cancers (thyroid, neuroendocrine, renal melanoma, and angiosarcoma). Common cancers, such as breast, colon, and lung, are hypovascular and thus poorly responsive to embolization.[98]

Embolization can be used for metastases not amenable to surgery or radiation. It is also used to reduce blood loss at the time of surgery. Pain relief can be experienced within 24 hours. Local pain, fever, and malaise may be experienced transiently post procedure. Serious complications (paraplegia, quadriplegia, dissection of the aorta) are seen in 1% to 2%.[98]

Celiac block is commonly performed for upper abdominal visceral pain.[101] The target is precrural and retrocrural spaces. Splanchnic blocks could be considered in those failing to respond to celiac block. Regional pain, hypotension, and diarrhea may occur post procedure. Most adverse effects are temporary.[101]

Neurolytic CNS blocks may benefit individuals with unilateral pain limited to a number of spinal segments.[102] Dorsal rhizotomy severs pain input at a particular level without producing motor deficits. This can be effective with brachial plexopathies due to superior sulcus lung cancers.[102] Commissural myelotomy disrupts pain and thermal fibers, which cross the midline in the anterior white commissure. This procedure will relieve intractable bilateral and midline pelvic and perineal pain.[102] Anterior cordotomy interrupts the anterior spinothalamic tracts, which contain pain and temperature fibers but no motor fibers. This reduces pain in the contralateral half of the body without motor deficits. Finally, thalamotomy relieves midline or bilateral pain in 80%. Pain recurs in 30%. Side effects include confusion, cognitive deficits, and disorientation.[102]

CONCLUSION

Cancer pain will be experienced by most with advanced cancer and a significant minority with early-stage disease. Pain can be related to treatment or may be due to comorbidities. Chronic pain is usually accompanied by transient flares of pain. Assessment is the key to management. Intensity and temporal pain pattern guide dosing strategies. Drug choices are based on the WHO three-step analgesic ladder. Those failing to achieve pain relief or who are experiencing side effects may undergo opioid switch or change in route, or may have adjuvant analgesic added. Nonpharmacologic approaches, including radiation, surgery, neurolytic blocks, and ablative procedures improve pain in those with relatively resistant opioid pain.

REFERENCES

1. Rustøen T, Fossci SD, Skarstein J, et al. The impact of demographics and disease-specific variables on pain in cancer patients. *J Pain Symptom Manage.* 2003;26:696–704.
2. Beck SL, Falkson G. Prevalence and management of cancer pain in South Africa. *J Pain Syst Manage.* 2001;94:75–84.
3. Strohbuecker B, Mayer H, Evers GC. Pain prevalence in hospitalized patients in a German university teaching hospital. *J Pain Symptom Manage.* 2005;29:498–506.
4. van den Beuken MHJ, de Rijke JM, Kessels AG, et al. Prevalence of pain in patients with cancer: a systematic review of the past 40 years. *Ann Oncol.* 2007;18:1437–1449.
5. Caraceni A, Portenoy RKa working group of the IASP Task Force on Cancer Pain. An international survey of cancer pain characteristics and syndromes. *Pain.* 1999;82:263–274.
6. Attal N, Fermanian C, Fermanian J, et al. Neuropathic pain: are there distinct subtypes depending on the aetiology or anatomical lesion? *Pain.* 2008;138:343–353.
7. D'Mello R, Dickenson AH. Spinal cord mechanisms of pain. *Br J Anaesth.* 2008;101:8–16.
8. Harvey VL, Dickenson AH. Mechanisms of pain in nonmalignant disease. *Curr Opin Support Palliat Care.* 2008;2:133–139.
9. Aurilio C, Pota V, Pace AC, et al. Ionic channels and neuropathic pain: physiopathology and applications. *J Cell Physiol.* 2007;215:8–14.
10. Rogers M, Tang L, Madge DJ, et al. The role of sodium channels in neuropathic pain. *Semin Develop Biol.* 2006;17:571–581.
11. Burian M, Geisslinger G. COX-dependent mechanisms involved in the antinociceptive action of NSAIDs at center and peripheral sites. *Pharmacol Ther.* 2005;107:139–154.
12. Murakami M, Kudo I. Prostaglandin E synthase: a novel drug target for inflammation and cancer. *Curr Pharmacol Design.* 2006;12:943–954.
13. Snyder SH. Opiate receptor revisited. *Anesthesiology.* 2007;107:659–661.
14. Pasternak GW. Molecular biology of opioid analgesia. *J Pain Symptom Manage.* 2005;29(5SS):S2–S9.
15. Trescot AM, Datta S, Lee M, et al. Opioid pharmacology. *Pain Physician.* 2008;11:S133–S153.
16. Urch CE, Donovan-Rodriguez T, Dickenson AH. Alterations in dorsal horn neurons in a rat

model of cancer-induced bone pain. *Pain.* 2003;106:347–356.

17. Carceni A, Zecca E, Martini C, et al. Gabapentin for breakthrough pain due to bone metastases. *Palliat Med.* 2008;22:392–393.

18. Regan JM, Peng P, Chan VWS. Neurophysiology of cancer pain: from the laboratory to the clinic. *Curr Rev Pain.* 1999;3:214–225.

19. Ji RR, Strichartz G. Cell signaling and the genesis of neuropathic pain. *Science.* 2004;252:14.

20. Finnerup NB, Sindrup S, Jensen T. Chronic neuropathic pain: mechanisms, drug targets and measurement. *Fundam Clin Pharmacol.* 2007;(21):129–136.

21. Caraceni A, Cherny N, Fainsinger R, et al. Pain measurement tools and methods in clinical research in palliative care: recommendations of an expert working group of the European Association of Palliative Care. *J Pain Symptom Manage.* 2002;(3):239–255.

22. Hjermstad MJ, Gibbins J, Haugen DF, et al. Pain assessment tools in palliative care: an urgent need for consensus. *J Palliat Med.* 2008;22:895–903.

23. Klepstad P, Hilton P, Moen J, et al. Self-reports are not related to objective assessments of cognitive function and sedation in patients with cancer pain admitted to a palliative care unit. *Palliat Med.* 2002;(6):513–519.

24. Turk DC, Dworkin RH, McDermott MP, et al. Analyzing multiple endpoints in clinical trials of pain treatments: IMMPACT recommendations. Initiative on methods, measurement, and pain assessment in clinical trials. *Pain.* 2008;(3):485–493.

25. Jenson MP, Karoly P, Braver S. The measurement of clinical pain intensity: a comparison of six methods. *Pain.* 1986;27:117–126.

26. Dworkin RH, Turk DC, McDermott MP, et al. Interpreting the clinical importance of group differences in chronic pain clinical trials: IMMPACT recommendations. *Pain.* 2009;146:238–244.

27. Farrar JT, Berlin JA, Strom BL. Clinically important changes in acute pain outcome measures: a validation study. *J Pain Symptom Manage.* 2003;25:406–411.

28. Dworkin RH, Turk DC, Wyrwich KW, et al. Interpreting the clinical importance of treatment outcomes in chronic pain clinical trials: IMMPACT recommendations. *J Pain.* 2008;(2):105–121.

29. Soderlund V. Radiological diagnosis of skeletal metastases. *Eur Radiol.* 1996;6:587–595.

30. Jacobson AF. Musculoskeletal pain as an indicator of occult malignancy: yield of bone scintigraphy. *Arch Intern Med.* 1997;157:105–109.

31. White AP, Kwon BK, Linskog DM, et al. Metastatic disease of the spine. *J Am Acad Orthop Surg.* 2006;14:587–588.

32. Rosenthal DI. Radiological diagnosis of bone metastases. *Cancer.* 1997;80:1595–1607.

33. Mahfouz AE, Hamm B, Mathieu D. Imaging of metastases to the liver. *Eur Radiol.* 1996;6:607–614.

34. Gould MK, Kuschner WG, Rydzak CE, et al. Test performance of positron emission tomography and computer tomography for mediastinal staging in patients with non-small-cell lung cancer: a methanalysis. *Ann Intern Med.* 2003;(22):879–892.

35. Pfister DG, Johnson DH, Azzoli C, et al. American Society of Clinical Oncology treatment of nonresectable non-small-cell lung cancer guidelines: update 2003. *J Clin Oncol.* 2004;22:330–353.

36. Pastorino V, Landoni C, Marchiano A, et al. Fluorodeoxyglucose uptake measured by positron emission tomography and standardized uptake value predicts long-term survival of CT screening detected lung cancer in heavy smokers. *J Thorac Oncol.* 2009;4:1352–1356.

37. Jost L. Management of cancer pain: ESMO clinical recommendations. *Ann Oncol.* 2007;18:92–94.

38. Hanks GW, de Conno F, Cherny N, et al. Morphine and alternative opioids in cancer pain: the EAPC recommendations. *Br J Cancer.* 2001;84:587–593.

39. Krakowski I, Theobald S, Balp L, et al. Summary version of the standards, options and recommendations for the use of analgesia for the treatment of nociceptive pain in adults with cancer (update 2002). *Br J Cancer.* 2003;89(suppl 1):S67–S72.

40. Ripamonti C, Tiziana C, Fagnoni E, et al. Normal-release oral morphine starting dose in cancer patients with pain. *Clin J Pain.* 2009;25:386–390.

41. Fallon M, Hanks G, Cherny N. Principles of control of cancer pain. *Brit Med J.* 2006;(7458):1022–1024.

42. Sawe J, Dahlstrom B, Rane A. Steady-state kinetics and analgesic effect of oral morphine in cancer patients. *Eur J Clin Pharmacol.* 1983;24:537–542.

43. Walsh D, Rivera NI, Davis MP, et al. Strategies for pain management: Cleveland Clinic Foundation guidelines for opioid dosing for cancer pain. *Support Cancer Ther.* 2004;1:157–164.

44. Walter C, Felden L, Lotsch J. Bioequivalence criteria for transdermal fentanyl generics. *Clin Pharmacokinet.* 2009;48:625–633.

45. Grond S, Radbruch L, Lehmann K. Clinical pharmacokinetics of transdermal opioids. *Clin Pharmacokinet.* 2000;38:59–89.

46. Foster D, Upton R, Christrup L, Popper L. Pharmacokinetics and pharmacodynamics of intranasal versus intravenous fentanyl in patients with pain after oral surgery. *Ann Pharmacother* 2008;42:1380–1387.

47. Portenoy RK, Hagen NA. Breakthrough pain: definition, prevalence and characteristics. *Pain.* 1990;41:273–281.

48. Zeppetella G, Ribeiro MDC. Opioids for the management of breakthrough (episodic) pain in cancer patients. Review. *The Cochrane Collaboration.* 2009;1–19.

49. Casuccio A, Mercadante S, Fulfaro F. Treatment strategies for cancer patients with breakthrough pain. *Expert Opin Pharmacol.* 2006;10:947–953.

50. Hagen NA, Biondo P, Stiles C. Assessment and management of breakthrough pain in cancer patients: current approaches and emerging research. *Curr Pain Headache.* 2008;12:241–248.

51. Davis MP, Weissman DE, Arnold RM. Opioid dose titration for severe cancer pain: a systematic evidence-based review. *J Palliat Med.* 2004;7:462–468.

52. Goodrich PA. Naloxone hydrochloride: a review. *AANA.* 1990;58:14–16.

53. Kerr D, Kelly AM, Dietze P, et al. Randomized controlled trial comparing the effectiveness and safety of intranasal and intramuscular naloxone for the treatment of suspected heroin overdose. *Addiction.* 2009;104:2067–2074.

54. Bradberry JC, Raebel MA. Continuous infusion of naloxone in the treatment of narcotic overdose. *Drug Intell Clin Pharmacol.* 1981;15:945–950.

55. Wanger K, Brough L, Macmillan I, et al. Intravenous vs. subcutaneous naloxone for out-of-hospital management of presumed opioids overdose. *Acad Emerg Med.* 1998;5:293–299.

56. Knotkova H, Fine PG, Portenoy RK. Opioid rotation: the science and the limitations of the equianalgesic dose table. *J Pain Symptom Manage.* 2009;(3Z):426–439.

57. Mercadante S. Recent progress in the pharmacotherapy of pain. *Expert Rev Anticancer Ther.* 2001;1:487–494.

58. Estfan B, LeGrand SB, Walsh D, et al. Opioid rotation in cancer patients: pros and cons. *Oncology.* 2005;19:511–516; 516-518; 521-523; 527-528.

59. Ahmedzai SH, Boland J. Opioids for chronic pain: molecular and genomic basis of actions and adverse effects. *Curr Opin Support Palliat Care.* 2007;1:117–125.

60. Anderson R, Saiers JH, Abram S, et al. Accuracy in equianalgesic dosing conversion dilemmas. *J Pain Symptom Manage.* 2001;(5):397–406.

61. Pereira J, Lawlor P, Vigano A, et al. Equianalgesic dose ratio for opioids, a critical review and proposals for long-term dosing. *J Pain Symptom Manage.* 2001;(2):672–687.

62. Shaheen P. Opioid equianalgesic tables: are they equally dangerous? *J Pain Symptom Manage.* 2009;38:409–417.

63. Fine P, Portenoy RK. Establishing "best practices" for opioid rotation: conclusions of an expert panel. *J Pain Symptom Manage.* 2009;38:418–425.

64. Mercadante S. Opioid poorly-responsive cancer pain. Part 3. Clinical strategies to improve opioid responsiveness. *J Pain Symptom Manage.* 2001;21:338–354.

65. DuPen SL. Epidural techniques for cancer pain management: when, why and how? *Curr Rev Pain.* 1999;3:183–189.

66. Buchheit T, Rauck R. Subarachnoid techniques for cancer pain therapy: when, why and how? *Curr Rev Pain.* 1999;3:198–205.

67. Eisenach JC, DuPen S, Dubois M, et al. Epidural clonidine analgesia for intractable cancer pain. *Pain.* 1995;61:391–399.

68. Newsome S, Frawley BK, Argoff CE. Intrathecal analgesia for refractory cancer pain. *Curr Pain Headache Rep.* 2008;12:249–256.

69. Finch PM, Roberts LJ, Price L, et al. Hypogonadism in patients treated with intrathecal morphine. *Clin J Pain.* 2000;16:251–254.

70. Rajagopal A, Vassilopoulou-Sellin R, Palmer JL, et al. Symptomatic hypogonadism in male survivors of cancer with chronic exposure to opioids. *Cancer.* 2004;100:851–858.

71. Marret E, Kurdi O, Zufferey P, et al. Effects of nonsteroidal anti-inflammatory drugs on patient-controlled analgesia morphine side effects. *Anesthesiology.* 2005;102:1249–1260.

72. McNicol E, Strassels SA, Goudas L, et al. NSAIDs or paracetamol, alone or combined with opioids, for cancer pain. *Cochrane Database Syst Rev.* 2005;(1):1–2.

73. Zelcer S, Kolesnikov Y, Kovalyshyn I, et al. Selective potentiation of opioid analgesia by nonsteroidal anti-inflammatory drugs. *Brain Res.* 2005;151–156.

74. Twycross R. The risks and benefits of corticosteroids in advanced cancer. *Drug Saf.* 1994;11:163–178.

75. Rousseau P. The palliative use of high-dose corticosteroids in three terminally ill patients with pain. *Am J Hospice Palliat Care.* 2001;18:343–346.

76. Woolridge JE, Anderson CM, Perry MC. Corticosteroids in advanced cancer. *Oncology.* 2001;15:225–234.

77. Lundstrom SH, Furst CJ. The use of corticosteroids in Swedish palliative care. *Acta Oncol.* 2006;45:430–437.

78. Gannon C, McNamara P. A retrospective observation of corticosteroid use at the end

of life in a hospice. *J Pain Symptom Manage.* 2002;24:328–334.

79. Lussier D. Adjuvant analgesics in cancer pain management. *Oncologist.* 2004;9:571–591.

80. Kong VK, Irwin MG. Adjuvant analgesics in neuropathic pain. *Eur J Anaesthesiol.* 2009;26:96–100.

81. Gilron I, Mitchell M. Combination pharmacotherapy for neuropathic pain: current evidence and future directions. *N Engl J Med.* 2005;5:823–830.

82. Gatti A. Controlled-released oxycodone and pregabalin in the treatment of neuropathic pain: results of a multi-center Italian study. *Eur Neurol.* 2009;61:129–137.

83. Doggrell SA. Pregabalin or morphine and gabapentin for neuropathic pain. *Expert Opin Pharmacol.* 2005;6:2535–2539.

84. Knotkova H, Pappagallo M. Adjuvant analgesics. *Anesthesiol Clin.* 2007;25:775–786.

85. Semenchuk MR, Sherman S, Davis B. Double-blind, randomized trial of bupropion SR for the treatment of neuropathic pain. *Neurology.* 2001;57:1583–1588.

86. Guay D. Oxcarbazepine, topiramate, zonisamide and levetiracetam: potential. *Am J Geriatr Pharmacol.* 2003;1:18–37.

87. Chesler E, Ritchie J, Kokayeff A, et al. Genotype-dependence of gabapentin and pregabalin sensitivity: the pharmacogenetic medication of

88. Challapali V, Tremont-Lukats IW. Systematic administration of local anesthetic agents to relieve neuropathic pain. *Cochrane Database Syst Rev.* 2005;(4): CCD003345.

89. Okon T. Ketamine: an introduction for the pain and palliative medicine physician. *Pain Physician.* 2007;10:493–500.

90. Wong R, Wiffin PJ. Bisphosphonates for the relief of pain secondary to bone metastases. *Cochrane Database Syst Rev.* 2006;(3):1–124.

91. Mancini I, Dumon JC, Body JJ. Efficacy and safety of ibandronate in the treatment of opioid-resistant bone pain associated with metastatic bone disease: a pilot study. *J Clin Oncol.* 2004;22:3587–3592.

92. Tsavaris N, Kopterides P, Kosmas C, et al. Analgesic activity of high-dose intravenous calcitonin in cancer patients with bone metastases. *Oncol Rep.* 2006;16:871–875.

93. Schiraldi GF, Soresi E, Locicero S, et al. Salmon calcitonin in cancer pain: comparison between two different treatment schedules. *Int J Clin Pharmacol Ther Toxicol.* 1987;25:229–232.

94. Mystakidou K, Befon S, Hondros K, et al. Continuous subcutaneous administration of high-dose salmon calcitonin in bone metastasis: pain control and beta-endorphin plasma levels. *J Pain Symptom Manage.* 1999;18:323–330.

95. Roth A, Kolaric K. Analgetic activity of calcitonin in patients with painful osteolytic metastases of breast cancer: results of a controlled randomized study. *Oncology.* 1986;43:283–287.

96. Martinez-Zapata R, Roque M, Alonso-Coello P, et al. Calcitonin for metastatic bone pain. *Cochrane Database Syst Rev.* 2006;(3) CD003233.

97. Callstrom MR, Charboneau JW, Goetz MP, et al. Image-guided ablation of painful metastatic bone tumors: a new and effective approach to a difficult problemv. *Skeletal Radiol.* 2006;35:1–15.

98. Sabharwal T, Salter R, Adam A, et al. Image-guided therapies in orthopedic oncology. *Orthop Clin North Am.* 2006;(1):105–112.

99. Buchbinder R, Osborne RH, Ebeling PR, et al. A randomized trial of vertebroplasty for painful osteoporotic vertebral fractures. *N Engl J Med.* 2009;361:557–568.

100. Bouza C, Lopez-Cuadrado T, Cediel P, et al. Balloon kyphoplasty in malignant spinal fractures: a systematic review and meta-analysis. *BMC Palliat Care.* 2009;8:12.

101. Yamamuro M, Kusaka K, Kato M, et al. Celiac plexus block in cancer pain management. *Exp Med.* 2000;192:1–18.

102. Lordon SP. Interventional approach to cancer pain. *Curr Pain Headache Rep.* 2002;6:202–206.

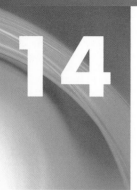

14 Cancer-related fatigue

Barbara F. Piper

Cancer-related fatigue (CRF) differs significantly from the usual sense of tiredness that healthy people experience.[1-3] In contrast, CRF is an unusual sense of tiredness that is not often relieved by a good night's sleep or by rest; symptoms are disproportionate to the degree of physical exertion,[4] and they interfere with functioning.[5] This type of unusual tiredness is known to precede or accompany most other major illnesses and treatments. All age groups can be affected, and it seldom occurs by itself. More often in cancer patients and in cancer survivors, it co-occurs or "clusters" with other symptoms, such as pain, depression, and insomnia.[6]

SIGNIFICANCE

CRF is one of the most common and distressing symptoms experienced by cancer patients[7] and is perceived by patients as being more distressing than pain, nausea, or vomiting.[8] It can negatively affect all aspects of a person's quality of life (QOL)[7] and can limit chemotherapy dosing and the timing and frequency of treatments.[9] For example, in some of the newer targeted agents such as the tyrosine kinase inhibitors sorafenib and sunitinib, and the mTOR inhibitor temsirolimus, fatigue is one of the major rate-limiting adverse events.[10,11] Fatigue may affect treatment adherence and survival.[12]

INCIDENCE AND PREVALENCE

Approximately 70% to 100% of cancer patients experience CRF at some time during diagnosis and treatment.[7] Although it is associated with all forms of cancer treatment, most information about its frequency and patterns over time comes from fatigue studies with patients undergoing chemotherapy and/or radiation therapy.[5]

CHEMOTHERAPY

Among patients receiving chemotherapy (CT), 80% to 90% report CRF, and its prevalence rates and patterns over time are thought to vary by specific CT agent, route of administration (IV vs. oral), and frequency (daily, weekly, monthly) and density of treatment cycles (weekly or every 2 weeks vs. once a month).[13] Less is known about CRF in patients receiving oral CT or the newer targeted CT agents being evaluated in early clinical drug trials.[5] A recent study in women treated for early-stage breast cancer found that fatigue increased significantly over time irrespective of the CT regimen (dose-dense taxane, dose-standard taxane, and dose-standard without taxane) from mild at baseline to moderate at treatments 4 and 8, falling back to mild 30 days after the last CT.[14] The data are conflicting as to whether women with breast cancer experience more fatigue at nadirs.[14]

RADIATION THERAPY

During external beam radiation therapy (RT), CRF is an almost universal occurrence, with 70% to 100% of patients experiencing a gradually increasing, cumulative pattern of CRF over time that peaks and plateaus, usually at 4 to 6 weeks into treatment, and gradually declines thereafter over time. Patients need to be forewarned about the possibility of experiencing this type of CRF pattern, as they may feel that their disease is getting worse instead of better, and may fear that their treatment is not working.[5,7] Despite this commonly observed pattern over time, not all RT patients exhibit this pattern. Thus, interindividual variability and predictors over time should be studied in patients receiving RT.[15] Most of what is known about CRF and RT comes from patients receiving 4 to 6 weeks of external beam RT. Few studies have examined how CRF patterns may vary over time from other forms of RT such as internally placed sources of RT (i.e., implants or brachytherapy), or in patients who receive shorter courses of RT for localized disease or symptoms such as bone pain in palliative care patients.[5] Increased CRF is reported when different therapies such as RT and CT are used in combination,[16] but these cross-sectional findings need to be confirmed in longitudinal studies.

OTHER FORMS OF TREATMENT

Few studies have examined fatigue in surgically treated cancer patients or in cancer patients when hospitalized. One study reported an increase in fatigue in cancer patients associated with a longer period of hospitalization.[17] In patients treated with biologic response modifiers or immunotherapy such as interleukin-2 and interferon-α, CRF can be dose-limiting.[5] A prevalence rate of 70% is reported with interferon.[18] Fatigue in cancer patients receiving hormonal therapy also has not been well studied.[18,19] In one hormone ablation study in men with prostate cancer, a prevalence rate of 14% of severe fatigue was reported at the beginning of the study. Fatigue severity and prevalence significantly increased over time between the beginning of treatment and 3 months later, when nearly two thirds of men were reporting severe CRF.[5,20]

TYPES AND STAGES OF CANCER

Few studies have compared CRF severity levels among patients with different types and stages of cancer. Increased levels of CRF severity are reported by patients with advanced malignancies[21] and in those who have other illnesses or comorbidities.[22] In patients with metastatic disease, for example, fatigue prevalence rates may exceed 75%.[5,7]

DEFINITIONS

SUBJECTIVE PERCEPTION AND IMPACT ON FUNCTIONING

Many definitions for CRF can be found in the literature.[5] The most commonly used is the National Comprehensive Cancer Network (NCCN) CRF definition, which states that CRF is a distressing persistent subjective sense of physical, emotional, and/or cognitive tiredness or exhaustion related to cancer or cancer treatment that is not proportional to recent activity and that interferes with usual functioning.[7] Thus, both the subjective perception of CRF and its impact on function are important definitional attributes that can be used to differentiate CRF from the usual sense of tiredness that healthy people experience.[5]

The words patients use to describe their perceptions of their CRF experiences may vary by language, by culture, and by the illness and treatment spectrum, such as during active treatment, survivorship (off active treatment with no evidence of disease), and palliative end-of-life care.[5] For example, symptoms such as weakness that can accompany CRF may more commonly occur in patients with advanced or incurable malignancies,[21] who also may be experiencing loss of appetite (anorexia), weight loss, and loss of muscle mass, whereas in earlier, more localized disease, weakness may not be a word that patients commonly use to describe their CRF experience.[5] Furthermore, the words that patients use to describe their fatigue experiences and the impact these experiences have on behavioral patterns (i.e., sleep quality, cognition, stamina, emotional reactivity, control over bodily processes, and social interaction) can be used to classify patients into tiredness, fatigue, and exhaustion groups.[23,24]

CASE DEFINITIONS

Consensus is emerging for clinicians and researchers to begin to develop and use a "case definition" for CRF to better classify patients experiencing CRF, and to enable comparisons across studies and populations.[25] For example, using a "cut score" of ≥ 4 on a 0 to 10 numeric rating scale (NRS) during the past week, where $0 =$ no fatigue and $10 =$ worst fatigue, and using established severity levels of $0 =$ none, 1 to $3 =$ mild, 4 to $6 =$ moderate, and 7 to $10 =$ severe,[7] are methods recommended by several investigators for clinical and research purposes.[26–28] Inherent in using a case definition to classify patients in this fashion is the need to better identify clinically significant fatigue in cancer patients that guides treatment planning and enables researchers to obtain meaningful estimates of the prevalence of fatigue.[29] More than one case definition for CRF may be needed to best capture and describe what constitutes clinically significant fatigue in subgroups of patients undergoing active treatment, in those who are disease free and no longer are receiving treatment (i.e., survivors), and in those who have advanced disease or may be receiving end-of-life palliative care.[24]

SYNDROME CRITERIA

In 1998, the first attempt to develop a case definition was proposed that included a set of diagnostic criteria for the syndrome of CRF.[30] These criteria were to be included in the U.S. version of the World Health Organization International Classification of Diseases-10 Clinical Modification (WHO ICD-10-CM) but were never submitted to the Centers for Disease Control and Prevention (CDC) (D. Pickett, personal communication, December 8, 2008). At a recent international CRF consensus conference,[31] it was acknowledged that these syndrome criteria unfortunately were not developed on the basis of a broad range of evidence.[30] They were designed to classify CT "cases" who were receiving every 2 week dosing cycles of CT, and may have "set the bar too high" for a CRF case definition, as many patients with CRF did not fit these criteria. Thus prevalence rates were far lower than expected.[5] Studies continue to evaluate the application of these CRF syndrome criteria in different cancer populations.[32–37]

UNDERLYING MECHANISMS

Despite the prevalence of CRF, little is known about its underlying mechanisms.[7] This area remains the subject of intense research interest and debate. Recent reviews[18,38–40] propose several possible mechanisms for CRF that include cytokine gene polymorphisms,[41–44] altered circadian rhythmicity,[12,18,45] immune dysregulation, serotonin and neurotransmitter dysregulation,[18,19] proinflammatory cytokines,[18] hypothalamic-pituitary-adrenal axis dysregulation,[18,39,46] vascular endothelial growth factors,[18] vagal afferent activation,[18] and disruption in adenosine triphosphate metabolism.[18]

Recently, teams working independently from one another have integrated these seemingly disparate underlying mechanisms into overarching conceptual models based on stressors, such as pain, cancer, its treatments, and other comorbidities, including psychological stress, that activate inflammation.[38,44,47,48] Cytokines released as part of the innate inflammatory immune response to these stressors alter the sleep-wake cycle. This in turn contributes to disruption in the neuroendocrine system, especially in the hypothalamic-pituitary-adrenal axis (HPA) and its related glucocorticoids.[38] This interaction results in unrestrained inflammation and increased release of proinflammatory cytokines, which interact with central nervous system (CNS) pathways that regulate behaviors. This leads to the pathophysiologic changes that underlie the behavioral manifestations of fatigue, depression, impaired sleep, and impaired cognitive function.[38]

The model put forth by Olson and colleagues[47] also includes central and peripheral nervous system mechanisms for muscle fatigue. In the past, these central and peripheral nervous system mechanisms have been limited by studies that have focused solely on their effects on muscle fatigue, have not included self-reports of fatigue (patient-reported outcomes [PROs]), and have not included cancer patients matched to healthy controls. Preliminary findings from recent preclinical studies[49] and review articles,[50–52] and studies in healthy subjects[53] and cancer patients,[54,55] are beginning to shed light on the importance of examining central fatigue mechanisms in cancer-related fatigue, and on examining the interactions among central, peripheral, and immune system mechanisms.[52] Clearly, more studies in this area are warranted.

Several molecular-genetic studies have examined genome-wide expression analyses[56] and single nucleotide polymorphisms (SNPs) (gene variants)[53] and their associations with CRF,[57] pain, depression, and insomnia phenotypes[42,43]; findings suggest that indeed an inflammatory process might be involved with the CRF phenotype. If studies can validate these proposed models and their underlying assumptions and propositions, and can replicate these preliminary gene-related findings, evidence may be available in the future for treatments to finally be targeted to specific underlying genetic variants and pathways producing the CRF phenotype.[5]

BARRIERS TO ASSESSMENT AND MANAGEMENT

Despite its frequency and negative impact, however, CRF remains underreported, underdiagnosed, and undertreated clinically.[7] Healthcare providers may not be routinely performing fatigue assessments in many institutions and oncology practice settings.[26,58–60] Numerous patient-, provider-, and system-related barriers hinder the translation of these guidelines into practice settings.[26,58]

For example, one study sponsored by the National Cancer Institute (NCI), designed to translate the NCCN CRF and pain guidelines into practice (R01-CA-115323) and known as the "Barriers" study, confirmed many of the barriers previously reported in the literature. The most frequent patient-related barrier was the patient's belief that the physician would ask about CRF if it was important; this was followed by the patient's desire to play the "good patient role" and not bring the subject up for discussion unless the physician did. Provider- and systems-related barriers included lack of documentation in the medical record for guideline adherence and lack of supportive care referrals[5] (Table 14-1).

When the intervention phase of the "Barriers" study, which included educational materials and teaching sessions for both patients and their providers,[26] was implemented, many patient-related barriers, including severity of CRF, were decreased over time compared with the usual care (control) group.[26]

This suggests that many patient-related barriers to the assessment and management of CRF, including its severity, can be reduced by patient and provider education.

PROVIDER ASSESSMENT

The NCCN CRF guidelines state that all patients must be assessed for the presence or absence of CRF at their first visit and at each subsequent visit. If CRF is present, the guidelines recommend that a simple 0 to 10 NRS be used to assess CRF intensity (0 = no fatigue, 10 = worst fatigue you can imagine). Patients can be asked directly, "How would you rate your fatigue on a scale of 0 to 10 over the past 7 days?" A 1 to 3 score indicates mild fatigue, a 4 to 6 score moderate fatigue, and a 7 to 10 score severe fatigue.[4,7] For patients who are unable to assign a number to their fatigue, using the words "none, mild, moderate, and severe" is recommended.[7]

In addition to this single-item, single-dimension scale recommended for practice settings, several other scales are now available to screen, assess, and measure the subjective perception of fatigue and its impact on functioning. These include additional single- and multi-item severity scales, as well as multidimensional, multi-item scales. Research is ongoing to develop a PRO version of the National Cancer Institute Common Terminology Criteria for Adverse Event Reporting (NCI-CTCAE)[61–63] and to further test fatigue items/scales that are part of the Patient-Reported Outcome Measurement System

Table 14-1 Barriers to translating/implementing National Comprehensive Cancer Network cancer-related fatigue guidelines into clinical practice

Patient-related	Provider-related	Setting-related
• May not want to "bother" the provider	• May not be aware of just how severe or common fatigue is in their patients unless patients bring up the subject for discussion	• Symptom assessment and the transition of evidence-based guidelines into practice settings are relatively new and have not been well studied.
• May view fatigue as just "something I have to live with"	• Fatigue is not routinely assessed in many clinical settings. Thus, it goes unreported, unassessed, and untreated.	• Pain is the only symptom required by the Joint Commission to be assessed, managed, and documented in clinical settings.
• May think that if they report fatigue, they may be viewed as a "complainer"	• May believe that CRF is not any different from usual tiredness	• Documentation of fatigue in medical records is not a common practice.
• May fear that their treatment may be negatively affected	• May believe that other symptoms, such as pain, nausea, or vomiting, are more important to treat	• Because of the lack of documentation, assessment of fatigue and its documentation are not viewed as practice priorities.
• May not realize how much CRF has personally affected them	• May not be comfortable initiating discussion about fatigue if they are unaware that effective treatments exist for fatigue, or if the underlying fatigue mechanisms are unknown	• As a consequence, providers are not reminded to document the presence, severity, or management of fatigue, particularly as patients transition between clinical settings (i.e., inpatient, outpatient, and office practice settings).
• May not realize how important it is to report fatigue to their provider		
• May fear that fatigue may mean that their cancer is getting "worse"		
• May bring up the subject of fatigue only when it becomes overwhelming and limits functioning	• May think that the guidelines may be too complex and are not feasible to implement in busy practice settings. Thus, there may be a lack of adherence to guideline documentation.	• It takes time to obtain a doctor's order for fatigue supportive care referrals (e.g., physical therapy, nutrition, psychological support, occupational therapy).
• May believe that if fatigue was important, their provider would bring the subject up for discussion		• Depending on the setting, such supportive care disciplines may not be available or may not be available in a timely fashion.
• May believe that fatigue is less important to discuss with their provider than how their cancer and/or treatment is going		• Referrals may be affected by the patient's type of healthcare coverage and reimbursement.
• Want to be the "good" patient and not bring fatigue up for discussion unless their provider does		

Adapted from Piper BF. Fatigue CCO Oncology in Practice. Available at http://inpractice.com.

(PROMIS).[64] To date, no one "best" scale has emerged. See recent reviews that describe these measures and their psychometric properties,[5,60] including one recent systematic review.[65]

BASELINE ASSESSMENT

Because baseline (beginning of treatment or at time of initial diagnosis) CRF severity levels have been shown to be predictive of severity levels over time in patients undergoing treatment,[66] it is important to assess and document these levels before patients begin treatment, and to repeat and compare these screening assessments periodically over time during treatment.[5] Because CRF can persist for months, even years, following treatment cessation in 21% to 35% of cancer survivors, repeated assessments are recommended.[7,9]

FOCUSED WORKUP

For patients who are experiencing moderate to severe levels of CRF (4 to 10 on the 0 to 10 NRS), further assessment of CRF and its possible underlying causes by the healthcare provider is indicated. The NCCN guidelines recommend that this focused workup should include a more in-depth CRF symptom history from the patient, noting when it first started; its timing, duration, and pattern over time; what makes it worse; what makes it better; and its impact on functioning. It is important to ask the patient what he perceives may be causing his fatigue, and whether he is experiencing any other symptoms such as pain, depression, insomnia, or change in functioning.[5] Part of this focused workup includes an assessment of the patient's current disease status and the type and length of cancer treatment planned, as well as its potential to cause CRF.[7] It is important to evaluate whether CRF is due to disease recurrence or progression, as treatment planning may be affected, and patients may be unnecessarily worried and will need reassurance whether or not this is the case.[5] A review of systems is important, as it serves to direct the physical examination and diagnostic testing.

DIFFERENTIAL DIAGNOSIS

In making the differential diagnosis of CRF, the provider tries to distinguish CRF from other diagnoses such as depression,[4] as the treatment may vary. It is essential to assess the presence of the more common contributing and treatable factors of CRF.[7] These factors include anemia, comorbidities and medication side effects, activity level and deconditioning, emotional distress (depression and/or anxiety), nutrition, pain, and sleep disturbance.[7]

TREATMENT

PROVIDER EDUCATION

Provider education about CRF is essential for effective CRF assessment and management. At one national symposium on CRF, approximately 50% of healthcare providers (mostly nurses), were only somewhat familiar with the NCCN CRF guidelines, and 41% were not at all familiar with them.[67] Similarly, in a recent national survey conducted by the NCCN of more than 1000 oncology clinicians, roughly one third were not aware of the CRF guidelines, and 34% of oncology specialist physicians (n = 293/863) were unaware of the guidelines, compared with 17% of advanced practitioners and nurses (n = 27/157). An additional 32% of oncologists were aware of the guidelines but had not accessed them in the past month.[68] These findings indicate that healthcare providers might benefit from more information about the existence of these CRF evidence-based guidelines and assistance in how to translate and implement them in their practice settings.

PATIENT/FAMILY EDUCATION

Similarly, patients and their family members need to receive education about CRF even before they start treatment to better prepare them for how to manage it should they experience it. Several studies have evaluated nurse-led patient educational programs focused on CRF during treatment.[26,69–74] All but one study[72] demonstrated decreased fatigue in the experimental groups receiving the educational intervention. The small sample size in the ineffective trial was thought to have affected its results.[72,75] Each of these studies included short educational interventions, consisting of three to four individual patient sessions lasting 10 to 60 minutes.[75] To a large extent, these studies contained the same elements, which included information about CRF, self-care or coping skills, and activity management, such as learning how to balance activities and rest.[75] Further evaluation of these educational programs is needed, especially in cancer survivors. Additional educational components specific to common factors that contribute to CRF are discussed under CRF treatment.

TREAT FATIGUE AS THE SIXTH VITAL SIGN

Findings from these patient educational studies suggest that educating cancer patients about CRF can empower them to better advocate for themselves; may give them self-care and coping strategies to use proactively in reporting and managing CRF; and may lead to decreased CRF. Patients need to be "coached" to treat CRF as the sixth vital sign (after temperature, pulse, respirations, blood pressure, and pain),[38,60] and to bring up the subject of CRF for discussion themselves with their healthcare provider, even if the provider does not do so on his own.

GENERAL EDUCATIONAL STRATEGIES

General educational strategies on how to manage CRF, such as energy conservation techniques[76] and distraction,[7] need to be included in these educational programs as well. Energy conservation techniques use a commonsense approach to help patients prioritize and pace activities, and to delegate less essential activities.[7,76] Daily or weekly diaries can inform patients about peak energy periods, allowing them to plan their activities accordingly.[7] Another general strategy to decrease fatigue includes the use of distraction techniques (e.g., games, music, reading, socializing).[7]

GENERAL TREATMENT PRINCIPLES FOR THE PROVIDER

Once the primary fatigue evaluation and focused workup are completed, it is important for the provider to consider general principles, in addition to education, that guide CRF treatment.

Treatment needs to be tailored to the patient.[7] Thus, treatment planning takes into consideration the patient's disease and treatment status. Does the patient have early-stage disease or recurrent, advanced-stage disease? What body systems are involved? Does the patient have any preexisting comorbidities, physical limitations, or deconditioning? Is the patient receiving active treatment with curative intent or maintenance therapy such as hormonal therapy during long-term survivorship without evidence of disease, or is he receiving end-of-life palliative care?

Treatment planning takes into account what most likely is the primary underlying cause of the fatigue, and whether multidisciplinary referrals to other healthcare providers or supportive care disciplines are needed.[7] Treatment usually is directed initially to one or more of the common and treatable factors of CRF (anemia, comorbidity and associated medications, activity level, emotional distress [anxiety, depression], nutritional problems, pain [and other symptoms, such as cognitive impairment, symptom clusters, and burden], and sleep disturbance). By the time a patient realizes that the fatigue has become unusual for him, CRF most likely is multicausal and will probably require multimodal combination therapies and referrals. If none of the common contributing and treatable factors is present, or if the patient continues to have moderate to severe fatigue despite treatment, additional workup and treatment planning must occur.[7] Each of these common contributing factors is discussed in greater depth in the following sections.

ANEMIA
Provider assessment

Decreased hematocrit[2] and hemoglobin levels are associated with CRF.[77] In one study, the degree of anemia (mild, moderate, severe) predicted fatigue severity ($P < .001$).[77] The NCCN CRF guidelines[7] identify anemia as one of CRF's common contributing and treatable factors. In many instances, however, anemia may be only a partial contributing factor, as the level of fatigue in cancer patients without anemia is greater than that reported for the general population at large.[77] Because both CRF and anemia can be multifactorial, the NCCN guidelines for cancer- and chemotherapy-related anemia[78] recommend assessing both subjective and objective symptoms associated with each, to better identify the underlying causes and to tailor treatment accordingly.

Anemia-related patient/family education

Patients need to be educated about the relationship between CRF and anemia, and that anemia is considered one of the common contributing and treatable factors of CRF. They need to receive information about possible underlying causes of anemia and how treatment may vary depending on a number of factors, including the underlying cause of anemia, and indications and rationale for the various types of anemia treatment, including iron supplements and their risks, benefits, and associated side effects.[7,78]

Anemia-related treatment

The anemia guidelines[78] suggest that it is unlikely, in the absence of objective signs and symptoms of anemia, that a patient's self-report of CRF alone would warrant intervention. However, if the patient is symptomatic and is evidencing fatigue and other signs and symptoms of anemia, such as a hemoglobin level <11 g/dl, then treatment will more likely be indicated. Correction of anemia within the context of CRF will depend on whether the anemia is cancer-related (non–treatment-related), treatment-related due to the myelosuppressive effects of CT, or due to other causes.[78] Anemia treatment will also depend on the goals of CT treatment (curative vs. noncurative), how rapidly the anemia must be corrected, and the presence of comorbidities.

COMORBIDITY

Despite the fact that comorbidity has been identified as one of the common contributing and treatable factors to CRF,[7] specific types of comorbidities and their medications have not undergone much investigation for their CRF association. Although more studies in this area are clearly needed, a few studies in cancer are beginning to report consistent and significant findings on how specific comorbidities such as arthritis[79] and an increase in the actual total number of comorbidities a patient has can increase CRF severity.[80]

Provider assessment

CRF guidelines recommend that each comorbidity be reviewed to determine whether any changes in the management of the comorbidity or its medications need to be made within the context of the patient's CRF.[7] These include comorbidities that affect cardiac, pulmonary, renal, hepatic, neurologic, and endocrine systems. Subclinical thyroid dysfunction can occur for many reasons[81] and may be present in cancer patients as well. Hypothyroidism may contribute to CRF and may be underdiagnosed in cancer patients.[82,83] Hypothyroidism is a frequent comorbidity that can result from specific cancer therapies such as RT directed toward the head and neck region[84] and total body irradiation administered before hematopoietic stem cell transplantation.[7] Some of the oral targeted agents also can produce this comorbidity.[85] Similarly, hypogonadism[86] and adrenal insufficiency need to be assessed for their CRF associations.[7]

All current medications, including over-the-counter, herbal, vitamins, minerals, and other supplements, need to be identified to determine whether the medications contribute to CRF and to drug-to-drug and drug-to-cancer treatment interactions. Different classes of medications, most notably narcotics, antiemetics, antidepressants, anticonvulsants, and antihistamines, can produce drowsiness and sedation that can contribute to CRF. Beta blockers are well known to produce fatigue as a side effect.[7] Any recent changes made in the medications patients have been taking need to be reassessed periodically over the course of their cancer treatment and disease trajectory, as their CRF patterns may change over time and may be affected by these changes.[5]

Comorbidity-related patient/family education

Patients need to receive education that comorbidities and medications are some of the common contributing and treatable factors associated with CRF. They need to be taught to report to their provider any changes in their comorbidity, its symptoms, or its management, including medication changes, as these can potentially affect CRF.[5]

Comorbidity-related treatment

If comorbidities and their associated treatments and medications are thought to affect CRF, then consideration needs to be given to altering the management of these comorbidities.[7] This may include a new comorbidity workup, a referral to an internist or specialist, and/or titrating or changing the patient's medication to determine what effects these changes may have on the patient's CRF. Often, consultation with a clinical pharmacist is helpful.[5]

ACTIVITY LEVEL

In cancer patients, cancer and treatment side effects such as CRF often result in decreased activity patterns and reductions in physical performance. As a consequence, deconditioning is common and is identified as one of the common contributing and treatable CRF factors.[7]

Provider assessment

Every cancer patient needs to have his activity levels assessed at baseline, when he is first diagnosed, and before treatment begins. Thereafter patients need to be periodically reassessed over time to identify changes in their exercise or activity patterns, and to identify whether any evidence indicates that deconditioning is present as a result of their malignancy, CRF, other comorbidities, treatments, or other symptoms such as pain. Patients need to be asked about their ability to perform activities of daily living. Have their activity and exercise patterns changed over time since they were diagnosed or began treatment, or since they developed CRF? What are the type, dose (intensity), duration, and frequency of their usual activity or exercise patterns? And how have these changed over time?[5]

Activity-related patient/family education

Patients need to be educated about the high risk of developing deconditioning, the multiple causes of deconditioning that can occur, and how deconditioning can lead to a downward spiral of secondary fatigue as a consequence. They need to be taught that deconditioning is one of the common contributing and treatable factors of CRF. Based on the strength of the evidence for exercise, patients need to be educated about the need to engage in moderate levels of physical activity during and after treatment.[7]

Exercise barriers

Despite this teaching, however, which was provided in the Barriers study previously mentioned,[26] one of the more persistent patient-related barriers in the intervention group was the belief that they should rest more when they were fatigued, and that exercise would increase rather than decrease their CRF despite evidence to the contrary. Being diagnosed with cancer constitutes a "teachable" moment.[87] Patients need to be educated not only about the barriers to exercise (patient-, provider-, and systems-related) (Table 14-2), but also about the benefits of exercise, which include prevention of disease recurrence; prevention and treatment of comorbidities such as diabetes, hypertension, and obesity; positive effects on sleep disturbance, depression, and cognition; the strong evidence suggesting that it has a role in reducing CRF in cancer patients and survivors.[5,7]

Table 14-2   Exercise barriers

Patient-related	Provider-related	Systems-related
• Believe that they should avoid exercise when tired	• Absence of evidence-based guidelines to follow, thus hesitant to prescribe exercise to their patients	• Currently, no evidence-based guidelines exist for exercise programs specific to cancer patients.
• Lack of time	• Fewer than 20% of medical oncologists recommend exercise for their patients.	• No position or policy statements regarding exercise have put forth by the American Society of Clinical Oncology (ASCO), the Oncology Nursing Society (ONS), or the American College of Sports Medicine (ACSM).
• Believe exercise causes fatigue		
• Decreased adherence rates over time in studies of exercise programs	• May be unaware that exercise has the strongest level of evidence supporting it as a fatigue therapy	
• Fear of side effects or adverse effects of exercise	• May be unaware of the many other benefits that exercise programs have for quality of life, disease recurrence, comorbidities, and symptoms	• The patient's insurance company may not cover referrals to physical therapy and/or occupational therapy.
• Do not know how to tailor exercise or activity patterns to their physical limitations, symptoms, treatment, or condition		• Physical therapy and/or occupational therapy may not be available in the clinical setting.
• May believe that they are too tired to exercise	• May be unaware that well-designed exercise programs far outweigh the negative consequences of inactivity	
• May not be aware of the various types of exercise that can be tailored to their current level of activity or fitness level	• May be unaware of just how powerful their recommendations for exercise can be for their patients	
• May be unaware of the positive benefits of exercise for disease-related side effects, risk for disease recurrence, and symptoms or comorbidities		
• May be unaware of the benefits of supportive care referrals to physical therapy or to occupational therapy		

Adapted from Piper BF. Fatigue CCO Oncology in Practice. Available at http://inpractice.com.

For patients not currently exercising, reassurance needs to be given that they will be able to start exercising initially at lower-intensity levels of activity, duration, and frequency. Progression will occur slowly over time as patients are taught how to monitor their own progress and are closely monitored by trained professionals. Patients need to be reassured that modifications in their exercise program will be made on the basis of changes in their condition, CRF, and other symptom profiles.[7]

Activity-related treatment

Providers may be hesitant to prescribe an exercise program for cancer patients without having evidence-based guidelines specific to cancer that they can follow.[88] Less than 20% of medical oncologists recommend exercise to their patients.[87,89] Providers may be unaware of just how powerful their recommendations for exercise prescriptions can be.[88,90] Maintaining or enhancing activity and exercise patterns in cancer patients has the highest level of evidence associated with decreasing CRF, as do psychosocial interventions.[7]

In a recent review of 57 nonpharmacologic randomized clinical trials (RCTs)[25] of exercise (physical activity, walking, yoga) and psychosocial interventions (counseling, stress management, and coping strategies), these interventions were equally and moderately effective in reducing CRF. This review suggested that multimodal therapy that combines these two types of interventions into an integrative intervention trial could be more likely to reduce CRF and improve vigor and vitality.[25] Although more study is needed in this area, walking and multimodal exercise programs appear to have the greatest potential for reducing CRF and enhancing vigor and vitality.[25] On the basis of these findings, it seems reasonable to encourage all patients to engage in a moderate level of physical activity during and after treatment cessation.[7,25]

For patients who are severely deconditioned, who are not currently exercising, or who have comorbidities (e.g., arthritis, COPD) or have undergone recent surgery for functional or anatomic issues, referral to healthcare providers or exercise specialists such as those involved in physical therapy, physical medicine, or rehabilitation should be considered.[7] Some evidence suggests that exercise may be beneficial in maintaining activity patterns and reducing or at least stabilizing CRF in patients with advanced disease at end of life as well.[7]

Types of exercise that may be tailored to the patient's condition include aerobic training, resistance or strength training, stretching or flexibility training,[25] balance training, and bed or chair exercises.[91] Exercise prescriptions should be tailored to the patient's age, gender, type and stage of disease, treatment status, and physical fitness level. Caution is needed in tailoring an exercise prescription for patients who have bone metastases, fever or infection, anemia, thrombocytopenia, neutropenia, or immunosuppression.[7]

EMOTIONAL DISTRESS

The NCCN Distress Guidelines[92] use the term "distress" in their definition because it is believed to be less stigmatizing than other terms that can be used to describe psychosocial problems such as anxiety and depression. In cancer patients, prevalence rates for depression range between 25% and 33%,[92] and anxiety can occur at all times and in all cancer patients.[93]

Emotional distress (i.e., anxiety and depression) is one of the common contributing factors of CRF.[7,17] Although CRF and depression are common concurrent symptoms in cancer patients,[7] one study in RT patients concluded that CRF and depression were independent conditions with different patterns over time.[94]

Provider assessment

The distress guidelines recommend asking cancer patients how their distress in the past week, including today, would be ranked on a 0 to 10 distress thermometer where scores ≥4 indicate clinically significant distress[92] that indicates that further workup and referrals may be needed. In addition, a checklist is provided for common problems that cancer patients can experience, such as practical, family, emotional, spiritual/religious, physical (symptoms), and memory/concentration items that patients can self-complete. It is recommended that this screening assessment be done initially at baseline before treatment is initiated, and that it be repeated periodically over time during and after treatment.

Distress-related patient/family education

Patients need to be taught about how CRF may be related to emotional distress, and that emotional distress is one of the common contributing and treatable factors of CRF. They need to be counseled about stress management techniques, about methods and resources that can help to reduce anxiety and depression, and that CRF is commonly associated with emotional distress often experienced when patients are experiencing cancer and its treatments, as well as during long-term survivorship and end-of-life care.

Distress-related treatment

Several nonpharmacologic, randomized clinical trials using psychosocial interventions such as participation in support groups, individual counseling sessions, and cognitive-behavioral training (identification and correction of inaccurate thoughts associated with depressed feelings using relaxation and enhancing problem-solving skills, and stress management training using a comprehensive coping strategy and a tailored behavioral intervention) have consistently shown that emotional distress can be reduced, and that CRF can be reduced when it is associated with depression or anxiety.[7,25,92] Supportive care referrals to other disciplines, including Nursing, Social Services, Psychology, and Chaplaincy/Pastoral Services, often are indicated and can be very beneficial. A variety of pharmacologic interventions to treat emotional distress are available; these include antianxiety medications and antidepressants. In one antidepressant study, depression was decreased, but the treatment had no effect on CRF.[95] For additional information, please refer to the NCCN Distress Guidelines[92] and the NCI's PDQ websites for anxiety[96] and depression.[97]

NUTRITION

In cancer patients, nutritional problems are common and can include alterations in the ability to process nutrients (impaired glucose, lipid, and protein metabolism), increased energy consumption (tumor consumption of and competition for nutrients, hypermetabolic state due to tumor growth, infection/fever, and dyspnea), decreased intake of energy sources (mucositis, nausea, vomiting, anorexia, early satiety, diarrhea, constipation, bowel obstruction, and cachexia),[98] and increased loss of micronutrients from CT agents (ifosfamide and cisplatin) that affect the kidneys.[7] It is estimated that 20% to 80% of cancer patients develop malnutrition during the course of their illness.[99] Although nutritional problems are one of the common contributing and treatable factors of CRF in cancer patients,[7] their relationships to CRF have not undergone much study.[5] Only two studies in cancer patients have examined these relationships, and both found no relationship between nutritional status and CRF.[100,101]

Provider assessment

Nutritional assessment within the context of CRF includes determining the presence of any unintentional weight gain or loss, and the extent to which the patient is experiencing nutritional problems such as fluid and electrolyte disturbances.[7] The degree to which CRF may be limiting the patient's ability to shop and prepare food needs to be assessed. Frequently, patients alter their dietary patterns when they receive a cancer diagnosis or experience disease recurrence, or during survivorship following treatment cessation.[87] They may take numerous over-the-counter supplements, vitamins, and other herbal remedies that may affect not only their nutritional status and their treatments, but also their CRF. The relationship between CRF and these over-the-counter supplements, vitamins, and other herbal remedies has not undergone much study.[5]

Nutrition-related patient/family education

All cancer patients need to be taught that nutritional problems are common in cancer and its treatments, and although not well studied, nutritional problems are one of the common contributable and treatable factors associated with CRF. Because of the lack of studies investigating relationships among nutritional status, nutritional problems, and CRF, counseling patients about general nutritional guidelines such as eating a balanced diet low in fat and high in vegetables and fruits as appropriate to their condition and the goals of their treatment seems to be a reasonable approach.[102] Patients also need to be taught to report nutritional problems as soon as they occur, especially if they start having problems with food shopping or preparing food because of CRF or changes in their economic situation.[5]

Nutrition-related treatment

When indicated by the patient's condition and goals of treatment, both pharmacologic and nonpharmacologic therapies may be considered to improve nutritional status. Treatment may include correction of fluid and electrolyte imbalances, use of nutritional supplements, nutritional therapies, and appetite stimulants, as well as referring the patient for a nutritional consultation.[7]

PAIN

Pain is one of the common contributing and treatable factors of CRF.[7] Pain commonly co-occurs with CRF, but may be more common in certain subgroups of patients. For example, one study found that women (vs. men), patients with late-stage cancer (vs. early-stage), patients with lung cancer (vs.

other solid tumors), and those with three or more comorbidities were more likely to experience pain and fatigue concurrently.[22] In the Barriers study, when usual care (Phase 1: n = 83) and intervention groups (Phase 2: n = 104) were combined for analysis (N = 187), 10.7% (N = 20) had pain only; 56.2% (N = 105) had fatigue only; and 33.2% (N = 62) had both symptoms.[26] In this study, women with breast cancer had significantly less pain at 3 months than those with prostate cancer, and, of importance, the higher the baseline pain intensity, the higher it was 3 months later. Again, this finding emphasizes the importance of assessing symptoms such as pain at baseline before treatment is started, and perhaps intervening earlier to prevent or lessen these symptom intensities over time.

Pain assessment

For assessment of pain in cancer patients, please see the NCCN Pain Guidelines.[103]

Pain-related patient/family education

In addition to education about pain, its causes, treatments, and associated side effects and their management, patients need to be taught that pain is a common contributing and treatable factor for CRF.[7] They need to be taught about barriers to effective pain assessment and management (Table 14-3).

In a recent review, patient educational interventions improved patient knowledge and attitudes about pain, and reduced average and worst pain intensity scores.[104] In the Barriers study, patients in the education intervention group demonstrated significantly greater improvement in pain knowledge scores and fewer patient-related barriers at 1 and 3 months after the intervention compared with the control group.[26] This suggests that these changes were sustained over time. Two persistent areas of lack of knowledge in the intervention group, however, included the belief that cancer pain can be treated only with medication, and the idea that pain medication can be stopped abruptly (i.e., instead of being titrated downward over time) if no longer needed.

Pain-related treatment

For information on management of pain, please refer to the NCCN Pain Guidelines.[105]

SYMPTOM CLUSTERS

Fatigue is thought to occur by itself rarely. More commonly, it is thought to co-occur or cluster with other symptoms such as pain, depression (i.e., emotional distress),[106] and insomnia.[6,17,107,108] Currently, emerging consensus suggests that a symptom cluster is defined as a grouping of at least two related, co-occurring symptoms that are stable (reproducible) and independent of other groupings.[109] This is an area of intense research interest.[110] Because the relationships among co-occurring symptoms can be complex, multivariate statistical procedures are used to classify patients and/or their symptoms into subgroups on the basis of empirical data.[24] Most symptom cluster studies to date have used cross-sectional designs[111] to validate symptom inventories,[24] with few exceptions.[112–114] It has been proposed that these symptom clusters may share a common underlying pathway or mechanism.[2,39,106,115] Thus, treatment of one or more of these symptoms might beneficially affect the other symptoms,[116]

Table 14-3 Barriers to translating/implementing into clinical practice the National Comprehensive Cancer Network's Adult Cancer Pain Guidelines

Patient-related	Provider-related	Systems-related
• Reluctance to report pain	• Failure to adequately assess the patient's pain	• Low referrals to supportive care services
• Fatalism about the possibility of achieving pain control	• Failure to recognize patient-related barriers to pain and its relief	• Regulatory structures that interfere with optimal pain management
• Fear of distracting their provider from treating their cancer	• Lack of knowledge about the principles of pain relief, side effect management, or understanding key concepts such as addiction, tolerance, dosing, and communication	• Inadequate reimbursement for pain services
• Belief that pain is always indicative of disease progression		• Lack of availability of pain consultative services
• Fears about becoming addicted		
• Belief that drowsiness or confusion caused by pain medication is difficult to control		
• Belief that chronic use of pain medications renders them ineffective later on	• Concerns about regulation of controlled substances	
• Belief that chronic use of pain medications may mask new pain or body changes	• Concerns about the adverse effects of pain medications	
• May be concerned about being the "good" patient and not a "complainer"		
• May be worried about side effects/adverse events		
• May not be aware of the need to maintain a constant blood level of pain medication in addition to using pain medication for breakthrough pain when experiencing chronic pain		

Adapted from Piper BF. Fatigue CCO Oncology in Practice. Available at http://inpractice.com.

including CRF.[7] The cumulative burden of these symptoms also is thought to contribute to or exacerbate CRF.[116] For a more in-depth discussion of design issues related to symptom cluster research[117,118] and the various types of multivariate statistical procedures and their indications, please see published reviews.[117–120]

COGNITIVE IMPAIRMENT

Another problem that cancer patients frequently experience, particularly when undergoing treatment, is cognitive impairment.[121] Signs and symptoms include forgetfulness, lack of mental clarity, and impaired concentration. Although relationships between CRF and cognitive impairment have not been well studied, attentional fatigue, that is, decreased capacity to concentrate or to direct attention, is considered one aspect of sensory CRF.[7] Use of attention-restoring interventions in women with breast cancer has positively affected concentration, problem solving, and the ability to direct attention on neurocognitive testing.[7] Bird watching and sitting in a park are examples of attention-restoring activities in natural environments.[122]

SLEEP DISTURBANCES

Sleep-wake disturbance is a general term used to describe perceived or actual alterations in nighttime sleep with concomitant daytime impairment.[123] This term is used when a specific diagnosis of a sleep disorder has not been made.[124] Although

a variety of sleep disturbances can occur in healthy adults and in adults with cancer, insomnia is the most common disorder that occurs in cancer patients.[125] Common descriptors of insomnia include problems falling asleep or staying asleep, early morning awakenings, an inability to fall back to sleep, and sleep described as nonrestorative or nonrefreshing, with some form of daytime impairment.[123,125] Insomnia is a serious issue in cancer patients because it associated with other symptoms such as CRF and pain during and after treatment. In one study, the co-occurrence of the symptom cluster of pain, fatigue, and insomnia in elderly cancer patients was associated with increased risk of death during the first year after the diagnosis.[126] Although most studies have assessed the relationship between CRF and sleep disturbance in women with breast cancer receiving CT, correlations have also been reported in patients undergoing RT and surgery, and in those with other malignancies.[127] Approximately 30% to 75% of cancer patients have sleep disturbances. As a consequence, sleep disturbances are identified as one of the common, contributing, and treatable factors of CRF.[7] Treating sleep disturbances by using cognitive-behavioral strategies in these patients is thought to reduce the incidence and prevalence of CRF.[127,128]

PROVIDER ASSESSMENT

Patients need to be asked at diagnosis, and periodically over time, whether they are experiencing any sleep disturbances such as falling asleep, staying asleep, early morning awakenings, inability to resume sleep, nonrefreshing or nonrestorative sleep, or daytime sleepiness.[123]

SLEEP-RELATED PATIENT/FAMILY EDUCATION

Patients need to receive education about how common sleep disturbances are in cancer patients, and that sleep disturbances are one of the common contributing and treatable factors of CRF.[7] Patients need to be taught to report disturbances to their providers and how to use some of the more common cognitive and behavioral therapies (CBTs) available to treat insomnia. These include stimulus control, such as going to bed when sleepy, sleep restriction, such as limiting total time in bed,[129] relaxation training, including complementary therapies, and sleep hygiene methods, such as avoiding caffeine after noontime.[7] Some of these CBTs are displayed in greater depth in Table 14-4. Patients also need to be taught about other interventions that can enhance sleep patterns, such as exercise and sleep medications, controlling other symptoms such as pain, and using complementary therapies to enhance relaxation before bedtime.[7]

SLEEP-RELATED TREATMENT

Nonpharmacologic therapies to manage sleep disturbances include the CBTs, complementary therapies, and exercise, as mentioned earlier. Some evidence suggests that these same therapies may also improve CRF,[7,130] but more study is needed. A wide variety of pharmacologic options are available, including the sedative-hypnotics, but little information can be obtained regarding their use in cancer patients or how they may affect CRF.[123] These medications are not without their own side effects, and concerns have been raised about drug-to-drug interactions when taken with tamoxifen or with selective serotonin reuptake inhibitors.[7,123,125] For further information on these sleep-enhancing medications, please see the National Cancer Institute's PDQ website on sleep disorders.[131] Consultation and referral to a sleep specialist may be indicated in some patients.

When indicated in medically induced fatigue such as opioid-induced sedation for pain, and when treating depression or cognitive impairment, psychostimulants can be considered.[132] NCCN CRF guidelines state that pharmacologic interventions for CRF remain investigational, but more evidence for methylphenidate[133] than for modafinil is available at present. These agents need to be used cautiously; optimal dosing and schedules have not been established.[7] When oncology physicians were asked about their use of psychostimulants,

---

Table 14-4 Strategies to enhance sleep, decrease insomnia, and possibly decrease CRF in adults

Sleep hygiene strategies	Stimulus control strategies	Relaxation strategies	Sleep restriction strategies	Other related strategies
• Avoid coffee, tea, chocolate, or caffeinated soft drinks before going to bed. • Avoid exercising 2 to 4 hours before bedtime. • Sleep in a dark, cool, quiet, and relaxing room. • Develop a "bedtime" ritual, such as having a warm drink such as milk before bedtime. • Avoid eating "heavy" meals before bedtime. • Avoid alcohol before going to bed, as it can help you fall asleep initially, but overall it will disrupt sleep patterns. • If you wake up during the night, keep the lights dim. • "Resist" behaviors that interfere with sleep. These are cognitive-behavioral strategies (CBTs).	• Use the bedroom only for sleep, with sexual activity the exception. • Avoid eating or watching television in bed. • Lie down or go to bed only when sleepy. • Limit naps to no more than two every day, with each lasting less than an hour. • If you do not fall asleep in 20 minutes after going to bed, read or get up out of bed, and do something nonstimulating. • Lie back down again when you feel drowsy. • Repeat as necessary. • "Ritualize" cues for sleep (CBT).	• Take a warm shower or bath before going to bed. • Listen to soothing music. • Use meditation, guided imagery, massage, progressive muscle relaxation, or other related strategies, such as mindfulness-based stress reduction, to decrease stress. • Tune out distractions by concentrating and focusing on your breathing and sensations in your extremities such as feelings of warmth or heaviness. • Relax and control tension.	• Avoid naps during the daytime if your nighttime sleep is disturbed. • Set an alarm clock to get up at the same time of day regardless of the amount of sleep you have had. • Limit the total time spent in bed. • Go to sleep at the same time each night. • "Regularize" or prioritize sleep-wake patterns (CBT).	• Keep yourself as active as possible during the day. • This might help promote sleep at night and decrease emotional distress such as depression and anxiety. • If you have other symptoms such as pain or fatigue, these can affect your sleep. • Talk to your provider about how best to manage these symptoms. • If you are worried, anxious, or depressed, talk with your healthcare provider about resources to help you cope with these concerns. • A variety of sleep medications (over-the-counter or prescribed) are available to help you sleep; ask your healthcare provider about which sleep medications would be best for you to take.

Adapted from Piper BF. Fatigue CCO Oncology in Practice. Available at http://inpractice.com.

45% (n = 388/863) indicated they do not use them for treating CRF in patients on active treatment or during follow-up (n = 389/863). More physicians used these agents for treating CRF at end-of-life.[68]

SUMMARY AND FUTURE DIRECTIONS

Cancer-related fatigue (CRF) is a complex, multicausal, and multidimensional sensation.[60] Both the intensity of CRF and its impact on functioning need to be assessed and measured in practice and research settings. It is suggested that different manifestations of CRF exist, and that they may vary by stage of disease and treatment trajectory (i.e., active treatment, survivorship [off treatment without evidence of disease], and palliative end-of-life care).[31] It is important to remember that the words patients use to describe CRF may vary by language and culture.[134] When CRF becomes unusual for patients, compared with the usual tiredness they experienced when healthy, it most likely has become chronic and has resulted from multiple causes. As a consequence, the condition most likely will require combination therapies directed toward alleviating it directly.[75] Provider and patient-family educational programs and supportive care referrals to other disciplines related to the NCCN CRF Guidelines are essential for effective assessment and management. More research is warranted to determine how best to translate and implement these educational programs and guidelines in practice and evaluate their impact on patient, provider, and setting outcomes.[58] Providers also need to appreciate the significant impact that their prescriptions and referrals have on patients making behavioral lifestyle changes such as diet and exercise.[135] Last, more research is needed to identify underlying mechanisms of CRF, so that treatments can be targeted and tailored accordingly.

WEB-BASED RESOURCES

Several Web-based resources can be used to enhance patient and provider education. These include the following: American Society of Clinical Oncology (ASCO): www.cancer.org; Lance Armstrong Foundation: www.livestrong.org; National Cancer Institute (NCI): http://www.nci.nih.gov/cancertopics/pdq/supportivecare (patients and healthcare professionals); National Comprehensive Cancer Network (NCCN): www.nccn.org (healthcare professionals) and www.nccn.com (patients); and Oncology Nursing Society (ONS): www.cancersymptoms.org.

REFERENCES

1. Gielissen MF, Knoop H, Servaes P, et al. Differences in the experience of fatigue in patients and healthy controls: patients' descriptions. *Health Qual Life Outcomes*. 2007;5:36.
2. Payne J, Piper BF, Rabinowitz I, et al. Biomarkers, fatigue, sleep, and depressive symptoms in women with breast cancer: a pilot study. *Oncol Nurs Forum*. 2006;33:775–783.
3. Wu HS, McSweeney M. Cancer-related fatigue: "it's so much more than just being tired". *Eur J Oncol Nurs*. 2007;11:117–125.
4. Jean-Pierre P, Figueroa-Moseley CD, Kohli S, et al. Assessment of cancer-related fatigue: implications for clinical diagnosis and treatment. *Oncologist*. 2007;12(suppl 1):11–21.
5. Piper BF. Cancer-related fatigue. 2009. Available from: http://www.clinicaloptions.com/inPractice/Oncology/Supportive_Care/ch48_SuppCare-Fatigue.aspx.
6. Barsevick AM. The concept of symptom cluster. *Semin Oncol Nurs*. 2007;23:89–98.
7. Berger AM, Abernethy AP, Atkinson A, et al. National Comprehensive Cancer Network (NCCN) clinical practice guidelines in oncology: cancer-related fatigue, v.1. 2010. Available from: http://www.nccn.org/professionals/physician_gls/PDF/fatigue.pdf.
8. Vogelzang NJ, Breitbart W, Cella D. Patient, caregiver, and oncologist perceptions of cancer-related fatigue: results of a tripart assessment survey. The Fatigue Coalition. *Semin Hematol*. 1997;34(suppl 2):4–12.
9. Hofman M, Ryan JL, Figueroa-Moseley CD, et al. Cancer-related fatigue: the scale of the problem. *Oncologist*. 2007;12(suppl 1):4–10.
10. Guevremont C, Alsaker A, Karakiewicz PI. Management of sorafenib, sunitinib, and temsirolimus toxicity in metastatic renal cell carcinoma. *Curr Opin Support Palliat Care*. 2009;3:170–179.
11. van der Veldt AAM, Boven E, Helgason HH, et al. Predictive factors for severe toxicity of sunitinib in unselected patients with advanced renal cell cancer. *Br J Cancer*. 2008;99:259–265.
12. Mormont MC, Waterhouse J, Bleuzen P, et al. Marked 24-h rest/activity rhythms are associated with better quality of life, better response, and longer survival in patients with metastatic colorectal cancer and good performance status. *Clin Cancer Res*. 2000;6:3038–3045.
13. Richardson A, Ream E, Wilson-Barnett J. Fatigue in patients receiving chemotherapy: patterns of change. *Cancer Nurs*. 1998;21:17–30.
14. Berger AM, Lockhart K, Agrawal S. Variability of patterns of fatigue and quality of life over time based on different breast cancer adjuvant chemotherapy regimens. *Oncol Nurs Forum*. 2009;36:563–570.
15. Dimsdale JE, Ancoli-Israel S, Ayalon L, et al. Taking fatigue seriously, II: variability in fatigue levels in cancer patients. *Psychosomatics*. 2007;48:247–252.
16. Woo B, Dibble SL, Piper BF, et al. Differences in fatigue by treatment methods in women with breast cancer. *Oncol Nurs Forum*. 1998;25:915–920.
17. Prue G, Rankin J, Allen J, et al. Cancer-related fatigue: a critical appraisal. *Eur J Cancer*. 2006;42:846–863.
18. Wang XS. Pathophysiology of cancer-related fatigue. *Clin J Oncol Nurs*. 2008;12(suppl 5):11–20.
19. Payne JK, Held J, Thorpe J, et al. Effect of exercise on biomarkers, fatigue, sleep disturbances, and depressive symptoms in older women with breast cancer receiving hormonal therapy. *Oncol Nurs Forum*. 2008;35:635–642.
20. Stone P, Hardy J, Huddart R, et al. Fatigue in patients with prostate cancer receiving hormone therapy. *Eur J Cancer*. 2000;36:1134–1141.
21. Teunissen SC, Wesker W, Kruitwagen C, et al. Symptom prevalence in patients with incurable cancer: a systematic review. *J Pain Symptom Manage*. 2007;34:94–104.
22. Given CW, Given B, Azzouz F, et al. Predictors of pain and fatigue in the year following diagnosis among elderly cancer patients. *J Pain Symptom Manage*. 2001;21:456–466.
23. Olson K. A new way of thinking about fatigue: a reconceptualization. *Oncol Nurs Forum*. 2007;34:93–98.
24. Piper BF, Cella D. Cancer-related fatigue: definitions and clinical subtypes. *J Natl Compr Cancer Netw*. 2010;8:958–966.
25. Kangas M, Bovbjerg DH, Montgomery GH. Cancer-related fatigue: a systematic and meta-analytic review of non-pharmacological therapies for cancer patients. *Psychol Bull*. 2008;134:700–741.
26. Borneman T, Koczywas M, Sun V, et al. Reducing patient barriers to pain and fatigue management. *J Pain Symptom Manage*. 2010;39:486–500.
27. Meeske K, Smith AW, Alfano CM, et al. Fatigue in breast cancer survivors two to five years post diagnosis: a HEAL study report. *Qual Life Res*. 2007;16:947–960.
28. Piper BF, Dodd MJ, Ream E, et al. Improving the clinical measurement of cancer treatment-related fatigue. In: Better health through nursing research: State of the science congress proceedings. Washington, DC: American Nurses' Association; 1999:99.
29. Lynch J, Mead G, Greig C, et al. Fatigue after stroke: the development and evaluation of a case definition. *J Psychosom Res*. 2007;63:539–544.
30. Cella D, Peterman A, Passik S, et al. Progress toward guidelines for the management of fatigue. *Oncology (Williston Park)*. 1998;12:369–377.
31. Jacobsen P. Cancer-related fatigue (CRF): Where is the evidence and where are the gaps? Can we achieve a case definition in our lifetime? Rome, Italy: Multinational Association of Supportive Care in Cancer (MASCC); 2009.

32. Bennett B, Goldstein D, Friedlander M, et al. The experience of cancer-related fatigue and chronic fatigue syndrome: a qualitative and comparative study. *J Pain Symptom Manage.* 2007;34:126–135.

33. Cella D, Davis K, Breitbart W, et al. Fatigue Coalition. Cancer-related fatigue: prevalence of proposed diagnostic criteria in a United States sample of cancer survivors. *J Clin Oncol.* 2001;19:3385–3391.

34. Fernandes R, Stone P, Andrews P, et al. Comparison between fatigue, sleep disturbance, and circadian rhythm in cancer inpatients and healthy volunteers: evaluation of diagnostic criteria for cancer-related fatigue. *J Pain Symptom Manage.* 2006;32:245–254.

35. Murphy H, Alexander S, Stone P. Investigation of diagnostic criteria for cancer-related fatigue syndrome in patients with advanced cancer: a feasibility study. *Palliat Med.* 2006;20:413–418.

36. Sadler IJ, Jacobsen P, Booth-Jones M, et al. Preliminary evaluation of a clinical syndrome approach to assessing cancer-related fatigue. *J Pain Symptom Manage.* 2002;23:406–416.

37. Van Belle S, Paridaens R, Evers G, et al. Comparison of proposed diagnostic criteria with FACT-F and VAS for cancer-related fatigue: proposal for use as a screening tool. *Support Care Cancer.* 2005;13:246–254.

38. Miller AH, Ancoli-Israel S, Bower JE, et al. Neuroendocrine-immune mechanisms of behavioral comorbidities in patients with cancer. *J Clin Oncol.* 2008;26:971–982.

39. Payne JK. A neuroendocrine-based regulatory fatigue model. *Biol Res Nurs.* 2004;6:141–150.

40. Ryan JL, Carroll JK, Ryan EP, et al. Mechanisms of cancer-related fatigue. *Oncologist.* 2007;12(suppl 1): 22–34.

41. Aouizerat BE, Miaskowski C, Dodd M, et al. Evidence of genetic association of a cytokine gene variation with sleep disturbance and fatigue in oncology patients and their family caregivers (FCs). *Oncol Nurs Forum.* 2007;34:171.

42. Aouizerat BE, Dodd M, Lee K, et al. Preliminary evidence of a genetic association between tumor necrosis factor alpha and the severity of sleep disturbance and morning fatigue. *Biol Res Nurs.* 2009;1:27–41.

43. Collado-Hidalgo A, Bower JE, Ganz PA, et al. Cytokine gene polymorphisms and fatigue in breast cancer survivors: early findings. *Brain Behav Immun.* 2008;22:1197–2000.

44. Reyes-Gibby CC, Wu X, Spitz M, et al. Molecular epidemiology, cancer-related symptoms, and cytokines pathway. *Lancet Oncol.* 2008;9: 777–785.

45. Innominato PF, Focan C, Gorlia T, et al. Circadian rhythm in rest and activity: a biological correlate of quality of life and a predictor of survival in patients with metastatic colorectal cancer. *Cancer Res.* 2009;69:4700–4707.

46. Rich T, Innominato PF, Boerner J, et al. Elevated serum cytokines correlated with altered behavior, serum cortisol rhythm, and dampened 24-hour rest-activity patterns in patients with metastatic colorectal cancer. *Clin Cancer Res.* 2005;11:1757–1764.

47. Olson K, Turner AR, Courneya KS, et al. Possible links between behavioral and physiological indices of tiredness, fatigue, and exhaustion in advanced cancer. *Support Care Cancer.* 2008;16:241–249.

48. Schubert C, Hong S, Natarajan L, et al. The association between fatigue and inflammatory marker levels in cancer patients: a quantitative review. *Brain Behav Immun.* 2007;21:413–427.

49. Capuruto EC, dos Santos RVT, Mello MT, et al. Effect of endurance training on hypothalamic serotonin concentration and performance. *Clin Exp Pharmacol Physiol.* 2009;36:189–191.

50. Chaudhuri A, Behan PO. Fatigue and basal ganglia. *J Neurol Sci.* 2000;179:34–42.

51. Chaudhuri A, Behan PO. Fatigue in neurological disorders. *Lancet.* 2004;363:978–988.

52. Laviano A, Meguid MM, Cascino A, et al. Tryptophan in wasting diseases: at the crossing between immune function and behavior. *Curr Opin Clin Nutr Metab Care.* 2009;12:392–397.

53. Maluchenko NV, Schegolkova JV, Kulikova MA, et al. Gender differences on association of serotonin transporter gene polymorphism with symptoms of central fatigue. *Bull Exp Biol Med.* 2009;147:462–465.

54. Weber MA, Krakowski-Roosen H, Schroder L, et al. Morphology, metabolism, microcirculation, and strength of skeletal muscles in cancer-related cachexia. *Acta Oncol.* 2009;48:116–124.

55. Yavuzsen T, Davis MP, Ranganathan VK, et al. Cancer-related fatigue: central or peripheral? *J Pain Symptom Manage.* 2009;38:587–596.

56. Landmark-Hoyvik H, Reinertsen KV, Loge JH, et al. Alterations of gene expression in blood cells associated with chronic fatigue in breast cancer survivors. *Pharmacogenom J.* 2009;9:333–340.

57. Sloan JA, Zhao CX. Genetics and quality of life. *Curr Probl Cancer.* 2006;30:255–260.

58. Borneman T, Piper BF, Sun VC, et al. Implementing the fatigue guidelines at one NCCN member institution: process and outcomes. *J Natl Compr Cancer Netw.* 2007;5:1092–1101.

59. Knowles G, Borthwick D, McNamara S, et al. Survey of nurses' assessment of cancer-related fatigue. *Eur J Cancer Care (Engl).* 2000;9:105–113.

60. Piper BF, Borneman T, Sun VC, et al. Cancer-related fatigue: role of oncology nurses in translating National Comprehensive Cancer Network assessment guidelines into practice. *Clin J Oncol Nurs.* 2008;12(suppl 5):37–47.

61. Basch E, Iasonos A, McDonough T, et al. Patient versus clinician symptom reporting using the National Cancer Institute Common Terminology for Adverse Events: results of a questionnaire-based study. *Lancet Oncol.* 2006;7:903–909.

62. Trotti A, Colevas D, Setser A, et al. Patient-reported outcomes and the evolution of adverse event reporting in oncology. *J Clin Oncol.* 2007;25:5121–5127.

63. Basch E, Jia X, Heller G, et al. Adverse symptom event reporting by patients vs clinicians: relationships with clinical outcomes. *J Natl Cancer Inst.* 2009;101:1624–1632.

64. Garcia SF, Cella D, Clauser SB, et al. Standardizing patient-reported outcomes assessment in cancer clinical trials: a patient-reported outcomes measurement information system initiative. *J Clin Oncol.* 2007;25:5106–5118.

65. Minton O, Stone P. A systematic review of the scales used for the measurement of cancer-related fatigue (CRF). *Ann Oncol.* 2009;20:17–25.

66. Wielgus KK, Berger AM, Hertzog M. Predictors of fatigue 30 days after completing anthracyclines plus taxane adjuvant chemotherapy for breast cancer. *Oncol Nurs Forum.* 2009;36:38–48.

67. Given B. Cancer-related fatigue: a brief overview of current nursing perspectives and experiences. *Clin J Oncol Nurs.* 2008;12(suppl 5):7–9.

68. NCCN survey identifies cancer-related fatigue as an area of need for education. July 6 2009. Available from: http://www.nccn.org/about/news/ebulletin/2009–07–06/survey.asp.

69. Barsevick AM, Whitmer K, Sweeney C, et al. A pilot study examining energy conservation for cancer treatment-related fatigue. *Cancer Nurs.* 2002;25:333–341.

70. Given B, Given CW, McCorkle R, et al. Pain and fatigue management: results of a nursing randomized clinical trial. *Oncol Nurs Forum.* 2002;29:949–956.

71. Ream E, Richardson A, Alexander-Dann C. Facilitating patients' coping with fatigue during chemotherapy-pilot outcomes. *Cancer Nurs.* 2002;25:300–308.

72. Godino C, Jodar L, Duran A, et al. Nursing education as an intervention to decrease fatigue perception in oncology patients. *Eur J Oncol Nurs.* 2006;10:150–155.

73. Armes J, Chalder T, Addington-Hall J, et al. A randomized controlled trial to evaluate the effectiveness of a brief, behaviorally oriented intervention for cancer-related fatigue. *Cancer.* 2007;110:1385–1395.

74. Yates P, Aranda S, Hargraves M, et al. Randomized controlled trial of an educational intervention for managing fatigue in women receiving adjuvant chemotherapy for early-stage breast cancer. *J Clin Oncol.* 2005;23:6027–6036.

75. Goedendorp MM, Gielissen MF, Verhagen CA, et al. Psychosocial interventions for reducing fatigue during cancer treatment in adults. *Cochrane Database Syst Rev.* 2009;(1) CD006953.

76. Barsevick AM, Dudley W, Beck S, et al. A randomized clinical trial of energy conservation for patients with cancer-related fatigue. *Cancer.* 2004;100:1302–1310.

77. Cella D, Lai JS, Chang CH, et al. Fatigue in cancer patients compared with fatigue in the general United States population. *Cancer.* 2002;94:528–538.

78. Rodgers GM, Becker PS, Bennett CL, et al. NCCN clinical practice guidelines in oncology: cancer and chemotherapy-induced anemia. Available from: http://www.nccn.org/professionals/physician_gls/PDF.

79. Belza BL. Comparison of self-reported fatigue in rheumatoid arthritis and controls. *J Rheumatol.* 1995;22:639–643.

80. Given B, Given C, Sikorskii A, et al. When compared with information interventions, are cognitive behavioral models more effective in assisting patients to manage symptoms? *Oncol Nurs Forum.* 2009;36:IV.

81. Biondi B, Cooper DS. The clinical significance of subclinical thyroid dysfunction. *Endocr Rev.* 2008;29:76–131.

82. Canaris GJ, Manowitz NR, Mayor G, et al. The Colorado thyroid disease prevalence study. *Arch Intern Med.* 2000;160:526–534.

83. Reddy A, Dash C, Leerapun A, et al. Hypothyroidism: a possible risk factor for liver cancer in patients with no known underlying cause of liver disease. *Clin Gastroenterol Hepatol.* 2007;5:118–123.

84. Smith GL, Smith BD, Giordano SH, et al. Risk of hypothyroidism in older breast cancer patients treated with radiation. *Cancer.* 2008;112:1371–1379.

85. Wolter P, Stefan C, Decallonne B, et al. The clinical implications of sunitinib-induced hypothyroidism: a prospective evaluation. *Br J Cancer.* 2008;99:448–454.

86. Strasser F, Palmer JL, Schover LR, et al. The impact of hypogonadism and autonomic dysfunction on fatigue, emotional function, and sexual desire in male patients with advanced cancer: a pilot study. *Cancer.* 2006;107:2949–2957.

87. Demark-Wahnefried W, Aziz NM, Rowland JH, et al. Riding the crest of the teachable moment: promoting long-term health after the diagnosis of cancer. *J Clin Oncol.* 2005;23:5814–5830.

88. Schwartz AL. Physical activity. *Semin Oncol Nurs.* 2008;24:164–170.

89. Blanchard CM, Stein KD, Baker F, et al. Association between current lifestyle behaviors and health-related quality of life in breast, colorectal, and prostate cancer survivors. *Psychol Health.* 2004;19:1–13.

90. Jones LW, Courneya KS, Fairey AS, et al. Effects of an oncologist's recommendation to exercise on self-reported exercise behavior in newly diagnosed breast cancer survivors: a single-blind, randomized controlled trial. *Ann Behav Med.* 2004;28:105–113.

91. Headley JA, Ownby KK, John LD. The effect of seated exercise on fatigue and quality of life in women with advanced breast cancer. *Oncol Nurs Forum.* 2004;31:977–983.

92. Holland JC, Andersen B, Breitbart WS, et al. National Comprehensive Cancer Network (NCCN) clinical practice guidelines in oncology: distress management. 2010. Available from: http://www.nccn.org/professionals/physician_gls/PDF/distress.pdf.

93. Stark D, Kiely M, Smith A, et al. Anxiety disorders in cancer patients: their nature, associations, and relation to quality of life. *J Clin Oncol.* 2002;20:3137–3148.

94. Smets EM, Visser MR, Willems-Groot AF, et al. Fatigue and radiotherapy: experience in patients 9 months following treatment. *Br J Cancer.* 1998;78:907–912.

95. Roscoe JA, Morrow GR, Hickok JT, et al. Effect of paroxetine hydrochloride (Paxil) on fatigue and depression in breast cancer patients receiving chemotherapy. *Breast Cancer Res Treat.* 2005;89:243–249.

96. Adjustment to cancer: anxiety and distress (PDQ). 2010. Available from: http://www.cancer.gov/cancertopics/pdq/supportivecare/adjustment/HealthProfessional.

97. Depression (PDQ). Available from: http://www.cancer.gov/cancertopics/pdq/supportivecare/depression/healthprofessional; 2010.

98. Fatigue (PDQ). Available from: http://www.cancer.gov/cancertopics/pdq/supportivecare/fatigue/HealthProfessional; 2010.

99. Kubrak C, Jensen L. Critical evaluation of nutrition screening tools recommended for oncology patients. *Cancer Nurs.* 2007;30:E1–E6.

100. Beach P, Siebeneck B, Buderer NF, et al. Relationship between fatigue and nutritional status in patients receiving radiation therapy to treat lung cancer. *Oncol Nurs Forum.* 2001;28:1027–1031.

101. Porock D, Beshears B, Hinton P, et al. Nutritional, functional, and emotional characteristics related to fatigue in patients during and after biochemotherapy. *Oncol Nurs Forum.* 2005;32:661–667.

102. Brown JK, Byers T, Doyle C, et al. Nutrition and physical activity during and after cancer treatment: an American Cancer Society guide for informed choices. *CA Cancer J Clin.* 2003;53:268–291.

103. Swarm R, Abernethy AP, Anghelescu DL, et al. National Comprehensive Cancer Network (NCCN) clinical practice guidelines in oncology adult cancer pain. 2009. Available from: http://www.nccn.org/professionals/physician_gls/PDF/pain.pdf.

104. Bennett MI, Bagnall AM, Jose Closs S. How effective are patient-based educational interventions in the management of cancer pain? Systematic review and meta-analysis. *Pain.* 2009;143:192–199.

105. NIH-state-of-the-science statement on symptom management in cancer: pain, depression, and fatigue. 2002. Available from: http://consensus.nih.gov/2002CancerPainDepressionFatigueSOSO22PDF.pdf.

106. Cleeland CS, Bennett GJ, Dantzer R, et al. Are the symptoms of cancer and cancer treatment due to a shared biologic mechanism? A cytokine-immunologic model of cancer symptoms. *Cancer.* 2003;97:2919–2925.

107. Dodd MJ, Miaskowski C, Lee KA. Occurrence of symptom clusters. *J Natl Cancer Inst Monogr.* 2004;32:76–78.

108. Dodd MJ, Cho MH, Cooper B, et al. Advancing our knowledge of symptom clusters. *J Support Oncol.* 2005;3(6 suppl 4):30–31.

109. Fan G, Filipczak L, Chow E. Symptom clusters in cancer patients: a review of the literature. *Curr Oncol.* 2007;14:173–179.

110. Barsevick AM. The elusive concept of the symptom cluster. *Oncol Nurs Forum.* 2007;34:971–980.

111. Walsh D, Rybicki L. Symptom clustering in advanced cancer. *Support Care Cancer.* 2006;14:831–836.

112. Gift AG, Strommel M, Jablonski A, et al. A cluster of symptoms over time in patients with lung cancer. *Nurs Res.* 2003;52:393–400.

113. Hayduk L, Olson K, Quan H, et al. Temporal changes in the causal foundations of palliative care symptoms. *Qual Life Res.* 2010;19:299–306.

114. Olson K, Hayduk L, Cree M, et al. The changing causal foundations of cancer-related symptom clustering during the final month of palliative care: a longitudinal study. *BMC Med Res Methodol.* 2008;8:1–11.

115. Musselman DL, Miller AH, Porter MR, et al. Higher than normal plasma interleukin-6 concentrations in cancer patients with depression: preliminary findings. *Am J Psychiatry.* 2001;158:1252–1257.

116. Cleeland CS, Reyes-Gibby CC. When is it justified to treat symptoms? Measuring symptom burden. *Oncology (Williston).* 2002;16(9 suppl 10):64–70.

117. Barsevick AM, Whitmer K, Nail LM, et al. Symptom cluster research: conceptual, design, measurement, and analysis. *J Pain Symptom Manage.* 2006;31:85–95.

118. Aktas A, Walsh D, Rybicki L. Symptom clusters: myth or reality? *Palliat Med.* 2010;24:373–385.

119. Kim HJ, Abraham IL. Statistical approaches to modeling symptom clusters in cancer patients. *Cancer Nurs.* 2008;31:E1–E10.

120. Skerman HM, Yates PM, Battistutta D. Multivariate methods to identify cancer-related symptom clusters. *Res Nurs Health.* 2009;32:345–360.

121. Hess LM, Insel KC. Chemotherapy-related change in cognitive function: a conceptual model. *Oncol Nurs Forum.* 2007;34:981–994.

122. Cimprich B, Ronis DL. An environmental intervention to restore attention in women with newly diagnosed breast cancer. *Cancer Nurs.* 2003;26:284 92; quiz 293–4.

123. Berger AM. Update on the state of the science: sleep-wake disturbances in adult patients with cancer. *Oncol Nurs Forum.* 2009;36:E165–E177.

124. Savard J, Simard S, Giguere I, et al. Randomized clinical trial on cognitive therapy for depression in women with metastatic breast cancer: psychological and immunological effects. *Palliat Support Care.* 2006;4:219–237.

125. Sateia MJ, Lang BJ. Sleep and cancer: recent developments. *Curr Oncol Rep.* 2008;10:309–318.

126. Kozachik SL, Bandeen-Roche K. Predictors of patterns of pain, fatigue, and insomnia during the first year after a cancer diagnosis in the elderly. *Cancer Nurs.* 2008;31:334–344.

127. Roscoe JA, Kaufman ME, Matteson-Rusby SE, et al. Cancer-related fatigue and sleep disorders. *Oncologist.* 2007;12(suppl 1):35–42.

128. Mitchell SA, Berger AM. Fatigue. In: Pine JWJ, ed. *Cancer: principles and practice of oncology.* 8th ed. Philadelphia, PA: Lippincott Williams and Wilkins; 2008:2710–2718.

129. Morin CM, Bootzin RR, Buysse DJ, et al. Psychological and behavioral treatment of insomnia: update of the recent evidence (1998–2004). *Sleep.* 2006;29:1398–1414.

130. Mustian KM, Morrow GR, Carroll JK, et al. Integrative nonpharmacologic behavioral interventions for the management of cancer-related fatigue. *Oncologist.* 2007;12(suppl 1):52–67.

131. Sleep disorders (PDQ). Available from: http://www.nci.nih.gov/cancertopics/pdq/supportivecare/sleepdisorders/HealthProfessional/; 2010.

132. Breitbart W, Alici Y. Pharmacologic treatment options for cancer-related fatigue: current state of clinical research. *Clin J Oncol Nurs.* 2008;12(suppl 5):27–36.

133. Minton O, Richardson A, Sharpe M, et al. A systematic review and meta-analysis of the pharmacological treatment of cancer-related fatigue. *J Natl Cancer Inst.* 2008;100:1155–1166.

134. Centeno CT, Carvajal A, San Miguel MT, et al. What is the best term in Spanish to express the concept of cancer-related fatigue? *J Palliat Med.* 2009;12:441–445.

135. Thomas R, Davies N. Lifestyle during and after cancer treatment. *Clin Oncol (R Coll Radiol).* 2007;19:616–627.

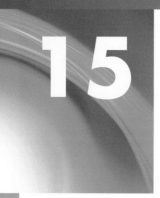

15 Cancer anorexia and cachexia

Shalini Dalal and Eduardo Bruera

One of the most common manifestations of advanced cancer is the development of a complex multifaceted metabolic syndrome, termed cancer cachexia. Because of the frequent presence of anorexia (or loss of appetite), it is also commonly referred to as the cancer anorexia-cachexia syndrome (CACS). Clinically, CACS is recognized by a constellation of symptoms that include unintentional weight loss, anorexia, early satiety, fatigue, and other symptoms such as nausea, dysphagia, and depressed mood of varying severity and duration. Weight loss in this context is the result of a combination of muscle and adipose tissue loss, and it occurs with or without decreased caloric intake. CACS is of great significance to cancer patients, in terms of both its high prevalence (50% at time of diagnosis, to more than 80% before death) and its consistent association with negative outcomes.[1,2] Studies on the same have demonstrated decreases in performance status scores, impairments in immunity, increased morbidity, and decreased tolerance to cancer therapies, all of which in turn predict treatment failure, diminished quality of life (QoL), and poor survival.[2-4] Cachexia is also associated with patient and family psychological distress.[5,6]

The anorexia-cachexia syndrome (ACS) is not unique to cancer but is central to many other conditions, such as autoimmune disorders, chronic obstructive pulmonary disease, chronic heart failure, infections such as human immunodeficiency virus and tuberculosis, and prolonged critical illnesses.[3,4] ACS in all these diverse disorders shares many similarities in terms of physical and psychosocial symptoms, adverse outcomes, and seemingly coordinated pathophysiologic mechanisms suggestive of a "common pathway" for deteriorating energy balance in end-stage disease. Although the pathogenesis of ACS is complex and is not fully understood, inflammation is a common theme that emerges from several studies on these disorders.[3,5,6] The presence of inflammation has been shown to be associated with abnormalities in endocrine functions, weight loss, and poor survival.[4] It is not surprising to note that cachexia in these conditions is referred to as "inflammatory cachexia," a term that helps distinguish it from starvation, where weight loss is not accompanied by inflammation. In starvation, weight loss occurs predominantly from depletion of adipose stores. The relative preservation of muscle protein is the result of finely coordinated regulatory processes that quickly come into play. By contrast, cachexia appears to involve defects in these homeostatic mechanisms, likely induced by inflammatory mediators, such that muscle protein depletion occurs early, along with adipose tissue wasting, and is irrespective of caloric intake. Further, the inflammatory process affects central appetite regulation. Differences between starvation and cachexia are shown in Table 15-1.

In this chapter, we will discuss how immune alterations lead to disruptions of normal regulatory mechanisms involved in energy balance in cancer patients, one of which may be applicable to other chronic disorders associated with wasting, and which offers practical approaches to the assessment and management of anorexia and cachexia in cancer patients.

MECHANISMS OF CANCER ANOREXIA-CACHEXIA SYNDROME

A common feature of advanced cancer is that the immune response fails to eradicate the tumor because of complex mechanisms of immune evasion that limit the protective host response. Such a particular tumor–host relationship results in the establishment of chronic systemic inflammation, during which a broad range of normal regulatory adaptive mechanisms become dysfunctional. This inflammatory state is accompanied by dysregulated production of a variety of inflammatory mediators (including cytokines) that induce disparate aberrations in key central and peripheral regulatory systems. In animal models, compelling data support the participation of proinflammatory cytokines, including interleukin (IL)-1β, IL-6, tumor necrosis factor (TNF)-α, and interferon-γ, in the genesis of CACS.[7] These cytokines are involved in mediating a wide range of systemic effects, including the hepatic acute phase protein response (APPR), hypermetabolism, adipose and skeletal muscle protein breakdown, and diminished appetite.[8–13] Furthermore, although not well understood, several circulating tumor-related factors, such as proteolysis-inducing factor (PIF) and lipid-mobilizing factor (LMF), are also believed to participate in muscle and adipose wasting, respectively.[14,15] Cachexia caused by these mechanisms is also referred to as *primary cachexia*. Figure 15-1 illustrates key components of cytokine-mediated CACS.[6]

In addition, weight loss in cancer patients can arise from one or multiple (common) coexisting symptoms that contribute to decreased nutritional intake. These symptoms, often referred to as "nutrition impact symptoms," include early satiety, nausea, anorexia, taste alterations, dry mouth, dysphagia, odynophagia, and constipation.[16] Some of these symptoms can be part of the primary cachexia process, or may arise as a result of side effects of cancer treatment. Further, psychological issues such as depressed mood, anxiety, and difficulty with coping are common in this patient population, and may possibly compromise appetite and oral intake. It is important to keep in mind that many patients may have coexisting comorbidities that could contribute to the total symptom burden experience. Weight loss resulting from these factors is referred to as *secondary cachexia*. Few studies have looked at the frequency of symptoms that contribute to secondary cachexia. One study reported dry mouth, belching, nausea, bad taste in the mouth, and constipation as most common and distressful to patients; all are associated with poorer QoL and performance status.[17] Another study reported anorexia, early satiety, and pain as most common among patients with gastrointestinal and lung cancers.[18] A recent review of 50 cachectic cancer patients followed in a cachexia clinic at a tertiary cancer hospital found a high frequency of such factors that were potentially contributing to cachexia, with the vast majority of patients presenting two or more factors.[19] Most common were early satiety, constipation, pain, and depression. Differences in studies could be attributed to differences in patient populations, stages of disease, cancer types, and treatment duration and frequency.

Table 15-1 Difference between starvation and cachexia

	Starvation	Cachexia
Mechanism	Calorie deficiency due to ↓ oral intake and/or ↑ loss (e.g., malabsorption)	More complex and regulated by cytokines
Body weight	↓	↓
Host metabolic response	Adaptive	Maladaptive
Acute phase protein response	No	Yes
Lean body mass	Conserved initially	↓
• Protein synthesis	↓↓↓	↓
• Protein degradation	↓↓↓	↑↑↑
Fat/adipose mass	↓↓↓	↓↓
Resting energy expenditure	↓↓↓	↑↑↑
Serum insulin	↓↓↓	↑↑↑
Serum cortisol	No change	↑↑
Effect of feeding	Appropriate nutrition may reverse these changes	Feeding does not reverse the macronutrient changes

Adapted from Kotler DP. Cachexia. Ann Intern Med 2000;133:622.
↓ denotes decrease; ↑ increase.

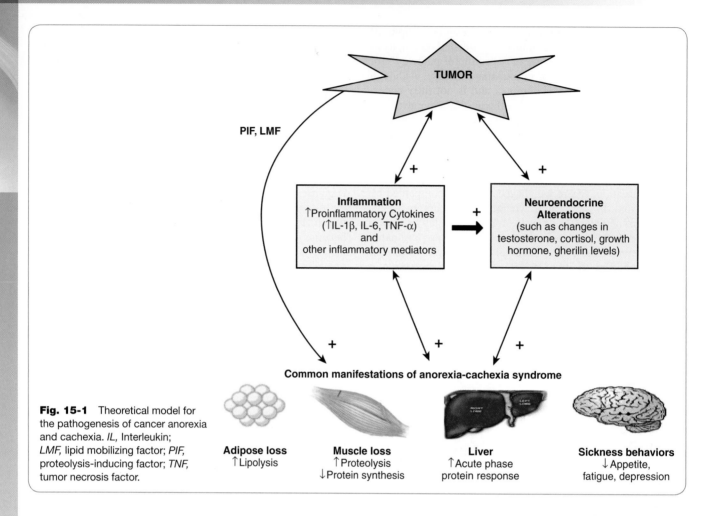

Fig. 15-1 Theoretical model for the pathogenesis of cancer anorexia and cachexia. *IL,* Interleukin; *LMF,* lipid mobilizing factor; *PIF,* proteolysis-inducing factor; *TNF,* tumor necrosis factor.

Thus it is important to keep in mind that in any given patient, cachexia is likely to result from a combination of primary and secondary mechanisms of cachexia, and a systematic approach to the identification of potentially reversible causes needs to be undertaken (discussed in the section on assessment of CACS).

ACUTE PHASE PROTEIN RESPONSE (APPR)

Approximately 50% of patients have an APPR at the time of cancer diagnosis.[20] Proinflammatory cytokines, in particular IL-6, appear to be involved in the generation of the hepatic APPR, resulting in an increase in acute phase proteins such as C-reactive protein (CRP) and fibrinogen, and a decrease in negative acute phase proteins such as albumin and transferrin. CRP is a sensitive and specific marker of systemic inflammation, and it has been shown to correlate with several aspects of CACS, including weight loss, hypermetabolism, reduced caloric intake, and anorexia, as well as poorer survival.[20–25]

EFFECTS OF IMMUNOLOGIC STRESS ON APPETITE REGULATION
Implications in advanced cancer

Neuroendocrine and endocrine responses to stress play an integral role in the maintenance of homeostasis. In general, these responses work toward inhibiting nonessential functions such as growth and reproduction in favor of maintenance and survival. Stress-induced reorganization of endocrine priorities results in activation of the hypothalamic-pituitary-adrenal (HPA) axis and the sympathetic nervous system (SNS), leading to increases in catabolic hormones, cortisol, and catecholamines, respectively. Although these adaptive responses are essential to coping and survival, the presence of long-term or chronic stressors elicits endocrine responses that become maladaptive, eventually leading to dysregulation across multiple physiologic systems such as the immune and cardiovascular systems, and the metabolic regulation of energy balance.[26–28]

Body weight, inevitably maintained by balancing food intake with energy expenditure, is regulated by the central nervous system (CNS). The hypothalamus in particular plays a central role in appetite regulation and energy expenditure, consisting of several nuclei that integrate a complex array of metabolic signals. Table 15-2 lists some of the most recognized peptides involved in the regulation of energy balance. The best characterized pathways are located in the arcuate nucleus (ARC), which includes two distinct populations of neurons, each with opposing effects. One population of neurons produces orexigenic peptides, agouti-related peptide (AgRP), and neuropeptide Y (NPY), and stimulates appetite. The second population produces anorexigenic peptides, pro-opiomelanocortin (POMC), and cocaine- and amphetamine-related transcript (CART), and inhibits appetite.[29] Neuronal projections from the ARC communicate with other key hypothalamic areas involved in feeding behaviors, such as the paraventricular (PVN), dorsomedial (DMN), and lateral hypothalamic nuclei. Projections to and from the brainstem, cortical areas, and reward pathways also may influence food intake.

The ARC, lacking an effective blood-brain barrier, is strategically positioned to integrate a number of peripheral signals controlling food intake. The NPY/AgRP and POMC/CART neuronal systems are therefore directly targeted by several metabolic signals, such as hormones secreted in proportion to body adiposity (such as insulin and leptin) and following a meal (ghrelin, cholecystokinin [CCK], and peptide YY).[29,30] As is shown in Figure 15-2, leptin, insulin, CCK, and peptide YY inhibit appetite and increase energy expenditure via their effects on POMC (activate) and NPY/AgRP (inhibition) systems, while ghrelin has an opposite effect. Activation of POMC-containing neurons results in cleavage of POMC into alpha-melanocyte stimulating hormone (α-MSH), which in turn activates melanocortin (MC) receptors (type 4 predominantly), leading to secretion of corticotropin-releasing factor (CRF) in the nearby paraventricular nucleus (PVN) region of the hypothalamus. CRF, in addition to its well-recognized effects on stimulating stress-related endocrine, autonomic, and behavioral responses, is a powerful endogenous anorectic and thermogenic agent.[31] These latter effects are mediated via its receptors, CRF-1 and CRF-2.[32] In contrast, activation of the NPY/AgRP system stimulates appetite by directly inhibiting

Table 15-2   Neuropeptides involved in appetite regulation

	Orexigenic	Anorexigenic
Central	Neuropeptide Y	Cocaine- and amphetamine-related transcript (CART)
	Melanin concentrating hormone (MCH)	Melanocortins (pro-opiomelanocortin [POMC])
	Orexins/hypocretins	Glucagon-like peptide
	Agouti-related peptide (AgRP)	Corticotropin-releasing factor (CRF)
	Galanin	Insulin
	Endogenous opioids	Serotonin
	Endocannabinoids	Neurotensin
Peripheral	Ghrelin	Peptide YY
		Cholecystokinin (CCK)
		Leptin
		Amylin
		Insulin
		Glucagon-like peptides
		Bombesin

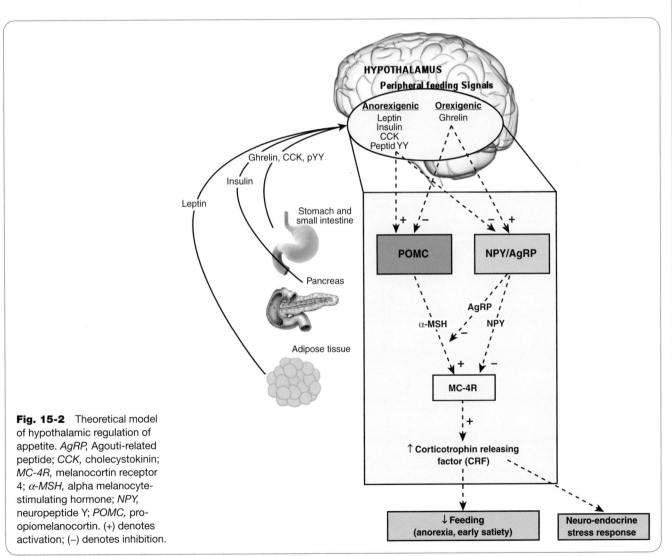

Fig. 15-2   Theoretical model of hypothalamic regulation of appetite. *AgRP,* Agouti-related peptide; *CCK,* cholecystokinin; *MC-4R,* melanocortin receptor 4; *α-MSH,* alpha melanocyte-stimulating hormone; *NPY,* neuropeptide Y; *POMC,* pro-opiomelanocortin. (+) denotes activation; (−) denotes inhibition.

the activation of MC-4 receptors (via NPY), or by blocking POMC neuronal signals (via AgRP). The unidirectional interaction between the NPY/AgRP and POMC neurons appears to be of potential significance, as it provides a tonic inhibition of POMC neurons whenever NPY/AgRP cells are active.[33,34]

The effects of stress on appetite are well recognized. Although not fully understood, complex immune-endocrine interplay is believed to mediate these effects. Proinflammatory cytokines (such as IL-1, TNF-α, and IL-6) play a predominant role, affecting food intake and energy homeostasis during infection and inflammation as part of a sickness response, via its effects in the CNS and gastrointestinal (GI) tract.[35] In animal models, such cytokines have been shown to suppress appetite and induce satiety via multiple mechanisms[36-38] (Fig. 15-3). Cytokines interact with appetite-regulating pathways by directly activating POMC neurons or by interfering with the release or function of orexigenic neuromediators. For instance, IL-1β antagonizes the effects of the orexigenic NPY,[39] which can be abolished by blocking the α-MSH receptor (MC-4).[35] Serotonin, a potent anorectic monoamine, is believed to be a critical link between cytokines and appetite pathways; its secretion in the brain is increased by IL-1β.[37] In the GI tract, cytokines mediate satiety by its effects on vagal afferents,

resulting in activation of mechanisms that mediate the sensation of fullness, such as impaired gastric accommodation or delayed antropyloric transit.[39] Cytokines also induce the release of CCK, glucagon, insulin, and leptin, all of which act as anorectic and satiety signals in the CNS.[35,39,40] Furthermore, cytokine-mediated alterations of the HPA axis and SNS lead to other manifestations of sickness behavior (such as depression or fatigue), autonomic instability, and elevations in resting energy expenditure (REE). Increased cortisol and catecholamine levels propagate catabolism in conjunction with other mechanisms in muscle and fat tissues.

SKELETAL MUSCLE LOSS

Skeletal muscle mass is maintained by a dynamic balance between anabolic (or hypertrophic) and catabolic (or atrophic) processes. The muscle wasting that occurs in catabolic states such as cancer results largely from loss of myofibrillar proteins (actin and myosin), which make up 60% to 70% of muscle protein.[41] Cachectic mediators such as proinflammatory cytokines and PIF, in concert with alterations in hormonal signals (glucocorticoids, insulin, insulin-like growth factor [IGF]), induce muscle wasting by reducing the rate of protein synthesis at the

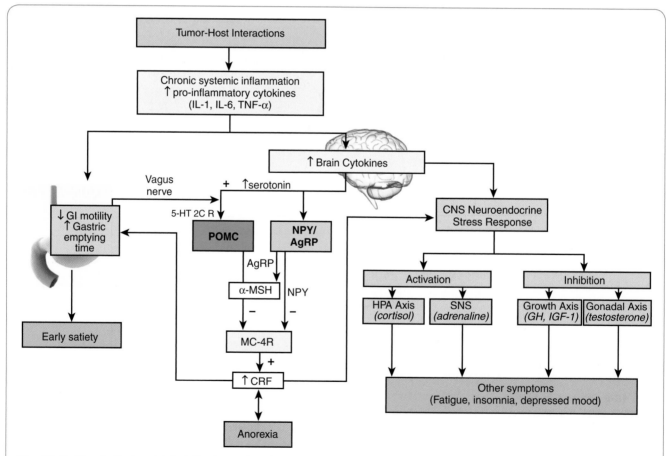

Fig. 15-3 Hypothetical model depicting interactions between the immune, neural, and endocrine systems in appetite regulation and symptoms commonly found in advanced stages of cancer. *AgRP,* Agouti-related peptide; *CRF,* corticotropin-releasing factor; *GH,* growth factor; *HPA,* hypothalamic-pituitary-adrenal; *IGF-1,* insulin-like growth factor 1; *IL,* interleukin; *MC-4R,* melanocortin receptor 4; *MSH,* melanocyte-stimulating hormone; *NPY,* neuropeptide Y; *POMC,* pro-opiomelanocortin; *SNS,* sympathetic nervous symptom; *TNF,* tumor necrosis factor.

level of protein translation (RNA content) and by stimulating protein catabolic mechanisms.[41–43] Of the myofibrillar proteins, the myosin heavy chain is the preferred substrate for degradation.[42] Two protein degradation mechanisms, calcium-dependent proteases or calpains (essential for the initial breakdown of myofibrillar proteins to actin and myosin) and the ubiquitin-proteosome pathway (UPP), are considered most important.[41–44] The UPP system has received the most intense scrutiny and involves a step-wise process of conjugation of target protein to activated ubiquitin, and its subsequent degradation by the 26S proteasome.[41] Activation of the UPP system has been demonstrated by ubiquitin E3 ligases, muscle RING finger-1 (MuRF1), and muscle atrophy F-Box (MAFBx) or atrogin-1.[45] A number of signaling pathways, upstream to the UPP, have been suggested to be pertinent to the wasting process. These include the nuclear factor (NF)-κ B, myostatin, and the dystrophin glycoprotein complex (DGC); as illustrated in Figure 15-4, they are believed to mediate their effects through activation of UPP.[46] Myostatin, an inhibitor of skeletal muscle mass, is a member of the transforming growth factor-β superfamily, and, like cytokine and PIF, it increases expression of UPP components. Activation of the NF-κB pathway occurs in response to inflammatory signals and induces muscle wasting, in part by increasing the expression of ubiquitin ligase MURF-1.[47,48]

As with protein degradation, several intracellular signaling mechanisms are involved in protein synthesis, of which signaling via AKT1 appears to play a major role.[49] Activation of Akt (as in response to anabolic signals, insulin, and IGF-1) results in inactivation of key transcription factors (Foxo) involved in the transcription of atrophic genes (e.g., MURF-1,

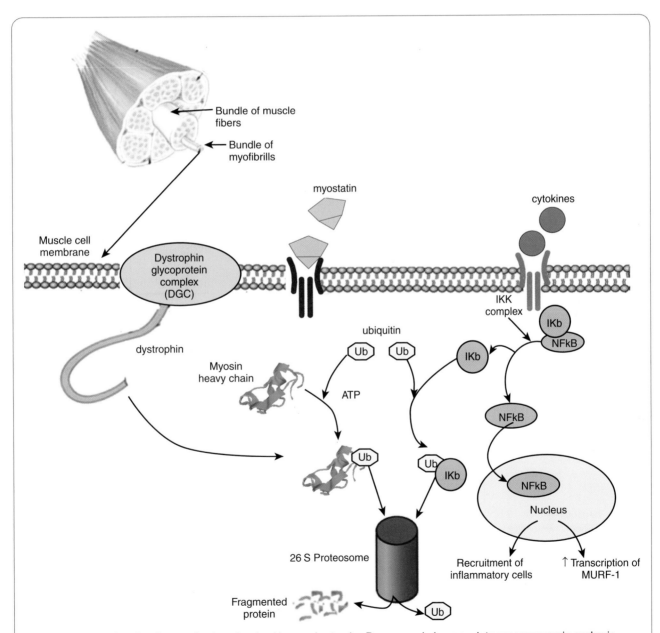

Fig. 15-4 Emerging signaling mechanisms involved in muscle atrophy. Recommended approach to cancer-anorexia-cachexia assessment and management. *ATP,* Adenosine-5′-triphosphate; *IKK,* IκB kinase; *MURF-1,* muscle-specific RING finger protein 1; *NF-κB,* nuclear factor-kappa b.

Atrogin). In cachexia, downregulation of insulin and IGF pathways leads to Akt inactivation, which removes the inhibitory influence of Foxo transcription factors.[50]

ADIPOSE TISSUE LOSS

Loss of a*dipose tissue* accounts for a large part of the dramatic weight loss observed in cancer patients.[51–54] Although the mechanism is not fully understood,[55,56] it appears to result from increased breakdown (lipolysis) and reduced energy storage (lipogenesis), with lipolysis believed to be of greater importance and independent of decreased oral intake.[52–59] An increase in lipolytic activity is demonstrated by high serum glycerol and hormone-sensitive lipase (HSL) mRNA expression in adipocytes in cancer patients.[51–54] As demonstrated in Figure 15-5, many factors have been suggested to promote the activation of HSL, the major rate-limiting enzyme of lipolysis. These include proinflammatory cytokines, catecholamines, LMF, natriuretic peptides, and tumor-derived lipolytic factor; they appear in contrast to insulin, which inhibits this process and functions as a lipogenic hormone.[60]

ASSESSMENT OF CANCER ANOREXIA-CACHEXIA SYNDROME (CACS)

As aforementioned, CACS is a complex and multifaceted syndrome that varies widely in its presentation, etiology (contributing factors), and impact on the patient. Although no two patients

are alike, a standardized approach to assessment should be adopted by the medical team, one that systematically assesses the various facets of the syndrome. We believe that such an assessment should be followed by a decision-making process that would help the medical team formulate an individualized treatment plan for nutritional care and cachexia management. An interdisciplinary and collaborative approach is highly encouraged, as is the use of validated assessment tools. Figure 15-1 depicts an approach to assessment and management that is used at University of Texas, M.D. Anderson Cancer Cachexia Center, and is discussed further in the following section.

NUTRITIONAL ASSESSMENT

The best approach to managing anorexia and cachexia in cancer patients is to begin early. Therefore, it is recommended that all cancer patients should ideally undergo nutritional screening at the time of cancer diagnosis to identify patients with and those at risk for malnutrition or cachexia. A number of validated nutritional screening assessment tools (such as the Malnutrition Screening Tool) are available and can be incorporated easily into the routine forms used in outpatient or inpatient clinical settings.

The Malnutrition Screening Tool (MST) is a quick and simple nutrition screening tool that has previously been validated for use in inpatients,[61] and in outpatient settings for patients receiving radiotherapy[62] or chemotherapy.[63] It is based on recent appetite and weight loss and is a strong predictor of nutritional status when compared with Subjective Global Assessment

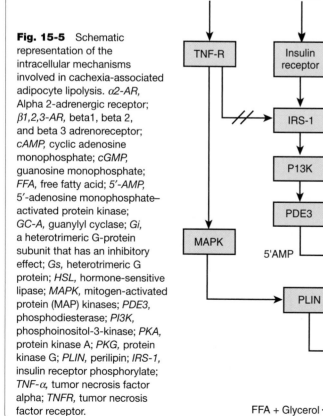
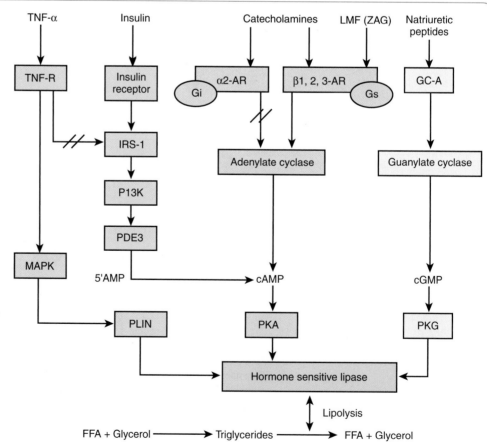

Fig. 15-5 Schematic representation of the intracellular mechanisms involved in cachexia-associated adipocyte lipolysis. *α2-AR,* Alpha 2-adrenergic receptor; *β1,2,3-AR,* beta1, beta 2, and beta 3 adrenoreceptor; *cAMP,* cyclic adenosine monophosphate; *cGMP,* guanosine monophosphate; *FFA,* free fatty acid; *5′-AMP,* 5′-adenosine monophosphate–activated protein kinase; *GC-A,* guanylyl cyclase; *Gi,* a heterotrimeric G-protein subunit that has an inhibitory effect; *Gs,* heterotrimeric G protein; *HSL,* hormone-sensitive lipase; *MAPK,* mitogen-activated protein (MAP) kinases; *PDE3,* phosphodiesterase; *PI3K,* phosphoinositol-3-kinase; *PKA,* protein kinase A; *PKG,* protein kinase G; *PLIN,* perilipin; *IRS-1,* insulin receptor phosphorylate; *TNF-α,* tumor necrosis factor alpha; *TNFR,* tumor necrosis factor receptor.

(SGA)[61,62] and Patient-Generated (PG)-SGA tools.[63] The MST can be completed by medical, nursing, dietetic, and administrative staff, or by the patient or caregiver, to identify those at risk of malnutrition to allow the initiation of appropriate nutritional support. For those patients who have a greater than low risk of malnutrition/cachexia, comprehensive nutritional assessment and consultation with a nutritionist are necessary.

Comprehensive nutritional assessment

A comprehensive assessment of nutritional status comprises several domains and focuses on obtaining a medical and nutritional history, symptom assessment, physical examination, functional status, anthropometric measurements, and laboratory data. Assessment of all these components is key in determining overall nutritional status and its impact on the patient, and in eliciting symptoms that may contribute to nutritional decline, formulating realistic treatment and nutritional interventions, and identifying future care needs.

Symptom assessment

Cancer patients may have one or multiple concurrent symptoms that potentially compromise oral intake. A multidimensional tool (such as the Edmonton Symptom Assessment Scale [ESAS]) can be used to assess for the presence and severity of common symptoms such as anorexia, nausea, depression, and fatigue. Careful history and assessment should be performed with attention to the mouth and gastrointestinal system that includes assessment of taste changes, dental issues, and the presence of early satiety and constipation.

Laboratory assessment

Several laboratory abnormalities are frequently noted in cachectic cancer patients, but none are specific enough to cachexia, each variously influenced by the status of cancer, related organ dysfunction, or treatment toxicities. For instance, anemia, iron deficiency, and low albumin are often present in patients with or without cachexia. In addition to poor nutritional intake, serum albumin can be low; along with liver function abnormalities, this may indicate the presence of liver dysfunction. It is also a "negative" acute phase protein in that it is reduced with chronic inflammation. Regardless of the underlying cause, a low serum albumin level has been shown to be an independent prognostic variable for survival in patients with cancer.[64] A high serum CRP is a well-established surrogate marker of inflammation that directly correlates with cachexia and poor outcomes. Patients with raised serum CRP levels have lower energy intake than those with normal levels,[65] and some evidence suggests that resting energy expenditure may be increased in these patients.[66] A normal CRP in a cachectic patient could indicate a predominance of secondary factors contributing to cachexia. Depending on the overall goals of care, laboratory studies may include a complete blood count, a metabolic and liver function panel, albumin, prealbumin, CRP, and vitamin and hormonal levels, if aberrations are suspected.

Anthropometrics and body composition assessment

In general, cancer cachexia in advanced stages is associated with loss of both adipose and lean body mass (LBM); however, in early stages, losses predominantly consist of LBM (most notably skeletal muscle). This contrasts with simple starvation, wherein LBM in early stages is relatively conserved.[67] The measurement of body composition is regarded as a gold standard of nutritional assessment in cachectic cancer patients. Several methods may be used to measure body composition: whole body potassium, densitometry, anthropometrics (e.g., triceps skinfold thickness [TSF], arm muscle area), bioelectrical impedance, phase angle and vector, magnetic resonance imaging and spectroscopy, and computed tomography (CT).[68–72] Most of these assessments are not practical because of cost or availability. Some of these methods (bioelectrical impedance, whole body potassium) do not directly distinguish skeletal muscle from other nonadipose tissues[22,73–75]; others, such as anthropometrics, are cumbersome and operator-dependent, making comparisons relatively imprecise upon repeat measurement. CT, which is emerging as the gold standard in body composition analysis,[76] is used routinely in cancer patients, but it has not been used consistently for this assessment. These imaging techniques allow for assessment of regional muscle and adipose tissue depots, including the separation of adipose tissue into subcutaneous and visceral compartments.[77–80] In cancer patients, with the standard incorporation of CT imaging in patient care, use of this modality for body composition analysis is most suitable, both from a practical standpoint and because of the precision of data that can be obtained. However, these methods have not been employed for this purpose, despite their wide availability and the importance attributed to lean tissue loss in the cancer cachexia literature. Several trials are currently evaluating their potential role in cachexia management. The emergence of obesity as a major health problem in the United States and the resulting increase in body mass index (BMI) over the past two decades make it particularly unreliable to diagnose cachexia on the basis of simple determination of weight or BMI. Reported ≥5% weight loss over the past 6 months or since cancer diagnosis should be considered a practical indication of cachexia even in patients who might appear normally nourished or obese, because sarcopenia may already be significantly present in these patients.

Validated nutrition assessment tools

Several nutritional assessment tools, usually presented as a questionnaire and comprising various variables associated with malnutrition, have been developed. The Subjective Global Assessment (SGA) is a validated nutritional assessment instrument that is based on patients' medical history and results of physical examination.[81] It has been applied successfully as a method of assessing nutritional status and predicting complications in a number of different patient groups, including cancer patients.[61,82] The Patient-Generated Subjective Global Assessment (PG-SGA), adapted from the SGA, was developed specifically for patients with cancer.[82,83] It includes additional questions including several related to the presence of nutritional symptoms and short-term weight loss. Some components of the form such as medical history can be completed by the patient using a check box format. The physical examination is then performed by a health professional, such as a physician, nurse, or dietitian. The scored PG-SGA[84] represents a further development of the PG-SGA and incorporates a numeric score; it also allows categorizing of patients into three categories—well-nourished, moderate or suspected malnourishment, or severely malnourished—based on their global assessment. The scored PG-SGA, unlike the SGA, which is categorical, is a continuous measure. The higher the score, the greater is the risk for malnutrition. A score ≥9 indicates a critical need for nutrition intervention. The scored PG-SGA has been validated for assessment of nutritional status in cancer patients.[85,86] It has been accepted by the Oncology Nutrition Dietetic Practice Group of the American Dietetic Association as the standard for nutrition assessment for patients with cancer. The scored PG-SGA can be used as a nutrition screen or as an assessment or outcome measure. However, because it must be conducted by a trained health professional, in health settings with limited dietetic resources, it is not typically used in practice, other than at some cancer centers.[87]

DECISION-MAKING PROCESS

After a multidimensional assessment as described above, it is important to have a frank discussion with the patient and caregivers about the goals of interventions and to define realistic outcomes (Fig. 15-6). The goals and outcomes of intervention will depend on the patient's cancer stage, comorbidities, and overall prognosis. It is important to discuss that the ensuing weight loss and wasting occur predominantly as the result of complex interactions between tumor and host that affect multiple organs and systems of the body (primary cachexia), and that no single therapy has been shown to be useful by itself. In addition to this primary cause of cachexia, a host of factors may be directly contributing or aggravating nutritional status (secondary cachexia); therefore an important purpose of therapeutic intervention would be to meticulously search and treat these potentially reversible causes. Furthermore,

although weight gain is a desired outcome, it should not be the primary outcome of treatment intervention. Studies suggest that weight stabilization is associated with improved QoL and survival, and it is an appropriate goal in advanced cancer patients who have life expectancy in months. For those patients whose life expectancy is limited to weeks or months, goals of therapy should focus on alleviating distressful symptoms.

INDIVIDUALIZED MULTIMODAL TREATMENT PLAN

Currently, no standard approach to the management of CACS is used. Likely because of the multifactorial and multidimensional nature of CACS, no single therapeutic agent to date has been shown to be consistently successful in treating all of the features of this syndrome. Because CACS varies in its presentation and in its impact on the patient, an individualized and multimodal therapeutic approach should be formulated for the patient, such that nutritional, exercise, and psychological supports are integrated with pharmacologic treatments (Fig. 15-7), all of which should be consistent with the goals and preferences of the patient/family unit.

NUTRITIONAL INTERVENTION

In cancer patients, nutrition intervention in the form of counseling, with or without high-protein energy supplementation, has been shown to improve QoL and symptoms, to increase oral intake, and to attenuate weight loss.[88–91] However, a recent systematic review did not find any benefit for survival.[92] Several national practice guidelines support nutritional counseling in cancer patients.[93,94] The key steps (ABCD) in nutritional counseling and are briefly discussed in the following section.

Assessment of current intake

In patients with advanced cancer dietary records, detailing of nutrient intakes and meal patterns for 3 consecutive days (including 1 weekend day) has been shown to adequately reflect current dietary intake.[95] However, depending on the setting, this may not be practical. Alternatively, patients can be asked to keep a record of their food and fluid intake (food diary) for 24 to 48 hours before their visit with the nutritionist. The nutritionist can review this record with the patient, and can assess for the frequency and size of meals, snacks, and beverages; the patient's dietary preferences; and food allergies. Recent changes in dietary patterns can also be noted. Energy and protein intake estimates can be calculated from the food intake and can serve as a baseline. For a 3-day calorie count, the average for 24 hours is obtained.

Barriers to nutritional intake

The nutritionist should seek to identify existing barriers to adequate dietary intake, including issues of food availability and preparation, companionship during meal times, relationships in the home, and physical and psychological symptoms that limit intake. Alterations in taste and the presence of mucositis, dysphagia, dry mouth, early satiety, bloating sensation, nausea, constipation, depressed mood, and anxiety are common causes of poor nutritional intake.

Multidimensional Assessment
- Medical and treatment history
- Nutritional history: current and in the past
- Symptoms: Physical and psychological symptoms
- Physical exam: attention to mouth and gastrointestinal symptoms
- Laboratory: Examples C-reactive protein, albumin
- Anthropometrics and body Composition

Decision Making Process
- Individualized goals
- Define realistic outcomes (improve body image, improve function, reduce symptoms, extend life expectancy)
- Determine prognosis and antineoplastic treatment
- Discuss challenges that may emerge in the future
- Consider patient/family attitudes
- Consider costs

Individualized Treatment Plan
- Manage treatable causes/aggravating factors
- Nutritional counseling
- Artificial nutrition if appropriate
- Pharmacological support
- Physical therapy/Exercise intervention

Fig. 15-6 Recommended approach to cancer anorexia-cachexia assessment and management.

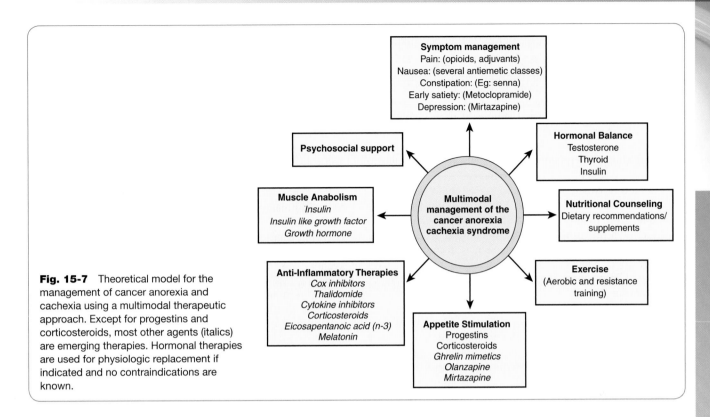

Fig. 15-7 Theoretical model for the management of cancer anorexia and cachexia using a multimodal therapeutic approach. Except for progestins and corticosteroids, most other agents (italics) are emerging therapies. Hormonal therapies are used for physiologic replacement if indicated and no contraindications are known.

Calculation of energy and protein requirements

The exact energy and protein needs of weight-losing cancer patients are not clear. In studies of cancer patients, energy intake in excess of 120 kJ/kg/day and protein intake in excess of 1.2 to 1.4 g/kg/day have been used for weight maintenance.[96,97] Because of high variation in basal energy requirements, an accurate method for measuring individual energy expenditure is indirect calorimetry. If indirect calorimetry is not available, energy intake in excess of 120 kJ/kg/day can be calculated for the patient.

Dietary recommendations

An individualized nutritional plan for the patient should be formulated on the basis of previous steps, patient preferences, and goals of care. The priority is to treat existing barriers to adequate nutritional intake while improving energy and protein intake. Patients' preferences for normal food versus use of nutritional supplements should be taken into account when formulating dietary recommendations. A Canadian study of dietary patterns in cachectic advanced cancer patients reported patient preference for normal foods, with an overwhelming majority (70%) of patients not using commercially available nutritional supplements.[98] The study also found that frequency of eating was as an important variable in total energy intake, and that greater total caloric intake was largely derived from the consumption of food outside of the three main meals of the day. A supportive environment for snacking behavior and use of snacks with high nutritional value were of importance.[98] The relationship of the nutritionist to the patient should not be imposing; rather, small efforts made by the patient and family should be validated. Frequent reinforcement and modification of care plans based on overall medical goals and tolerance may be required.

SYMPTOM MANAGEMENT

Treatment of symptoms that cause or aggravate poor nutritional intake should be a priority. As mentioned, advanced cancer patients may have one or multiple concurrent symptoms that compromise oral intake. Some of these are discussed in the following paragraphs.

Nausea, early satiety, and constipation

These are extremely common symptoms in cachectic cancer patients. Various factors, such as opioids, other medications, chemotherapy, radiation, metabolic disturbances, and tumor location, may contribute to nausea. The cause(s) of nausea could be secondary to chemotherapy and radiation and may respond to 5-serotonin (HT)$_3$ receptor antagonists. Clinicians are urged to review their institutional or national guidelines for management of cancer treatment–induced nausea or vomiting. Agents with antidopaminergic and/or antihistaminic effects are frequently used as an antiemetic. In presence of early satiety, oral metoclopramide is preferred because of its prokinetic effects in the stomach. Constipation frequently occurs in cancer patients, especially if they are on opioids or anticholinergic medications, and may contribute to early satiety and/or nausea. Laxatives such as senna, bisacodyl, magnesium citrate, and polyethylene glycol 3350 can be initiated and dose titrated to ensure regular bowel movements.

Anorexia

A number of agents from diverse drug classes with proposed appetite stimulant properties have been studied for their use in cancer patients. Unfortunately, as discussed later, only two of these—progestins (such as megestrol acetate) and corticosteroids—have shown beneficial effects on appetite, but they have not been shown to halt cachexia and are associated with significant side effects.

MEGESTROL ACETATE

Megestrol acetate has demonstrated dose-dependent improvements (starting at 160 mg/day) in appetite, fatigue, and general well-being in up to 60 % of patients.[99] Symptomatic improvement in appetite occurs in less than 1 week; however, weight gain may take several weeks, and it happens in less than a quarter of treated patients. Unfortunately, this weight gain is predominantly due to fat or fluid rather than lean body mass. Common side effects include hypertension, hyperglycemia, fluid retention, and thrombosis. If patients are started on megestrol that is not found to be of benefit, the dose should be gradually decreased, as adrenal insufficiency may result from continued use. Stress dose corticosteroids should be given to those patients admitted for an acute illness. Consideration should also be given to monitoring testosterone levels because profound hypogonadism is a common treatable side effect. Megestrol should be avoided in patients with a history of deep venous thrombosis, pulmonary embolism, or severe cardiac disease.

CORTICOSTEROIDS

Corticosteroids have been shown to improve appetite and food intake.[100] These effects are usually limited to a couple of weeks, and the side effects of these drugs increase dramatically over time. Therefore, corticosteroids should generally be reserved for patients with limited life expectancy (less than 6 weeks). No dose has been established for corticosteroids. In studies, doses of prednisone ranging from 20 to 40 mg or equivalent doses of dexamethasone have been used.

CANNABINOIDS

Dronabinol, a synthetic cannabinoid, is approved by the U.S. Food and Drug Administration (FDA) for anorexia related to acquired immunodeficiency syndrome (AIDS) and chemotherapy-induced nausea and emesis. In cancer patients with anorexia, some studies have shown it to be beneficial, but weight did not improve.[101,102] The effects of dronabinol on cachexia appear to be limited. A large trial showed no clinical benefit when used alone or in combination with megestrol acetate.[103] Furthermore, the use of dronabinol is limited by undesirable CNS side effects, such as sedation, confusion, and perceptual disturbance.[104] These side effects are of special concern in advanced cancer patients, as they may also be using opioids.

Depression

Depressed mood can lead to decreased oral intake and should be managed with counseling and antidepressants if indicated. Anecdotal evidence suggests that mirtazapine, an antidepressant, improves appetite and weight gain; it is currently undergoing study in cancer patients.

Mucositis, xerostomia, and odynophagia

These symptoms are commonly reported by patients undergoing combined chemoradiation treatment and are frequently severe enough to require treatment interruptions or delays. These symptoms may also occur secondary to fungal or viral infection and should be appropriately treated. Symptomatic treatment includes maintaining oral hygiene and using opioids for pain and local analgesics such as xyloxylin preparations. Patients who have severe symptoms and are nutritionally compromised may benefit from parenteral or enteral nutrition, as described in the next section.

THERAPIES DIRECTED AT UNDERLYING MECHANISMS OF CACS

Several agents that target immune and/or endocrine pathways believed to be involved in the pathophysiology of CACS are being explored for the treatment of CACS. Several commercially available agents have undergone preliminary investigation in cancer patients and await further research. These include antiinflammatory therapies such as cyclooxygenase (COX)-2 inhibitors,[105,106] thalidomide,[107] and eicosapentaenoic acid n-3 (EPA)[108]; anabolic agents such as oxandrolone[109] and insulin[110]; melatonin[111]; ghrelin mimetics[112]; and the atypical antipsychotic olanzapine.[113,114] Anticytokine therapies with agents targeting TNF-α, infliximab,[115] or etanercept[116] have not been shown to improve anorexia, weight, QoL, or survival. These negative findings may be explained in part by the redundant role of these cytokines. Clinical trials targeting other inflammatory cytokines (IL-1β and IL-6) are awaited.[117]

In the context of combined approaches for treatment of CACS, few preliminary trials have been encouraging.[118] Results from other ongoing trials are eagerly awaited.[119,120] An interim analysis (125 patients) on one of these trials[119] found the combination regimen arm to be most effective. In this study, patients were randomized to one of the following five arms: progestins, EPA (2 g/day), L-carnitine, thalidomide, or all of these. Because this is a preliminary finding, results should be considered with caution.

Other promising therapies that are currently being investigated include myostatin inhibition, selective androgen receptor modulators (SARMs), and MC-4 receptor antagonists.[121]

EXERCISE

In cancer patients, exercise has been shown to improve physical function, fatigue, and body composition.[122] In these trials,[122] exercise interventions were primarily aerobic in nature. Resistance training has been shown to attenuate cancer-induced muscle wasting and protein depletion in tumor-bearing rats.[123] In one clinical trial in cancer patients that incorporated high-intensity resistance training with aerobic exercise,[124] increased muscle strength and improved fitness were noted in those patients who were able to participate for 9 hours/wk. A lengthy and complex exercise regimen may not be achievable in patients with more advanced disease or with low performance status, and in such patients, performing a lower-intensity regimen using inexpensive equipment (exercise bands) at home is more likely to encourage adherence. Consultation with a physical therapist should be considered to help formulate an individualized therapy plan.

IS THERE A ROLE FOR ENTERAL OR PARENTERAL NUTRITION?

Although it would seem intuitively that caloric replacement via artificial means (enteral or parenteral routes) would help improve nutritional status in weight-losing advanced cancer patients, a large body of evidence collectively suggests that for most patients, artificial nutrition does not improve patient survival, performance status, QoL, treatment toxicity, or psychological well-being.[125–127] Furthermore, these studies have suggested that routine use of nutritional support in patients with advanced incurable cancer is associated with a higher risk of treatment-related complications. However, enteral nutrition via gastrostomy tubes may be appropriate for patients with a predominant starvation component because of dysphagia or obstruction caused by the primary location of their tumors (such as cancer of the esophagus, head, and neck) or treatment complications (such as radiation-induced severe mucositis or esophagitis), and if they have an estimated life expectancy that would allow expected benefit. Aspiration pneumonia, nausea, and diarrhea are some of the complications of enteral nutrition therapy. Overall, if bowel functioning is normal, no additional benefit of parenteral versus enteral feeding is known. In rare cases, home total parenteral nutrition (TPN) can be associated with long-term survival. A retrospective single-institution study of home TPN[128] identified 16 cancer patients over a 20-year period who survived a year or longer. Most of the tumors were carcinoid, and QoL data were not assessed. One recent randomized prospective study[129] of patients with primarily gastrointestinal tumors suggested a trend toward increased survival in patients who received TPN. If artificial nutrition is considered, patients must be made aware of inherent risks associated with its use.

MONITORING RESPONSE TO THERAPY

Ongoing attention to optimal management of symptoms remains a key component of the monitoring process. As was mentioned previously, although weight gain is a desired outcome, it should not be the sole focus of intervention. In patients with advanced cancer and predominantly primary cachexia, weight stabilization is associated with improved QoL and survival; this is an appropriate goal for advanced cancer patients who have life expectancy in months. For patients whose life expectancy is limited to weeks or months, goals of therapy should focus on alleviating distressful symptoms. In this setting, additional measures of nutritional assessment are less important than indicators of QoL, such as activity level, stamina, mood, and sense of well-being. Visceral proteins are not likely to improve in patients with advanced disease. Further, body weight may not accurately reflect changes in nutritional status due to the presence of ascites or edema.

SUMMARY

Alterations in nutritional status are common in cancer patients. Complex tumor–host interactions resulting in an aberrant metabolic host response and symptoms related to tumor burden or the effects of treatment often lead to debilitating weight loss and wasting. Attention to nutritional status should begin early, at the time of cancer diagnosis, and should continue throughout the cancer trajectory. Patients vary widely in their presentation. Efforts to maintain adequate nutrition require effective control of symptoms that contribute to poor intake. A standardized approach of assessment should be followed by a decision-making process that would help in formulating an individualized plan for cachexia management. When oral intake is consistently inadequate, decisions regarding the use of enteral or parenteral nutrition must take into consideration the prognosis, treatment goals, and views of the patient. Finally, all therapeutic interventions should aim to preserve or improve QoL according to the wishes of the patient.

REFERENCES

1. Ma GAH. Prevalence and pathophysiology of cancer cachexia. In: Portenoy RK, ed. *Topics in palliative care.* New York: Oxford University Press; 1998:91–129.

2. Dewys WD, Begg C, Lavin PT, et al. Prognostic effect of weight loss prior to chemotherapy in cancer patients. Eastern Cooperative Oncology Group. *Am J Med.* 1980;69:491–497.

3. Kotler DP. Cachexia. *Ann Intern Med.* 2000;133:622–634.

4. Morley JE, Thomas DR, Wilson MM. Cachexia: pathophysiology and clinical relevance. *Am J Clin Nutr.* 2006;83:735–743.

5. Anker SD, Coats AJ. Cardiac cachexia: a syndrome with impaired survival and immune and neuroendocrine activation. *Chest.* 1999;115:836–847.

6. MacDonald N, Easson AM, Mazurak VC, et al. Understanding and managing cancer cachexia. *J Am Coll Surg.* 2003;197:143–161.

7. Barton BE. IL-6-like cytokines and cancer cachexia: consequences of chronic inflammation. *Immunol Res.* 2001;23:41–58.

8. O'Riordain MG, Falconer JS, Maingay J, et al. Peripheral blood cells from weight-losing cancer patients control the hepatic acute phase response by a primarily interleukin-6 dependent mechanism. *Int J Oncol.* 1999;15:823–827.

9. Zhou W, Jiang ZW, Tian J, et al. Role of NF-kappaB and cytokine in experimental cancer cachexia. *World J Gastroenterol.* 2003;9:1567–1570.

10. Wigmore SJ, Fearon KC, Maingay JP, et al. Effect of interleukin-2 on peripheral blood mononuclear cell cytokine production and the hepatic acute phase protein response. *Clin Immunol.* 2002;104:174–182.

11. Costelli P, Bossola M, Muscaritoli M, et al. Anticytokine treatment prevents the increase in the activity of ATP-ubiquitin- and Ca(2+)-dependent proteolytic systems in the muscle of tumour-bearing rats. *Cytokine.* 2002;19:1–5.

12. Llovera M, Garcia-Martinez C, Agell N, et al. TNF can directly induce the expression of ubiquitin-dependent proteolytic system in rat soleus muscles. *Biochem Biophys Res Commun.* 1997;230:238–241.

13. Baracos V, Rodemann HP, Dinarello CA, et al. Stimulation of muscle protein degradation and prostaglandin E2 release by leukocytic pyrogen (interleukin-1): a mechanism for the increased degradation of muscle proteins during fever. *N Engl J Med.* 1983;308:553–558.

14. Todorov P, Cariuk P, McDevitt T, et al. Characterization of a cancer cachectic factor. *Nature.* 1996;379:739–742.

15. Todorov PT, McDevitt TM, Meyer DJ, et al. Purification and characterization of a tumor lipid-mobilizing factor. *Cancer Res.* 1998;58:2353–2358.

16. Baracos VE. Cancer-associated cachexia and underlying biological mechanisms. *Annu Rev Nutr.* 2006;26:435–461.

17. Tong H, Isenring E, Yates P. The prevalence of nutrition impact symptoms and their relationship to quality of life and clinical outcomes in medical oncology patients. *Support Care Cancer.* 2009;17:83–90.

18. Khalid U, Spiro A, Baldwin C, et al. Symptoms and weight loss in patients with gastrointestinal and lung cancer at presentation. *Support Care Cancer.* 2007;15:39–46.

19. Del Fabbro E, Dalal S, Delgado M, et al. Secondary vs. primary cachexia in patients with advanced cancer. *J Clin Oncol (Meeting Abstracts).* 2007;25:9128.

20. Falconer JS, Fearon KC, Ross JA, et al. Acute-phase protein response and survival duration of patients with pancreatic cancer. *Cancer.* 1995;75:2077–2082.

21. Marsik C, Kazemi-Shirazi L, Schic kbauer T, et al. C-reactive protein and all-cause mortality in a large hospital-based cohort. *Clin Chem.* 2008;54:343–349.

22. McMillan DC, Watson WS, Preston T, et al. Lean body mass changes in cancer patients with weight loss. *Clin Nutr*. 2000;19:403–406.

23. Maltoni M, Caraceni A, Brunelli C, et al. Prognostic factors in advanced cancer patients: evidence-based clinical recommendations—a study by the Steering Committee of the European Association for Palliative Care. *J Clin Oncol*. 2005;23:6240–6248.

24. Scott HR, McMillan DC, Forrest LM, et al. The systemic inflammatory response, weight loss, performance status and survival in patients with inoperable non-small cell lung cancer. *Br J Cancer*. 2002;87:264–267.

25. Karakiewicz PI, Hutterer GC, Trinh QD, et al. C-reactive protein is an informative predictor of renal cell carcinoma-specific mortality: a European study of 313 patients. *Cancer*. 2007;110:1241–1247.

26. Glaser R, Kiecolt-Glaser JK. Stress-induced immune dysfunction: implications for health. *Nat Rev Immunol*. 2005;5:243–251.

27. Antoni MH, Lutgendorf SK, Cole SW, et al. The influence of bio-behavioural factors on tumour biology: pathways and mechanisms. *Nat Rev Cancer*. 2006;6:240–248.

28. McEwen BS. Sex, stress and the hippocampus: allostasis, allostatic load and the aging process. *Neurobiol Aging*. 2002;23:921–939.

29. Levin BE. Metabolic sensing neurons and the control of energy homeostasis. *Physiol Behav*. 2006;89:486–489.

30. Korner J, Aronne LJ. The emerging science of body weight regulation and its impact on obesity treatment. *J Clin Invest*. 2003;111:565–570.

31. Richard D, Huang Q, Timofeeva E. The corticotropin-releasing hormone system in the regulation of energy balance in obesity. *Int J Obes Relat Metab Disord*. 2000;24(suppl 2):S36–S39.

32. Smagin GN, Howell LA, Ryan DH, et al. The role of CRF2 receptors in corticotropin-releasing factor- and urocortin-induced anorexia. *Neuroreport*. 1998;9:1601–1606.

33. Horvath TL. The hardship of obesity: a soft-wired hypothalamus. *Nat Neurosci*. 2005;8:561–565.

34. Cone RD. Anatomy and regulation of the central melanocortin system. *Nat Neurosci*. 2005;8:571–578.

35. Wong S, Pinkney J. Role of cytokines in regulating feeding behaviour. *Curr Drug Targets*. 2004;5:251–263.

36. Davis MP, Dreicer R, Walsh D, et al. Appetite and cancer-associated anorexia: a review. *J Clin Oncol*. 2004;22:1510–1517.

37. Laviano A, Russo M, Freda F, et al. Neurochemical mechanisms for cancer anorexia. *Nutrition*. 2002;18:100–105.

38. Inui A. Cancer anorexia-cachexia syndrome: are neuropeptides the key? *Cancer Res*. 1999;59:4493–4501.

39. Plata-Salaman CR. Central nervous system mechanisms contributing to the cachexia-anorexia syndrome. *Nutrition*. 2000;16:1009–1012.

40. Turrin NP, Plata-Salaman CR. Cytokine-cytokine interactions and the brain. *Brain Res Bull*. 2000;51:3–9.

41. Mitch WE, Goldberg AL. Mechanisms of muscle wasting: the role of the ubiquitin-proteasome pathway. *N Engl J Med*. 1996;335:1897–1905.

42. Acharyya S, Ladner KJ, Nelsen LL, et al. Cancer cachexia is regulated by selective targeting of skeletal muscle gene products. *J Clin Invest*. 2004;114:370–378.

43. Baracos VE. Regulation of skeletal-muscle-protein turnover in cancer-associated cachexia. *Nutrition*. 2000;16:1015–1018.

44. Argiles JM, Busquets S, Lopez-Soriano FJ. The pivotal role of cytokines in muscle wasting during cancer. *Int J Biochem Cell Biol*. 2005;37:2036–2046.

45. Bodine SC, Latres E, Baumhueter S, et al. Identification of ubiquitin ligases required for skeletal muscle atrophy. *Science*. 2001;294:1704–1708.

46. Acharyya S, Guttridge DC. Cancer cachexia signaling pathways continue to emerge yet much still points to the proteasome. *Clin Cancer Res*. 2007;13:1356–1361.

47. Langen RC, Schols AM, Kelders MC, et al. Inflammatory cytokines inhibit myogenic differentiation through activation of nuclear factor-kappaB. *FASEB J*. 2001;15:1169–1180.

48. Cai D, Frantz JD, Tawa Jr NE, et al. IKKbeta/NF-kappaB activation causes severe muscle wasting in mice. *Cell*. 2004;119:285–298.

49. Glass DJ. Signalling pathways that mediate skeletal muscle hypertrophy and atrophy. *Nat Cell Biol*. 2003;5:87–90.

50. Brunet A, Bonni A, Zigmond MJ, et al. Akt promotes cell survival by phosphorylating and inhibiting a Forkhead transcription factor. *Cell*. 1999;96:857–868.

51. Drott C, Persson H, Lundholm K. Cardiovascular and metabolic response to adrenaline infusion in weight-losing patients with and without cancer. *Clin Physiol*. 1989;9:427–439.

52. Zuijdgeest-van Leeuwen SD, van den Berg JW, Wattimena JL, et al. Lipolysis and lipid oxidation in weight-losing cancer patients and healthy subjects. *Metabolism*. 2000;49:931–936.

53. Legaspi A, Jeevanandam M, Starnes Jr HF, et al. Whole body lipid and energy metabolism in the cancer patient. *Metabolism*. 1987;36:958–963.

54. Shaw JH, Wolfe RR. Fatty acid and glycerol kinetics in septic patients and in patients with gastrointestinal cancer: the response to glucose infusion and parenteral feeding. *Ann Surg*. 1987;205:368–376.

55. Esper DH, Harb WA. The cancer cachexia syndrome: a review of metabolic and clinical manifestations. *Nutr Clin Pract*. 2005;20:369–376.

56. Tijerina AJ. The biochemical basis of metabolism in cancer cachexia. *Dimens Crit Care Nurs*. 2004;23:237–243.

57. Kalra PR, Tigas S. Regulation of lipolysis: natriuretic peptides and the development of cachexia. *Int J Cardiol*. 2002;85:125–132.

58. Hyltander A, Daneryd P, Sandstrom R, et al. Beta-adrenoceptor activity and resting energy metabolism in weight losing cancer patients. *Eur J Cancer*. 2000;36:330–334.

59. Klein S, Wolfe RR. Whole-body lipolysis and triglyceride-fatty acid cycling in cachectic patients with esophageal cancer. *J Clin Invest*. 1990;86:1403–1408.

60. Zhang HH, Halbleib M, Ahmad F, et al. Tumor necrosis factor-alpha stimulates lipolysis in differentiated human adipocytes through activation of extracellular signal-related kinase and elevation of intracellular cAMP. *Diabetes*. 2002;51:2929–2935.

61. Ferguson M, Capra S, Bauer J, et al. Development of a valid and reliable malnutrition screening tool for adult acute hospital patients. *Nutrition*. 1999;15:458–464.

62. Ferguson ML, Bauer J, Gallagher B, et al. Validation of a malnutrition screening tool for patients receiving radiotherapy. *Australas Radiol*. 1999;43:325–327.

63. Isenring E, Cross G, Daniels L, et al. Validity of the malnutrition screening tool as an effective predictor of nutritional risk in oncology outpatients receiving chemotherapy. *Support Care Cancer*. 2006;14:1152–1156.

64. Evans WK, Nixon DW, Daly JM, et al. A randomized study of oral nutritional support versus ad lib nutritional intake during chemotherapy for advanced colorectal and non-small-cell lung cancer. *J Clin Oncol*. 1987;5:113–124.

65. Wigmore SJ, Plester CE, Ross JA, et al. Contribution of anorexia and hypermetabolism to weight loss in anicteric patients with pancreatic cancer. *Br J Surg*. 1997;84:196–197.

66. Falconer JS, Fearon KC, Plester CE, et al. Cytokines, the acute-phase response, and resting energy expenditure in cachectic patients with pancreatic cancer. *Ann Surg*. 1994;219:325–331.

67. Minnesota University Laboratory of Physiological Hygiene, Keys AB. *The biology of human starvation*. Minneapolis, MN: University of Minnesota Press; 1950.

68. Lukaski HC. Methods for the assessment of human body composition: traditional and new. *Am J Clin Nutr*. 1987;46:537–556.

69. Jensen MD. Research techniques for body composition assessment. *J Am Diet Assoc*. 1992;92:454–460.

70. van der Kooy K, Seidell JC. Techniques for the measurement of visceral fat: a practical guide. *Int J Obes Relat Metab Disord*. 1993;17:187–196.

71. Ohsuzu F, Kosuda S, Takayama E, et al. Imaging techniques for measuring adipose-tissue distribution in the abdomen: a comparison between computed tomography and 1.5-tesla magnetic resonance spin-echo imaging. *Radiat Med*. 1998;16:99–107.

72. Pontiroli AE, Pizzocri P, Giacomelli M, et al. Ultrasound measurement of visceral and subcutaneous fat in morbidly obese patients before and after laparoscopic adjustable gastric banding: comparison with computerized tomography and with anthropometric measurements. *Obes Surg*. 2002;12:648–651.

73. Jatoi A, Daly BD, Hughes VA, et al. Do patients with nonmetastatic non-small cell lung cancer demonstrate altered resting energy expenditure? *Ann Thorac Surg*. 2001;72:348–351.

74. Moley JF, Aamodt R, Rumble W, et al. Body cell mass in cancer-bearing and anorexic patients. *JPEN J Parenter Enteral Nutr*. 1987;11:219–222.

75. Pichard C, Kyle UG. Body composition measurements during wasting diseases. *Curr Opin Clin Nutr Metab Care*. 1998;1:357–361.

76. Pietrobelli A, Wang Z, Heymsfield SB. Techniques used in measuring human body composition. *Curr Opin Clin Nutr Metab Care*. 1998;1:439–448.

77. Heymsfield SB, Wang Z, Baumgartner RN, et al. Human body composition: advances in models and methods. *Annu Rev Nutr*. 1997;17:527–558.

78. Mitsiopoulos N, Baumgartner RN, Heymsfield SB, et al. Cadaver validation of skeletal muscle measurement by magnetic resonance imaging and computerized tomography. *J Appl Physiol*. 1998;85:115–122.

79. Janssen I, Heymsfield SB, Wang ZM, et al. Skeletal muscle mass and distribution in 468 men and women aged 18–88 yr. *J Appl Physiol*. 2000;89:81–88.

80. Janssen I, Ross R. Effects of sex on the change in visceral, subcutaneous adipose tissue and skeletal muscle in response to weight loss. *Int J Obes Relat Metab Disord*. 1999;23:1035–1046.

81. Detsky AS, McLaughlin JR, Baker JP, et al. What is subjective global assessment of nutritional status? *JPEN J Parenter Enteral Nutr*. 1987;11:8–13.

82. Ottery FD. Rethinking nutritional support of the cancer patient: the new field of nutritional oncology. *Semin Oncol*. 1994;21:770–778.

83. Ottery FD. Definition of standardized nutritional assessment and interventional pathways in oncology. *Nutrition.* 1996;12:S15–19.

84. Ottery FD. *Patient generated subjective global assessment.* Chicago, IL: The American Diabetic Association; 2000.

85. Bauer J, Capra S, Ferguson M. Use of the scored Patient-Generated Subjective Global Assessment (PG-SGA) as a nutrition assessment tool in patients with cancer. *Eur J Clin Nutr.* 2002;56:779–785.

86. Persson C, Sjoden PO, Glimelius B. The Swedish version of the patient-generated subjective global assessment of nutritional status: gastrointestinal vs urological cancers. *Clin Nutr.* 1999;18:71–77.

87. Vigano A, Trutschnigg B, Morais JA, et al. Use of the scored Patient-Generated Subjective Global Assessment (PG-SGA) to characterize cachexia in newly diagnosed advanced cancer patients. *J Clin Oncol (Meeting Abstracts).* 2009;27:9574.

88. Ollenschlager G, Thomas W, Konkol K, et al. Nutritional behaviour and quality of life during oncological polychemotherapy: results of a prospective study on the efficacy of oral nutrition therapy in patients with acute leukaemia. *Eur J Clin Invest.* 1992;22:546–553.

89. Ovesen L, Allingstrup L, Hannibal J, et al. Effect of dietary counseling on food intake, body weight, response rate, survival, and quality of life in cancer patients undergoing chemotherapy: a prospective, randomized study. *J Clin Oncol.* 1993;11:2043–2049.

90. Ravasco P, Monteiro-Grillo I, Vidal PM, et al. Dietary counseling improves patient outcomes: a prospective, randomized, controlled trial in colorectal cancer patients undergoing radiotherapy. *J Clin Oncol.* 2005;23:1431–1438.

91. Isenring EA, Capra S, Bauer JD. Nutrition intervention is beneficial in oncology outpatients receiving radiotherapy to the gastrointestinal or head and neck area. *Br J Cancer.* 2004;91:447–452.

92. Davies AA, Davey Smith G, Harbord R, et al. Nutritional interventions and outcome in patients with cancer or preinvasive lesions: systematic review. *J Natl Cancer Inst.* 2006;98:961–973.

93. Ladas EJ, Sacks N, Meacham L, et al. A multidisciplinary review of nutrition considerations in the pediatric oncology population: a perspective from children's oncology group. *Nutr Clin Pract.* 2005;20:377–393.

94. Bauer JDAS, Davidson WL, Hill JM, Brown T, Isenring EA, et al. Evidence based practice guidelines for the nutritional management of cancer cachexia. *Nutri Diet.* 2006;63:S3–132.

95. Posner BM, Martin-Munley SS, Smigelski C, et al. Comparison of techniques for estimating nutrient intake: the Framingham Study. *Epidemiology.* 1992;3:171–177.

96. Bauer JD, Capra S. Nutrition intervention improves outcomes in patients with cancer cachexia receiving chemotherapy—a pilot study. *Support Care Cancer.* 2005;13:270–274.

97. Davidson W, Ash S, Capra S, et al. Weight stabilisation is associated with improved survival duration and quality of life in unresectable pancreatic cancer. *Clin Nutr.* 2004;23:239–247.

98. Hutton JL, Martin L, Field CJ, et al. Dietary patterns in patients with advanced cancer: implications for anorexia-cachexia therapy. *Am J Clin Nutr.* 2006;84:1163–1170.

99. Pascual Lopez A, Roque i Figuls M, Urrutia Cuchi G, et al. Systematic review of megestrol acetate in the treatment of anorexia-cachexia syndrome. *J Pain Symptom Manage.* 2004;27:360–369.

100. Yavuzsen T, Davis MP, Walsh D, et al. Systematic review of the treatment of cancer-associated anorexia and weight loss. *J Clin Oncol.* 2005;23:8500–8511.

101. Walsh D, Nelson KA, Mahmoud FA. Established and potential therapeutic applications of cannabinoids in oncology. *Support Care Cancer.* 2003;11:137–143.

102. Lane M, Vogel CL, Ferguson J, et al. Dronabinol and prochlorperazine in combination for treatment of cancer chemotherapy-induced nausea and vomiting. *J Pain Symptom Manage.* 1991;6:352–359.

103. Jatoi A, Windschitl HE, Loprinzi CL, et al. Dronabinol versus megestrol acetate versus combination therapy for cancer-associated anorexia: a North Central Cancer Treatment Group study. *J Clin Oncol.* 2002;20:567–573.

104. Beal JE, Olson R, Lefkowitz L, et al. Long-term efficacy and safety of dronabinol for acquired immunodeficiency syndrome-associated anorexia. *J Pain Symptom Manage.* 1997;14:7–14.

105. Lundholm K, Daneryd P, Korner U, et al. Evidence that long-term COX-treatment improves energy homeostasis and body composition in cancer patients with progressive cachexia. *Int J Oncol.* 2004;24:505–512.

106. Lai V, George J, Richey L, et al. Results of a pilot study of the effects of celecoxib on cancer cachexia in patients with cancer of the head, neck, and gastrointestinal tract. *Head Neck.* 2008;30:67–74.

107. Gordon JN, Trebble TM, Ellis RD, et al. Thalidomide in the treatment of cancer cachexia: a randomised placebo controlled trial. *Gut.* 2005;54:540–545.

108. Fearon KC, Von Meyenfeldt MF, Moses AG, et al. Effect of a protein and energy dense N-3 fatty acid enriched oral supplement on loss of weight and lean tissue in cancer cachexia: a randomised double blind trial. *Gut.* 2003;52:1479–1486.

109. Lesser DC, Sharp S, Choksi J, et al. A phase III randomized study comparing the effects of oxandrolone (Ox) and megestrol acetate (Meg) on lean body mass (LBM), weight (wt) and quality of life (QOL) in patients with solid tumors and weight loss receiving chemotherapy. *J Clin Oncol.* 2008;26(suppl) Abstract 9513.

110. Lundholm K, Korner U, Gunnebo L, et al. Insulin treatment in cancer cachexia: effects on survival, metabolism, and physical functioning. *Clin Cancer Res.* 2007;13:2699–2706.

111. Lissoni P, Paolorossi F, Tancini G, et al. Is there a role for melatonin in the treatment of neoplastic cachexia? *Eur J Cancer.* 1996;32A:1340–1343.

112. Neary NM, Small CJ, Wren AM, et al. Ghrelin increases energy intake in cancer patients with impaired appetite: acute, randomized, placebo-controlled trial. *J Clin Endocrinol Metab.* 2004;89:2832–2836.

113. Braiteh FDS, Dalal S, Khuwaja H, et al. Phase I pilot study of the safety and tolerability of olanzapine (OZA) for the treatment of cachexia in patients with advanced cancer. *J Clin Oncol.* 2008;26(suppl): Abstract 20529.

114. Navari RM. Treatment of cancer-related anorexia with olanzapine and megestrol acetate. *J Clin Oncol.* 2008;26(suppl) Abstract 9576.

115. Jatoi A, Ritter HL, Dueck A, et al. A placebo-controlled, double-blind trial of infliximab for cancer-associated weight loss in elderly and/or poor performance non-small cell lung cancer patients (N01C9). *Lung Cancer.* 2010;68:234–239.

116. Jatoi A, Dakhil SR, Nguyen PL, et al. A placebo-controlled double blind trial of etanercept for the cancer anorexia/weight loss syndrome: results from N00C1 from the North Central Cancer Treatment Group. *Cancer.* 2007;110:1396–1403.

117. Alder Biopharmaceuticals I. A phase II study to determine the safety, efficacy and pharmacokinetics of multiple intravenous doses of ALD518 80 mg, 160 mg, and 320 mg versus placebo administered to patients with non-small cell lung cancer-related fatigue and cachexia. In: ClinicalTrials.gov. Bethesda, MD: National Library of Medicine; 2000. Available from: http://clinicaltrials. gov/ct2/results?term=ClinicalTrials. gov+Identifier%3A++NCT00866970.

118. Mantovani G, Madeddu C, Maccio A, et al. Cancer-related anorexia/cachexia syndrome and oxidative stress: an innovative approach beyond current treatment. *Cancer Epidemiol Biomarkers Prev.* 2004;13:1651–1659.

119. Mantovani G, Maccio A, Madeddu C, et al. Randomized phase III clinical trial of five different arms of treatment for patients with cancer cachexia: interim results. *Nutrition.* 2008;24:305–313.

120. M. D. Anderson Cancer Center. An exploratory trial of a multimodal treatment strategy for cancer cachexia. In: ClinicalTrials.gov. Bethesda, MD: National Library of Medicine; 2000. Available from: http://clinicaltrials.gov/ct2/show/NCT00625 742?term=nct00625742&rank=1.

121. Mantovani G, Madeddu C. Cancer cachexia: medical management. *Support Care Cancer.* 2009; August 18, [Epub ahead of print].

122. Conn VS, Hafdahl AR, Porock DC, et al. A meta-analysis of exercise interventions among people treated for cancer. *Support Care Cancer.* 2006;14:699–712.

123. al-Majid S, McCarthy DO. Resistance exercise training attenuates wasting of the extensor digitorum longus muscle in mice bearing the colon-26 adenocarcinoma. *Biol Res Nurs.* 2001;2:155–166.

124. Adamsen L, Quist M, Midtgaard J, et al. The effect of a multidimensional exercise intervention on physical capacity, well-being and quality of life in cancer patients undergoing chemotherapy. *Support Care Cancer.* 2006;14:116–127.

125. Klein S, Koretz RL. Nutrition support in patients with cancer: what do the data really show? *Nutr Clin Pract.* 1994;9:91–100.

126. Koretz RL, Avenell A, Lipman TO, et al. Does enteral nutrition affect clinical outcome? A systematic review of the randomized trials. *Am J Gastroenterol.* 2007;102:412–429 quiz 468.

127. McGeer AJ, Detsky AS, O'Rourke K. Parenteral nutrition in cancer patients undergoing chemotherapy: a meta-analysis. *Nutrition.* 1990;6:233–240.

128. Hoda D, Jatoi A, Burnes J, et al. Should patients with advanced, incurable cancers ever be sent home with total parenteral nutrition? A single institution's 20-year experience. *Cancer.* 2005;103:863–868.

129. Lundholm K, Daneryd P, Bosaeus I, et al. Palliative nutritional intervention in addition to cyclooxygenase and erythropoietin treatment for patients with malignant disease: effects on survival, metabolism, and function. *Cancer.* 2004;100:1967–1977.

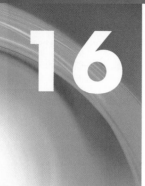

16 Dyspnea in supportive oncology

David C. Currow and Amy P. Abernethy

Dyspnea remains one of the most feared symptoms, with sufferers graphically describing the sense that they are fighting for each breath, or even that each breath feels like their last. These descriptions reflect the physical and psychological aspects of the subjective sensation of breathlessness. Every aspect of a person's being can be affected by the sensation, including relationships, mobility, sleep, social interactions, and the sense of absolute threat to one's existence. Dyspnea in people with advanced disease is also an independent predictor of poorer prognosis, with dyspneic adults in a palliative care program twice as likely to die (hazard ratio, 2.04; 95% confidence interval [CI], 1.26–3.31; $P < .01$).[1] Higher levels of symptom distress predict poorer survival, reflecting the severity of underlying causative factors and the overall impact that this distressing symptom has on one's personhood.[2]

MAGNITUDE AND SEVERITY OF DYSPNEA

Breathlessness is a prevalent and distressing problem, especially for people with cancer. Starting with basic prevalence rates in the community as a whole, irrespective of health service utilization, background rates run at 9%; 1 in 300 people are housebound because of breathlessness.[3,4] In a recent prospective consecutive cohort study, dyspnea was a major symptom for the majority of people with advanced cancer, with incidence increasing dramatically in the last weeks of life despite palliation.[5] In people with advanced cancer, the original National Hospice Study data revealed that prevalence rates were greater than 50%, especially late in life; subsequent studies confirmed these findings.[6,7] Prevalence rates quoted vary, which likely is related to when the estimates are taken in the disease trajectory.[8–10] The total burden of dyspnea in people with advanced cancer therefore is a combination of the background levels of dyspnea for comorbid illnesses, the direct effects of cancer on the respiratory system, and the systemic effects of cancer such as cachexia.[5] In people with cancer, dyspnea remains one of the symptoms most likely to worsen as death approaches,[5,11] whether health care is delivered in the community or in the hospital.[12,13]

Because the predictable prevalence of breathlessness is at least one in two people with advanced cancer, irrespective of the primary site of disease, it is imperative to have evidence-based management strategies available. Given the multiple factors in the origin of breathlessness, potential interventions must cover a wide range of mechanisms. No single intervention will predictably deal with all aspects, and, after a careful evaluation of the patient, a multimodal approach will almost certainly be necessary.

It is not surprising to note that dyspnea can generate a breathlessness-anxiety-breathlessness-anxiety cycle that is difficult to break. Other emotions that drive such a cycle include anger and fear. Studies of people with advanced cancer reported a significant relationship between intensity of breathlessness and both anxiety and panic.[14] The psychological distress for the person who is breathless and for those who are watching the breathless person is almost palpable in many clinical encounters.[7,13] For many people with advanced cancer, severe breathlessness feels as though they are fighting for their last breath, thereby threatening a person's very existence. It is therefore understandable that dyspnea is associated with significant existential distress for many people.[15]

MECHANISMS OF DYSPNEA

A fundamental challenge in the management of breathlessness is that it is a subjective sensation, and wide variations between individuals are noted in their interpretation of the symptom and response to interventions. For example, although it would be clinically convenient to have a direct correlation of the intensity of breathlessness with worsening hypoxemia, wide variation is seen in the rating of the sensation as blood oxygenation falls. Physiologic factors have consistently shown poor correlation with the sensation of breathlessness.

A wide range of factors can lead to a common pathway that a patient describes as breathlessness. Such plurality is not a layperson's misinterpretation of breathlessness, but an honest reflection of the many ways in which the sensation can be generated and interpreted. Factors such as underlying pathophysiologies (patients rarely have a single mechanism causing breathlessness), one's psychological status, and the way one expresses illness behavior in a cultural setting can all influence how breathlessness is perceived and subsequently expressed. Ultimately, the sensation is the sum of the insult(s), transmission, interpretation, and expression of the symptom. Families and clinical staff may hear multiple interpretations of the symptom, reflective of these variable inputs. Such a sensation therefore involves the physical, emotional, spiritual, and social aspects of a person.[16]

At the most fundamental level, dyspnea can be considered a mismatch between the afferent pathways (stimulated by insults such as hypoxemia, hypercarbia, stretch receptors, or changes in acid-base balance) and the efferent response.[16] Although such a concept has been characterized by several titles, including "neuroventilatory dissociation" and "efferent-reafferent dissociation," the basic concept of stimuli/response mismatch explains the sensation and the responses that many people manifest.[17] The response mismatch can occur because of increasing ventilator impedance or demand, abnormal respiratory neural or muscular responses, or central factors such as anxiety. This gives rise to the potential for a series of complex interactions between coexisting causes and the sensation ultimately experienced by the person with dyspnea.

Because advancing age is a common risk factor among chronic complex illnesses, many people with cancer have comorbid cardiorespiratory or neuromuscular diseases that contribute to breathlessness. Understanding the relative contribution of all underlying factors will allow focus on any reversible or modifiable causes and will point to additional disease-focused investigations as needed.

Contrary to individuals with obvious underlying causes for their breathlessness, a substantial population of people with cancer have no evidence of primary or secondary cancer in their lungs and no other obvious comorbid cause other than advancing cachexia. In fact, in advanced cancer, this is the most frequently encountered scenario for increasing breathlessness as death approaches[5]; clinically, the breathlessness

appears out of proportion to documentable cardiorespiratory disease. Given both the intensity and the prevalence of this presentation, it is imperative that clinicians respect the reported level of breathlessness. Such an apparent mismatch between perceived sensation and objective measures should not limit symptomatic interventions once all reasonable efforts have been made to address reversible causes.

Although reversible causes of dyspnea are being attended, the symptom still must be controlled. Once all reversible causes have been addressed, residual dyspnea is termed refractory or intractable.[18]

ASSESSING DYSPNEA

The management of dyspnea requires palliation of the symptom in parallel with a systematic search for reversible causes. For most people, this will involve evaluating the potential contribution of a number of factors because rarely is one single simple cause identified.

A careful history is crucial to understanding the trajectory of breathlessness, the temporal relationships to its evolution, and its impact on the person. The more acute the onset, the more likely it is that a single dominant cause can be identified, and often some reversible aspect is more likely as well.

Physical examination in someone with cancer and worsening dyspnea requires attention to the local (e.g., obstruction of a bronchus, pleural effusion) and systemic (e.g., cachexia, thromboembolic disease) effects of cancer and other comorbidities (e.g., evidence of chronic obstructive pulmonary disease [COPD], cardiac failure). Emphasis is placed on factors that are potentially reversible, on quantifying the extent of disease, and on thoughtfully prognosticating the effects of disease progression. Necessary investigations predominantly focus on the history and examination, but careful assessment of oxygenation at rest and on exertion is likely to provide useful information for most people; more invasive or extensive tests are rarely needed.

Assessment of the symptom of breathlessness can include the use of formal tools such as visual analog or numeric rating scales, categorical scales (Likert scales), or a mixture of scales such as the Borg scale.[19] Questions associated with these scales can include breathlessness now, or worst or best breathlessness over a period of time. Dimensions of dyspnea to consider include its intensity and its unpleasantness or both.[20] These scales are clearly subjective, but they are reliable, valid, and responsive to change over time. Subjective scales are meaningful in the context of an intensely subjective experience and have poor individual correlation to the physiologic parameters that clinicians can objectively measure.

Scales that explore the ability to exercise before the onset of breathlessness include the modified Medical Research Council Dyspnea Scale or the Dyspnea Exertion Scale. Such scales, although more objective, complement but do not replace subjective assessments. More recently, the Cancer Dyspnea Scale (CDS) provides a specific measure of the impact of breathlessness in someone with cancer; assessed domains include effort, anxiety, and discomfort.[21] This scale has good face and construct validity, and the English language version has been validated in a variety of clinical settings. The functional impact of dyspnea can direct the need for additional support in the community, including cooking, cleaning, and shopping services. Other symptoms that require equally careful assessment in the presence of ongoing breathlessness include fatigue, insomnia, anxiety, and depression.

To quantify the impact of breathlessness on the person's day-to-day function can, the clinician use of formal assessments of activities of daily living (Lawton Instrumental Activities of Daily Living Scale),[22] assessments global functioning (Australian Modified Karnofsky Performance Scale),[23] or measures of exercise tolerance before breathlessness supervenes (3- or 6-Minute Walk Test). In people with more severe compromise, functional evaluation can include isometric exercises or, for those with the most severe impairment, reading aloud. Although not useful for predicting breathlessness, such assessment provides a baseline for future comparison.

Change from baseline in both subjective and objective measures of breathlessness is the most important way of tracking this symptom across time. The rate of this change may be important in the perception of the symptom and its ultimate impact on the way the person functions and the way he or she deals with the emotional sequelae of this debilitating symptom.

EVIDENCE-BASED INTERVENTIONS FOR DYSPNEA MANAGEMENT

MEDICAL GASES

Oxygen helps to relieve breathlessness in severely hypoxemic people (partial pressure of oxygen in arterial blood [PaO_2] < 55 mm Hg) and those with evidence of secondary compromise from hypoxia (e.g., cor pulmonale and PaO_2 < 60 mmHg) and should be made available for these individuals. Recent technological advances make portability more practical with the advent of liquid oxygen delivery systems. Despite the expense, this is allowing greater mobility for people who are oxygen dependent.

More broadly, oxygen is routinely made available with a low threshold to people who are breathless, regardless of PaO_2. In a Canadian study, more than 40% of people receiving domiciliary oxygen therapy (n = 237) did not meet the local guidelines for home oxygen.[24] Both Canadian and Australian clinician surveys have identified that even in nonhypoxemic people, oxygen is commonly prescribed.[25,26] The evidence base for this, and the net clinical benefit in day-to-day practice, is questionable.[4] Further, evidence that the palliative prescription of oxygen in the community may often be driven by caregivers rather than by patients creates an interesting dilemma for clinicians.[27] A desire to be able to do something to help relieve breathlessness is understandable, but oxygen, whether from a concentrator or a cylinder, is not something that patients want to be reliant on unless absolutely necessary. Palliative oxygen is often prescribed in the hope that it will provide symptomatic relief of breathlessness, irrespective of the person's partial pressure of oxygen.

Two systematic reviews of available studies challenge the net clinical benefits of this pattern of prescribing. Booth et al, in 2003, reviewed the literature for a number of conditions for which palliative oxygen is prescribed, including cancer and COPD. Most studies were relatively small and included a short duration of oxygen administration. Blinding was variable, and crossover studies had no or short washout periods. Results did not point systematically to benefit across these populations.

A 2008 meta-analysis of randomized controlled trials conducted only in cancer cohorts included full datasets from five studies; although the same methodologic issues were identified, synthesized analysis of patient-level data demonstrated that in those who were not profoundly hypoxemic, the symptomatic benefit derived from supplementary oxygen was limited.[28] None of these studies focused on people who qualified for long-term domiciliary oxygen, nor on people who had been documented to desaturate with exertion. The studies in this meta-analysis included people offered short-term oxygen when at rest or on a 6-minute walk test. All were crossover studies. No differences in breathlessness or exercise tolerance were noted (when measured), nor did consistent blinded preferences favor oxygen when the studies were combined.[29–31] When these original data were brought into a single analysis, no net symptomatic nor clinical benefit was identified (standardized mean difference [SMD], −0.09; 95% confidence interval, −0.22 to 0.04; $P = .16$).[28]

A novel study looked at the use of Heliox 28, which is a mixture of 28% oxygen and 72% helium, in people with moderate to severe COPD.[32] Helium is a very small element, and it has different laminar flow properties than nitrogen, the dominant gas in air. This three-arm crossover study included a 6-minute walk test and compared the benefit of supplemental oxygen at 28% versus Heliox 28 or medical air. At rest, people had significantly higher partial pressures of oxygen. During the 6-minute walk test, participants on Heliox 28 had less dyspnea with increased distances covered (Heliox 28, 214 m [standard deviation {SD}, 9.6] vs. 28% oxygen, 175 m [SD, 11.2] vs. medical air, 129 m [SD, 10.3]), with better oxygen saturation. The availability and expense of this unique gas currently make its widespread use impractical, but it does point to an innovative way of addressing the problem of breathlessness.

Abernethy et al[32a] conducted an adequately powered, international, randomized, controlled, parallel-arm, double-blind study of palliative oxygen versus medical air delivered through nasal prongs at 2 liters/min, ideally for longer than 15 hours/day. Eligible participants did not qualify for domiciliary oxygen. Average scores for "breathlessness now," "worst breathlessness in the last 24 hours," and "best breathlessness in the last 24 hours" did not differ clinically nor statistically between groups. Further, no differences in quality of life were noted between the two groups. Breathlessness on both gases improved over the 1-week period of the study, reflecting findings of earlier studies reporting that any movement of gas across the face seems to be of benefit; for this reason, medical air was not deemed a "placebo" in this study. Of note, participants with the most severe breathlessness seemed to derive the greatest benefit from oxygen over medical air (numeric rating scale of 7 to 10/10), and those randomized to oxygen tended toward better morning scores for breathlessness, assuming that most people chose nighttime as the major time at which oxygen was used.

Clinically, what recommendations can be made from currently available evidence? First, the study by Abernethy et al[32a] has shown that patients are very discerning about their continued use of oxygen even with evidence of clinical benefit, given the perceived burden of the intervention. Caregivers may well seek to influence such prescribing. Given the ability of patients to carefully define net benefit, it could be argued that people who are breathless should be offered a therapeutic trial of oxygen, especially if that breathlessness is severe. Ideally, this could take the form of a formal "n of 1" trial, but the logistics of this are potentially difficult to justify.[33]

NONPHARMACOLOGIC INTERVENTIONS

Given the complexity of the origin of breathlessness for many people with cancer, management demands a multimodal approach. Although statistically and clinically significant improvements can be obtained for some people using pharmacologic interventions or oxygen, many people's experience with these interventions warrants approaches that complement them. Nonpharmacologic interventions may be used alone or in combination with existing pharmacologic therapies. A systematic review has addressed the quality and breadth of nonpharmacologic techniques.[19] The focus in this review was on both malignant and nonmalignant disease. The ability to extrapolate from nonmalignant causes to cancer may be valid for some interventions (activity pacing) and not others (pursed-lip breathing, which is more associated with obstructive patterns of lung disease). As with all systematic reviews, the reviewers are limited by the work that has been done to inform the question, and the subcomponent of the larger meta-analysis that relates directly to cancer is limited to a handful of studies.[34]

In lung cancer, Sola and colleagues systematically reviewed nine studies for nonpharmacologic interventions.[35] Nurse-led interventions showed benefit with reduced distress and better maintained function for lung cancer patients. Counseling may help to reduce distress, but additional studies are needed.

Breathing techniques

In advanced cancer, patients may have some ability to improve breathing by positioning. As cachexia worsens systemic muscle function, some people gain partial relief of the effort of breathing by sitting and leaning forward. By supporting their upper body weight with their arms, patients may be able to improve the efficiency of respiratory muscles for inspiration because they are at a greater mechanical advantage in this position.[16] This position may help to increase the effective use of the diaphragm and may reduce the use of accessory muscles.[36]

For people with a small airway obstructive component to their breathing, pursed-lip breathing may provide some benefits. This is likely to be of benefit particularly to people with a significant history of tobacco smoking and lung cancer. For expiration, leaving only a small aperture for the lips and exhaling slowly creates backpressure, keeping smaller airways open longer and thus preventing dynamic airway collapse.[37] Use of this intervention requires that the patient be cognitively intact and able to practice at times other than when breathlessness is particularly bad.

Emotional and social support

The diagnosis of cancer, and particularly the realization that this cancer is not going to be cured and is likely to lead to death, is for many people the most challenging news that they will ever face. Beyond the diagnosis, the daily challenge of having breathlessness controlled sufficiently to feel that every breath is not one's last, and to feel that there is some level of control in life, is even more important than when a person is healthy. Additionally, the breathless person often reflects on a "social death" as friends and family are confronted by their own helplessness in the face of uncontrolled breathlessness and shy away. This is a time of life when loss of mastery will worsen fear, and concerns about future worsening breathlessness will create understandable anxiety. People with breathlessness report poorer levels of quality of life.[38]

Existing evidence-based guidelines for the psychological support of people with cancer provide excellent guidance for practitioners.[39] Careful evaluation by a clinical psychologist experienced in dealing with anxiety is a reasonable first step in providing care for people with breathlessness; these healthcare professionals can assess the contribution of anxiety or other emotions to the sensation of dyspnea. Targeted interventions from the broader psychology literature can then be offered to the person.

Caregivers and breathlessness

Individuals in the presence of someone with refractory breathlessness cannot help but be aware of their own inability to make a substantial difference in how that person is feeling. For the patient, their presence is usually better than their absence, but ultimately this is a symptom that can be lessened but not relieved, and the abject sense of helplessness in the caregiver creates its own set of needs for support. This is especially the case in the setting where family and friends are providing care.

The range of responses to the role of caregiving is predictably broad. Evidence is extrapolated from data on COPD. Qualitative data by two separate teams have generated similar caregiver needs in the setting of someone with refractory dyspnea: It is an anxious role that limits other activities and contact with people other than immediate householders and the patient; the role has a constancy that is burdensome; and the role changes the dynamic of the preexisting relationship between the patient and caregiver.[40,41] Such consequences require acknowledgment by clinicians and, when possible, support directed at caregivers.

Models for improving service delivery

Two models for improving the provision of breathlessness interventions have been evaluated in randomized controlled trials. Bredin[42] et al evaluated a nurse-led outpatient-based intervention for breathlessness palliation in a multisite study, which provided between three and eight clinical visits. The multimodal intervention incorporated counseling, breathing retraining, relaxation, and coping/adaptation strategies for dealing with breathlessness. The intervention group positively benefited with an improved sense of mastery and reduced breathlessness.[42] This has led to some changes in the way services are delivered, but the long-term effectiveness of the strategy has not been reported. More recently, a Breathlessness Intervention Service (BIS) model has been described, which adapts some key elements of pulmonary rehabilitation to the palliative setting. In pilot data, clinically meaningful reductions in distress as a result of breathlessness have been identified.[43]

PHARMACOLOGIC INTERVENTIONS

Although modifying the underlying cause(s) of breathlessness relies heavily on pharmacologic interventions, this chapter focuses on the symptomatic treatment of refractory dyspnea irrespective of the pathology that generated it. These systemic approaches have a rapidly evolving evidence base that allows improved confidence regarding not only the clinical efficacy of medications for the symptomatic treatment of breathlessness, but also their longer-term effectiveness and safety. As with many areas of clinical practice, much of what can be brought into cancer practice needs to be extrapolated from diseases other than cancer.[44]

Systemic opioids

Low-dose, regular systemic opioids have been shown to reduce refractory breathlessness in people with a range of underlying pathologies, but predominantly in people with COPD and cancer. The opioid used almost exclusively in these studies has been morphine. A systematic review reflects a net clinical benefit in favor of morphine over placebo.[45] It is important to note that a recent position statement from the American College of Chest Physicians explicitly endorses, for the first time, the use of individually titrated opioids in the control of breathlessness for people with advanced cardiorespiratory diseases.[46]

New work outlining the mechanisms through which opioids may palliate breathlessness continues to grow. Existing data support reduced ventilator responses to rising partial pressures of carbon dioxide; reducing levels of oxygenation reduces response to inspiratory flow, resistive loading, and exercise, and decreases oxygen consumption.[47-51] More recent work in a group of volunteers with moderate to severe COPD confirms a central role for endogenous opioids that does not contribute to a reduction in work effort. In a crossover study in people who were opioid naïve, participants were randomly administered normal saline or naloxone (a centrally acting opioid antagonist). Work effort to 75% of individual maximum work effort was no different with either arm, but breathlessness was far worse with the naloxone arm.[17]

Although concerns about respiratory depression have been raised, no case reports have been forthcoming. Instead, concerns are extrapolated from the population of opioid-naïve people who are given opioids in the acute setting, generally at much higher doses than in studies for the reduction of refractory dyspnea.[52,53] Such extrapolation is not evidence-based practice, but it does highlight the need for careful pharmacovigilance studies.

A meta-analysis of controlled trials in the palliation of breathlessness with opioids showed a net clinical benefit. Unfortunately, many of these studies were single-dose studies with relatively few participants, and this may lower the estimated benefit.[45] The overall pooled effect size (-0.31; 95% CI, -0.50 to -0.13; $P = .0008$) translated to a reduction of approximately 16% of breathlessness intensity over and above the control arm. These data include two small underpowered studies in people with cancer and breathlessness.[33]

A randomized, double-blind, adequately powered, crossover study of 48 participants was conducted at the same time. In this study, the primary endpoints included the point at which participants reached steady state. Outcomes reflected the same magnitude of benefit. This was achieved with a once-daily sustained-release morphine dose of 20 mg. Peak benefit coincided with peak plasma concentrations. No reported episodes of respiratory compromise were reported in either study[18]; however, constipation was more likely when on opioids despite regular aperients.

In addition to morphine, dihydrocodeine has been shown to reduce breathlessness in four placebo-controlled trials using differing dosing schedules and durations of study.[44] Equally, it must be noted that the meta-analysis of nebulized morphine is not supported by currently available data.[45]

Psychotropic medications

Given the complex origin of the sensation of breathlessness, it is reasonable to assume that psychotropic medications may demonstrate some benefits. Medications from this class that have been reported from systematic observations include benzodiazepines, phenothiazines, and selective serontonin reuptake inhibitors. Of these, the most convincing data support the use of oral promethazine as a second-line agent if systemic opioids cannot be used.[44] For selective serontonin reuptake inhibitors, a potential mechanism of action has been identified in the brainstem.[54] To support this clinical observation, one small, blinded, randomized trial of paroxetine supports additional studies in this setting.[55] The other case series suggests symptomatic benefit even in people whose breathlessness is not primarily driven by anxiety.[56]

For benzodiazepines, despite their widespread use in this setting and the understandable rationale behind this, a recent systematic review of the small number of studies in the area does not conclude that any benefits are derived across populations studied from their widespread use.[57] In specific circumstances, it is reasonable to consider an individually tailored n-of-1 study, but beyond this, these medications cannot be recommended at this time. In someone with an overwhelming component of anxiety, the use of alprazolam or clonazepam allows choice between short- and long-acting agents, respectively.

The other anxiolytic with a small quantity of data to support further investigation is buspirone, also a serotonergic agent. Two studies have been conducted in populations with and without anxiety. They are small studies and suggest that additional studies may be warranted.[58,59]

Inhaled furosemide

Although known for its diuretic properties, furosemide has been suggested as a potential intervention for dyspnea because of its potential to prevent bronchoconstriction in susceptible individuals[60-62] and to limit vagally mediated afferent signals. Inhaled furosemide appears to prolong breath-holding and to slow the development of discomfort during loaded breathing.[63] Whether the primary benefit is symptom control or modification of the course of the illness is not known. A recent systematic review suggested that data are insufficient to allow any conclusion about the current role of inhaled furosemide in the relief of breathlessness.[64]

CURRENT EVIDENCE-BASED THERAPEUTIC OPTIONS

Breathlessness in cancer remains a distressing symptom.[65] At this time, the use of nonpharmacologic interventions for breathlessness, including a nurse-led clinic and specific interventions such as activity pacing, have received support. The use of low-dose, regular opioids is also supported by level I evidence. Several emerging candidate medications should be further evaluated in randomized, controlled clinical trials.

REFERENCES

1. Hardy JR, Turner R, Saunders M, et al. Prediction of survival in a hospital-based continuing care unit. *Eur J Cancer.* 1994;30A:284–288.

2. Chang VT, Thaler HT, Polyak TA, et al. Quality of life and survival: the role of multidimensional symptom assessment. *Cancer.* 1998;83:173–179.

3. Hammond EC. Some preliminary findings on physical complaints from a prospective study of 1,064,004 men and women. *Am J Publ Health.* 1964;54:11–23.

4. Currow DC, Plummer JL, Crockett A, et al. A community population survey of prevalence and severity of dyspnea in adults. *J Pain Symptom Manage.* 2009;38:533–545.

5. Currow DC, Smith J, Davidson PM, et al. Do the trajectories of dyspnea differ in prevalence and intensity by diagnosis at the end of life? A consecutive cohort study. *J Pain Symptom Manage.* 2010;39:680–690.

6. Reuben DB, Mor V. Dyspnea in terminally ill cancer patients. *Chest.* 1986;89:234–236.

7. Dudgeon DJ, Kristjanson L, Sloan JA, et al. Dyspnea in cancer patients: prevalence and associated factors. *J Pain Symptom Manage.* 2001;21:95–102.

8. Vainio A, Auvinen A. Prevalence of symptoms among patients with advanced cancer: an international collaborative study. Symptom Prevalence Group. *Journal Pain Symptom Manage.* 1996;12:3–10.

9. Coyle N, Adelhardt J, Foley KM, et al. Character of terminal illness in the advanced cancer patient: pain and other symptoms during the last four weeks of life. *J Pain Symptom Manage.* 1990;5:83–93.

10. Reuben DB, Mor V, Hiris J. Clinical symptoms and length of survival in patients with terminal cancer. *Arch Intern Med.* 1988;148:1586–1591.

11. Mercadante S, Casuccio A, Fulfaro F. The course of symptom frequency and intensity in advanced cancer patients followed at home. *J Pain Symptom Manage.* 2000;20:104–112.

12. Tsai J-S, Wu C-H, Chiu T-Y, et al. Symptom patterns of advanced cancer patients in a palliative care unit. *Palliat Med.* 2006;20:617–622.

13. Chiu T-Y, Hu W-Y, Lue B-H, et al. Dyspnea and its correlates in Taiwanese patients with terminal cancer. *J Pain Symptom Manage.* 2004;28:123–132.

14. Dudgeon DJ, Lertzman M, Dudgeon DJ, et al. Dyspnea in the advanced cancer patient. *J Pain Symptom Manage.* 1998;16:212–219.

15. Edmonds P, Higginson I, Altmann D, et al. Is the presence of dyspnea a risk factor for morbidity in cancer patients? *J Pain Symptom Manage.* 2000;19:15–22.

16. Anon. Dyspnea: mechanisms, assessment, and management: a consensus statement. American Thoracic Society. *Am J Respir Crit Care Med.* 1999;159:321–340.

17. Mahler DA, Murray JA, Waterman LA, et al. Endogenous opioids modify dyspnea during treadmill exercise in patients with COPD. *Eur Respir J.* 2009;33:771–777.

18. Abernethy AP, Currow DC, Frith P, et al. Randomised, double blind, placebo controlled crossover trial of sustained release morphine for the management of refractory dyspnea. *Br Med J.* 2003;327:523–528.

19. Bausewein C, Booth S, Gysels M, et al. Non-pharmacological interventions for breathlessness in advanced stages of malignant and non-malignant diseases. *Cochrane Database Syst Rev.* 2008;(2): CD005623.

20. O'Donnell De, Banzett RB, Carrieri-Kohlman V, et al. Pathophysiology of dyspnea in chronic obstructive pulmonary disease: a roundtable. *Proc Am Thorac Soc.* 2007;4:145–168.

21. Tanaka K, Akechi T, Okuyama T, et al. Development and validation of the Cancer Dyspnea Scale: a multidimensional, brief, self-rating scale. *Br J Cancer.* 2000;82:800–805.

22. Abrams WB, Beers MH, Berkow R. The Merck manual of geriatrics. 2nd ed. Whitehouse Station, NJ: Merck Research Laboratories; 1995.

23. Abernethy AP, Shelby-James TM, Fazekas BS, et al. The Australian-modified Karnofsky Performance Status (AKPS) scale: a revised scale for contemporary palliative care clinical practice. *BMC Pall Care.* 2005;4:7.

24. Guyatt GH, McKim DA, Austin P, et al. Appropriateness of domiciliary oxygen delivery. *Chest.* 2000;118:1303–1308.

25. Stringer E, McParland C, Hernandez P. Physician practices for prescribing supplemental oxygen in the palliative care setting. *J Palliat Care.* 2004;20:303–307.

26. Abernethy AP, Currow DC, Frith PA, et al. Prescribing palliative oxygen: a clinician survey of expected benefit and patterns of use. *Palliat Med.* 2005;19:165–172.

27. Currow DC, Christou T, Smith J, et al. Do terminally ill people who live alone miss out on home oxygen treatment? An hypothesis generating study? *J Palliat Med.* 2008;11:1015–1022.

28. Uronis HE, Currow DC, McCrory DC, et al. Oxygen for relief of dyspnea in mildly- or non-hypoxaemic patients with cancer: a systematic review and meta-analysis. *Br J Cancer.* 2008;98:294–299.

29. Philip J, Gold M, Milner A, et al. A randomized, double-blind, crossover trial of the effect of oxygen on dyspnea in patients with advanced cancer. *J Pain Symptom Manage.* 2006;32:541–550.

30. Bruera E, Sweeney C, Willey J, et al. A randomized controlled trial of supplemental oxygen versus air in cancer patients with dyspnea. *Palliat Med.* 2003;17:659–663.

31. Booth S, Kelly MJ, Cox NP, et al. Does oxygen help dyspnea in patients with cancer? *Am J Respir Crit Care Med.* 1996;153:1515–1518.

32. Ahmedzai SH, Laude E, Robertson A, et al. A double-blind, randomised, controlled Phase II trial of Heliox28 gas mixture in lung cancer patients with dyspnea on exertion. *Br J Cancer.* 2004;90:366–371.

32a. Abernethy AP, McDonald CF, Frith PA, et al. Effect of palliative oxygen versus medical (room) air in relieving breathlessness in patients with refractory dyspnea: a double-blind randomised controlled trial (NCT00327873). *Lancet.* 2010;376:784–793.

33. Bruera E, Schoeller T, MacEachern T. Symptomatic benefit of supplemental oxygen in hypoxemic patients with terminal cancer: the use of the N of 1 randomized controlled trial. *J Pain Symptom Manage.* 1992;7:365–368.

34. Zhao I, Yates P. Non-pharmacological interventions for breathlessness management in patients with lung cancer: a systematic review. *Palliat Med.* 2008;22:693–701.

35. Solà I, Thompson E, Subirana M, et al. Non-invasive interventions for improving well-being and quality of life in patients with lung cancer. *Cochrane Database Syst Rev.* 2004;(4): CD004282.

36. Sharp JT, Drutz WS, Moisan T, et al. Postural relief of dyspnea in severe chronic obstructive pulmonary disease. *Am J Rev Respir Dis.* 1980;122:201–211.

37. Tiep BL, Burns M, Kao D, et al. Pursed lips breathing training using ear oximetry. *Chest.* 1986;90:218–221.

38. Smith EL, Hann DM, Ahles TA, et al. Dyspnea, anxiety, body consciousness, and quality of life in patients with lung cancer. *J Pain Symptom Manage.* 2001;21:323–329.

39. Anon. *Clinical practice guidelines for the psychosocial care of adults with cancer.* Sydney, Australia: National Breast Cancer Centre; 2003.

40. Booth S, Anderson H, Swannick M, et al. The use of oxygen in the palliation of breathlessness: a report of the expert working group of the Scientific Committee of the Association of Palliative Medicine. *Respir Med.* 2004;98:66–77.

41. Seamark DA, Blake SD, Seamark CJ, et al. Living with severe chronic obstructive pulmonary disease (COPD): perceptions of patients and their carers. An interpretative phenomenological analysis. *Palliat Med.* 2004;18:619–625.

42. Bredin M, Corner J, Krishnasamy M, et al. Multicentre randomised controlled trial of nursing intervention for breathlessness in patients with lung cancer. *BMJ.* 1999;318:901–904.

43. Farquhar M, Higginson IJ, Fagan P, et al. Results of a pilot investigation into a complex intervention for breathlessness in advanced chronic obstructive pulmonary disease (COPD): brief report. *Palliat Support Care.* 2010;1–7. [Epub ahead of print].

44. Viola R, Kiteley C, Lloyd NS, et al. The management of dyspnea in cancer patients: a systematic review. *Support Care Cancer.* 2008;16:329–337.

45. Jennings AL, Davies AN, Higgins JP, et al. A systematic review of the use of opioids in the management of dyspnea. *Thorax.* 2002;57:939–944.

46. Mahler DA, Selecky PA, Harrod CG, et al. American College of Chest Physicians consensus statement on the management of dyspnea in patients with advanced lung or heart disease. *Chest.* 2010;137:674–691.

47. Eckenhoff JE, Oech SR. The effects of narcotics and antagonists upon respiration and circulation in man: a review. *Clin Pharmacol Ther.* 1960;1:483–524.

48. Santiago TV, Pugliese AC, Edelman NH. Control of breathing during methadone addiction. *Am J Med.* 1977;62:347–354.

49. Weil JV, McCullough RE, Kline JS, et al. Diminished ventilatory response to hypoxia and hypercapnia after morphine in normal man. *N Engl J Med.* 1975;292:1103–1106.

50. Kryger MH, Yacoub O, Dosman J, et al. Effect of meperidine on occlusion pressure responses to hypercapnia and hypoxia with and without external inspiratory resistance. *Am Rev Respir Dis.* 1976;114:333–340.

51. Santiago TV, Johnson J, Riley DJ, et al. Effects of morphine on ventilatory response to exercise. *J Appl Physiol Respir Environ Exerc Physiol.* 1979;47:112–118.

52. Currow DC, Abernethy AP, Frith P. Morphine for management of refractory dyspnea. *Br Med J.* 2003;327:1288–1289.

53. Pauwels RA, Buist AS, Calverley PM, et al. Global strategy for the diagnosis, management, and prevention of chronic obstructive pulmonary disease. NHLBI/WHO Global Initiative for Chronic Obstructive Lung

Disease (GOLD) Workshop summary. *Am J Respir Crit Care Med.* 2001;163:1256–1276.

54. Mueller RA, Lundberg DB, Breese GR, et al. The neuropharmacology of respiratory control. *Pharmacol Rev.* 1982;34:255–285.

55. Lacasse Y, Beaudoin L, Rousseau L, et al. Randomized trial of paroxetine in end-stage COPD. *Monaldi Arch Chest Dis.* 2004;61:140–147.

56. Smoller JW, Pollack MH, Systrom D, et al. Sertraline effects on dyspnea in patients with obstructive airways disease. *Psychosomatics.* 1998;39:24–29.

57. Simon ST, Higginson IJ, Booth S, et al. Benzodiazepines for the relief of breathlessness in advanced malignant and non-malignant diseases in adults. *Cochrane Database Syst Rev.* 2010;(1): CD007354.

58. Singh NP, Despars JA, Stansbury DW, et al. Effects of buspirone on anxiety levels and exercise tolerance in patients with chronic airflow obstruction and mild anxiety. *Chest.* 1993;103:800–804.

59. Argyropoulou P, Patakas D, Koukou A, et al. Buspirone effect on breathlessness and exercise performance in patients with chronic obstructive pulmonary disease. *Respiration.* 1993;60:216–220.

60. Bianco S, Vaghi A, Robuschi M, et al. Prevention of exercise-induced bronchoconstriction by inhaled frusemide. *Lancet.* 1988;2:252–255.

61. Bianco S, Pieroni MG, Refini RM, et al. Protective effect of inhaled furosemide on allergen-induced early and late asthmatic reactions. *N Engl J Med.* 1989;321:1069–1073.

62. Robuschi M, Gambaro G, Spagnotto S, et al. Inhaled frusemide is highly effective in preventing ultrasonically nebulised water bronchoconstriction. *Pulm Pharmacol.* 1989;1:187–191.

63. Nishino T, Ide T, Sudo T, et al. Inhaled furosemide greatly alleviates the sensation of experimentally induced dyspnea. *Am J Respir Crit Care Med.* 2000;161:1963–1967.

64. Newton PJ, Davidson PM, Macdonald P, et al. Nebulized furosemide for the management of dyspnea: does the evidence support its use? *J Pain Symptom Manage.* 2008;36:424–441.

65. Booth S, Silvester S, Todd C, et al. Breathlessness in cancer and chronic obstructive pulmonary disease: using a qualitative approach to describe the experience of patients and carers. *Palliat Support Care.* 2003;1:337–344.

Malignant dysphagia: Evaluation and endoscopic treatment

Nikhil Banerjee and Douglas G. Adler

Swallowing is a complex act consisting of coordinated activity involving mouth, pharynx, larynx, and esophagus. Swallowing comprises four phases: oral preparatory, oral propulsive, pharyngeal, and esophageal.[1] Dysphagia is defined as difficulty swallowing solids, liquids, or both.

Malignant dysphagia is the impaired transfer of solids and/or liquids through the esophagus into the stomach caused by malignant mechanical obstruction, which may be intrinsic or extrinsic to the esophagus.[1,2] Typical symptoms include retrosternal discomfort and progressive dysphagia, initially with solids, progressing to liquids.[3] Complications involve aspiration, nutritional deficiencies, weight loss, difficulty handling secretions and drooling, and family and psychosocial issues centered on the inability to eat.

This chapter focuses on current diagnosis and management of malignant esophageal dysphagia with an emphasis on the therapeutic interventions performed to improve dysphagia in patients with advanced malignancies. All therapies can be used in conjunction with traditional chemotherapy and/or radiation therapy. Gastrointestinal therapeutic interventions, including enteral feeding tubes, argon plasma coagulation, laser therapy, photodynamic therapy, and esophageal stents, will be reviewed.

MALIGNANT ESOPHAGEAL DYSPHAGIA

Anatomic structures involved in dysphagia include the esophagus, the lower esophageal sphincter, and the stomach cardia. Disturbances in these sites typically impair swallowing through mechanical obstruction and/or motility disturbances.[4] Malignant esophageal dysphagia (hereafter referred to as malignant dysphagia) is defined as dysphagia due to cancer invasion of these structures.

Most individuals with malignant dysphagia have advanced incurable cancer, and a large percentage of these patients have unresectable malignancies, making the goals of care palliative.[5] A dysphagia scoring system (DSS) has been developed that assesses symptomatic outcomes of therapies designed to palliate causes of malignant dysphagia.[6] The DSS has a numeric scale that stratifies the severity of swallowing difficulties from no dysphagia to inability to swallow saliva. The DSS should be repeated at multiple time points postintervention to gauge the outcomes of interventions (Table 17-1).

Malignant dysphagia is most commonly the result of squamous carcinoma or adenocarcinoma of the esophagus or gastric cardia[7] (Fig. 17-1). Lung cancer, liposarcoma, and lymphoma are the most common extragastrointestinal cancers to cause extrinsic compression and invade the esophagus.[8–10] Lung cancer in fact is responsible for one third to one half of extrinsic causes of malignant dysphagia; these tumors directly invade the esophagus as well (Fig. 17-2). Lung cancers are also a frequent cause of malignant tracheoesophageal fistulas; this poses special problems in management.[11,12]

DIAGNOSIS

Patients with dysphagia typically undergo evaluation of the structure and function of the esophagus. A barium esophagram fills and coats the lining of the esophagus, stomach, and duodenum, which is visualized and images captured via fluoroscopy. Double-contrast barium esophagrams (DCBEs) are particularly useful for detecting carcinoma and other structural lesions such as paraneoplastic achalasia.[13] DCBE has greater than 95% sensitivity in detecting esophageal cancers.[14] Esophageal cancers have characteristic appearances on endoscopy and DCBE that help in their diagnosis.[15–19] Malignant lesions can be circumferential with an apple-core appearance or may have a partially circumferential configuration that appears as a mural filling defect on contrast studies. Early-stage squamous carcinoma and adenocarcinoma of the esophagus are not reliably found with barium studies. The location

Table 17-1   Dysphagia scoring system

0	Able to eat normal diet/no dysphagia
1	Able to swallow some solid foods
2	Able to swallow only semisolid foods
3	Able to swallow liquids only
4	Unable to swallow anything/total dysphagia

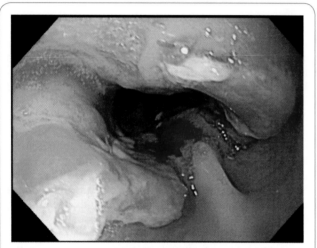

Fig. 17-1   Representative esophageal adenocarcinoma arising in the distal esophagus.

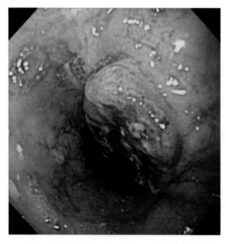

Fig. 17-2   Endoscopic image of lung cancer directly invading the esophagus.

of cancer within the esophagus provides some evidence as to the type of cancer.[20] In general, squamous cell cancers of the esophagus tend to occur in the proximal to mid esophagus, and adenocarcinomas tend to occur in the distal esophagus, although exceptions to this rule can be encountered.

Barium studies are also able to detect esophago-respiratory fistulas and the length and grade of stricture.[21,22] Obstruction and/or displacement of the esophagus by lung malignancies can be visualized with dilute oral barium used for chest computed tomography (CT) scans.[23]

Esophagogastroduodenoscopy (EGD) should be performed in all patients with dysphagia to assess the type of obstruction (tumor- or treatment-related stricture) and is the gold standard when evaluating dysphagia. EGD visualizes esophagus, stomach, and duodenum and identifies tumors, strictures, polyps, diverticuli, ulcers, candidiasis, viral esophagitis, and inflammatory lesions. High-quality color images and biopsies of any pathologic lesions are obtained. EGD is also the most commonly used modality for therapeutic interventions such as esophageal dilation, tumor ablative therapies, and stent placement.[24] Endoscopically, malignancies tend to manifest as fungating, friable, often ulcerated lesions that partially or totally obstruct the lumen.

NUTRITION

Weight loss and poor nutritional status are serious problems faced by patients with malignant dysphagia.[23,25] Malnutrition is present in more than 75% of patients at the time of diagnosis and is predictive of early mortality with esophageal cancer.[26,27] Feeding may be enteral (EN) or parenteral (TPN), according to the function of the gut and the success of the intervention. EN is less expensive and is better managed at home than TPN. EN maintains gut integrity by stimulating normal gut physiologic processes; it maintains the gut immune response and reduces the risk of infection better than TPN.[28–31]

Feeding tubes

Placement of feeding tubes (via orogastric, nasogastric, or percutaneous gastrostomy) provides enteral access to deliver nutrients, hydration, and medication when obstruction prevents adequate oral intake. Nasoenteric tubes (NETs) are useful for short-term nutritional support (typically less than 30 days) and are placed at the bedside, or via endoscopy with or without fluoroscopy.[32]

Patients requiring longer-duration enteral feeding access (months) should be considered for percutaneous endoscopic gastrostomy (PEG) or jejunostomy (PEJ) tube placement. PEG is widely practiced and well tolerated by most individuals for prolonged nutritional supplementation. PEG tubes allow for gastric decompression in the case of small-bowel obstruction and are placed endoscopically, surgically, or radiologically with equal effectiveness; most commonly though PEG tubes are placed endoscopically because of ease of access.

Patients with gastroesophageal reflux disease (GERD), at high aspiration risk, or who have gastric dysmotility warrant consideration of percutaneous jejunal tubes (PEJ).[33] Jejunal tubes can include gastrojejunostomy tubes (a PEG tube with an internal jejunal extension) (PEGJ) or may be directly placed via percutaneous endoscopic jejunostomy (DPEJ). Gastrojejunostomy tubes are placed fluoroscopically, and direct jejunal feeding tubes are placed by surgical techniques. DPEJ tubes are very useful as a source of calories in weaning patients from TPN; this simplifies hospital discharge after esophagectomy.[34] Specifically, DPEJ allows enteral feeding even in the presence of postoperative complications such as anastomotic leaks, fistulas, sepsis, respiratory insufficiency, and aspiration, which precludes oral intake and leads to dependence on TPN.[35] Evidence for the risk of aspiration pneumonia with gastric feeding is conflicting as compared with postpyloric feeding, where the risk is not increased. Meta-analyses have suggested that postpyloric feeding decreases rates of aspiration pneumonia and gastroesophageal regurgitation. Persistent aspiration of oral secretions in patients fed by gastric delivery and jejunal delivery may continue despite successful interventions.[36–40]

ENDOSCOPIC TREATMENT OPTIONS FOR PATIENTS WITH MALIGNANT DYSPHAGIA
Ablative techniques

Lasers, argon plasma coagulation, and photodynamic therapy are means by which malignant obstructions are treated endoscopically in an attempt to enlarge luminal diameter, thereby improving oral intake in patients with malignant dysphagia.

Neodymium:yttrium-aluminum-garnet (Nd:YAG) lasers and argon plasma coagulation (APC) devices are shown to reduce tumor bulk, recanalize lumina, and improve swallowing.[41] Using specialized endoscopic catheters, Nd:YAG laser light is directly applied to tumor tissue. APC is used to ablate tissue via destructive coagulation using a stream of high-energy ionized argon gas to deliver thermal energy to the tissues. Similar to Nd:YAG, APC is done under direct vision through EGD.[42]

Lasers and APC have successfully relieved dysphagia for many years. Lasers are more commonly used in Europe than in the United States, largely because of cost and availability. Laser ablation is successful in most circumstances, but almost all patients require multiple treatment sessions before achieving significant relief from dysphagia.[43] Retreatment every 1 to 2 months may be necessary to prevent reocclusion.[44]

Complications of bleeding, perforation, and fistula formation are similar for both laser therapy and APC, although lasers are more likely than APC to cause perforation.[45–47] Both techniques can be combined with radiation therapy, resulting in higher patency rates and longer periods between treatments.[48]

In a case series involving 46 patients with malignant strictures of the esophagus and gastric cardia who underwent APC, 16 with early localized esophagogastric cancers were alive and four were disease-free at a median follow-up of 21 months. Individuals required a median of two APC sessions. Four patients with locally advanced cancer were disease free after the first treatment at multiple time points. APC was successful in palliating dysphagia-related tumor invasion in and around the stent interstices in 13 of 14 patients. In all patients, stent patency was restored with the first treatment, and only three required repeat treatments.[49] A pilot study found APC to be effective in restoring lumen patency in nearly all individuals, requiring a mean number of 3.3 treatment sessions.[50] Recent studies using newer, higher-powered APC devices have shown effectiveness in palliating malignant obstructions, with a mean/maximum number of 2 and 5 sessions, respectively.[51,52]

Photodynamic therapy (PDT) is another technique that causes local tissue destruction in an attempt to recanalize obstructed lumina and improve dysphagia. PDT uses a special light-guide catheter that generates light at specific wavelengths to activate (in the presence of molecular oxygen) certain dyes known as photosensitizers. The photosensitizers are given systemically and concentrate in tumor tissue, possibly as the result of poor lymphatic drainage from these sites. Porfimer sodium is currently FDA approved for this purpose in the United States; outside of the United States, aminolevulonic acid (ALA) is also used as a photosensitizer.[53]

The antitumor effects of PDT result from the combination of direct tumor cell photo damage, destruction of tumor vasculature, and activation of the host immune response. This differs from thermal methods in terms of delivery, uniformity, and immediacy of effect (several hours after treatment with PDT as opposed to immediate tissue destruction with lasers and APC).

PDT is comparable to Nd:YAG laser treatment in effectiveness, with fewer treatment sessions and serious complications such as perforation.[54] Esophageal peristalsis and respiratory motion of the chest are challenges to correctly positioning the light source within, for a uniform light distribution.[55] Irregularities in the surface of the esophagus/tumor create areas of excessive light exposure or inadequate exposure. Areas that are overexposed to light are at risk for subsequent stricture formation, and undertreated areas are at risk for recurrent tumor.[56] Modern PDT light-delivery systems use elastic balloon catheters as fiber-centering devices to promote delivery of the desired light intensity to the targeted region.[57,58] The most common complication of PDT is the development of esophageal stricture during healing.[59,60]

A common toxicity with PDT is skin photosensitivity.[61,62] This is due to the photosensitizer's predilection to collect in skin. Patients undergoing PDT must scrupulously avoid sun exposure because dermal reactions are painful, and in some circumstances severe, producing signs and symptoms similar to extensive sunburn. Photosensitivity risk lasts for approximately 1 month after treatment, although photoreactions are reported as late as 72 days after treatment.[63]

Esophageal stents

In general, oral nutrition is preferred whenever possible because it promotes a more normal lifestyle for patients, enhances nutritional intake, and can improve quality of life. Esophageal stents are used to recanalize an obstructed esophagus and allow restoration of oral feeding. Stenting allows rapid restoration intake of food, water, and medication. Esophageal stents are commonly used to close malignant tracheoesophageal fistulas, which result from tumor invasion or chemoradiation, or as a complication of surgery.[64,65]

Two main types of self-expandable stents are currently in use: self-expanding metal stents (SEMSs) and self-expanding plastic stents (SEPSs). SEMS are made from a variety of metals and alloys, including nitinol (nickel-titanium alloy), stainless steel, and cobalt chromium-nickel alloy, and may be coated with silicon or polyurethane. All currently available SEMS are at least partially coated to prevent tumor ingrowth through stent interstices. Through endoscopic and fluoroscopic techniques, stents are placed most commonly by gastroenterologists, and to a lesser extent by interventional radiologists and surgeons.[66,67] Stents are generally deployed under endoscopic and fluoroscopic guidance, but some stents can be deployed under endoscopic guidance alone[68] (Fig. 17-3).

SEMSs are permanent prostheses that are most commonly placed as palliative devices in patients with unresectable disease. Studies designed to look at both pre-stenting and post-stenting outcomes in malignant dysphagia patients have shown SEMSs to both reduce the dysphagia score and create a significant improvement in quality of life.[69,70] The uncovered portion of an SEMS (typically short segments of the stent at the proximal and distal ends of the device) expands into the tumor, with stent incorporation into the submucosal surface of the esophageal wall occurring in as few as 18 days.[71] Modern partially covered stents are at less risk of obstruction by tumor in-growth but have an associated increased risk of migration. Current studies suggest a relatively low migration rate with covered SEMSs of approximately 8%; however, risk of migration can be increased by as much as 50% when the stent is placed over an anastomotic site.[72,73]

Early complications of SEMS placement include perforation (2%–6%), hemorrhage (2%–14%), chest pain (15%–27%), stent migration (3%–13%), and the possibility of recurrent or unresolved dysphagia (4%–34%).[74–76] Late complications can include tumor in-growth, tumor overgrowth, delayed migration, and food impaction. Many patients will have some degree of temporary chest discomfort after stent placement; this typically resolves within 7 to 10 days. All patients with an esophageal stent should be placed on a prophylactic proton pump inhibitor to reduce the risk of reflux esophagitis, which can be painful.[77,78]

Larger-diameter stents reduce the risk of recurrent dysphagia from stent migration, tissue overgrowth, or food obstruction. However, as compared with smaller-diameter stents, they may pose increased risk of hemorrhage, perforation, fever, and fistula. Both have similar efficacy in improving the initial dysphagia score; the 18-mm SEMS had equal effectiveness but less pain than the 24-mm SEMS.[79,80]

SEPSs were developed as an alternative to SEMSs for palliation of malignant dysphagia. Potential advantages of this newer generation of stents include decreased rate of tissue in-growth, new stricture formation, increased levels of radial expansion that potentially reduce the need for dilation at the time of insertion, and the option of elective removal.[81–87] SEPSs are less expensive than SEMSs, but they have efficacy.[88] Stent properties are more appealing by allowing stent placement at the time of diagnosis, with subsequent removal after therapy to minimize stent-related complications.

Only one SEPS is commercially available in the United States: the Polyflex stent (Boston Scientific, Natick, MA). The Polyflex stent consists of polyester netting covered completely by a silicone membrane. The Polyflex stent as the representative SEPS is comparable to SEMS in relieving dysphagia.[89,90] Larger studies have demonstrated similar improvements in dysphagia and in rates of stent migration. Migration rates are slightly higher than those reported with SEMS.[88,91,92]

Polyflex stents were placed before chemoradiation therapy and surgery in six patients with malignant obstruction. This allowed five patients to maintain oral nutrition. These stents could be removed endoscopically without complications.[93] A more recent prospective study involved 13 patients with locally advanced esophageal cancer who underwent Polyflex stent placement at the time of endoscopic ultrasound (EUS). These patients could maintain oral feeding while undergoing neoadjuvant therapy and had significant decreases in mean dysphagia score at (1, 2, 3, and 4 weeks) after stent placement. It is feasible to place polyflex stents at the time of EUS, combining cancer staging and palliative stenting into a single procedure.[94]

SEPSs are well suited for sealing anastomotic leaks after esophageal surgery for benign and malignant diseases; they are commonly used to treat anastomotic strictures in patients with esophageal cancer following esophagectomy.[95] Questions regarding the use and timing of SEPSs in patients with anastomotic strictures remain unanswered. Some patients can be managed by dilation, others require placement of a temporary SEPS, and still others ultimately require placement of a permanent SEMS.[95,96]

Disadvantages of SEPSs include an anatomically wide and cumbersome delivery system that may require more frequent predeployment esophageal dilation than is commonly used with SEMS.[97] SEPSs also appear to have higher stent migration

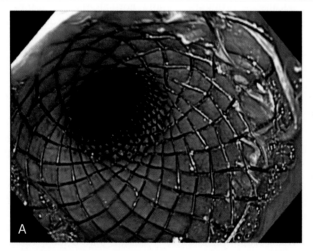 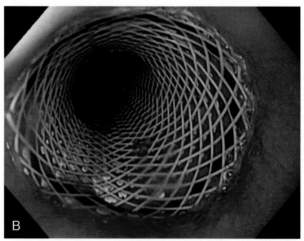

Fig. 17-3 A, Endoscopic image of a fully deployed esophageal self-expanding metal stent (SEMS). **B,** Endoscopic image of a fully deployed esophageal self-expanding plastic stent (SEPS; Polyflex stent).

rates than SEMSs because of the fully coated nature of the device, which prevents the stent from embedding into the surrounding esophagus, as is commonly seen with SEMS.

CONCLUSION

Enteral nutrition is an important option for patients with malignant dysphagia who are to undergo surgery, radiation, chemotherapy, or a combination of treatments. PEG, PEJ, and esophageal stents remain the current standard for palliation of malignant dysphagia. SEMSs and SEPSs produce similar relief from dysphagia. Nd:YAG lasers, APC, and PDT offer an ablation-based approach to reducing tumor bulk. Ablative therapies can be used in combination with esophageal stents. PEG and PEJ tubes are viable alternatives to deliver nutrition but do not restore oral intake and are less desirable overall.

REFERENCES

1. Dodds WJ, Logemann JA, Stewart ET. Radiologic assessment of abnormal oral and pharyngeal phases of swallowing. *AJR Am J Roentgenol.* 1990;154:965–974.
2. Dhir V, Vege SS, Mohandas KM, et al. Dilation of proximal esophageal strictures following therapy for head and neck cancer: Experience with Savary Gilliard dilators. *J Surg Oncol.* 1996;63:187.
3. Castell DO, Donner MW. Evaluation of dysphagia: A careful history is crucial. *Dysphagia.* 1987;2:65.
4. Palmer JB, Drennan JC, Baba M. Evaluation and treatment of swallowing impairments. *Am Fam Physician.* 2000;15;61:2453–2462.
5. Mougey A, Adler DG. Esophageal stenting for the palliation of malignant dysphagia. *J Support Oncol.* 2008;6:267–273.
6. Mellow MH, Pinkas H. Endoscopic laser therapy for malignancies affecting the esophagus and gastroesophageal junction. Analysis of technical and functional efficacy. *Arch Intern Med.* 1985;145:1443–1446.
7. DiBaise JK, Quigley EM. Tumor-related dysmotility. Gastrointestinal dysmotility syndromes associated with tumors. *Dig Dis Sci.* 1998;43:1369.
8. Kamby C, Vejborg I, Kristensen B, et al. Metastatic pattern in recurrent breast cancer. Special reference to intrathoracic recurrences. *Cancer.* 1988;62:2226–2233.
9. Sobel JM, Lai R, Mallery S, et al. The utility of EUS-guided FNA in the diagnosis of metastatic breast cancer to the esophagus and the mediastinum. *Gastrointest Endosc.* 2005;61:416–420.
10. Kassis ES, Belani CP, Ferson PF, et al. Hodgkin's disease presenting with a bronchoesophageal fistula. *Ann Thorac Surg.* 1998;66:1409–1410.
11. Spechler SJ. AGA technical review on treatment of patients with dysphagia caused by benign disorders of the distal esophagus. *Gastroenterology.* 1999;117:233.
12. Baltayiannis N, Magoulas D, Bolanos N, et al. Expandable wallstents for treatment of tracheoesophageal fistulas of malignant origin. *J BUON.* 2006;11:457–462.
13. Levine MS, Rubesin SE. Diseases of the esophagus: diagnosis with esophagography. *Radiology.* 2005;237:414–427.
14. Levine MS, Chu P, Furth EE, et al. Carcinoma of the esophagus and esophagogastric junction: sensitivity of radiographic diagnosis. *AJR Am J Roentgenol.* 1997;168:1423–1426.
15. Levine MS, Dillon EC, Saul SH, et al. Early esophageal cancer. *AJR Am J Roentgenol.* 1986;146:507–512.
16. Gloyna RE, Zornoza J, Goldstein HM. Primary ulcerative carcinoma of the esophagus. *AJR Am J Roentgenol.* 1977;129:599–600.
17. Yates CW, LeVine MA, Jensen KM. Varicoid carcinoma of the esophagus. *Radiology.* 1977;122:605–608.

18. Levine MS, Halvorsen RA. Carcinoma of the esophagus. In: Gore RM, Levine MS, eds. *Textbook of gastrointestinal radiology.* 2nd ed. Philadelphia: Saunders; 2000:403–433.
19. Itai Y, Kogure T, Okuyama Y, et al. Superficial esophageal carcinoma: radiological findings in double-contrast studies. *Radiology.* 1978;126:597–601.
20. Keen SJ, Dodd GD, Smith JL. Adenocarcinoma arising in Barrett esophagus: pathologic and radiologic features. *Mt Sinai J Med.* 1984;51:442–450.
21. Deb S, Ali MB, Fonseca P. Congenital bronchoesophageal fistula in an adult. *Chest.* 1998;114:1784–1786.
22. Pregun I, Hritz I, Tulassay Z, et al. Peptic esophageal stricture: medical treatment. *Dig Dis.* 2009;27:31–37.
23. Gale ME, Birnbaum SB, Gale DR, et al. Esophageal invasion by lung cancer: CT diagnosis. *J Comput Assist Tomogr.* 1984;8:694–698.
24. Varadarajulu S, Eloubeidi MA, Patel RS, et al. The yield and the predictors of esophageal pathology when upper endoscopy is used for the initial evaluation of dysphagia. *Gastrointest Endosc.* 2005;61:804.
25. Bower MR, Martin 2nd RC. Nutritional management during neoadjuvant therapy for esophageal cancer. *J Surg Oncol.* 2009;100:82–87.
26. Riccardi D, Allen K. Nutritional management of patients with esophageal and esophagogastric junction cancer. *Cancer Control.* 1999;6:64–72.
27. Lecleire S, Di Fiore F, Antonietti M, et al. Undernutrition is predictive of early mortality after palliative self-expanding metal stent insertion in patients with inoperable or recurrent esophageal cancer. *Gastrointest Endosc.* 2006;64:479–484.
28. Braga M, Gianotti L, Nespoli L, et al. Nutritional approach in malnourished surgical patients: a prospective randomized study. *Arch Surg.* 2002;137:174–180.
29. Braga M, Gianotti L, Vignali A, et al. Artificial nutrition after major abdominal surgery: impact of route of administration and composition of the diet. *Crit Care Med.* 1998;26:24–30.
30. Bozzetti F. Nutrition and gastrointestinal cancer. *Curr Opin Clin Nutr Metab Care.* 2001;4:541–546.
31. Braunschweig CL, Levy P, Sheean PM, et al. Enteral compared with parenteral nutrition: a meta-analysis. *Am J Clin Nutr.* 2001;74:534–542.
32. Kirby D, Delegge M, Flemming C. American gastroenterological association technical review on tube feeding for enteral nutrition. *Gastroenterology.* 1995;108:1282–1301.
33. Shike M, Latkany L. Direct percutaneous endoscopic jejunostomy. *Gastrointest Endosc Clin N Am.* 1998;8:569–580.
34. Schattner M. Enteral nutritional support of the patient with cancer: route and role. *J Clin Gastroenterol.* 2003;36:297–302.

35. Bueno JT, Schattner MA, Barrera R, et al. Endoscopic placement of direct percutaneous jejunostomy tubes in patients with complications after esophagectomy. *Gastrointest Endosc.* 2003;57:536–540.
36. Marik PE, Zaloga GP. Gastric versus postpyloric feeding: a systematic review. *Crit Care.* 2003;7:46–50.
37. Montecalvo M, Steger K, Farber H. Nutritional outcome and pneumonia in critical care patients randomized to gastric versus jejunal tube feedings. *Crit Care Med.* 1992;20:1377–1387.
38. Heyland D, Drover J, MacDonald S, et al. Effect of postpyloric feeding on gastroesophageal regurgitation and pulmonary microaspiration: results of a randomized controlled trial. *Crit Care Med.* 2001;29:1495–1501.
39. Lien H, Chang C, Chen G. Can percutaneous endoscopic jejunostomy prevent gastroesophageal reflux in patients with preexisting esophagitis? *Am J Gastroenterol.* 2000;95:3439–3443.
40. Kadakia S, Sullivan H, Starnes E. Percutaneous endoscopic gastrostomy or jejunostomy and the incidence of aspiration in 79 patients. *Am J Surg.* 1993;164:114–118.
41. Fleischer D, Kessler F, Haye O, et al. YAG laser therapy for carcinoma of the esophagus: a new palliative approach. *Am J Surg.* 1982;143:280–283.
42. Dumot JA, Greenwald BD. Argon plasma coagulation, bipolar cautery, and cryotherapy: ABC's of ablative techniques. *Endoscopy.* 2008;40:1026–1032.
43. Ponec RJ, Kimmey MB. Endoscopic therapy of esophageal cancer. *Surg Clin North Am.* 1997;77:1197–1217.
44. Lightdale C, Heier SK, Marcon NE, et al. Photodynamic therapy with porfimer sodium versus thermal ablation therapy with Nd:YAG laser for palliation of esophageal cancer: a multicenter randomized trial. *Gastrointest Endosc.* 1995;42:507–512.
45. Krasner N, Beard J. Laser irradiation of tumours of the oesophagus and gastric cardia. *Br Med J (Clin Res Ed).* 1984;288:829.
46. Gossner L, Ell C. Malignant strictures: thermal treatment. *Gastrointest Endosc Clin N Am.* 1998;8:493–501.
47. Pereira-Lima JC, Busnello JV, Saul C, et al. High power setting argon plasma coagulation for the eradication of Barrett's esophagus. *Am J Gastroenterol.* 2000;95:1661–1668.
48. Alexander P, Mayoral W, Reilly 3rd HF, et al. Endoscopic Nd:YAG laser with aggressive multimodality therapy for locally advanced esophageal cancer. *Gastrointest Endosc.* 2002;55:674–679.
49. Akhtar K, Byrne JP, Bancewicz J, et al. Argon beam plasma coagulation in the management of cancers of the esophagus and stomach. *Surg Endosc.* 2000;14:1127–1130.

50. Wahab PJ, Mulder CJ, den Hartog G, et al. Argon plasma coagulation in flexible gastrointestinal endoscopy: pilot experiences. *Endoscopy.* 1997;29:176–181.

51. Manner H, May A, Rabenstein T, et al. Prospective evaluation of a new high-power argon plasma coagulation system (hp-APC) in therapeutic gastrointestinal endoscopy. *Scand J Gastroenterol.* 2007;42:397–405.

52. Manner H, May A, Faerber M, et al. Safety and efficacy of a new high power argon plasma coagulation system (hp-APC) in lesions of the upper gastrointestinal tract. *Dig Liver Dis.* 2006;38:471–478.

53. Filip AG, Clichici S, Daicoviciu D, et al. Photodynamic therapy–indications and limits in malignant tumors treatment. *Rom J Intern Med.* 2008;46:285–293.

54. Monga SP, Wadleigh R, Sharma A, et al. Intratumoral therapy of ciplatin/epinephrine injectable gel for palliation patients with obstructive esophageal cancer. *Am J Clin Oncol.* 2000;23:386–392.

55. Gossner L, May A, Sroka R, et al. A new long-range through-the-scope balloon applicator for photodynamic therapy in the esophagus and cardia. *Endoscopy.* 1999;31:370–376.

56. Wang KK. Current status of photodynamic therapy of Barrett's esophagus. *Gastrointest Endosc.* 1999;49(suppl):20–23.

57. van den Bergh H. On the evolution of some endoscopic light delivery systems for photodynamic therapy. *Endoscopy.* 1998;30:392–407.

58. Panjehpour M, Overholt BF, Haydek JM. Light sources and delivery devices for photodynamic therapy in the gastrointestinal tract. *Gastrointest Endosc Clin North Am.* 2000;10:513–532.

59. Luketich JD, Christie NA, Buenaventura PO, et al. Endoscopic photodynamic therapy for obstructing esophageal cancer: 77 cases over a 2-year period. *Surg Endosc.* 2000;14:653–657.

60. Overholt BF, Panjehpour M. Photodynamic therapy for Barrett's esophagus. *Gastrointest Endosc Clin North Am.* 1997;7:207–220.

61. Likier HM, Levine JG, Lightdale CJ. Photodynamic therapy for completely obstructing esophageal carcinoma. *Gastrointest Endosc.* 1991;37:75–78.

62. Lightdale CJ, Heier SK, Marcon NE, et al. Photodynamic therapy with porfimer sodium versus thermal ablation therapy with Nd:YAG laser for palliation of esophageal cancer: a multicenter randomized trial. *Gastrointest Endosc.* 1995;42:507–512.

63. Heier SK, Rothman KA, Heier LM, et al. Photodynamic therapy for obstructing esophageal cancer: light dosimetry and randomized comparison with Nd:YAG laser therapy. *Gastroenterology.* 1995;109:63–72.

64. Sarper A, Oz N, Cihangir C, et al. The efficacy of self-expanding metal stents for palliation of malignant esophageal strictures and fistulas. *Eur J Cardiothorac Surg.* 2003;23:794–798.

65. Agustsson T, Nilsson M, Henriksson G, et al. Treatment of postoperative esophagorespiratory fistulas with dual self-expanding metal stents. *World J Surg.* 2009;33:1224–1228.

66. Winkelbauer FW, Schöfl R, Niederle B, et al. Palliative treatment of obstructing esophageal cancer with nitinol stents: value, safety, and long-term results. *AJR Am J Roentgenol.* 1996;166:79–84.

67. Neyaz Z, Srivastava DN, Thulkar S, et al. Radiological evaluation of covered self-expandable metallic stents used for palliation in patients with malignant esophageal strictures. *Acta Radiol.* 2007;48:156–164.

68. Rathore OI, Coss A, Patchett SE, et al. Direct-vision stenting: the way forward for malignant oesophageal obstruction. *Endoscopy.* 2006;38:382–384.

69. Ross WA, Alkassab F, Lynch PM, et al. Evolving role of self-expanding metal stents in the treatment of malignant dysphagia and fistulas. *Gastrointest Endosc.* 2007;65:70–76.

70. Maroju NK, Anbalagan P, Kate V, et al. Improvement in dysphagia and quality of life with self-expanding metallic stents in malignant esophageal strictures. *Indian J Gastroenterol.* 2006;25:62–65.

71. Bethge N, Sommer A, Gross U, et al. Human tissue responses to metal stents implanted in vivo for the palliation of malignant stenoses. *Gastrointest Endosc.* 1996;43:596–602.

72. Binmoeller KF, Maeda M, Lieberman D, et al. Silicone-covered expandable metallic stents in the esophagus: an experimental study. *Endoscopy.* 1992;24:416–420.

73. Ko HK, Song HY, Shin JH, et al. Fate of migrated esophageal and gastroduodenal stents: experience in 70 patients. *J Vasc Interv Radiol.* 2007;18:725–732.

74. Bethge N, Knyrim K, Wagner HJ, et al. Self-expanding metal stents for palliation of malignant esophageal obstruction—a pilot study of eight patients. *Endoscopy.* 1992;24:411–415.

75. Ko HK, Song HY, Shin JH, et al. Fate of migrated esophageal and gastroduodenal stents: experience in 70 patients. *J Vasc Interv Radiol.* 2007;18:725–732.

76. Tomaselli F, Maier A, Sankin O, et al. Ultraflex stent—benefits and risks in ultimate palliation of advanced, malignant stenosis in the esophagus. *Hepatogastroenterology.* 2004;51:1021–1026.

77. Homann N, Noftz MR, Klingenberg-Noftz RD, et al. Delayed complications after placement of self-expanding stents in malignant esophageal obstruction: treatment strategies and survival rate. *Dig Dis Sci.* 2008;53:334–340.

78. Wang MQ, Sze DY, Wang ZP, et al. Delayed complications after esophageal stent placement for treatment of malignant esophageal obstructions and esophagorespiratory fistulas. *J Vasc Interv Radiol.* 2001;12:465–474.

79. Verschuur EM, Steyerberg EW, Kuipers EJ, et al. Effect of stent size on complications and recurrent dysphagia in patients with esophageal or gastric cardia cancer. *Gastrointest Endosc.* 2007;65:592–601.

80. Shenfine J, McNamee P, Steen N, et al. A pragmatic randomised controlled trial of the cost-effectiveness of palliative therapies for patients with inoperable oesophageal cancer. *Health Technol Assess.* 2005;iii,1–121.

81. Repici A, Conio M, De Angelis C, et al. Temporary placement of an expandable polyester silicone-covered stent for treatment of refractory benign esophageal strictures. *Gastrointest Endosc.* 2004;60:513–519.

82. Evrard S, Le Moine O, Lazaraki G, et al. Self-expanding plastic stents for benign esophageal lesions. *Gastrointest Endosc.* 2004;60:894–900.

83. Schubert D, Scheidbach H, Kuhn R, et al. Endoscopic treatment of thoracic esophage anastomotic leaks by using silicone-covered, self-expanding polyester stents. *Gastrointest Endos.* 2005;61:891–896.

84. Müldner A, Reinshagen K, Wüstner M, et al. Modified self-expanding plastic stent for the treatment of refractory benign esophageal strictures. *Endoscopy.* 2005;37:925.

85. Costamagna G, Shah A, Tringali A, et al. Prospective evaluation of a new self-expanding plastic stent for inoperable esophageal strictures. *Surg Endosc.* 2003;17:891–895.

86. Petruzziello L, Costamagna G. Stenting in esophageal strictures. *Dig Dis.* 2002;20:154–166.

87. Gelbmann CM, Ratiu NL, Rath HC, et al. Use of self-expandable plastic stents for the treatment of esophageal perforations and symptomatic anastomotic leaks. *Endoscopy.* 2004;36:695–699.

88. Conigliaro R, Battaglia G, Repici A, et al. Polyflex stents for malignant oesophageal and oesophagogastric stricture: a prospective, multicentric study. *Eur J Gastroenterol Hepatol.* 2007;19:195–203.

89. Ott C, Ratiu N, Endlicher E, et al. Self-expanding Polyflex plastic stents in esophageal disease: various indications, complications, and outcomes. *Surg Endosc.* 2007;21:889–896.

90. Radecke K, Gerken G, Treichel U. Impact of a self-expanding, plastic esophageal stent on various esophageal stenoses, fistulas, and leakages: a single-center experience in 39 patients. *Gastrointest Endosc.* 2005;61:812–818.

91. Szegedi L, Gál I, Kósa I, et al. Palliative treatment of esophageal carcinoma with self-expanding plastic stents: a report on 69 cases. *Eur J Gastroenterol Hepatol.* 2006;18:1197–1201.

92. Johnson E, Enden T, Noreng HJ, et al. Survival and complications after insertion of self-expandable metal stents for malignant oesophageal stenosis. *Scand J Gastroenterol.* 2006;41:252–256.

93. Siddiqui AA, Loren D, Dudnick R, et al. Expandable polyester silicon-covered stent for malignant esophageal strictures before neoadjuvant chemoradiation: a pilot study. *Dig Dis Sci.* 2007;52:823–829.

94. Adler DG, Fang J, Wong R, et al. Placement of Polyflex stents in patients with locally advanced esophageal cancer is safe and improves dysphagia during neoadjuvant therapy. *Gastrointest Endosc.* 2009;70:614–619.

95. Langer FB, Wenzl E, Prager G, et al. Management of postoperative esophageal leaks with the Polyflex self-expanding covered plastic stent. *Ann Thorac Surg.* 2005;79:398–403; discussion 404.

96. Gelbmann CM, Ratiu NL, Rath HC, et al. Use of self-expandable plastic stents for the treatment of esophageal perforations and symptomatic anastomotic leaks. *Endoscopy.* 2004;36:695–699.

97. Szegedi L, Gál I, Kósa I, et al. Palliative treatment of esophageal carcinoma with self-expanding plastic stents: a report on 69 cases. *Eur J Gastroenterol Hepatol.* 2006;18:1197–1201.

Constipation during active cancer therapy: Diagnosis and management

Nigel P. Sykes

Active treatment for cancer is often a gruelling experience, marked by a range of distressing symptoms, including fatigue, nausea, vomiting, and hair loss, in degrees varying according to the therapeutic regimen and the supportive measures that are put in place. To these symptoms may be added diarrhea or, conversely, constipation, the subject of this chapter.

DEFINITION

Constipation can be defined in terms of measurable physical variables. For the purposes of gastroenterologic research into idiopathic constipation, a consensus statement on the level of variables that constitute constipation has been drawn up in the Rome Criteria, now in their third iteration.[1] To satisfy the key parts of the definition of constipation, a patient should have had for at least 3 months two or more of the following: straining during at least 25% of defecations, a sensation of anorectal obstruction during at least 25% of defecations, lumpy or hard stools at least 25% of the time, and fewer than three bowel movements per week.

However, people differ in the weights they give to different aspects of this symptom cluster and the length of time over which these have to persist before they consider themselves constipated. Therefore, patients may consider themselves constipated when a doctor using the Rome Criteria would not.[2] The importance of constipation in the context of cancer is as a symptom rather than a disease, and it is therefore appropriate that we should be hearing patients' complaints of constipation and understanding what they mean by them, rather than trying to validate their opinion by comparison with external norms.

At the same time, it is apparent that not all patients recognize in themselves bowel dysfunction that would meet the definition of constipation. Noguera et al[3] found that 13% of their sample had signs and symptoms of constipation but had no complaints about their bowel function. For this reason, they suggest that in cancer, constipation might more appropriately be described as a syndrome rather than a symptom. Both conceptualizations have value.

DIAGNOSIS

The primary evidence for a diagnosis of constipation in cancer care should be the patient's complaint of the problem, illuminated by the patient's account of how key aspects of his bowel function, such as frequency and completeness of defecation, straining at stool, and abdominal or rectal discomfort, have changed from his previous norm. Exceptions include the minority who do not identify constipation in themselves, even though it might be causing symptoms such as nausea, vomiting, or abdominal pain, and those with fecal impaction that has led to overflow, who may complain of diarrhea or fecal or urinary incontinence. The assessing clinician should always be alert to constipation as a possible cause of any of these symptoms, especially in the very young or the very old.

Patients' perceptions of their constipation can be formally assessed with a visual analog (VAS), or adjectival scales or questionnaires. Discrete response modification of the VAS and of an adjectival scale has been found to have validity and to be easy to use in a palliative care setting.[4] Because active cancer treatment may be associated with diarrhea rather than with constipation, as may efforts to relieve constipation, it is appropriate that any subjective measure of bowel function includes the ability to assess not only constipation but diarrhea as well. This is easily arranged with VAS and adjectival scales but is lacking in the questionnaires that have been validated only for the assessment of constipation.

Among questionnaires, the Constipation Assessment Scale (CAS) of McMillan and Williams has particular relevance for a population undergoing active treatment for cancer in that it was validated by its ability to distinguish between constipation experienced by patients taking morphine and those on a course of vinca alkaloid chemotherapy. The assumption was that opioid-induced constipation would be the more severe. The CAS is an eight-item scale with an average completion time of 2 minutes,[5] but it measures only constipation.

The PAC-SYM (Patient Assessment of Constipation—Symptoms) and the PAC-QOL (Patient Assessment of Constipation—Quality of Life) are related questionnaires directed at the patient's perspective on constipation.[6] The PAC-SYM has three subscales related to stool symptoms, rectal symptoms, and abdominal symptoms, and has been validated in a large (n = 216) sample of chronically constipated subjects but not in a cancer or palliative care population. The PAC-QOL is a constipation-specific quality-of-life measure. The PAC-SYM contains no assessment of diarrhea, although the PAC-QOL has a bowel frequency rating. This tool recognizes that the reason for symptom control is to enable a sense of improved well-being, and the results of interventions may lack clinical relevance if this cannot be demonstrated. McCrea et al[7] placed emphasis on this in their recent review of self-report measures of constipation. However, the issue remains that an absence of constipation does not necessarily imply normal bowel function if a measurement instrument cannot assess diarrhea.

Aspects of bowel function that are objectively measurable by direct assessment are stool frequency and form. Simply counting the number of occasions when some stool has been passed may be misleading in making a diagnosis of the presence or absence of constipation: A frequent loose stool may indicate not diarrhea but severe constipation leading to rectal impaction, with overflow of liquid stool from behind the impacted mass. What is more helpful is to count only episodes of formed stool leading to a sense of reasonably complete rectal evacuation. The basis of comparison is the individual's previous normal pattern, as the range of normal bowel movement frequency is very wide, ranging from 3 to 21 stools per week.[8]

The shape of the stools is a guide to their consistency and has been shown to be correlated with bowel transit time in both idiopathic constipation and palliative care cancer populations.[9,10] With the aid of illustrated charts (Fig. 18-1), patients can estimate stool form reliably for themselves as an adjunct to recording stool frequency.

More invasive methods of constipation assessment exist, but these are of questionable clinical value in oncology. An exception is seen when the combination of abdominal examination to detect fecal masses and rectal examination to detect fecal impaction has not been sufficiently revealing; a plain abdominal radiograph will indicate the extent of colonic fecal loading and may help distinguish severe constipation from malignant obstruction. Scoring systems for radiologic assessment of constipation exist, even within cancer care,[11] but they have been heavily criticized for their unreliability.[12]

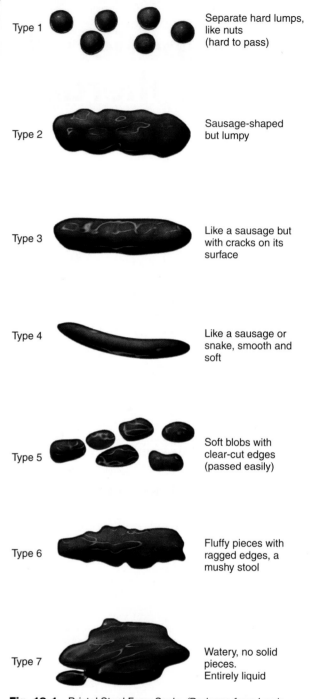

Type 1	Separate hard lumps, like nuts (hard to pass)
Type 2	Sausage-shaped but lumpy
Type 3	Like a sausage but with cracks on its surface
Type 4	Like a sausage or snake, smooth and soft
Type 5	Soft blobs with clear-cut edges (passed easily)
Type 6	Fluffy pieces with ragged edges, a mushy stool
Type 7	Watery, no solid pieces. Entirely liquid

Fig. 18-1 Bristol Stool Form Scale. *(Redrawn from Lewis SJ, Heaton KW. Stool form scale as a useful guide to intestinal transit time. Scand J Gastroenterol 1997;32:920–924.)*

PREVALENCE AND PATHOPHYSIOLOGY

In the general population, around 10% will report that they have constipation. A survey of 93 cancer palliative care inpatients conducted by the author indicated that until they became ill, their bowel function had been typical of the population as a whole. When healthy, just 16% had had any significant difficulty with constipation, and in only 6% had it been persistent. Yet since the onset of their illness, 54% had been constipated at least half the time. Around 50% of patients admitted to a hospice report constipation, but this is certainly short of the true figure in that a proportion will already be taking effective doses of laxatives. Even non–terminally ill cancer patients have increased constipation as one of the indicators distinguishing them from a healthy control group.[13]

Cancer is therefore associated with a marked increase in the likelihood of being constipated. To see why this might be so, it would be helpful to summarize normal gut physiology.

NORMAL INTESTINAL PHYSIOLOGY

Gut contents spend 2 to 4 hours in the small bowel, whereas transit time through the colon is usually 24 to 48 hours and may be considerably longer: Nearly half of a hospice population had transit times of between 4 and 12 days.[10]

About 7 liters of fluid is secreted into the gut each day, to which is added at least 1.5 liters of dietary fluid. Most of this is reabsorbed by the small bowel, especially the jejunum, but more than a liter is left to enter the colon. As daily stool water content is around 200 ml and the difference between constipation and diarrhea in terms of fluid excretion is only about 100 ml/day, the fine tuning of fluid absorption by the colon is very important in maintaining a convenient bowel habit.

NEURAL CONTROL OF INTESTINAL ACTIVITY

Intestinal physiology is complex, involving neural, endocrine, and luminal sources of modulation. Neural control has both intrinsic and extrinsic elements. Cell bodies of the intrinsic nervous system lie in the submucosal ganglia (Meissner's plexus) and the myenteric ganglia (Auerbach's plexus). Broadly speaking, the submucosal plexus is concerned with the modulation of fluid and electrolyte transport, and the myenteric plexus with control of motility, with additional effects on vascular tone and immune responses. Peristalsis occurs as a response to distention of the gut wall and to chemical stimulation of the mucosa by substances such as bile salts or short-chain fatty acids. Its continuance even in chronically denervated bowel shows it to be an intrinsic function of the intestinal neuromuscular system.

The primary neurotransmitters in the intrinsic intestinal neural system seem to be common across species. Acetylcholine (ACh) is the primary neurotransmitter of excitatory motor neurons, but the same neurons also contain tachykinins, and only blockade of both types of receptors completely abolishes excitatory transmission. Inhibitory neurons similarly have co-transmitters, but how these work together remains unclear. Nitric oxide (NO) is probably the primary inhibitory neurotransmitter, but adenosine triphosphate (ATP) and vasoactive intestinal peptide (VIP) are also key contributors to transmission.

Effects on the muscle from excitatory or inhibitory motor neurons are relayed through the interstitial cells of Cajal, which are electrically coupled to the muscle. As well as being intermediaries in the neural pathways to gut muscle, the interstitial cells of Cajal have a pacemaker function that generates the characteristic cyclic activity of gut muscle.

Another key intestinal neurotransmitter is serotonin (5-HT). This is released by the epithelial enterochromaffin cells, which act as sensory transducers to trigger peristaltic or sensory reflexes in response to luminal stimuli. Of the many 5-HT receptor types, those essential for motility are the $5\text{-HT}_{(1P)}$ type, through which submucosal intrinsic primary afferent neurons are stimulated, and 5-HT_4 receptors, which reinforce activity in prokinetic reflex pathways.[14]

The enteric nervous system is influenced by the sympathetic and parasympathetic divisions of the extrinsic nervous system. Sympathetic inflow exerts an inhibitory effect via noradrenaline. Parasympathetic fiber activity promotes peristalsis and increases local blood flow and gut fluid secretion.

PATTERNS OF INTESTINAL MOTILITY

The small intestine has two patterns of activity that between them regulate the speed of gastric emptying in response to epithelial sensitivity to the pH, osmolarity, and chemical composition of the luminal contents. The interdigestive pattern contains the migrating motor complex, in which intense rhythmic contractions of the circular muscle periodically proceed distally along the gut to clear the lumen and reduce bacterial growth. Soon after eating, the interdigestive pattern is replaced by the fed pattern, in which contractile activity is ongoing. About half of these contractions propagate distally for a shorter or a longer distance, both mixing and propelling the small intestinal contents.

The large bowel also displays two main types of motility, but it has no regular sequence of motor patterns such as the migrating motor complex seen in the small bowel. Most colonic contractile activity takes the form of segmental activity.[15] This consists of irregular waves of contraction occurring singly or in bursts. The purpose of the segmental component of large bowel motility appears to be to mix the luminal contents, facilitating absorption of water and nutrients while gradually moving them toward the rectum.

About 6 times per day, high-amplitude propagated contractions occur, corresponding to the phenomenon long known as "mass movements," in which large quantities of intestinal contents are propelled distally over significant distances. High-amplitude contractions are associated with defecation and precede the expulsion of stools; hence they are thought to be one of the major initiators of this process.

INTESTINAL FLUID HANDLING

Bowel function reflects the state of intestinal motility and of intestinal fluid handling, which is the net result of a dynamic state of absorption and secretion in the gut wall. Most secretion occurs from the mucosal crypt cells, and absorption takes place in the villous cells. Through the enteric nervous system, mechanical stimulation of mucosal sensory neurons activates secretion and stimulates blood flow and smooth muscle contraction. 5-HT, substance P, and neurokinins 1 and 2 are involved on the sensory side of the reflex, and VIP is the secretomotor neurotransmitter.[16] The presumed physiologic importance of this linkage consists of enhancement of digestion through greater mixing and dilution of luminal contents, and increased absorption that accompanies an increase in motility. Secretion is principally the result of the active transport of chloride and bicarbonate ions through apical chloride channels.[17]

CAUSES OF CONSTIPATION

Most research into constipation has been carried out in otherwise healthy people who have a functional bowel disorder. For most cancer patients, constipation is related to the onset of their disease. The potential causes of this change in bowel habit can be considered under three headings:

- Factors arising from treatment of the illness
- Factors arising directly from the cancer itself
- Factors associated with the illness but not directly due to it

For patients undergoing active cancer treatment, certain chemotherapy regimens commonly have constipation as an adverse effect, which is said to be a reflection of the drug's neurotoxicity. The cytotoxic agents most commonly associated with constipation are platinum compounds, which affect up to 70% of patients in this way, and vinca alkaloids, with which 35% of users have been reported to become constipated.[18] Both of these classes of drugs cause frequent sensory neuropathies, and it is understandable that research into patterns of nerve damage that they cause has focused on these. The platinum agents damage the neuronal cell body, resulting in anterograde axonal degeneration. The neuropathy can be delayed in its onset, being most severe 3 to 6 months after treatment has stopped, and it can be long lasting, with up to 55% persistence after 15 years.[19] Whether this is the same for the autonomic or myenteric neuropathy to which platinum-related constipation is attributed is not clear. However, a trial of nortriptyline for cisplatin-induced peripheral neuropathy found that the tricyclic increased constipation compared with placebo, but it had little effect on neuropathic discomfort, suggesting that the two aspects of neurotoxicity have different intensities, time courses, or, perhaps, mechanisms.[20]

The cytotoxic action of vinca alkaloids derives from their inhibition of microtubule formation, which destabilizes the mitotic spindle. The neuropathy they cause, which is more likely than with other cytotoxic drugs to cause motor, autonomic, and sensory symptoms, has been shown to be associated with microtubule disruption and consequent blockade of axonal transport through alterations in the cytoskeletal structure of the axon. A direct axonal toxicity effect may be reflected in the relatively rapid improvement in symptoms sometimes seen when treatment ceases.

The taxanes, particularly paclitaxel, have shown a distal sensory neuropathy as a significant dose-limiting factor. This is again attributed to microtubule disruption. Because the taxanes are often given in combination with platinum compounds, the relative neurotoxic effects of the two classes of drugs can be difficult to disentangle, but when given on its own, paclitaxel has been associated with only mild constipation,[21,22] and neither paclitaxel nor docetaxel reversed the diarrhea caused by 5-fluorouracil when given in combination with it.[23]

Among more recently introduced cancer chemotherapies, thalidomide, which acts as an immunomodulatory agent, and

the cell cycle inhibitor bortezomib—both used for multiple myeloma—have precipitated painful sensory neuropathies in 75% and 30% of patients, respectively.[19] An association with increased prevalence of constipation is also noted: 55% (8% severe, i.e., grade 3) for thalidomide and 42% (2% severe) for bortezomib. Lenalidomide, an analog of thalidomide, has shown a level of constipation similar to that of bortezomib.[24] Thalidomide and lenalidomide appear to cause ganglion damage leading to axonal degeneration, whereas multiple mechanisms, including demyelination, microtubule disruption, and inhibition of cytokines and transcription factors, are likely to be involved in the neurotoxicity seen with bortezomib.

A degree of constipation is widely reported in trials of other chemotherapy agents, including apoptosis inducers[25] and recombinant human monoclonal antibodies.[26] In most cases, the severity of constipation attributed to the medication is mild, and several medications can also be associated with diarrhea. This fact and their disparate mechanisms make it uncertain whether the relationship between drug use and symptoms is a causative one. Even in the case of those drugs with an established tendency to cause neuropathies, investigations of the mechanisms involved have not so far led to effective ways to prevent neurotoxicity from occurring.

The complexity of the intestinal serotinergic receptors has already been noted, and although they can also cause diarrhea, constipation is the most common side effect of 5-HT$_3$ antagonist antiemetics, whose introduction revolutionized the control of chemotherapy-induced emesis. The class prototype, ondansetron, has been associated with constipation in up to 23% of users.[27] Its antidiarrheal effects have been proposed as a helpful adjunct to its antiemesis for patients undergoing abdominal radiotherapy.[28] Granisetron has been associated with similar levels of constipation, showing a degree of dose-response relationship,[29] and constipation has also been noted with tropisetron.[30]

Control of pain and other symptoms of cancer must run alongside active treatment of the disease. Opioids remain the most effective family of analgesics for cancer pain but are strongly associated with constipation. In advanced cancer, the use of morphine and other opioids is probably the most important single constipating factor that can be isolated, but a background of widespread constipation arises from debility. Sixty-three percent of advanced cancer patients not taking morphine required laxatives—a figure similar to that reported in the ill elderly—but 87% of those receiving morphine needed them and used a higher average dose.[31]

A physiologic role of intrinsic opioids in the regulation of intestinal function is suggested by the presence of opioid receptors in the bowel and by its extrinsic nervous supply, and by the ability of opioid antagonists to speed gut transit in the absence of exogenous opioids.[32] The neural action of opioids, whether intrinsic or extrinsic, is always to suppress neuronal excitability. Their functional effect is to reduce peristaltic propulsion, because their inhibition of enteric interneurons prevents the integration needed for contractions to be propulsive.

As well as having effects on peristalsis, opioids cause constipation through changes in intestinal fluid handling. In part, these changes result simply from an increase in time available for water absorption because of slowing of the passage of luminal contents. In addition, the presence of opioids causes inhibition of secretomotor neurons, so that less fluid enters the gut. The result is drier, harder, and smaller stools that are more difficult to pass.[33] An additional factor is that opioids reduce sensations of gut distention, including distention of the rectum. This may help to precipitate fecal impaction, especially in older patients in whom rectal sensitivity may already be impaired as a result of aging.

Most opioids are probably similar in their constipating potency. However, evidence suggests that transdermal fentanyl is somewhat less constipating than morphine[34] or oxycodone[35]; the same is probably true of other lipophilic opioids such as buprenorphine and alfentanil that require only relatively small doses to be given to achieve CNS penetration. Reduction in laxative use has been reported after changing from morphine to methadone,[36] and lower laxative requirements are associated with the use of methadone as compared with morphine or hydromorphone.[37] This has been attributed to the fact that the effects of methadone are only partially mediated through opioid receptors as a result of its N-methyl-d-aspartate (NMDA) receptor activity. Tramadol, another opioid with NMDA antagonist properties, is said to be significantly less constipating than morphine but is a significantly less potent analgesic.

A second group of constipation-inducing drugs frequently used in cancer supportive and palliative care consists of those with anticholinergic effects; tricyclics, antihistamines, and neuroleptics all come under this category. Given the role of ACh as the chief stimulant neurotransmitter for peristalsis, it is not hard to see how their constipating effect arises.

FACTORS ARISING DIRECTLY FROM THE CANCER ITSELF

The most common direct constipating effect of cancer is invasion of the gut wall to cause narrowing or obstruction of the lumen, or functional obstruction as a result of tumor infiltration damage to enteric nerves and muscle. Impaired gut motility can also arise from damage to the external neural input to the bowel, through tumor compression of the nerve along its course or weakening of vertebral bodies by metastases, giving rise to spinal cord compression.

Alternatively, the intestinal neural network can be affected as a paraneoplastic phenomenon, particularly in association with small cell carcinoma of the lung and carcinoid tumors.[38] An autoimmune mechanism is implicated, and investigations in small cell lung cancer patients have established a clear link between the presence of polyclonal immunoglobulin (Ig)G antibodies that react with neuronal nuclear proteins in the central nervous system and gastrointestinal paraneoplastic syndromes. It is proposed that damage arises from an immune response to tumor antigens that are also present in neural cells. Affected small cell lung cancer patients tend to have limited stage disease that is sensitive to chemotherapy, and eradication of the tumor is the most effective form of symptom relief. If this is not possible, some patients have required colectomy.

Paraneoplastic constipation is not usually an isolated finding but is accompanied by other neurologic symptoms. In particular, autonomic dysfunction is an underrecognized nonmetastatic manifestation of cancer that may exacerbate constipation in some individuals.[39]

Case report evidence indicates that malignant tumors may cause constipation through the secretion of chemical mediators that have an inhibitory effect on peristalsis. For instance,

severe constipation associated with a carcinoid tumor immunohistochemically positive for peptide YY was relieved by tumor resection.[40] Constipation occurring with small cell lung cancer has been corrected by using the somatostatin analog octreotide, also implying excessive levels of an intrinsic mediator of motility as a cause of impaired intestinal transit.[41]

Hypercalcemia of malignant disease is associated with worsening of constipation. Calcium plays an important part in excitation-contraction coupling of muscle, as well as in stimulus-secretion coupling, in most exocrine and endocrine glands. Although the mechanism is not precisely understood, it is not surprising that disturbance of extracellular calcium levels should have widespread effects on tissue excitability, including intestinal contractility and fluid handling.

FACTORS ASSOCIATED WITH THE ILLNESS BUT NOT DIRECTLY DUE TO IT

Around 75% of cancer patients are over age 60, and whatever influences due to their cancer that may be acting to precipitate constipation are subject to age-related factors that may slow bowel function. A link between advancing age and constipation or increased use of laxatives has been found by some studies[42] but not others.[8] However, a 37% loss of enteric neurons has been found in the colon of people older than 65 years of age compared with those younger than 35,[43] which could contribute to the lengthened colon transit times that have been reported in elderly people and could make this group more susceptible to other constipating factors. Age-associated reduction in rectal sensitivity might predispose to constipation through lack of awareness of a full rectum and hence progression to fecal impaction.[44] Not all parts of the gut are equally affected by aging: Small intestinal transit changes little, as does absorptive or secretory capacity.

Both cancer and its treatment are commonly debilitating, reducing mobility and both dietary and fluid intake. Because colonic mass movements, the chief form of propulsive contractility in the large bowel, are associated with physical activity,[45] it is likely that a reduction in mobility will impair them and contribute to constipation. Evidence from humans suggests faster transit times[46] and more colonic propulsive activity after exercise. However, in healthy adults, constipation is only weakly correlated with the level of physical activity, with increasing exercise being much more likely to improve well-being than to reduce constipation.[47] In a cancer population, the prime motivation for physical rehabilitation will be enhancement of quality of life, with any improvement in constipation being a side benefit.

Many palliative care patients have a degree of anorexia.[48] This tends to result in a reduction in the overall amount of food consumed and a preferential fall in intake of higher-fiber foods. Colonic mass movements are influenced by activity and are associated with food intake, reflecting the action of the gastrocolic reflex by which gastric distention stimulates colonic motility. Also, the intestine contracts if distended; because fiber contributes largely to the bulk of food residues, this source of stimulation of gut activity will be diminished by food with a low fiber content.

Dietary fiber supplementation increases stool weight and decreases transit time in both normal and constipated adults.[49] Unfortunately, the amount of fiber required for effect can be large[42] and can be unpalatable to a cancer population.[50] The effect of fiber on bowel function relies on adequate fluid intake[51] and the amount of fiber itself. Ensuring a daily water intake of at least 1.5 to 2 liters has been shown to have a positive effect complementary to that of dietary fiber in increasing stool frequency and reducing the use of laxatives in healthy adults.[52] If daily fluid volume is diminished, fiber will be less effective, and in this situation, some preparations can give rise to a gelatinous mass in the intestinal tract capable of precipitating or completing an intestinal obstruction.[53] Hence for reasons of both efficacy and safety, a reliance on fiber for the relief of constipation in cancer, particularly in more advanced disease, is inappropriate.

TREATMENT

Little research has been done on the management of constipation in cancer patients, and most of what has been studied is related to palliative care in advanced disease and, particularly, opioid-induced constipation. For patients undergoing active cancer treatment, the AIM (Assessment, Information, and Management) nursing initiative to improve the relief of chemotherapy toxicities includes constipation in its scope.[24,54] A multiplicity of local guidelines have been generated that are principally aimed at cancer palliative care.[55–57] A pan-European consensus guidance document has recently been produced for the same audience[58] (Fig. 18-2). Although not primarily aimed at patients receiving active cancer treatment, these documents are more relevant to their needs than are guidelines that cover the whole of constipation or chronic idiopathic constipation.[59] However, constipation is an area where adherence to guidelines has been shown to be poor even when locally promoted and endorsed,[60] raising doubt as to whether they are an effective way of improving practice.

Most of these guidelines have a common pattern, derived from research where it exists and otherwise from clinical experience, that seems to have bred overall agreement across practitioners in different locations. The first step is to include bowel function in routine patient assessment. A complaint of constipation should then evoke enquiry about not only what symptoms the person is experiencing now, such as decreased stool frequency, straining or pain at defecation, incomplete evacuation, and the need for digital assistance in defecation, but also the pattern of bowel habit they have been used to in the past, bearing in mind that the range of normality is wide. On the other hand, a report of diarrhea, loose stools, or onset of fecal or urinary incontinence should attract diagnostic steps, most importantly abdominal and rectal examination, to exclude severe constipation that has led to fecal impaction with overflow.

A broad approach to symptom management will set the best context for relief of constipation. Thus tackling pain and breathlessness with the aid of both drugs and physiotherapy will maximize mobility; control of nausea and provision of a tailored diet containing as much fiber as tolerable will maximize dietary intake; encouragement of fluids will minimize dehydration; and the sum effect of all these interventions will be to normalize as far as possible the working environment of the gut.

Despite these measures, many patients—most by the later stages of cancer—will need drug assistance to avoid constipation. Some will wish to use nonpharmacologic methods initially or on an ongoing basis. Herbal remedies may contain the same types of chemicals as pharmaceutical laxatives and so will have similar effectiveness, albeit less predictable because less standardized. However, little or no evidence has been found for other complementary treatment approaches, whose principal contribution is likely to be geared to the overall sense of well-being of patients rather than to specific relief of their constipation. The best support has been obtained for abdominal massage, which can equal the effect of a regular laxative regimen but at a significantly greater cost in terms of staff time.[61]

It seems generally accepted that it is worth classifying the predominant action of laxative agents as softening the stool or stimulating peristalsis, and that, although initially a softening laxative alone may be adequate, more severe constipation tends to respond best to a combination of the two types. This conclusion originates from clinical experience but has received some experimental support from a comparison of stimulant and softening laxatives given alone or in combination in a model of opioid-induced constipation. In this study, the combination resulted in fewest adverse effects, such as colic, and the least medication burden.[62] This is not to claim that a combination of stimulant and softening laxatives is more effective than either type alone at relieving constipation; any of the laxatives tried could restore bowel function if a sufficient volume was swallowed and side effects were endured with enough stoicism. A systematic review of laxative use in the elderly came to a similar conclusion, finding that any laxative would increase bowel frequency by about 1.4 stools/wk compared with placebo.[63] Given the lack of evidence of true differences in efficacy, the choice of laxative should be strongly influenced by patient preference and by cost.

STIMULANT LAXATIVES

Examples include senna, bisacodyl, danthron, and sodium picosulfate. These drugs differ principally in the extent to which they require activation by colonic bacteria and are subject to hepatic recirculation. They all act on the myenteric plexus to stimulate intestinal contraction. Concerns about carcinogenicity with continued use appear to be unsupported in practice.[64] However, danthron is subject to a limited license in some countries for this reason and has the potential to cause perianal skin rash in incontinent patients.

$5-HT_4$ agonists, of which tegaserod is currently licensed in some countries, may also be considered stimulant laxatives because they increase motility by reinforcing normal enteric neuronal stimulation of peristalsis.[65] Whether they are effective in situations where the enteric nervous system is damaged, as in some cases of cancer-related constipation, has not been demonstrated.

SOFTENING LAXATIVES

All these preparations primarily soften the stool, making it easier to pass, but they do so by different mechanisms.

- *Osmotic* agents retain water within the gut lumen. Sugars, such as lactulose, act in their native form in the small bowel before they are broken down by colonic flora to organic acids, whose pH-lowering effect is speculated to enhance motility and secretion. In practice, lactulose is a relatively

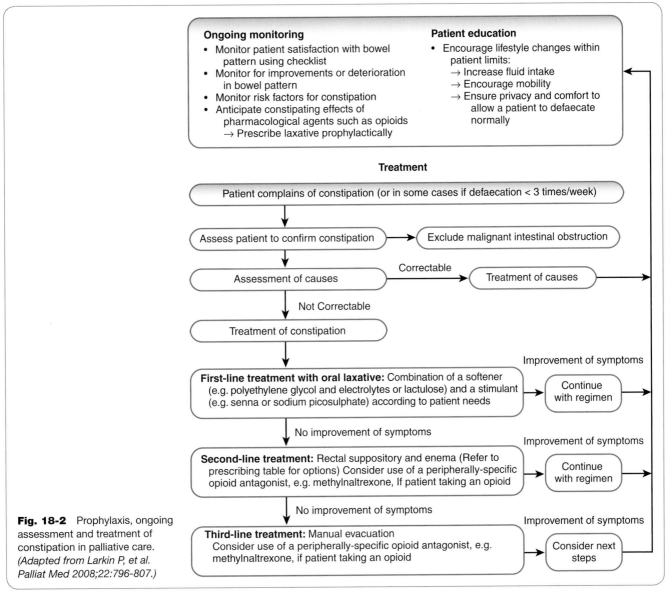

Fig. 18-2 Prophylaxis, ongoing assessment and treatment of constipation in palliative care. *(Adapted from Larkin P, et al. Palliat Med 2008;22:796-807.)*

weak laxative that gives rise to flatulence in about 20% of patients. Conversely, inorganic osmotic substances such as magnesium hydroxide or sulphate are not absorbed and so maintain their osmotic potency throughout the intestine. They appear capable of stimulating peristalsis and at higher doses cause a pronounced purgative effect.

- *Surfactants* such as docusate or poloxamer increase water penetration of the stools. Docusate also promotes water, sodium, and chloride secretion in the jejunum and colon; a clinical impression suggests that at higher doses, it may stimulate peristalsis.

- *Macrogols* render water unabsorbable by the gut. Their effect therefore depends on the volume of water in which they are dissolved. Secondarily, this contributes to stimulation of gut contraction as a reflex response to distention. Macrogols have been shown to be an effective oral treatment for fecal impaction, but this may require the daily consumption of a liter of the solution, which not all patients can tolerate.[66]

- *Chloride channel activators* include lubiprostone, which to date is the only example of this mode of action. Acting on

type 2 chloride channels on the apical surface of the luminal epithelium, it increases secretions without electrolyte disturbance. A secondary effect on motility is claimed, and small and large bowel transit is accelerated.[67]

- *Bulk-forming agents* increase the size of stools in part by providing material that resists bacterial breakdown and hence remains in the gut, and in part by providing a substrate for bacterial growth and gas production. Effective in mild constipation, they are less helpful in cancer patients, as they need to be taken with at least 200 to 300 ml water, which, together with their consistency, is unacceptable to many people who feel unwell. If taken with inadequate water, a viscous mass may result, which can complete an incipient malignant obstruction. Their effectiveness in severe constipation is doubtful.

The key to using general laxatives such as those mentioned above is to titrate the dose against response. This implies that some disciplined follow-up of patients' perception of their bowel function is in place, preferably assisted by recording the frequency and types of bowel actions passed. A softening laxative alone may be adequate initially, but for more resistant constipation, the addition of a stimulant agent is likely to be needed, although a macrogol may be capable of meeting the challenge if a sufficiently high dose can be tolerated.

RECTAL LAXATIVES

If oral laxatives are inadequate, recourse can include rectal interventions such as suppositories, enemas, or, in the last resort and with appropriate analgesia and sedation, manual evacuation of the rectum. Anything introduced into the rectum may induce defecation via the anocolic reflex, but suppositories may have an osmotic softening action (glycerine or sodium phosphate) or may stimulate peristalsis (bisacodyl). Enemas may lubricate (olive or arachis oils) or soften via osmotic (sorbitol, sodium phosphate, sodium citrate) or surfactant (sodium docusate, sodium lauryl, or alkyl sulphoacetate) actions. Attention to laxative dosing can halve the use of enemas and suppositories.[68] This is important not only because of the staff time involved but also because rectal laxatives are widely disliked; only 17% prefer suppositories or enemas to oral laxatives. Nevertheless, it has been reported that among late-stage cancer patients, 72% have received suppositories and 65% an enema, with no less than 40% continuing to receive them on an ongoing basis.[69]

SPECIFIC THERAPIES FOR OPIOID-INDUCED CONSTIPATION

Limitations of existing general laxatives have led to interest in finding specific agents for opioid-induced constipation. Because the constipating action of opioids is predominantly peripheral in man, mediated via opioid receptors in the gut itself, an opioid antagonist could prevent or relieve this, provided it did not reach the opioid receptors in the central nervous system responsible for analgesia. Two preparations are currently licensed for this indication. Methylnaltrexone is a quaternary derivative of the mu-opioid antagonist naltrexone; the modification to the molecule confers on it a polarity that prevents it from crossing the blood-brain barrier. It is administered by subcutaneous injection and, in a series of 134 patients who were taking regular opioids and had advanced disease, just over half with cancer, was significantly ($P < .0001$) more likely than placebo to induce a bowel action. The median time to response was 0.5 hours.[70] A patient who responded to an initial dose of methylnaltrexone had a 57% to 100% chance of responding to subsequent doses. For patients who had not responded to the first dose, the chance of a bowel movement response to a second dose was 35%, and for those who had not responded to either of the first two doses, a 26% response rate to a third dose was reported.[71] If no response has been obtained after three methylnaltrexone doses, it is appropriate to seek other remedies. The overall response rate in this sample was about 50%, probably indicating the important role of other constipating factors even when opioids are involved. The observed adverse effects did not suggest any methylnaltrexone antagonism of central effects of opioids.

Methylnaltrexone appears appropriate to use when constipation is associated with opioid use, when it has not been satisfactorily controlled with general laxatives by mouth, and an enema or suppositories are being considered (see Fig. 18-2). For a few people, methylnaltrexone may become their routine therapy for constipation, but the excess cost over existing laxatives is considerable, and it seems likely that for most patients, the role of methylnaltrexone will be to remove an accumulation of stool and allow a fresh start to be made on laxative therapy to establish an effective regimen.

Naloxone is the best-established mu-opioid antagonist, but earlier work with this drug, used orally for opioid-induced constipation, found an unacceptable incidence of precipitation of opioid withdrawal or return of pain, despite having only 1% to 3% bioavailability by this route.[72] However, an oral sustained-release combination of oxycodone and naloxone in a fixed 2:1 dose ratio has been licensed as an analgesic with the claimed advantage in the United States of reducing the risk of opioid abuse, and in Europe of reducing the risk of opioid-induced constipation. Evidence suggests that it reduces the subjective severity of constipation and increases bowel movement frequency.[73] Within the narrow dose range tested and licensed, no significant excess of opioid withdrawal effects has occurred, perhaps as a result of the lower peak of naloxone absorption achieved with the sustained-release mechanism rather than the immediate-release formulation employed in previous studies. It might be noted that the low oral bioavailability of naloxone depends on rapid metabolism by the liver; in hepatic impairment, blood levels can be very much greater. The oxycodone/naloxone preparation has been studied in an otherwise healthy population with chronic pain, whose liver function might be expected to be intact, rather than in people with cancer, in whom it might not be intact. At present, it appears wise to be selective when using an oxycodone/naloxone combination in patients with cancer.

CONCLUSION

Most people with cancer do not start out with constipation, but many will experience it as a result of factors related to the disease or its treatment. Constipation has been reported to rank with pain as a source of distress in cancer,[74] is associated with depression in cancer patients,[75] and is linked with higher healthcare costs.[76] Proper assessment and management of this condition is therefore an intrinsic part of adequate supportive care for cancer patients, whatever their disease stage. Many treatments are available, but evidence indicates that they are all too often inadequately applied. For the subset of patients in whom opioids are an important factor in their constipation, specific therapy is now available that could improve comfort substantially in selected patients, but again, only if the condition is sought out and a management plan formulated that has regard for the individuality of the person concerned and is followed by ongoing monitoring of its success.

REFERENCES

1. Longstreth GF, Thompson WG, Chey WD, et al. Functional bowel disorders. *Gastroenterology.* 2006;130:1480–1491.
2. Probert CSJ, Emmett PM, Cripps HA, et al. Evidence for the ambiguity of the word constipation: the role of irritable bowel syndrome. *Gut.* 1994;35:1455–1458.
3. Noguera A, Centeno C, Librada S, et al. Screening for constipation in palliative care patients. *J Palliat Med.* 2009;12:915–920.
4. Sykes NP. Methods for clinical research in constipation. In: Max M, Lynn J, eds. Interactive textbook on clinical symptom research. Bethesda, MD: National Institutes of Dental and Craniofacial Research; 2001. Available at: http://painconsortium. nih.gov/symptomresearch/chapter_3/sec5/ cnss5popadjectivals.htm.
5. McMillan SC, Williams FA. Validity and reliability of the Constipation Assessment Scale. *Cancer Nurs.* 1989;12:183–188.
6. Frank L, Kleinman L, Farup C, et al. Psychometric validation of a constipation assessment questionnaire. *Scand J Gastroenterol.* 1999;34:870–877.
7. McCrea GL, Miaskowski C, Stotts NA, et al. Review article: self-report measures to evaluate constipation. *Aliment Pharmacol Ther.* 2008;27:638–648.
8. Connell AM, Hilton C, Irvine G, et al. Variation in bowel habit in two population samples. *Br Med J.* 1965;ii:1095–1099.
9. O'Donnell LJD, Virjee J, Heaton KW. Detection of pseudodiarrhoea by simple clinical assessment of intestinal transit rate. *Br Med J.* 1990;300:439–440.
10. Sykes NP. Methods of assessment of bowel function in patients with advanced cancer. *Palliat Med.* 1990;4:287–292.
11. Bruera E, Suarez-Almazor M, Velasco A, et al. The assessment of constipation in terminal cancer patients admitted to a Palliative Care Unit. *J Pain Symptom Manage.* 1994;9:515–519.
12. Jackson CR, Lee RE, Wylie AB, et al. Diagnostic accuracy of the Barr and Blethyn radiological scoring systems for childhood constipation assessed using colonic transit time as the gold standard. *Pediatr Radiol.* 2009;39:664–667.
13. Trabal J, Leyes P, Forga MT, et al. Quality of life, dietary intake and nutritional status assessment in hospital admitted cancer patients. *Nutr Hosp.* 2006;21:505–510.
14. Gershon MD. Review article: serotonin receptors and transporters—roles in normal and abnormal gastrointestinal motility. *Aliment Pharmacol Ther.* 2004;20(suppl 7):3–14.
15. Bassotti G, de Roberto G, Castellani D, et al. Normal aspects of colorectal motility and abnormalities in slow transit constipation. *World J Gastroenterol.* 2005;11:2691–2696.
16. Cooke HJ, Sidhu M, Wang YZ. Activation of 5-HT1P receptors on submucosal afferents subsequently triggers VIP neurons and chloride secretion in the guinea-pig colon. *J Autonom Nerv Syst.* 1997;66:105–110.
17. Banks MR, Farthing MJ. Fluid and electrolyte transport in the small intestine. *Curr Opin Gastroenterol.* 2002;18:176–181.
18. Smith S. Evidence-based management of constipation in the oncology patient. *Eur J Oncol Nurs.* 2001;5:18–25.
19. Park SB, Krishnan AV, Lin C, et al. Mechanisms underlying chemotherapy-induced neurotoxicity and the potential for neuroprotective strategies. *Curr Med Chem.* 2008;15:3081–3094.

20. Hammack JE, Michalak JC, Loprinzi CL, et al. Phase III evaluation of nortriptyline for alleviation of symptoms of cis-platinum-induced peripheral neuropathy. *Pain.* 2002;98:195–203.
21. Hirai Y, Hasumi K, Onose R, et al. Phase II trial of 3-h infusion of paclitaxel in patients with adenocarcinoma of endometrium: Japanese Multicenter Study Group. *Gynecol Oncol.* 2004;94:471–476.
22. Byrd L, Thistlethwaite FC, Clamp A, et al. Weekly paclitaxel in the treatment of recurrent ovarian carcinoma. *Eur J Gynaecol Oncol.* 2007;28:174–178.
23. Park SH, Lee WK, Chung M, et al. Paclitaxel versus docetaxel for advanced gastric cancer: a randomized phase II trial in combination with infusional 5-fluorouracil. *Anticancer Drugs.* 2006;17:225–229.
24. Smith LC, Bertolotti P, Curran K, et al. Gastrointestinal side effects associated with novel therapies in patients with multiple myeloma: consensus statement of the IMF Nurse Leadership Board. *Clin J Oncol Nurs.* 2008;12(suppl 37–52):1092–1095.
25. Kitzen JJ, de Jonge MJA, Lamers CH, et al. Phase I dose-escalation study of F60008, a novel apoptosis inducer, in patients with advanced solid tumours. *Eur J Cancer.* 2009;45:1764–1772.
26. Motl S. Bevacizumab in combination chemotherapy for colorectal and other cancers. *Am J Health-Syst Pharm.* 2005;62:1021–1032.
27. Chiou T-J, Tzeng W-F, Wang W-S, et al. Comparison of the efficacy and safety of oral granisetron plus dexamethasone with intravenous ondansetron plus dexamethasone to control nausea and vomiting induced by moderate/severe emetogenic chemotherapy. *Chinese Med J (Taipei).* 2000;63:729–736.
28. Henriksson R, Lomberg H, Israelsson G, et al. The effect of ondansetron on radiation-induced emesis and diarrhoea. *Acta Oncol.* 1992;31:767–769.
29. Martoni A, Piana E, Strocchi E, et al. Comparative crossover trial of two intravenous doses of Granisetron (1 mg vs 3 mg) + Dexamethasone in the prevention of acute Cis-platinum-induced emesis. *Anticancer Res.* 1998;18(4 B):2799–2803.
30. Otten J, Hachimi-Idrissi S, Balduck N, et al. Prevention of emesis by tropisetron (Navoban) in children receiving cytotoxic therapy for solid malignancies. *Semin Oncol.* 1994;21(suppl 9):17–19.
31. Sykes NP. The relationship between opioid use and laxative use in terminally ill cancer patients. *Palliat Med.* 1998;12:375–382.
32. Yuan CS, Doshan H, Charney MR, et al. Tolerability, gut effects and pharmacokinetics of methylnaltrexone following repeated intravenous administration in humans. *J Clin Pharmacol.* 2005;45:538–546.
33. Bannister JJ, Davison P, Timms JM, et al. Effect of stool size and consistency on defecation. *Gut.* 1987;28:1246–1250.
34. Radbruch L, Sabatowski R, Loick G, et al. Constipation and the use of laxatives: a comparison between transdermal fentanyl and oral morphine. *Palliat Med.* 2000;14:111–119.
35. Ackerman SJ, Knight T, Schein J, et al. Risk of constipation in patients prescribed fentanyl transdermal system or oxycodone hydrochloride controlled-release in a California Medicaid population. *Consult Pharm.* 2004;19:118–132.
36. Daeninck PJ, Bruera E. Reduction in constipation and laxative requirements following opioid

rotation to methadone. *J Pain Symptom Manage.* 1999;18:303–309.
37. Mancini IL, Hanson J, Neumann CM, et al. Opioid type and other predictors of laxative dose in advanced cancer patients: a retrospective study. *J Palliat Med.* 2000;3:49–56.
38. Jun S, Dimyan M, Jones KD, et al. Obstipation as a paraneoplastic presentation of small cell lung cancer: case report and literature review. *Neurogasterenterol Motil.* 2005;17:16–22.
39. Walsh D, Nelson KA. Autonomic nervous system dysfunction in advanced cancer. *Support Care Cancer.* 2002;10:523–528.
40. Utsumi N, Havasaka T, et al. Ovarian carcinoid exhibiting double function. *Pathol Int.* 2003;53:191–194.
41. Sorhaug S, Steinshamn SL, Waldum HL. Octreotide treatment for paraneoplastic intestinal pseudo-obstruction complicating SCLC. *Lung Cancer.* 2005;48:137–140.
42. Richmond JP, Wright ME. Review of the literature on constipation to enable development of a constipation risk assessment scale. *Clin Effect Nurs.* 2004;8:11–25.
43. Gomes OA, de Souza RR, Liberti EA. A preliminary investigation of ageing on the nerve cell number in the myenteric ganglia of the human colon. *Gerontology.* 1997;43:210–217.
44. Read NW, Abouzekry I, Read MG, et al. Anorectal function in elderly patients with faecal impaction. *Gastroenterology.* 1985;89:959–966.
45. Holdstock DJ, Misiewicz JJ, Smithy T, et al. Propulsion (mass movements) in the human colon and its relationship to meals and somatic activity. *Gut.* 1970;11:91–99.
46. Cordain L, Latin RW, Behnke JJ. The effects of an aerobic running program on bowel transit time. *J Sport Med.* 1986;26:101–104.
47. Tuteja AK, Talley NJ, Joos SK, et al. Is constipation associated with decreased physical activity in normally active subjects? *Am J Gastroenterol.* 2005;100:124–129.
48. Addington-Hall J, McCarthy M. Dying from cancer: results of a national population based investigation. *Palliat Med.* 1995;9:295–305.
49. Muller-Lissner SA. Effect of wheat bran on weight of stool and gastrointestinal transit time. *Br Med J.* 1988;296:615–617.
50. Mumford SP. Can high fibre diets improve the bowel function in patients on radiotherapy ward? In: Twycross RG, Lack SA, eds. *Control of alimentary symptoms in far advanced cancer.* London: Churchill Livingstone; 1986:183.
51. Ouellet LL, Turner TR, Pond S, et al. Dietary fiber and laxation in postop orthopaedic patients. *Clin Nurs Res.* 1996;5:428–440.
52. Anti M, Pignataro G, Armuzzi A, et al. Water supplementation enhances the effect of high-fiber diet on stool frequency and laxative consumption in adult patients with functional constipation. *Hepatogastroenterology.* 1998;45:727–732.
53. Waud SP. Fecal impaction due to a hygroscopic gum laxative. *Am J Digest Dis.* 1940;7:297–298.
54. Moore K, Johnson G, Fortner BV, et al. New procedures implemented for assessment, information and management of chemotherapy toxicities in community oncology clinics. *Clin J Oncol Nursing.* 2008;12:229–238.
55. Cambridge and Huntingdon Palliative Care Group. Factsheet 12 on palliative care: constipation. 2008. February, Available at: www.arthurrankhouse.nhs. uk/documents/Factsheets/Factsheet_12.pdf.

56. Pan-Glasgow Palliative Care Algorithm Group. Constipation in palliative care. 2007. June, Available at: http://www.palliativecareggc.org.uk/uploads/file/guidelines/algorithms/Constipation.pdf.

57. Scragg SFife Palliative Care Guidelines Group. Guidelines for the control of constipation in patients with cancer. 2008. December, Available at: www.fifeadtc.scot.nhs.uk/.../Control_of_Constipation_in_Patients_with_Cancer.pdf.

58. Larkin P, Sykes N, Centeno C, et al. The management of constipation in palliative care: clinical practice recommendations. *Palliat Med.* 2008;22:796–807.

59. Constipation World Gastroenterology Organisation. World Gastroenterology Organisation practice guidelines. 2007. Available at: http://www.worldgastroenterology.org/assets/downloads/en/pdf/guidelines/05_constipation.pdf.

60. Lanza P, Carey M. The impact of opioid and laxative prescribing habits on constipation in the primary care setting before and after the introduction of SIGN 44: control of pain in patients with cancer. *Primary Health Care Research and Development.* 2006;7:3–9.

61. Emly M, Cooper S, Vail A. Colonic motility in profoundly disabled people: a comparison of massage and laxative therapy in the management of constipation. *Physiotherapy.* 1998;84:178–183.

62. Sykes NP. A volunteer model for the comparison of laxatives in opioid-induced constipation. *J Pain Symptom Manage.* 1997;11:363–369.

63. Petticrew M, Watt I, Sheldon T. Systematic review of the effectiveness of laxatives in the elderly. *Health Technol Assess.* 1997;1:1–52.

64. Nusko G, Schneider B, Schneider I, et al. Anthranoid laxative use is not a risk factor for colorectal neoplasia: results of a prospective case control study. *Gut.* 2000;46:651–655.

65. Kamm MA, Muller-Lissner S, Talley NJ, et al. Tegaserod for the treatment of chronic constipation: a randomised, double-blind, placebo-controlled trial. *Am J Gastroenterol.* 2005;100:362–372.

66. Culbert P, Gillett H, Ferguson A. Highly effective new oral therapy for faecal impaction. *Br J Gen Pract.* 1998;48:1599–1600.

67. Camilleri M, Bharucha AE, Ueno R, et al. Effect of a selective chloride channel activator, lubiprostone, on gastrointestinal transit, gastric sensory, and motor functions in healthy volunteers. *Am J Physiol Gastrointest Liver Physiol.* 2006;290:G942–G947.

68. Sykes NP. A clinical comparison of laxatives in a hospice. *Palliat Med.* 1991;5:307–314.

69. Droney J, Ross J, Gretton S, et al. Constipation in cancer patients on morphine. *Support Care Cancer.* 2008;16:453–459.

70. Thomas J, Karver S, Cooney GA, et al. A randomised, placebo-controlled trial of subcutaneous methylnaltrexone for the treatment of opioid-induced constipation in patients with advanced illness. *N Engl J Med.* 2008;358:2332–2334.

71. Chamberlain BH, Cross K, Winston JL, et al. Methylnaltrexone treatment of opioid-induced constipation in patients with advanced illness. *J Pain Symptom Manage.* 2009;38:683–690.

72. Sykes NP. Using oral naloxone in the management of opioid bowel dysfunction. In: Yuan CS, ed. *Handbook of opioid bowel syndrome.* New York: Haworth; 2005:175–195.

73. Vondrackova D, Leyendecker P, Meissner W, et al. Analgesic efficacy and safety of oxycodone in combination with naloxone as prolonged release tablets in patients with moderate to severe chronic pain. *J Pain.* 2008;9:1144–1154.

74. Dunlop GM. A study of the relative frequency and importance of gastrointestinal symptoms and weakness in patients with far advanced cancer: student paper. *Palliat Med.* 1989;4:37–44.

75. Mystakidou K, Tsilika E, Parpa E, et al. Assessment of anxiety and depression in advanced cancer patients and their relationship with quality of life. *Qual Life Res.* 2005;14:1825–1833.

76. Candrilli SD, Davis KL, Iyer S. Impact of constipation on opioid use patterns, health care resource utilization, and costs in cancer patients on opioid therapy. *J Pain Palliat Care Pharmacother.* 2009;23:231–241.

Insomnia

19

Josée Savard

PREVALENCE

Sleep disturbances are among the most common symptoms reported by cancer patients. Early cross-sectional studies, mainly conducted in the posttreatment phase, revealed that between 30% and 50% of cancer patients report sleep difficulties. More recent epidemiologic evidence from large-scale longitudinal studies suggests that these rates may be even higher in patients undergoing cancer treatment, at least in certain subgroups of patients. Overall, rates reported in cancer patients appear to be at least 2 to 3 times higher than in the general population. Only a few studies have been conducted to objectify these subjective complaints of poor sleep in cancer patients using polysomnography or actigraphy. These studies have identified several sleep impairments associated with cancer that are consistent with an insomnia disorder.

SUBJECTIVE MEASURES
Cross-sectional studies

Dozens of cross-sectional studies have assessed the presence of sleep impairments in cancer patients. The findings of these surveys have been summarized in several review papers.[1,2] Overall, they suggest that 30% to 50% of cancer patients complain of sleep difficulties, and that nearly 20% meet the diagnostic criteria for an insomnia syndrome, although this last issue has received much less attention. However, these studies were characterized by several limitations, including the use of small, convenient samples and of sleep measures composed of one or a small number of items, and the fact that sleep was often assessed in the posttreatment phase, in many cases, several years later. Also, because of their cross-sectional nature, these studies do not provide any information on the natural course of sleep impairments (incidence, remission, persistence) throughout the cancer care trajectory and beyond.

Longitudinal studies

In recent years, an increasing number of longitudinal studies on the psychosocial aspects of cancer treatments have integrated measures of sleep disturbances. It is difficult to draw general conclusions because some of these studies found a general decrease in sleep disturbances over time,[3,4] and others revealed relatively stable scores.[5,6] Moreover, the vast majority of these studies used small samples of patients with specific cancer sites. They also assessed sleep at different phases of the cancer trajectory and in patients receiving various treatment regimens, making comparisons across studies virtually impossible. Besides, most studies used sleep quality items from general quality of life (e.g., EORTC Quality of Life Questionnaire) or physical symptoms questionnaires (e.g., Symptom Distress Scale), which do not distinguish the presence of clinically significant sleep impairments.

Therefore, large-scale longitudinal studies, conducted in patients with heterogeneous cancer sites, were clearly needed to better assess the differential prevalence of insomnia across cancer sites and its evolution over time. Our research team has just completed such a study in 991 nonmetastatic patients awaiting surgery for mixed cancer sites (breast, 47.0%; prostate, 27.1%; gynecologic, 11.9%; head and neck, 2.3%; urinary and gastrointestinal, 8.2%; other, 3.4%). Patients were assessed at baseline (T1; i.e., during the perioperative phase) and 2 (T2), 6 (T3), 10 (T4), 14 (T5), and 18 (T6) months later. Results on the first two time points were recently published.[7] At T1, 59.5% had insomnia symptoms; among these, 28.5% of patients met the diagnostic criteria for an insomnia syndrome, established using a phone interview. Patients were considered to have an insomnia syndrome when they met the criteria listed in Table 19-1, or when they were using a hypnotic medication 3 or more nights/wk for at least 1 month. Although these rates decreased to 48.4% and 22.2%, respectively, at T2, they remained much higher than in the general population. Findings indicated an overall incidence rate of 18.6%, a persistence rate of 68.0%, and a remission rate of 32.0% between T1 and T2. Together, these data suggest that insomnia is particularly prevalent in the perioperative phase. Whether these elevated rates at the time of surgery are attributable to the surgery per se (e.g., hospitalization, postsurgery pain) or to the psychological reaction to the surgical procedure or the cancer diagnosis established not too long beforehand remains to be investigated.

Our study also revealed striking differences across cancer sites, with breast (T1, 69.6%; T2, 59.6%) and gynecologic (T1, 68.2%; T2, 49.4%) cancer patients having the highest prevalence rates of insomnia symptoms, and prostate cancer patients having the lowest (T1, 37.8%; T2, 27.8%). Given that gender does not appear to fully explain these differences, based on complementary analyses performed, the reasons for these differential rates have yet to be found. Incidence rates from T1 to T2 ranged from 11.1% (prostate) to 28.6% (head

and neck), whereas remission rates during the same interval ranged from 25.6% (breast) to 44.8% (prostate). The greater incidence of insomnia reported in patients with head and neck cancer could be explained by their poorer prognosis, psychological reactions to possible surgical complications (e.g., loss of voice, facial disfigurement), or intense nicotine withdrawal.

In another large-scale prospective study, Palesh and her collaborators[8] assessed the presence of insomnia in 823 patients scheduled to receive at least four cycles of chemotherapy for various types of cancer (all stages). Participants completed a depression questionnaire (Hamilton Depression Inventory) that contained six questions assessing sleep difficulties, on day 7 of cycles 1 and 2 of chemotherapy. The insomnia syndrome was defined as difficulty falling asleep, difficulty staying asleep, and/or early morning awakenings (at least 30 minutes each) on at least 3 nights a week for 2 weeks. This more liberal definition (not taking into account insomnia-related functioning impairments), coupled with the fact that the information was derived from a questionnaire rather than from a diagnostic interview, yielded greater prevalence rates. At cycle 1, 79.6% of patients displayed insomnia symptoms, including the 43.0% who met the criteria for an insomnia syndrome—rates that decreased to 68.3% and 35.2%, respectively, at cycle 2. Among good sleepers at cycle 1, 34.6% developed insomnia symptoms at cycle 2 (of which 10% developed an insomnia syndrome).

When cancer sites (i.e., breast, gynecologic, hematologic, lung, gastrointestinal) were compared, the prevalence of insomnia symptoms was seen to be greatest in breast cancer patients, followed closely by gynecologic cancer patients. Prevalence of the insomnia syndrome was highest in patients with lung cancer and lowest in those with a gastrointestinal malignancy. No significant difference was noted between men and women, but patients who were younger than 58 years of age had a significantly greater prevalence of insomnia symptoms than their older counterparts, and Caucasian individuals were found to have significantly more insomnia.

Very little research has assessed the prevalence of sleep disturbances in patients with advanced cancer. A longitudinal study conducted in 209 terminally ill cancer patients in Japan showed that 15.3% of patients had sleep disturbances, and 29.2% had subthreshold disturbance at the moment of registration at a palliative care unit.[9] The presence of sleep disturbance was determined using the insomnia/hypersomnia item of the Structured Clinical Interview for DSM-III-R. These rates increased to 25.9% and 36.5%, respectively, at the time of admission to the unit (follow-up assessment), which took place on average 58 days later (range, 7 to 622 days). A change in sleep status was observed in 67.1% of patients between the two time points; sleep deteriorated (45.9%) more frequently than it improved (21.2%). Sleep disturbance at baseline was associated with younger age, the presence of diarrhea, and the fact of living alone, and the increase in psychological distress over time was predictive of sleep disturbance at follow-up.

OBJECTIVE MEASURES

A few studies have used objective measures—polysomnography (PSG) or actigraphy—to characterize the sleep disturbances of cancer patients. An early study compared PSG

Table 19-1 Diagnostic criteria for an insomnia syndrome

1. Sleep-onset latency (i.e., time to fall asleep) or wake after sleep onset (i.e., nocturnal awakenings) >30 minutes at least 3 nights per week

2. Sleep efficiency (total sleep time/total time spent in bed × 100) <85%

3. Duration ≥ 1 month

4. Insomnia-related impaired daytime functioning or marked distress

Adapted from Morin, 1993.[16]

recordings of patients with breast or lung cancer, patients with insomnia, and volunteers with no sleep problems. Results indicated that insomnia patients had the shortest total sleep time, but that lung cancer patients had the longest sleep-onset latency, the least sleep efficiency, and the greatest wake time during the night.[10]

Actigraphy is a noninvasive, continuous, ambulatory measure of rest-activity rhythms obtained with a device worn on the wrist. Studies comparing cancer patients versus healthy controls on actigraphic measures have consistently shown less contrast between daytime and nighttime activity in cancer patients—a pattern indicative of circadian disruption.[11] In a study conducted by Ancoli-Israel et al[12] that included 85 women with breast cancer, 72-hour actigraphic recording before the start of chemotherapy demonstrated a mean total sleep time of 6 hours, with only 76% of the night spent asleep. Moreover, the women napped for about 1 hour a day on average. Another study, which investigated sleep and sleep-wake rhythms in 130 breast cancer patients about to receive chemotherapy, reported similar findings.[13] On average, patients slept 6.6 hours, were awake for 62 minutes during the night, had a sleep efficiency of 86%, and napped for 64 minutes during the day.

Taken together, these data suggest that rest-activity patterns are altered in cancer patients even before they receive adjuvant treatments. Recent evidence suggests that these pretreatment disturbances are further aggravated by chemotherapy. In the same sample described above,[12] breast cancer patients wore a wrist actigraph for 72 consecutive hours at baseline, as well as at weeks 1, 2, and 3 of cycles 1 and 4 of chemotherapy. All circadian rhythm measures, with the exception of one, were significantly more impaired during the first week of each chemotherapy cycle relative to baseline.[14] Although circadian variables approached baseline values during weeks 2 and 3 of cycle 1, most remained significantly more impaired during weeks 2 and 3 of cycle 4, suggesting that repeated administration of chemotherapy results in progressively worse and more enduring impairments in sleep-wake activity rhythms.

PATHOPHYSIOLOGY

According to Spielman's model,[15] three categories of etiologic factors are involved in the development of insomnia: (1) predisposing factors, or enduring traits that increase the individual's general vulnerability to develop insomnia; (2) precipitating factors, or situational conditions that trigger the onset of insomnia; and (3) perpetuating factors, or variables that contribute to the maintenance of insomnia over time. As Figure 19-1 shows, predisposing factors are insufficient in themselves to cause insomnia (they do not exceed the insomnia threshold). Rather, they provide an enriched soil for the future development of insomnia episodes, which generally will be triggered by the occurrence of stressful situations (precipitating factors). In many cases, insomnia is situational, and sleep normalizes after precipitating factors have faded away, or the person has adapted to their more enduring presence. Conversely, insomnia may develop a chronic course; this is most likely to occur when the person adopts maladaptive sleep behaviors and entertains faulty cognitions about sleep (perpetuating factors). Few

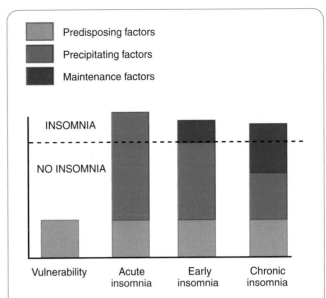

Fig. 19-1 The 3 P model. *(Adapted and reproduced with the kind permission of Springer Science and Business Media.)*

data have been published on the specific causative factors of cancer-related insomnia, but they are likely to be very similar to those of primary insomnia. These factors will be briefly enumerated, but factors specific to cancer will be the primary focus (see also Table 19-2).

PREDISPOSING FACTORS

Factors that have been found to increase vulnerability to primary insomnia include the following: hyperarousability trait (i.e., individual's predisposition to cognitive arousal), being female (twice the prevalence), aging (i.e., insomnia increases with age), marital status, a personal and familial history of insomnia, antecedents of psychological disorders, and medical comorbidity.[16]

In the specific context of cancer, research has found that insomnia, on the contrary, is more prevalent in younger patients,[8,17] perhaps because these individuals display the highest levels of psychological distress. Results about the comorbidity of insomnia with depression and anxiety disorders have revealed that, although these disorders often co-occur, insomnia frequently arises in the absence of such mood disturbances. One study conducted in prostate cancer survivors found that 54.4% of patients with sleep disturbances (and 45.8% with an insomnia syndrome) had no comorbid depression or anxiety symptoms (defined by a score of 8 or higher on the Hospital Anxiety and Depression Scale subscales).[18] More recently, Savard et al[7] investigated several potential risk factors for the incidence of insomnia between baseline (T1) and 2-month assessment (T2) in a heterogeneous group of patients scheduled to undergo cancer surgery. Among good sleepers at T1, those who were female and with a hyperarousability trait had increased risk for developing insomnia symptoms at T2. However, when females and males with a urinary or gastrointestinal cancer (the only cancer site with both genders represented) were considered, no significant difference

Table 19-2 Potential risk factors for insomnia comorbid with cancer

Predisposing factors	Precipitating factors	Perpetuating factors
Hyperarousability trait	Psychological reaction (e.g., depressive/ anxiety symptoms) to:	Maladaptive sleep behaviors
Being a woman	Initial diagnosis	Excessive amount of time spent in bed
Younger age	Recurrence diagnosis	Irregular sleep-wake schedule
Personal and familial history of insomnia	Progression	Napping
Antecedents of a psychiatric disorder (e.g., depressive or anxiety disorders)	Adjuvant treatments	Engaging in sleep-interfering activities in the bedroom
	Surgery	Faulty beliefs and attitudes about sleep
	Psychological reactions (e.g., mutilating surgery)	Unrealistic sleep requirement expectations
	Hospitalization (e.g., environment, changes in sleep routine)	Faulty causal attributions
	Side effects (e.g., pain)	Misattribution/amplification of perceived consequences of insomnia
	Radiation therapy	Decreased perception of control/ predictability of sleep
	Changes in circadian rhythms	Faulty beliefs about sleep-promoting practices
	Chemotherapy	
	Side effects (e.g., nausea/vomiting) and medications used (e.g., antiemetics)	
	Menopausal symptoms (e.g., hot flashes)	
	Changes in circadian rhythms	
	Hormone therapy	
	Menopausal symptoms (e.g., hot flashes)	
	Pain	
	Delirium	

Adapted from Savard J, Morin CM. 2001.[1]

in prevalence rates of insomnia was found. This suggests that this apparent gender effect may be accounted for, at least in part, by other factors.

PRECIPITATING FACTORS

Insomnia is generally precipitated by stressful life events such as job loss/work stress, separation/divorce, death of a loved one, and medical conditions.[16] Illnesses such as cancer represent a potentially potent precipitating factor for insomnia. In fact, cancer does not represent a single event; rather, it is characterized by a succession of severe stressors, each of which can serve as a precipitating factor for insomnia. Insomnia can be triggered at any point during the cancer process: at initial diagnosis, at the time of surgery, during treatment, at the time of diagnosis and treatment of a recurrence, and during the palliative and terminal stages of the disease.[1]

Oncologic treatments may increase the risk to develop insomnia through their emotional impact, their direct physiologic effects, or their side effects. For example, some types of surgery, particularly those involving adverse esthetic effects (e.g., total mastectomy) or a functional loss (e.g., colostomy), produce greater levels of psychological distress,[19] which, in turn, might increase the risk for insomnia. This hypothesis needs empirical validation because one study found no difference in the frequency of sleep disturbances between women who were treated with a disfiguring mastectomy and those treated with lumpectomy for their breast cancer.[20] It is important to note that hospitalization in itself can also trigger sleep disturbances[21] because of environmental factors (e.g., noise, bed discomfort, administration of medications during sleeping periods), as well as psychological and behavioral factors (e.g., anxiety, modification of sleep routine).

Comparative studies of insomnia as a function of various adjuvant cancer treatments are lacking, and very few longitudinal studies have looked at the evolution of insomnia throughout cancer care. One study found that breast cancer patients who had received radiotherapy reported more sleep disturbance 4 months after surgery compared with women who had not, but this difference disappeared at 13 months post surgery.[20] A study cited earlier suggested that repeated administration of chemotherapy for breast cancer was associated with increased perturbation of sleep-wake rhythms[14] assessed with actigraphy. The reasons for this deleterious effect of chemotherapy have yet to be established but are likely to involve both behavioral and physiologic mechanisms. On the behavioral side, patients receiving chemotherapy are likely to nap more during the day to recuperate and spend less time outside, thus limiting their exposition to natural daylight, which can alter their circadian rhythms. Chemotherapy side effects (nausea/vomiting) and medications that are used to prevent them can also contribute to the development of sleep disturbances. For instance, insomnia is a well-known side effect of dexamethasone, a corticosteroid commonly used for that purpose.[22,23]

In women, the estrogen deficiency produced by chemotherapy and hormone therapy (e.g., tamoxifen, arimidex) causes the occurrence of premature menopause (in premenopausal and perimenopausal women) or the aggravation of menopausal symptoms (in postmenopausal women), particularly hot flashes (HFs), that can interfere with sleep. Abrupt cessation of hormone replacement therapy (HRT), which is routinely recommended to breast cancer patients because of a heightened risk for cancer recurrence, may also exacerbate climacteric symptoms.[24] HFs are also frequently reported by men with prostate cancer treated with androgen-deprivation therapy (i.e., bilateral orchiectomy, gonadotropin-releasing hormone analogs, antiandrogens).[25]

Several lines of evidence have linked menopausal symptoms with sleep disturbances in the general population. For instance, studies have revealed that HFs occurring during the menopause transition are associated with the development of insomnia symptoms,[26,27] and that hormone replacement therapy is associated with improved sleep—an effect that may be explained by the alleviation of HFs and sweating.[28–30]

Studies that have used objective recordings of sleep (i.e., polysomnography) and HFs (i.e., sternal skin conductance) have revealed conflicting findings,[28,31–35] but recent evidence from the breast cancer literature supports the relationship between objectively recorded nocturnal HFs and sleep disturbances. The study by Savard et al[36] of 24 breast cancer survivors showed that the 10-minute periods around HFs had more wake time and more stage changes to lighter sleep than other 10-minute periods during the night. In addition, compared with nights without, nights with HFs had a significantly higher percentage of wake time, a lower percentage of stage 2 sleep, and a longer rapid eye movement (REM) latency. A more recent investigation conducted in 56 women undergoing treatment for breast cancer revealed that slower and longer HFs, but not increased HF frequency, were associated with several sleep impairments (e.g., greater total wake time, poorer sleep efficiency, higher number of awakenings).[36a]

Insomnia can also be precipitated by cancer pain. It has been estimated that 30% to 50% of ambulatory cancer patients or patients undergoing antineoplastic treatment and 60% to 80% of advanced cancer patients experience pain.[37–39] In addition, approximately 10% to 25% of cancer patients have pain unrelated to their illness.[37] In a sample of ambulatory lung and colon cancer patients experiencing pain, 56% reported that sleep was significantly impaired because of pain. Likewise, 59%[40] and 67%[41] of cancer patients referred to a pain clinic reported sleep disturbance, and patients experiencing more severe pain reported more sleep disturbance.[40] Pain affects both the initiation and the maintenance of sleep.[42,43]

Finally, delirium, occurring mostly in terminal cancer, is another condition that may precipitate sleep disturbances. In a study conducted in patients with advanced cancer admitted to an acute palliative care unit, delirium was present in 42% on admission and developed in 45% of remaining patients later during the hospitalization.[44] Sleep disturbances represent a typical clinical feature of delirium and are most frequently characterized by daytime sleepiness, nighttime agitation, difficulty falling asleep, and, in some cases, complete reversal of the sleep-wake cycle.[45,46]

When assessing the contributions of several potential risk factors for cancer-related insomnia, Savard et al[7] found that good sleepers at baseline who experienced an increase in anxiety symptoms, who had undergone cancer surgery and were being treated for head and neck cancer, were at significantly greater risk of developing insomnia 2 months later.

PERPETUATING FACTORS

Although some precipitating factors of insomnia, such as cancer-related pain, may be chronic in nature, individual responses to the sleep problem determine in large part whether the sleep disturbance will cease or become chronic. According to a cognitive-behavioral conceptualization of insomnia,[16] the most salient conditions maintaining insomnia are maladaptive sleep habits and dysfunctional cognitions about sleep. Both types of factors are believed to exert their negative effects by increasing arousal (i.e., physiologic, cognitive, and emotional) and performance anxiety (i.e., the pressure to sleep); this occurs in direct opposition to the relaxation state required for sleep (Fig. 19-2).

Individuals with chronic insomnia tend to spend too much time in bed, nap during the day, and have an irregular sleep-wake schedule to compensate for sleep loss. Although these sleep habits can be effective in the short term to cope with acute sleep loss and fatigue, they desynchronize the sleep-wake cycle in the long run. These maladaptive sleep behaviors are particularly frequent in cancer patients, who are encouraged to get rest and sleep to recuperate from their cancer treatments.[47–49] This may explain in part why cancer patients appear to be at higher risk for developing chronic insomnia. In addition, individuals with persistent insomnia, possibly including those with cancer, tend to engage in sleep-interfering activities in their bedroom that serve as cues for staying awake rather than inducing sleep (e.g., watching TV, listening to music, eating, working, or reading in the bed or the bedroom). These behaviors tend to weaken the association (i.e., deconditioning) between certain normally sleep-inducing stimuli (e.g., bed, bedtime, bedroom) and sleep.[16]

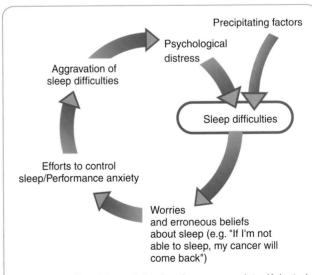

Fig. 19-2 The vicious circle of performance anxiety. *(Adapted and reproduced with the author's permission [C.M. Morin]).*

Individuals with insomnia entertain a number of faulty beliefs and attitudes about sleep and sleeplessness that may contribute to maintaining their problem over time.[16] These cognitions can be grouped into the following categories: (1) unrealistic sleep requirement expectations (e.g., "I need 8 hours of sleep to feel refreshed and to function well during the day"); (2) faulty causal attributions (e.g., "I feel that insomnia is basically the result of aging"); (3) misattribution or amplification of the perceived consequences of insomnia (e.g., "My chronic insomnia may have serious consequences for my physical health"); (4) decreased perception of control and predictability of sleep (e.g., "I have lost control over my ability to sleep"); and (5) faulty beliefs about sleep-promoting practices (e.g., "When I have trouble getting to sleep, I should stay in bed and try harder"). Cancer patients also entertain specific erroneous beliefs about sleep, including "If I don't sleep well, my cancer will come back," which may induce great levels of arousal and performance anxiety ("I really need to sleep tonight") as bedtime approaches (Fig. 19-2).

To our knowledge, only the longitudinal study by Savard et al[7] has investigated the role of behavioral and cognitive factors in the maintenance of insomnia comorbid with cancer. In this study, the persistence of insomnia from baseline to the 2-month evaluation was significantly predicted by higher baseline levels and increases from T1 to T2 in dysfunctional beliefs about sleep, cognitive monitoring of sleep-related threat (e.g., calculate the number of hours that one hopes to get), and maladaptive sleep behaviors. Although additional studies are warranted, these findings support the applicability of Spielman's model in explaining the development of insomnia in cancer patients.

DIAGNOSIS

INSOMNIA DIAGNOSIS

No consensual definition of insomnia is exists. In the 4th edition of the *Diagnostic and Statistical Manual of Mental Disorders—Revised* (DSM-IV-R),[45] primary insomnia is defined by the following: (1) a complaint of difficulty initiating or maintaining sleep, or of nonrestorative sleep, for at least 1 month; and (2) the sleep disturbance (or associated daytime fatigue) causes clinically significant distress or impairment in social, occupational, or other important areas of functioning. In addition, to establish a diagnosis of primary insomnia, the sleep disturbance should not occur exclusively during the course of another sleep disorder (e.g., breathing-related sleep disorder) or a psychiatric disorder (e.g., major depression), and should not be due to the direct physiologic effects of a substance or a general medical condition (e.g., cancer).

Up until the last National Institutes of Health state-of-the-science conference on chronic insomnia in adults, which was held in 2005,[50] insomnia that was occurring in the context of another medical or psychological condition was called *secondary insomnia*. Because of difficulty in establishing the causal role of medical and psychological conditions in the development of insomnia, it has been agreed to favor utilization of the term *comorbid insomnia*.

Clinical researchers commonly add some specificity to the criteria used to diagnose an insomnia disorder. In our own work, and based on the definition proposed by Morin,[16] difficulties initiating sleep or maintaining sleep are defined by sleep-onset latency, awakening after sleep onset or early awakening of at least 30 minutes, and sleep efficiency (i.e., ratio of total sleep time to total time spent in bed) lower than 85%. Additionally, these difficulties have to be present at least three nights per week (see Table 19-1).

DIFFERENTIAL DIAGNOSIS

Several other sleep disorders may arise with a chief complaint of insomnia. Before a diagnosis of insomnia can be established, a differential diagnosis needs to be undertaken. No fewer than 88 different diagnoses of sleep-wake disorders are included in the most recent version of the *International Classification of Sleep Disorders.*[51] Sleep apnea syndromes, sleep-related movement disorders, circadian rhythm disorders, parasomnias, and narcolepsy are examples of disorders that may lead to a subjective complaint of insomnia. After a clinical interview reveals the possible presence of one of these disorders, a polysomnographic evaluation will be essential to confirm the diagnosis (except for restless legs syndrome).

Scarce evidence suggests that other sleep disorders such as obstructive sleep apnea (OSA) and periodic limb movements disorder (PLMS) may affect cancer patients at a higher rate relative to the general population. In the study of Silberfarb et al cited above,[10] a higher prevalence of PLMS was found in lung and breast cancer patients as compared with insomnia patients and healthy volunteers, but no difference in OSA was noted. Two recent small-scale studies (17 to 33 patients) revealed a prevalence of OSA ranging from 12% to 91.7% in patients with head and neck cancer.[52,53] Sleep-disordered breathing appears to be frequent in patients with brain tumors, with tumor removal resulting in a significant decrease in the apnea-hypopnea index.[54] Larger and prospective studies are warranted to better assess the prevalence of these disorders across cancer sites, and to investigate to what extent they are caused by the cancer itself or by the cancer treatment.

Causes of other sleep disorders such as sleep-disordered breathing and periodic limb movement disorders are believed to be more biological in nature, although psychological factors may play a role in their aggravation. It is beyond the scope of this chapter to comprehensively review the cause of all sleep disorders. Each disorder has its own pathophysiology, and it is unknown whether etiologic factors are the same in the context of cancer. Risk factors of sleep-disordered breathing (e.g., obstructive sleep apnea) include obesity, male gender (and female after menopause), familial antecedents, aging, craniofacial anatomy, and alcohol and sedative use.[55] The risk of presenting with a sleep-related movement disorder (e.g., periodic limb movement disorder) is increased in individuals with familial antecedents and in women, and is often associated with other medical conditions such as anemia, peripheral neuropathy, rheumatoid arthritis, fibromyalgia, and kidney failure.[56]

Sleep apnea syndromes

Sleep apnea is characterized by episodes of impaired breathing during sleep. Cessation of breathing can result from obstruction of the upper airway (obstructive sleep apnea) or temporary loss of ventilatory effort (central sleep apnea). The most common symptoms of sleep apnea, many of which patients are unaware, include loud snoring, pauses in breathing during sleep, restless and fragmented sleep (nocturnal awakenings), and excessive daytime sleepiness. Use of continuous positive airway pressure (CPAP) devices is the most effective treatment for sleep apnea.

Sleep-related movement disorders

Restless legs syndrome is characterized by an uncomfortable aching sensation in the legs, accompanied by an irresistible urge to move them. Walking or stretching of the legs usually alleviates the symptoms. This unpleasant sensation occurs at rest at any time during the day, but is usually worse at bedtime, thus leading to prolonged sleep-onset latency. The restless legs syndrome often coexists with the periodic limb movement disorder, a disorder that consists of repetitive, highly stereotyped movements of the limbs (legs and arms) occurring during sleep. Sleep fragmentation and excessive daytime sleepiness are common consequences of this disorder. Treatment for these two conditions is mostly pharmacologic (e.g., ropinirole, levodopa).

Circadian rhythm sleep disorders

These disorders have in common a misalignment between the individual's sleep-wake rhythm and the sleep-wake schedule that is desired or regarded as the societal norm. In the delayed sleep phase type, more prevalent in young adults, sleep onset is delayed until late in the night (e.g., 3:00 am) with consequent difficulties waking up in the morning. Conversely, in the advanced sleep phase type, which is more frequent in the elderly, the patient falls asleep in the early evening (e.g., 8:00 pm) and wakes up early in the morning or even in the middle of the night. In both cases, sleep is usually not interrupted during the sleeping episode. It is essential to distinguish these disorders from insomnia, because treatment will involve alternative options (chronotherapy, light therapy, melatonin).

Narcolepsy

Narcolepsy is a rare hereditary condition that is characterized by excessive daytime sleepiness, uncontrollable and recurrent sleep attacks throughout the day, sleep paralysis, hypnagogic hallucinations, and cataplexy. Typically, narcolepsy develops during adolescence or early adulthood, and excessive daytime sleepiness is the first symptom to occur. Pharmacologic options for this disorder include stimulants (e.g., modafinil) and sodium oxybate. Scheduled napping and sleep hygiene can be of some utility.

Parasomnias

Finally, insomnia must be differentiated from parasomnia. Parasomnias are characterized by abnormal behaviors during sleep that are readily detectable and include sleepwalking, sleep talking, sleep terrors, nightmares, and REM sleep behavior disorder. Parasomnias do not necessarily lead to a complaint of insomnia, although it may be present in their most severe forms.

PHARMACOLOGIC MANAGEMENT

FREQUENCY OF USE

Hypnotic medications are by far the most common treatment option used in both primary and comorbid insomnia. In a recent epidemiologic study of 2001 individuals randomly selected from the general population, 11.0% of all respondents reported that they had used a prescribed medication in the past year—a rate that increased to 33.2% in patients with an insomnia syndrome.[57]

Early studies conducted in the context of cancer have been carried out mostly on hospitalized patients with advanced cancer. In a group of more than 1500 hospitalized cancer patients, hypnotics were the most frequent form of psychotropic prescriptions, accounting for 48% of total prescriptions.[58] In 85% of cases, the hypnotic was prescribed for poor sleep. Similarly, a study of more than 200 cancer inpatients revealed that 44% of the prescriptions given were for hypnotic medications.[59]

More recently, Paltiel et al[60] observed that 25.7% of all 909 surveyed patients (53.8% outpatients; 31% with advanced cancer) reported that they had used a tranquilizer or a sleeping pill (undistinguished) during the previous week. The highest rate of 42.5% was found among lung cancer patients. Similar rates of utilization have been reported in ambulatory settings. In a study conducted by Davidson et al,[17] 21.5% of 982 patients reported using a tranquilizer/sleeping pill, but their reasons for using these medications were not documented. Finally, a survey conducted in 1984 cancer patients revealed that 22.6% were currently using a sleep-promoting medication.[61] The mean duration of use was 58.1 months, and, in most cases, a benzodiazepine with recognized hypnotic properties was prescribed.

DESCRIPTION OF AVAILABLE MEDICATIONS

Several classes of medications are used for the treatment of insomnia. These include benzodiazepines that are specifically marketed as hypnotics (e.g., flurazepam, temazepam, triazolam), several other benzodiazepines that are marketed as anxiolytics (e.g., lorazepam, clonazepam, oxazepam), and newer nonbenzodiazepine hypnotics (e.g., zolpidem, eszopiclone, zaleplon). These latest medications have more selective or specific hypnotic effects and fewer residual effects the next day. A melatonin agonist receptor (ramelteon) also is now available to treat insomnia. Some antidepressant medications (those with sedating properties, such as trazodone, amitriptyline, and mirtazapine) can be of some utility in the treatment of insomnia in depressed patients, although they tend to induce more residual daytime sedation. Other medications that may be prescribed for insomnia include sedating antipsychotics (quetiapine, olanzapine).

EFFICACY

No study has yet assessed the efficacy of hypnotic medications specifically in oncology. However, scarce available evidence suggests that eszopiclone and zolpidem are effective for insomnia that is comorbid with some psychological (e.g., depression, generalized anxiety disorder) and medical (e.g., perimenopausal and postmenopausal insomnia) conditions.[62]

In primary insomnia, numerous placebo-controlled studies have supported the efficacy of benzodiazepines and non-benzodiazepine hypnotics for the short-term management of insomnia. More precisely, meta-analyses of the available literature indicated notable improvements in the number of awakenings (ds = 0.65–1.00), total sleep time (ds = 0.71–0.76), and sleep quality ratings (ds = 0.62–1.30), but smaller treatment effects on sleep-onset latency (ds = 0.28–0.56) and wake time after sleep onset (d = 0.29).[63,64] These effects translated into increases in sleep duration of 61.8 minutes and reductions of only 4.2 minutes in sleep-onset latency, on average, compared with placebo.[65]

However, little evidence of long-term efficacy has been found with prolonged use of hypnotics, as most trials have had a duration shorter than 35 days. In the United States, eszopiclone is the only hypnotic that has been approved by the Food and Drug Administration for the long-term management of insomnia (not available in Canada). Placebo-controlled studies found 6 months of nightly eszopiclone to be effective in primary insomnia.[66,67] Although this medication appears to be well tolerated and not associated with the development of tolerance with long-term use, additional comparative studies are needed to assess its relative efficacy and safety.[68]

LIMITATIONS

The use of hypnotic medications is associated with a number of risks and limitations. Long-acting agents (e.g., flurazepam, quazepam) can produce residual effects the next day, including daytime drowsiness, dizziness or light-headedness, and psychomotor and cognitive impairments.[69,70] Other important limitations of hypnotic medications include their risks of tolerance (i.e., reduction of efficacy with prolonged usage and need to increase the dosage to maintain therapeutic effects) and dependence (particularly psychological dependence), which are associated with prolonged usage.[16,69,71] Modification of the sleep architecture, including increased stage 2 and REM sleep latency, and decreased slow-wave sleep are associated with long-term benzodiazepine use.[72]

These limitations have led some sleep experts to recommend using hypnotic medications primarily for situational and transient insomnia and using the lowest effective dosage of hypnotics for the shortest period of time. Treatment should start with a small dosage, with a subsequent gradual increase only if necessary. Generally, it is recommended that the treatment duration should not exceed 4 weeks to avoid the development of tolerance and to minimize the risk of dependency. Then, if the problem persists or is recurrent, the main intervention should be nonpharmacologic.[73,74]

NONPHARMACOLOGIC MANAGEMENT

EFFICACY OF COGNITIVE-BEHAVIORAL THERAPY (CBT)
Primary insomnia

Cognitive-behavioral therapy (CBT) is now considered the treatment of choice for primary insomnia, especially when chronic.[70] The efficacy of CBT for primary insomnia has been demonstrated in numerous randomized clinical trials.

Meta-analyses of the available literature[64,75,76] revealed effect sizes generally falling into the moderate to large range: sleep-onset latency (0.76–0.88), sleep quality ratings (0.94–1.20), duration of awakenings (0.19–0.65), total sleep time (0.42–0.62), and number of awakenings (0.53–1.30). It is interesting to note that one of these meta-analyses compared the magnitude of treatment effects of CBT and pharmacotherapy and found no difference, except for sleep-onset latency, which was most importantly reduced after CBT.[64]

A few studies have compared head-to-head the efficacy of pharmacologic and psychological treatments for primary insomnia. A placebo-controlled study by Morin et al[77] contrasted the efficacy of CBT versus acute treatment of temazepam, singly and combined, in older individuals with primary insomnia. Posttreatment data revealed significantly greater sleep improvements in the three active treatment conditions compared with the placebo group. A trend, albeit nonsignificant, favored the combination of medication and CBT. At follow-up, patients who received CBT had a better sustainment of treatment effects than those treated with medication alone, and those treated with the combination had more variable outcomes. More recently, Morin and his collaborators[78] evaluated the added value of medication (zolpidem) over CBT alone for the acute treatment of persistent primary insomnia and found this effect to be only modest. Another goal of this study was to assess the effects of various maintenance treatments at a 6-month follow-up. The best long-term outcome was obtained in patients treated initially with the combined treatment, followed by CBT alone, which suggests that the maintenance of treatment effects is better when medication is discontinued. In sum, although some inconsistencies are apparent in results obtained with the combination of psychological and pharmacologic treatments, the existing literature appears to support the view that CBT is at least as efficacious as pharmacotherapy, and that CBT has the advantage of leading to sleep improvements that are more durable over time.

Among the various strategies that have been tested, relaxation, stimulus control, sleep restriction, and multimodal treatments (i.e., combining several approaches) have generally been found to be efficacious psychological interventions, whereas sleep hygiene education appeared to produce only modest gains when used alone.[64,75,79,80] The efficacy of cognitive therapy as a stand-alone treatment for insomnia has not been established yet, but a preliminary study found significant sleep improvements post treatment, which were maintained at a 12-month follow-up.[81] In addition, studies that have incorporated cognitive restructuring of a multicomponent treatment have shown some therapeutic benefits associated with its use.[82]

Insomnia comorbid with cancer

Although the efficacy of CBT appears to be well established, most published studies have excluded patients with comorbid psychological or medical disorders. It is only recently that researchers have begun to specifically investigate the efficacy of CBT in patients with comorbid insomnia. Available data suggest that CBT is as efficacious in these patients as in primary insomnia. The efficacy of this treatment has been supported in patients with insomnia comorbid with chronic pain,[83] fibromyalgia,[84] and mixed medical and psychiatric conditions,[85] and in older adults with mixed medical disorders.[86] In cancer, the first studies—uncontrolled, nonrandomized, or conducted in small samples of cancer patients—found that CBT for insomnia was associated with improvement in most subjective sleep parameters and some aspects of quality of life, along with reduced psychological distress.[87–89] These promising results were then corroborated by the first controlled and randomized trial conducted in 57 breast cancer survivors.[90] In this study, 6-week CBT for insomnia administered in small groups was associated with significantly greater improvement on several subjective sleep indices (sleep efficiency, sleep-onset latency, wake time after sleep onset, insomnia severity), greater reduction of psychological distress and use of hypnotic medications, and greater improvement in global quality of life compared with a waiting-list control condition at post treatment. In addition, these treatment effects were well sustained up to a 12-month follow-up (see Fig. 19-3).

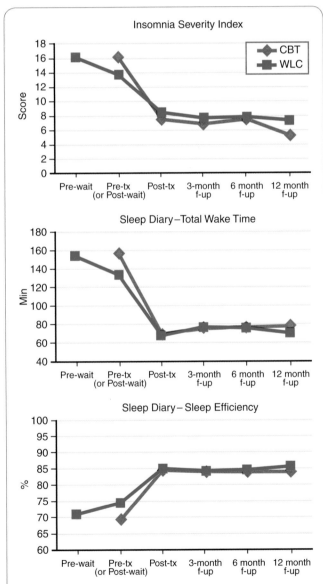

Fig. 19-3 Results of a study conducted by Savard et al (2005) on the efficacy of cognitive-behavioral therapy (CBT) for insomnia in breast cancer survivors. *CBT,* Cognitive-behavioral therapy; *tx,* treatment; *f-up,* follow-up; *WLC,* waiting-list control condition.

Description of CBT components

In recent years, research into primary and comorbid insomnia has mostly evaluated the efficacy of a multimodal approach combining behavioral (stimulus control, sleep restriction, relaxation), cognitive (cognitive restructuring), and educational (sleep hygiene) strategies. The common goal of these strategies is to modify the behavioral and cognitive factors that are believed to play a significant role in the maintenance of sleep difficulties over time, including cognitive and physiological arousal, maladaptive sleep habits, and dysfunctional cognitions (beliefs, automatic thoughts) about sleep (Table 19-3).[16] It would appear that no contraindication occurs when any of these strategies is used in cancer patients. However, all studies published to date were conducted in patients who had completed their cancer treatment, many months or even years before. Hence, the applicability of these techniques (especially sleep restriction) during the course of cancer treatments has yet to be determined. Of note, very few researchers have adapted the content of CBT for insomnia to cancer patients, and the additional benefit of these modifications has never been assessed (e.g., addition of fatigue management component). It is therefore unknown whether some adaptations might increase the efficacy/applicability of this intervention in oncology.

STIMULUS CONTROL THERAPY

Stimulus control therapy is aimed at reassociating the bed and the bed environment with sleep (rather than being associated with sleeplessness) and establishing a regular sleep-wake rhythm. Original instructions include the following: (1) Go to bed only when sleepy; (2) when unable to fall asleep or go back to sleep within 15 to 20 minutes, get out of bed and leave the bedroom, and return to bed only when sleepy; (3) use the bed/bedroom only for sleep and sexual activities (e.g., do not watch TV, listen to the radio, eat, or read in bed); (4) arise at the same time every morning; and (5) do not nap during the day.[91] In addition to these instructions, patients may be recommended to (1) set aside at least an hour to relax before going to bed (to reduce activation and ease the appearance of sleepiness); and (2) establish a presleep routine to be used every night (which eventually will become a sleep-inducing stimulus).

Totally avoiding day napping can be challenging—if not impossible—for many sick individuals, especially when they are receiving medical treatments that affect their energy level and require physical recuperation. In our own work with cancer patients, we have relaxed this rule and allow patients who need it to take naps under certain conditions: Naps should be taken before 3 pm and for a maximum duration of 60 minutes, in the bed. Following these instructions reduces the likelihood that naps may impair sleep quality on the upcoming night and contributes to reinforcing the association between the bedroom environment and sleep.[16]

SLEEP RESTRICTION

Sleep restriction is aimed at curtailing the time in bed to the actual sleep time, which creates mild sleep deprivation (facilitating sleep onset) and results in more consolidated and more efficient sleep.[92] In the first phase of this intervention, the amount of time spent in bed is restricted to the actual amount of time asleep based on sleep diaries completed at baseline. However, it is generally prohibited to fix a sleep window at lower than 5 hours to avoid excessive daytime sleepiness.

Table 19-3 Summary of CBT components

Intervention	Goals	Procedures
Stimulus control therapy	• Reassociate temporal (bedtime) and environmental (bed and bedroom) stimuli with rapid sleep onset. • Establish a regular circadian sleep-wake rhythm.	Set aside at least an hour before going to bed to relax. Develop a ritual to do before going to bed. Go to bed only when sleepy. When unable to fall asleep or go back to sleep within 15 to 20 minutes, get out of bed and leave the bedroom, and return to bed only when sleepy. Maintain a regular arising time in the morning. Use the bed/bedroom for sleep and sex only (do not watch TV, listen to the radio, eat, or read in bed). Do not nap during the day.
Sleep restriction	• Curtail time in bed to actual sleep time, thereby creating mild sleep deprivation, which results in more consolidated and more efficient sleep.	Restrict the amount of time spent in bed to the actual amount of time asleep; time in bed is progressively increased as sleep efficiency improves.
Relaxation training	• Reduce somatic and cognitive arousal interference with sleep.	Progressive muscle relaxation, autogenic training, biofeedback, imagery training, hypnosis, meditation.
Cognitive therapy	• Change dysfunctional beliefs and attitudes about sleep and insomnia that exacerbate arousal and performance anxiety.	Identify sleep cognitive distortions (mainly by self-monitoring), challenge the validity of sleep cognitions (by using probing questions such as "What evidence supports this idea? Is there an alternative explanation?"); reframe dysfunctional cognitions into more adaptive thoughts by using cognitive restructuring techniques (e.g., decatastrophizing, reattribution, reappraisal, attention shifting).
Sleep hygiene education	• Change health practices and environmental factors that interfere with sleep.	Avoid stimulants (e.g., caffeine, nicotine) and alcohol around bedtime. Do not eat heavy or spicy meals too close to bedtime. Exercise regularly but not too late in the evening. Maintain a dark, quiet, and comfortable sleep environment.

Adapted from Savard J, Morin CM. 2001.[1]

During the course of treatment, time in bed is progressively adjusted, each week, as sleep efficiency changes, until the patient's optimal sleep time is reached. Time spent in bed may be increased by 20 to 30 minutes when sleep efficiency exceeds 85%, may be reduced by the same amount when sleep efficiency is lower than 80%, or may be kept stable when sleep efficiency falls to between 80% and 85%.

COGNITIVE RESTRUCTURING

With cognitive restructuring, patients are taught how to identify and restructure dysfunctional thoughts and beliefs about their sleep difficulties that are believed to be instrumental in maintaining insomnia over time, mainly through the deleterious effects of performance anxiety. This is accomplished by guiding the patient to identify maladaptive sleep cognitions, challenging their validity, and reframing them into more adaptative (realistic) substitutes.[16,93] Dysfunctional beliefs that are addressed in the context of cancer include those typically observed in insomnia patients from the general population and those that are more specific to their condition (e.g., "If I'm not able to sleep well, my cancer will come back"; Table 19-4). Participants should be encouraged to generalize the use of cognitive restructuring to other anxiety-provoking thoughts that might induce arousal and interfere with sleep.

Table 19-4 Example of cognitive restructuring of an erroneous belief common in cancer patients with insomnia.

Situation	Automatic thoughts	Emotions, %	Alternative (realistic) thoughts	Emotions, %
Wide awake in the middle of the night, I think about my difficulties sleeping.	"If my difficulties sleeping persist, I am going to have a cancer recurrence."	Anxiety, 100%	"I have no evidence that insomnia alone can cause a cancer recurrence. Cancer is a multifactorial disease that is influenced by several factors. I know good sleepers who have had a cancer recurrence and others who have been in remission for years, despite sleeping poorly." "This thought brings me a lot of anxiety, which aggravates my trouble sleeping." "One of the worst consequences of insomnia is sleepiness, and that will help me sleep tomorrow." "I need to focus on what I can do to improve my sleep, such as not staying in bed worrying when I am awake, rather than on the possible consequences of sleeping poorly."	Anxiety, 20%

SLEEP HYGIENE

Sleep hygiene consists of providing information about the effects of environmental factors and health behaviors on sleep. Specific instructions may vary but generally include the following: (1) Avoid caffeine at least 4 to 6 hours before bedtime, and smoking at bedtime and during nocturnal awakenings (both are stimulants); (2) limit alcohol consumption during the evening (this may facilitate sleep onset but may fragment sleep during the night); (3) avoid heavy and spicy meals and eating foods that activate gastrointestinal functioning (e.g., uncooked fruits and vegetables), and limit ingestion of liquids close to bedtime; (4) exercise regularly, but not too close to bedtime because of its activating effect; and (5) keep the bedroom dark, quiet, and comfortable, and avoid extreme temperatures.

RELAXATION

Many forms of relaxation have been used in the treatment of insomnia. Some are aimed at reducing physiologic arousal (e.g., progressive muscular relaxation), but others mainly target cognitive arousal (e.g., imagery training, meditation). In spite of empirical evidence supporting the efficacy of this approach, some disagreement is ongoing as to whether this is an essential component of CBT for insomnia, because this question has never been directly investigated. In addition, relaxation needs regular practice, ideally on a daily basis, to be effective, and this procedure sometimes may have a paradoxical effect, exacerbating performance anxiety and insomnia, particularly in patients with marked cognitive hyperarousability.

FATIGUE MANAGEMENT

Because of the elevated prevalence of cancer-related fatigue and its possible comorbidity with sleep disturbances,[94] we added a brief fatigue management component to our randomized controlled trial of CBT for insomnia comorbid with breast cancer.[90] First, a multifactorial model of fatigue was presented to illustrate the role of physiologic, emotional, cognitive, and behavioral factors in fatigue. Also, the distinction between somnolence and fatigue was discussed. Most important, patients were encouraged to increase their level of physical activity to short-circuit the vicious cycle of fatigue → decreased level of activity → physical deconditioning → increased fatigue.[95] From our data, it is impossible to determine whether the addition of these strategies translated into greater treatment efficacy. Actually, fatigue appeared to be one of the few symptoms that did not improve more notably in CBT patients compared with patients in the waiting-list condition. This lack of significant effect on fatigue may be due to the brevity of this treatment component in our study, and may suggest the need to offer a more intensive intervention for this seemingly resistant symptom (e.g., adding cognitive restructuring of fatigue catastrophization). It could also be that insomnia and fatigue are not as highly correlated as is commonly believed. Future studies are needed for researchers to gain a better understanding of the relationship between sleep disturbances and fatigue in cancer patients, and to determine whether adding fatigue management to CBT for insomnia is beneficial in terms of treatment outcomes.

ACCESSIBILITY OF CBT FOR INSOMNIA COMORBID WITH CANCER

In spite of strong evidence supporting its efficacy for insomnia comorbid with cancer, accessibility to CBT for insomnia remains extremely limited. Only a few cancer centers are staffed by mental health professionals formally trained in the psychological management of insomnia. In addition, the significant number of sessions that usually constitute CBT-I and the costs associated with it preclude its implementation as a part of routine cancer care.

To improve dissemination of this treatment, Espie and his collaborators[96] evaluated the effectiveness of CBT administered by oncologic nurses who were trained beforehand and received regular supervision during the course of the study. At post treatment, CBT patients had a significantly greater reduction in sleep-onset latency and in wake after sleep onset, as well as a significantly larger increase in sleep efficiency, when assessed subjectively, than patients in the usual care condition (without CBT).

Although these results are very encouraging, they are limited by the fact that the nurses involved in this study were liberated from a certain proportion of their usual tasks to administer CBT for insomnia, an option that is fairly unlikely in most clinical settings. It is therefore important to develop other intervention formats, requiring less therapist contact, to ensure broader dissemination of CBT for insomnia in cancer patients. The efficacy of self-administered CBT for insomnia is well established in the context of primary insomnia. The interventions tested have taken the form of written material treatment (i.e., bibliotherapy) with or without therapist guidance,[97–99] and video,[100] television,[101] and Web-based training programs.[102] Research has revealed that self-help interventions are more efficacious in treating insomnia than a no-treatment condition,[98–100] and they are as efficacious as professionally administered interventions.[97]

With this goal in mind, our research team recently developed a self-administered CBT for cancer-related insomnia, which consists of a 60-minute video and six short booklets. A pilot study of 11 breast cancer patients showed that this intervention format was well accepted by the women.[103] Moreover, significant improvements were noted at post treatment, which were well sustained 3 months later. A large controlled and randomized clinical study of 300 breast cancer patients is under way to confirm these preliminary findings and assess the cost-effectiveness ratio of this self-help intervention compared with professionally administered CBT for insomnia.

CONCLUSION

Insomnia is highly prevalent in cancer patients. Although insomnia may be precipitated by an array of cancer-related factors that are difficult to change (e.g., nocturnal hot flashes), its persistence over time is most importantly explained by modifiable behavioral and cognitive factors, such as maladaptive sleep behaviors and dysfunctional cognitions about sleep. Hypnotic medications (benzodiazepines and nonbenzodiazepines) are the most commonly used strategies for cancer-related insomnia, often for prolonged periods of time. Although a handful of studies have shown some promise in the long-term use of eszopiclone for primary insomnia, evidence is lacking for long-term use of other hypnotic drugs. Moreover, utilization of these medications is associated with a number of side effects and risks, especially when used on a long-term basis and in older adults. CBT directly targets factors that are believed to be involved in the maintenance of insomnia over time and has minimal risks. Accumulating evidence supports its efficacy for insomnia comorbid with cancer, in improving sleep, relieving psychological distress, and enhancing overall quality of life. In addition, treatment effects associated with CBT last well beyond its termination.

REFERENCES

1. Savard J, Morin CM. Insomnia in the context of cancer: a review of a neglected problem. *J Clin Oncol.* 2001;19:895–908.
2. Fiorentino L, Ancoli-Israel S. Sleep dysfunction in patients with cancer. *Curr Treat Options Neurol.* 2007;9:337–346.
3. Cooley ME, Short TH, Moriarty HJ. Symptom prevalence, distress, and change over time in adults receiving treatment for lung cancer. *Psychooncology.* 2003;12:694–708.
4. Kenefick AL. Patterns of symptom distress in older women after surgical treatment for breast cancer. *Oncol Nurs Forum.* 2006;33:327–335.
5. Ahlberg K, Ekman T, Gaston-Johansson F. The experience of fatigue, other symptoms and global quality of life during radiotherapy for uterine cancer. *Int J Nurs Stud.* 2005;42:377–386.
6. Hickok JT, Morrow GR, Roscoe JA, et al. Occurrence, severity, and longitudinal course of twelve common symptoms in 1129 consecutive patients during radiotherapy for cancer. *J Pain Symptom Manage.* 2005;30:433–442.
7. Savard J, Villa J, Ivers H, et al. Prevalence, natural course, and risk factors of insomnia comorbid with cancer over a 2-month period. *J Clin Oncol.* 2009;27:5233–5239.
8. Palesh OG, Roscoe JA, Mustian KM, et al. Prevalence, demographics, and psychological associations of sleep disruption in cancer patients: University of Rochester Cancer Center Community Clinical Oncology Program. *J Clin Oncol.* 2010;28:292–298.
9. Akechi T, Okuyama T, Akizuki N, et al. Associated and predictive factors of sleep disturbance in advanced cancer patients. *Psychooncology.* 2007;16:888–894.
10. Silberfarb PM, Hauri PJ, Oxman TE, et al. Assessment of sleep in patients with lung cancer and breast cancer. *J Clin Oncol.* 1993;11:997–1004.
11. Pati AK, Parganiha A, Kar A, et al. Alterations of the characteristics of the circadian rest-activity rhythm of cancer in-patients. *Chronobiol Int.* 2007;24:1179–1197.
12. Ancoli-Israel S, Liu L, Marler MR, et al. Fatigue, sleep, and circadian rhythms prior to chemotherapy for breast cancer. *Supportive Care Cancer.* 2006;14:201–209.
13. Berger AM, Farr LA, Kuhn BR, et al. Values of sleep/wake, activity/rest, circadian rhythms, and fatigue prior to adjuvant breast cancer chemotherapy. *J Pain Symptom Manage.* 2007;33:398–409.
14. Savard J, Liu L, Natarajan L, et al. Breast cancer patients have progressively impaired sleep-wake activity rhythms during chemotherapy. *Sleep.* 2009;32:1155–1160.
15. Spielman AJ, Glovinsky P. Case studies in insomnia. In: Hauri PJ, ed *The varied nature of insomnia.* New York: Plenum Press; 1991:1–15.
16. Morin CM. *Insomnia: psychological assessment and management.* New York, NY: The Guilford Press; 1993.

17. Davidson JR, MacLean AW, Brundage MD, et al. Sleep disturbance in cancer patients. *Soc Sci Med.* 2002;54:1309–1321.
18. Savard J, Simard S, Hervouet S, et al. Insomnia in men treated with radical prostatectomy for prostate cancer. *Psychooncology.* 2005;14:147–156.
19. Jacobsen PB, Roth AJ, Holland JC. Surgery. In: Holland JC, ed. *Psycho-oncology.* New York, NY: Oxford University Press; 1998:257–268.
20. Omne-Pontén M, Holmberg L, Burns T, et al. Determinants of the psycho-social outcome after operation for breast cancer: results of a prospective comparative interview study following mastectomy and breast conservation. *Eur J Cancer.* 1992;28A:1062–1067.
21. Sheely LC. Sleep disturbances in hospitalized patients with cancer. *Oncol Nurs Forum.* 1996;23:109–111.
22. Cassileth PA, Lusk EJ, Torri S, et al. Antiemetic efficacy of dexamethasone therapy in patients receiving cancer chemotherapy. *Arch Intern Med.* 1983;143:1347–1349.
23. Ling MHM, Perry PJ, Tsuang MT. Side effects of corticosteroid therapy: psychiatric aspects. *Arch Gen Psychiatry.* 1981;38:471–477.
24. Carpenter JS. State of the science: hot flashes and cancer. Part 2: Management and future directions. *Oncol Nurs Forum.* 2005;32:969–978.
25. Engstrom CA. Hot flashes in prostate cancer: state of the science. *Am J Men's Health.* 2008;2:122–132.
26. Nelson HD. Menopause. *Lancet.* 2008;371:760–770.
27. National Institute of Health. NIH State-of-the-Science Conference statement on management of menopause-related symptoms. *NIH Consens State Sci Statements.* 2005;22:1–38.
28. Erlik Y, Tataryn IV, Meldrum DR, et al. Association of waking episodes with menopausal hot flushes. *JAMA.* 1981;245:1741–1744.
29. Hachul H, Bittencourt LR, Andersen ML, et al. Effects of hormone therapy with estrogen and/or progesterone on sleep pattern in postmenopausal women. *Int J Gynaecol Obstet.* 2008;103:207–212.
30. Polo-Kantola P, Erkkola R, Helenius H, et al. When does estrogen replacement therapy improve sleep quality? *Am J Obstet Gynecol.* 1998;178:1002–1009.
31. Freedman RR, Roehrs TA. Lack of sleep disturbance from menopausal hot flashes. *Fertil Steril.* 2004;82:138–144.
32. Freedman RR, Roehrs TA. Effects of REM sleep and ambient temperature on hot flash-induced sleep disturbance. *Menopause.* 2006;13:576–583.
33. Gonen R, Sharf M, Lavie P. The association between mid-sleep waking episodes and hot flushes in post-menopausal women. *J Psychosom Obstet Gynecol.* 1986;5:113–117.
34. Woodward S, Freedman RR. The thermoregulatory effects of menopausal hot flashes on sleep. *Sleep.* 1994;17:497–501.
35. Carpenter JS, Elam J, Ridner S, et al. Sleep, fatigue, and depressive symptoms in breast cancer survivors

and matched healthy women experiencing hot flashes. *Oncol Nurs Forum.* 2004;31:591–598.
36. Savard J, Davidson JR, Ivers H, et al. The association between nocturnal hot flashes and sleep in breast cancer survivors. *J Pain Symptom Manage.* 2004;27:513–522.
36a. Savard MH, Savard J, Caplette-Gingras A, et al. The association between hot flash characteristics and polysomnographic and spectral measures of sleep among breast cancer patients. *Sleep* Submitted for publication.
37. Belgrade MJ. Control of pain in cancer patients. *Postgrad Med.* 1989;85:319–329.
38. Portenoy RK, Miransky J, Thaler HT, et al. Pain in ambulatory patients with lung or colon cancer. *Cancer.* 1992;70:1616–1624.
39. Taddeini L, Rotschafer JC. Pain syndromes associated with cancer. *Postgrad Med.* 1984;75:101–108.
40. Grond S, Zech D, Diefenbach C, et al. Prevalence and pattern of symptoms in patients with cancer pain: a prospective evaluation of 1635 cancer patients referred to a pain clinic. *J Pain Symptom Manage.* 1994;9:372–382.
41. Tsui SL, Tong WN, Lam CS, et al. Cancer pain management: a recent experience by anaesthesiologists in a teaching hospital in Hong Kong. *Acta Anaesthesiol Scand.* 1994;32:193–201.
42. Dorrepaal KL, Aaronson NK, Van Dam FSAM. Pain experience and pain management among hospitalized cancer patients. *Cancer.* 1989;63:593–598.
43. Strang P. Emotional and social aspects of cancer pain. *Acta Oncol.* 1992;31:323–326.
44. Lawlor PG, Gagnon B, Mancini IL, et al. Occurrence, causes, and outcome of delirium in patients with advanced cancer: a prospective study. *Arch Intern Med.* 2000;160:786–794.
45. American Psychiatric Association. *Diagnostic and statistical manual of mental disorders, text revision.* 4th ed. Washington, DC: American Psychiatric Association; 2000.
46. Breitbart W, Cohen KR. Delirium. In: Holland JC, ed. *Psycho-oncology.* New York NY: Oxford University Press; 1998:564–575.
47. Graydon JE, Bubela N, Irvine D, et al. Fatigue-reducing strategies used by patients receiving treatment for cancer. *Cancer Nurs.* 1995;18:23–28.
48. Irvine DM, Vincent L, Graydon JE, et al. Fatigue in women with breast cancer receiving radiation therapy. *Cancer Nurs.* 1998;21:127–135.
49. Richardson A, Ream EK. Self-care behaviours initiated by chemotherapy patients in response to fatigue. *Int J Nurs Stud.* 1997;34:35–43.
50. National Institutes of Health. *Manifestations and management of chronic insomnia in adults.* Bethesda, MD: National Institutes of Health State-of-the-Science Conference; 2005:1–22.
51. American Academy of Sleep Medicine. *International classification of sleep disorders, revised: diagnostic and coding manual.* Chicago, IL: American Academy of Sleep Medicine; 2001.

52. Nesse W, Hoekema A, Stegenga B, et al. Prevalence of obstructive sleep apnoea following head and neck cancer treatment: a cross-sectional study. *Oral Oncol.* 2006;42:108–114.

53. Payne RJ, Hier MP, Kost KM, et al. High prevalence of obstructive sleep apnea among patients with head and neck cancer. *J Otolaryngol.* 2005;34:304–311.

54. Pollak L, Shpirer I, Rabey JM, et al. Polysomnography in patients with intracranial tumors before and after operation. *Acta Neurol Scand.* 2004;109.

55. Guilleminault C, Bassiri A. Clinical features and evaluation of obstructive sleep apnea-hypopnea syndrome and upper airway resistance syndrome. In: Kryger MH, Roth T, Dement WC, eds. *Principles and practice of sleep medicine.* Philadelphia: Elsevier Saunders; 2005:1043–1052.

56. Montplaisir J, Allen RP, Walters AS, et al. Restless legs syndrome and periodic limb movements during sleep. In: Kryger MH, Roth T, Dement WC, eds. *Principles and practice of sleep medicine.* Philadelphia: Elsevier Saunders; 2005:839–851.

57. Morin CM, LeBlanc M, Daley M, et al. Epidemiology of insomnia: prevalence, self-help treatments, consultations, and determinants of help-seeking behaviors. *Sleep Med.* 2006;7:123–130.

58. Derogatis LR, Feldstein M, Morrow G, et al. A survey of psychotropic drug prescriptions in an oncology population. *Cancer.* 1979;44:1919–1929.

59. Stiefel FC, Kornblith AB, Holland JC. Changes in the prescription patterns of psychotropic drugs for cancer patients during a 10-year period. *Cancer.* 1990;65:1048–1053.

60. Paltiel O, Marzec-Bogulawska A, Soskolne V, et al. Use of tranquilizers and sleeping pills among cancer patients is associated with a poorer quality of life. *Qual Life Res.* 2004;13:1699–1706.

61. Casault L, Savard J, Ivers H, et al. Utilization of hypnotic medication in the context of cancer: Predictors and frequency of use. *Supportive Care in Cancer.* Submitted for publication.

62. Neubauer DN. Current and new thinking in the management of comorbid insomnia. *Am J Manag Care.* 2009;15(suppl):S24–S32.

63. Nowell PD, Mazumdar S, Buysse DJ, et al. Benzodiazepines and zolpidem for chronic insomnia: a meta-analysis of treatment efficacy. *JAMA.* 1997;278:2170–2177.

64. Smith MT, Perlis ML, Park A, et al. Comparative meta-analysis of pharmacotherapy and behavior therapy for persistent insomnia. *Am J Psychiatry.* 2002;159:5–11.

65. Holbrook AM, Crowther R, Lotter A, et al. Meta-analysis of benzodiazepine use in the treatment of insomnia. *Can Med Assoc J.* 2000;162:225–233.

66. Krystal AD, Walsh JK, Laska E, et al. Sustained efficacy of eszopiclone over 6 months of nightly treatment: results of a randomized, double-blind, placebo-controlled study in adults with chronic insomnia. *Sleep.* 2003;26:793–799.

67. Walsh JK, Krystal AD, Amato DA, et al. Nightly treatment of primary insomnia with eszopiclone for six months: effect on sleep, quality of life, and work limitations. *Sleep.* 2007;30:959–968.

68. Hair PI, McCormack PL, Curran MP. Eszopiclone: a review of its use in the treatment of insomnia. *Drugs.* 2008;68:1415–1434.

69. Hall N. Taking policy action to reduce benzodiazepine use and promote self-care among seniors. *J Appl Gerontol.* 1998;17:318–351.

70. National Institutes of Health. National Institutes of Health State of the Science Conference statement on manifestations and management of chronic insomnia in adults, June 13-15, 2005. *Sleep.* 2005;28:1049–1057.

71. Morin CM. Psychological and pharmacological treatments for insomnia. In: Sammons M, Schmidt NB, eds. *Combining psychological and pharmacological treatments for mental disorders: a guide for psychologists.* Washington, DC: American Psychological Association; 2001.

72. Poyares D, Guilleminault C, Ohayon MM, et al. Chronic benzodiazepine usage and withdrawal in insomnia patients. *J Psychiatric Res.* 2004;38:327–334.

73. Morin CM. Combined therapeutics for insomnia: should our first approach be behavioral or pharmacological? *Sleep Med.* 2006;7(suppl 1):S15–S19.

74. National Institutes of Health. NIH releases statement on behavioral and relaxation approaches for chronic pain and insomnia. *Am Fam Physician.* 1996;53:1877–1880.

75. Morin CM, Culbert JP, Schwartz SM. Nonpharmacological interventions for insomnia: a meta-analysis of treatment efficacy. *Am J Psychiatry.* 1994;151:1172–1180.

76. Murtagh DR, Greenwood KM. Identifying effective psychological treatments for insomnia: a meta-analysis. *J Consult Clin Psychol.* 1995;63:79–89.

77. Morin CM, Colecchi C, Stone J, et al. Behavioral and pharmacological therapies for late-life insomnia: a randomized controlled trial. *JAMA.* 1999;281:991–999.

78. Morin CM, Vallières A, Guay B, et al. Cognitive behavioral therapy, singly and combined with medication, for persistent insomnia: a randomized controlled trial. *JAMA.* 2009;301:2005–2015.

79. Irwin MR, Cole JC, Nicassio PM. Comparative meta-analysis of behavioral interventions for insomnia and their efficacy in middle-aged adults and in older adults 55+ years of age. *Health Psychol.* 2006;25:3–14.

80. Morin CM, Bootzin RR, Buysse DJ, et al. Psychological and behavioral treatment of insomnia: update of the recent evidence (1998–2004). *Sleep.* 2006;29:1398–1414.

81. Harvey AG, Sharpley AL, Ree MJ, et al. An open trial of cognitive therapy for chronic insomnia. *Behav Res Ther.* 2007;45:2491–2501.

82. Morin CM, Savard J, Blais FC. Cognitive therapy for late-life insomnia. In: Lichstein KL, Morin CM, eds. *Treatment of late-life insomnia.* Thousand Oaks, CA: Sage Publications; 2000:207–230.

83. Currie SR, Wilson KG, Pontefract AJ, et al. Cognitive-behavioral treatment of insomnia secondary to chronic pain. *J Consult Clin Psychol.* 2000;68:407–416.

84. Edinger JD, Wohlgemuth WK, Krystal AD, et al. Behavioral insomnia therapy for fibromyalgia patients: a randomized clinical trial. *Arch Int Med.* 2005;165:2527–2535.

85. Lichstein KL, Wilson NM, Johnson CT. Psychological treatment of secondary insomnia. *Psychol Aging.* 2000;15:232–240.

86. Rybarczyk B, Lopez M, Benson R, et al. Efficacy of two behavioral treatment programs for comorbid geriatric insomnia. *Psychol Aging.* 2002;17:288–298.

87. Davidson JR, Waisberg JL, Brundage MD, et al. Nonpharmacologic group treatment of insomnia: a preliminary study with cancer survivors. *Psychooncology.* 2001;10:389–397.

88. Quesnel C, Savard J, Simard S, et al. Efficacy of cognitive-behavioral therapy for insomnia in women treated for nonmetastatic breast cancer. *J Consult Clin Psychol.* 2003;71:189–200.

89. Simeit R, Deck R, Conta-Marx B. Sleep management training for cancer patients with insomnia. *Support Care Cancer.* 2004;12:176–183.

90. Savard J, Simard S, Ivers H, et al. Randomized study on the efficacy of cognitive-behavioral therapy for insomnia secondary to breast cancer: I, Sleep and psychological effects. *J Clin Oncol.* 2005;23:6083–6095.

91. Bootzin RR, Epstein D, Wood JM. Stimulus control instructions. In: Hauri IP, ed. *Case studies in insomnia.* Vols 19–28. New York: Plenum Press; 1991.

92. Spielman AJ, Saskin P, Thorpy MJ. Treatment of chronic insomnia by restriction of time in bed. *Sleep.* 1987;10:45–56.

93. Belanger L, Savard J, Morin CM. Clinical management of insomnia using cognitive therapy. *Behav Sleep Med.* 2006;4:179–198.

94. Savard J, Ancoli-Israel S. Sleep and fatigue in cancer patients. In: Kryger MH, Roth T, Dement W, eds. *Principles and practice of sleep medicine.* 5th ed. St. Louis: Elsevier Saunders; 2011, pp 1416–1421.

95. Sharpe MC. Cognitive-behavioral therapy for patients with chronic fatigue syndrome: How? In: Demitrack MA, Abbey SE, eds. *Chronic fatigue syndrome: an integrative approach to evaluation and treatment.* New York: The Guilford Press; 1996:240–262.

96. Espie CA, Fleming L, Cassidy J, et al. Randomized controlled clinical effectiveness trial of cognitive behavior therapy compared with treatment as usual for persistent insomnia in patients with cancer. *J Clin Oncol.* 2008;26:4651–4658.

97. Bastien CH, Morin CM, Ouellet MC, et al. Cognitive-behavioral therapy for insomnia: comparison of individual therapy, group therapy, and telephone consultations. *J Consult Clin Psychol.* 2004;72:653–659.

98. Mimeault V, Morin CM. Self-help treatment for insomnia: bibliotherapy with and without professional guidance. *J Consult Clin Psychol.* 1999;67:511–519.

99. Morin CM, Beaulieu-Bonneau S, LeBlanc M, et al. Self-help treatment for insomnia: a randomized controlled trial. *Sleep.* 2005;28:1319–1327.

100. Riedel BW, Lichstein KL, Dwyer WO. *Sleep* compression and sleep education for older insomniacs: self-help versus therapist guidance. *Psychol Aging.* 1995;10:54–63.

101. Oosterhuis A, Klip EC. The treatment of insomnia through mass media, the results of a televised behavioral training programme. *Soc Sci Med.* 1997;45:1223–1229.

102. Ström L, Pettersson R, Andersson G. Internet-based treatment for insomnia: a controlled evaluation. *J Consult Clin Psychol.* 2004;72:113–120.

103. Savard J, Villa J, Simard S, et al. Feasibility of a self-help treatment for insomnia comorbid with cancer. *Psychooncology.* In press.

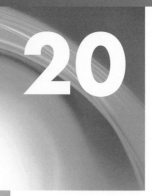

20 Itch complicating malignant diseases

Zbigniew Zylicz and Małgorzata Krajnik

Itch (prurigo, pruritus) is an unpleasant cutaneous sensation that provokes scratching. Although this old definition dating from the 17th century is still valid, in the clinical sense it can be nuanced slightly. Itch can also be sensed on the surface of the skin as mucous membranes (e.g., conjunctiva, mouth, vagina), and itch does not always provoke scratching. Some people experience severe itch but never scratch. Their suffering is probably no less because of this. And some people experience intense pleasure while gently scratching. Itch is an atavistic phenomenon from the earlier stages of evolution; it is useful to clear the surface of haired skin of insects and their excrement, toxins, and dirt by scratching. In nearly hairless human beings, itching does not have a specific function, and the neuronal representation in the spinal cord of itch neurons is much smaller than of those conveying pain.[1]

Mild itch is a common feature in both health and disease. However, moderate to severe itch is a rare but dreaded symptom accompanying a number of very diverse conditions.[1,2] Most of the patients who suffer severe itch wish they could have pain instead: "at least something could be done about this." Severe itch is so rare, and its physiopathology so diverse, that few drugs have been developed specifically to treat particular itch symptoms. Few controlled trials on itch have been conducted, and many of them were too underpowered to prove their point. Most therapies for itch are of an empirical nature, although some are now supported by a considerable amount of evidence.

CLASSIFICATION OF ITCH

Two classifications of severe chronic itch have been proposed until now.[1,3] The first classification by Twycross et al.[1] is based on the presumed mechanisms of the onset of the symptom. In this classification, which is similar to the classification of pain, the authors assume that three main mechanisms are involved in itch. First is the *pruritoceptive itch* (an analogy to nociceptive), which is caused by activation of the peripheral nerve endings of dedicated types of nerve fibers (see later). The other main type of itch is caused by *neurogenic* mechanisms. The nervous system is intact, but an imbalance between the neurotransmitters causes or disinhibits itch. These conditions may be reversible or amenable to pharmacologic treatment, provided that a new balance between the neurotransmitters can be found. The third category is the *neuropathic itch,* which is caused by disruption of the integrity and functioning of the nervous system. This disturbance may be peripheral (e.g., a peripheral nerve lesion due to surgery) or central (e.g., brain metastasis, stroke, abscess). Initially, peripheral disorders may be exacerbated by central extension of the disease, better known as sensitization.[4] Itch from this category is mostly irreversible. When the drugs used to depress itch are discontinued, the itch returns. In addition, another category of *psychogenic itch* can probably be seen as a subset of *neurogenic itch,* and the category of *mixed pruritus* is best represented by the multifactorial itch that complicates chronic kidney disease and dialysis.

This mechanism-oriented classification is controversial because the cause of itch remains unknown in many situations, and precise mechanism-oriented classification is impossible. Above all, the subcategory of *neurogenic itch* is believed to be misleading and difficult to differentiate from *neuropathic itch.* A more recent classification, endorsed by the International Forum for the Studies of Itch (IFSI), is believed to be more clinical and of practical use.[3] Itch is categorized as *itch in dermatologic disorders,* with primary skin disease, where skin inflammation (dermatosis) is the primary and predominant feature. Examples of these diseases are psoriasis, atopic dermatitis, xeroderma, and urticaria. It is believed that in many but not all of these diseases, histamine plays an important role in the origin of itch. The other main category is the itch encountered in the course of systemic diseases, where the skin is primarily intact. In this category, one finds renal and hepatic impairment and malignancies, both hematologic and solid tumors. In this category, skin involvement is usually secondary and is the result of persistent scratching and lichenification of the skin. Several dermatologic conditions are recognized as symptoms accompanying malignancies; most of these, however, are rare and play a role in early diagnosis. In itch with intact skin (the old name being *prurigo sine materia*), histamine plays a much lesser role than in dermatologic types of itch. Another main category is *neuropathy,* both central and peripheral. *Psychogenic itch* is yet another category where psychiatric disorders such as pruritic somatoform pruritus, delusions, and depression are in the foreground. Similar to previous classifications, two categories have been identified: mixed and unknown.

Another part of the classification is the recognition that itch may be generalized, which is most often the case in systemic disorders, or localized, most often in neuropathy, where the itch is limited to the area served by one single nerve. More often, itch appears initially in some typical areas of the skin. This is characteristic of the dermatologic disorders and forms a basis for the clinical recognition of these diseases. Itch may evolve over time, starting as a localized phenomenon (e.g., post-herpetic pruritus), but extends to other areas because of spinal cord sensitization.[5]

EPIDEMIOLOGY OF ITCH IN MALIGNANT DISEASES

Few true epidemiologic studies of itch have been conducted.[6] Among all patients seeking medical attention for pruritus, the prevalence of an underlying systemic disease has been reported to be 10% to 50%.[7,8] Pruritus without primary skin involvement is thought to be an interesting phenomenon, as it precedes the diagnosis of malignancy. However, when patients with unexplained itch are followed for a longer

time, only a few of them will be diagnosed with malignancies. For 6 years Paul and Jansen.[9] followed 125 patients with unexplained generalized itch. Two thirds of these patients continued to suffer from pruritus. In four patients (3.2%), malignancies were diagnosed during the initial investigation; four others (3.2%) were diagnosed with malignancy during the follow-up period. In another more recent study, Afifi et al.[10] followed 95 patients for 5 years while they were suffering from pruritus without primary skin involvement. In 40% of the patients, a systemic disease was diagnosed in the course of the study. Hematologic malignancies were most common (7%), among them myeloma, Hodgkin's disease, and myeloproliferative syndromes. Cancer was diagnosed in one individual (1%). In both studies, the incidence of cancers did not vary much from the expected incidence for sex- and age-matched populations. However, in both studies, significance was reached for hematologic malignancies. Itch is a leading symptom in 30% of patients with Hodgkin's disease,[11] and the presence of itch has a negative prognostic value for Hodgkin's disease.[12,13] In polycythemia rubra vera, this percentage approaches 50%.[14]

Taking it from another angle, Kilic et al.[15] investigated 700 patients with newly diagnosed cancer for the presence of cutaneous manifestations: Three hundred sixteen patients (45%) had cutaneous manifestations; xerosis without itch was the feature in 59 (8.4%), and generalized pruritus without dermatoses in 41 (5.9%). Again, pruritus was most common among hematologic malignancies (6/87), gastrointestinal cancers (10/107), lung cancers (5/130), breast cancers (7/80), genitourinary cancers (4/84), cerebral tumors (2/17), and sarcomas (2/77). In a study by Sommer et al.,[16] among 263 patients referred to the specialist center interested in the diagnosis and treatment of itch, four had non-Hodgkin's lymphoma and one patient with prostate cancer was suffering from pruritus. If both studies are taken as true, this means that only a few patients with itch are referred to specialist centers, and we are missing substantial numbers of them. It may also reflect the fact that most of the itch that accompanies malignancies responds to chemotherapy and radiotherapy, and referral for symptomatic treatment is not yet needed. The results of these studies leave us with an uncomfortable feeling that the needs of patients with itch in the course of malignancies are not being addressed effectively.

Another issue arising from these data is that patients with chronic unexplained itch, especially the variety without primary skin involvement, should be periodically investigated for hematologic malignancies in particular.[17–19] Itch accompanying malignancies with dermatoses has been reviewed many times previously [20–23] and will not be discussed here. Recognition of dermatoses contributes to the diagnosis of malignancy. However, it must be pointed out here that although pruritus without dermatosis may precede the diagnosis of malignancy by months to years (hematologic malignancies) or weeks to months (solid tumors), skin dermatoses related to malignancy (with or without itch) tend to appear at the moment of diagnosis or develop later in the course of disease (Table 20-1).

The intensity of itch symptoms tends to increase when the course of a disease can no longer be modified. However, the overall incidence of severe itch in palliative care remains very low and is certainly less than 1% (Z. Zylicz, unpublished).

Table 20-1 Pruritus may complicate the following malignant diseases (in decreasing order of frequency)

Cutaneous T-cell lymphomas
- Mycosis fungoides
- Sézary syndrome

Polycythemia rubra vera

Hodgkin's lymphoma (with and without cholestasis)

Myeloproliferative diseases
- Multiple myeloma
- Waldenström macroglobulinemia
- Chronic myeloid leukemia
- Benign gammopathies

Solid tumors (very rare)
- Breast, stomach, lung, prostate, nasopharynx, pharynx, other

of these interneurons may be modified by endogenous and exogenous opioids administered spinally. It is interesting to note that the activation of μ-opioid receptors (MORs) results in analgesia but also in the facilitation of itch. Activation of κ-opioid receptors (KORs) results in analgesia and inhibition of itch.[31,32] This serves as the basis for the action of the recently introduced κ agonist nalfurafine in the treatment of different types of itch.[33] Interaction between MORs and KORs probably explains opioid-induced itch after spinal administration of morphine,[34,35] but not itch after systemic administration.[34] On the segmental level, the activity of the itch-conveying neurons is modified by serotonergic (5-HT$_3$) and dopaminergic (D$_2$) receptors and prostaglandins, gamma-aminobutyric acid (GABA), and glycine receptors.[35] Involvement of these receptors forms the basis of future therapies. Irritation of the peripheral nociceptors can inhibit itch in the spinal cord. These nociceptors are identical to those that are stimulated by scratching; the mechanism has been exploited in so-called cutaneous field stimulation[36–38] (Fig. 20-1).

NEUROPHYSIOLOGY OF CHRONIC ITCH

For decades, histamine released from skin mast cells was regarded as the most important and only mechanism of itch.[24] Injections of histamine under the skin cause an axon reflex reaction (flare) and severe itch. Histamine released from the mast cells reacts with specific receptors (*pruritoceptors*) on the nerve endings of the mechano-insensitive subset of C fibers (H$_1$, H$_3$, and H$_4$).[25] This type of itch is responsive to antihistamines. It is now well established that a tropical plant, cowhage (*Mucuna pruriens*), evokes a histamine-independent itch through its spiculae.[26] The active agent inducing itch has been identified as mucunain protease, which activates host PAR-2 and PAR-4 receptors on the mechano-sensitive C fibers.[27–29] Cowhage spiculae produce severe pruritus but without skin flare. This is important for understanding why antihistamines are usually ineffective in the treatment of many types of itch, especially those without apparent cutaneous reaction to histamine. In the spinal cord, itch neurons end in the lamina-I area of the dorsal horn and switch over to second order neurons similar to those that convey pain.[26] Both itch and pain neurons are connected by interneurons that are activated by pain and may inhibit itch. This is the predominant mechanism behind inhibition of pruritus by scratching (nociception).[30] The activity

PRURITIC SYNDROMES ENCOUNTERED IN THE COURSE OF MALIGNANT DISEASE

DRY SKIN (XEROSIS)

Dry skin (xerosis) has been recognized as a cause of itch for many decades. Dry skin may result from inflammation, dehydration, lack of protecting skin fats, or exposure to wind and sunlight. It is a specific but frequent symptom in many diseases, but it also occurs in healthy elderly people.[39,40] Dry skin accompanies many diseases, malignancies among them.[15] However, in a study by Kilic et al.,[15] patients suffering from xerosis were distinct from those suffering from generalized pruritus. No overlap between populations was noted. Older patients suffer from xerosis because of age-related changes in skin biology, and itch may result in this group from the acquired abnormality of keratinization.[41] Changes in the skin, inflammation, and especially breaks in the skin sensitize nerve endings of C-unmyelinated, itch-conveying neurons.[42] It is no surprise that skin moisturizers are seen as important for the treatment of every type of itch.[43] Providing skin with a thin and slippery fat layer not only prevents skin from drying but also prevents further damage during scratching. Skin moisturizers break the vicious cycle of itch-scratching-sensitization-more itch.[43]

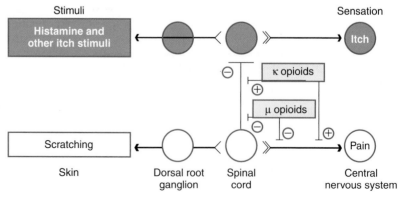

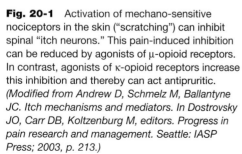

Fig. 20-1 Activation of mechano-sensitive nociceptors in the skin ("scratching") can inhibit spinal "itch neurons." This pain-induced inhibition can be reduced by agonists of μ-opioid receptors. In contrast, agonists of κ-opioid receptors increase this inhibition and thereby can act antipruritic. (*Modified from Andrew D, Schmelz M, Ballantyne JC. Itch mechanisms and mediators. In Dostrovsky JO, Carr DB, Koltzenburg M, editors. Progress in pain research and management. Seattle: IASP Press; 2003, p. 213.*)

Skin moisturizers should be applied to the skin several times a day, and not only after bathing. To prevent drying, patients should not bathe or shower with hot water and should not use rough towels. This removes the rest of the protective fat layer and also increases skin inflammation.

ITCH OF CHOLESTASIS

The most common severe pruritic condition in advanced disease is the itch of cholestasis.[1] Cholestasis may be caused by intrahepatic metastases, tumor infiltration of the liver, and obstruction of the common bile duct by pancreatic cancer and secondary tumors in the liver hilus. For decades, accumulation of bile acids in the skin was thought to be responsible for this phenomenon.[44–46] However, the correlation between plasma concentrations of bile acids and itch is poor,[47,48] and the current consensus is that bile acids probably play a minor role in this syndrome.[49] Pruritogen(s) or their components or activators are synthesized in the cholestatic liver and excreted with bile.[49] Their retention in the liver and enterohepatic absorption are responsible for itch. Pruritogen(s) is/are metabolized in the liver by CYP enzymes.

Bile drainage

Successful bile drainage through endoscopy-placed stents in the common bile duct relieves jaundice and in many cases relieves itch.[50,51] The evidence for itch relief after stenting is scant and controversial. A meta-analysis of endoscopic techniques for bile drainage stated only that "the drainage improves quality of life including itch."[52] However, after stenting, the presumptive pruritogen would still be reabsorbed from the duodenum and would be responsible for the reappearance of itch. In some cases after stenting, only transient relief of itch is observed. The now rarely performed percutaneous bile drainage[53] and the recently more fashionable nasobiliary drainage[54–56] may be better alternatives. When the biliary system is drained externally, ion exchange resins are ineffective because there is nothing to bind in the gut. Another disadvantage of ion exchange resins even with patent bile ducts is their palatability, particularly cholestyramine.

Rifampicin

A treatment for the itch of cholestasis is the use of rifampicin.[57–60] It is thought that rifampicin may interfere with the metabolism of pruritogen(s), including bile acids,[61] through the induction of microsomal enzymes (CYP3A4)[49] and may promote the 6-alpha-hydroxylation and subsequent 6-alpha-glucuronidation of toxic bile salts.[62] Even though the relationship between bile acids and pruritus is doubted, the increased metabolic conversion may reduce the putative and still unknown pruritogen(s). On the other hand, the induction of cytochrome reduces enzymes, but other drugs such as carbamazepine are not known to relieve pruritus. Rifampicin is only rarely used in the context of palliative care, as rifampicin hepatotoxicity is increased in emaciated and cachectic cancer patients.[63–65]

Opioid agonists and antagonists

Cholestasis induces synthesis of endogenous opioids in the liver.[66] These opioid peptides influence hormones and neurotransmitters in the distant organs. An imbalance of opioid peptides and increased opioidergic tone serve as the basis for the use of opioid antagonists in the treatment of itch.[67–70] Increased opioidergic tone in the central nervous system may be responsible not only for itch, but also for analgesia.[71,72] Blocking the latter with naloxone will alleviate itch but will also unmask pain.[73,74] Very low continuous infusions of naloxone (3 μg/kg/24 hr) have been tried with success.[75,76] Oral naltrexone in tablet form (50 mg) is too high a dose and will inevitably reverse analgesia. Unconfirmed reports have used oral methylnaltrexone to block endogenous opioids at the skin level and reduce itch, as this drug is peripherally restricted by peripheral opioid receptors on the C-fiber nerve endings.[77]

Alternatives to opioid receptor blockers at the primary site of action include buprenorphine for the treatment of cholestatic itch. Buprenorphine has a high affinity for μ-opioid receptors and thus makes them unavailable for binding endogenous pruritogenic opioids. The use of buprenorphine for this purpose was reported in a small trial by Juby et al.[78] Although sublingual buprenorphine exhibited toxicity in patients with cholestatic pruritus, the availability of transdermal patches has renewed interest in buprenorphine. Several case reports have suggested benefit of this drug against itch.[79–81] However, critical analysis of these cases suggests that it is not buprenorphine alone, but the combination of buprenorphine and an ultra-low dose of naloxone, that provides benefit.

The recently introduced opioid κ-agonist nalfurafine has proved to be effective in animal models.[82,83] This drug, which until now has been tested only in patients with uremic itch, is very promising with cholestatic pruritus in advanced disease.

Serotonin reuptake inhibitors

Various selective serotonin reuptake inhibiting (SSRI) antidepressant drugs have been investigated in cholestatic pruritus. In two trials by Zylicz et al.[84] and Ständer et al.,[85] few patients with cholestatic pruritus were included; most evidence can be distilled from the trial by Mayo et al.[86] In this trial, sertraline was found to be efficacious against cholestatic pruritus of primary biliary cirrhosis and was proposed as the first-line treatment in this condition. Slow titration prevents nausea and vomiting as seen in the trial by Zylicz et al.[84] Pruritus is usually relieved within days, but the optimal benefits are seen after a couple of weeks.[85] If cholestasis cannot be relieved by bile drainage, tachyphylaxis to SSRIs is frequently observed (Zylicz, unpublished). This was not a problem in primary biliary cirrhosis, where no acute retention of a putative pruritogen(s) occurs.[87] The mechanism of action is unclear. On the one hand, SSRIs are thought to influence the processing of pain and pruritus in the spinal cord.[88] SSRIs may also act on peripheral serotonin receptors in the skin.[89] SSRIs may be useful drugs, but their use is limited in malignancy-related cholestasis.

Serotonin receptor antagonists

Antagonists to serotonin 5-HT$_3$ receptors such as ondansetron, tropisetron, and granisetron are reported to relieve itch from various conditions.[90–94] These drugs are most effective when pruritus is accompanied by nausea.[90] Despite a plethora of case reports, controlled trials have not confirmed the benefits of these drugs in cholestatic pruritus[93] or uremic pruritus.[95] Benefits are seen in the case of spinal opioid-induced pruritus.[90,94,96,97]

WHEN A PATIENT CANNOT SWALLOW

A frequent problem in advanced cancer is the inability to swallow in the last days of life, when the itch can be at its worst. Transdermal buprenorphine, with or without naloxone, and intravenous 5-HT$_3$ antagonists can be tried, although their benefits are not well established (see earlier). An alternative is parenteral intravenous lignocaine.[98,99] Palliative lignocaine is equally effective as parenteral lignocaine when administered via continuous subcutaneous infusion (unpublished). Doses need to be titrated upward from 100 mg/24 hr. Alternatively, 5% lidocaine patches are used on the skin, where the itch is localized. A eutectic mixture of local anesthetic agents also may be useful.[100]

Miscellaneous

In the past, it was reported that the itch of cholestasis responds to administration of androgens.[101] Androgens increase the threshold for pain and itch, while estrogens decrease it. No reports have confirmed these findings. In intractable itch of cholestasis in terminal illness, propofol has been used to depress spinal conveyance of both itch and pain.[102,103] This treatment is used as a last resort therapy when sedation is a welcome option.

What does not work

Histamine is a potent pruritogen and is synthesized in mast cells by the decarboxylation of histidine. Multiple factors are able to release histamine from the mast cells. Morphine releases histamine, and this is not reversible by naloxone.[104,105] The only histamine-related skin reactions are the wheal and itch after an intradermal injection of morphine and, sometimes, itch and redness along a vein after intravenous injection of morphine. Bile acids are able to release histamine from the mast cells, albeit at very high concentrations only.[106,107] Antihistamines have little effect on cholestatic itch and play only a minor role in the mechanism generating pruritus of cholestasis.[49,69] Gabapentin is very effective in the treatment of uremic itch and complicating hemodialysis,[108,109] but is ineffective in cholestatic pruritus.[110]

UREMIC PRURITUS

Uremic pruritus is very rare in cancer. This type of itch is most prevalent in patients on hemodialysis and less so in patients with chronic renal insufficiency.[111] Virtually no pruritus is seen in acute renal insufficiency. Occasionally, patients with multiple myeloma who are hemodialyzed for chronic renal failure will have severe pruritus.[112,113] Uremic pruritus is known to be multifactorial, and its complex nature and treatment have been reviewed extensively in the past.[114,115] Among therapies tried for uremic itch, gabapentin at a low dose has been found to be effective.[109,116–119] Nalfurafine, a κ-opioid receptor agonist, is very promising also.[32,33]

Localized uremic itch is treated with tacrolimus ointment[120] or capsaicin cream.[121,122]

PARANEOPLASTIC PRURITUS

In a study by Kilic et al.[15] (41/700), all patients suffered from paraneoplastic itch. This study is difficult to interpret, as at least some paraneoplastic itches are accompanied by dermatoses, and itch without dermatosis is rare. Pruritic dermatoses associated with malignancies have been reviewed several times elsewhere,[123–125] and antipruritic therapy in these cases should be aimed at decreasing skin inflammation.

Paraneoplastic itch without skin involvement is common with hematologic malignancies but is much less common in cancers and sarcomas.[1] A series of patients with solid tumors was described by Cormia and Domonkos in 1965,[126] and in this unique and still unchallenged publication, the authors described criteria for paraneoplastic itch. Itch may precede the diagnosis of malignancy. The period of itch before the diagnosis may be very long in hematologic disorders (months to years) but is usually much shorter (weeks to months) with solid tumors. Treatment of the underlying cancer may be the single most effective remedy for paraneoplastic itch, and the reappearance of itch may herald recurrence. Itch has a tendency to become more intense when cancer is advanced. Some patients in advanced stages may suffer both from the itch due to their disease and from itch as a complication of the treatment. Thus, one may suffer several different types of pruritus.

Until now, no specific treatments were recommended for paraneoplastic itch. In a controlled trial by Zylicz et al.,[84] paroxetine was used for palliation of intractable itch in different groups of patients. Among those recruited for this trial, 17/26 (65%) had malignancies. Paroxetine was effective in approximately 30% of all patients; patients with paraneoplastic pruritus responded more often than patients without malignancies. These results were confirmed by a trial by Ständer et al.[85] Both Zylicz et al.[84] and Ständer et al.[85] reported that paraneoplastic itch accompanying lymphomas responded less well to SSRIs than paraneoplastic itch from solid tumors. However, paroxetine was effective in the treatment of itch accompanying polycythemia vera.[127,128] The long-term effects in this latter disease are promising only when cytoreductive therapy is continued (Tefferi, personal communication)—something that is not possible or is uncommon in advanced solid tumors.

Antihistamines are ineffective in treating paraneoplastic pruritus. However, interest in these drugs has recently increased after high doses of nonsedating antihistamines were introduced.[129,130] In intractable pruritus, high-dose antihistamines should be tried, given alone or in combination with other drugs.

NEUROPATHIC ITCH

Neuropathic itch is defined as itch caused by a primary lesion or dysfunction of the central or afferent peripheral nervous system.[131] This type of itch is chronic and persistent. Itch fibers are mostly histamine-insensitive, mechano-sensitive C fibers, which is the reason why this type of itch is insensitive to antihistamines and is associated with sensory changes. Itch may coexist with pain in the same area. The involved area may have paresthesias, allodynia, and hyperalgesia. In addition to pruritus, the involved area may show hyperknesis, which means an itch in response to innocuous stimuli that usually do not provoke itch. The area of itch may also include motor or autonomous damage. Secondary changes to the skin such as prurigo nodularis or lichenification are apparent if itch has existed for a long time. The site of itch may be hyperpigmented as the result of chronic inflammation.[132]

Total nerve fiber loss in an area of skin is rarely associated with itch. However, neuropathic itch is invariably associated with substantial loss of nerve fibers in the epidermis and papillary dermis.[133,134] Itch experienced after mastectomy is thought to be analogous to phantom pain, generated from the central neural signals proximal to the damage.[131] More often, the area of involvement is the result of partial nerve damage or compression of peripheral nerves. Frequently, this damage is due to herpetic infection (post-herpetic itch [PHI]),[135] nerve root compression by spinal metastases, tumor growth into the spinal cord,[136,137] or trauma.[138] It starts in one area, usually served by one nerve or nerve root, and extends later as a consequence of spinal cord sensitization. Painful stimuli can also be experienced as itch through the same process.[5] Less frequently, damage to areas in the brain causes itch distributed in the areas characteristic for such damage. The itch, therefore, may have a hemibody distribution if it results from abscess,[139] stroke,[140,141] or brain metastasis or primary brain tumor.[142]

POST-HERPETIC ITCH

Post-herpetic itch (PHI) is described in detail by Liddell[143] and Oaklander et al.[135,144] In the past, it was thought that PHI was uncommon; however, among 153 patients with shingles, 48% reported itch, with some reporting severe itch. This was confirmed later in another study by the same author.[145] Patients with shingles in head and neck dermatomes are more likely to develop PHI. Many patients with PHI have subclinical herpetic infection, without typical skin lesions. A common feature of PHN and PHI neuropathy is loss of skin nerve fibers consistent with loss of sensation to cold and warmth.[146] No specific trials of drugs for pruritus in PHI have been conducted, but the best guesses for drug benefit are gabapentin and pregabalin.[147-149] Other therapies worth trying are topical local anesthetics such as a eutectic mixture of local anesthetics (EMLA cream) and 5% lidocaine patch. Capsaicin cream (0.025%) can also be used.[150]

BRACHIORADIAL PRURITUS

Brachioradial pruritus (BP) is experienced in the dorsolateral arm, shoulder, and neck.[151-153] In most individuals with this disorder, compression of the spine at the level of C5-C8 is seen on magnetic resonance imaging (MRI).[154,155] Spinal tumors, both primary and secondary, especially those accompanied by multiple sensory changes, cause pruritus. Denervated skin is more sensitive to sunlight, and the mechanisms of BP were thought to be caused by increased light sensitivity.[156] Reduction in skin nerve fibers results in insensitivity to cold or warmth, which explains the "ice pack sign."[157] Treatment is similar to that for other neuropathies, and the best results, although not confirmed in controlled trials, are obtained with gabapentin and pregabalin.[158,159] In benign compression, gentle manipulation was also found to be effective.[160]

NOTALGIA PARESTHETICA

Notalgia paresthetica (NP) is a similar syndrome to BP that occurs at a different level of the spine, most often at the level of T2-T6,[161] which results in subscapular itch. Typically, it is not the nerve roots that are impinged but posterior primary rami of the intercostal nerves; thus itch and hyperalgesia are frequently limited to paravertebral parts of the dermatomes.[161] The state of impingement lies outside the spine, and spasm of the paraspinal muscles can be blamed. Although an increase in nerve fiber density within the skin was previously reported,[162]

in chronic cases, decreased nerve density is more likely to be observed.[132] Treatment is similar to that for other neuropathies, although in benign cases, vertebral manipulation results in decreased spasm of the paraspinal muscles, which is very effective (Zylicz, unpublished).

CHEIRALGIA PARESTHETICA

Cheiralgia paresthetica is a pruritic syndrome that is confined to the radial aspect of the lower arm and is caused by entrapment of the radial nerve.[163] It is a peripheral neuropathy caused by diabetes[164,165] or by handcuffs.[166]

TRIGEMINAL TROPHIC SYNDROME

Trigeminal trophic syndrome (TTS) is a rare condition caused by damage to the trigeminal nuclei or nerves, which is manifested by numbness, burning pain, and a crawling sensation. Physical signs include excoriations on face and damage to the nasal ala. TTS most often results from ablation of the Gasserian ganglion. This procedure is frequently performed for pain control; tumors infiltrating the Gasserian ganglion will have the same effect. Treatment is the same as for other neuropathies: carbamazepine and gabapentin.[167]

CENTRAL PRURITIC NEUROPATHIC SYNDROMES

Nearly all localized brain disease may produce itch.[168] This includes brain abscesses, tumors, strokes, scars, and Creutzfeldt-Jakob disease. Multiple sclerosis plaques will also generate itch. The affected area depends on localization of the lesion in the brain. For example, poststroke pruritus may be apparent as hemibody pruritus. No specific treatment is different from treatment provided for painful peripheral neuropathy; the usual drugs are gabapentin, carbamazepine, 5% lidocaine patches, and, in the most severe cases, intravenous lidocaine.

DRUG-INDUCED ITCH

Many drugs induce itch.[169] These reactions are divided into itch related to histamine release and histamine skin reactions (urticaria) and itch independent of histamine, without primary skin reactions. Histamine-related skin reactions appear within hours or days after drug initiation, although in some cases, this may be delayed and may be apparent even a week after discontinuation of the drug. This is frequently the case with amoxicillin. Some of the drugs used for chemotherapy cause yet another reaction, which is rare—itching neuropathy. These neuropathies develop slowly and take months before they are clinically apparent. It is important to note the temporal relationships. Another important step is to identify whether the suspected drug is on the list of notorious itch inducers (Table 20-2). The drug is discontinued or is replaced by other drugs from the same class.

Most often, drug-induced itch will be generalized. Rapid injection of intravenous dexamethasone will produce an annoying itch around the perineum.[170] This itch disappears rapidly upon completion of the IV injection. Heparins produce itch around the site of an injection,[171] probably through local extravasation and subsequent induration and inflammation.

Table 20-2 Drugs and treatment methods that may cause itch without skin histamine reaction (alphabetically)

Allopurinol	Insulin
Amiodarone	Isotretinoin
Amitriptyline	Ketoconazole
Ampicillin	Metronidazole
Aspirin	Miconazole
Atenolol	Morphine
Bleomycin	Niacin
Butorphanol	NSAIDs
Captopril	Estrogens
Cephalosporins	Oral contraceptives
Clonidine	Phenolphthalein
Colchicine	Polymyxin B
Colistin	Photochemotherapy (PUVA)
Coumarins	Probenecid
Dexamethasone	Progestagens
Diazoxide	Propylthiouracil
Dobutamine	Quinidine
Enalapril	Starch, hydroxyethylstarch
Fentanyl	Sulfonamides
Furosemide	Sulfonylureas
Gold salts	Suramin
Heparins	Vitamin B complex
Hydrochlorothiazide	Warfarin
Imipramine	

From Zylicz Z, Twycross R, Jones EA. *Pruritus in advanced disease.* Oxford: Oxford University Press; 2004.

NSAIDs, Nonsteroidal antiinflammatory drugs; *PUVA,* psoralen and ultraviolet A therapy.

Itch may be due to the vehicle and not to the drug. Changing to another product may result in resolution. Itch induced by opioids is discussed separately in the next section.

OPIOID-INDUCED PRURITUS

Opioid-induced itch is divided into two different phenomena[34]: itch related to spinal opioids (epidural and intrathecal) and itch produced by systemic opioids.

Spinal opioids

Approximately 60% of patients receiving spinal opioids without an antipruritic drug will experience pruritus.[172]

Estrogens increase susceptibility to pruritus, especially during pregnancy.[173,174] Pruritus due to intrathecal opioids occurs within minutes in the case of fentanyl and within hours with morphine. Morphine needs to be transported cephalad to produce itch.[175] Itch becomes less common with subsequent doses, which may be the reason why patients treated for pain long term with spinal opioids do not suffer from pruritus.[176,177] Pruritus due to intrathecal morphine is usually limited to the face, neck, and/or upper thorax, and is especially centered in the facial areas innervated by the trigeminal nerve. Rarely does it appear as generalized pruritus.[178] Opioid-induced itching is probably neurogenic in origin, resulting from a spinal reflex transmitted through a medullary itch center proximal to the spinal nucleus of the trigeminal nerve.[179,180] Transmission is blocked by small amounts of local anesthetic added to spinal opioid.[175] The spinal nucleus of the trigeminal nerve and the medullary dorsal horn are rich in μ-opioid receptors, which, if stimulated, evoke segmental itch.[180] Opioids have an excitatory effect on central ascending neuronal tracts, resulting in activation of serotonergic pathways. Another hypothesis is that opioids block inhibitory transmitter glycine and GABA release.[181] Local effects of opioids within the spinal cord are amplified by prostaglandins.[182]

The most effective treatment, as evidenced by randomized controlled trials, is naloxone (given intravenously or epidurally) in low enough doses, below those needed to reverse analgesia.[183,184] Another option is κ-opioid receptor agonists, especially when the need to avoid compromising analgesia is mandatory. Several clinical trials have confirmed the effectiveness of nalbuphine (a μ-opioid receptor partial agonist and a κ-opioid receptor agonist).[185] Benefits have been observed with intranasal butorphanol (a strong κ-opioid receptor agonist and a weak μ-opioid receptor antagonist).[186] Ondansetron, a 5-HT$_3$ receptor antagonist, relieves pruritus associated with intrathecal and epidural morphine.[97,187] The effects of ondansetron on pruritus induced by intrathecal fentanyl are still debated.[188,189] The addition of local anesthetics controls opioid-induced neuroexcitation—a fact that has been known for many years by anesthetists and was recently confirmed in a meta-analysis of controlled trials.[190] Similar effects are seen with propofol.[191] The benefit of intravenous droperidol in epidural morphine-induced pruritus is disputed.[192,193] Another valuable suggestion, not verified by controlled trials, is the use of diclofenac and tenoxicam.[182,194]

Spinal opioids are rarely used without local anesthetics; this means that in everyday practice, spinal opioid–induced pruritus is rarely seen. It is more of a problem when opioids are used for perioperative and postoperative analgesia and treatment.

Pruritus induced by systemic opioids

The incidence of pruritus with systemic administration in adults is much lower than after spinal administration at approximately 1%.[181] Prevalence is increased in children with cancer treated with morphine (28%).[195] Unlike epidural or intrathecal opioids, systemic opioids provide a generalized itch. The mechanism underlying itch is completely different from those caused by spinal opioids. The mechanism is both peripheral and central. In some situations, pruritus evoked by systemic opioids is mediated by opioid receptors and is reversed by naloxone; in others, naloxone is ineffective. Certain opioids evoke histamine release from mast cells and produce histamine-related pruritus.[196] The failure of naloxone to prevent histamine release from human mast cells (by morphine) suggests that it is not mediated by opioid receptors. Plasma concentrations of histamine are increased after intravenous administration of morphine but not with intravenous fentanyl and epidural morphine.[197] In histamine-related pruritus, it makes sense to rotate opioids or administer H₁-antihistamines.

Most pruritus with systemic opioids does not involve histamine and is reversed by naloxone. This type of itch is common with fentanyl. Pruritus that results from activation of opioid receptors may be decreased by an opioid switch, that is, administration of a μ-opioid receptor antagonist, a κ-opioid receptor agonist, or a partial μ-opioid receptor agonist.

If not effective, ondansetron or propofol restores central inhibition of itch by modulating serotonergic transmission.[198] When opioid switching or H₁-antihistamines are not effective, paroxetine is a good and practical choice.[199]

CONCLUSION

Itch or pruritus is a common problem for patients with cancer and has diverse causes. Treatments are various and complicated. Relatively few data are derived from controlled studies; this makes it difficult to formulate a rational choice of therapy. With improved understanding of the phenomenon of itch, new therapies are becoming available.

REFERENCES

1. Twycross R, Greaves MW, Handwerker H, et al. Itch: scratching more than the surface. *QJM.* 2003;96:7–26.
2. Krajnik M, Zylicz Z. Understanding pruritus in systemic disease. *J Pain Symptom Manage.* 2001;21:151–168.
3. Ständer S, Weisshaar E, Mettang T, et al. Clinical classification of itch: a position paper of the International Forum for the Study of Itch. *Acta Derm Venereol.* 2007;87:291–294.
4. D'Mello R, Dickenson AH. Spinal cord mechanisms of pain. *Br J Anaesth.* 2008;101:8–16.
5. Ikoma A, Fartasch M, Heyer G, et al. Painful stimuli evoke itch in patients with chronic pruritus: central sensitization for itch. *Neurology.* 2004;62:212–217.
6. Weisshaar E, Dalgard F. Epidemiology of itch: adding to the burden of skin morbidity. *Acta Derm Venereol.* 2009;89:339–350.
7. Kantor GR. Evaluation and treatment of generalized pruritus. *Cleve Clin J Med.* 1990;57:521–526.
8. Kantor GR, Lookingbill DP. Generalized pruritus and systemic disease. *J Am Acad Dermatol.* 1983;9:375–382.
9. Paul R, Jansen CT. Itch and malignancy prognosis in generalized pruritus: a 6-year follow-up of 125 patients. *J Am Acad Dermatol.* 1987;16:1179–1182.
10. Afifi Y, Aubin F, Puzenat E, et al. [Pruritus sine materia: a prospective study of 95 patients]. *Rev Med Interne.* 2004;25:490–493.
11. Alexander LL. Pruritus and Hodgkin's disease. *JAMA.* 1979;241:2598–2599.
12. Feiner AS, Mahmood T, Wallner SF. Prognostic importance of pruritus in Hodgkin's disease. *JAMA.* 1978;240:2738–2740.
13. Gobbi PG, Attardo-Parrinello G, Lattanzio G, et al. Severe pruritus should be a B-symptom in Hodgkin's disease. *Cancer.* 1983;51:1934–1936.
14. Diehn F, Tefferi A. Pruritus in polycythaemia vera: prevalence, laboratory correlates and management. *Br J Haematol.* 2001;115:619–621.
15. Kilic A, Gul U, Soylu S. Skin findings in internal malignant diseases. *Int J Dermatol.* 2007;46:1055–1060.
16. Sommer F, Hensen P, Bockenholt B, et al. Underlying diseases and co-factors in patients with severe chronic pruritus: a 3-year retrospective study. *Acta Derm Venereol.* 2007;87:510–516.
17. Lober CW. Should the patient with generalized pruritus be evaluated for malignancy? *J Am Acad Dermatol.* 1988;19:350–352.
18. Hiramanek N. Itch: a symptom of occult disease. *Aust Fam Physician.* 2004;33:495–499.
19. Moses S. Pruritus. *Am Fam Physician.* 2003;68:1135–1142.
20. Sneddon IB. Cutaneous manifestations of visceral malignancy. *Postgrad Med J.* 1970;46:678–685.
21. Costache M, Simionescu O, Sajin M, et al. Cutaneous metastasis carcinoma: case report and pathological considerations. *Rom J Morphol Embryol.* 2007;48:177–180.
22. Cahill J, Sinclair R. Cutaneous manifestations of systemic disease. *Aust Fam Physician.* 2005;34:335–340.
23. Lee A. Skin manifestations of systemic disease. *Aust Fam Physician.* 2009;38:498–505.
24. Kosteletzky F, Namer B, Forster C, et al. Impact of scratching on itch and sympathetic reflexes induced by cowhage *(Mucuna pruriens)* and histamine. *Acta Derm Venereol.* 2009;89:271–277.
25. Ständer S, Weisshaar E, Luger TA. Neurophysiological and neurochemical basis of modern pruritus treatment. *Exp Dermatol.* 2008;17:161–169.
26. Namer B, Carr R, Johanek LM, et al. Separate peripheral pathways for pruritus in man. *J Neurophysiol.* 2008;100:2062–2069.
27. Lamotte RH, Shimada SG, Green BG, et al. Pruritic and nociceptive sensations and dysesthesias from a spicule of cowhage. *J Neurophysiol.* 2009;101:1430–1443.
28. Reddy VB, Iuga AO, Shimada SG, et al. Cowhage-evoked itch is mediated by a novel cysteine protease: a ligand of protease-activated receptors. *J Neurosci.* 2008;28:4331–4335.
29. Johanek LM, Meyer RA, Friedman RM, et al. A role for polymodal C-fiber afferents in nonhistaminergic itch. *J Neurosci.* 2008;28:7659–7669.
30. Schmelz M, Schmidt R, Bickel A, et al. Specific C-receptors for itch in human skin. *J Neurosci.* 1997;17:8003–8008.
31. Ko MC, Lee H, Song MS, et al. Activation of kappa-opioid receptors inhibits pruritus evoked by subcutaneous or intrathecal administration of morphine in monkeys. *J Pharmacol Exp Ther.* 2003;305:173–179.
32. Ko MC, Husbands SM. Effects of atypical kappa-opioid receptor agonists on intrathecal morphine-induced itch and analgesia in primates. *J Pharmacol Exp Ther.* 2009;328:193–200.
33. Nakao K, Mochizuki H. Nalfurafine hydrochloride: a new drug for the treatment of uremic pruritus in hemodialysis patients. *Drugs Today (Barc).* 2009;45:323–329.
34. Reich A, Szepietowski JC. Opioid-induced pruritus: an update. *Clin Exp Dermatol.* 2009;35:2–6.
35. Ganesh A, Maxwell LG. Pathophysiology and management of opioid-induced pruritus. *Drugs.* 2007;67:2323–2333.
36. Nilsson HJ, Psouni E, Carstam R, et al. Profound inhibition of chronic itch induced by stimulation of thin cutaneous nerve fibres. *J Eur Acad Dermatol Venereol.* 2004;18:37–43.
37. Wallengren J. Cutaneous field stimulation of sensory nerve fibers reduces itch without affecting contact dermatitis. *Allergy.* 2002;57:1195–1199.
38. Yosipovitch G, Fleischer A. Itch associated with skin disease: advances in pathophysiology and emerging therapies. *Am J Clin Dermatol.* 2003;4:617–622.
39. Thaipisuttikul Y. Pruritic skin diseases in the elderly. *J Dermatol.* 1998;25:153–157.
40. Fleischer Jr AB. Pruritus in the elderly: management by senior dermatologists. *J Am Acad Dermatol.* 1993;28:603–609.
41. Long CC, Marks R. Stratum corneum changes in patients with senile pruritus. *J Am Acad Dermatol.* 1992;27:560–564.
42. Kobayashi H, Kikuchi K, Tsubono Y, et al. Measurement of electrical current perception threshold of sensory nerves for pruritus in atopic dermatitis patients and normal individuals with various degrees of mild damage to the stratum corneum. *Dermatology.* 2003;206:204–211.
43. Yosipovitch G, Hundley JL. Practical guidelines for relief of itch. *Dermatol Nurs.* 2004;16:325–328; quiz 9.
44. Bergasa NV. Update on the treatment of the pruritus of cholestasis. *Clin Liver Dis.* 2008;12:219–234.
45. Rosenthal E, Diamond E, Benderly A, et al. Cholestatic pruritus: effect of phototherapy on pruritus and excretion of bile acids in urine. *Acta Paediatr.* 1994;83:888–891.
46. Jones EA, Bergasa NV. The pruritus of cholestasis: from bile acids to opiate agonists. *Hepatology.* 1990;11:884–887.
47. Ghent CN, Bloomer JR, Klatskin G. Elevations in skin tissue levels of bile acids in human cholestasis: relation to serum levels and topruritus. *Gastroenterology.* 1977;73:1125–1130.
48. Freedman MR, Holzbach RT, Ferguson DR. Pruritus in cholestasis: no direct causative role for bile acid retention. *Am J Med.* 1981;70:1011–1016.
49. Kremer AE, Beuers U, Oude-Elferink RP, et al. Pathogenesis and treatment of pruritus in cholestasis. *Drugs.* 2008;68:2163–2182.
50. Luman W, Cull A, Palmer KR. Quality of life in patients stented for malignant biliary obstructions. *Eur J Gastroenterol Hepatol.* 1997;9:481–484.

51. Ballinger AB, McHugh M, Catnach SM, et al. Symptom relief and quality of life after stenting for malignant bile duct obstruction. *Gut.* 1994;35:467–470.

52. Hammarstrom LE. Role of palliative endoscopic drainage in patients with malignant biliary obstruction. *Dig Surg.* 2005;22:295–304.

53. Pollock TW, Ring ER, Oleaga JA, et al. Percutaneous decompression of benign and malignant biliary obstruction. *Arch Surg.* 1979;114:148–151.

54. Singh V, Bhalla A, Sharma N, et al. Nasobiliary drainage in acute cholestatic hepatitis with pruritus. *Dig Liver Dis.* 2009;41:442–445.

55. Stapelbroek JM, van Erpecum KJ, Klomp LW, et al. Nasobiliary drainage induces long-lasting remission in benign recurrent intrahepatic cholestasis. *Hepatology.* 2006;43:51–53.

56. Hofmann AF, Huet PM. Nasobiliary drainage for cholestatic pruritus. *Hepatology.* 2006;43:1170–1171.

57. Price TJ, Patterson WK, Olver IN. Rifampicin as treatment for pruritus in malignant cholestasis. *Support Care Cancer.* 1998;6:533–535.

58. Karas JA, Pillay DG, Sturm AW. Rifampicin and pruritus. *S Afr Med J.* 1998;88:807.

59. Airede AK, Weerasinghe HD. Rifampicin and the relief of pruritus of hepatic cholestatic origin. *Acta Paediatr.* 1996;85:887–888.

60. Gregorio GV, Ball CS, Mowat AP, et al. Effect of rifampicin in the treatment of pruritus in hepatic cholestasis. *Arch Dis Child.* 1993;69:141–143.

61. Galeazzi R, Lorenzini I, Orlandi F. Rifampicin-induced elevation of serum bile acids in man. *Dig Dis Sci.* 1980;25:108–112.

62. Miguet JP, Mavier P, Soussy CJ, et al. Induction of hepatic microsomal enzymes after brief administration of rifampicin in man. *Gastroenterology.* 1977;72:924–926.

63. Tandon P, Rowe BH, Vandermeer B, et al. The efficacy and safety of bile Acid binding agents, opioid antagonists, or rifampin in the treatment of cholestasis-associated pruritus. *Am J Gastroenterol.* 2007;102:1528–1536.

64. Bachs L, Pares A, Elena M, et al. Effects of long-term rifampicin administration in primary biliary cirrhosis. *Gastroenterology.* 1992;102:2077–2080.

65. Prince MI, Burt AD, Jones DE. Hepatitis and liver dysfunction with rifampicin therapy for pruritus in primary biliary cirrhosis. *Gut.* 2002;50:436–439.

66. Jones EA, Weissenborn K. Neurology and the liver. *J Neurol Neurosurg Psychiatry.* 1997;63:279–293.

67. Bergasa NV. The pruritus of cholestasis. *J Hepatol.* 2005;43:1078–1088.

68. Jones EA, Neuberger J, Bergasa NV. Opiate antagonist therapy for the pruritus of cholestasis: the avoidance of opioid withdrawal-like reactions. *QJM.* 2002;95:547–552.

69. Jones EA, Bergasa NV. Evolving concepts of the pathogenesis and treatment of the pruritus of cholestasis. *Can J Gastroenterol.* 2000;14:33–40.

70. Jones EA, Zylicz Z. Treatment of pruritus caused by cholestasis with opioid antagonists. *J Palliat Med.* 2005;8:1290–1294.

71. Nelson L, Vergnolle N, D'Mello C, et al. Endogenous opioid-mediated antinociception in cholestatic mice is peripherally, not centrally, mediated. *J Hepatol.* 2006;44:1141–1149.

72. Zyliez Z, Krajnik M. What has dry cough in common with pruritus? Treatment of dry cough with paroxetine. *J Pain Symptom Manage.* 2004;27:180–184.

73. Bergasa NV, Alling DW, Vergalla J, et al. Cholestasis in the male rat is associated with naloxone-reversible antinociception. *J Hepatol.* 1994;20:85–90.

74. Lonsdale-Eccles AA, Carmichael AJ. Opioid antagonist for pruritus of cholestasis unmasking bony metastases. *Acta Derm Venereol.* 2009;89:90.

75. Zylicz Z, Krajnik M. Managing severe pruritus in cancer patients. *Eur J Pall Care.* 2007;14:93–95.

76. Zylicz Z, Stork N, Krajnik M. Severe pruritus of cholestasis in disseminated cancer: developing a rational treatment strategy: a case report. *J Pain Symptom Manage.* 2005;29:100–103.

77. Yuan CS, Foss JF, O'Connor M, et al. Efficacy of orally administered methylnaltrexone in decreasing subjective effects after intravenous morphine. *Drug Alcohol Depend.* 1998;52:161–165.

78. Juby LD, Wong VS, Losowsky MS. Buprenorphine and hepatic pruritus. *Br J Clin Pract.* 1994;48:331.

79. Krajnik M, Adamczyk A, Zylicz Z. Transdermal buprenorphine ameliorated pruritus complicating advanced hepatocellular cancer. *Adv Palliat Med.* 2007;6:83–86.

80. Reddy L, Krajnik M, Zylicz Z. Transdermal buprenorphine may be effective in the treatment of pruritus in primary biliary cirrhosis. *J Pain Symptom Manage.* 2007;34:455–456.

81. Marinangeli F, Guetti C, Angeletti C, et al. Intravenous naloxone plus transdermal buprenorphine in cancer pain associated with intractable cholestatic pruritus. *J Pain Symptom Manage.* 2009;38:e5–e8.

82. Inan S, Cowan A. Nalfurafine, a kappa opioid receptor agonist, inhibits scratching behavior secondary to cholestasis induced by chronic ethynylestradiol injections in rats. *Pharmacol Biochem Behav.* 2006;85:39–43.

83. Umeuchi H, Kawashima Y, Aoki CA, et al. Spontaneous scratching behavior in MRL/lpr mice, a possible model for pruritus in autoimmune diseases, and antipruritic activity of a novel kappa-opioid receptor agonist nalfurafine hydrochloride. *Eur J Pharmacol.* 2005;518:133–139.

84. Zylicz Z, Krajnik M, Sorge AA, et al. Paroxetine in the treatment of severe non-dermatological pruritus: a randomized, controlled trial. *J Pain Symptom Manage.* 2003;26:1105–1112.

85. Ständer S, Bockenholt B, Schurmeyer-Horst F, et al. Treatment of chronic pruritus with the selective serotonin re-uptake inhibitors paroxetine and fluvoxamine: results of an open-labelled, two-arm proof-of-concept study. *Acta Derm Venereol.* 2009;89:45–51.

86. Mayo MJ, Handem I, Saldana S, et al. Sertraline as a first-line treatment for cholestatic pruritus. *Hepatology.* 2007;45:666–674.

87. Browning J, Combes B, Mayo MJ. Long-term efficacy of sertraline as a treatment for cholestatic pruritus in patients with primary biliary cirrhosis. *Am J Gastroenterol.* 2003;98:2736–2741.

88. Cross SA. Pathophysiology of pain. *Mayo Clin Proc.* 1994;69:375–383.

89. Berendsen HH, Broekkamp CL. A peripheral 5-HT1D-like receptor involved in serotonergic induced hindlimb scratching in rats. *Eur J Pharmacol.* 1991;194:201–208.

90. George RB, Allen TK, Habib AS. Serotonin receptor antagonists for the prevention and treatment of pruritus, nausea, and vomiting in women undergoing cesarean delivery with intrathecal morphine: a systematic review and meta-analysis. *Anesth Analg.* 2009;109:174–182.

91. Bonnet MP, Marret E, Josserand J, et al. Effect of prophylactic 5-HT3 receptor antagonists on pruritus induced by neuraxial opioids: a quantitative systematic review. *Br J Anaesth.* 2008;101:311–319.

92. Layegh P, Mojahedi MJ, Malekshah PE, et al. Effect of oral granisetron in uremic pruritus. *Indian J Dermatol Venereol Leprol.* 2007;73:231–234.

93. Jones EA, Molenaar HA, Oosting J. Ondansetron and pruritus in chronic liver disease: a controlled study. *Hepatogastroenterology.* 2007;54:1196–1199.

94. Kyriakides K, Hussain SK, Hobbs GJ. Management of opioid-induced pruritus: a role for 5-HT3 antagonists? *Br J Anaesth.* 1999;82:439–441.

95. Weisshaar E, Dunker N, Rohl FW, et al. Antipruritic effects of two different 5-HT3 receptor antagonists and an antihistamine in haemodialysis patients. *Exp Dermatol.* 2004;13:298–304.

96. Charuluxananan S, Somboonviboon W, Kyokong O, et al. Ondansetron for treatment of intrathecal morphine-induced pruritus after cesarean delivery. *Reg Anesth Pain Med.* 2000;25:535–539.

97. Iatrou CA, Dragoumanis CK, Vogiatzaki TD, et al. Prophylactic intravenous ondansetron and dolasetron in intrathecal morphine-induced pruritus: a randomized, double-blinded, placebo-controlled study. *Anesth Analg.* 2005;101:1516–1520.

98. Watson WC. Intravenous lignocaine for relief of intractable itch. *Lancet.* 1973;1:211.

99. Villamil AG, Bandi JC, Galdame OA, et al. Efficacy of lidocaine in the treatment of pruritus in patients with chronic cholestatic liver diseases. *Am J Med.* 2005;118:1160–1163.

100. Shuttleworth D, Hill S, Marks R, et al. Relief of experimentally induced pruritus with a novel eutectic mixture of local anaesthetic agents. *Br J Dermatol.* 1988;119:535–540.

101. Lloyd-Thomas HG, Sherlock S. Testosterone therapy for the pruritus of obstructive jaundice. *Br Med J.* 1952;2:1289–1291.

102. Borgeat A, Wilder-Smith O, Mentha G, et al. Propofol and cholestatic pruritus. *Am J Gastroenterol.* 1992;87:672–674.

103. Borgeat A, Wilder-Smith OH, Mentha G. Subhypnotic doses of propofol relieve pruritus associated with liver disease. *Gastroenterology.* 1993;104:244–247.

104. Risdahl JM, Huether MJ, Gustafson KV, et al. Morphine alteration of histamine release in vivo. *Adv Exp Med Biol.* 1995;373:161–168.

105. Veien M, Szlam F, Holden JT, et al. Mechanisms of nonimmunological histamine and tryptase release from human cutaneous mast cells. *Anesthesiology.* 2000;92:1074–1081.

106. Quist RG, Ton-Nu HT, Lillienau J, et al. Activation of mast cells by bile acids. *Gastroenterology.* 1991;101:446–456.

107. Clements WD, O'Rourke DM, Rowlands BJ, et al. The role of mast cell activation in cholestatic pruritus. *Agents Actions.* 1994;41: Spec No:C30–1.

108. Manenti L, Vaglio A. Gabapentin use in chronic uraemic itch is in line with emerging pathogenetic hypothesis. *Nephrol Dial Transplant.* 2007;22:3669–3670.

109. Naini AE, Harandi AA, Khanbabapour S, et al. Gabapentin: a promising drug for the treatment of uremic pruritus. *Saudi J Kidney Dis Transpl.* 2007;18:378–381.

110. Bergasa NV, McGee M, Ginsburg IH, et al. Gabapentin in patients with the pruritus of cholestasis: a double-blind, randomized, placebo-controlled trial. *Hepatology.* 2006;44:1317–1323.

111. Szepietowski JC, Salomon J. Uremic pruritus: still an important clinical problem. *J Am Acad Dermatol.* 2004;51:842–843.

112. Chang SL, Lai PC, Cheng CJ, et al. Bullous amyloidosis in a hemodialysis patient is myeloma-associated rather than hemodialysis-associated amyloidosis. *Amyloid.* 2007;14:153–156.

113. Innes A, Cuthbert RJ, Russell NH, et al. Intensive treatment of renal failure in patients with myeloma. *Clin Lab Haematol.* 1994;16:149–156.

114. Mettang T, Pauli-Magnus C. The pathophysiological puzzle of uremic pruritus—insights and speculations from therapeutic and epidemiological studies. *Perit Dial Int.* 2000;20:493–494.

115. Mettang T, Pauli-Magnus C, Alscher DM. Uraemic pruritus—new perspectives and insights from recent trials. *Nephrol Dial Transplant.* 2002;17:1558–1563.

116. Gunal AI, Ozalp G, Yoldas TK, et al. Gabapentin therapy for pruritus in haemodialysis patients: a randomized, placebo-controlled, double-blind trial. *Nephrol Dial Transplant.* 2004;19:3137–3139.

117. Manenti L, Vaglio A, Costantino E, et al. Gabapentin in the treatment of uremic itch: an index case and a pilot evaluation. *J Nephrol.* 2005;18:86–91.

118. Razeghi E, Eskandari D, Ganji MR, et al. Gabapentin and uremic pruritus in hemodialysis patients. *Ren Fail.* 2009;31:85–90.

119. Vila T, Gommer J, Scates AC. Role of gabapentin in the treatment of uremic pruritus. *Ann Pharmacother.* 2008;42:1080–1084.

120. Kuypers DR, Claes K, Evenepoel P, et al. A prospective proof of concept study of the efficacy of tacrolimus ointment on uraemic pruritus (UP) in patients on chronic dialysis therapy. *Nephrol Dial Transplant.* 2004;19:1895–1901.

121. Tarng DC, Cho YL, Liu HN, et al. Hemodialysis-related pruritus: a double-blind, placebo-controlled, crossover study of capsaicin 0.025% cream. *Nephron.* 1996;72:617–622.

122. Weisshaar E, Dunker N, Gollnick H. Topical capsaicin therapy in humans with hemodialysis-related pruritus. *Neurosci Lett.* 2003;345:192–194.

123. Braverman IM. Skin manifestations of internal malignancy. *Clin Geriatr Med.* 2002;18:1–19.

124. Rajagopal R, Arora PN, Ramasastry CV, et al. Skin changes in internal malignancy. *Indian J Dermatol Venereol Leprol.* 2004;70:221–225.

125. Ridgway HB. Skin signs of internal malignancy. *Am Fam Physician.* 1978;17:123–129.

126. Cormia FE, Domonkos AN. Cutaneous reactions to internal malignancy. *Med Clin North Am.* 1965;49:655–680.

127. Tefferi A. Polycythemia vera: a comprehensive review and clinical recommendations. *Mayo Clin Proc.* 2003;78:174–194.

128. Tefferi A, Fonseca R. Selective serotonin reuptake inhibitors are effective in the treatment of polycythemia vera-associated pruritus. *Blood.* 2002;99:26–27.

129. Schulz S, Metz M, Siepmann D, et al. Antipruritic efficacy of a high-dosage antihistamine therapy: results of a retrospectively analysed case series. *Hautarzt.* 2009;60:564–568.

130. Stander S. Rational symptomatic therapy for chronic pruritus. *Hautarzt.* 2006;57:403–410.

131. Yosipovitch G, Samuel LS. Neuropathic and psychogenic itch. *Dermatol Ther.* 2008;21:32–41.

132. Savk E, Dikicioglu E, Culhaci N, et al. Immunohistochemical findings in notalgia paresthetica. *Dermatology.* 2002;204:88–93.

133. Wallengren J, Sundler F. Brachioradial pruritus is associated with a reduction in cutaneous innervation that normalizes during the symptom-free remissions. *J Am Acad Dermatol.* 2005;52:142–145.

134. Wallengren J, Tegner E, Sundler F. Cutaneous sensory nerve fibers are decreased in number after peripheral and central nerve damage. *J Am Acad Dermatol.* 2002;46:215–217.

135. Oaklander AL. Mechanisms of pain and itch caused by herpes zoster (shingles). *J Pain.* 2008;9:S10–18.

136. Dey DD, Landrum O, Oaklander AL. Central neuropathic itch from spinal-cord cavernous hemangioma: a human case, a possible animal model, and hypotheses about pathogenesis. *Pain.* 2005;113:233–237.

137. Magilner D. Localized cervical pruritus as the presenting symptom of a spinal cord tumor. *Pediatr Emerg Care.* 2006;22:746–747.

138. Crane DA, Jaffee KM, Kundu A. Intractable pruritus after traumatic spinal cord injury. *J Spinal Cord Med.* 2009;32:436–439.

139. Sullivan MJ, Drake Jr ME. Unilateral pruritus and Nocardia brain abscess. *Neurology.* 1984;34:828–829.

140. Kimyai-Asadi A, Nousari HC, Kimyai-Asadi T, et al. Poststroke pruritus. *Stroke.* 1999;30:692–693.

141. Shapiro PE, Braun CW. Unilateral pruritus after a stroke. *Arch Dermatol.* 1987;123:1527–1530.

142. Adreev VC, Petkov I. Skin manifestations associated with tumours of the brain. *Br J Dermatol.* 1975;92:675–678.

143. Liddell K. Letter: Post-herpetic pruritus. *Br Med J.* 1974;4:165.

144. Oaklander AL, Cohen SP, Raju SV. Intractable postherpetic itch and cutaneous deafferentation after facial shingles. *Pain.* 2002;96:9–12.

145. Oaklander AL, Bowsher D, Galer B, et al. Herpes zoster itch: preliminary epidemiologic data. *J Pain.* 2003;4:338–343.

146. Rowbotham MC, Yosipovitch G, Connolly MK, et al. Cutaneous innervation density in the allodynic form of postherpetic neuralgia. *Neurobiol Dis.* 1996;3:205–214.

147. Sonnett TE, Setter SM, Campbell RK. Pregabalin for the treatment of painful neuropathy. *Expert Rev Neurother.* 2006;6:1629–1635.

148. Tassone DM, Boyce E, Guyer J, et al. Pregabalin: a novel gamma-aminobutyric acid analogue in the treatment of neuropathic pain, partial-onset seizures, and anxiety disorders. *Clin Ther.* 2007;29:26–48.

149. Yesudian PD, Wilson NJ. Efficacy of gabapentin in the management of pruritus of unknown origin. *Arch Dermatol.* 2005;141:1507–1509.

150. Summey Jr BT, Yosipovitch G. Pharmacologic advances in the systemic treatment of itch. *Dermatol Ther.* 2005;18:328–332.

151. Lane JE, McKenzie JT, Spiegel J. Brachioradial pruritus: a case report and review of the literature. *Cutis.* 2008;81:37–40.

152. Crevits L. Brachioradial pruritus—a peculiar neuropathic disorder. *Clin Neurol Neurosurg.* 2006;108:803–805.

153. Barry R, Rogers S. Brachioradial pruritus—an enigmatic entity. *Clin Exp Dermatol.* 2004;29:637–638.

154. Cohen AD, Masalha R, Medvedovsky E, et al. Brachioradial pruritus: a symptom of neuropathy. *J Am Acad Dermatol.* 2003;48:825–828.

155. Goodkin R, Wingard E, Bernhard JD. Brachioradial pruritus: cervical spine disease and neurogenic/neuropathic pruritus. *J Am Acad Dermatol.* 2003;48:521–524.

156. Fisher DA. Brachioradial pruritus: a recurrent solar dermopathy. *J Am Acad Dermatol.* 1999;41:656–658.

157. Bernhard JD, Bordeaux JS. Medical pearl: the ice-pack sign in brachioradial pruritus. *J Am Acad Dermatol.* 2005;52:1073.

158. Winhoven SM, Coulson IH, Bottomley WW. Brachioradial pruritus: response to treatment with gabapentin. *Br J Dermatol.* 2004;150:786–787.

159. Scheinfeld N. The role of gabapentin in treating diseases with cutaneous manifestations and pain. *Int J Dermatol.* 2003;42:491–495.

160. Tait CP, Grigg E, Quirk CJ. Brachioradial pruritus and cervical spine manipulation. *Australas J Dermatol.* 1998;39:168–170.

161. Massey EW, Pleet AB. Localized pruritus-notalgia paresthetica. *Arch Dermatol.* 1979;115:982–983.

162. Springall DR, Karanth SS, Kirkham N, et al. Symptoms of notalgia paresthetica may be explained by increased dermal innervation. *J Invest Dermatol.* 1991;97:555–561.

163. Ehrlich W, Dellon AL, Mackinnon SE. Classical article: cheiralgia paresthetica (entrapment of the radial nerve). [A translation in condensed form of Robert Wartenberg's original article published in 1932]. *J Hand Surg Am.* 1986;11:196–199.

164. Lazzarino LG, Nicolai A, Toppani D. A case of cheiralgia paresthetica secondary to diabetes mellitus. *Ital J Neurol Sci.* 1983;4:103–106.

165. Massey EW, O'Brian JT. Cheiralgia paresthetica in diabetes mellitus. *Diabetes Care.* 1978;1:365–366.

166. Massey EW, Pleet AB. Handcuffs and cheiralgia paresthetica. *Neurology.* 1978;28:1312–1313.

167. Hancox JG, Wittenberg GF, Yosipovitch G. A patient with nasal ulceration after brain surgery. *Arch Dermatol.* 2005;141:796–798.

168. Canavero S, Bonicalzi V, Massa-Micon B. Central neurogenic pruritus: a literature review. *Acta Neurol Belg.* 1997;97:244–247.

169. Zylicz Z. Clinical assessment of patients with pruritus. In: Zylicz Z, Twycross R, Jones EA, eds. *Pruritus in advanced disease.* Oxford: Oxford University Press; 2004:33.

170. Perron G, Dolbec P, Germain J, et al. Perineal pruritus after i.v. dexamethasone administration. *Can J Anaesth.* 2003;50:749–750.

171. Tuneu A, Moreno A, de Moragas JM. Cutaneous reactions secondary to heparin injections. *J Am Acad Dermatol.* 1985;12:1072–1077.

172. Kjellberg F, Tramer MR. Pharmacological control of opioid-induced pruritus: a quantitative systematic review of randomized trials. *Eur J Anaesthesiol.* 2001;18:346–357.

173. Kelly MC, Carabine UA, Mirakhur RK. Intrathecal diamorphine for analgesia after caesarean section: a dose finding study and assessment of side-effects. *Anaesthesia.* 1998;53:231–237.

174. Fuller JG, McMorland GH, Douglas MJ, et al. Epidural morphine for analgesia after caesarean section: a report of 4880 patients. *Can J Anaesth.* 1990;37:636–640.

175. Asokumar B, Newman LM, McCarthy RJ, et al. Intrathecal bupivacaine reduces pruritus and prolongs duration of fentanyl analgesia during labor: a prospective, randomized controlled trial. *Anesth Analg.* 1998;87:1309–1315.

176. Arner S, Rawal N, Gustafsson LL. Clinical experience of long-term treatment with epidural and intrathecal opioids—a nationwide survey. *Acta Anaesthesiol Scand.* 1988;32:253–259.

177. Cousins MJ, Mather LE. Intrathecal and epidural administration of opioids. *Anesthesiology.* 1984;61:276–310.

178. White MJ, Berghausen EJ, Dumont SW, et al. Side effects during continuous epidural infusion of morphine and fentanyl. *Can J Anaesth.* 1992;39:576–582.

179. Scott PV, Fischer HB. Intraspinal opiates and itching: a new reflex? *Br Med J (Clin Res Ed)*. 1982;284:1015–1016.

180. Thomas DA, Williams GM, Iwata K, et al. The medullary dorsal horn: a site of action of morphine in producing facial scratching in monkeys. *Anesthesiology*. 1993;79:548–554.

181. Ballantyne JC, Loach AB, Carr DB. Itching after epidural and spinal opiates. *Pain*. 1988;33:149–160.

182. Colbert S, O'Hanlon DM, Galvin S, et al. The effect of rectal diclofenac on pruritus in patients receiving intrathecal morphine. *Anaesthesia*. 1999;54:948–952.

183. Choi JH, Lee J, Bishop MJ. Epidural naloxone reduces pruritus and nausea without affecting analgesia by epidural morphine in bupivacaine. *Can J Anaesth*. 2000;47:33–37.

184. Jeon Y, Hwang J, Kang J, et al. Effects of epidural naloxone on pruritus induced by epidural morphine: a randomized controlled trial. *Int J Obstet Anesth*. 2005;14:22–25.

185. Somrat C, Oranuch K, Ketchada U, et al. Optimal dose of nalbuphine for treatment of intrathecal-morphine induced pruritus after caesarean section. *J Obstet Gynaecol Res*. 1999;25:209–213.

186. Dunteman E, Karanikolas M, Filos KS. Transnasal butorphanol for the treatment of opioid-induced pruritus unresponsive to antihistamines. *J Pain Symptom Manage*. 1996;12:255–260.

187. Pirat A, Tuncay SF, Torgay A, et al. Ondansetron, orally disintegrating tablets versus intravenous injection for prevention of intrathecal morphine-induced nausea, vomiting, and pruritus in young males. *Anesth Analg*. 2005;101:1330–1336.

188. Wells J, Paech MJ, Evans SF. Intrathecal fentanyl-induced pruritus during labour: the effect of prophylactic ondansetron. *Int J Obstet Anesth*. 2004;13:35–39.

189. Korhonen AM, Valanne JV, Jokela RM, et al. Ondansetron does not prevent pruritus induced by low-dose intrathecal fentanyl. *Acta Anaesthesiol Scand*. 2003;47:1292–1297.

190. Meylan N, Elia N, Lysakowski C, et al. Benefit and risk of intrathecal morphine without local anaesthetic in patients undergoing major surgery: meta-analysis of randomized trials. *Br J Anaesth*. 2009;102:156–167.

191. Charuluxananan S, Kyokong O, Somboonviboon W, et al. Nalbuphine versus propofol for treatment of intrathecal morphine-induced pruritus after cesarean delivery. *Anesth Analg*. 2001;93:162–165.

192. Horta ML, Ramos L, Goncalves ZR. The inhibition of epidural morphine-induced pruritus by epidural droperidol. *Anesth Analg*. 2000;90:638–641.

193. Carvalho JC, Mathias RS, Senra WG, et al. Systemic droperidol and epidural morphine in the management of postoperative pain. *Anesth Analg*. 1991;72:416.

194. Colbert S, O'Hanlon DM, Chambers F, et al. The effect of intravenous tenoxicam on pruritus in patients receiving epidural fentanyl. *Anaesthesia*. 1999;54:76–80.

195. Mashayekhi SO, Ghandforoush-Sattari M, Routledge PA, et al. Pharmacokinetic and pharmacodynamic study of morphine and morphine 6-glucuronide after oral and intravenous administration of morphine in children with cancer. *Biopharm Drug Dispos*. 2009;30:99–106.

196. Hermens JM, Ebertz JM, Hanifin JM, et al. Comparison of histamine release in human skin mast cells induced by morphine, fentanyl, and oxymorphone. *Anesthesiology*. 1985;62:124–129.

197. McLelland J. The mechanism of morphine-induced urticaria. *Arch Dermatol*. 1986;122:138–139.

198. Krajnik M. Opioid-induced pruritus. In: Zylicz Z, Twycross R, Jones EA, eds. *Pruritus in advanced disease*. Oxford: Oxford University Press; 2004:84.

199. Zylicz Z, Smits C, Krajnik M. Paroxetine for pruritus in advanced cancer. *J Pain Symptom Manage*. 1998;16:121–124.

21

Lymphedema management

Sumner A. Slavin, Carolyn C. Schook, and Arin K. Greene

PREVALENCE AND PATHOPHYSIOLOGY

Lymphedema is chronic, progressive swelling following injury or anomalous development of the peripheral lymphatic system. Fluid accumulates in the superficial, interstitial space, causing enlargement of the subcutaneous tissue; over time, adipose and fibrous tissues further increase limb volume. Extremities are most commonly affected, followed by genitalia. Complications include functional disability, psychosocial morbidity, infection, skin changes, and, rarely, malignant transformation. Primary lymphedema affects 10% of patients with lymphedema; the incidence is 1.2 per 100,000 persons younger than 20 years old (Table 21-1).[1] Secondary lymphedema results from an acquired lymphatic insult such as malignancy, excision of lymph nodes, radiation, penetrating trauma, or infection. Until recently, lymphedema was not routinely recognized or managed as part of cancer-related care. Although lymphedema remains a progressive, incurable disease, advances in nonoperative and operative management are able to slow its progression, prevent complications, and improve symptoms.

PREVALENCE

As many as 140 to 250 million persons are affected with lymphedema worldwide.[2] A majority of patients reside in Third World countries and suffer from a parasitic infection (e.g., *Wuchereria bancrofti*).[2] In the United States and Europe, 1.4 per 1000 persons has lymphedema, usually secondary to malignancy.[3,4] Lymphedema commonly affects the lower extremity (90%), the upper extremity (10%), and the genitalia (<1%), although almost any body part can be involved (e.g., face, trunk, breast). Upper extremity lymphedema following breast cancer treatment is the most common cause of lymphedema in the United States. The incidence is approximately 30% at 2 years subsequent to breast cancer treatment, although rates range from 2% to 89%.[5–10] The exact burden of cancer-associated lymphedema, however, is unknown because of different definitions of lymphedema, lengths of follow-up, and treatment bias (patients with worse disease receive more aggressive management and follow-up) (Fig. 21-1).

Table 21-1 Lymphedema classification

Primary (idiopathic)		Secondary injury to lymphatics (axilla, groin)	
Type	*Characteristics*	*Cause*	*Examples*
Congenital	Onset in infancy Milroy disease (inherited)	Infection	Parasite *(Wuchereria bancrofti)*
Praecox	Pediatric onset Meige disease (inherited)	Iatrogenic	Lymphadenectomy Radiation
Tarda	Adult onset	Trauma	Penetrating
		Malignancy	Compression Metastasis

The incidence of lymphedema is related to cancer stage; advanced disease doubles the risk of developing lymphedema.[11] The extent of breast resection and of axillary lymph node dissection is also a strong predictor of lymphedema. For example, the prevalence of lymphedema after modified radical mastectomy is 7.5 times higher than following partial mastectomy.[12] Similarly, removal of more than 15 axillary lymph nodes increases the rate of lymphedema tenfold compared with excision of fewer than 5 nodes.[13,14] Sentinel lymph node biopsy reduces the prevalence of lymphedema (0.5%) compared with axillary lymph node dissection (16%).[15]

Radiation is another risk factor for breast cancer–related lymphedema.[12,16] When the posterior axilla is included in the radiation field, the risk of lymphedema doubles compared with radiation of the breast and supraclavicular nodes only.[17] Breast-conserving surgery with radiation reduces the risk of lymphedema compared with mastectomy (32.0% vs. 49.2%, respectively).[11]

Lower extremity or genital lymphedema is a complication of treatment for pelvic malignancy in 10% to 69% of patients.[18–20] Lower extremity lymphedema occurs in 20% to 30% of patients with ovarian, cervical, and endometrial cancer treated with pelvic lymph node dissection.[21,22] Lower

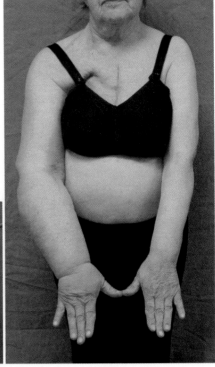
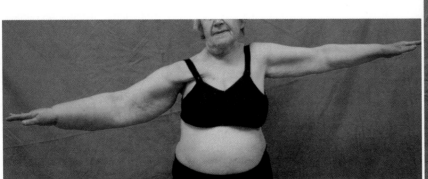

Fig. 21-1 Secondary lymphedema of the upper extremity. An 82-year-old female with right upper extremity lymphedema 2 years after mastectomy, radiation therapy, and lymphadenectomy for breast cancer. Note inability to completely abduct the right shoulder.

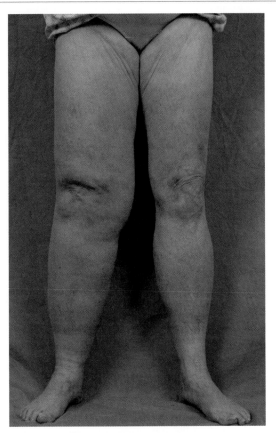

Fig. 21-2 Secondary lymphedema of the lower extremity. A 56-year-old woman with unilateral lower extremity 14 years after hysterectomy, bilateral oophorectomy, and lymphadenectomy for ovarian cancer. The patient has had approximately 50 hospitalizations for infection and has been placed on prophylactic penicillin.

extremity and genital lymphedema rates decrease when inguinal sentinel lymph node biopsy (SLNB) is performed instead of lymphadenectomy (1.9% vs. 25.5%).[23] Postoperative radiation to inguinal nodes for cervical or uterine cancer increases the risk of lymphedema by 13%[21] (Fig. 21-2).

PATHOPHYSIOLOGY

Lymphatic vessels are endothelium-lined channels arising from outpouchings of veins. Poorly defined basement membranes facilitate protein and lipid diffusion.[24] Both superficial and deep lymphatics travel parallel to the venous system within the extremities. Superficial lymphatics, which lack valves, drain into the deep, valved lymphatic vessels below the muscular fascia.[25] Deep lymphatic vessels travel adjacent to large subfascial veins.[26] Lymph nodes connect the superficial and deep lymphatic systems. The thoracic duct drains lower extremities, left trunk, and left upper extremity into the left subclavian vein. The right lymphatic duct empties the head and neck, right upper extremity, and right thorax into the right subclavian vein.[24] Additional lymphoid tissue is found in the gastrointestinal tract, tonsils, spleen, and thymus. Lymphatics

are not present in brain, bone marrow, cartilage, cornea, central nervous system, intralobar liver, muscle, or tendon.[24,27]

Lymphatic vasculature serves three functions: (1) proteinaceous fluid (lymph) transport, (2) fat absorption, and (3) immunologic defense.[24] Peripheral lymphatics transport fluid and proteins from the interstitial space back into the vascular system. Muscle contractions, venous pulsations, and variations in intra-abdominal and intrathoracic pressure stimulate proximal lymph flow.[24] Between 2 and 8 L of blood and between 10% and 50% of high-molecular-weight proteins are returned to the venous circulation daily by the lymphatic system.[28,29] Intestinal lymphatics transmit digested fat (chyle) into the venous circulation via the thoracic duct.[24] Lymphatic tissue provides immunologic defense by clearing and presenting foreign material in lymph nodes, as well as by producing antibodies.[24]

Lymphatic channel or node dysfunction from malformation or injury causes lymph accumulation in the superficial interstitial space. Elevated intralymphatic pressure leads to valvular incompetence, decreased proximal flow, and subcutaneous fluid collections.[28] Spillage of intravascular proteins raises extracellular oncotic pressure and expands interstitial edema. Compensatory mechanisms, such as increased macrophage activity and spontaneous lymphatico-venous shunts, prevent swelling until 80% of lymphatic flow has been reduced.[26] Once proteinaceous lymph fluid collects in the interstitial compartment, subsequent inflammation induces fibrosis and further lymphatic injury. Lymph stagnation increases infection after minor trauma as the result of impaired immunosurveillance, decreased oxygen delivery to the integument, and a proteinaceous environment favorable to bacterial growth. With chronic fluid stasis, subcutaneous adipose tissue hypertrophies, and the amount of fat in the extremity increases by 73%; this further expands the extremity.[30]

MORBIDITY

Thirty percent of patients with lymphedema will have on average one infection each year; one fourth will require hospitalization.[3] Inflammation and fibrosis lead to integument induration and hyperkeratosis. Decreased range of motion causes poor work performance and psychosocial morbidity.[3,31] Women with breast cancer-related lymphedema score lower on quality-of-life measures than breast cancer survivors without lymphedema.[32,33] Sarcoma is a rare complication of chronic lymphedema (0.5%) and is associated with long-term, severe disease.[34,35] Several hundred cases of Stewart-Treves syndrome (lymphangiosarcoma following mastectomy for breast-cancer) have been reported with an average survival is 19 months.[35–38] Because this malignancy is resistant to chemotherapy and radiation, amputation is the treatment of choice.[39]

DIAGNOSIS
History and physical examination

Ninety percent of patients with lymphedema are diagnosed by history and physical examination (Fig. 21-3). Documentation of past medical history includes previous operations, nodal dissections, radiation therapy, penetrating trauma, and comorbidities (heart, liver, and renal disease). Onset and duration of swelling also are noted, and patients usually describe a history of recurrent infection. Lymphedema typically occurs 6 to 9 months after breast cancer treatment, and in 80% of patients by 24 months.[6,40,41] Travel to filariasis-endemic areas should be ruled out. Physical

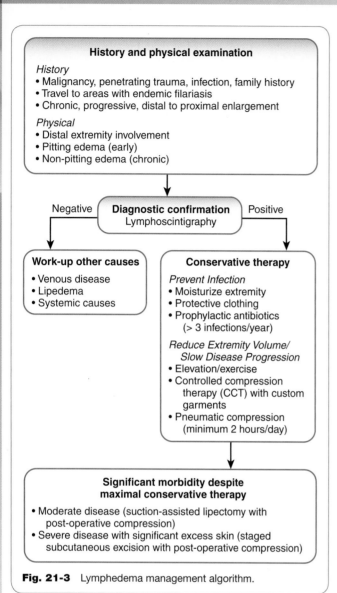

History and physical examination

History
• Malignancy, penetrating trauma, infection, family history
• Travel to areas with endemic filariasis
• Chronic, progressive, distal to proximal enlargement

Physical
• Distal extremity involvement
• Pitting edema (early)
• Non-pitting edema (chronic)

Negative ← **Diagnostic confirmation** → Positive
Lymphoscintigraphy

Work-up other causes
• Venous disease
• Lipedema
• Systemic causes

Conservative therapy

Prevent Infection
• Moisturize extremity
• Protective clothing
• Prophylactic antibiotics
  (> 3 infections/year)

*Reduce Extremity Volume/
Slow Disease Progression*
• Elevation/exercise
• Controlled compression
  therapy (CCT) with custom
  garments
• Pneumatic compression
  (minimum 2 hours/day)

**Significant morbidity despite
maximal conservative therapy**
• Moderate disease (suction-assisted lipectomy with
  post-operative compression)
• Severe disease with significant excess skin (staged
  subcutaneous excision with post-operative compression)

Fig. 21-3 Lymphedema management algorithm.

examination identifies the location of swelling and skin quality (see Fig. 21-1). Swelling involves the distal extremity (including hands and feet) and migrates proximally over time. Edema in early stages is painless and pitting, and has minimal pigment changes. With chronicity, adipose depositions and fibrosis cause nonpitting edema and a positive Stemmer sign (the inability to grasp the base of the second toe or finger).[42,43]

Imaging

When history and physical examination are equivocal for lymphedema, lymphoscintigraphy can confirm the diagnosis. Lymphoscintigraphy evaluates lymphatic function after Tc99m-labeled antimony sulfur or albumin is injected into the distal subcutaneous tissue of the affected body part. It is 92% sensitive and 100% specific for lymphedema.[44] Proximal migration of the radiolabeled protein will be visualized toward the lymph node basin under normal conditions.[20,44] Lymphedema will delay transport and dermal backflow at the site of injection.[20,36,44]

Lymphangiography involves the direct injection of lymphatic channels with radiopaque contrast dye. Lymphangiography is rarely performed because it is technically difficult and less accurate than lymphoscintigraphy. Patients can develop allergic reactions to the contrast dye, lymphangitis (19%), or worsening lymphedema (32%).[45] Lymphangiography is rarely used to identify a localized anatomic obstruction.

Magnetic resonance imaging (MRI) and computed tomography (CT) are neither sensitive nor specific for lymphedema. Lymphedema appears as thickened skin and subcutaneous tissue with a "honey-comb" pattern.[46] MRI can illustrate the extent of adipose hypertrophy for surgical planning, particularly for suction-assisted lipectomy (Table 21-2). CT is rarely indicated because it has inferior soft tissue resolution compared with MRI and exposes the patient to radiation. Ultrasound of lymphedematous tissue shows nonspecific thickening, but will evaluate venous thrombosis.[36] Biopsy is not useful in the diagnosis of lymphedema because histopathology consists of nonspecific inflammation.

Differential diagnosis

Lymphedema is differentiated from other causes of swelling because it is localized to an extremity or genitalia with the distal limb most severely involved. In addition, lymphedema is progressive, chronic, and associated with a high risk for infection. Edema from congestive heart failure, liver disease, protein-wasting enteropathies, and renal insufficiency, in contrast, cause symmetric, bilateral extremity swelling (see Fig. 21-3). Bilateral limb enlargement also occurs secondary to obesity, chronic venous insufficiency, and lipedema. Venous disease causes hyperpigmentation, ulceration, pitting edema, and varicosities, and in general spares hands or feet. Lipedema primarily involves

Table 21-2 Differential diagnosis of a swollen extremity

	Lymph-edema	Venous stasis	Lipedema	Systemic edema
Foot/Hand affected	+	±	-	+
Bilateral	±	±	+	+
Pain	±	+	+	-
Pigment change	±	+	-	-
Pitting edema	±	+	-	+
Response to diuretics	-	±	-	+
Ulceration	-	+	-	-
Delayed lymph flow (lymphoscintigram)	+	-	-	-
Increased skin thickness (CT/MRI)	+	-	-	-
Increased adipose tissue (CT/MRI)	+	-	+	-

CT, Computed tomography; *MRI,* magnetic resonance imaging.

the legs of pubertal females and not the feet; patients have tenderness and a negative Stemmer sign.[47] Deep vein thrombosis (DVT) and malignancy cause localized, unilateral extremity swelling. In contrast to lymphedema, DVT has an acute onset and is associated with erythema and pain. Malignancy should be considered if swelling occurs with skin changes, a mass, or systemic symptoms (e.g., weight loss, malaise).

MANAGEMENT

Historically, lymphedema has not been well understood. Physician referral for specialized care often is poor; 60% of patients managed at lymphedema clinics are self-referred.[20] Patients are seldom provided information or guidance as to how to manage lymphedema when undergoing a procedure that has a significant risk for postoperative lymphedema.[48–50] Long-term, interdisciplinary care of patients with lymphedema is required because of its chronic and progressive course. Few dedicated lymphedema clinics are available that offer medical and surgical care. At our lymphedema program, plastic surgery, nuclear medicine, radiology, and rehabilitation specialists provide consultation, diagnostic services, and treatment options to patients of all ages. All individuals with a suspected diagnosis of lymphedema should be referred to a specialized center for current, comprehensive management.

CLINICAL MONITORING

Clinicians should monitor disease progression and treatment response annually using circumferential and water displacement measurements of the edematous limb. Water displacement is more accurate for determining volume than circumferential recordings; tape measurements provide data for specific anatomic sites of lymphedema on the extremity. Disease severity is graded by volume differences between the affected and the contralateral extremity: <10%, mild; 10% to 30%, moderate; and >30%, severe.[27] Cellulitis should be treated at onset with oral antibiotics; intravenous therapy and hospitalization may be required. Daily prophylactic antibiotics should be given to patients experiencing three or more episodes of cellulitis per year.

Blood pressure monitoring and venipuncture are safe to perform in a lymphedematous extremity if a normal limb is unavailable.[51] Blood pressure cuff monitoring should not be problematic because pneumatic pressures over 100 mm Hg are used to treat lymphedema (the blood pressure cuff may improve lymph drainage). Venipuncture should not increase the risk of cellulitis because sterile skin is penetrated. Venipuncture is commonly performed with lymphoscintigraphy, which does not increase the risk of infection.[51]

NONOPERATIVE MANAGEMENT

ACTIVITIES OF DAILY LIVING

Patients should wash and moisturize the extremity regularly to prevent desiccation and subsequent skin breakdown and cellulitis. Shoes and long-sleeved clothing are worn to avoid incidental trauma; walking barefoot should be avoided.

Elevation provides a temporary, small reduction in swelling; patients should raise the affected extremity when convenient.[52,53] Exercise, including weight lifting, does not worsen lymphedema and might improve symptoms.[54]

STATIC COMPRESSION

Compression is the first-line treatment for lymphedema (Table 21-3). Compression garments provide only transient volume reduction; swelling recurs if therapy is stopped, thus lifelong compliance is required.[55] Pressure improves extremity volume by (1) increasing lymph transport, (2) decreasing capillary filtration, (3) opening collapsed vessels, (4) reducing interstitial pressure, and/or (5) widening the vessel wall by direct injury (Fig. 21-4).

A variety of garments, either single or multilayer, provide a proximal pressure gradient along the extremity. Single stockings (30–80 mm Hg) reduce limb volume by 4% to 8%, and multilayer bandaging (MLB) is twice as effective.[36,52,56] Layered garments that are progressively tightened (controlled compression therapy [CCT]) decrease limb volume by 47% over 1 year.[57]

Custom-fitted garments are superior to commercially produced stockings.[57] We apply one Level 3 sleeve (30 mm Hg) for the upper extremity and use two layers for lower extremities (a Level 3 garment is placed first, followed by a Level 2 stocking [20 mm Hg]). Garments are worn continuously but may be removed for social functions or bathing. Individuals should have several stockings prescribed, so they may be worn while others are cleaned. Washing will tighten the garment, thus providing increased compression, even as the elastic loosens over

Table 21-3 Nonoperative management		
Treatment	**Advantages**	**Disadvantages**
Elevation and exercise	Minimal efficacy Home treatment No cost	
Static compression	Moderate/good efficacy Home treatment	Low compliance
Pneumatic compression	Good efficacy Home treatment High compliance	
Manual lymphatic drainage	Minimal efficacy	Limited to mild/moderate disease Time-intensive/inconvenient for patient Patient reliant on therapist
Combination therapy Decongestive lymphatic therapy (DLT) Complex physical therapy (CPT) Complex decongestive physiotherapy (CDP)	Good efficacy Home treatment (maintenance phase)	Time-intensive/inconvenient for patient Patient reliant on therapist

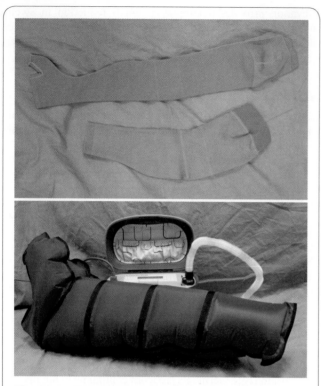

Fig. 21-4 First-line therapy for lymphedema. *Top,* Custom-fitted static compression garments. *Bottom,* Pneumatic compression device.

time. Alternatively, the stockings may be taken in by placing a seam. As the leg volume decreases, tighter measurements are made, and smaller garments are prescribed (CCT). New custom stockings are usually required every 6 months. Because garments and bandaging can be uncomfortable and unattractive in social settings, compliance is often poor.

MASSAGE THERAPY

Manual lymphatic drainage (MLD), performed by a trained therapist, utilizes gentle massage to stimulate proximal lymphatic flow. MLD improves quality of life but minimally reduces extremity volume (≈10%). This is equivalent to static garments without CCT.[52,58,59] MLD does not improve volume reduction when added to a static compression regimen.[59] MLD may be helpful in managing early or mild disease but is less likely to

be effective with chronic lymphedema.[33] Disadvantages of massage therapy include (1) substantial time burden for patients, (2) reliance on a provider for treatment, and (3) cost of therapy.

PNEUMATIC COMPRESSION

Pneumatic compression devices supply intermittent pressure through an inflatable sleeve. The alternating inflation/deflation pattern varies widely across models (Table 21-4). Multichambered sleeves apply sequential pressures by inflating distal chambers first, then more proximal chambers. Sequential pressure with eight compartments is more effective than single-compartment, nonsequential pressure (32.6% volume decrease vs. 0.4% volume increase when applied over 2 hours).[60] A sequential device provides a pressure gradient that applies greater force in distal chambers and lesser force in proximal chambers. Additional design variables include pulsating peristaltic-like inflation, valves to prevent backflow, and distal release during proximal inflation. All pumps allow adjustment of applied pressures; some devices allow for customized chamber pressure and inflation cycle time. Pneumatic compression therapy ranges from simple (nonprogrammable, nonsequential, nongradient pressure) to complex (programmable, sequential, gradient, peristaltic pressure).

Most studies demonstrate that pneumatic compression reduces limb volume by one quarter to two thirds; other studies suggest a more modest improvement (3%–7% volume decrease).[60-64] Results depend on device technology, outcome measures, and treatment regimen. Although pneumatic compression is effective, long-term, randomized controlled trials have not been conducted. Advantages of pneumatic compression include (1) efficacy, (2) simplicity, (3) convenience in that therapy is delivered at home, and (4) treatment that is not dependent on a therapist. We recommend a minimum of 2 hours of pneumatic compression daily. Alternatively, patients should undergo controlled compression therapy (CCT) with static garments when not using a pneumatic pump.

COMBINATION NONOPERATIVE THERAPY

A combination of compressive regimens is more effective than a single intervention.[52,64,65] Formal programs have been developed that combine skin care, manual lymphatic drainage (MLD), compression bandaging, and exercise, as well as decongestive lymphatic therapy (DLT), complex physical therapy (CPT), and complex decongestive physiotherapy (CDP). These programs typically consist of two phases: (1) treatment (phase I), and (2)

Table 21-4 Pneumatic compression devices

Device category	Compartment(s)	Pressure gradient	Examples
Nonsequential, nongradient	Single	None	Huntleigh Flowtron Hydroven 3
Sequential, nongradient	Multiple	None	Lympha Press Petite Basic System
Sequential, gradient	Multiple	Distal > Proximal	Bio Compression Sequential Circulator 3008 NormaTec Compression Device

Sequential: Multichambered sleeve that inflates distal chambers first, then more proximal chambers.
Gradient: Multichambered sleeve that applies greater force in distal chambers and lesser force in proximal chambers.

maintenance (phase II). Phase I lasts up to 4 weeks at an outpatient facility. Phase II includes self-treatment at home with the goal to maintain volume reduction achieved during phase I. Patients are managed largely as outpatients. Although limb volume is reported to be reduced by 19% to 68% with combined therapy, these studies have small sample sizes and unclear inclusion criteria.[52,66,67] DLT plus pneumatic compression is reported to decrease limb volume to a greater extent than DLT alone (45% vs. 26%).[68] Disadvantages of these programs include significant patient time commitment, effort, and expense.

PHARMACOTHERAPY

Drug therapy has not been established for lymphedema. Although the benzopyrone, coumarin, is an immunomodulator that causes minor volume reductions, it is associated with hepatotoxicity.[36,52,69] Coumarin is not recommended because of its minimal efficacy and potential morbidity. Diuretics, which are ineffective for lymphedema, are used for conditions that cause systemic fluid overload (e.g., congestive heart failure), but they may worsen lymphedema by increasing the concentration of interstitial protein.

OPERATIVE MANAGEMENT

Surgical treatment of lymphedema is considered when conservative measures fail to improve the condition of patients who are experiencing significant morbidity from their lymphedema (Table 21-5). However, no operation is curative, and lifelong postoperative compression is still required to prevent reexpansion of the limb. The severity of lymphedema is the product of the amount of lymph production (load) and the ability to transport lymph fluid to venous circulation (drainage). Physiologic procedures create new lymphatic connections to enhance drainage. Excisional procedures remove affected tissues to decrease load. Although physiologic techniques attempt to correct the underlying lymphatic defect, long-term benefits are modest. Suction-assisted lipectomy and staged excision of subcutaneous tissue are our preferred operative interventions because of their superior long-term benefits.

PHYSIOLOGIC PROCEDURES
Microsurgery

Microsurgical creation of lymphatico-venous connections has been used to improve proximal lymphatic flow. One retrospective review of patients with secondary lymphedema treated with lymphatico-venous anastomoses (LVA) reported objective improvement in only 42% and average volume reduction of 44%.[70] Anastomotic patency was 66% after 12 weeks. The best results were seen in patients with early disease and distal anastomoses (wrist/ankle level), and when microsurgery was combined with an excisional procedure.[70]

More recently, proximal LVA at the inguinal and mid arm regions were attempted in both primary and secondary lymphedema.[71–73] Long-term improvement occurred in 83% of patients, with an average reduction of 75% in excess volume over a 30-year period.[73] The infection rate decreased in 87% of patients.[73] Both primary and secondary lymphedema were treated successfully with this procedure. However, 17% of patients had less than 50% volume reduction.[73]

Table 21-5 Operative management

Physiologic technique	Advantages	Disadvantages
Lymphatico-venous anastomosis	Moderate efficacy Minimal morbidity One stage	Limited to mild/moderate disease Requires functional veins and lymphatics Does not remove excess adipose tissue
Flap transposition		Unclear efficacy Does not remove excess adipose tissue Significant morbidity

Excisional technique	Advantages	Disadvantages
Suction-assisted lipectomy	Good efficacy Reliable volume reduction Minimal morbidity One stage	Not indicated in advanced disease
Staged subcutaneous excision	Good efficacy Reliable volume reduction Effective for advanced disease	Moderate morbidity Two stages
Charles procedure	Good efficacy Reliable volume reduction Effective for advanced disease One stage	Poor cosmesis, chronic wound instability Significant morbidity

Because of concern that the quality of proximal lymphatic vessels is unreliable and cutaneous venous pressure is too high to allow for forward flow through a lymphovenous connection, a "super" microlymphaticovenular procedure has been developed by creating small, distal, subdermal lymphatico-venous anastomoses.[74] After 3 years, no anastomotic failures were observed, and two thirds of patients had a greater than 4 cm circumferential reduction with postoperative compression.[75,76] Patients with both primary and secondary lymphedema were included. Advanced lymphedema showed inferior improvement after 1 year (41% excess volume reduction) compared with mild/moderate disease (55.6% excess volume reduction).[75–77]

Microsurgical procedures demonstrate good benefits, but long-term volume reduction is unpredictable. Contrary to earlier studies, LVA has proven successful in primary lymphedema.[73,76] The contribution of postoperative static compression to microsurgical outcomes is unclear. LVA appears to be beneficial for patients with mild to moderate lymphedema but does not correct adipose hypertrophy in chronic disease; thus complete normalization of extremity volume is not achievable. LVA requires functional veins, a lymphatic-to-venous pressure gradient, and patent lymphatic vessels.[36,64,72] If they are to be effective, LVA anastomoses should be done before significant fibrosis has occurred, as is seen in advanced disease.[71,73]

Flap transposition

Flap transpositions attempt to connect superficial lymphatics to the deep system. The Thompson procedure buries a de-epithelialized dermal flap into the muscle compartment in an effort to allow superficial tissues to drain through deep structures.[78–80] Improved lymphatic flow has not been documented with this technique; clinical improvement is likely secondary to the excisional step of the procedure. Myocutaneous and omental flap transposition have variable efficacy.[81–83] Omental flaps have been associated with substantial donor-site morbidity without evidence of long-term success.[84]

Early transfer of pedicle flaps does not maintain the initial reduction. Instead, significant operative morbidity, including donor-site lymphedema, has been reported.[85–91] Initial improvements in extremity volume are likely to occur from the excisional component of the procedure, and not as the result of lymphatic drainage.[89,91] Recent animal and small human studies have demonstrated potential benefits of using pedicle rectus abdominal muscle flaps.[92,93] Return of lymphatic function has been demonstrated in free flaps in humans; however, free-tissue transfer has not been utilized clinically to treat lymphedema.[92] Currently, flap transpositions are infrequently performed because efficacy is established. Flap transpositions have greater morbidity than LVA or excisional procedures.

Other physiologic procedures

Removal of fascial strips to allow drainage from superficial to deep compartments has not proved beneficial.[94–97] Early attempts at lymph node/venous shunts were also unsuccessful.[73] A newer technique, lymph node transplantation with an inguinal free flap to the affected axilla, has shown benefit in patients who were more than 5 years postoperative; 62.5% of patients were able to discontinue conservative treatment.[98] A sheep model of lymph node transplantation has demonstrated restoration of lymphatic function after reimplantation of vascularized lymph nodes into a nodal excision site.[99] Although it has not been studied comprehensively in humans, vascularized lymph node transfer may prevent lymphedema in patients undergoing high-risk procedures for lymphedema. Other potential applications include inguinal lymph node transfer with deep inferior epigastric perforator (DIEP) breast reconstruction following mastectomy. However, patients are at risk for donor-site lymphedema secondary to the lymph node harvest; excision of even one node (i.e., sentinel lymph node biopsy) can cause lymphedema.[15]

EXCISIONAL PROCEDURES

Although physiologic procedures decrease extremity volume by improving proximal lymph flow, they do not eliminate hypertrophied adipose tissue or fibrotic skin in chronic disease.[30,57] Consequently, excision of the suprafascial compartment is more popular than physiologic methods because of (1) greater limb size reduction, (2) more consistent results, and (3) the fact that all patients (mild, moderate, or severe lymphedema) are potential candidates. Because the underlying disease is not cured, patients require lifelong compression to minimize limb edema, inflammation, and recurrent adipose production.

Suction-assisted lipectomy

Suction-assisted lipectomy (SAL) is currently our first-line operative intervention for lymphedema because of its superior efficacy, consistent results, and low morbidity.[30,57,100–106] This technique removes the hypertrophied, subcutaneous adipose tissue present in chronic lymphedema. Liposuction also increases cutaneous blood flow and lowers the annual risk of cellulitis by 30%; quality of life is substantially improved.[107,108] Lymphatics are not injured by SAL, and lymph flow is not affected.[102,107]

Although the initial use of SAL produced modest benefits, good results are now achievable when modern liposuction techniques (circumferential suctioning, tumescence, and power-assisted cannulas) are used.[101,103,105,109,110] Prospective studies of SAL combined with CCT for upper extremity lymphedema show an overall volume reduction of 106% after 1 year, with no recurrence after 15 years.[57,100,101,111] SAL for the lower extremity achieves 75% volume reduction at 18 months of follow-up.[104]

Complete reduction in extremity volume is difficult to achieve in severe disease because of extensive fibrosis.[55] However, SAL provides excellent volume reduction with minimal morbidity and short recovery in patients with moderate disease. The ideal candidate for SAL has moderate disease; patients with minor disease do not require operative intervention, and those with severe lymphedema usually require skin excision. Preoperative MRI is obtained to document excess adipose tissue before the procedure is performed. If significant skin excess is predicted after SAL, the patient may be better served by staged subcutaneous excision.

Staged subcutaneous excision

Staged subcutaneous excision is the preferred operative treatment for severe lymphedema with extensive fibrosis and excess skin. The medial subcutaneous tissues and the muscle fascia are excised and covered by vascularized skin flaps.[95,112–115] Resection of lateral subcutaneous tissues is performed 3 months later.[113] Follow-up at 14 years shows significant improvement in limb size in 79% of patients, as well as a reduction in the risk of infection.[113] Some physiologic benefits also might occur because flow is improved, as can be seen on postoperative lymphoscintigraphy.[113] Disadvantages, compared with SAL, include a two-stage approach, extended hospital stays, long incisions, and greater operative morbidity.

Charles procedure

The Charles procedure removes skin, subcutaneous tissue, and muscle fascia circumferentially, followed by skin graft coverage of the underlying muscle.[116] Although lymphedema rarely recurs, lymphorrhea, hyperkeratosis, and poor cosmesis are common, especially if split-thickness grafts are used.[117] This method is rarely performed because of poor wound healing, hypertrophic scarring, sensory loss, and poor cosmesis.[113,117–119] A modified Charles procedure with negative-pressure dressings and delayed, split-thickness skin grafting from excised tissue has a more favorable outcome with less morbidity.[120] However, this approach should be used only for end-stage disease after other options have been exhausted.

REFERENCES

1. Smeltzer DM. Primary lymphedema in children and adolescents: a follow-up study and review. *Pediatrics.* 1985;76:206–218.

2. WHO, ECR. Lymphatic filariasis. Fourth report of the WHO Expert Committee on Filariasis. *World Health Organ Tech Rep Ser.* 1984;702:3–112.

3. Moffatt CJ. Lymphoedema: an underestimated health problem. *QJM.* 2003;96:731–738.

4. Rockson SG. Estimating the population burden of lymphedema. *Ann N Y Acad Sci.* 2008;1131:147–154.

5. Hayes SC. Lymphedema after breast cancer: incidence, risk factors, and effect on upper body function. *J Clin Oncol.* 2008;26:3536–3542.

6. Stout Gergich NL. Preoperative assessment enables the early diagnosis and successful treatment of lymphedema. *Cancer.* 2008;112:2809–2819.

7. Langbecker D. Treatment for upper-limb and lower-limb lymphedema by professionals specializing in lymphedema care. *Eur J Cancer Care (Engl).* 2008;17:557–564.

8. Segerstrom K. Factors that influence the incidence of brachial oedema after treatment of breast cancer. *Scand J Plast Reconstr Surg Hand Surg.* 1992;26:223–227.

9. Erickson VS. Arm edema in breast cancer patients. *J Natl Cancer Inst.* 2001;93:96–111.

10. Petrek JA. Incidence of breast carcinoma-related lymphedema. *Cancer.* 1998;83:2776–2781.

11. Dayangac M. Precipitating factors for lymphedema following surgical treatment of breast cancer: implications for patients undergoing axillary lymph node dissection. *Breast J.* 2009;15:210–211.

12. Park JH. Incidence and risk factors of breast cancer lymphoedema. *J Clin Nurs.* 2008;17:1450–1459.

13. Abu-Rustum NR. The incidence of symptomatic lower-extremity lymphedema following treatment of uterine corpus malignancies: a 12-year experience at Memorial Sloan-Kettering Cancer Center. *Gynecol Oncol.* 2006;103:714–718.

14. Yen TW. A contemporary, population-based study of lymphedema risk factors in older women with breast cancer. *Ann Surg Oncol.* 2009;16:979–988.

15. McLaughlin SA. Prevalence of lymphedema in women with breast cancer 5 years after sentinel lymph node biopsy or axillary dissection: patient perceptions and precautionary behaviors. *J Clin Oncol.* 2008;26:5220–5226.

16. Kissin MW. Risk of lymphoedema following the treatment of breast cancer. *Br J Surg.* 1986;73:580–584.

17. Hayes SB. Does axillary boost increase lymphedema compared with supraclavicular radiation alone after breast conservation? *Int J Radiat Oncol Biol Phys.* 2008;72:1449–1455.

18. Podratz KC. Carcinoma of the vulva: analysis of treatment and survival. *Obstet Gynecol.* 1983;61:63–74.

19. de Hullu JA. What doctors and patients think about false-negative sentinel lymph nodes in vulvar cancer. *J Psychosom Obstet Gynaecol.* 2001;22:199–203.

20. Szuba A. The third circulation: radionuclide lymphoscintigraphy in the evaluation of lymphedema. *J Nucl Med.* 2003;44:43–57.

21. Tada H. Risk factors for lower limb lymphedema after lymph node dissection in patients with ovarian and uterine carcinoma. *BMC Cancer.* 2009;9:47.

22. Gould N. Predictors of complications after inguinal lymphadenectomy. *Gynecol Oncol.* 2001;82:329–332.

23. Van der Zee AG. Sentinel node dissection is safe in the treatment of early-stage vulvar cancer. *J Clin Oncol.* 2008;26:884–889.

24. Seifter J, Ratner A, Sloane D. *Concepts in medical physiology.* Philadelphia: Lippincott; 2005.

25. Crockett D. Lymphatic anatomy and lymphedema. *J Plast Surg.* 1965;18:12.

26. McCarthy JG. *Plastic surgery.* Philadelphia: WB Saunders; 1990.

27. Weinzweig J. *Plastic surgery secrets plus.* St Louis: Mosby; 2009.

28. Mathes SJ. *Plastic surgery.* St Louis: Elsevier; 2006.

29. Stanton AW. Recent advances in breast cancer-related lymphedema of the arm: lymphatic pump failure and predisposing factors. *Lymphat Res Biol.* 2009;7:29–45.

30. Brorson H. Breast cancer-related chronic arm lymphedema is associated with excess adipose and muscle tissue. *Lymphat Res Biol.* 2009;7:3–10.

31. Ahmed RL. Lymphedema and quality of life in breast cancer survivors: the Iowa Women's Health Study. *J Clin Oncol.* 2008;26:5689–5696.

32. Swenson KK. Case-control study to evaluate predictors of lymphedema after breast cancer surgery. *Oncol Nurs Forum.* 2009;36:185–193.

33. McNeely ML. The addition of manual lymph drainage to compression therapy for breast cancer related lymphedema: a randomized controlled trial. *Breast Cancer Res Treat.* 2004;86:95–106.

34. Schirger A. Postoperative lymphedema: etiologic and diagnostic factors. *Med Clin North Am.* 1962;46:1045–1050.

35. Brady MS. Post-treatment sarcoma in breast cancer patients. *Ann Surg Oncol.* 1994;1:66–72.

36. Szuba A. Lymphedema: classification, diagnosis and therapy. *Vasc Med.* 1998;3:145–156.

37. Aygit AC. Lymphangiosarcoma in chronic lymphoedema: Stewart-Treves syndrome. *J Hand Surg [Br].* 1999;24:135–137.

38. Woodward AH. Lymphangiosarcoma arising in chronic lymphedematous extremities. *Cancer.* 1972;30:562–572.

39. Stewart NJ. Lymphangiosarcoma following mastectomy. *Clin Orthop Relat Res.* 1995;135–141.

40. Norman SA. Lymphedema in breast cancer survivors: incidence, degree, time course, treatment, and symptoms. *J Clin Oncol.* 2009;27:390–397.

41. Hayes SC. Lymphedema following breast cancer. *J Clin Oncol.* 2009;27:2890; author reply 2890.

42. Stemmer R. Stemmer's sign—possibilities and limits of clinical diagnosis of lymphedema. *Wien Med Wochenschr.* 1999;149:85–86.

43. Stemmer R. A clinical symptom for the early and differential diagnosis of lymphedema. *Vasa.* 1976;5:261–262.

44. Gloviczki P. Noninvasive evaluation of the swollen extremity: experiences with 190 lymphoscintigraphic examinations. *J Vasc Surg.* 1989;9:683–689; discussion 690.

45. O'Brien BM. Effect of lymphangiography on lymphedema. *Plast Reconstr Surg.* 1981;68:922–926.

46. Duewell S. Swollen lower extremity: role of MR imaging. *Radiology.* 1992;184:227–231.

47. Rudkin GH. Lipedema: a clinical entity distinct from lymphedema. *Plast Reconstr Surg.* 1994;94:841–847; discussion 848–9.

48. Ridner SH. Pretreatment lymphedema education and identified educational resources in breast cancer patients. *Patient Educ Couns.* 2006;61:72–79.

49. Towers A. The psychosocial effects of cancer-related lymphedema. *J Palliat Care.* 2008;24:134–143.

50. Paskett ED. Breast cancer-related lymphedema: attention to a significant problem resulting from cancer diagnosis. *J Clin Oncol.* 2008;26:5666–5667.

51. Greene AK. Blood pressure monitoring and venipuncture in the lymphedematous extremity. *Plast Reconstr Surg.* 2005;116:2058–2059.

52. Moseley AL. A systematic review of common conservative therapies for arm lymphoedema secondary to breast cancer treatment. *Ann Oncol.* 2007;18:639–646.

53. Swedborg I. Lymphoedema post-mastectomy: is elevation alone an effective treatment? *Scand J Rehabil Med.* 1993;25:79–82.

54. Schmitz KH. Weight lifting in women with breast-cancer-related lymphedema. *N Engl J Med.* 2009;361:664–673.

55. Brorson H. Complete reduction of lymphoedema of the arm by liposuction after breast cancer. *Scand J Plast Reconstr Surg Hand Surg.* 1997;31:137–143.

56. Badger CM. A randomized, controlled, parallel-group clinical trial comparing multilayer bandaging followed by hosiery versus hosiery alone in the treatment of patients with lymphedema of the limb. *Cancer.* 2000;88:2832–2837.

57. Brorson H. Liposuction combined with controlled compression therapy reduces arm lymphedema more effectively than controlled compression therapy alone. *Plast Reconstr Surg.* 1998;102:1058–1067; discussion 1068.

58. Williams AF. A randomized controlled crossover study of manual lymphatic drainage therapy in women with breast cancer-related lymphoedema. *Eur J Cancer Care (English Language Edition).* 2002;11:254–261.

59. Andersen L. Treatment of breast-cancer-related lymphedema with or without manual lymphatic drainage—a randomized study. *Acta Oncol.* 2000;39:399–405.

60. Bergan J. A comparison of compression pumps in the treatment of lymphedema. *Vasc Surg.* 1998;32.

61. Richmand DM. Sequential pneumatic compression for lymphedema: a controlled trial. *Arch Surg.* 1985;120:1116–1119.

62. Zelikovski A. The mobile pneumatic arm sleeve: a new device for treatment of arm lymphedema. *Lymphology.* 1985;18:68–71.

63. Kim-Sing C. Postmastectomy lymphedema treated with the Wright linear pump. *Can J Surg.* 1987;30:368–372.

64. Tiwari A. Differential diagnosis, investigation, and current treatment of lower limb lymphedema. *Arch Surg.* 2003;138:152–161.

65. Didem K. The comparison of two different physiotherapy methods in treatment of lymphedema after breast surgery. *Breast Cancer Res Treat.* 2005;93:49–54.

66. Koul R. Efficacy of complete decongestive therapy and manual lymphatic drainage on treatment-related lymphedema in breast cancer. *Int J Radiat Oncol Biol Phys.* 2007;67:841–846.

67. Ko DS. Effective treatment of lymphedema of the extremities. *Arch Surg.* 1998;133:452–458.

68. Szuba A. Decongestive lymphatic therapy for patients with breast carcinoma-associated lymphedema: a randomized, prospective study of a role for adjunctive intermittent pneumatic compression. *Cancer.* 2002;95:2260–2267.

69. Kligman L. The treatment of lymphedema related to breast cancer: a systematic review and evidence summary. *Support Care Cancer*. 2004;12:421–431.

70. O'Brien BM. Long-term results after microlymphaticovenous anastomoses for the treatment of obstructive lymphedema. *Plast Reconstr Surg*. 1990;85:562–572.

71. Campisi C. Long-term results after lymphatic-venous anastomoses for the treatment of obstructive lymphedema. *Microsurgery*. 2001;21:135–139.

72. Campisi C. Lymphatic microsurgery for the treatment of lymphedema. *Microsurgery*. 2006;26:65–69.

73. Campisi C. Microsurgery for treatment of peripheral lymphedema: long-term outcome and future perspectives. *Microsurgery*. 2007;27:333–338.

74. Nagase T. Treatment of lymphedema with lymphaticovenular anastomoses. *Int J Clin Oncol*. 2005;10:304–310.

75. Koshima I. Supermicrosurgical lymphaticovenular anastomosis for the treatment of lymphedema in the upper extremities. *J Reconstr Microsurg*. 2000;16:437–442.

76. Koshima I. Long-term follow-up after lymphaticovenular anastomosis for lymphedema in the leg. *J Reconstr Microsurg*. 2003;19:209–215.

77. Koshima I. Minimal invasive lymphaticovenular anastomosis under local anesthesia for leg lymphedema: is it effective for stage III and IV? *Ann Plast Surg*. 2004;53:261–266.

78. Thompson N. Buried dermal flap operation for chronic lymphedema of the extremities: ten-year survey of results in 79 cases. *Plast Reconstr Surg*. 1970;45:541–548.

79. Thompson N. Surgical treatment of chronic lymphoedema of the lower limb with preliminary report of new operation. *Br Med J*. 1962;2:1567–1573.

80. Thompson N. The surgical treatment of chronic lymphoedema of the extremities. *Surg Clin North Am*. 1967;47:445–503.

81. Goldsmith HS. Relief of chronic lymphedema by omental transposition. *Ann Surg*. 1967;166:573–585.

82. Goldsmith HS. Omental transposition in primary lymphedema. *Surg Gynecol Obstet*. 1967;125:607–610.

83. Classen DA. Free muscle flap transfer as a lymphatic bridge for upper extremity lymphedema. *J Reconstr Microsurg*. 2005;21:93–99.

84. Goldsmith HS. Long term evaluation of omental transposition for chronic lymphedema. *Ann Surg*. 1974;180:847–849.

85. Gillies H. The treatment of lymphoedema by plastic operation. *Br Med J*. 1935;1:96.

86. Gillies H. The lymphatic wick. *Proc R Soc Med*. 1950;43:1054.

87. Smith JW. Selection of appropriate surgical procedures in lymphedema: introduction of the hinged pedicle. *Plast Reconstr Surg Transplant Bull*. 1962;30:10–31.

88. Kinmonth JB. Primary lymphoedema; clinical and lymphangiographic studies of a series of 107 patients in which the lower limbs were affected. *Br J Surg*. 1957;45:1–9.

89. Kinmonth JB. Comments on operations for lower limb lymphoedema. *Lymphology*. 1975;8:56–61.

90. Clodius L. Problems of microsurgery in lymphedema. *Handchir Mikrochir Plast Chir*. 1982;14:79–82.

91. Mowlem R. The treatment of lymphoedema. *Br J Plast Surg*. 1948;1:48–55.

92. Slavin SA. Return of lymphatic function after flap transfer for acute lymphedema. *Ann Surg*. 1999;229:421–427.

93. Parrett BM. The contralateral rectus abdominis musculocutaneous flap for treatment of lower extremity lymphedema. *Ann Plast Surg*. 2009;62:75–79.

94. Kondoleon. *Zentralbl Chir*. 1912;39:1022.

95. Sistrunk WE. Further experiences with the Kondoleon operation for elephantiasis. *JAMA*. 1918;71:800.

96. Weinstein M. Elephantiasis and the Kondoleon operation: a 20-year postoperative follow-up. *Am J Surg*. 1950;79:327–331, illust.

97. Green TM. Elephantiasis and the Kondoleon operation. *Ann Surg*. 1920;71:28–31.

98. Becker C. Postmastectomy lymphedema: long-term results following microsurgical lymph node transplantation. *Ann Surg*. 2006;243:313–315.

99. Tobbia D. Experimental assessment of autologous lymph node transplantation as treatment of postsurgical lymphedema. *Plast Reconstr Surg*. 2009;124:777–786.

100. Brorson H. Liposuction in arm lymphedema treatment. *Scand J Surg*. 2003;92:287–295.

101. Brorson H. Controlled compression and liposuction treatment for lower extremity lymphedema. *Lymphology*. 2008;41:52–63.

102. Brorson H. Liposuction reduces arm lymphedema without significantly altering the already impaired lymph transport. *Lymphology*. 1998;31:156–172.

103. Eryilmaz T. Suction-assisted lipectomy for treatment of lower-extremity lymphedema. *Aesthetic Plast Surg*. 2009;33:671–673.

104. Greene AK. Treatment of lower extremity lymphedema with suction-assisted lipectomy. *Plast Reconstr Surg*. 2006;118:118e–121e.

105. Sando WC. Suction lipectomy in the management of limb lymphedema. *Clin Plast Surg*. 1989;16:369–373.

106. Brorson H. Adipose tissue in lymphedema: the ignorance of adipose tissue in lymphedema. *Lymphology*. 2004;37:175–177.

107. Brorson H. Liposuction gives complete reduction of chronic large arm lymphedema after breast cancer. *Acta Oncol*. 2000;39:407–420.

108. Brorson H. Quality of life following liposuction and conservative treatment of arm lymphedema. *Lymphology*. 2006;39:8–25.

109. Louton RB. The use of suction curettage as adjunct to the management of lymphedema. *Ann Plast Surg*. 1989;22:354–357.

110. O'Brien BM. Liposuction in the treatment of lymphoedema: a preliminary report. *Br J Plast Surg*. 1989;42:530–533.

111. Brorson H. Adipose tissue dominates chronic arm lymphedema following breast cancer: an analysis using volume rendered CT images. *Lymphat Res Biol*. 2006;4:199–210.

112. Homans J. The treatment of elephantiasis of the legs: a preliminary report. *N Engl J Med*. 1936;215:1099.

113. Miller TA. Staged skin and subcutaneous excision for lymphedema: a favorable report of long-term results. *Plast Reconstr Surg*. 1998;102:1486–1498; discussion 1499–501.

114. Miller TA. Surgical management of lymphedema of the extremity. *Plast Reconstr Surg*. 1975;56:633–641.

115. Miller TA. The management of lymphedema by staged subcutaneous excision. *Surg Gynecol Obstet*. 1973;136:586–592.

116. *A system of treatment*. London: J & A Churchill Ltd; 1912.

117. Miller TA. Charles procedure for lymphedema: a warning. *Am J Surg*. 1980;139:290–292.

118. Mavili ME. Modified Charles operation for primary fibrosclerotic lymphedema. *Lymphology*. 1994;27:14–20.

119. Dellon AL. The Charles procedure for primary lymphedema: long-term clinical results. *Plast Reconstr Surg*. 1977;60:589–595.

120. van der Walt JC. Modified Charles procedure using negative pressure dressings for primary lymphedema: a functional assessment. *Ann Plast Surg*. 2009;62:669–675.

Nonestrogenic management of hot flashes

Jason M. Jones, Deirdre R. Pachman, and Charles L. Loprinzi

22

PREVALENCE AND PATHOPHYSIOLOGY

PREVALENCE

Hot flashes are sudden intense warm sensations over the upper chest, neck, and face commonly associated with red, blotchy skin and profuse sweating. They are frequently accompanied by anxiety and palpitations. Episodes typically last from 2 to 4 minutes and can occur frequently throughout the day. These episodes can have a significant impact on quality of life, including negative effects on work, recreation, and sleep[1] The scope of the problem is wide, with nearly 75% of all menopausal woman suffering from hot flashes.[2]

Patients with cancer may be more prone to developing hot flashes. Chemotherapy can cause ovarian failure, referred to as chemotherapy-induced premature menopause. This occurs because chemotherapy causes depletion of follicles, resulting in decreased production of estradiol. Estradiol feedback on the pituitary gland is lost, and follicle-stimulating hormone (FSH) and luteinizing hormone (LH) levels rise, resulting in a menopause-like syndrome. Alkylating agents are the chemotherapeutic agents most frequently associated with premature menopause. Cancer survivors may also experience premature menopause secondary to pelvic radiation.[3]

Breast cancer survivors are at higher risk for menopause-induced symptoms. Many of these patients take tamoxifen or aromatase inhibitors, each of which have been associated with hot flashes.[4] Tamoxifen-induced hot flashes, on average, develop and increase over a 2- to 3-month period and then gradually diminish.[5] In some patients, the negative effect on quality of life leads to decreased compliance with taking tamoxifen.[6,7] Another reason for hot flashes in premenopausal women with breast cancer is therapeutic ovarian suppression related to surgical ovarian ablation or luteinizing hormone releasing factor agonists/antagonists.

Although traditionally hot flashes have been described in women, they are also a frequent problem in men with prostate cancer. It has been reported that 60% to 80% of such patients have hot flashes associated with androgen ablation therapy.[8–10]

PATHOPHYSIOLOGY

The pathophysiology of hot flashes is complex and is not completely understood. The thermoregulatory nucleus in the medial preoptic area of the hypothalamus is believed to be responsible for control of the core body temperature.[11] The core body temperature is maintained in a homeostatic range, known as the *thermoregulatory zone.*[12] When the core temperature exceeds the upper limit of normal of the thermoregulatory zone, vasodilation and perspiration are triggered as a compensatory response to lower temperature. Women with frequent hot flashes have been shown to have thermoregulatory zones that are narrower than those in women without hot flashes. In these women, even small changes in core body temperature—as little as 0.01° C—have been noted to trigger hot flash episodes.[13,14]

The thermoregulatory zone is regulated by complex neuroendocrine pathways and is influenced by levels of norepinephrine, serotonin, estrogen, testosterone, and endorphins. The proposed model of this interaction is shown in Figure 22-1.[12] Many of these pathways have become targets for therapy.

In normal premenopausal females, the anterior pituitary gland releases FSH and LH, and this causes monthly maturation of ovarian follicles. After menopause, oophorectomy, or ovarian dysfunction, no follicles remain to produce estrogen. This causes lack of feedback on the pituitary and adjustment of the thermoregulatory zone; gonadotropin hormones remain elevated, and women experience menopausal symptoms.

It is important to distinguish between relatively abrupt lowering of serum estrogen concentrations versus chronically low estrogen concentrations. Patients experiencing abrupt withdrawal of estrogen, such as oophorectomy in premenopausal women or natural menopause, may develop hot flashes.[11] In contrast, patients with gonadal dysgenesis who have low levels of endogenous estrogen levels do not experience hot flashes. However, if these women are started on estrogen replacement and then have it withdrawn, they develop hot flashes.[11]

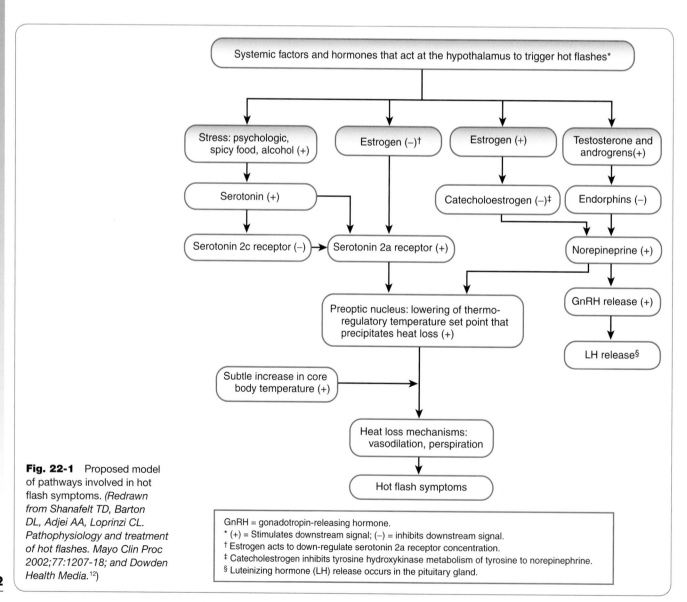

Fig. 22-1 Proposed model of pathways involved in hot flash symptoms. (*Redrawn from Shanafelt TD, Barton DL, Adjei AA, Loprinzi CL. Pathophysiology and treatment of hot flashes. Mayo Clin Proc 2002;77:1207-18; and Dowden Health Media.*[12])

GnRH = gonadotropin-releasing hormone.
* (+) = Stimulates downstream signal; (−) = inhibits downstream signal.
† Estrogen acts to down-regulate serotonin 2a receptor concentration.
‡ Catecholestrogen inhibits tyrosine hydroxykinase metabolism of tyrosine to norepinephrine.
§ Luteinizing hormone (LH) release occurs in the pituitary gland.

PHARMACOLOGIC MANAGEMENT/BASIC PRINCIPLES OF DRUG THERAPY

HOT FLASH MEASUREMENT AND EVALUATION

Hot flash data in most trials have been collected with the use of hot flash diaries. Patients are asked to report each episode and to delineate the severity as "mild," "moderate," "severe," or "very severe." After trial completion, efficacy is evaluated by reduction of hot flash frequency as an absolute reduction or as percent reduction from baseline. Some studies have used a hot flash score. This is calculated by assigning 1 point for every mild hot flash, 2 points for every moderate hot flash, 3 points for every severe hot flash, and 4 points for every very severe hot flash. The advantage of using the hot flash score over frequency alone is that it accounts for changes in severity.[15] However, comparable results has been seen when hot flash frequency is compared with hot flash score.[15–17] The validity and reliability of collecting and analyzing data through this method have been supported through the use of toxicity data, reported quality of life, patient drug preferences during crossover trials, and repeatability.[15]

Multiple tools and devices have been developed to physiologically evaluate hot flashes. These typically have measured sweating episodes and temperature changes associated with hot flashes. Detection of sweating episodes has been shown to be well correlated with reported hot flashes in the laboratory setting.[18] However, these devices may overestimate hot flashes in real-life settings.[19,20] This overestimation is likely due to the lack of a mechanism to differentiate sweating and temperature changes secondary to exertion versus a hot flash. A recent editorial concluded that hot flash diaries should continue to be the gold standard as patients report clinically significant symptoms.[21] Further work on physiologic measurements of sweating episodes is needed before they can be relied on in clinical trials.

HORMONAL THERAPY

Estrogen therapy has long been considered the primary treatment for hot flashes and continues to be the most effective therapy. It has been shown to reduce hot flash symptoms by as much as 80% to 90%.[22] However, estrogen is considered to be contraindicated in patients with coronary artery disease, breast cancer, venous thromboembolism, and uterine cancer. The Women's Health Initiative demonstrated an increased risk of CHD, stroke, pulmonary embolism, and invasive breast cancer in women receiving hormonal therapy.[23] However, benefits of estrogen included a 37% reduction in colon cancer and a 24% reduction in bone fractures. No significant change in risk of endometrial cancer was appreciated. These results have caused the use of estrogen therapy in breast cancer patients to become more controversial. One randomized controlled trial of hormone therapy (HT) in breast cancer survivors was stopped because the risk of breast cancer was increased in patients receiving HT.[24] However, another recent randomized controlled trial found no increase in the risk of breast cancer recurrence with hormone therapy.[25] Until the role of estrogen therapy in breast cancer patients is clearly defined, many patients and their physicians choose to avoid

estrogen. This has helped to fuel the investigation of alternative medications and methods to treat hot flashes.

Progesterone analogs were initially examined as a treatment for hot flashes in pilot studies during the 1970s and 1980s. On the basis of promising data, randomized control trials were performed with several agents. Megestrol acetate was tested at a dose of 40 mg daily in women with a history of breast cancer and in men with prostate cancer receiving androgen ablation therapy. Both men and women showed about a 75% to 80% reduction in hot flashes, compared with a 20% to 25% reduction in patients receiving placebo.[17] Follow-up at 3 years showed that one third of the patients had continued treatment with megestrol acetate and were experiencing fewer hot flashes than those who had stopped taking the medication.[26] Daily megestrol acetate doses of 20 mg are equally as efficacious as 40 mg.[27]

Depomedroxyprogesterone (DMPA) is a long-acting, intramuscular progestational agent that has shown to be similar to oral megestrol acetate, but it offers the advantage of injections that last weeks to months as compared with daily oral dosing with megestrol acetate.[28] Months after the initial dose, a subset of patients asked for repeat dosing.

Progesterone cream has been studied; however, its efficacy in treating hot flashes is controversial. Healthy postmenopausal women using progesterone cream had an 83% reduction in hot flashes compared with 19% with placebo.[29] However, a recent double-blind randomized controlled trial of progesterone cream versus placebo in postmenopausal women found no significant difference in hot flash control.[30]

Although progesterone analogs are clearly effective against hot flashes, many practitioners are concerned about the safety of using these agents. Trepidation is primarily centered on in vitro studies showing epithelial cell proliferation, which would be of hypothetical concern in cancer patients.[31] Additionally, it has been reported that megestrol caused elevation of prostate-specific antigen (PSA) level in patients receiving treatment for prostate cancer.[32] Nonetheless, progesterone analogs, such as megestrol acetate and medroxyprogesterone acetate, have been used to treat breast cancer. Overall, the association between progesterone and increased breast cancer risk is still unclear. Before using progesterone analogs, patients should be counseled about the potential risks and ongoing debate regarding these issues.

NONHORMONAL AGENTS

The potential for serious side effects and complications secondary to hormonal therapy has led to investigations of nonhormonal agents for the treatment of hot flashes. This area has grown over the past 20 years and has included multiple classes of nonhormonal therapies and various complementary medicines and nonmedication approaches. The remainder of this chapter will explore these new treatments in detail.

Newer antidepressants

It was observed in the 1990s that some patients had a decrease in hot flashes when started on antidepressants. Randomized placebo-controlled trials subsequently established antidepressants as an acceptable alternative to hormonal therapy. A pooled analysis of all published randomized trials through December 2007 provides supporting evidence as to the benefits of antidepressants.[33]

VENLAFAXINE

Venlafaxine is a serotonin-norepinephrine reuptake inhibitor (SNRI) that inhibits reuptake of serotonin, norepinephrine, and dopamine. A pilot study was performed in 28 patients with a history of breast cancer or undergoing androgen deprivation for prostate cancer. Patients reported a 55% reduction in hot flashes.[34] In addition, symptoms of fatigue, diaphoresis, and difficulty sleeping improved. At the completion of the study, 64% of participants chose to continue treatment with venlafaxine.

Randomized controlled trials have been performed to evaluate the efficacy of venlafaxine. A large placebo-controlled, double-blind, randomized trial was performed in patients with a history of breast cancer.[16] Hot flash diaries were used to measure frequency and associated symptoms as the outcome. One hundred ninety-one patients received placebo or venlafaxine 37.5 mg/day, 75 mg/day, or 150 mg/day. After 4 weeks, a 27% reduction in hot flashes occurred in the placebo arm, 37% in the 37.5-mg/day arm, 61 % in the 75-mg/day arm, and 61% in the 150-mg/day arm. The 75-mg/day dose was superior to the 37.5-mg/day dose but was similar to the 150-mg/day dose. The 150-mg/day dose was associated with greater toxicities.

Side effects, consisting of dry mouth, nausea, constipation, and decreased appetite, were generally mild. Sexual dysfunction occurs in about 2% of subjects taking venlafaxine.[35] However, in this trial, patients on venlafaxine tended to have improved libido, compared with those on placebo. It was speculated that this benefit might be due to decreased fatigue and improved sleep as a result of improved nighttime hot flashes.

A subsequent placebo-controlled trial evaluated the efficacy of venlafaxine in postmenopausal females, and confirmed the positive effect of venlafaxine on hot flashes.[36] However, results were difficult to interpret, as no hot flashes were recorded at baseline.[37]

A randomized trial designed to compare DMPA versus venlafaxine involved 94 patients assigned to extended-release venlafaxine 37.5 mg/day for a week, and then 75 mg/day thereafter, and 94 patients randomized to 400 mg IM injection of DMPA.[38] After 6 weeks, patients on the DMPA arm reported a 79% reduction in hot flash frequency, and patients on the venlafaxine arm reported a 55% reduction. Initially, patients on the venlafaxine arm reported increased nausea, appetite loss, dizziness, dry mouth, constipation, and sleepiness; however, no significant differences were seen after 6 weeks.

Patients should be placed on the extended-release formulation, 37.5 mg daily, for 1 week, and the dose should then be increased to extended-release 75 mg daily. Patients should be counseled about temporary gastrointestinal side effects, which improve after 1 to 2 weeks. No benefit is seen with the dose to 150 mg/day if hot flashes are not responsive to 75 mg/day.

DESVENLAFAXINE

Desvenlafaxine is the succinate salt form of the active metabolite of venlafaxine and improves temperature dysregulation in animal models.[39,40] Animal studies have supported the use of desvenlafaxine for vasomotor symptoms.

A randomized controlled trial assigned 77 patients to placebo and 141, 145, 137, and 120 patients to desvenlafaxine 50 mg/day, 100 mg/day, 150 mg/day, and 200 mg/day, respectively.[41] Placebo reduced hot flashes by 51%, which was not significantly different

from the 54% reduction in the 50-mg/day arm. Significant reductions of 64%, 60%, and 60% occurred in the 100-mg/day, 150-mg/day, and 200-mg/day arms, respectively. Toxicities included dry mouth, asthenia, nausea, insomnia, and somnolence, which resolved after 1 week.

Another recent randomized controlled trial allocated 150 patients to 100 mg daily, 151 to 150 mg daily, and 151 to placebo.[42] After 12 weeks, 65% and 67% had reductions in hot flash frequency in the 100-mg and 150-mg arms, respectively. These were significantly better than the 51% reduction in the placebo arm.

The recommended starting dose of desvenlafaxine is 50 mg daily for the first 3 days of treatment, increased to 100 mg daily on day 4. Doses greater than 100 mg daily have not been shown to improve responses. The side effect profile of desvenlafaxine is similar to that of venlafaxine and includes dry mouth, nausea, somnolence, and asthenia. These symptoms typically resolve after 1 week of therapy.

PAROXETINE

Paroxetine mainly inhibits reuptake of serotonin and has little effect on the reuptake of norepinephrine or dopamine. The first pilot study of paroxetine for hot flashes included 30 breast cancer survivors and showed a 67% reduction in hot flashes.[43] Another pilot study of 13 patients reported to have hot flashes "quite a bit" or "extremely severe" at baseline noted a reduction in hot flashes by 38%.[44]

A double-blind, randomized, controlled trial enrolled primarily breast cancer survivors; 151 patients were assigned to placebo, 10 mg of paroxetine, or 20 mg of paroxetine.[45] Patients on 10 mg reported a 41% reduction in hot flash frequency compared with 14% on placebo. Patients on 20 mg daily reported a 52% reduction in hot flashes. No significant difference in hot flashes was observed between the 10-mg and 20-mg doses. The only significant side effect in the paroxetine arm was nausea.

Another randomized controlled trial of paroxetine involved a cross section of menopausal women and enrolled 56 to placebo, 51 to 12.5 mg/day, and 58 to 25 mg/day.[46] The 12.5-mg/day dose reduced hot flash frequency from 7.1 to 3.8 per day. Patients on 25 mg had 6.4 hot flashes daily at baseline and 3.2 daily at the end of the trial. Patients on placebo had a baseline frequency of 6.6 daily and 4.8 hot flashes daily at the conclusion. Both doses of paroxetine were significantly superior to placebo, but no difference was noted between doses.

A pilot study in men undergoing androgen ablation for prostate cancer showed a 50% reduction in hot flash frequency with paroxetine.[47] Patients were started on 12.5 mg daily and were gradually increased to 37.5 mg daily by the end of the trial. After 4 weeks, a 50% reduction in hot flash frequency was seen, with a 56% reduction in hot flash score. To date, no randomized trials have examined paroxetine in men.

Paroxetine is a strong inhibitor of the cytochrome P450 2D6 isotype (CYP2D6), an enzyme that is important for tamoxifen metabolism, to the active metabolite endoxifen.[48] Paroxetine appears to decrease the effectiveness of tamoxifen.

Patients should be started on controlled-release paroxetine 10 mg daily, which is to be increased to up to 20 mg daily. Side effects include gastrointestinal symptoms, with the most prominent being nausea.

FLUOXETINE

Fluoxetine, a selective serotonin reuptake inhibitor (SSRI), was anecdotally reported in the 1990s to reduce hot flashes. A phase III crossover study of fluoxetine for the treatment of hot flashes was performed.[49] In this trial, 81 women were assigned to placebo or fluoxetine 20 mg daily. During the first period before crossover, patients on fluoxetine recorded 42% and 50% reductions in hot flash frequency and score, respectively; patients on placebo reported 31% and 36% reductions. Reported toxicities included nausea, loss of appetite, sleeplessness, fatigue, nervousness, and constipation.

A subsequent randomized trial assigned patients to placebo, fluoxetine, or citalopram.[50] This trial is marred by the fact that no baseline hot flash data were collected for comparison and stratification.[37] The reduction in events was calculated from the first recordings in the diary on day 1 of active treatment. In multiple trials, antidepressants were observed to cause a rapid reduction in hot flashes. In fact, hot flashes were reduced by 31% during the first day of venlafaxine therapy.[37]

Fluoxetine appears to be at least mildly effective with minimal toxicities but is not used often for this indication, as other antidepressants appear to work better. In addition, fluoxetine is contraindicated with the use of tamoxifen because it is a significant inhibitor of CYP2D6.

CITALOPRAM

By the early 2000s, newer antidepressants were shown to be an effective alternative to hormonal therapy for the treatment of hot flashes. However, some patients do not tolerate SSRIs, and others may be able to tolerate certain SSRIs or SNRIs better than others. In addition, concern for SSRI interactions with tamoxifen led to the decision to test citalopram because it has little CYP2D6 inhibitory activity. Citalopram is an alternate if a patient does not tolerate venlafaxine or paroxetine.[51]

A pilot study was performed in 26 patients with a history of breast cancer. Four weeks of treatment reduced hot flashes by 58%.[52] A randomized trial divided 254 patients into 4 arms: placebo and citalopram 10 mg, 20 mg, or 30 mg daily.[53] At the conclusion of the study, hot flash frequency was reduced by 46%, 43%, and 50% in patients receiving 10 mg, 20 mg, and 30 mg of citalopram, respectively. Patients on placebo had a 20% reduction. No significant negative side effects were seen with citalopram.

A randomized trial included placebo, fluoxetine, and citalopram arms, but baseline data were not recorded, thus marring the study.

Citalopram should be considered for treatment in patients whose hot flashes do not respond to other antidepressants. A pilot trial was performed in patients who had inadequate relief on venlafaxine.[54] Twenty-two patients were evaluable, and at the end of 4 weeks, a 53% reduction in hot flash scores was reported. These results provide some evidence that citalopram may be an alternative treatment for those with poorly responsive hot flashes on other standard SSRIs. Randomized trials will need to be done to confirm this observation.

Citalopram is started at 10 mg daily for the treatment of hot flashes. No evidence indicates that its benefits are dose related.

SSRIs and CYP2D6

In recent years, the role of tamoxifen metabolites has become more completely understood. 4-Hydroxy-N-desmethyl tamoxifen, also known as endoxifen, is the active metabolite of tamoxifen needed for anticancer activity. N-desmethyl tamoxifen is oxidized to endoxifen by cytochrome P450 enzyme CYP2D6.[55] Older SSRIs are inhibitors of CYP2D6 that lower endoxifen levels.[48] Paroxetine and fluoxetine are strong inhibitors of CYP2D6, and venlafaxine is a weak inhibitor that does not appear to substantially reduce endoxifen levels.[56] Data regarding the effects of citalopram on this enzyme are scarce, but it does not appear to be a clinically significant inhibitor. If a patient is on tamoxifen, venlafaxine is the best antidepressant option for hot flashes, and citalopram may be considered a second option if venlafaxine is not effective or is not tolerated.

Anticonvulsants

GABAPENTIN

Gabapentin has been used traditionally as an anticonvulsant and an analgesic for neuropathic pain. It is structurally related to the neurotransmitter gamma-aminobutyric acid (GABA). However, overall, its mechanism of action remains unknown, although recent evidence supports GABA as a calcium channel blocker. It is not thought to bind to GABA receptors, it is not a GABA receptor agonist, and it does not inhibit GABA uptake.[57]

In a case series of six patients, gabapentin caused an 89% reduction in hot flashes.[58] Gabapentin offers an advantage over SSRIs in that it is not metabolized, is not known to interfere with CYP2D6, and has few drug interactions. In addition, gabapentin targets different mechanisms that may precipitate hot flashes, and therefore might be useful to treat refractory hot flashes.

A pilot study was performed in 20 women.[59] After a baseline measurement of hot flashes, patients were started on 300 mg/day for 1 week, titrated by 300-mg/day increments weekly to a goal dose of 900 mg/day in three divided doses. A 66% reduction in hot flash frequency was observed.

Two randomized placebo-controlled trials have been reported. The first trial randomized 59 postmenopausal women to receive gabapentin 900 mg/day or placebo.[60] After 12 weeks of treatment, gabapentin reduced hot flash frequency by 45% and hot flash score by 54%. Patients on placebo had reductions of 29% and 31% for the same measures, respectively. After 12 weeks, a second phase consisting of open label treatment was started, and doses were increased up to 2700 mg/day. After 5 weeks with increased doses, 54% and 67% reductions from baseline were noted in frequency and score, respectively. Side effects included somnolence, dizziness, and rash.

The other trial involved 420 women with a history of breast cancer, who were divided into three arms: placebo, 300 mg/day, and 900 mg/day in three divided doses.[61] After 8 weeks, the 900-mg/day arm had a 44% reduction in hot flash frequency, whereas 15% and 30% reductions were reported in the placebo and 300-mg/day arms, respectively. A statistically significant reduction in hot flashes occurred with 900 mg/day.

A small, randomized, controlled trial compared high-dose gabapentin, conjugated estrogens, and placebo.[62] Reductions of 71% and 72% were reported in the gabapentin and estrogen groups, respectively, compared with a 54% reduction with placebo. Although this suggested that gabapentin, at a high dose of 2400 mg daily, was comparable with estrogens, the treatment arms each included only 20 patients, and so were subject to type II error. The 20% improvement over the placebo arm is comparable with what was observed in other randomized trials. Thus, the dose-response question regarding gabapentin and hot flashes has not been adequately addressed.

A subsequent trial evaluated the effectiveness of gabapentin in patients whose hot flashes were inadequately responsive to antidepressant therapy. Ninety-one eligible patients were assigned to continue with the antidepressant while starting gabapentin, or to discontinue their antidepressant while starting gabapentin. After 5 weeks, each group had about a 50% reduction in hot flashes.[59]

Limited evidence is available to give direction to the management of hot flashes in men. For men who prefer to avoid hormonal therapy, gabapentin is a viable alternative. A randomized, placebo-controlled trial performed in men with prostate cancer undergoing androgen ablation therapy enrolled 214 men divided into 4 arms: placebo and gabapentin 300 mg/day, 600 mg/day, and 900 mg/day.[63] After 4 weeks, reductions in hot flashes were reported in 22%, 23%, 32%, and 46% of the placebo, 300-mg/day, 600-mg/day, and 900-mg/day arms, respectively. Patients receiving 900 mg/day of gabapentin had a significantly better response compared with placebo. These results are similar to those reported in women. Side effects were generally mild.

Gabapentin is effective at reducing hot flashes in both men and women with a history of cancer and should be used in patients who are concerned about hormonal therapy for hot flashes, or in those for whom contraindications are known. A pooled analysis of randomized trials also supports this premise.[33] Gabapentin is started at a dose of 300 mg daily for 1 week and is increased to 300 mg twice daily the next week. The goal is 300 mg 3 times daily. Higher doses may be even more effective, but this has not been confirmed by large prospective, randomized, controlled trials.

PREGABALIN

Pregabalin is a newer anticonvulsant related to gabapentin. Pregabalin could represent a beneficial treatment for hot flashes similar to gabapentin, with a longer half-life and fewer tablets. A pilot trial of six patients showed a 65% median reduction in hot flashes.[64]

A double-blind, randomized, controlled trial of pregabalin involved 163 patients divided into three arms: placebo or pregabalin 75 mg twice daily or 150 mg twice daily.[65] Patients were started on 50 mg daily, increased at weekly intervals to 50 mg twice daily, then 75 mg twice daily, and finally 150 mg twice daily. After 6 weeks of treatment, reductions from baseline of 36%, 60%, and 61% were seen in the placebo, 75 mg twice daily, and 150 mg twice daily arms, respectively. Toxicities included dizziness at both doses and cognitive dysfunction with the higher dose. Other side effects included weight gain, sleepiness, and blurred vision. Toxicities were substantially greater with the higher dose.

Pregabalin is an effective drug for the treatment of hot flashes. No difference in effectiveness has been noted between lower and higher doses. Pregabalin is started at 50 mg daily, increased at weekly intervals to 50 mg twice daily and finally to 75 mg twice daily.

Other centrally acting medications
CLONIDINE

Clonidine is a centrally acting alpha-2 adrenergic agonist that was first investigated for the treatment of hot flashes in the 1970s.[66–68] Clonidine raises hot flash threshold by reducing norepinephrine release.[69] A large, randomized, controlled trial of transdermal clonidine was conducted in women with a history of breast cancer that enrolled 110 patients divided into two arms: placebo and 0.1-mg transdermal clonidine patch.[70] After 5 weeks, hot flashes were reduced by 44% in the clonidine arm, compared with a 27% reduction in the placebo group. Side effects included dry mouth, constipation, pruritus, and drowsiness. Side effects from treatment outweighed benefits.

Another randomized controlled trial compared placebo versus oral clonidine in women with a history of breast cancer who were receiving tamoxifen.[71] A total of 194 patients were assigned to placebo or clonidine 0.1 mg daily. After 8 weeks, a 38% reduction occurred in the clonidine group versus a 24% reduction in the placebo group. Side effects were generally mild; the only statistically significant difference was greater sleeping problems with clonidine.

Transdermal clonidine was also examined in post-orchiectomy men treated for prostate cancer.[72] In a double-blind, randomized, controlled trial of 70 patients, clonidine did not significantly reduce hot flashes compared with placebo.

Clonidine is moderately effective in women with a history of breast cancer who are taking tamoxifen, but does not appear to be very effective in the treatment of hot flashes in men. The side effect profile needs to be considered before clonidine is prescribed. The clonidine dose for hot flashes is 0.1 mg daily.

BELLERGAL

Bellergal is a combination of phenobarbital, ergotamine tartrate, and alkaloids of belladonna. It has antimuscarinic effects and was originally used as eye drops for pupil dilation. A randomized controlled trial in the 1960s evaluated patients by asking them to describe their hot flashes on bellergal as "success" or "failure" of treatment, and to rate them as absent, moderate, or severe.[73] Bellergal decreased hot flashes compared with placebo. Another randomized controlled trial in the 1980s showed a significant reduction in hot flashes with bellergal after 2 weeks of treatment.[74] However, after 8 weeks, the difference between treatment and placebo disappeared with reductions of 68% and 75%, respectively. Toxicity in both trials was significant, with more than 30% withdrawing because of side effects, which included dry mouth, dizziness, rash, and sleepiness. Bellergal is no longer available in the United States.

Complimentary agents
VITAMIN E

Vitamin E is an antioxidant that was originally reported to reduce hot flashes in the 1940s.[75,76] In addition, popular women's journals recommended 400 to 800 IU of vitamin E daily for menopausal symptoms.

A crossover, randomized, placebo-controlled trial of women with a history of breast cancer used vitamin E 800 IU/day divided into two doses.[77] After 4 weeks, similar reductions in vitamin E and placebo were noted. However, secondary endpoint data from the crossover of this study demonstrated a statistically significant reduction with vitamin E. The overall reduction was about one hot flash per day, which may not be clinically significant. This was demonstrated when patients were asked which medication they preferred after the crossover of the trial; 32% chose vitamin E, and 29% preferred placebo. No significant side effects were noted with vitamin E.

It may be reasonable to consider vitamin E because it may relieve hot flashes, is inexpensive, and has no side effects or drug interactions. Vitamin E has been reported to be potentially harmful in recent years, but this was refuted in a recent meta-analysis; no evidence of increased cancer risk was obtained.[78] Vitamin E is started at 400 IU twice daily.

BLACK COHOSH

Black cohosh, also known as *Cimicifuga racemosa*, is a member of the buttercup family used by American Indians for the treatment of various female ailments.[79] Small, randomized trials performed in Europe reported improvements in vasomotor symptoms.[80–82] Several pilot trials in the United States, including one that enrolled 21 patients, reported a 50% reduction in hot flash frequency from baseline.[83] A randomized controlled trial enrolled 132 patients. Patients in the black cohosh group experienced a 17% reduction in hot flash frequency from baseline after 4 weeks, compared with a 26% reduction with placebo. Other randomized trials have reported similar results.[84,85] Recent reports have described serious side effects associated with black cohosh, including liver failure.[86] Current evidence argues against the use of black cohosh for hot flashes.

Phytoestrogens

The prevalence of hot flashes in women has been shown to be lower in Southeast Asians than in Caucasians.[87] One hypothesis is that Southeast Asian women have diets high in phytoestrogens.[88] Two types of phytoestrogens—isoflavones and lignans—have been shown to compete for binding at estrogen receptors, and binding to estrogen receptors is thought to be a potential treatment for hot flashes.[89] To date, trials have been performed using isoflavones such as soy and red clover extract. Most have shown no benefit over placebo. Ongoing studies are using lignans such as flaxseed. These studies will clarify the benefits or lack of benefits of soy, red clover, and flaxseed.

SOY

Numerous trials have examined the effects of soy isoflavones on vasomotor symptoms. These have been heterogeneous with regard to dosing and medicinal forms. Several trials have been conducted in women with breast cancer.[90–93] A double-blind, placebo-controlled, randomized trial of soy isoflavone 150 mg daily was performed in 177 patients with breast cancer.[92] This study failed to show any difference in hot flash frequency or score. Several subsequent studies evaluating patients with hot flashes and a history of breast cancer have supported these results.[90,91,93] Several meta-analyses have been performed to examine the use of soy. One meta-analysis did show a 5% reduction in hot flashes over placebo.[94] However, this finding should be viewed cautiously because of potential publication bias, and because a large trial in breast cancer patients showing numerically more hot flashes with soy was excluded from the meta-analysis. The relevance of a 5% reduction in

hot flashes must be questioned. A more recent meta-analysis included studies with cancer patients and menopausal patients and concluded that evidence does not support the use of soy in the treatment of hot flashes.[95] The treatment of hot flashes with soy products is not recommended.

RED CLOVER ISOFLAVONE EXTRACT

Red clover isoflavone extract is another phytoestrogen that was believed to be promising in the treatment of hot flashes. However, multiple randomized controlled trials have reported negative results. The largest of these trials enrolled 252 patients.[96] Patients receiving red clover extract had a 41% reduction compared with a 36% reduction with placebo. No significant side effects were seen. Most trials have reported similar results.[97,98] A meta-analysis combining six trials did not show benefit with red clover extract.[95] Red clover isoflavone extract is not recommended for hot flashes.

FLAXSEED

Flaxseed, also known as linseed, is an exceptionally rich source of lignin, which has estrogen receptor affinity and is considered a possible treatment for hot flashes.[88] It is structurally similar to estradiol and tamoxifen and has been reported to possibly inhibit tumor activity in estrogen-positive breast cancer.[99] The interaction between flaxseed and tamoxifen is not entirely clear.

The potential for cancer-suppressing, nonestrogen treatment of hot flashes makes flaxseed an intriguing therapy. A pilot trial showed promise, with a 50% reduction in hot flash frequency in 31 women taking 40 g of crushed flaxseed daily.[100] The only published report to date describes a randomized controlled trial that used flaxseed muffins and soy muffins versus placebo.[88] A significant reduction in hot flashes was observed in those eating the flaxseed muffins. However, the primary outcome in this trial was a Menopause-Specific Quality of Life Scale (MENQOL) score—not hot flash frequency or severity. Therefore, at this time, it is difficult to interpret the impact of flaxseed on hot flashes. A placebo-controlled, double-blind, randomized trial examining the utility of flaxseed for treating hot flashes completed its accrual goal in December 2009. Results should be forthcoming shortly.

NONPHARMACOLOGIC MANAGEMENT
Acupuncture

Acupuncture has been used in Asia for more than 2500 years. It has been deemed safe and effective for the treatment of chronic pain and chemotherapy-induced nausea and vomiting.[101] Several pilot studies have suggested that acupuncture may be an effective treatment for hot flashes without a major risk of side effects.[102–104] Multiple randomized controlled trials have been conducted to evaluate possible benefits. A randomized placebo-controlled trial paired 103 patients into acupuncture versus sham acupuncture groups.[56,105] After 6 weeks, 60% and 62% of residual hot flashes were present in the acupuncture and sham arms, respectively. At 12 weeks, 72% of residual hot flashes were present in the acupuncture group, and 55% in the sham group. Similar results were reported in another trial, which enrolled breast cancer patients.[106] In this study, patients receiving acupuncture had a reduction in hot flashes from 8.6 to 6.2. Those undergoing the sham procedure had a reduction from 10.0 to 7.6. A recent systematic review consisting of 11 randomized controlled trials concluded that no evidence can be found for the use of acupuncture for hot flashes.[107]

Several variables make it difficult to study acupuncture. First, acupuncture should be performed by experienced practitioners. Inexperience may lead to incorrect performance of the procedure and essentially sham procedures. If patients undergoing this incorrect procedure are included in the active treatment arm, then acupuncture may wrongfully be construed as ineffective. Second, a sham procedure is often used as the placebo and can produce a physiologic response. A sham procedure usually involves "incorrect" positioning of needles or placement of noninvasive needles in correct locations. Acupuncture is not recommended for the treatment of hot flashes.

Stellate ganglion block

A stellate ganglion block is a procedure commonly used in pain medicine for the treatment of pain syndromes and vascular insufficiency. It is performed by a posterior approach just lateral to the C6 vertebra. When the anterior portion is reached, local anesthetic is injected, inducing a sympathectomy, which often results in Horner's syndrome. A case series report in 2005 suggested that stellate ganglion blocks had marked effects in reducing hot flashes.[108] The same investigators then conducted a pilot trial of stellate ganglion block in 13 breast cancer survivors and again reported a significant decrease in hot flashes.[109] A more recent pilot trial performed by another group involved eight women with a history of breast cancer.[110] Patients received one stellate ganglion block after a baseline week. After 6 weeks, an approximate 55% reduction in hot flash frequency occurred. In all trials, no significant adverse events related to the procedure were noted.

The mechanism by which the stellate ganglion block reduces hot flashes is unclear. It is proposed that the efficacy of this procedure is the result of a central nervous system effect in areas of the brain that appear to be responsible for temperature regulation.[111]

Preliminary results are encouraging, and upcoming trials will define the role and efficacy of this novel treatment for hot flashes. If randomized trials demonstrate benefit for a stellate ganglion block in the treatment of hot flashes, it will be an alternative therapy for patients who cannot tolerate medications for the treatment of hot flashes, or who do not benefit from other medications.

BEHAVIORAL MODIFICATIONS

PACED RESPIRATIONS

Behavioral therapy has become increasingly popular because of its potential benefit with no substantial side effects. Few data are available, but trials thus far have been encouraging, showing as much as a 50% reduction in hot flashes.[112] Another trial did not show a change in frequency but noted a decrease in severity.[113] In addition, in pilot trials, positive effects on vasomotor symptoms were reported with yoga.[114] Trials are ongoing, and it is hoped that they will demonstrate that this modality will offer benefit to patients with hot flashes.

HYPNOSIS

Hypnosis is another behavioral therapy that is being investigated for the treatment of hot flashes. Hypnosis places patients in a state of deep relaxation and uses suggestion and mental imagery to alter perception, memory, or mood. It has been used successfully to increase relaxation, reduce anxiety, and reduce distress in patients with breast cancer.[115,116] In addition, hypnosis has been shown to improve sleep.[117] Anxiety and psychosocial symptoms have been associated with hot flashes. It is believed that hypnosis may reduce hot flash symptoms and/or improve quality of life. A pilot study of self-hypnosis showed a reduction in hot flash score by 68%.[118] Additional studies are ongoing and may show hypnosis as an alternative for those wishing to avoid pharmacologic therapy.

PHYSICAL MEASURES

Finally, evidence indicates that some easily done things can help hot flashes.[11] These include using a fan, wearing loose-fitting clothing, sipping cold drinks, and lowering room temperature. Additional suggestions include dietary modifications

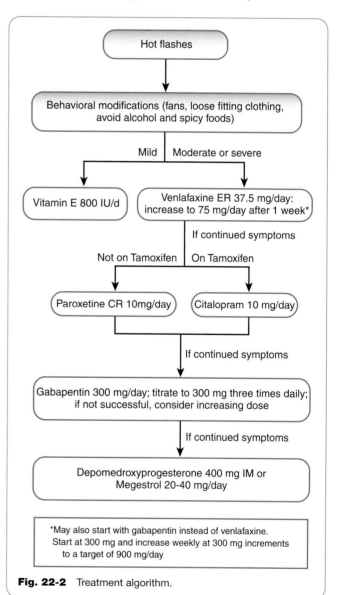

Fig. 22-2 Treatment algorithm.

such as eliminating alcohol and spicy foods. Although evidence is limited, behavioral modification is still a reasonable first-line treatment for patients with mild hot flashes.[119]

CONCLUSION AND RECOMMENDATIONS

An increasing number of treatment options can be used for hot flashes in patients electing to avoid estrogen replacement. Most trials have been conducted in women, but a growing number of trials are being performed in men.

Figure 22-2 presents an algorithm for the treatment approach for hot flashes in women. Patients should be educated on potential behavioral modifications that might be helpful, including wearing loose-fitting clothing, sipping cold drinks, lowering room temperature, and avoiding alcohol and spicy food in the diet. If hot flashes are generally mild, a patient may try vitamin E 400 IU twice daily. For moderate or severe hot flashes, patients could be started on extended-release venlafaxine 37.5 mg, increased to 75 mg daily after 1 week. If the patient continues to have residual hot flashes, a trial of an alternative antidepressant is appropriate. If the patient is not taking tamoxifen, then paroxetine 10 mg with a maximum dose of 20 mg, or citalopram at a dose of 10 mg daily, can be used. If the patient is taking tamoxifen, then paroxetine should be avoided and citalopram can be considered. If the patient continues to have refractory hot flashes, then gabapentin can be initiated at 300 mg daily. This can be increased to twice daily and three times daily at weekly increments. Alternatively, instead of starting with an antidepressant, it would be reasonable to start with gabapentin and switch to an antidepressant if gabapentin does not work. Pregabalin can be used as an alternative to gabapentin at doses of 50 mg daily titrated at weekly intervals to 50 mg twice daily and finally to 75 mg twice daily. The main disadvantage is that pregabalin is more expensive than gabapentin. If hot flashes persist, progestins can be considered. Megestrol acetate at 20 to 40 mg daily for 1 month with a decrease to 20 mg thereafter can be successful. Alternatively, a one-time 400-mg depomedroxyprogesterone intramuscular injection can diminish hot flash symptoms for weeks to months. If progestins are used, the unknown risks should be discussed with the patient.

Figure 22-2 can also be used as an algorithm for the treatment approach to hot flashes in men, with an understanding that not as much evidence is available. Nonetheless, a recent editorial suggests that more similarities than differences exist between male and female hot flashes.[120] If this is accepted, it could be stated that it is reasonable to treat hot flashes similarly in both genders, unless compelling evidence suggests that something that works for one sex may not work for the other.

Thus, a variety of alternative treatment options are available for hot flashes, other than estrogen therapy. These options should continue to grow and improve as new treatment strategies are developed and studied.

REFERENCES

1. Hoda D, Perez DG, Loprinzi CL. Hot flashes in breast cancer survivors. *Breast J.* 2003;9:431–438.
2. McKinlay SM, Jefferys M. The menopausal syndrome. *Br J Prev Soc Med.* 1974;28:108–115.
3. Ataya K, Moghissi K. Chemotherapy-induced premature ovarian failure: mechanisms and prevention. *Steroids.* 1989;54:607–626.
4. Nabholtz JM. Long-term safety of aromatase inhibitors in the treatment of breast cancer. *Ther Clin Risk Manag.* 2008;4:189–204.
5. Loprinzi CL, Zahasky KM, Sloan JA, et al. Tamoxifen-induced hot flashes. *Clin Breast Cancer.* 2000;1:52–56.
6. Powles T, Eeles R, Ashley S, et al. Interim analysis of the incidence of breast cancer in the Royal Marsden Hospital tamoxifen randomised chemoprevention trial. *Lancet.* 1998;352:98–101.
7. Veronesi U, Maisonneuve P, Costa A, et al. Prevention of breast cancer with tamoxifen: preliminary findings from the Italian randomised trial among hysterectomised women. Italian Tamoxifen Prevention Study. *Lancet.* 1998;352:93–97.
8. Charig CR, Rundle JS. Flushing: long-term side effect of orchiectomy in treatment of prostatic carcinoma. *Urology.* 1989;33:175–178.
9. Lanfrey P, Mottet N, Dagues F, et al. [Hot flashes and hormonal treatment of prostate cancer]. *Prog Urol.* 1996;6:17–22.
10. Schow DA, Renfer LG, Rozanski TA, et al. Prevalence of hot flushes during and after neoadjuvant hormonal therapy for localized prostate cancer. *South Med J.* 1998;91:855–857.
11. Casper RF, Yen SS. Neuroendocrinology of menopausal flushes: an hypothesis of flush mechanism. *Clin Endocrinol (Oxf).* 1985;22:293–312.

12. Shanafelt TD, Barton DL, Adjei AA, et al. Pathophysiology and treatment of hot flashes. *Mayo Clin Proc.* 2002;77:1207–1218.
13. Freedman RR, Krell W. Reduced thermoregulatory null zone in postmenopausal women with hot flashes. *Am J Obstet Gynecol.* 1999;181:66–70.
14. Freedman RR, Norton D, Woodward S, et al. Core body temperature and circadian rhythm of hot flashes in menopausal women. *J Clin Endocrinol Metab.* 1995;80:2354–2358.
15. Sloan JA, Loprinzi CL, Novotny PJ, et al. Methodologic lessons learned from hot flash studies. *J Clin Oncol.* 2001;19:4280–4290.
16. Loprinzi CL, Kugler JW, Sloan JA, et al. Venlafaxine in management of hot flashes in survivors of breast cancer: a randomised controlled trial. *Lancet.* 2000;356:2059–2063.
17. Loprinzi CL, Michalak JC, Quella SK, et al. Megestrol acetate for the prevention of hot flashes. *N Engl J Med.* 1994;331:347–352.
18. Freedman RR. Laboratory and ambulatory monitoring of menopausal hot flashes. *Psychophysiology.* 1989;26:573–579.
19. Carpenter JS, Andrykowski MA, Freedman RR, et al. Feasibility and psychometrics of an ambulatory hot flash monitoring device. *Menopause.* 1999;6:209–215.
20. Carpenter JS, Monahan PO, Azzouz F. Accuracy of subjective hot flush reports compared with continuous sternal skin conductance monitoring. *Obstet Gynecol.* 2004;104:1322–1326.
21. Loprinzi CL, Barton DL. Gadgets for measuring hot flashes: have they become the gold standard? *J Support Oncol.* 2009;7:136–137.
22. Notelovitz M, Lenihan JP, McDermott M, et al. Initial 17beta-estradiol dose for treating vasomotor symptoms. *Obstet Gynecol.* 2000;95:726–731.

23. Rossouw JE, Anderson GL, Prentice RL, et al. Risks and benefits of estrogen plus progestin in healthy postmenopausal women: principal results From the Women's Health Initiative randomized controlled trial. *JAMA.* 2002;288:321–333.
24. Holmberg L, Anderson H. HABITS (hormonal replacement therapy after breast cancer—is it safe?), a randomised comparison: trial stopped. *Lancet.* 2004;363:453–455.
25. von Schoultz E, Rutqvist LE. Menopausal hormone therapy after breast cancer: the Stockholm randomized trial. *J Natl Cancer Inst.* 2005;97:533–535.
26. Quella SK, Loprinzi CL, Sloan JA, et al. Long term use of megestrol acetate by cancer survivors for the treatment of hot flashes. *Cancer.* 1998;82:1784–1788.
27. Goodwin JW, Green SJ, Moinpour CM, et al. Phase III randomized placebo-controlled trial of two doses of megestrol acetate as treatment for menopausal symptoms in women with breast cancer: Southwest Oncology Group Study 9626. *J Clin Oncol.* 2008;26:1650–1656.
28. Bertelli G, Venturini M, Del Mastro L, et al. Intramuscular depot medroxyprogesterone versus oral megestrol for the control of postmenopausal hot flashes in breast cancer patients: a randomized study. *Ann Oncol.* 2002;13:883–888.
29. Leonetti HB, Longo S, Anasti JN. Transdermal progesterone cream for vasomotor symptoms and postmenopausal bone loss. *Obstet Gynecol.* 1999;94:225–228.
30. Benster B, Carey A, Wadsworth F, et al. A double-blind placebo-controlled study to evaluate the effect of progestelle progesterone cream on postmenopausal women. *Menopause Int.* 2009;15:63–69.

31. Hofseth LJ, Raafat AM, Osuch JR, et al. Hormone replacement therapy with estrogen or estrogen plus medroxyprogesterone acetate is associated with increased epithelial proliferation in the normal postmenopausal breast. *J Clin Endocrinol Metab.* 1999;84:4559–4565.

32. Sartor O, Eastham JA. Progressive prostate cancer associated with use of megestrol acetate administered for control of hot flashes. *South Med J.* 1999;92:415–416.

33. Loprinzi CL, Sloan J, Stearns V, et al. Newer antidepressants and gabapentin for hot flashes: an individual patient pooled analysis. *J Clin Oncol.* 2009;27:2831–2837.

34. Loprinzi CL, Pisansky TM, Fonseca R, et al. Pilot evaluation of venlafaxine hydrochloride for the therapy of hot flashes in cancer survivors. *J Clin Oncol.* 1998;16:2377–2381.

35. *Physician's desk reference.* Editor Ed Series Montvale, NJ: Medical Economic Data; 1995.

36. Evans ML, Pritts E, Vittinghoff E, et al. Management of postmenopausal hot flushes with venlafaxine hydrochloride: a randomized, controlled trial. *Obstet Gynecol.* 2005;105:161–166.

37. Loprinzi CL, Barton DL, Sloan JA, et al. Newer antidepressants for hot flashes—should their efficacy still be up for debate? *Menopause.* 2009;16:184–187.

38. Loprinzi CL, Levitt R, Barton D, et al. Phase III comparison of depomedroxyprogesterone acetate to venlafaxine for managing hot flashes: North Central Cancer Treatment Group Trial N99C7. *J Clin Oncol.* 2006;24:1409–1414.

39. Deecher DC, Alfinito PD, Leventhal L, et al. Alleviation of thermoregulatory dysfunction with the new serotonin and norepinephrine reuptake inhibitor desvenlafaxine succinate in ovariectomized rodent models. *Endocrinology.* 2007;148:1376–1383.

40. Deecher DC, Beyer CE, Johnston G, et al. Desvenlafaxine succinate: a new serotonin and norepinephrine reuptake inhibitor. *J Pharmacol Exp Ther.* 2006;318:657–665.

41. Speroff L, Gass M, Constantine G, et al. Efficacy and tolerability of desvenlafaxine succinate treatment for menopausal vasomotor symptoms: a randomized controlled trial. *Obstet Gynecol.* 2008;111:77–87.

42. Archer DF, Seidman L, Constantine GD, et al. A double-blind, randomly assigned, placebo-controlled study of desvenlafaxine efficacy and safety for the treatment of vasomotor symptoms associated with menopause. *Am J Obstet Gynecol.* 2009;200:172 e1–17310.

43. Stearns V, Isaacs C, Rowland J, et al. A pilot trial assessing the efficacy of paroxetine hydrochloride (Paxil) in controlling hot flashes in breast cancer survivors. *Ann Oncol.* 2000;11:17–22.

44. Weitzner MA, Moncello J, Jacobsen PB, et al. A pilot trial of paroxetine for the treatment of hot flashes and associated symptoms in women with breast cancer. *J Pain Symptom Manage.* 2002;23:337–345.

45. Stearns V, Slack R, Greep N, et al. Paroxetine is an effective treatment for hot flashes: results from a prospective randomized clinical trial. *J Clin Oncol.* 2005;23:6919–6930.

46. Stearns V, Beebe KL, Iyengar M, et al. Paroxetine controlled release in the treatment of menopausal hot flashes: a randomized controlled trial. *JAMA.* 2003;289:2827–2834.

47. Loprinzi CL, Barton DL, Carpenter LA, et al. Pilot evaluation of paroxetine for treating hot flashes in men. *Mayo Clin Proc.* 2004;79:1247–1251.

48. Stearns V, Johnson MD, Rae JM, et al. Active tamoxifen metabolite plasma concentrations after coadministration of tamoxifen and the selective serotonin reuptake inhibitor paroxetine. *J Natl Cancer Inst.* 2003;95:1758–1764.

49. Loprinzi CL, Sloan JA, Perez EA, et al. Phase III evaluation of fluoxetine for treatment of hot flashes. *J Clin Oncol.* 2002;20:1578–1583.

50. Suvanto-Luukkonen E, Koivunen R, Sundstrom H, et al. Citalopram and fluoxetine in the treatment of postmenopausal symptoms: a prospective, randomized, 9-month, placebo-controlled, double-blind study. *Menopause.* 2005;12:18–26.

51. Lash TL, Pedersen L, Cronin-Fenton D, et al. Tamoxifen's protection against breast cancer recurrence is not reduced by concurrent use of the SSRI citalopram. *Br J Cancer.* 2008;99:616–621.

52. Barton DL, Loprinzi CL, Novotny P, et al. Pilot evaluation of citalopram for the relief of hot flashes. *J Support Oncol.* 2003;1:47–51.

53. Barton DL, Sloan JA, Stella PJ, et al. A phase III trial evaluating three doses of citalopram for hot flashes: NCCTG trial N05C9. *J Clin Oncol.* 2009;(suppl). Abstract 9538.

54 Caxrpenter LA, Loprinzi C, Flynn PJ, et al. *Pilot evaluation of citalopram for alleviation of hot flashes in women with inadequate hot flash control with venlafaxine.* Presented at: 2005 Annual Meeting of the American Society of Clinical Oncology. Abstract 8061.

55. Dehal SS, Kupfer D. CYP2D6 catalyzes tamoxifen 4-hydroxylation in human liver. *Cancer Res.* 1997;57:3402–3406.

56. Jin Y, Desta Z, Stearns V, et al. CYP2D6 genotype, antidepressant use, and tamoxifen metabolism during adjuvant breast cancer treatment. *J Natl Cancer Inst.* 2005;97:30–39.

57. Loprinzi C, Barton D, Sloan J, et al. Pilot evaluation of gabapentin for treating hot flashes. *Mayo Clin Proc.* 2002;77:1155–1163.

58. Guttuso Jr TJ. Gabapentin's effects on hot flashes and hypothermia. *Neurology.* 2000;54:2161–2163.

59. Loprinzi CL, Kugler JW, Barton DL, et al. Phase III trial of gabapentin alone or in conjunction with an antidepressant in the management of hot flashes in women who have inadequate control with an antidepressant alone: NCCTG N03C5. *J Clin Oncol.* 2007;25:308–312.

60. Guttuso Jr T, Kurlan R, McDermott MP, et al. Gabapentin's effects on hot flashes in postmenopausal women: a randomized controlled trial. *Obstet Gynecol.* 2003;101:337–345.

61. Pandya KJ, Morrow GR, Roscoe JA, et al. Gabapentin for hot flashes in 420 women with breast cancer: a randomised double-blind placebo-controlled trial. *Lancet.* 2005;366:818–824.

62. Reddy SY, Warner H, Guttuso Jr T, et al. Gabapentin, estrogen, and placebo for treating hot flushes: a randomized controlled trial. *Obstet Gynecol.* 2006;108:41–48.

63. Loprinzi CL, Dueck AC, Khoyratty BS, et al. A phase III randomized, double-blind, placebo-controlled trial of gabapentin in the management of hot flashes in men (N00CB). *Ann Oncol.* 2009;20:542–549.

64. Presant CA. Palliation of vasomotor instability (hot flashes) using pregabalin. *Community Oncol.* 2007;4:83–84.

65. Loprinzi CL, Qin R, Baclueva EP, et al. Phase III, randomized, double-blind, placebo-controlled evaluation of pregabalin for alleviating hot flashes, N07C1. *J Clin Oncol.* 2010;28:641–647.

66. Clayden JR, Bell JW, Pollard P. Menopausal flushing: double-blind trial of a non-hormonal medication. *Br Med J.* 1974;1:409–412.

67. Laufer LR, Erlik Y, Meldrum DR, et al. Effect of clonidine on hot flashes in postmenopausal women. *Obstet Gynecol.* 1982;60:583–586.

68. Schindler AE, Muller D, Keller E, et al. Studies with clonidine (Dixarit) in menopausal women. *Arch Gynecol.* 1979;227:341–347.

69. Freedman RR, Dinsay R. Clonidine raises the sweating threshold in symptomatic but not in asymptomatic postmenopausal women. *Fertil Steril.* 2000;74:20–23.

70. Goldberg RM, Loprinzi CL, O'Fallon JR, et al. Transdermal clonidine for ameliorating tamoxifen-induced hot flashes. *J Clin Oncol.* 1994;12:155–158.

71. Pandya KJ, Raubertas RF, Flynn PJ, et al. Oral clonidine in postmenopausal patients with breast cancer experiencing tamoxifen-induced hot flashes: a University of Rochester Cancer Center Community Clinical Oncology Program study. *Ann Intern Med.* 2000;132:788–793.

72. Loprinzi CL, Goldberg RM, O'Fallon JR, et al. Transdermal clonidine for ameliorating post-orchiectomy hot flashes. *J Urol.* 1994;151:634–636.

73. Lebherz TB, French L. Nonhormonal treatment of the menopausal syndrome. A double-blind evaluation of an autonomic system stabilizer. *Obstet Gynecol.* 1969;33:795–799.

74. Bergmans MG, Merkus JM, Corbey RS, et al. Effect of Bellergal Retard on climacteric complaints: a double-blind, placebo-controlled study. *Maturitas.* 1987;9:227–234.

75. Christy C. Vitamin E in menopause. *Am J Obstet Gynecol.* 1945;50:84–87.

76. Finkler R. The effect of vitamin E in the menopause. *J Clin Endocrinol Metab.* 1949;9:89–94.

77. Barton DL, Loprinzi CL, Quella SK, et al. Prospective evaluation of vitamin E for hot flashes in breast cancer survivors. *J Clin Oncol.* 1998;16:495–500.

78. Bardia A, Tleyjeh IM, Cerhan JR, et al. Efficacy of antioxidant supplementation in reducing primary cancer incidence and mortality: systematic review and meta-analysis. *Mayo Clin Proc.* 2008;83:23–34.

79. Wade C, Kronenberg F, Kelly A, et al. Hormone-modulating herbs: implications for women's health. *J Am Med Womens Assoc.* 1999;54:181–183.

80. Lieberman S. A review of the effectiveness of Cimicifuga racemosa (black cohosh) for the symptoms of menopause. *J Womens Health.* 1998;7:525–529.

81. Liske E, Wustenberg P. Therapy of climacteric complaints with cimicguga racemosa: herbal medicine with clinically proven evidence. *Menopause.* 1998;5:250.

82. Pepping J. Black cohosh: Cimicifuga racemosa. *Am J Health Syst Pharm.* 1999;56:1400–1402.

83. Pockaj BA, Loprinzi CL, Sloan JA, et al. Pilot evaluation of black cohosh for the treatment of hot flashes in women. *Cancer Invest.* 2004;22:515–521.

84. Newton KM, Reed SD, LaCroix AZ, et al. Treatment of vasomotor symptoms of menopause with black cohosh, multibotanicals, soy, hormone therapy, or placebo: a randomized trial. *Ann Intern Med.* 2006;145:869–879.

85. Reed SD, Newton KM, LaCroix AZ, et al. Vaginal, endometrial, and reproductive hormone findings: randomized, placebo-controlled trial of black cohosh, multibotanical herbs, and dietary soy for vasomotor symptoms: the Herbal Alternatives for Menopause (HALT) Study. *Menopause.* 2008;15:51–58.

86. Joy D, Joy J, Duane P. Black cohosh: a cause of abnormal postmenopausal liver function tests. *Climacteric.* 2008;11:84–88.

87. Haines CJ, Chung TK, Leung DH. A prospective study of the frequency of acute menopausal symptoms in Hong Kong Chinese women. *Maturitas.* 1994;18:175–181.

88. Lewis JE, Nickell LA, Thompson LU, et al. A randomized controlled trial of the effect of dietary soy and flaxseed muffins on quality of life and hot flashes during menopause. *Menopause.* 2006;13:631–642.

89. Adlercreutz H, Mousavi Y, Clark J, et al. Dietary phytoestrogens and cancer: in vitro and in vivo studies. *J Steroid Biochem Mol Biol.* 1992;41:331–337.

90. MacGregor CA, Canney PA, Patterson G, et al. A randomised double-blind controlled trial of oral soy supplements versus placebo for treatment of menopausal symptoms in patients with early breast cancer. *Eur J Cancer.* 2005;41:708–714.

91. Nikander E, Kilkkinen A, Metsa-Heikkila M, et al. A randomized placebo-controlled crossover trial with phytoestrogens in treatment of menopause in breast cancer patients. *Obstet Gynecol.* 2003;101:1213–1220.

92. Quella SK, Loprinzi CL, Barton DL, et al. Evaluation of soy phytoestrogens for the treatment of hot flashes in breast cancer survivors: a North Central Cancer Treatment Group Trial. [see comment]. *J Clin Oncol.* 2000;18:1068–1074.

93. Secreto G, Chiechi LM, Amadori A, et al. Soy isoflavones and melatonin for the relief of climacteric symptoms: a multicenter, double-blind, randomized study. *Maturitas.* 2004;47:11–20.

94. Messina MJ, Loprinzi CL. Soy for breast cancer survivors: a critical review of the literature. *J Nutr.* 2001;131(11 suppl):3095S–310108S.

95. Nelson HD, Vesco KK, Haney E, et al. Nonhormonal therapies for menopausal hot flashes: systematic review and meta-analysis. *JAMA.* 2006;295:2057–2071.

96. Tice JA, Ettinger B, Ensrud K, et al. Phytoestrogen supplements for the treatment of hot flashes: the Isoflavone Clover Extract (ICE) Study: a randomized controlled trial. *JAMA.* 2003;290:207–214.

97. Atkinson C, Warren RM, Sala E, et al. Red-clover-derived isoflavones and mammographic breast density: a double-blind, randomized, placebo-controlled trial [ISRCTN42940165]. *Breast Cancer Res.* 2004;6:R170–179.

98. Baber RJ, Templeman C, Morton T, et al. Randomized placebo-controlled trial of an isoflavone supplement and menopausal symptoms in women. *Climacteric.* 1999;2:85–92.

99. Chen J, Hui E, Ip T, et al. Dietary flaxseed enhances the inhibitory effect of tamoxifen on the growth of estrogen-dependent human breast cancer (mcf-7) in nude mice. *Clin Cancer Res.* 2004;10:7703–7711.

100. Pruthi S, Thompson SL, Novotny PJ, et al. Pilot evaluation of flaxseed for the management of hot flashes. *J Soc Integr Oncol.* 2007;5:106–112.

101. Conference NC. Acupuncture. *JAMA.* 1998;280:1518–1524.

102. Dong H, Ludicke F, Comte I, et al. An exploratory pilot study of acupuncture on the quality of life and reproductive hormone secretion in menopausal women. *J Altern Complement Med.* 2001;7:651–658.

103. Porzio G, Trapasso T, Martelli S, et al. Acupuncture in the treatment of menopause-related symptoms in women taking tamoxifen. *Tumori.* 2002;88:128–130.

104. Wyon Y, Lindgren R, Lundeberg T, et al. Effects of acupuncture on climacteric vasomotor symptoms, quality of life, and urinary excretion of neuropeptides among postmenopausal women. *Menopause.* 1995;2:3–12.

105. Vincent A, Barton DL, Mandrekar JN, et al. Acupuncture for hot flashes: a randomized, sham-controlled clinical study. *Menopause.* 2007;14:45–52.

106. Deng G, Vickers A, Yeung S, et al. Randomized, controlled trial of acupuncture for the treatment of hot flashes in breast cancer patients. *J Clin Oncol.* 2007;25:5584–5590.

107. Cho SH, Whang WW. Acupuncture for vasomotor menopausal symptoms: a systematic review. *Menopause.* 2009;16:1065–1073.

108. Lipov E, Lipov S, Stark JT. Stellate ganglion blockade provides relief from menopausal hot flashes: a case report series. *J Womens Health (Larchmt).* 2005;14:737–741.

109. Lipov EG, Joshi JR, Sanders S, et al. Effects of stellate-ganglion block on hot flushes and night awakenings in survivors of breast cancer: a pilot study. *Lancet Oncol.* 2008;9:523–532.

110. Pachman D, Barton D, Carns PE, et al. Pilot evaluation of a stellate ganglion block for the treatment of hot flashes. *Support Care Cancer.* 2010 May 23 [Epub ahead of print].

111. Lipov EG, Lipov S, Joshi JR, et al. Stellate ganglion block may relieve hot flashes by interrupting the sympathetic nervous system. *Med Hypotheses.* 2007;69:758–763.

112. Freedman RR, Woodward S. Behavioral treatment of menopausal hot flushes: evaluation by ambulatory monitoring. *Am J Obstet Gynecol.* 1992;167:436–439.

113. Irvin JH, Domar AD, Clark C, et al. The effects of relaxation response training on menopausal symptoms. *J Psychosom Obstet Gynaecol.* 1996;17:202–207.

114. Carson JW, Carson KM, Porter LS, et al. Yoga of Awareness program for menopausal symptoms in breast cancer survivors: results from a randomized trial. *Support Care Cancer.* 2009;17:1301–1309.

115. Bridge LR, Benson P, Pietroni PC, et al. Relaxation and imagery in the treatment of breast cancer. *BMJ.* 1988;297:1169–1172.

116. Gruber BL, Hersh SP, Hall NR, et al. Immunological responses of breast cancer patients to behavioral interventions. *Biofeedback Self Regul.* 1993;18:1–22.

117. Elkins G. Consulting about insomnia: hypnotherapy, sleep hygiene, and stimulus-control instructions. In: Matthews WJ, ed. *Current thinking and research in brief therapy.* New York: Brunner/Mazel; 1997.

118. Elkins G, Marcus J, Stearns V, et al. Randomized trial of a hypnosis intervention for treatment of hot flashes among breast cancer survivors. *J Clin Oncol.* 2008;26:5022–5026.

119. North American Menopause Society. Treatment of menopause-associated vasomotor symptoms: position statement of The North American Menopause Society. *Menopause.* 2004;11:11–33.

120. Loprinzi CL, Wolf SL. Hot flushes: mostly sex neutral? *Lancet Oncol.* 2010;11:107–108.

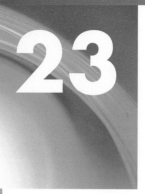

23 Xerostomia

Arjan Vissink, Fred K. L. Spijkervet, Siri Beier Jensen, and Michael T. Brennan

Worldwide, head and neck cancer affects many patients each year. Most of these patients undergo radiotherapy, which plays a pivotal role in the curative treatment of head and neck cancer, either as single-modality treatment or in combination with surgery and/or chemotherapy.[1] The overall 5-year survival for squamous cell carcinoma of the oral cavity is about 80% for the early stages of oral cancer and about 35% for locally advanced stages.

Despite the beneficial effects of radiotherapy in locoregional tumor control, the damage inflicted to normal tissues

surrounding the tumor may cause severe complications. Tissues at risk include the salivary glands, which generally are co-irradiated during the treatment of head and neck cancer. This chapter focuses on the clinical signs and symptoms and the clinical management of radiation-induced salivary gland injury, because resulting hyposalivation and xerostomia are among the most frequent and severe long-term side effects of radiotherapy in the head and neck region. Additionally, salivary gland hypofunction and xerostomia may be sequelae of other radiation regimens (e.g., iodine treatment of thyroid cancer, preconditioning total body irradiation in hematopoietic stem cell transplantation for the treatment of hematologic malignancies), although to a much lesser extent.[2,3]

SYMPTOMS OF SALIVARY GLAND HYPOFUNCTION

Dry mouth is rarely an isolated symptom. Usually, it is accompanied by other oral and systemic complaints. The oral symptoms primarily accrue from chronic salivary gland hypofunction that induces, over time, a decrease in the amount and composition of the oral fluids that bathe and protect the oral tissues and contribute to the alimentary and masticatory functions of saliva. Patients may complain of dryness that is present throughout their oral cavity or of dryness that is localized to select areas of the mouth (e.g., the lips, cheeks, tongue, palate, floor of the mouth and throat). Patients may also complain of difficulty with chewing, swallowing, and speaking. The general complaint and the severity of oral dryness are not always related to a decrease in the flow rate of saliva, however.[4] In about a quarter of the patients complaining of moderate to severe oral dryness, the mouth might even appear moist on clinical inspection.

Patients with dry mouth often complain of gastroesophageal reflux disease. Most patients carry bottles of water or other fluids with them at all times to aid speaking and swallowing and for their overall oral comfort. Patients also often have a bottle or glass of water beside their bed. The mucosa may be sensitive to spicy or coarse foods. This limits patients' enjoyment of meals and may compromise their nutrition or nutritional status.[5–7] Mild to modest oral pain is also common.

Overall, salivary gland hypofunction and xerostomia induced by radiation therapy may have a major deteriorating impact on patients' quality of life, which is most pronounced during a period of 6 months after irradiation, followed by some improvement up to 2 years after treatment.[8–10]

CLINICAL EXAMINATION

Most patients with advanced salivary gland hypofunction have obvious signs of mucosal dryness.[11,12] The lips often appear cracked, peeling, and atrophic (Fig. 23-1). The lips may even appear furrowed or lobulated, similar to dry soil in an arid climate. The buccal mucosa may be pale and corrugated in appearance (Figs. 23-2 and 23-3); the tongue may be smooth and reddened, with loss of some of the dorsal papillae (Fig. 23-4). Patients may report that their lips stick to their teeth. Others may report that their "tongue cleaves to the roof of their mouth." A marked increase in erosion and dental caries often occurs, particularly recurrent lesions and decay on root surfaces, and even cusp tip involvement

(Fig. 23-5). The decay may be progressive, even in the presence of vigilant oral hygiene (Fig. 23-6). With diminished salivary output, greater accumulations of food debris tend to occur in the interproximal regions, especially where recession has occurred.[13]

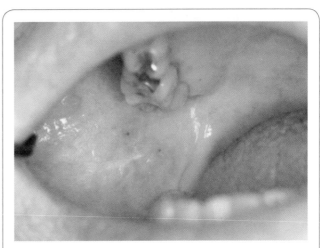

Fig. 23-3 Hyperkeratinized buccal mucosa and petechiae due to dryness-related mechanical irritation and trauma during speaking and eating.

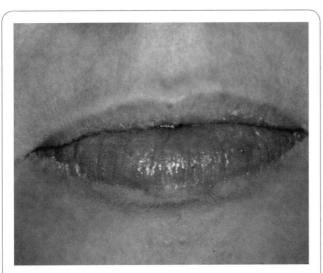

Fig. 23-1 Cracked lips.

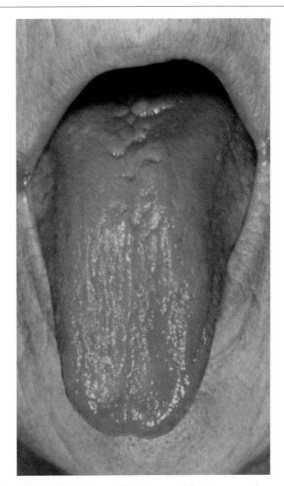

Fig. 23-4 Dry surface of the dorsum of the tongue and angular cheilitis.

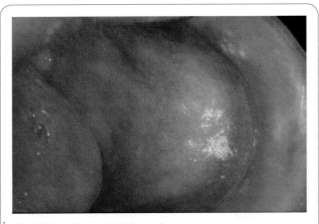

Fig. 23-2 Dry and pale buccal mucosa.

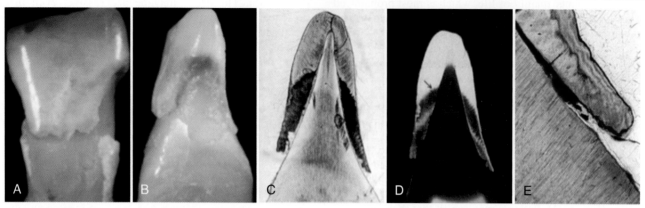

Fig. 23-5 Mandibular incisor extracted within 1 year after radiation therapy for head and neck cancer. **A** and **B,** Facial and distal surfaces shown macroscopically. **C,** Unstained section shows gap formation between dentin and remaining enamel. **D,** Microradiograph shows demineralization of the dentin core and remaining enamel. Spread of the most incisal enamel lesion *(arrow)* indicates that demineralization has started from the gap. **E,** Gram-stained section shows an accumulation of bacteria in the gap between the dentin and the enamel. *(Modified after Jensen SB, Dynesen AW. Histopathologic studies on teeth from irradiated patients [in Danish]. Danish Dent J 1998;102:408–414.)*

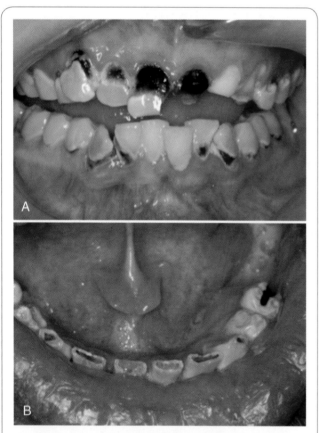

Fig. 23-6 Hyposalivation-related dental caries. **A,** Severe destruction of the cervical area of the teeth may lead to amputation of the crown. **B,** Involvement of the incisal edges of the teeth.

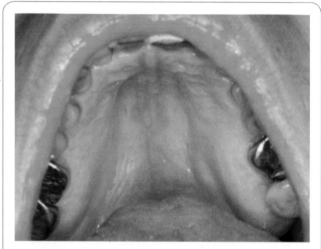

Fig. 23-7 Red erythematous patches on the oral mucosa are a sign of oral candidiasis.

Oropharyngeal candidiasis is frequently present. Because of the reduced salivary flow and the changed salivary composition, colonization defense in the oral cavity has changed. The change in colonization defense is accompanied by a higher level of colonization with *Candida* spp.

As a result, patients with xerostomia may easily develop a fungal infection of the oral mucosa. Oral candidiasis may appear as red, erythematous patches on the oral mucosa (e.g., beneath dentures), or it may appear as white, curd-like mucocutaneous lesions on any surface (thrush) (Figs. 23-7 and 23-8). Fungal lesions of the corners of the mouth (angular cheilitis; Fig. 23-9) are more likely to occur in patients with dry mouth who wear dentures and have a posterior bite collapse.[13]

It is important to assess whether saliva can be expressed from the main excretory ducts. Normally, saliva can be "milked" from each major gland by compression of the glands or by bimanual palpation, and by pushing the fluid contained within them to the gland orifices. The consistency of the secretions should be examined. Expressed saliva should be clear, watery, and copious. Viscous or scant secretions suggest chronically reduced function. In addition, the remaining secretory potential of the salivary glands has to be assessed. This can be done easily by applying a gustatory or tactile stimulant. If an

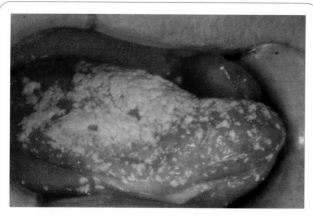

Fig. 23-8 White, curd-like mucocutaneous lesions on the tongue are a sign of oral candidiasis.

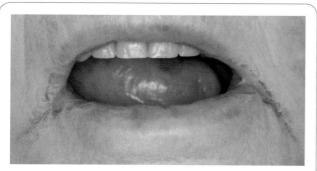

Fig. 23-9 Angular cheilitis.

increase in salivary flow is observed, it may be worthwhile to prescribe pharmacologic sialagogue, or to use gustatory or tactile stimulants. If no increase in salivary flow is observed, only frequent moistening of the mouth (e.g., with saliva substitutes) is an option.[13]

PREVENTION AND TREATMENT

CAN RADIATION INJURY TO SALIVARY GLAND TISSUE BE REDUCED?

In humans, depending on localization of radiation portals, a rapid decrease in the salivary flow rate is observed during the first week of radiotherapy; after this, a gradual decrease continues to less than 10% of the initial flow rate[14–16] (Fig. 23-10). Recently, it was shown that no threshold dose exists for reduced parotid gland function after radiotherapy, and that the median toxic dose (TD50) is probably equal to 40 Gy,[17] and thus is comparable to the TD50 (39 Gy) for submandibular gland function.[18] The lower TD50 for parotid gland function in some studies is probably due to few data in the critical dose range (30–40 Gy).

Strategies to reduce radiation injury to salivary gland tissue

At present, prevention of radiation damage to salivary glands is best accomplished by meticulous treatment planning and beam arrangement designed to spare as much of the parotid and submandibular glands as possible. A reasonable option to reduce radiation damage to salivary glands includes sparing one of the parotid and submandibular glands by using three-dimensional treatment planning and conformal dose-delivery techniques, in particular, intensity-modulated radiotherapy (IMRT).

IMRT allows more accurate delivery of a specific radiation dosage and dose distribution to the tumor and thereby brings about the possibility of better sparing of surrounding tissues (e.g., major salivary glands). Indeed, general consensus from randomized controlled trials and from cohort, case-control, and cross-sectional studies provides supporting evidence that parotid-sparing IMRT decreases the prevalence and severity of salivary gland hypofunction and xerostomia.[19] In addition, saliva secretion from spared salivary glands has the potential of increasing over time after therapy, unlike when similar tumors were treated by conventional radiotherapy.[8,10,20–28] As such,

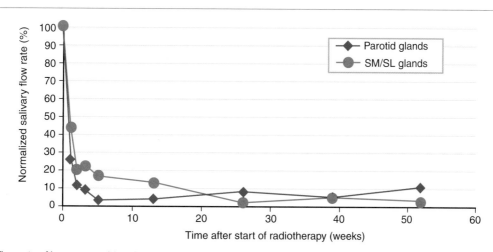

Fig. 23-10 Flow rate of human parotid and submandibular-sublingual (SM/SL) saliva as a function of time after the start of radiotherapy (conventional fractionation schedule: 2 Gy per day, 5 days per week, total dose 60–70 Gy). The parotid, submandibular, and sublingual glands are located in the treatment portal. Initial flow rates were set to 100%. *(Modified after Burlage FR, Coppes RP, Meertens H, et al. 2001.[16])*

potential benefits derived from IMRT for salivary gland function, xerostomia, and xerostomia-related quality of life are most pronounced late (≥6 months) after radiotherapy, and result in improvement in xerostomia-related quality of life over time, as assessed up to 2 years after therapy.[8–10,14,20,21,23–25,27–35] However, although IMRT, when compared with two-dimensional radiotherapy, results in significant reductions in patient- and observer-rated xerostomia, about 40% of patients still complain of xerostomia.[36]

SURGICAL TRANSFER OF THE SUBMANDIBULAR GLAND

In selected patients, a preventive strategy to reduce radiation-induced salivary gland hypofunction and xerostomia might be surgical transfer of one submandibular gland to the submental space not included in the radiation portal.[37–39] If all major salivary glands are to be included in the radiation portal, this approach may be of relevance in oropharyngeal and hypopharyngeal/laryngeal cancer patients before irradiation, and where the contralateral submandibular gland, or the side with clinically negative cervical lymph nodes in midline primaries, can be surgically translocated to the submental space. Furthermore, it should be ensured that the submental space can be kept excluded from the radiation portal. In patients who qualify for such an approach, surgical transfer of one submandibular gland has been shown to be superior to the administration of oral pilocarpine in the management of radiation-induced xerostomia.[40]

RADIOPROTECTORS

Direct radioprotection may be achieved with the use of amifostine, an oxygen radical scavenger, when systemically administered during radiation treatment.[41–43] Amifostine is preferentially accumulated in certain tissues, including the salivary glands, making these tissues less sensitive to radiation damage. The various cohort studies and randomized clinical trials performed thus far have revealed that amifostine has the potential to reduce complaints of xerostomia during and after radiation treatment. The results of the various studies included were not concurrent, however, in that some studies showed a significant benefit of amifostine treatment on patients' experience of acute and late xerostomia, although the effect may be minor,[44] and in other studies, the effect just reached significance.[41,42,45–47] In addition, other studies showed a beneficial effect only for some acute and late time points assessed.[48,49] Moreover, although many studies showed a beneficial effect on xerostomia, most studies failed to show that amifostine treatment resulted in less of a radiation-induced drop in salivary flow rate.[41,42,49–51] Furthermore, although amifostine has the potential to reduce xerostomia during and after radiation treatment, a significant proportion of patients continue to experience xerostomia. Finally, intravenous administration of amifostine is accompanied by many side effects, but recently, subcutaneous administration of amifostine has been shown to be a well-tolerated alternative.[52,53]

Tempol might serve as an alternative to amifostine. Tempol is a stable nitroxide that has been shown to be a radioprotector in vivo and in vitro.[54] Tempol is thought to provide radioprotection via several mechanisms, including oxidizing transition metals, mimicking superoxide dismutase activity, and scavenging free radicals. In experimental models, Tempol was shown to protect salivary glands against radiation damage and to reduce irradiation-induced salivary gland hypofunction while not protecting tumor tissue,[55–57] which has been reported as a potentially undesirable effect of amifostine.[58] Further development and consideration of Tempol for human clinical trials are indicated at the current time point.

PILOCARPINE DURING RADIOTHERAPY

Pilocarpine is a cholinergic parasympathomimetic agent with mainly nonselective muscarinic action but with mild beta-adrenergic activity. Pilocarpine has been shown to enhance salivary secretion by stimulating muscarinic receptors on the surfaces of salivary gland cells, thereby reducing the sensation of dry mouth in patients in whom some functional salivary gland tissue has been preserved.[59]

Administration of pilocarpine or pure cholinergic sialagogues to stimulate any residual function of the salivary gland post radiotherapy is worthwhile to a limited extent (see section on management of radiation-induced salivary gland hypofunction), as the functional gain ceases as soon as administration of the sialagogue is stopped.[60–62] Evidence suggests that a more persistent effect can be observed when oral pilocarpine HCl is administered before radiotherapy and is continued during radiotherapy, although not all studies have proved such a sparing effect on salivary gland function.

Several studies have reported no statistically significant differences between patients treated with placebo and those treated with oral pilocarpine HCl during radiotherapy with regard to xerostomia.[63–69] A problem associated with most of these studies is that a wide range of cumulative doses was applied, and thus the potentially beneficial effects of pilocarpine could be confounded (i.e., patients were subjected to a low cumulative dose [radiation effects are reversible], and patients were subjected to a very high cumulative dose [radiation damage is so severe that no sparing effect of pilocarpine is to be expected]). In one large study, unstimulated whole salivary flow rates were significantly increased at 3 and 6 months in patients who received pilocarpine HCl, although no significant differences in xerostomia were reported.[68] On the other hand, other studies found no improvement in salivary gland function (unstimulated/stimulated whole salivary flow rates and scintigraphy) in patients taking pilocarpine HCl during radiotherapy.[63,67] In addition, no significant differences were found between patients who had received oral pilocarpine HCl and a placebo group with regard to submandibular/sublingual flow rates.[69] It is important to note that the submandibular glands in this study were removed as a part of the head and neck dissection procedure or had been exposed to high cumulative doses (>60 Gy). However, results from the latter study indicate that the efficacy of oral pilocarpine HCl was dependent on the dose distributed to the parotid glands (i.e., in patients in whom the mean parotid dose exceeded 40 Gy, pilocarpine HCl significantly spared parotid gland function flow and reduced xerostomia, which became particularly significant after 12 months).[69] The adverse effects reported in the various studies were generally mild to moderate; this also favors oral pilocarpine as an agent to be considered when the goal of treatment is reduction of radiation damage to salivary gland tissue.

The protective effects of pilocarpine HCl on salivary gland function are not fully understood. One theory suggests that pilocarpine HCl acts by causing depletion of secretory granules in serous cells, thereby reducing the extent of radiation-induced salivary gland damage.[70] Others suggest that pilocarpine exerts stimulatory actions on minor salivary glands outside the radiation field.[71,72]

OTHER PREVENTIVE AGENTS

Other preventive agents include pretreatment or concurrent radiotherapy administration of insulin-like growth factor 1 (IGF-1) and keratinocyte growth factor (KGF). Both agents have been studied in mice. The rationale for the use of IGF-1 is to suppress apoptosis, as p53-dependent apoptosis has been proposed to contribute to radiation-induced salivary gland dysfunction.[73] p53 −/− mice do not induce apoptosis and preserve salivary function after treatment with therapeutic doses of radiation.[73] This study suggests that the p53 small molecule inhibitor, pifithrin-α, could be temporarily used to spare the salivary glands from radiation-induced apoptosis. Subcutaneous administration of KGF, before or directly after irradiation, also reduced radiation-induced hyposalivation.[75] When used before radiation, KGF induced salivary gland stem/progenitor cell proliferation, increasing the stem and progenitor cell pool. This did not change the relative radiation sensitivity of these cells, but, as a consequence, absolute higher numbers of stem/progenitor cells and acinar cells survived after radiation.

MANAGEMENT OF RADIATION-INDUCED SALIVARY GLAND DYSFUNCTION

STIMULATION OF RESIDUAL FUNCTION

When radiation damage has occurred and patients report xerostomia, the next step is to apply a salivary stimulant—a gustatory or tactile stimulant (Table 23-1) or a pharmacologic sialagogue (Table 23-2). Irradiated areas that are still able to produce some saliva and untreated portions of salivary glands are the targets of these sialagogues.

Table 23-1 Gustatory and tactile sialagogues*

Acid-tasting substances
   Acidic (sugar-free) sweets
   Acidic or effervescent drinks (lemon juice, citric acid, buttermilk)
   Citric acid crystals
   Cotton-wool gauze soaked in a citric acid and glycerin solution
   Lemon pastilles
   Lemon slices
   Vitamin C tablets
Miscellaneous substances
   Dried pieces of reed root (Calami rhizoma)
   Sugar-free chewing gum
   Sugar-free sweets
   Vegetables or fruits

*Not all substances are recommended in dentulous patients, as acidic products may induce demineralization of dental hard tissues.

Table 23-2 Pharmacologic sialagogues

Anetholetrithione

Benzapyrone

Bethanechol chloride

Carbachol

Cevimeline*

Folia Jaborandi and Tinctura Jaborandi

Neostigmine, neostigmine bromide, pyridostigmine bromide, destigmine bromide

Nicotinamide and nicotine acid

Pilocarpine hydrochloride,* pilocarpine nitrate

Potassium iodide

Trithioparamethoxyphenylpropene

*Only these agents have been approved for relief of xerostomia in humans after having undergone substantial controlled clinical testing.

With regard to gustatory and tactile stimulation, no general consensus can be extracted from the literature, because addressed topics in various studies are sporadic within the field of salivary gland hypofunction and xerostomia as sequelae of cancer therapies. Small studies indicated that sucking on acidic candy and salivary-stimulating lozenges led to an increase in whole saliva secretion and improvement in oral dryness,[76,77] respectively, whereas an oral antimicrobial lozenge administered to reduce acute radiation toxicity (i.e., mucositis) did not influence xerostomia during radiation treatment.

With regard to pharmacologic substances, data from randomized clinical trials and from before and after studies indicate that oral administration of pilocarpine HCl (most often, a dose of 5 mg 3 or 4 times daily is used) is effective in the treatment of radiation-induced xerostomia in patients with head and neck cancer.[61,62,72,78–80] Approximately 50% of patients will benefit from oral pilocarpine treatment post radiotherapy.[61,62,79] Optimum results were obtained with continuous treatment for longer than 8 weeks with doses higher than 2.5 mg 3 times a day.[61,62,79] Also, topical administration of pilocarpine HCl in the form of a candy-like pastille[81] or a lozenge[82] was shown to be more effective than placebo treatment in alleviating symptoms of post-radiation xerostomia. In several studies, improvement in oral dryness did not correlate with improvements in whole and/or parotid salivary flow rates,[61,72,81] however, which could be ascribed to a significant stimulatory action of pilocarpine HCl on minor (predominantly mucous) salivary glands and/or better preserved functional capacity of these glands.

Adverse effects were common in relation to treatment with pilocarpine, but were generally reported as mild or of moderate severity.[61,62,79] Nevertheless, some patients had to withdraw from trials because of adverse effects (6%–15%), and the adverse effects, but not the response rates, were dose dependent.[61,62] The most common adverse effects at a standard dose of 5 mg 3 times daily included sweating (15%–55%), headache (15%), urinary frequency (14%), vasodilation (12%), dizziness (10%), dyspepsia (10%), lacrimation (10%), and nausea (6%–20%).[61,62,79,80]

Although often not very prominent, the adverse effects of pilocarpine are of clinical relevance in that observed improvement in radiation-induced xerostomia and salivary gland function declines after cessation of treatment with pilocarpine.[61,62] Consequently, pilocarpine has to be administered on a lifelong basis, which can be problematic because of its adverse effects. Thus, oral pilocarpine HCl should be administered with caution, and close medical monitoring should be provided to patients with cardiovascular diseases such as hypertension and arrhythmia, as well as to those with pulmonary diseases such as asthma, chronic bronchitis, or chronic obstructive pulmonary disease. Contraindications for pilocarpine HCl include narrow-angle glaucoma, uncontrolled asthma, and gastric ulcer.[83,84] The interaction of pilocarpine HCl with other medications, especially with agents with parasympathetic and beta-adrenergic effects, may preclude its use.

As an alternative for pilocarpine, cevimeline HCl can be used. Cevimeline HCl is a relatively new cholinergic agonist with high affinity for muscarinic M3 receptors, which are present predominantly on salivary gland cells. It has minimal adverse effects on organs such as heart and lungs. It has been shown that cevimeline HCl was generally well tolerated, and oral administration of 30 to 45 mg 3 times daily for 52 weeks improved xerostomia (response rate of 59% at the final visit)[85] and significantly increased unstimulated, but not stimulated, whole salivary flow rate.[85] About 70% experienced adverse effects, most of which were mild to moderate.[86] The most common adverse effect was sweating, followed by dyspepsia.

Acupuncture

Stimulation of residual salivary secretory capacity by acupuncture has shown promising results in head and neck radiotherapy patients.[87,88] The effects of acupuncture treatment on secretion of whole saliva and related symptoms are sustained for at least 6 months,[88–90] and additional acupuncture therapy can maintain this improvement for up to 3 years.[89] Moreover, Deng et al.[91] showed that acupuncture was associated with neuronal activation that was absent during sham acupuncture.

Electrostimulation

Augmentation of salivary reflexes through the application of an electrical stimulus to the oral mucosa has been shown to result in a significant increase in salivary flow and to alleviate xerostomia-related symptoms.[92] In a sham-controlled, double-blind, multicenter study, a stimulating device mounted on an individualized intraoral removable appliance caused a significant decrease in oral dryness (as measured with a built-in wetness sensor) and had beneficial effects on the patients' subjective condition.[93]

Hyperbaric oxygen treatment

Studies suggest that irradiated head and neck cancer patients receiving hyperbaric oxygen treatment as part of the treatment/prevention of osteoradionecrosis have a decrease in xerostomia following hyperbaric oxygen treatment.[94–96] Because these studies show methodologic limitations, additional studies are

needed to confirm whether the lesser degree of xerostomia experienced by patients can be (completely) attributed to hyperbaric oxygen treatment or whether other phenomena play a significant role.

Insufficient effect of stimulation

When stimulation of residual secretion is insufficient to relieve patients' complaints, the clinician is left with a purely *symptomatic approach*. The most common approach is the frequent use of water. A critical disadvantage of moistening oral surfaces with water and mouthwashes to relieve xerostomia is the necessity for frequent application because of poor retention properties.[97] For this reason, complex saliva substitutes have been developed, which contain agents that impart viscosity and keep soft tissues moist. These substitutes may be based on carboxymethylcellulose (CMC),[98] mucin,[99] or xanthan gum.[100] Mucin-containing and xanthan gum–containing saliva substitutes are usually preferred over CMC-containing substitutes, both by patients with Sjögren's syndrome and by those with radiation-induced xerostomia.[100–103] When compared with CMC substitutes, mucin-containing and xanthan gum–containing substitutes have superior rheologic and wetting properties.[100,104,105] In addition to the more "liquid-like" saliva substitutes, additional "gel-like" saliva substitutes have been developed, of which the polyglycerylmethacrylate-based substitute holds promise,[106,107] particularly when used at night, and when daily activities are performed at a low level.

Although it has proved effective in many studies, patients often object to the taste or inconvenience of using artificial saliva[100] and frequently return to the use of water. Furthermore, the success of artificial saliva usage is strictly dependent on adequate instructions, and great variation in the ability to tolerate artificial salivas has been noted among patients.[100] Because of this variability, it is worthwhile to use different types of saliva substitutes in a particular patient, so the most effective substitute for that patient can be selected.[100,108,109] Based on the literature, the following recommendations for the treatment of hyposalivation have been proposed[106,110]:

- *Severe hyposalivation:* A saliva substitute with gel-like properties should be used during the night, and when daily activities are at a low level. During the day, a saliva substitute with properties resembling the viscoelasticity of natural saliva, such as substitutes that have xanthan gum and mucin (particularly bovine submandibular mucin) as a base, should be applied.
- *Moderate hyposalivation:* If gustatory, tactile, or pharmacologic stimulation of residual salivary secretion does not provide sufficient amelioration, saliva substitutes with rather low viscoelasticity, such as those that have carboxymethylcellulose, hydroxypropylmethylcellulose, mucin (porcine gastric mucin), or low concentrations of xanthan gum as a base, are indicated. During the night or other periods of severe oral dryness, the application of a gel is helpful.
- *Slight hyposalivation:* Gustatory, tactile, or pharmacologic stimulation of residual secretion is the treatment of choice. Little amelioration is to be expected from the use of saliva substitutes.

FUTURE MANAGEMENT STRATEGIES FOR RADIATION-DAMAGED SALIVARY GLANDS

May new radiation techniques result in less xerostomia?

A prerequisite for preventing xerostomia with new radiation-delivery techniques such as IMRT is the existence of dose-volume effect relationships between relevant organs at risk and xerostomia. Numerous studies have showed a significant relationship between mean dose in the parotid gland and the probability of a reduction in parotid flow.[17,18,29,111-114] Limited clinical data exist regarding the dose to the submandibular glands and submandibular flow.[18,33] Although most studies focus on salivary flow, other endpoints related to salivary function, such as patient-rated xerostomia and physician-rated RTOG (Radiation Therapy Oncology Group) xerostomia, are probably of even greater clinical relevance. The problem with these clinical endpoints is that the incidence at which they occur depends not only on dose distribution to the parotid glands, but on that to other major and minor salivary glands as well.[8,114a]

Is gene therapy the answer?

No single therapeutic solution has been identified for radiation-induced salivary gland hypofunction, and, to date, no treatment has resulted in restoration of function lost during irradiation. However, in some patients, gene therapy might provide a therapeutic option for this enigmatic oral problem. The ultimate gene transfer strategy as adopted by Baum et al.[115] included four key elements: (1) a hypothesis as to how a gene transfer event could elicit fluid secretion from surviving (primarily duct) epithelial cells in an irradiated salivary gland, (2) an appropriate gene to transfer that would facilitate the hypothesized fluid secretion mechanism, (3) a safe and reliable vector to carry the selected gene into the salivary glands, and (4) a convenient way to administer the vector to the salivary glands.[116] Because few acinar cells survive radiation, little to no primary fluid secretion remains. Furthermore, duct cells are considered relatively water impermeable because they lack a water channel in their plasma membranes.

Theoretically, for fluid movement to occur across a duct cell, the cell must have generated an osmotic gradient (lumen > interstitium) and must have facilitated a water permeability pathway (water channel) within the plasma membrane to allow water to follow the osmotic gradient. Delporte et al.[116] reasoned that duct cells could generate such an osmotic gradient in the absence of significant primary fluid secretion, but that they had no water permeability pathway in their luminal plasma membranes. However, surviving duct cells could serve as water-secreting cells if a pathway for water transport was inserted into the duct cell membranes.

The first water channel protein that was characterized and cloned was human aquaporin-1 (hAQP1).[117] On the basis of its promising properties, a recombinant serotype 5 adenoviral vector encoding hAQP1, that is, AdhAQP1, was constructed.[116] Although this vector can transfer genes to target cells, it cannot replicate. The vector is delivered to salivary glands via intraductal cannulation through the orifice of the main excretory duct, which is accessible through the mouth. Currently, a phase I study is under way in individuals with salivary gland hypofunction to see whether hAQP1 gene transfer is safe and effective in humans (http://www.clinical-trials.gov/ct/show/NCT00372320).

Is stem cell therapy a reasonable approach?

In general, radiation-induced organ failure is caused mainly by impaired replacement of differentiated functional cells resulting from sterilization of their progenitor/stem cells. Tissue damage due to radiotherapy, therefore, is, in part, a function of cell turnover rates. Cells with a high turnover rate respond earlier to radiation damage than those with lower rates. In this regard, as noted earlier, the high radiosensitivity of salivary glands is an anomaly, because their secretory cells have a low turnover rate of ≈60 days. It is the remaining, viable stem cells that determine the capacity for regeneration and hence the extent of late radiation injury.[118]

It is important to note that salivary glands exhibit a substantial regenerative capacity. The repopulation of acinar cells probably originates in undamaged stem/progenitor cells. Acinar cells also "disappear" following irradiation. Here, recovery is dependent on the radiation dose and on the number of remaining viable stem cells.[119] Enhanced proliferation of surviving stem/progenitor cells, as observed, for example, after prophylactic pilocarpine treatment,[69,120,121] aids recovery and reduces radiation-induced hyposalivation. These findings indicate that salivary glands can undergo renewal if enough stem cells survive the injury caused by radiation. If not enough stem cells survive, transplantation of undamaged (donor) stem cells could enable the gland to regenerate. Often, after irradiation, ductal cells proliferate and duct compartments remain relatively intact. They could serve as a natural engraftment place for transplanted cells. This makes the salivary gland an ideal organ for experimental stem cell therapy.

EPILOGUE

Dry mouth (xerostomia) and salivary gland hypofunction are common complaints among patients treated with cancer therapy for head and neck tumors. The subjective complaint of dry mouth can have a significant impact on quality of life, and numerous oral problems resulting from decreased salivary function can occur. Early recognition of these oral manifestations (e.g., dental caries, fungal infection) is important to minimize their impact. Various prevention and management strategies for xerostomia have been evaluated. Although many pharmacologic approaches have shown a positive response in the treatment of xerostomia, the benefits are mostly temporary, and xerostomia returns without long-term use. In general, a combination of treatment strategies is necessary for long-term management. Future strategies may include gene therapy or stem cell therapy to manage this often irreversible cancer therapy side effect.

REFERENCES

1. Hunter KD, Parkinson EK, Harrison PR. Profiling early head and neck cancer. *Nat Rev Cancer*. 2005;5:127–135.

2. Dahllöf G, Bågesund M, Ringdén O. Impact of conditioning regimens on salivary function, caries-associated microorganisms and dental caries in children after bone marrow transplantation: a 4-year longitudinal study. *Bone Marrow Transplant*. 1997;20:479–483.

3. Hyer S, Kong A, Pratt B, et al. Salivary gland toxicity after radioiodine therapy for thyroid cancer. *Clin Oncol (R Coll Radiol)*. 2007;19:83–86.

4. Fox PC, Busch KA, Baum BJ. Subjective reports of xerostomia and objective measures of salivary gland performance. *J Am Dent Assoc*. 1987;115:581–584.

5. Dormenval V, Budtz-Jørgensen E, Mojon P, et al. Associations between malnutrition, poor general health and oral dryness in hospitalized elderly patients. *Age Ageing*. 1998;27:123–128.

6. Hay KD, Morton RP, Wall CR. Quality of life and nutritional studies in Sjogren's syndrome patients with xerostomia. *N Z Dent J*. 2001;97:128–131.

7. Walls AW, Steele JG. The relationship between oral health and nutrition in older people. *Mech Ageing Dev*. 2004;125:853–857.

8. Eisbruch A, Kim HM, Terrell JE, et al. Xerostomia and its predictors following parotid-sparing irradiation of head-and-neck cancer. *Int J Radiat Oncol Biol Phys*. 2001;50:695–704.

9. Jabbari S, Kim HM, Feng M, et al. Matched case-control study of quality of life and xerostomia after intensity-modulated radiotherapy or standard radiotherapy for head-and-neck cancer: initial report. *Int J Radiat Oncol Biol Phys*. 2005;63:725–731.

10. Pow EH, Kwong DL, McMillan AS, et al. Xerostomia and quality of life after intensity-modulated radiotherapy vs. conventional radiotherapy for early-stage nasopharyngeal carcinoma: initial report on a randomized controlled clinical trial. *Int J Radiat Oncol Biol Phys*. 2006;66:981–991.

11. Fox PC, van der Ven PF, Sonies BC, et al. Xerostomia: evaluation of a symptom with increasing significance. *J Am Dent Assoc*. 1985;110:519–525.

12. Guggenheimer J, Moore PA. Xerostomia: etiology, recognition and treatment. *J Am Dent Assoc*. 2003;134:61–69.

13. Sreebny LM, Vissink A. *Dry mouth. The malevolent symptom: a clinical guide*. Ames, Iowa: Wiley-Blackwell; 2010.

14. Liu RP, Fleming TJ, Toth BB, et al. Salivary flow rates in patients with head and neck cancer 0.5 to 25 years after radiotherapy. *Oral Surg Oral Med Oral Pathol*. 1990;70:724–729.

15. Valdez IH, Wolff A, Atkinson JC, et al. Use of pilocarpine during head and neck radiation therapy to reduce xerostomia and salivary dysfunction. *Cancer*. 1993;71:1848–1851.

16. Burlage FR, Coppes RP, Meertens H, et al. Parotid and submandibular/sublingual flow during high dose radiotherapy. *Radiother Oncol*. 2001;61:271–274.

17. Dijkema T, Raaijmakers CPJ, Ten Haken RK, et al. Parotid gland function after radiotherapy: the combined Michigan and Utrecht experience. *Int J Radiat Oncol Biol Phys*. 2010;78:449–453.

18. Murdoch-Kinch CA, Kim HM, Vineberg KA, et al. Dose-effect relationship for the submandibular salivary glands and implications for their sparing by intensity modulated radiotherapy. *Int J Radiat Oncol Biol Phys*. 2008;72:373–382.

19. Jensen SB, Pedersen AML, Vissink A, et al. A systematic review of salivary gland hypofunction and xerostomia induced by cancer therapies: prevalence, severity and impact on quality of life. *Support Care Cancer*. 2010;18:1039–1060.

20. Lin A, Kim HM, Terrell JE, et al. Quality of life after parotid-sparing IMRT for head-and-neck cancer: a prospective longitudinal study. *Int J Radiat Oncol Biol Phys*. 2003;57:61–70.

21. Blanco AI, Chao KS, El Naqa I, et al. Dose-volume modeling of salivary function in patients with head-and-neck cancer receiving radiotherapy. *Int J Radiat Oncol Biol Phys*. 2005;62:1055–1069.

22. Saarilahti K, Kouri M, Collan J, et al. Intensity modulated radiotherapy for head and neck cancer: evidence for preserved salivary gland function. *Radiother Oncol*. 2005;74:251–258.

23. de Arruda FF, Puri DR, Zhung J, et al. Intensity-modulated radiation therapy for the treatment of oropharyngeal carcinoma: the Memorial Sloan-Kettering Cancer Center experience. *Int J Radiat Oncol Biol Phys*. 2006;64:363–373.

24. Hsiung CY, Ting HM, Huang HY, et al. Parotid-sparing intensity-modulated radiotherapy (IMRT) for nasopharyngeal carcinoma: preserved parotid function after IMRT on quantitative salivary scintigraphy, and comparison with historical data after conventional radiotherapy. *Int J Radiat Oncol Biol Phys*. 2006;66:454–461.

25. Liu WS, Kuo HC, Lin JC, et al. Assessment of salivary function change in nasopharyngeal carcinoma treated by parotid-sparing radiotherapy. *Cancer J*. 2006;12:494–500.

26. Liu WS, Lee SP, Lee JK, et al. Factors influencing the parotid function in nasopharyngeal carcinoma treated with parotid-sparing radiotherapy. *Jpn J Clin Oncol*. 2006;36:626–631.

27. Li Y, Taylor JM, Ten Haken RK, et al. The impact of dose on parotid salivary recovery in head and neck cancer patients treated with radiation therapy. *Int J Radiat Oncol Biol Phys*. 2007;67:660–669.

28. Kam MK, Leung SF, Zee B, et al. Prospective randomized study of intensity-modulated radiotherapy on salivary gland function in early-stage nasopharyngeal carcinoma patients. *J Clin Oncol*. 2007;25:4873–4879.

29. Eisbruch A, Ten Haken RK, Kim HM, et al. Dose, volume and function relationships in parotid salivary glands following conformal and intensity-modulated irradiation of head and neck cancer. *Int J Radiat Oncol Biol Phys*. 1999;45:577–587.

30. Sultanem K, Shu HK, Xia P, et al. Three-dimensional intensity-modulated radiotherapy in the treatment of nasopharyngeal carcinoma: the University of California-San Francisco experience. *Int J Radiat Oncol Biol Phys*. 2000;48:711–722.

31. Chao KS, Deasy JO, Markman J, et al. A prospective study of salivary function sparing in patients with head-and-neck cancers receiving intensity-modulated or three-dimensional radiation therapy: initial results. *Int J Radiat Oncol Biol Phys*. 2001;49:907–916.

32. Chao KS, Majhail N, Huang CJ, et al. Intensity-modulated radiation therapy reduces late salivary toxicity without compromising tumor control in patients with oropharyngeal carcinoma: a comparison with conventional techniques. *Radiother Oncol*. 2001;61:275–280.

33. Kam MK, Teo PM, Chau RM, et al. Treatment of nasopharyngeal carcinoma with intensity-modulated radiotherapy: the Hong Kong experience. *Int J Radiat Oncol Biol Phys*. 2004;60:1440–1450.

34. Anand AK, Chaudhoory AR, Shukla A, et al. Favourable impact of intensity-modulated radiation therapy on chronic dysphagia in patients with head and neck cancer. *Br J Radiol*. 2008;81:865–871.

35. Seung S, Bae J, Solhjem M, et al. Intensity-modulated radiotherapy for head-and-neck cancer in the community setting. *Int J Radiat Oncol Biol Phys*. 2008;72:1075–1081.

36. Vergeer MR, Doornaert PA, Rietveld DH, et al. Intensity-modulated radiotherapy reduces radiation-induced morbidity and improves health-related quality of life: results of a nonrandomized prospective study using a standardized follow-up program. *Int J Radiat Oncol Biol Phys*. 2009;74:1–8.

37. Jha N, Seikaly H, Harris J, et al. Prevention of radiation induced xerostomia by surgical transfer of submandibular salivary gland into the submental space. *Radiother Oncol*. 2003;66:283–289.

38. Seikaly H, Jha N, Harris JR, et al. Long-term outcomes of submandibular gland transfer for prevention of postradiation xerostomia. *Arch Otolaryngol Head Neck Surg*. 2004;130:956–961.

39. Al-Qahtani K, Hier MP, Sultanum K, et al. The role of submandibular salivary gland transfer in preventing xerostomia in the chemoradiotherapy patient. *Oral Surg Oral Med Oral Pathol Oral Radiol Endod*. 2006;101:753–756.

40. Jha N, Seikaly H, Harris J, et al. *Head Neck*. 2009;31:234–243.

41. Brizel DM, Wasserman TH, Henke M, et al. Phase III randomized trial of amifostine as a radioprotector in head and neck cancer. *J Clin Oncol*. 2000;18:3339–3345.

42. Wasserman TH, Brizel DM, Henke M, et al. Influence of intravenous amifostine on xerostomia, tumor control, and survival after radiotherapy for head-and-neck cancer: 2-year follow-up of a prospective, randomized, phase III trial. *Int J Radiat Oncol Biol Phys*. 2005;63:985–990.

43. Hensley ML, Hagerty KL, Kewalramani T, et al. American Society of Clinical Oncology 2008 clinical practice guideline update: use of chemotherapy and radiation therapy protectants. *J Clin Oncol*. 2009;27:127–145.

44. Vacha P, Fehlauer F, Mahlmann B, et al. Randomized phase III trial of postoperative radiochemotherapy ± amifostine in head and neck cancer. Is there evidence for radioprotection? *Strahlenther Onkol*. 2003;179:385–389.

45. Antonadou D, Pepelassi M, Synodinou M, et al. Prophylactic use of amifostine to prevent radiochemotherapy-induced mucositis and xerostomia in head-and-neck cancer. *Int J Radiat Oncol Biol Phys*. 2002;52:739–747.

46. Karacetin D, Yucel B, Leblebicioglu B, et al. A randomized trial of amifostine as radioprotector in the radiotherapy of head and neck cancer. *J BUON*. 2004;9:23–26.

47. Buntzel J, Glatzel M, Mucke R, et al. Influence of amifostine on late radiation- toxicity in head and neck cancer—a follow-up study. *Anticancer Res*. 2007;27:1953–1956.

48. Kouloulias VE, Kouvaris JR, Kokakis JD, et al. Impact on cytoprotective efficacy of intermediate interval between amifostine administration and

radiotherapy: a retrospective analysis. *Int J Radiat Oncol Biol Phys.* 2004;59:1148–1156.

49. Buentzel J, Micke O, Adamietz IA, et al. Intravenous amifostine during chemoradiotherapy for head-and-neck cancer: a randomized placebo-controlled phase III study. *Int J Radiat Oncol Biol Phys.* 2006;64:684–691.

50. Rudat V, Meyer J, Momm F, et al. Protective effect of amifostine on dental health after radiotherapy of the head and neck. *Int J Radiat Oncol Biol Phys.* 2000;48:1339–1343.

51. Veerasarn V, Phromratanapongse P, Suntornpong N, et al. Effect of amifostine to prevent radiotherapy-induced acute and late toxicity in head and neck cancer patients who had normal or mild impaired salivary gland function. *J Med Assoc Thai.* 2006;89:2056–2067.

52. Ozsahin M, Betz M, Matzinger O, et al. Feasibility and efficacy of subcutaneous amifostine therapy in patients with head and neck cancer treated with curative accelerated concomitant-boost radiation therapy. *Arch Otolaryngol Head Neck Surg.* 2006;132:141–145.

53. Law A, Kennedy T, Pellitteri P, et al. Efficacy and safety of subcutaneous amifostine in minimizing radiation-induced toxicities in patients receiving combined-modality treatment for squamous cell carcinoma of the head and neck. *Int J Radiat Oncol Biol Phys.* 2007;69:1361–1368.

54. Soule BP, Hyodo F, Matsumoto K, et al. The chemistry and biology of nitroxide compounds. *Free Radic Biol Med.* 2007;42:1632–1650.

55. Vitolo JM, Cotrim AP, Sowers AL, et al. The stable nitroxide tempol facilitates salivary gland protection during head and neck irradiation in a mouse model. *Clin Cancer Res.* 2004;10:1807–1812.

56. Cotrim AP, Sowers AL, Lodde BM, et al. Kinetics of tempol for prevention of xerostomia following head and neck irradiation in a mouse model. *Clin Cancer Res.* 2005;11:7564–7568.

57. Cotrim AP, Hyodo F, Matsumoto K, et al. Differential radiation protection of salivary glands versus tumor by Tempol with accompanying tissue assessment of Tempol by magnetic resonance imaging. *Clin Cancer Res.* 2007;13:4928–4933.

58. Brizel DM, Overgaard J. Does amifostine have a role in chemoradiation treatment? Lancet Oncol. 2003;4:378–381.

59. Fox PC, Atkinson JC, Macynski AA, et al. Pilocarpine treatment of salivary gland hypofunction and dry mouth (xerostomia). Arch Intern Med. 1991;151:1149–1152.

60. Greenspan D, Daniels TE. Effectiveness of pilocarpine in postradiation xerostomia. Cancer. 1987;59:1123–1125.

61. Johnson JT, Ferretti GA, Nethery WJ, et al. Oral pilocarpine for post-irradiation xerostomia in patients with head and neck cancer. N Engl J Med. 1993;329:390–395.

62. LeVeque FG, Montgomery M, Potter D, et al. A multicenter, randomized, double-blind, placebo-controlled, dose-titration study of oral pilocarpine for treatment of radiation-induced xerostomia in head and neck cancer patients. J Clin Oncol. 1993;11:1124–1131.

63. Mateos JJ, Setoain X, Ferre J, et al. Salivary scintigraphy for assessing the protective effect of pilocarpine in head and neck irradiated tumours. Nucl Med Commun. 2001;22:651–656.

64. Sangthawan D, Watthanaarpornchai S, Phungrassami T. Randomized double blind, placebo-controlled study of pilocarpine administered during head and neck irradiation to reduce xerostomia. J Med Assoc Thai. 2001;84:195–203.

65. Warde P, O'Sullivan B, Aslanidis J, et al. A Phase III placebo-controlled trial of oral pilocarpine in patients undergoing radiotherapy for head-and-neck cancer. Int J Radiat Oncol Biol Phys. 2002;54:9–13.

66. Fisher J, Scott C, Scarantino CW, et al. Phase III quality-of-life study results: impact on patients' quality of life to reducing xerostomia after radiotherapy for head-and-neck cancer—RTOG 97-09. Int J Radiat Oncol Biol Phys. 2003;56:832–836.

67. Gornitsky M, Shenouda G, Sultanem K, et al. Double-blind randomized, placebo-controlled study of pilocarpine to salvage salivary gland function during radiotherapy of patients with head and neck cancer. Oral Surg Oral Med Oral Pathol Oral Radiol Endod. 2004;98:45–52.

68. Scarantino C, LeVeque F, Swann RS, et al. Effect of pilocarpine during radiation therapy: results of RTOG 97-09, a phase III randomized study in head and neck cancer patients. J Support Oncol. 2006;4:252–258.

69. Burlage FR, Roesink JM, Faber H, et al. Optimum dose range for the amelioration of long term radiation-induced hyposalivation using prophylactic pilocarpine treatment. Radiother Oncol. 2008;86:347–353.

70. Zimmerman RP, Mark RJ, Tran LM, et al. Concomitant pilocarpine during head and neck irradiation is associated with decreased posttreatment xerostomia. Int J Radiat Oncol Biol Phys. 1997;37:571–575.

71. Valdez JH, Atkinson JC, Ship JA, et al. Major salivary gland function in patients with radiation-induced xerostomia: flow rates and sialochemistry. Int J Radiat Oncol Biol Phys. 1993;25:41–47.

72. Horiot JC, Lipinski F, Schraub S, et al. Post-radiation severe xerostomia relieved by pilocarpine: a prospective French cooperative study. Radiother Oncol. 2000;55:233–239.

73. Avila JL, Grundmann O, Burd R, et al. Radiation-induced salivary gland dysfunction results from p53-dependent apoptosis. Int J Radiat Oncol Biol Phys. 2009;73:523–529.

74. Reference deleted in proofs.

75. Lombaert IM, Brunsting JF, Wierenga PK, et al. Keratinocyte growth factor prevents radiation damage to salivary glands by expansion of the stem/progenitor pool. Stem Cells. 2008;31:2007–2034.

76. Senahayake F, Piggott K, Hamilton-Miller JM. A pilot study of Salix SST (saliva-stimulating lozenges) in post-irradiation xerostomia. Curr Med Res Opin. 1998;14:155–159.

77. Jensdottir T, Nauntofte B, Buchwald C, et al. Effects of sucking acidic candies on saliva in unilaterally irradiated pharyngeal cancer patients. Oral Oncol. 2006;42:317–322.

78. Davies AN, Singer J. A comparison of artificial saliva and pilocarpine in radiation-induced xerostomia. J Laryngol Otol. 1994;108:663–665.

79. Rieke JW, Hafermann MD, Johnson JT, et al. Oral pilocarpine for radiation-induced xerostomia: integrated efficacy and safety results from two prospective randomized clinical trials. Int J Radiat Oncol Biol Phys. 1995;31:661–669.

80. Chitapanarux I, Kamnerdsupaphon P, Tharavichitkul E, et al. Effect of oral pilocarpine on post-irradiation xerostomia in head and neck cancer patients: a single-center, single-blind clinical trial. J Med Assoc Thai. 2008;91:1410–1415.

81. Hamlar DD, Schuller DE, Gahbauer RA, et al. Determination of the efficacy of topical oral pilocarpine for postirradiation xerostomia in patients with head and neck carcinoma. Laryngoscope. 1996;106:972–976.

82. Nyarady Z, Nemeth A, Ban A, et al. A randomized study to assess the effectiveness of orally administered pilocarpine during and after radiotherapy of head and neck cancer. Anticancer Res. 2006;26:1557–1562.

83. Daniels TE, Wu AJ. Xerostomia—clinical evaluation and treatment in general practice. J Calif Dent Assoc. 2000;28:933–941.

84. Bernardi R, Perin C, Becker FL, et al. Effect of pilocarpine mouthwash on salivary flow. Braz J Med Biol Res. 2002;35:105–110.

85. Chambers MS, Jones CU, Biel MA, et al. Open-label, long-term safety study of cevimeline in the treatment of postirradiation xerostomia. Int J Radiat Oncol Biol Phys. 2007;69:1369–1376.

86. Chambers MS, Posner M, Jones CU, et al. Cevimeline for the treatment of postirradiation xerostomia in patients with head and neck cancer. Int J Radiat Oncol Biol Phys. 2007;68:1102–1109.

87. Blom M, Dawidson I, Fernberg JO, et al. Acupuncture treatment of patients with radiation-induced xerostomia. Oral Oncol Eur J Cancer. 1996;32B:182–190.

88. Wong RKW, Jones GW, Sagar SM, et al. study in the use of acupuncture-like transcutaneous nerve stimulation in the treatment of radiation-induced xerostomia in head-and-neck cancer patients treated with radical radiotherapy. Int J Radiat Oncol Biol Phys. 2003;57:472–480.

89. Blom M, Lundeberg T. Long-term follow-up of patients treated with acupuncture for xerostomia and the influence of additional treatment. Oral Dis. 2000;6:15–24.

90. Braga FP, Sugaya NN, Hirota SK, et al. The effect of acupuncture on salivary flow rates in patients with radiation-induced xerostomia. Minerva Stomatol. 2008;57:343–348.

91. Deng G, Hou BL, Holodny AI, et al. Functional magnetic resonance imaging (fMRI) changes and saliva production associated with acupuncture at L1–2 acupuncture point: a randomized controlled study. BMC Complementary Alternative Med. 2008;8:137.

92. Weiss WW, Brenman HS, Katz P, et al. Use of an electric stimulator for the treatment of dry mouth. J Oral Maxillofac Surg. 1986;44:845–850.

93. Strietzel FP, Martín-Granizo R, Fedele S, et al. Electrostimulating device in the management of xerostomia. Oral Dis. 2007;13:206–213.

94. Gerlach NL, Barkhuysen R, Kaanders JH, et al. The effect of hyperbaric oxygen therapy on quality of life in oral and oropharyngeal cancer patients treated with radiotherapy. Int J Oral Maxillofac Surg. 2008;37:255–259.

95. Harding SA, Hodder SC, Courtney DJ, et al. Impact of perioperative hyperbaric oxygen therapy on the quality of life of maxillofacial patients who undergo surgery in irradiated fields. Int J Oral Maxillofac Surg. 2008;37:617–624.

96. Teguh DN, Levendag PC, Noever I, et al. Early hyperbaric oxygen therapy for reducing radiotherapy side effects: early results of a randomized trial in oropharyngeal and asopharyngeal cancer. Int J Radiat Oncol Biol Phys. 2009;75:711–716.

97. Levine MJ. Development of artificial salivas. Crit Rev Oral Biol Med. 1993;4:279–286.

98. Matzker J, Schreiber J. [Synthetic saliva in the treatment of hyposialies, especially in radiation sialadenitis]. Z Laryngol Rhinol Otol. 1972;51:422–428.

99. Gravenmade EJ, Roukema PA, Panders AK. The effect of mucin-containing artificial saliva on severe xerostomia. Int J Oral Surg. 1974;3:435–439.

100. Van der Reijden WA, Van der Kwaak H, Vissink A, et al. Treatment of xerostomia with polymer-based

saliva substitutes in patients with Sjögren's syndrome. *Arthritis Rheum.* 1996;39:57–69.

101. Vissink A, Gravenmade EJ, Panders AK, et al. A clinical comparison between commercially available mucin- and CMC-containing saliva substitutes. *Int J Oral Surg.* 1983;12:232–238.

102. Visch LL, Gravenmade EJ, Schaub RM, et al. A double-blind crossover trial of CMC- and mucin-containing saliva substitutes. *Int J Oral Maxillofac Surg.* 1986;15:395–400.

103. Jellema AP, Langendijk H, Bergenhenegouwen L, et al. The efficacy of Xialine in patients with xerostomia resulting from radiotherapy for head and neck cancer: a pilot-study. *Radiother Oncol.* 2001;59:157–160.

104. Vissink A, Waterman HA, Gravenmade EJ, et al. Rheological properties of saliva substitutes containing mucin, carboxymethylcellulose or polyethylenoxide. *J Oral Pathol.* 1984;13:22–28.

105. Vissink A, De Jong HP, Busscher HJ, et al. Wetting properties of human saliva and saliva substitutes. *J Dent Res.* 1986;65:1121–1124.

106. Regelink G, Vissink A, Reintsema H, et al. Efficacy of a synthetic polymer saliva substitute in reducing oral complaints of patients suffering from irradiation-induced xerostomia. *Quintessence Int.* 1998;29:383–388.

107. Epstein JB, Emerton S, Le ND, et al. A double-blind crossover trial of Oral Balance gel and Biotene toothpaste versus placebo in patients with xerostomia following radiation therapy. *Oral Oncol.* 1999;35:132–137.

108. Samarawickrama DYD. Saliva substitutes: how effective and safe are they? *Oral Dis.* 2002;8:177–179.

109. Momm F, Guttenberger R. Treatment of xerostomia following radiotherapy: does age matter? *Support Care Cancer.* 2002;10:505–508.

110. Oh DJ, Lee JY, Kim YK, et al. Effects of carboxymethylcellulose (CMC)-based artificial saliva in patients with xerostomia. *Int J Oral Maxillofac Surg.* 2008;37:1027–1031.

111. Kaneko M, Shirato H, Nishioka T, et al. Scintigraphic evaluation of long-term salivary function after bilateral whole parotid gland irradiation in radiotherapy for head and neck tumour. *Oral Oncol.* 1998;34:140–146.

112. Roesink JM, Moerland MA, Battermann JJ, et al. Quantitative dose-volume response analysis of changes in parotid gland function after radiotherapy in the head-and-neck region. *Int J Radiat Oncol Biol Phys.* 2001;51:938–946.

113. Semenenko VA, Li XA, Lyman-Kutcher-Burman NTCP. model parameters for radiation pneumonitis and xerostomia based on combined analysis of published clinical data. *Phys Med Biol.* 2008;53:737–755.

114. Ortholan C, Chamorey E, Benezery K, et al. Modeling of salivary production recovery after radiotherapy using mixed models: determination of optimal dose constraint for IMRT planning and construction of convenient tools to predict salivary function. *Int J Radiat Oncol Biol Phys.* 2009;73:178–186.

114a. Jellema AP, Doornaert P, Slotman BJ, et al. Does radiation dose to the salivary glands and oral cavity predict patient-rated xerostomia and sticky saliva in head and neck cancer patients treated with curative radiotherapy? *Radiother Oncol.* 2005;77:164–171.

115. Baum BJ, Zheng C, Cotrim AP, et al. Aquaporin-1 gene transfer to correct radiation-induced salivary hypofunction. In: Beitz E, ed. *Aquaporins: Handbook of experimental pharmacology.* Berlin Heidelberg: Springer-Verlag; 2009:403.

116. Delporte C, O'Connell BC, He X, et al. Increased fluid secretion after adenovira-mediated transfer of the aquaporin-1 cDNA to irradiated rat salivary glands. *Proc Natl Acad Sci U S A.* 1997;94:3268–3273.

117. Preston GM, Agre P. Isolation of the cDNA for erythrocyte integral membrane protein of 28 kilodaltons: member of an ancient channel family. *Proc Natl Acad Sci U S A.* 1991;88:1110–1114.

118. Konings AWT, Coppes RP, Vissink A. On the mechanism of salivary gland radiosensitivity. *Int J Radiat Oncol Biol Phys.* 2005;62:1187–1194.

119. Lombaert IM, Brunsting JF, Wierenga PK, et al. Rescue of salivary gland function after stem cell transplantation in irradiated glands. *PLoS ONE.* 2008;3:e2063.

120. Burlage FR, Faber H, Kampinga HH, et al. Enhanced proliferation of acinar and progenitor cells by prophylactic pilocarpine treatment underlies the observed amelioration of radiation injury to parotid glands. *Radiother Oncol.* 2009;90:253–256.

121. Burlage FR, Roesink JM, Kampinga HH, et al. Protection of salivary function by concomitant pilocarpine during radiotherapy: a double-blind, randomized, placebo-controlled study. *Int J Radiat Oncol Biol Phys.* 2008;70:14–22.

Bisphosphonates and RANKL antibodies in breast carcinoma with bone metastases

Ingo J. Diel

24

It is estimated that 60,000 women in Germany will be confronted with a breast cancer diagnosis in 2010 (in the United States, ≈220,500). The number of women who will die of this disease in this same time frame is about 18,000 (in the United States, ≈42,000). And even if the numbers for Germany are only estimates, because of inadequate record keeping, the mortality rate is about 20% to 25%, which is comparable with other Western countries with similar diagnostic and treatment provisions.

The primary cause of morbidity and mortality in breast cancer is distant metastases and resulting organ failure. The primary sites for metastases are the skeleton, lungs, and liver. Bone metastases are found in 75% to 80% of all women who die of breast cancer, and in one half of these cases, the skeleton is the target organ for metastases. In Germany, about 11,000 to 12,000 patients are affected annually by bone metastases.

BONE METASTASES

Bone metastases in principle can be precipitated by any malignant tumor. It is interesting to note, though, that a very small number of cancers are responsible for about 90% of all bone metastases. Included in this group are breast cancer, prostate cancer, lung and thyroid cancer, and, lastly, renal cell cancer. Two types of bone metastases are radiologically detectable: osteolytic metastases that destroy bone, and osteoblastic metastases that permeate bone with inferior new tissue. The two types can occur simultaneously, sometimes even in the same bone. In women with breast cancer, osteolytic metastases are predominant (≈70%) when compared with blastic metastases (≈30%).

Almost all patients (>90%) experience at least one episode with severe bone pain that requires treatment. The second most common complication in breast cancer with skeletal metastasis is pathologic fractures, that is, fractures that occur spontaneously or after minor trauma (≈25%). However, fractures from "out of the blue" are rare. Often the preceding bone pain is incorrectly interpreted, and the diagnosis is missed. The nihilistic attitude that for years has been widespread in follow-up care for those with breast cancer has had an impact. Because the disease in the metastasized state is seen as incurable, and an early diagnosis does not demonstrably contribute to longer survival, the physical examination is limited with regard to bone metastases to percussion of the spinal column 1 to 2 times per year. The fact that a pathologic fracture is a worst-case scenario for the patient is often deliberately ignored. Spinal compression syndrome is a specific complication that occurs in conjunction with pathologic fractures (<5%). Pinching of the spinal cord or spinal nerves typically occurs after fractures of the vertebral bodies. This complication must be viewed as an absolute emergency and requires immediate surgical decompression and stabilization, followed by radiation therapy.

Another complication that many years ago was still very frequent has become in the meantime, at least in breast cancer, a rarity—hypercalcemia. A disturbance that may be accompanied by many symptoms (electrolyte shifts and central nervous complications, among others) and may remain untreated can be fatal. Broad and early use of bisphosphonates has led worldwide to a dramatic decrease in the incidence of

243

hypercalcemia. Breast cancer patients with bone metastases can live for a long time. Even if average survival time is only 3 years following diagnosis of metastasis, every caregiver knows of women who have survived for 8 years or longer. The time frame depends on many things: the age of the patient, the biology of the primary tumor, the types of specimens and metastases to other organs, and the involvement and experience of the caregiver.

PATHOGENESIS OF BONE METASTASIS

Bone metastases develop similarly to other metastases, but they have some unique characteristics that are not associated with other metastases (i.e., other processes follow). Initially, the primary tumor gives off cells in nutritive vessels. With many carcinomas, this occurs at an early, clinically unapparent stage (e.g., breast cancer). The process of tumor cell proliferation has not been adequately researched. It is known however that the process is very ineffective because very few of the cells produced have metastatic potential. Most are destroyed or are successfully fought off by the immune system.[1,2]

It is known that tumor cells that are detectable in the bone marrow can remain for years in this foreign environment as so-called "dormant cells." Similar to terrorist "sleepers" the cells can remain in the foreign environment to some day complete their fatal destructive work. How tumor cells become virulent is unknown. Some researchers surmise that tumor cells linger at a low proliferation level, and their growth is limited by T cells, until this immunologic protection breaks down for a variety of reasons, and uncontrolled growth is permitted. These cells may correspond to the currently hotly debated breast cancer stem cells.

DESTRUCTION OF BONES BY METASTASIS

If the barriers for tumor suppression are penetrated, then the host organism and tumor cells work closely together in the formation of bone metastases. As in a vicious circle, tumor cells and bones support each other and are in a constant "malignant"

dialogue with each other (Fig. 24-1).[3,4] In simple terms, the following happens: In their proliferation, no longer limited metastatic cells secrete osteoclast-activating substances. This ability is supposedly genetically determined (seed). The best known paracrine-secreted substance is the PTHrP. Parathyroid hormone–related protein (PTHrP) binds to the parathyroid hormone (PTH) receptor of the osteoblasts. This on the other hand emits RANK-Ligand (RANKL), which binds to the receptor activator of nuclear factor κ-B (RANK) in osteoclasts and increases the fusion and activity of bone-resorbing cells. Simultaneously, the regulating effect of osteoprotegerin (OPG) is reduced (see previous chapter on bone health). Activated osteoclasts destroy the bone (tumor cells alone only rarely can do this). When the bone matrix degrades, previously stored growth factors (e.g., transforming growth factor [TGF]-beta, insulin-like growth factor [IGF], platelet-derived growth factor [PDGF], among many others) that promote proliferation among metastatic cells are released. In this insidious way, the metastasis creates the area in which it can secondarily infiltrate.

Decoding of this mechanism opens up new types of treatment that counteract the destruction of bone. Not just bisphosphonates belong to the osteoclast inhibitor medication class; recently, antibodies were noted to block RANKL (similar to osteoprotegerin), cathepsin K inhibitors, and *src*-kinase inhibitors.

TREATMENT WITH BISPHOSPHONATES

Bone metastases can be treated surgically and locally with radiation therapy. Included among the systemic options are chemotherapy antibody treatment and antihormone treatment. Classical pain treatment and treatment with radioisotopes can be used as part of the arsenal to fight bone metastases, as can anti-osteolytic treatment with bisphosphonates.[5,6]

Bisphosphonates are chemically related to pyrophosphate and together are part of the polyphosphate family. Polyphosphates were already developed in the nineteenth century by the laundry detergent industry as de-scalers for

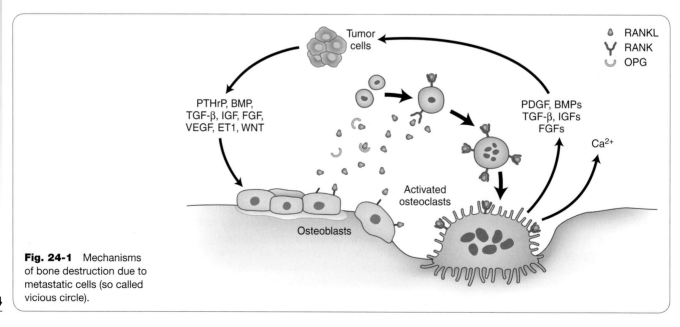

Fig. 24-1 Mechanisms of bone destruction due to metastatic cells (so called vicious circle).

PTHrP, BMP, TGF-β, IGF, FGF, VEGF, ET1, WNT

Tumor cells

PDGF, BMPs TGF-β, IGFs FGFs

Ca²⁺

RANKL
RANK
OPG

Osteoblasts

Activated osteoclasts

tubes, among others (softener). The first bisphosphonate, which also is still used therapeutically (etidronate), stems from this time period. Therapeutic efficacy in the fight against hypercalcemic conditions was developed toward the end of the 1960s. Since that time, clinical development has advanced, and bisphosphonates are now used as treatment for bone metastases, osteoporosis, and Paget's disease of the bone, and for other diseases that are accompanied by an increase in bone metabolism.

In contrast to pyrophosphates that have a P-O-P bond and are relatively unstable, bisphosphonates have a carbon atom between the two phosphorous atoms. Free valences on the C-atom enable a variety of molecules with their side chains that are characteristic of the various bisphosphonates. Clodronate is relatively simply constructed with two chlorine atoms attached to a carbon atom. The newer bisphosphonates, with somewhat complex side chains, exceed the binding capacity (to the bony matrix) of etidronate and clodronate, but they also have a different range of side effects. To assert that the new, "more potent" bisphosphonates are basically better is more relevant to marketing than to science. The advantage of the newer substances lies in its shorter intravenous administration time.

Until a few years ago, the mechanism of action for bisphosphonates at the molecular level was unexplained. The anti-osteolytic effect was seen—quite correctly—in reduction of osteoclastic activity. Today, we know that this effect primarily forms the basis of induction of apoptotic processes.[7,8] The aminobisphosphonates (e.g., pamidronate, ibandronate, risedronate, alendronate, zoledronate) competitively inhibit geranylation and farnesylation in mevalonate metabolism, which on the other hand, is significant for cholesterol synthesis (statins have a very similar effect, but they interfere with a different step in the synthesis pathway and accumulate in the liver). In this way, the effect and function of GTP-binding proteins are suspended, and this is interrupted by the intracellular signal transfer (Fig. 24-2).[9] With the non-aminobisphosphonates (e.g., clodronate, tiludronate, etidronate), apoptosis (and necrosis) is achieved through intracellular accumulation of toxic metabolites of adenosine triphosphate (ATP).[10] Regrettably, this apoptotic effect can also be seen in cells of the intestinal mucosa and in renal tubule cells.

Bisphosphonates can be administered orally and parenterally. However, absorption through the intestinal mucosa is ineffective and is dependent on food composition. For this reason, oral bisphosphonates must be taken on an empty stomach, and calcium-rich meals and drinks must be avoided for 30 to 60 minutes; otherwise, chelates may form. All in all, resorption rates are between 0.5% and 5%. Initially, this is meaningless, except that tablets in comparison with parenterally administered bisphophonates must be given in higher doses (similarly to antibiotics).

Regardless of the route of administration, bisphosphonates are stored on the calcium apatite of the mineralized bone matrix (30%–70%) or are excreted unmetabolized by the kidneys. In areas with increased "bone turnover," uptake is particularly high (principle of skeletal scintigraphy with technetium bound to bisphosphonate). Osteoclasts take up bisphosphonates with microsequestration from the bone matrix. Bisphosphonates on the other hand induce in osteoclasts the previously described apoptotic processes.

Bisphosphonates for anti-osteolytic treatment of bone metastases

For no other tumor entity are as many data on bisphosphonate treatment available as for breast cancer. Clodronate, pamidronate, ibandronate, and zoledronate are all approved in Germany.

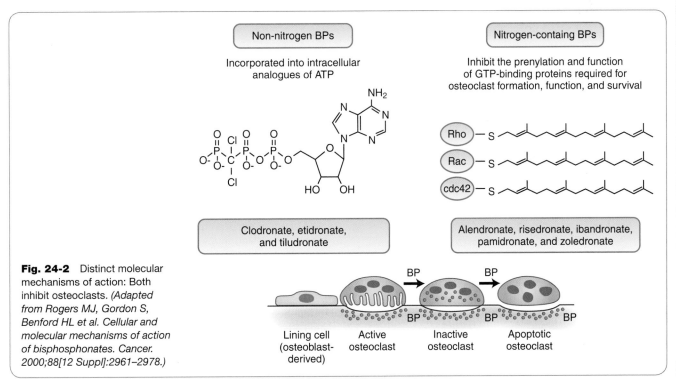

Fig. 24-2 Distinct molecular mechanisms of action: Both inhibit osteoclasts. (*Adapted from Rogers MJ, Gordon S, Benford HL et al. Cellular and molecular mechanisms of action of bisphosphonates. Cancer. 2000;88[12 Suppl]:2961–2978.*)

Clodronate is a first-generation bisphosphonate that can be administered intravenously (1500 mg over 4 hours every 3–4 weeks) or orally (1600 mg/day). Intravenous administration is suitable for normalization of hypercalcemia and to reduce skeletal complications, but because of the long infusion time and the large number of molecules, it is not used frequently.

Oral clodronate also decreases the rate of skeletal complications, but is not very effective against hypercalcemia or for acute bone pain (Fig. 24-3).[11] The scope of application lies primarily in preventing these complications (asymptomatic metastases) and in providing adjuvant treatment to avoid subsequent metastases. It is absolutely not true that oral bisphosphonates have poor efficacy only because they are poorly absorbed enterally (clodronate 3%, aminobisphosphonates less than 1%). Oral and intravenous bisphosphonates have been shown to be equally good at reducing skeletal events.

For many years, pamidronate has been given as standard treatment for carcinoma with bone metastasis. Because oral treatment has been shown to be too toxic, only the intravenous form is used in Germany as in most countries (90 mg over 2 hours, every 3–4 weeks). Pamidronate decreases all skeletal complications, except for the incidence of vertebral fractures.

Pamidronate was the first aminobisphosphonate approved for treatment of tumor osteolysis. Pamidronate is more potent than clodronate, and this is attributed to the strong affinity of the drug for hydroxylapatite on the bone surface. The broadest use of pamidronate was as interval therapy at a dose of 90 mg every 4 weeks. Intravenously administered bisphosphonates are 100% bioavailable and do not depend on individual intestinal resorption rates, which, in contrast, may be affected by meal times and calcium-rich components.

The reference study on the use of IV pamidronate was published in December 1996 by Hortobagyi et al. (Fig. 24-4).[12] In this multicenter, double-blind, placebo-controlled study, pamidronate, as well as chemotherapy, was administered to patients with osteolytic destruction (n = 382) at a dose of 90 mg IV every 4 weeks, or placebo was given (for 1 year = 12 cycles). In the pamidronate group, the appearance of extravertebral fractures was significantly reduced, as were bone pain and the need for radiation therapy. Nevertheless, no reduction in vertebral fractures was noted. In a follow-up study with a

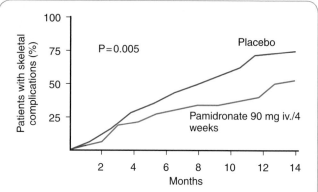

Fig. 24-4 Reduction in skeletal complications with pamidronate. (*Data fraom Hortobagyi GN, Theriault RL, Porter L, et al.[12]*)

significantly longer follow-up time, the effects of pamidronate were confirmed.[13,14]

It is interesting to note that approval studies for pamidronate compared with placebo showed a life-prolonging effect in the subgroup of premenopausal patients (24.6 vs. 15.7 months). Similar observations were made with multiple myoloma.[15]

Ibandronate is a highly potent third-generation bisphosphonate that has been approved for intravenous use since November 2003 for the treatment of bone metastases in breast cancer.[16] It has been available as oral treatment for osteolysis since April 2004. Studies on parenteral use were conducted by using 2 and 6 mg IV versus placebo in 462 patients with breast cancer with skeletal metastases over 2 years.[17] Although 6 mg of ibandronate compared with placebo significantly reduced skeletal complications, this was not evident with 2 mg. With 6 mg, a significant reduction in vertebral, but not in extravertebral, fractures occurred. On the other hand, the best effectiveness can be verified by avoidance of radiation therapy. Furthermore, the 6-mg dose led to significant lengthening of the time period until the first skeletal complications appeared, and to a lasting reduction in bone pain over 24 months (Fig. 24-5). This study showed excellent results in terms of improved quality of life for affected patients in all areas measured (based on the EORTC-QLQ-C30-questionnaire) and reduced need for pain medication[18] (Fig. 24-6). Three large comparative studies were performed for approval of oral ibandronate. In all three studies, 50 mg versus 20 mg versus placebo were tested, respectively. In total, 999 patients with breast cancer with bone metastasis were included.[19–21] Results of these studies were roughly comparable. With the (approved) dose of 50 mg, a significant reduction in bone pain and in all skeletal events was achieved (Fig. 24-7).

Zoledronate is one of the most potent bisphosphonates used in oncology; for ethical reasons, in the phase III study of breast cancer and multiple myeloma, it was no longer tested against placebo, but rather against 90 mg pamidronate IV. In the treatment of hypercalcemia, it was shown that zoledronate had a 10% higher response rate, and the time until hypercalcemia recurred was increased.[22] No other drug was tested before approval for the treatment of metastases in such a large number of patients with breast cancer (n = 1130). Zoledronate was administered over 12 months in an equivalence study against 90 mg pamidronate at doses of 4 mg and 8 mg in patients with skeletal metastases.[23] Results of the

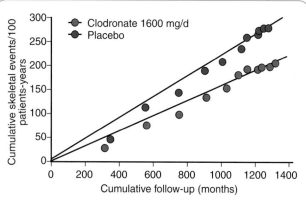

SRE: Placebo *vs.* Clodronate (/100 pt years) : 305 *vs* 219 p < 0.001
*hypercalcaemia, fractures, radiotherapy for bone pain

Fig. 24-3 Long-term decrease in all skeletal-related events (SRE)* with clodronate. (*Data from Paterson AHG, Powles TJ, Kanis JA, et al.[11]*)

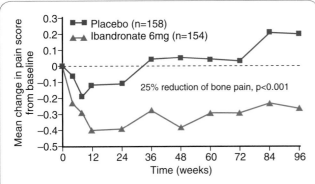

Fig. 24-5 Long-term bone pain relief (up to 2 years) with intravenous ibandronate. *(Data from Diel IJ, Body JJ, Lichinitser MR, et al.[18])*

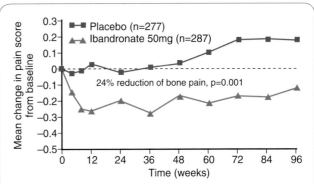

Fig. 24-7 Long-term bone pain relief (up to 2 years) with oral ibandronate. *(Data from Body JJ, Diel IJ, Bell R, et al. Oral ibandronate improves bone pain and preserves quality of life in patients with skeletal metastases due to breast cancer. Pain. 2004:111:306–312.)*

comparative study showed no differences in efficacy in the short term between pamidronate and zoledronate (Fig. 24-8). Both drugs demonstrated significant pain reduction. The 8-mg dose in particular led to increased serum creatinine in some patients; therefore, for the rest of the study, the 8-mg group was switched to 4 mg, and the length of the infusion was increased to 15 minutes. In the final analysis, renal toxicity from 4 mg given over 15 minutes was in the same range as with 90 mg of pamidronate.

In a long-term analysis of the approval study over 25 months in patients with breast cancer, a reduction of 20% in skeletal complications was reported with 4 mg of zoledronate compared with 90 mg of pamidronate.[24,25] Similarly, as with other bisphosphonates, this effect was achieved primarily by reducing necessary radiation treatment. This is a clear indication that the more potent drug (in comparison with pamidronate) is more effective in acute events, such as bone pain and hypercalcemia. In the prevention of pathologic fractures, this does not appear to be the case.

These results were underscored by the results of an individual placebo-controlled study with zoledronate (Japan) that was published in May 2005.[26] In this study, 114 patients with breast cancer with skeletal metastases were treated with 4 mg of

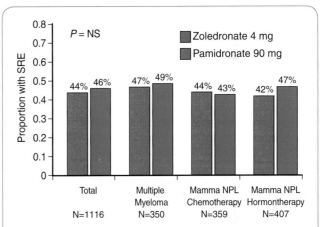

Fig. 24-8 Reduction in skeletal-related events with zoledronate. *(Data from Rosen LS, Gordon D, Kaminski M, et al.[23])*

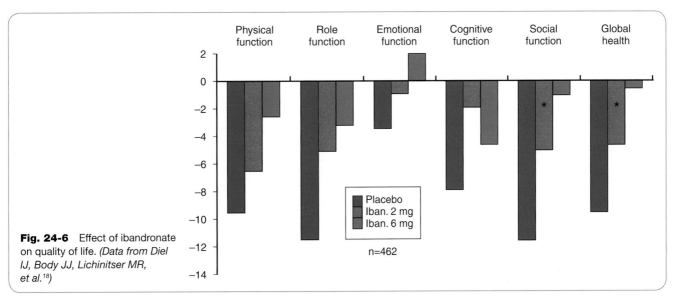

Fig. 24-6 Effect of ibandronate on quality of life. *(Data from Diel IJ, Body JJ, Lichinitser MR, et al.[18])*

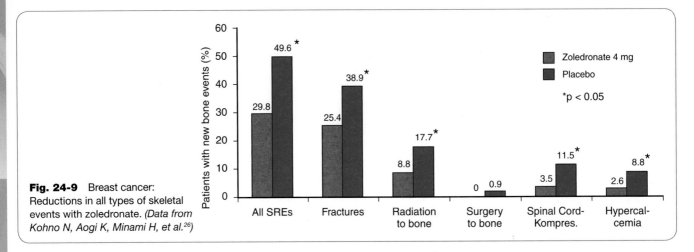

Fig. 24-9 Breast cancer: Reductions in all types of skeletal events with zoledronate. (*Data from Kohno N, Aogi K, Minami H, et al.[26]*)

zoledronate every 4 weeks for 1 year; another 114 women received placebo infusions. A significant reduction in all evaluated skeletal complications was noted with zoledronate (Fig. 24-9). Pain reduction with 4 mg of zoledronate was shown impressively and over the long term, whereas pain intensity in the placebo group significantly increased over time ($P < .05$) (Fig. 24-10).

Side effects of bisphosphonates

If you want to understand the side effects of bisphosphonates, you first must be familiar with the mechanism of action of the drug class.[8] This is also relevant for most side effects. As described previously, bisphosphonates induce apoptotic processes in osteoclasts. But this effect is visible not only in osteoclasts and macrophages, but also in the corresponding accumulation in the intestinal mucosa and in the kidney tubules.

With bisphosphonates, the distinction is made between infrequent and frequent adverse effects (Table 24-1). Clinically active oncologists at least should be familiar with those encoun-

Table 24-1	Side effects of bisphosphonates

A. Frequent side effects
- Infusion-related events (acute phase reaction)
- Renal toxicity/deterioration
- GI side effects (gastritis, diarrhea)
- Osteonecrosis of the jaw

B. Rare side effects (selected)
- Hypocalcemia (symptomatic)
- Ocular side effects (retinitis, uveitis, scleritis)
- Asthmatic attacks (sensitive to aspirin)
- Skin rashes
- Phlebitis
- Alteration of taste

tered most frequently, including the acute phase response, gastrointestinal disturbances, nephrotoxic complications, and, recently, osteonecrosis of the jawbone (Table 24-2).

ACUTE PHASE REACTION AND GASTROINTESTINAL SIDE EFFECTS

A large number of flu-like symptoms and findings are classified by the term *acute phase reaction* (also called "flu-like syndrome" in English); these include especially subfebrile temperatures, leukocytosis, abnormal fatigue, and muscle and bone pain.[27] These responses are seen exclusively in intravenously administered aminobisphosphonates (zoledronate, ibandronate, and pamidronate) and typically appear after the first infusion, at a frequency of up to 30%. This type of side effect is not life-threatening, but often is perceived by the patient as very stressful and rarely leads to interruption of parenteral treatment. Symptoms as a rule regress at the latest after 48 hours and respond well to nonsteroidal antirheumatics and antipyretic measures.

Bisphosphonate-induced side effects in the gastrointestinal tract are seen—of course—exclusively during oral treatment. All sections from the lower esophagus to the colon may be affected. Ulcerations in the stomach, duodenum, and esophagus have been described. However, abdominal pain, flatulence, and diarrhea are much more common.[28,29] In the presence of intolerable symptoms, the switch should be made to an intravenous bisphosphonate.

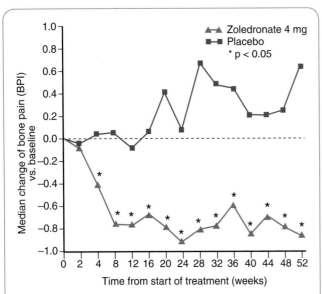

Fig. 24-10 Breast cancer: Significant reduction in bone pain with zoledronate versus placebo. (*Data from Kohno N, Aogi K, Minami H, et al.[26]*)

Table 24-2 Synopsis of the most frequent side effects of bisphosphonates

Drug	Acute phase	Nephrotoxic	Upper GI	Diarrhea	ONJ
Clodronate IV	0	+	0	0	?
Clodonate 800 (×2)	0	0	+	++	0
Clodronate 520 (×2)	0	0	+	++	0
Ibandronate 6 mg IV	++	0	0	0	+
Ibandronate 50 mg	0	0	+	0	(+)
Zoledronate 4 mg IV	++	++	0	0	++
Pamidronate 90 mg IV	++	++	0	0	++
Alendronate	0	0	++	+	+
Risedronate	0	0	+	+	(+)
Etidronate	0	0	(+)	(+)	0

GI, Gastrointestinal; *ONJ,* osteonecrosis of the jaw.

RENAL TOXICITY

Almost no side effect in the last few years has led to such heated discussion as the question about renal toxicity from bisphosphonates. To be sure, all bisphosphonates can damage the tubule system, but significant differences have been noted between the individual drugs. Bisphosphonates are stored in the bones following oral or parenteral administration (30%–60%) or are excreted renally unmetabolized. Influx into the tubule cells is passive and depends only on serum concentration and protein binding. An active, limited transportation mechanism forms the basis for excretion into the lumen. If this mechanism is overburdened, an accumulation of bisphosphonates can occur in the tubule cells with induction of apoptotic processes.[30–32] No evidence of renal complications has been noted with oral bisphosphonates given at therapeutic doses.

The following is recommended to avoid kidney damage: (1) Adhere strictly to recommended measures in the package insert; (2) maintain good hydration; and (3) reduce dose if an increase in creatinine (i.e., restricted calculated clearance) occurs.

OSTEONECROSES OF THE JAWBONE

Osteonecroses of the mandible and the maxilla (osteonecrosis of the jaw [ONJ]) during treatment with bisphosphonates was first described in 2003, even if reference to earlier manifestations was made retrospectively in publications.[33,34] In Germany, since the creation of a central registry for osteonecroses of the jawbone at the Charité Hospital in Berlin until mid 2010, more than 1000 cases have been registered; every week, 3 to 5 new cases are reported[35] (www.charite.de/zmk). Among 932 evaluated cases with malignancies, 37% had breast cancer, 14% prostate cancer, and 12% multiple myeloma, and 37% were divided among other tumor entities. Most osteonecroses (85%) appeared in the first 4 years of treatment (personal communication, Professor D. Felsenberg). More than 68% of registered patients were treated with zoledronate, 17% with

pamidronate, and 8.5% with ibandronate; most others were treated with a sequence of the named bisphosphonates. Cases while on oral therapy are rare, and osteonecrosis of the jaw while on clodronate is unknown.[36]

In the meantime, it is assumed that jaw necroses represent the final stage of osteomyelitis, which has occurred previously. Macrophages and osteoclasts originate from the same stem cell line and are inhibited by bisphosphonates, so that defense mechanisms are suppressed and existing infections are able to spread. Whether the antiangiogenetic effect of bisphosphonates is pathophysiologically relevant is still unclear.

A dental procedure precedes most jawbone osteonecroses. Even though it has not been proven, studies indicate that with manipulation of teeth or the jawbone that is associated with an increased rate of turnover, bisphosphonate treatment should be interrupted for 2 months. Because treatment of jawbone osteonecroses is unusually complicated, cleaning of teeth and all potential focuses of inflammation should be performed as prophylaxis before long-term treatment is started. When in doubt, inspection of the oral cavity within the context of tumor follow-up is appropriate.

RESEARCH ON PREVENTION OF SKELETAL METASTASES

Even if preventive use of bisphosphonates for metastasis prophylaxis has occasionally been shown in animal studies, clinical studies of metastasized breast cancer have been disappointing.[37–40] However in a small study, Elooma demonstrated a reduction in new bone metastases with clodronate in cases of breast cancer with skeletal metastases.[41] Another study published by Kanis et al. showed that patients with distant or locally advanced breast cancer (without skeletal metastases) developed fewer skeletal metastases with preventive clodronate treatment.[42]

Adjuvant use of clodronate was tested in two smaller studies and in one large study. The first publication was put forth by Diel et al., from Heidelberg. In this study, 302 patients with primary breast cancer and disseminated tumor cells in the marrow were randomized and were treated orally with 1600 mg clodronate or were simply monitored.[43,44] After a median follow-up time of 3 years, the incidence of skeletal and visceral metastases in the treated group of patients decreased, and total length of survival increased. In a reanalysis with a median follow-up time of 109 months, it was shown that adjuvant use of oral clodronate led to a long-term decrease in mortality[45] (Fig. 24-11). Nevertheless, after this period of time, no further significant reduction in the incidence of bone and visceral metastases could be established. This might

mean that in some patients, early use of bisphosphonates may achieve long-term healing, but in many others, the relatively short duration of treatment (only 2 years) led to a delay in metastasis.

A study by Saarto et al., from Helsinki, showed completely contradictory results.[46] Here, no differences in the incidence of bone metastases were found in either group, but rather an increase in the frequency of visceral metastases and an increase in mortality were reported. The 10-year analysis, which was published in 2004, showed no significant changes.[47] Experts assert that the reason for the negative result may lie in the unequal distribution of patients with negative receptor status. Primarily, significantly more patients with negative receptor status were treated in the clodronate group, and treatment of these patients consisted predominantly of endocrine therapy, and not chemotherapy. A second problem is the breaches in protocol that led to the exclusion of at least 15 patients, in whom distant metastases were discovered after inclusion in the study. This reduced the number of evaluated patients to 282. Another issue was increased mortality in the group treated with bisphosphonates. No explanation other than coincidence or the previously mentioned breaches in protocol was provided for this negative effect. In no other placebo-controlled study with bisphosphonates given as treatment for bone metastases was an increase in mortality reported, not even in patients treated for a long time. No biological-pharmacologic explanation for such an effect was suggested.

The third study, by Powles et al., which not only was a multicenter study but was double blind and placebo controlled,[48] is extremely interesting. In the end, 1076 patients with primary breast cancer with no other risks were evaluated. Also in this study, 1600 mg of clodronate versus placebo was used over 2 years. The study showed a significant reduction in bone metastases during 2 treatment years, but not after that time. However, a significant reduction in mortality was reported after a follow-up period (clodronate, n = 98; placebo, n = 129; P = .047) (Fig. 24-12). Powles et al. were able to show in their new analysis that patients with

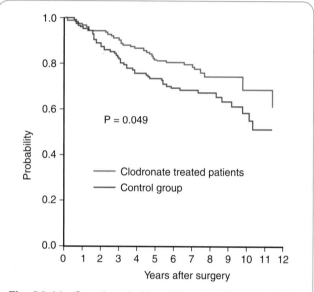

Fig. 24-11 Overall survival (m = 97 months). (Data from Diel IJ, Schuetz F, Jaschke A, et al.[45])

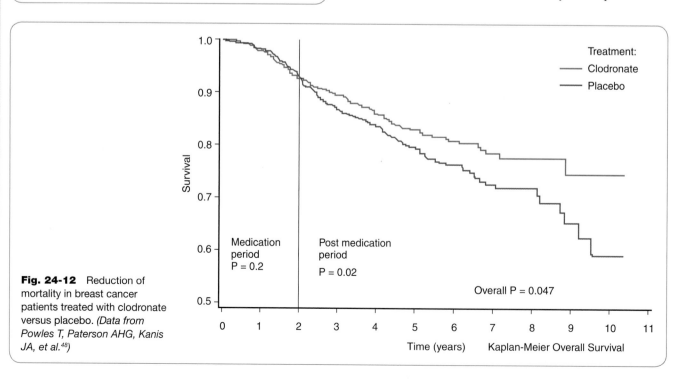

Fig. 24-12 Reduction of mortality in breast cancer patients treated with clodronate versus placebo. (Data from Powles T, Paterson AHG, Kanis JA, et al.[48])

high risk of relapse will benefit from adjuvant clodronate treatment.[49] When women with a good to very good prognosis were excluded from a subgroup analysis (stage I), and only patients in stages II and III were evaluated, the group treated with clodronate showed significant advantages in terms of survival free of metastases and total survival (Figs. 24-13 and 24-14). Among stage II patients, 20 women had to be treated to avoid bone metastases in 1 of them; in women with stage III, only 6; in women with stage 1, no advantage was assigned to treatment with clodronate (number needed to treat [NNT] for stages I–III). This result can be viewed as confirmation of findings of the Heidelberg study, into which exclusively high-risk women with tumor cells in the bone marrow were accepted.

In 2001, the National Surgical Adjuvant Breast and Bowel Project (NSABP) with the B-34 protocol published a fourth clodronate study (www.nsabp.pitt.edu), in which patients with primary breast cancer (although 75% were in stage I) were randomized and received 1600 mg of clodronate orally or placebo for 3 years, in addition to adjuvant systemic treatment. The recruiting process was already complete for this study (n = 3200). First results are expected in 2011. Another study (Southwest Oncology Group [SWOG] SO307) compared the efficacy of adjuvant clodronate, ibandronate, and zoledronate. The AZURE (Adjuvant Treatment with Zoledronic Acid to Reduce Recurrence) study investigated zoledronate given with longer administration intervals. Results of these clinical studies will finally explain whether normalization of bone metabolism leads to a reduction in later bone metastases, and whether an IV treatment interval leads to the same results as continuous oral bisphosphonate administration.

DEVELOPMENT OF ANTIBODIES AGAINST RANKL

Soon after discovery of the RANK/RANKL/OPG System in the mid 90s, the first recombinant proteins for inhibition of the signaling pathway were developed. The first clinical trials with OPG in postmenopausal women with osteoporosis showed a significant decline in the bone resorption marker with unaffected organic markers. This effect occurred quickly and effectively after subcutaneous injection of OPG.

However, the development of denosumab (AMG 162), which proved to be more effective in decreasing the resorption marker at a lower dose, led to the first systematic trials in people. Denosumab is a fully human monoclonal antibody against RANK-Ligand; it was generated by immunization of xenomice with human RANKL-protein. The immunoglobulin (Ig)G_2 antibody (AMG 162) has an extremely high affinity for human RANK-Ligand and does not bind to TNF or TRAIL (tumor necrosis factor–related apoptosis-inducing ligand).

The human antibody denosumab works similarly to osteoprotegerin (Fig. 24-15). This means that it interrupts the signal transfer to RANK on osteoclasts and to monocytic precursor

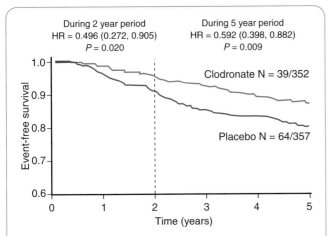

Fig. 24-13 Oral clodronate significantly reduces the incidence of bone metastasis (stage II/III disease). *(Data from Powles T, Paterson A, McCloskey E, et al.*[49]*)*

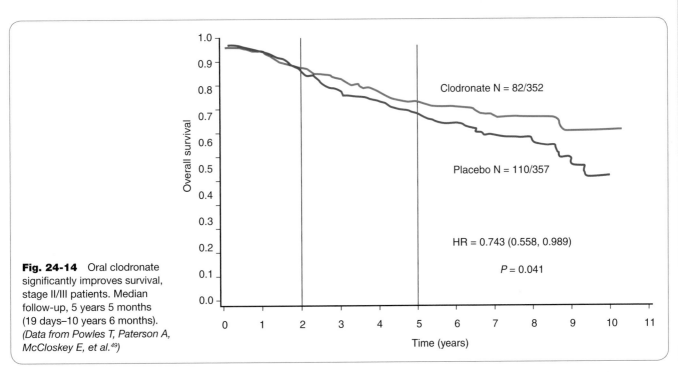

Fig. 24-14 Oral clodronate significantly improves survival, stage II/III patients. Median follow-up, 5 years 5 months (19 days–10 years 6 months). *(Data from Powles T, Paterson A, McCloskey E, et al.*[49]*)*

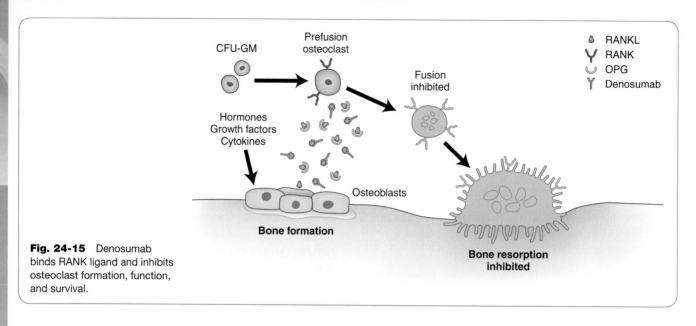

Fig. 24-15 Denosumab binds RANK ligand and inhibits osteoclast formation, function, and survival.

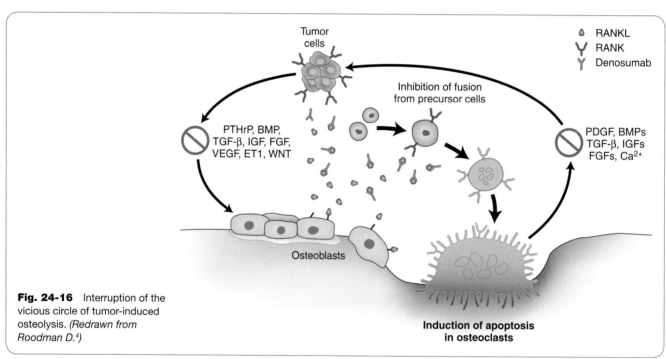

Fig. 24-16 Interruption of the vicious circle of tumor-induced osteolysis. *(Redrawn from Roodman D.[4])*

cells. In this way, fusion of osteoclasts is inhibited and inhibits the activity of mature polynuclear giant cells.[50,51] Through this mechanism of action, not only is the "vicious circle" of metastasis-induced bone destruction interrupted (Fig. 24-16), but bone resorption in primary and secondary osteoporosis is increased. Currently, 20,000 patients are being treated with denosumab in clinical studies. Most patients had nonmalignant diseases (osteoporosis, rheumatoid arthritis, among others). In oncology, phase I and II studies have been completed and published. The results on TTI (tumor-therapy-induced) osteoporosis have been published and/or presented at conferences. Approval studies (phase III) have ended in the meantime. Data on trials for the treatment of bone metastases have been evaluated and have been presented at conferences. The use of RANKL antibodies, such as denosumab, thus made sense in both metabolic and malignant bone diseases.

DOSE-FINDING STUDIES WITH DENOSUMAB IN ONCOLOGY

The first dose-finding study was published in 2006 by Body et al.[52] In this study, 29 patients with breast cancer with bone metastases and 25 patients with multiple myeloma after randomization received 0.1, 0.3, 1.0, or 3.0 mg/kg of denusomab SC (escalated or constant) or pamidronate 90 mg IV. Treatment success was measured by the reduction in serum and urine values of N-telopeptides. Results showed a decrease comparable with pamidronate but sustainable of bone resorption markers (84 days at the highest dose). The rate of side effects was less than that with pamidronate.

A second study published by Lipton et al.[53] pursued a similar concept with the goal of reducing bone resorption markers (uNTx/Cr) as surrogate parameters for osteoclast inhibition, but also for the appearance of skeletal complications (fractures, necessity for surgery, and radiation treatment among others). Patients with breast cancer with bone metastasis were included in the study (n = 255). After randomization, study participants were treated with 30, 120, or 180 mg denusomab (SC) every 4 weeks, or they received the drug in a dose of 60 or 180 mg every 12 weeks. In a third arm, patients received a standard osteoprotective treatment with an intravenously administered bisphosphonate (usually zoledronate or pamidronate). Treatment duration was 25 weeks, followed by a follow-up period of another 32 weeks.

Results of the reduction in urine telopeptides in the denosumab-treated group were comparable with those in the bisphosphonate group: 9% of patients had skeletal complications while on antibody treatment, but 16% while on bisphosphonate treatment. As a consequence of this study, the individual treatment dose for patients with skeletal metastases was set at 120 mg subcutaneously. In a third published study by Fizazi et al.,[54] the administration interval was especially addressed in the study design. Patients received the usual bisphosphonate treatment (n = 37) or denosumab (but 180 mg) every 4 weeks (n = 38) or every 12 weeks (n = 36). On the other hand, the degradation fragments from collagen metabolism (NTx/Cr) were surrogate markers for expected effectiveness in the urine. The results clearly showed that monthly administration led to significant suppression of bone metabolism in more patients than occurred in patients who received only the antibodies every 3 months. Both groups showed superiority compared with the bisphosphonate group, also regarding the speed of onset. This rapidly appearing effect can be easily explained because interruption of the signal pathway by RANKL antibodies is not tied to incorporation of the drug with osteoclasts (as with bisphosphonates). The outcome of cited phase II studies was establishment of the dose at 120 mg every 4 weeks in subsequent phase III studies.

Denosumab in the treatment of breast cancer with skeletal metastasis

In breast cancer with bone metastases, denusomab was tested in a phase III study at a dose of 120 mg subcutaneously every 4 weeks (n = 1026) against zoledronate 4 mg IV every 4 weeks (n = 1020). The target criterion was the reduction of skeletal complications in the respective treatment arms (primary: time to first SRE/noninferiority; secondary: time to first SRE [skeletal-related event] superiority and to first and subsequent SREs). After a median follow-up period of 17 months, the first analysis of study results was undertaken.[55] Patients who were treated with denusomab, in comparison with those who were treated with bisphosphonate, had significantly less frequent skeletal complications (hazard ratio [HR], 0.77; P = .001) and a longer interval until the appearance of the first event (HR, 0.82; P = .01) (Fig. 24-17). The superiority of the antibodies in the "multiple-event analysis" appeared especially clear when not only the first complications were evaluated, but also any subsequent ones. In the group treated with denusomab, only 474 events occurred, but in the group treated with zoledronate, 608 complications were evaluated (Fig. 24-18). However, no differences in overall survival were reported (HR, 0.95; P = .49). Assessment of side effects showed a decrease in the number of acute phase responses in patients on denosumab (10.4%), compared with those treated with zoledronate (27.3%). Also, renal complications occurred less often on antibody treatment (4.9%) in comparison with bisphosphonate treatment (8.5%). It was astonishing that the frequency of jaw necrosis in the denosumab group (2%) was similar and not significantly different from that observed in the bisphosphonate group (1.4%) (Table 24-3). This astonishment resulted from the fact that established theories about the development of osteonecroses until that point were heavily focused on the mechanism of action of bisphosphonates. The study at least showed prospectively for the first time that the incidence of jawbone osteonecrosis for the previously mentioned time period was between 1% and 2%.

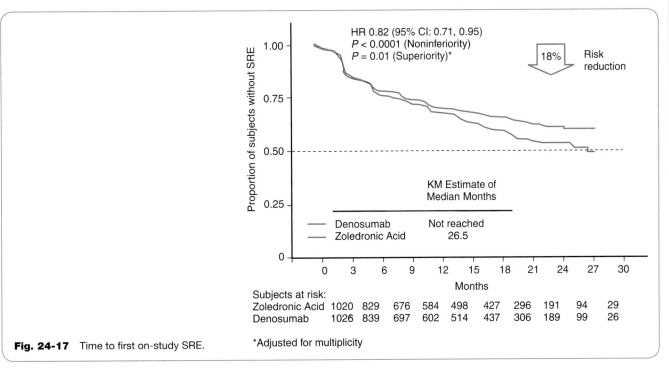

Fig. 24-17 Time to first on-study SRE.   *Adjusted for multiplicity

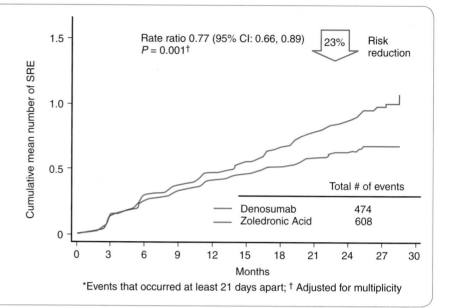

Fig. 24-18 Time to first and subsequent on-study SRE* (multiple-event analysis).

*Events that occurred at least 21 days apart; † Adjusted for multiplicity

Table 24-3 Adverse events

Event, n (%)	Zoledronic acid (N = 1013)	Denosumab (N = 1020)
Overall adverse events (AEs)	985 (97)	977 (96)
Serious AEs (SAEs)	471 (46)	453 (44)
Acute phase reactions*	277 (27.3)	106 (10.4)
Pyrexia	116 (11.5)	9 (0.9)
Bone pain	36 (3.6)	13 (1.3)
Chills	36 (3.6)	3 (0.3)
Arthralgia	32 (3.2)	15 (1.5)
Influenza-like disease	23 (2.3)	5 (0.5)
Myalgia	22 (2.2)	7 (0.7)
Flushing	3 (0.3)	0 (0.0)
Adverse events related to renal toxicity	86 (8.5)	50 (4.9)
SAEs related to renal toxicity	15 (1.5)	2 (0.2)
Osteonecrosis of the jaw (ONJ)†	14 (1.4)	20 (2.0)

*Within 3 days following investigational product administration.
†$P = .39$.

Denosumab for treatment of bone metastases in solid tumors and multiple myeloma (without breast and prostate cancer)

The study design and study goals were identical to those in the trial for breast cancer. A total of 886 patients received denosumab to reduce skeletal events, and 890 received zoledronic acid every 4 weeks. About 700 patients had non–small cell lung carcinoma (NSCLC), and 180 had multiple myeloma. The remaining 900 patients had various other tumor entities. Results with regard to the primary study goal were comparable with those seen with breast cancer.[56] In other words, the time until the first complication was lengthened by denosumab (HR, 0.84; $P = .0007$/noninferiority). But this was not the case for the secondary goal of superiority ($P = .06$; adjusted). The differences noted in research findings related to breast cancer can be explained by the great variety in the study population with respect to the original tumor and the relatively short survival time for patients with a diagnosis of lung cancer (NSCLC = 688; SCLC = 109). Also in this study, no significant differences in total survival and progress-free survival were observed. A similar picture is seen in the list of side effects and complications as in patients with breast cancer with bone metastasis. Among patients treated with zoledronate, 11 had jawbone osteonecrosis (1.3%), and among those treated with denosumab, 10 cases of jawbone osteonecrosis were documented (1.1%).

Denosumab for the treatment of bone metastases from prostate cancer

The results of the pivotal study for denosumab in the treatment of bone metastases due to prostate cancer were presented at the ASCO meeting 2010 in Chicago. In this trial, 1901 men with castrate-resistant prostate cancer and at least one proven bone metastasis were treated with denosumab (n = 950) or zoledronic acid (n = 951). Patients' characteristics were well balanced in both groups (e.g., age, ECOG status, previous skeletal events). First and second study objectives could be reached, comparable to the study in breast cancer patients. The superiority of denosumab compared with zoledronic acid could be shown both with regard to the time to first skeletal complication (HR 0.82; 95% CI 0.71; 0.95, reduction of the relative risk 18%), and up to the first and the following complication (HR 0.82; 95% CI 0.71; 0.94, RR reduction 18%). In the multiple event analysis for the denosumab-treated collective, 494 events were counted, and for the zoledronate-treated group, 585 events. As in the studies of patients with breast cancer and of patients with solid tumors and multiple myeloma, the survival times were the same for both treatment arms. Similar to the two other pivotal trials (breast and solid tumors), the incidence of cases with osteonecrosis of the jaw was not significantly different for both groups. In the antibody-treated group, 22 men were affected from this side effect; in contrast, only 12 men in the group treated with zoledronic acid were affected.[57]

CONCLUSION

In three large, randomized, comparative studies, denosumab showed significant improvement in reduction of skeletal events when compared with zoledronate in patients with breast cancer with bone metastases and with solid tumors/ multiple myeloma (and prostate cancer will be presented this year). Treatment with the antibody is accompanied by a decreased frequency of side effects, which is typical for treatment with zoledronic acid. No difference was noted in either group in the appearance of jawbone osteonecrosis—a seldom occurring but severe complication. Denusomab differs from bisphosphonates in its more rapid onset and in the rapid reversibility of its effects. Moreover, an advantage was seen with monthly subcutaneous injection over IV infusion treatment with bisphosphonates. In the future, denosumab could serve as a sensible addition to the arsenal used to treat bone metastases and may replace treatment with bisphosphonates over the long term.

REFERENCES

1. Mundy GR. Metastasis to bone: causes, consequences and therapeutic opportunities. *Nat Rev.* 2002;2:584–593.
2. Chambers AF, Groom AC, MacDonald IC. Dissemination and growth of cancer cells in metastatic sites. *Nat Rev.* 2002;2:563–572.
3. Roodman GD. Biology of osteoclast activation in cancer. *J Clin Oncol.* 2001;19:3562–3571.
4. Roodman GD. Mechanisms of bone metastasis. *N Engl J Med.* 2004;350:1655–1664.
5. Diel IJ, Seegenschmiedt H. Therapie von Skelettmetastasen. In: Schmoll H, Höffken K, Possinger K, HRSG. *Kompendium internistische Onkologie.* New York: Springer Verlag; 2005:994.
6. Diel IJ, Solomayer EF, Bastert G. Treatment of metastatic bone disease in breast cancer: bisphosphonates. *Clin Breast Cancer.* 2000;1:43–51.
7. Rodan GA, Fleisch H. Bisphosphonates: mechanisms of action. *J Clin Invest.* 1996;97:2692–2696.
8. Rogers MJ, Frith JC, Luckman SP, et al. Molecular mechanism of action of bisphosphonates. *Bone.* 1999;24:73S–79S.
9. Luckman SP, Hughes DE, Coxon FP, et al. Nitrogen-containing bisphosphonates inhibit the mevalonate pathway and prevent post-translational prenylation of GTP-binding proteins, including RAS. *J Bone Miner Res.* 1998;13:581–589.
10. Selander KS, Mönkkönen J, Karhukorpi EK, et al. Characteristics of clodronate-induced apoptosis in osteoclasts and macrophages. *Mol Pharmacol.* 1996;50:1127–1138.
11. Paterson AHG, Powles TJ, Kanis JA, et al. Double-blind controlled trial of oral clodronate in patients with bone metastases from breast cancer. *J Clin Oncol.* 1993;11:59–65.
12. Hortobagyi GN, Theriault RL, Porter L, et al. Efficacy of pamidronate in reducing skeletal complications in patients with breast cancer and lytic bone metastases. *N Engl J Med.* 1996;335:1785–1791.
13. Hortobagyi GN, Theriault RL, Lipton A, et al. Long-term prevention of skeletal complications of metastatic breast cancer with pamidronate. *J Clin Oncol.* 1998;16:2038–2044.
14. Theriault RL, Lipton A, Hortobagyi GN, et al. Pamidronate reduces skeletal morbidity in woman with advanced breast cancer and lytic bone lesions: a randomized, placebo-controlled trial. *J Clin Oncol.* 1999;17:846–854.
15. Lipton A, Theriault RL, Hortobagyi GN. Pamidronate prevents skeletal complications and is effective palliative treatment in woman with breast carcinoma and osteolytic bone metastases: long-term follow-up of two randomized, placebo-controlled trials. *Cancer.* 2000;34:2021–2026.
16. Ralston SH, Thiébaud D, Herrmann Z, et al. Dose-response study of ibandronate in the treatment of cancer-associated hypercalcaemia. *Br J Cancer.* 1997;75:295–300.
17. Body JJ, Diel IJ, Lichinitser MR, et al. Intravenous ibandronate reduces the incidence of skeletal complications in patients with breast cancer and bone metastases. *Ann Oncol.* 2003;14:1399–1405.
18. Diel IJ, Body JJ, Lichinitser MR, et al. Improved quality of life for long-term treatment with the bisphosphonate ibandronate in patients with metastatic bone disease due to breast cancer. *Eur J Cancer.* 2004;40:1704–1712.
19. Body JJ, Diel IJ, Lichinitser M, et al. Oral ibandronate reduces the risk of skeletal complications in breast cancer patients with metastatic bone disease: results from two randomized, placebo-controlled phase III studies. *Br J Cancer.* 2004;90:1133–1137.
20. Tripathy D, Lichinitser M, Lazarev A, et al. Oral ibandronate for the treatment of metastatic bone disease in breast cancer: efficacy and safety results from a randomized, double-blind, placebo-controlled trial. *Ann Oncol.* 2004;15:743–750.
21. Body JJ, Diel IJ, Bell R, et al. Oral ibandronate improves bone pain and preserves quality of life in patients with skeletal metastases due to breast cancer. *Pain.* 2004;111:306–312.
22. Major P, Lortholary A, Hon J, et al. Zoledronic acid is superior to pamidronate in the treatment of hypercalcemia of malignancy: a pooled analysis of two randomized, controlled clinical trials. *J Clin Oncol.* 2001;19:558–567.
23. Rosen LS, Gordon D, Kaminski M, et al. Zoledronic acid versus pamidronate in the treatment of skeletal metastases in patients with breast cancer or osteolytic lesions of multiple myeloma: a phase III, double-blind comparative trial. *Cancer J.* 2001;7:377–387.
24. Rosen LS, Gordon D, Kaminski M, et al. Long-term efficacy and safety of zoledronic acid compared with pamidronate disodium in the treatment of skeletal complications in patients with advanced multiple myeloma or breast cancer. *Cancer.* 2003;98:1735–1744.
25. Rosen LS, Gordon DH, Dugan W, et al. Zoledronic acid is superior to pamidronate for the treatment of bone metastases in breast carcinoma patients with at least one osteolytic lesion. *Cancer.* 2004;100:36–43.
26. Kohno N, Aogi K, Minami H, et al. Zoledronic acid significantly reduces skeletal complications compared with placebo in Japanese women with bone metastases from breast cancer: a randomized, placebo-controlled trial. *J Clin Oncol.* 2005;23:3314–3321.
27. Thiebaud D, Sauty A, Burckhardt P, et al. An in vitro and in vivo study of cytokines in the acute-phase response associated with bisphosphonates. *Calcif Tissue Int.* 1997;61:386–392.
28. De Groen PC, Lubbe DF, Hirsch LJ, et al. Esophagitis associated with the use of alendronate. *N Engl J Med.* 1996;335:1016–1021.
29. Marshall JK. The gastrointestinal tolerability and safety of oral bisphosphonates. *Expert Opin Drug Saf.* 2002;1:71–78.
30. Markowitz GS, Appel GB, Fine PL, et al. Collapsing focal segmental glomerulosclerosis following treatment with high-dose pamidronate. *J Am Soc Nephrol.* 2001;12:1164–1172.
31. Markowitz GS, Fine PL, Stack JI, et al. Toxic acute tubular necrosis following treatment with zoledronate (Zometa). *Kidney Int.* 2003;64:281–289.
32. Pfister T, Atzpodien E, Bauss F. The renal effects of minimally nephrotoxic doses of ibandronate and zoledronate following single and intermittent intravenous administration in rats. *Toxicology.* 2003;191:159–167.
33. Marx RE. Pamidronate (Aredia) and Zoledronate (Zometa) induced avascular necrosis of the jaws: a growing epidemic. *J Oral Maxillofac Surg.* 2003;61:1115–1117.
34. Ruggiero SL, Mehrota B, Rosenberg TJ, et al. Osteonecrosis of the jaws associated with the use of bisphosphonates: a review of 63 cases. *J Oral Maxillofac Surg.* 2004;62:527–534.
35. Felsenberg D, Hoffmeister B, Amling M, et al. Kiefernekrosen nach hoch dosierter Bisphosphonattherapie. *Dtsch Ärzteblatt.* 2006;103:A3078–3080.
36. Diel IJ, Fogelman I, Hoffmeister B, et al. Pathophysiology, risk factors and management of bisphosphonate-associated osteonecrosis of the jaw: is there a diverse relationship of amino- and non-amino-bisphosphonates? *Crit Rev Oncol.* 2007;64:198–207.
37. Diel IJ, Mundy GR. Bisphosphonates in the adjuvant treatment of cancer: experimental evidence and first clinical results. *Br J Cancer.* 2000;82:1381–1386.
38. Paterson AHG. The role of adjuvant therapy with bisphosphonates in cancer. *Am J Cancer.* 2004;3:25–39.

39. Yoneda T, Michigami T, Yi B, et al. Actions of bisphosphonate on bone metastasis in animal models of breast carcinoma. *Cancer.* 2000;88:2979–2988.

40. Mundy G. Bisphosphonates as anticancer drugs. *Exp Opin Invest Drugs.* 1999;8:2009–2015.

41. Elomaa I, Blomqvist C, Porkka L, et al. Clodronate for osteolytic metastases due to breast cancer. *Biomed Pharmacother.* 1988;42:111–116.

42. Kanis JA, Powles TJ, Paterson AHG, et al. Clodronate decreases the frequency of skeletal metastases in women with breast cancer. *Bone.* 1996;19:663–667.

43. Diel IJ, Solomayer EF, Costa SD, et al. Reduction in new metastases in breast cancer with adjuvant clodronate treatment. *N Engl J Med.* 1998;339:357–363.

44. Diel IJ. Bisphosphonates in the prevention of bone metastases: current evidence. *Semin Oncol.* 2001;28:75–80.

45. Diel IJ, Schuetz F, Jaschke A, et al. Adjuvant oral clodronate improves the overall survival of primary breast cancer patients with micrometastases to the bone marrow—a long term follow-up. *Ann Oncol.* 2008;19:2007–2011.

46. Saarto T, Blomqvist C, Virkkunen P, et al. Adjuvant clodronate treatment does not reduce the frequency of skeletal metastases in node-positive breast cancer patients: 5-year results of a randomized controlled trial. *J Clin Oncol.* 2001;19:10–17.

47. Saarto T, Vehmanen L, Virkkunen P, et al. Ten-year follow-up of a randomized controlled trial of adjuvant clodronate treatment in node-positive breast cancer patients. *Acta Oncol.* 2004;43:650–656.

48. Powles TJ, Paterson AHG, Kanis JA, et al. Randomized, placebo-controlled trial of clodronate in patients with primary operable breast cancer. *J Clin Oncol.* 2002;20:3219–3224.

49. Powles T, Paterson A, McCloskey E, et al. Reduction in bone relapse and improved survival with oral clodronate for adjuvant treatment of operable breast cancer. *Breast Cancer Res.* 2006;8:1–7.

50. Lacey DL, Timms E, Tan HL, et al. Osteoprotegerin ligand is a cytokine that regulates osteoclast differentiation and activation. *Cell.* 1998;93:165–176.

51. Hofbauer LC, Heufelder AE. Role of receptor activator of nuclear factor-kappa B ligand and osteoprotegerin in bone cell biology. *J Mol Med.* 2001;79:243–253.

52. Body JJ, Facon T, Coleman RE, et al. A study of the biological receptor activator of nuclear factor-kappa B ligand inhibitor, denusomab, in patients with multiple myeloma or bone metastases from breast cancer. *Clin Cancer Res.* 2006;12:1221–1228.

53. Lipton A, Steger GG, Figueroa J, et al. Randomized active-controlled Phase II study of denusomab efficacy and safety in patients with breast cancer-related bone metastases. *J Clin Oncol.* 2007;25:4431–4437.

54. Fizazi K, Lipton A, Mariette X, et al. Randomized Phase II trial of denosumab in patients with bone metastases from prostate cancer, breast cancer, or other neoplasms after intravenous bisphophonates. *J Clin Oncol.* 2009;27:1564–1571.

55. Stopeck AT, Lipton A, Body JJ, et al. Denosumab compared with zoledronic acid for the treatment of bone metastases in patients with advanced breast cancer: a randomized double-blind study. *J Clin Oncol.* 2010;10;28:5132–5139.

56. Henry D, von Moos R, Vadhan-Raj S, et al. A double-blind, randomized study of denosumab versus zoledronic acid for the treatment of bone metastases in patients with advanced cancer (excluding breast and prostate cancer) or multiple myeloma. *Eur J Cancer.* 2009;(suppl 7):20.

57. Fizazi K, Carducci M, Smith M, et al. Denosumab compared with zoledronic acid for the treatment of bone metastases in patients with castrate-resistant prostate cancer. *J Clin Oncol.* 2010;(suppl 18):LBA 4507.

MANAGEMENT OF COMPLICATIONS IN THE PALLIATIVE SETTING

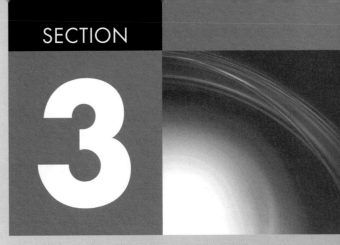

SECTION OUTLINE

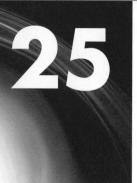

25 Management of nausea and vomiting in patients with advanced cancer*

Paul A. Glare and Tanya Nikolova

Nausea and vomiting not occurring as side effects of chemotherapy or radiation therapy represent a prevalent and complex multicausal problem in patients with advanced cancer, are associated with high levels of distress, and significantly impair quality of life.[1,2] The primary method of treatment is pharmacologic. Current practice recommends antiemetic drug selection based on three factors: (1) the presumed cause of the nausea, (2) knowledge of the neuropharmacology of the emetogenic pathways, and (3) matching the supposed emetogenic stimulus with the drug most likely to block that stimulus.[3] However, because the emetic pathway is complex, because often no cause is identifiable or multiple causes are operating, and because many antiemetics work on multiple receptors, this approach has its detractors who prefer empirical prescribing of broad-spectrum agents. The aim of this chapter is to review the status of these two approaches in this changing field and to review nonsurgical interventions in patients with inoperable cancer and obstructive nausea and vomiting.

DEFINITIONS OF NAUSEA AND VOMITING IN ADVANCED CANCER

A prerequisite to the assessment and treatment of nausea and vomiting is being clear on the definitions of these and related terms, which are often poorly understood and used incorrectly.[4]

Nausea is an entirely subjective experience defined simply as "the sensation (or sensations) that immediately precede vomiting." Patients state that they feel as if they are about to vomit, or they use such terms as "queasy" or "sick to the stomach."

*Other than chemotherapy/radiation therapy–induced emesis.

Vomiting, in contrast, is a highly specific physical event, defined as "the rapid, forceful evacuation of gastric contents in retrograde fashion from the stomach up to and out of the mouth." Vomiting usually, but not always, is preceded by nausea. Nausea is followed by retching—repetitive active contraction of the abdominal musculature—which generates a pressure gradient that leads to evacuation of stomach contents, the most clearly recognized component of vomiting. Retching may occur in isolation without discharge of gastric contents from the mouth; this is referred to as "dry heaves." It is important to emphasize that vomiting is a complex physiologic process that includes both involuntary and voluntary components.

Unlike retching and vomiting, regurgitation is a passive process that consists of the retrograde flow of esophageal contents into the mouth. Acid regurgitation, for example, is a cardinal symptom of gastroesophageal reflux. Regurgitation also occurs with esophageal obstruction and dysphagia.

Rumination, a phenomenon that may easily be confused with vomiting, is the effortless regurgitation of recently ingested food into the mouth, followed by re-chewing and re-swallowing or spitting out. This passive phenomenon is not preceded by nausea and does not include the various physical events associated with vomiting. It is a type of eating disorder that typically begins within minutes of a meal, is usually repetitive, and is rarely associated with retching.

Dyspepsia is a vague term, most commonly defined as chronic or recurrent pain or discomfort centered in the upper abdomen.[5,6] Two types of dyspepsia have been distinguished: structural (acid-related) and functional (dysmotility-related). Nausea and vomiting may be associated with dyspepsia but are not central to its definition. Nausea is the symptom most commonly reported by patients with functional dyspepsia. Functional dyspepsia may be associated with cancer (cancer-associated dyspepsia syndrome [CADS]).[7] Early satiety and postprandial fullness are other features of dyspepsia.

INCIDENCE, PREVALENCE, AND CHARACTERISTICS OF NAUSEA AND VOMITING IN ADVANCED CANCER

Nausea and vomiting are common problems in advanced cancer, affecting some 33% of individuals, ranging from 16% to 60% across various studies of seriously ill patients.[8–10] In one study, where 50% of patients had nausea and/or vomiting, 62% had both, 34% had isolated nausea, and 4% had isolated vomiting.[11]

Similar to pain, nausea is progressive in advanced cancer, present in 36% upon entering a palliative care service,[12–14] in 62% at 1 to 2 months before death,[15,16] and in 71% in the final week of life.[17,18] Although nausea and vomiting have been reported to affect only 14% during the last few days of life,[19–21] these reports may underestimate its true prevalence, as dying patients with deteriorating cognitive and physical status may be unable to report such symptoms reliably.[22] In fact, although 32% of patients experienced nausea on admission to a palliative care unit, 98% developed nausea requiring treatment at some time during admission (average length of stay, 25 days).[23] Studies have also reported a curvilinear relationship between nausea and performance status, with nausea reported to be highest when a Karnofsky rating (on a scale from 0–100) is 40, decreasing as performance status declines.[24] The presence of nausea in patients with advanced cancer has been associated with shortened survival.[25]

Reports vary with regard to severity, frequency, and distress caused by nausea and vomiting in advanced cancer. One study reported that 25% of patients admitted to a tertiary palliative care unit had nausea ratings >50 on a 0 (none) to 100 (worst possible) scale.[26] A longitudinal study of advanced cancer patients admitted for pain treatment reported that on average, patients experienced nausea on about one quarter of assessment days,[27] but in a palliative care unit, nausea was present all or most of the time in 45% of cases. A large Australian study of almost 3000 consecutive patients from five inpatient and community palliative care services found that 20% had reported the presence of nausea sometime during the past week.[28] An additional 600 patients unable to provide a self-report had nausea reported by caregiver proxies in 21% of cases. A subset of those experiencing nausea used a numeric rating scale (0 = no nausea to 10 = extreme nausea) to report mean average nausea scores during the past 24 hours of 3.03 (standard deviation [SD] = 2.67) and mean worst nausea scores of 4.12 (SD = 3.38). More than 40% rated the impact of nausea on general activity and emotional well-being in the past week at >5 on a similar scale. For most, the experience of nausea was chronic, and patients had experienced nausea for a median of 7 weeks (range, 1–468 weeks).[28]

Similar to pain,[29] nausea and vomiting are said to be frequently undertreated; in an older U.S. study, only one third of patients with nausea were prescribed antiemetics.[30] More recently, an audit of the symptom profile of 82 advanced cancer patients admitted to an Australian teaching hospital found an improved situation, with nausea reported in 26 (32%) respondents, antiemetics prescribed in 52 (68%) respondents, and antiemetics taken by 32 (39%) respondents. However, paradoxically, patients reporting moderate to severe nausea often missed out on treatment, underscoring the need for greater attention to the education of hospital staff in assessment and treatment of nausea.[31]

CAUSES OF NAUSEA AND VOMITING IN PATIENTS WITH CANCER

Multiple causes may be implicated in the development of nausea in advanced cancer, and for a number of patients, these factors may coexist. Experienced clinicians are able to identify a cause in approximately two thirds to three quarters of cases.[11,32,33] The taxonomy used for classifying causes of pain in patients with cancer—tumor, side effect of therapy, debilitation, and/or an unrelated comorbid condition—can be applied equally to nausea and vomiting. An abbreviated list is shown in Table 25-1. Certain demographic and clinical factors predict the development of nausea in supportive care patients, whatever the cause. These include female gender[34]; age younger than 65 years[34]; specific tumor types such as gynecologic, stomach, esophageal, and breast cancers[14]; the presence of metastases in the lung, pleura, or peritoneum[35]; gastrointestinal symptoms such as local pathology or intestinal obstruction[36]; and opioid medication.[27]

Table 25-1 Assessment of the advanced cancer patient with nausea and vomiting

History

  Quality: nausea, vomiting, retching, regurgitation

  Duration

  Persistent or intermittent

  Intensity

  Associated vomiting, nature of vomitus, relief from vomiting

  Associated pain, altered bowel habit

  Aggravating factors: sight/smell of food, worse after eating, movement

  Temporal factors: worse in morning

  Relieving factors (e.g., vomiting)

  Drug history: opioids, NSAIDs, antibiotics

  Anticancer treatment

Physical examination

  Abdomen: organomegaly, other masses, bowel sounds (ileus or mechanical obstruction), rectal examination

  Other: signs of sepsis, metabolic abnormalities (liver failure, renal failure, hypercalcemia), neurologic signs

Investigations

  Radiology: AXR, CT scan/MRI

  Laboratory tests: sepsis, renal failure, hypercalcemia

AXR, Abdominal X-ray; *CT,* computed tomography; *MRI,* magnetic resonance imaging; *NSAIDs,* nonsteroidal antiinflammatory drugs.

ASSESSMENT OF NAUSEA IN PATIENTS WITH CANCER

When nausea and vomiting are assessed in the patient with advanced cancer, four concurrent goals are pursued: (1) to clarify whether the problem is nausea, vomiting, or regurgitation; (2) to determine the cause, which may be treatable/reversible; (3) to document intensity, frequency, and associated distress; and (4) to direct the choice of antiemetic therapy. Although the clinician makes a comprehensive assessment of nausea and vomiting, the patient should be the prime assessor of intensity and distress caused by it, if he or she is well enough to do so. As is the case with pain, caregivers may underestimate and family members may overestimate the severity of nausea.[37-39] If possible, an objective measure of nausea, based on the patient's self-report, should be obtained with a tool such as the Memorial Symptom Assessment Schedule, the Edmonton Symptom Assessment Scale, or the McGill Nausea Scale.[40-42]

It is always important to remember that symptoms of advanced cancer such as nausea are more than monodimensional physical problems. The psychological, social, and spiritual effects of the symptom also need to be addressed. Cognitive, emotional, sociocultural, and physical factors can alter pain tolerance, and it is likely that the same applies to nausea. What is bearable to one person may be intolerable to another. It is important to distinguish between the intensity of nausea and how much distress it causes. It has been noted that the proportion of patients who describe a symptom as intense or frequent tends to be greater than the proportion reporting the symptom as distressing.[41] A psychosocial evaluation is a key part of the patient assessment.[43]

The patient history is the cornerstone when the causes of nausea and vomiting are elicited, with the putative mechanism being supported by a focused physical examination and review of any relevant data (e.g., recent blood work and imaging). The psychosocial assessment completes the evaluation (Table 25-2).

The history aims to (1) clarify whether nausea, vomiting, and regurgitation are occurring together or in isolation; (2) rule out associated problems such as reflux, gastric irritation, and constipation; and (3) review the home medication list. The history should include sentinel details that aid in determination of the causative mechanism, such as the following:

- Intermittent nausea associated with early satiety and postprandial fullness or bloating, relieved by vomiting that usually is small volume, occasionally is forceful, and may contain food (suggesting gastroparesis)
- Intermittent nausea associated with crampy abdominal pain and altered bowel habit, relieved by vomiting that may become large volume and bilious or feculent (suggesting bowel obstruction)
- Persistent nausea, aggravated by the sight and smell of food, unrelieved by vomiting (suggesting that chemical causes are activating the chemoreceptor trigger zone)
- Early morning nausea and vomiting associated with headache (suggesting raised intracranial pressure)
- Nausea aggravated by movement, including motion sickness or even just turning the head (suggesting vestibular component)
- Anxiety associated with nausea and vomiting (suggesting a cortical component)

The importance of regularly reassessing nausea and the effects of antiemetics and other treatment strategies cannot be overemphasized. The timing of reassessment depends on individual circumstances, but ideally the patient who requires antiemetic drugs should be reevaluated at least every 24 hours until the symptom is controlled, then less frequently to ensure that control is maintained. Recurrence or exacerbation of the symptom may require a full reevaluation of the nausea, as discussed earlier. As for cancer pain, sudden severe nausea, especially if associated with vomiting, should be recognized by all professional caregivers as a medical emergency, and the patient should be assessed without delay.

BARRIERS TO NAUSEA ASSESSMENT

For nausea to be accurately assessed and thereby appropriately managed, caregivers must be aware of the complexities of, and barriers to, effective nausea assessment. These include the subjective nature of nausea and its associated distress, underestimation of the importance of nausea and vomiting by caregivers, the lack of a clearly defined language of nausea, and communication barriers between caregivers and patient, but these have not been studied as they have for pain.[44]

OUTCOMES OF COMPREHENSIVE NAUSEA ASSESSMENT

As mentioned previously, a cause can be identified in most patients, and more than one cause has been identified in 15% to 25% cases.[11,33] The most common cause tends to be impaired gastric emptying (occurring in 35%–45% of patients), followed by chemical causes (30%–40%) and bowel obstruction (10%–30%).[11,33] Other causes shown in Table 25-1, such as raised intracranial pressure or vestibular changes, occurred in <15% of cases in these series.

NAUSEA AND SYMPTOM CLUSTERS

Because patients with advanced cancer often experience multiple symptoms, nausea and vomiting rarely occur in isolation. Symptom clusters are defined as two or more concurrent symptoms that are related and may or may not have a common cause. In the cancer patient, nausea can be a part of a constellation of symptoms with a common origin. For example, nausea will occur, along with abdominal discomfort, anorexia, early satiety, postprandial fullness, bloating, and/or constipation, in patients with gut dysmotility due to peritoneal disease. The clinical importance of this is that if a patient is nauseated, then concurrent problems such as constipation need to be ruled out or treated, and in anorectic patients, nausea should be evaluated and treated with the aim of improving intake.

It has been observed that certain cancer symptoms frequently occur together with no obvious common cause, and those symptoms can independently predict changes in patient function, treatment failure, and post-therapeutic outcomes. A review of early studies of symptom clusters in inpatients or those with early-stage cancers, or a single cancer type or metastatic site, found a gastrointestinal cluster consisting of nausea and vomiting as the only cluster common to two of the studies.[45] The severity of this cluster increased when patients were treated with chemotherapy. Method disparities with regard to assessment tools used, statistical analyses performed, and populations studied hampered this review. A study exploring symptom clusters among 1336 outpatients with different advanced cancers attending the Oncology Palliative Care Clinics at Princess Margaret Hospital from January 2005 to October 2007 found that the three most distressing symptoms were fatigue, poor general well-being, and decreased appetite.[46] Two major symptom clusters were identified, one of which included nausea with fatigue, drowsiness, decreased appetite, and dyspnea. Within the various primary cancer sites, differences in the pattern of symptom clusters were seen. Cancer symptom cluster research is still in its infancy, but multiple symptoms clearly affect prognosis, quality of life, and functional status. Treatments directed at symptom clusters rather than at individual symptoms may provide greater therapeutic benefit.

APPROACHES TO THE PHARMACOLOGIC TREATMENT OF NAUSEA IN PATIENTS WITH CANCER

As mentioned in the Introduction, two different approaches are used to select drugs to treat nausea and vomiting in advanced cancer: mechanistic and empirical. The mechanistic approach is taught by most specialists in supportive and palliative care, and aims to identify the cause of a symptom and remove it if possible. Even in patients with advanced, incurable cancer, a reversible cause for nausea and vomiting may be identifiable, for example, when it is due to drug toxicity, bowel obstruction, constipation, or hypercalcemia. When the cause is irreversible, or while waiting for cause-specific treatment to take effect, a variety of pharmacologic and nonpharmacologic

Table 25-2 Causes of nausea and vomiting in terminally ill cancer patients

Syndrome	Examples
Gastric stasis	Cancer-related • Carcinoma of stomach • Hepatomegaly or ascites ("squashed stomach") • Paraneoplastic neuropathy Treatment-related • Drug-induced (e.g., opioids) Comorbidities • Dyspepsia • Gastritis (including drug-related, e.g., NSAIDs) • Diabetic gastroparesis
Biochemical	Cancer-related • Hypercalcemia • Liver metastases • Obstructive uropathy • Bowel obstruction • "Toxins" (anorexia-cachexia syndrome) Treatment-related • Drugs: opioids, chemotherapy Comorbidities • Organ failure • Infection • Drugs: antibiotics, SSRIs
Raised intracranial pressure	Cancer-related • Brain tumor • Cerebral secondary • Meningeal disease
Vestibular	Cancer-related • Cerebral secondary Treatment-related • Drugs (e.g., opioids) Comorbidities • Motion sickness, vestibular problems
Bowel obstruction/ dysmotility	Cancer-related • Bowel, primary • Intra-abdominal secondary (e.g., peritoneal disease) • Ascites Treatment-related • Adhesions Debility • Constipation
Other	• Anxiety

NSAIDs, Nonsteroidal antiinflammatory drugs; *SSRIs,* selective serotonin reuptake inhibitors.

methods are available to alleviate sensations of nausea and suppress the urge to vomit. Pharmacologic agents are chosen according to our current understanding of the neuropharmacology of the so-called "emetic pathway."[47] The main impetus for investigating the structures and receptors involved in this pathway has been the problem of nausea and vomiting caused by highly emetogenic chemotherapy agents such as cisplatin. Although the chemotherapy-induced emesis (CTIE) paradigm is quite different from that of chronic nausea, the results of this basic scientific research have been applied to the management of drug selection for nausea in advanced cancer.

Structures involved in the pathway include the stomach, bowel, and vagus nerve and several structures in the central nervous system (CNS). These CNS structures include (1) the chemoreceptor trigger zone (CTZ), located in the floor of the fourth ventricle outside the blood-brain barrier, (2) the vestibular nucleus, (3) the vomiting center, located in the medulla, and (4) the cerebral cortex. These CNS structures contain large numbers of receptors for one or more of the specific neurotransmitters that are believed to carry emetic messages from the periphery, around the pathway, and back to the periphery again. These neurotransmitters include (but may not be restricted to) dopamine, serotonin, histamine, acetylcholine, and the endogenous opioids.

Drug selection for controlling nausea and vomiting is based on blockade of receptors in the structure on which the cause of the nausea and vomiting is acting. The receptors at which the various drugs are known to work are shown in Table 25-3. This mechanistic approach to antiemetic drug selection is a complex process that requires integration of multiple sources of basic science (knowledge of the emetic pathway and its neuropharmacology) and clinical acumen (the putative cause, inferred from elicited symptoms and signs, and review of laboratory and imaging results).

Thus, the mechanistic approach may be perceived as arcane, the cause is often unidentifiable or multifactorial, and, as indicated in Table 25-3, many available drugs act on multiple receptors. Therefore, an empirical approach, which dispenses with the complexities of the emetogenic pathway and makes drug selection arbitrary, is now being advocated by some palliative care experts, and fits more closely with current practice in oncology. Serotonin antagonists and lorazepam are often prescribed in this way for chronic nausea. The effectiveness of mechanistic and empirical approaches to prescribing antiemetics has been evaluated, with similar rates of nausea control achieved by both. No study has directly addressed the question of whether one approach is superior to the other. Toxicity of antiemetics is rarely reported in supportive care studies.

Three uncontrolled studies of the mechanistic approach involving some 200 heterogeneous episodes found that symptoms were controlled in 60% to 90% cases, and residual symptoms were generally mild.[11,33,48] A number of other studies (controlled and uncontrolled) that looked at specific syndromes such as CADS and opioid-induced nausea (OIN) also support utilizing a mechanistic approach. On the other hand, three randomized trials and one uncontrolled trial in North America and Europe have evaluated the empirical approach.[7,23,49,50] These studies are difficult to synthesize, and none was placebo-controlled; metoclopramide (at standard low doses) was effective in 30% to 40% of cases. Other agents, including a dopamine antagonist (in one out of two studies) and a serotonin antagonist (in one study), were superior.

In summary, consistent evidence from observational studies indicates that the mechanistic approach is highly effective,[33,48] although this type of study design is prone to bias. These studies were carried out in palliative care units (PCUs) by experts, and in approximately 20% of cases involved drugs not available in the United States (e.g., cyclizine, methotrimeprazine). It does not appear to matter whether an algorithm is used when drugs are prescribed on the basis of the mechanism.

Drug toxicity is a frequent cause of nausea and vomiting in patients with advanced cancer, and OIN is a dose-limiting side effect of opioid therapy in approximately one third of cases. OIN can be approached in various ways. Providing antiemetic cover until tolerance develops has been the traditional approach. Opioids may cause nausea through a variety of mechanisms, including gastric stasis and activation of the CTZ. Consequently, a prokinetic agent or an antidopaminergic drug would usually be prescribed. In patients in whom vomiting is present that may preclude the adequate absorption

Table 25-3 Receptor site affinities of commonly used antiemetics

Drug	Dopamine antagonist	Histamine antagonist	Acetylcholine (muscarinic) antagonist	5-HT$_2$ antagonist	5-HT$_3$ antagonist	5-HT$_4$ agonist
Chlorpromazine	dark gray	dark gray	light gray	light gray		
Cisapride						Black
Cyclizine		dark gray	dark gray			
Domperidone	dark gray					
Haloperidol	Black					
Hyoscine			Black			
Levomepromazine	dark gray	Black	dark gray	Black		
Metoclopramide	dark gray				dark gray	dark gray
Ondansetron					Black	
Prochlorperazine	dark gray	light gray				
Promethazine	dark gray	Black	dark gray			

Adapted from references 53, 85, and 169.
Key: Black, High affinity for receptor; *dark gray,* moderate affinity; *light gray,* low affinity; *white,* no known affinity.

of oral medications, agents need to be made available by non-oral routes. In recent years, the availability of a variety of strong opioids in a range of formulations and doses as an alternative to morphine has meant that opioid rotation is another alternative to prescribing antiemetics for OIN.[51]

DRUGS FOR TREATING NAUSEA AND VOMITING
Prokinetic agents

In patients with nausea and dyspepsia, gastric stasis and/or delayed gastric emptying is likely to occur, and prokinetic agents are the drugs of first choice. These agents stimulate the motility of the upper gastrointestinal tract in various ways: by activating the cholinergic system in the gut wall, by releasing acetylcholine from enteric neurons via activation of $5-HT_4$ receptors, by blocking $5-HT_3$ receptors,[52,53] by activating the motilin receptor,[54] or by releasing the dopaminergic "brake" on gastric emptying.[55] The prokinetic effects of these agents will be blocked by agents with antimuscarinic properties (e.g., antihistamines), so these agents should not be prescribed together. Prokinetic agents should not be used when stimulation of muscular contractions might adversely affect the gut, for example, in complete bowel obstruction, in gastrointestinal hemorrhage and perforation, or immediately post surgery.

PHARMACOLOGY OF PROKINETIC AGENTS

Metoclopramide activates $5-HT_4$ receptors, antagonizes $5-HT_3$ receptors, and antagonizes central and peripheral D_2 receptors to release the "dopamine brake." It works on the stomach and proximal small bowel but has little effect on colonic motility. The pharmacokinetics of metoclopramide and of most other antiemetics discussed in this chapter is summarized in Table 25-4.

The dose of metoclopramide for gastroparesis is 10 mg given 3 to 4 times daily PO/IV, a half hour before meals and at bedtime (maximum daily dose, 100 mg). The pediatric dose is 0.1 mg/kg/dose given every 6 to 8 hours PO/IV/SC.[56] At high doses (10 mg every 6 hours PO/IV, or 0.5–1 mg/kg/dose PO/IV in children), metoclopramide is also a central D_2 antagonist, similar to haloperidol (see next section). Dose reductions are recommended in moderate to severe renal impairment (50% decrease with creatinine clearance [CrCl] of 10–40, with 75% reduction if <10)[57,58] and in the elderly. The most common side effects are restlessness, drowsiness, and fatigue. Extrapyramidal symptoms (EPSs), including acute dystonic reactions and tardive dyskinesia, may occur. Acute reactions are dose-related but are most troublesome in children and young adults. Pretreatment with diphenhydramine is recommended when high-dose metoclopramide is used in these populations.[56] Metoclopramide carries a Food and Drug Administration (FDA) black box warning regarding tardive dyskinesia, which is related to the duration of treatment and the cumulative dose. Administration beyond 12 weeks is not recommended. Metoclopramide should be avoided in patients taking sirolimus or tacrolimus, as metoclopramide may increase their absorption, leading to toxicity. It does not appear to interact with standard chemotherapies.

Unfortunately, alternative prokinetic agents to metoclopramide are currently limited. Cisapride is more potent than metoclopramide and is able to increase the motility of the entire length of the gastrointestinal tract.[59-61] It is a pure $5-HT_4$ receptor agonist that is devoid of any D_2 antagonist activity.[53] It had to be withdrawn from the U.S. market 10 years ago because of problems with corrected QT interval (QTc) prolongation[62,63] and other arrhythmias, aggravated by the fact that it was prone to many drug interactions via CYP3A4 that increased its blood levels.

Domperidone is a dopamine antagonist that does not readily cross the blood-brain barrier (BBB),[64] so it acts only at peripheral dopamine receptors to release the "dopaminergic brake." Because it does not act centrally, EPSs are much less likely with domperidone than with metoclopramide. The doses are similar to those of metoclopramide at 10 to 20 mg 3 or 4 times daily PO. In children, the dose is 0.2 to 0.4 mg/kg/dose every 6 hours PO, but it is not commonly used in pediatrics. Parenteral domperidone is not available, having been withdrawn in the 1980s because of the risk of cardiac toxicity.[65] Sulpiride is a dopamine blocker used for some psychotic and other psychiatric disorders. It also has prokinetic properties, but a pharmacologic profile that is somewhat different from metoclopramide and domperidone, and has been studied in patients with advanced cancer and dyspeptic symptoms.[66] Itopride is a new D_2 antagonist with anti-acetylcholinesterase effects. None of these drugs is available in the United States.

Erythromycin has recently emerged as a potential gastrointestinal prokinetic agent. Research into the mechanism of the well-recognized gastrointestinal side effects of erythromycin demonstrated that erythromycin increases gastrointestinal motility via stimulation of the receptor for the upper gastrointestinal peptide motilin.[54] $5-HT_3$ receptors may also be involved in this process.[67] The dose is 250 mg 3 times daily PO (the suspension has better kinetics than the tablet form) or 250 to 500 mg/t.i.d. IV. Aside from its effects on the GI tract, the adverse effects of erythromycin include impaired hepatic function and QTc prolongation. For this reason, it should be avoided in patients on certain tyrosine kinase inhibitors (e.g., dasatinib, imatinib, lapatinib, sunitinib) and the immunosuppressants tacrolimus and sirolimus. No renal dose adjustment is needed. It has also been suggested that mirtazapine may have prokinetic properties.[68]

EVIDENCE FOR EFFICACY OF PROKINETICS IN CHRONIC NAUSEA OF ADVANCED CANCER

Two small, placebo-controlled trials have investigated the effectiveness of metoclopramide.[7,69] The results are conflicting, as one study showed it was superior for CADS,[7] the other that it was not for OIN.[69] A randomized trial of empirical use of levosulpiride versus metoclopramide found that levosulpiride was superior and effective in approximately 80% of cases.[66] Erythromycin has been shown to be effective in non-malignant conditions such as diabetic gastroparesis,[70] but evidence for its use in advanced cancer is limited. It is effective in patients undergoing subtotal gastrectomy, with significant improvement in gastric half-emptying time and increased clustered waves resembling a migrating motor complex (MMC).[71] However, in patients who had total gastrectomy, no improvement was noted in jejunal half-emptying or MMCs. Nor does erythromycin appear to alter clinically important outcomes related to postoperative ileus,[72] including patients undergoing resection for colorectal cancer.[73]

Table 25-4 Pharmacokinetics of selected antiemetic drugs

Drug	BA(%)	Onset, hours	T_{max}, hours	$t_{1/2}$, hours	Duration, hours
Chlorpromazine[170]	10-69	–	PO: 2-4 IM: 0.5-1	8-35	>24
Cisapride[61]	40-50	0.5-1	1-2	7-10	12-16
Cyclizine[171]		<2	2.0	7, 24	4-6
Dexamethasone[109]	61-86	8-24	1-2	4	36-54
Domperidone[55,64,172,173]	13-17	0.5	0.5	7.5-16	8-16
Haloperidol[87]	60-65	PO: >1 SC: 0.15-0.25	PO: 1.7-6 IM: 0.3-0.5	14-36	–
Hyoscine butylbromide[173]	8-10	PO: 1-2 SC: 0.25-0.5	–	5-6	–
Hyoscine hydrobromide[174]	N/A	SL: 0.15-0.25	0.15-0.5	5-6	0.25-10
Levomepromazine[96]	50	0.5	PO: 1-3 IM 0.5-1.5	15-30	12-24
Metoclopramide[175]	32-100	IV: 0.01-0.05 IM: 0.15-0.25 PO: 0.5-1	<1	4-6	1-2
Octreotide[176,177]	N/A		<0.5	1.5	8-12
Olanzapine[178]	60-80		PO: 5-8 IM: 0.25-0.75	21-54	
Prochlorperazine[179,180]	12.5		1.5-5	6.8-9	
Promethazine[181,182]	25		PO: 2-3	10-14	4-12
Serotonin antagonists					
• Dolasetron[183,184]	76		IV: 0.6 PO: 1.4	6.6-8.8	
• Granisetron[185]	60		PO: 2	10-12	
• Ondansetron[186-188]	60-70		IV: 0.1 PO: 0.5-2	2.5-5.4	
• Palonosetron[189,190]	N/A			40	
• Tropisetron[75,76]	60-100		PO: 1-1.3	8-40	

$t_{1/2}$, Half-life; T_{max}, time to maximum concentration.

BA, oral bioavailability.

5-HT₃ receptor antagonists (5-HT₃-RAs)

The 5-HT$_3$-RAs appear to exert their antiemetic effects via blockade of 5-HT$_3$ receptors both peripherally, on the enterochromaffin cells of the enteric nervous system, and centrally, in the nucleus tractus solitarius and the CTZ.[74] The 5-HT$_3$-RAs block the amplifying effects of serotonin (also known as 5-HT) on the vagal nerve, which feeds into the emetic center. Because these agents work centrally and peripherally, are familiar to oncologists, and have few clinically important drug interactions with chemotherapeutic agents or side effects, they are widely used in U.S. supportive oncology as first-line antiemet-

ics. On the other hand, in United Kingdom–based palliative care algorithms, 5HT$_3$-RAs are generally reserved as third-line agents for refractory cases, primarily because they are nonformulary on account of cost. 5-HT$_3$-RAs have also been shown to be effective in bowel obstruction and renal failure, both of which are also associated with excess 5-HT release.

PHARMACOLOGY

Four 5-HT$_3$-RAs are available in the United States: ondansetron, granisetron, dolasetron, and palonosetron. Doses for ondansetron in chronic nausea are 4 to 8 mg given once or twice a day in adults, and 0.15 mg/kg/dose every 8 hours PO/

IV (max 8 mg/dose) in children.[56,75,76] Side effects of these agents are usually mild and transient, with constipation being the main problem in palliative care patients.[77] All 5-HT$_3$-RAs are metabolized by cytochrome P450 isoenzymes, although the extent of metabolism and the specific isoenzymes involved differ for each drug. This has potentially clinically significant implications for patients receiving multiple medications. The 5-HT$_3$-RAs may decrease the efficacy of tramadol. They should be used with caution with drugs that prolong the QTc interval. In severe hepatic impairment, the maximum dose is 8 mg/day.[78]

It is noteworthy that several other antiemetics have activity at serotonin receptors. Metoclopramide is a weak 5-HT$_3$-RA and a 5-HT$_4$ agonist (for its prokinetic effect). Cisapride is a more potent 5-HT$_4$ agonist than metoclopramide without 5-HT$_3$ antagonist activity. Olanzapine has activity at 5-HT$_{2A}$, 5-HT$_{2c}$, and 5-HT$_3$. The antidepressant mirtazapine also works as a 5-HT$_3$-RA.[68] Levomepromazine is a potent 5-HT$_2$ antagonist but has no activity at the 5-HT$_3$ (or 5-HT$_4$) receptor. Anecdotal experience from the United Kingdom indicates that 5-HT$_2$ antagonism is important for controlling nausea.

EVIDENCE FOR USE OF 5-HT$_3$-RAs IN ADVANCED CANCER

Although high-level evidence is available for the use of 5-HT$_3$-RA agents in chemotherapy-induced emesis,[79] evidence of benefit for refractory nausea in palliative and supportive care is less strong.[50,69,80] Two randomized trials have investigated the use of 5-HT$_3$-RAs in advanced cancer.[50,69] One was an international, multicenter study comparing ondansetron 24 mg/day, metoclopramide 10 mg 3 times daily, and placebo in 90 patients with advanced cancer with OIN.[69] No significant differences were noted between any of the treatment groups, and treatment with metoclopramide and ondansetron was no more effective than placebo; partial control of nausea was achieved in 48% of patients on ondansetron, in 52% of patients on metoclopramide, and in 33% of patients on placebo. Ondansetron was more effective than placebo (48% vs. 33%) for emesis (less so for nausea), but the difference was not significant. The other randomized trial compared tropisetron (not available in the United States) with conventional antiemetics (metoclopramide and chlorpromazine) for any cause of nausea and found that tropisetron was much more effective than the other agents. No clinical trials have investigated these agents in chronic nausea of advanced cancer, but one case series of ondansetron showed rigorous outcome assessment for its efficacy as a second-line agent.[81]

Dopamine receptor antagonists

Control of nausea and vomiting through stimulation of the CTZ by chemical or toxic events such as hypercalcemia, renal failure, and drug toxicity may be achieved by inhibiting the dopamine type 2 (D$_2$) receptors found there. Phenothiazines and other antipsychotics (haloperidol, olanzapine) are used for this purpose; their antiemetic effects are proportionate to their antidopaminergic activity.[82] These agents also exhibit some prokinetic activity via blockade of peripheral dopamine receptors to release the dopaminergic "brake" on gastric emptying and are used in malignant bowel obstruction (MBO).

PHARMACOLOGY OF THE D$_2$ ANTAGONISTS

Prochlorperazine is a phenothiazine derivative with a broad spectrum of activity, so it causes sedation, hypotension (by alpha-1-adrenergic blockade), and anticholinergic side effects, although not to as great an extent as chlorpromazine.[83] Prochlorperazine also produces vagal blockade in the gastrointestinal tract. The antiemetic dose of prochlorperazine is 5 to 10 mg 3 to 4 times daily orally, 25 mg 2 to 3 times per day rectally, or 5 to 10 mg every 3 to 4 hours intramuscularly or IV (to a maximum of 40 mg daily). In children, the dose is 0.2 mg/kg/dose every 8 to 12 hours PO/slow IV (maximum, 15 mg/day),[84] but it is not commonly used as an antiemetic in pediatric palliative care, especially in children younger than 2 years of age.

In supportive oncology, prochlorperazine and the other D$_2$ antagonists should be avoided in patients on tyrosine kinase inhibitors because of their additive effects on QTc prolongation. Prochlorperazine should be avoided in patients with absolute neutrophil count (ANC) <1000 because of the risk of neutropenia. Reduced doses are recommended in the elderly, and a black box warning gives notice about precipitating psychosis in demented patients. Caution is advised in those with hepatic impairment, and dose reduction is also recommended. Extrapyramidal symptoms (EPSs) are uncommon with prochlorperazine. Other risks include neuroleptic malignant syndrome and respiratory depression. General precautions include epilepsy, glaucoma, and prostate hyperplasia.

Haloperidol is a more potent and competitive blocker of postsynaptic D$_2$ receptors than prochlorperazine.[85] It is widely used in palliative care as an antiemetic, although very little evidence supports its efficacy for this purpose,[86] and it is not FDA-approved for this purpose. Antiemetic doses are lower than antipsychotic doses: 1.5 to 5 mg 2 or 3 times daily PO or 1 to 2 mg every 8 to 12 hours SC/IV, or 2 to 10 mg per day via continuous subcutaneous infusion (CSCI). In pediatric nausea, 0.01 to 0.05 mg/kg/day PO/IV/SC or via CSCI (max 0.15 mg/kg/day) is recommended.[84] As with the phenothiazines, QTc prolongation and agranulocytosis are also risks with haloperidol. It is less likely to cause sedation or hypotension than the phenothiazines, but it causes more EPSs. Other side effects include the neuroleptic malignant syndrome. Caution and dose reduction are recommended in patients with severe hepatic impairment. Haloperidol is a substrate of CYP3A4 and an inhibitor and stimulator of CYP2D6, but this appears to be of little clinical significance.[87] Coadministration of carbamazepine, phenytoin, phenobarbital, rifampicin, or quinidine may affect the clinical pharmacokinetics of haloperidol.

Chlorpromazine is a phenothiazine with broad-spectrum (D$_2$, histamine [H$_1$], alpha-1-adrenergic, and cholinergic [M$_{1-5}$]) receptor antagonist properties.[85] The usual antiemetic dose is 10 to 25 mg every 4 to 6 hours orally or 25 to 50 mg 4 to 6 times per day IV. In children, the dose is 0.5 to 1 mg/kg/dose every 4 to 6 hours PO/IV (max 40 mg/day in children <5 years, 75 mg/day in children 5 to 12 years), although it is not commonly used in pediatric populations.[84] Dose reduction should be considered in patients with liver dysfunction and in the elderly. Dose-limiting sedation is a problem but may be useful in a distressed, dying patient. Other side effects, including confusion, respiratory depression, EPSs, and anticholinergic effects, are common. Similar to all phenothiazines, it may affect the QTc interval and the white count and may lower seizure thresholds.

Olanzapine is an atypical antipsychotic with high affinity for multiple dopamine (D_1, D_2, D_4), serotonin (5-HT$_{2A}$, 5-HT$_{2C}$, 5-HT$_3$), alpha-1-adrenergic, H_1, and M_{1-5} receptors.[88,89] It has been used as an antiemetic in palliative care.[90] Olanzapine does not cause QTc prolongation at conventional doses but has been reported to do so at high doses.[91] It may affect the white count. It causes fewer EPSs than other antipsychotics[92,93]; the main side effects are somnolence and weight gain. Dry mouth, constipation, increased appetite, agitation, hyperglycemia, and edema have also been reported.[93] The antiemetic dose of olanzapine in adults is 2.5 to 10 mg/day PO. Dosing is not established in children, although it has been used in adolescents.[56]

Levomepromazine is available in the United Kingdom and Australia, but it is no longer available in the United States. A broad-spectrum phenothiazine (antagonist at D_2, H_1, alpha-1-adrenergic, M_{1-5}, and 5-HT$_2$ but not 5-HT$_3$ receptors), it is utilized as second- or third-line therapy for refractory nausea and vomiting in British palliative care.[94] Compared with chlorpromazine, it is said to produce more analgesia[95] but is more sedative and more likely to cause postural hypotension.[94] The dose is 6.25 to 25 mg twice a day, or 25 to 50 mg/day, via CSCI. Levomepromazine has limited data available for use in pediatrics, but doses of 0.25 to 1 mg/kg/dose given once to twice daily PO/IV/SC (max 25 mg/24 hours) or 0.1 to 0.4 mg/kg/day via CSCI (max 12.5 to 25 mg/24 hours, depending on age) have been used. Anticholinergic effects, confusion, hallucinations, and dystonic reactions are rare. It may prolong the QT interval and should be administered cautiously in patients with renal or hepatic impairment.[96]

EVIDENCE FOR USE OF ANTIDOPAMINERGIC DRUGS IN CHRONIC NAUSEA OF ADVANCED CANCER

Although haloperidol is frequently used by palliative care physicians for nausea or vomiting, systematic reviews in 2001 and again in 2009 found no randomized controlled trials of haloperidol for this purpose in this population, and were successful in retrieving only case reports and case series.[86,97] Randomized controlled trials have investigated the use of haloperidol in postoperative nausea and vomiting and gastrointestinal disorders, and as prophylaxis against nausea and vomiting associated with radiotherapy and chemotherapy. A recent meta-analysis calculated that the number needed to treat (NNT) for haloperidol 2 mg to prevent postoperative nausea or vomiting compared with placebo was 4,[98] although it is unclear how these studies apply to supportive oncology populations. Haloperidol was part of the therapeutic platform in a randomized controlled trial of steroids for MBO,[99] and data are available from uncontrolled trials of various agents, including haloperidol, using the mechanistic approach.[33,48] Where outcome data are available, haloperidol is effective in approximately 80% of cases.[33,48]

Supportive care data for other dopamine antagonists are even more limited. In a large randomized controlled trial of empirical prescribing of various drug combinations,[50] the chlorpromazine-containing combinations were effective only 20% to 30% of the time. No data are available for the use of prochlorperazine in advanced cancer of various causes, although old studies showed it to be significantly less effective than high-dose metoclopramide for CTIE.[100] Two small cases series, with subjective outcome assessment, consistently indicate that olanzapine appears to be effective in refractory

cases.[101] In an uncontrolled trial of the mechanistic approach, some 12% received levomepromazine first-line, apparently successfully; another two patients were switched to it when they did not respond to other agents.[33] In case series, it was effective in 60% to 80% cases.[37,102]

Antihistaminic agents (promethazine, cyclizine)

Only the first generation of piperazine class H_1 antagonists appear to be antiemetic, and they work by blocking H_1 receptors in the vomiting center of the medulla,[103] the vestibular nucleus, and the CTZ.[104] These agents may also have variable antimuscarinic activity, blocking the cholinergic receptors on intestinal muscle fibers.[55] This results in decreased tone and peristalsis of gut smooth muscle and counteracts the effects of prokinetic drugs such as metoclopramide.[105] The antimuscarinic activity also reduces mucosal secretory activity, which is helpful in bowel obstruction.

PHARMACOLOGY OF ANTIHISTAMINE ANTIEMETICS

Promethazine is widely prescribed for motion sickness and vestibular disorders; it also can help with raised intracranial pressure. It has little anticholinergic activity. The antiemetic dose is 12.5 to 25 mg PO/IV every 4 to 6 hours (maximum 100 mg/day). The pediatric dose is 0.125 to 0.5 mg/kg/dose every 6 hours PO/IV (maximum 25 mg/dose).[84] The main side effect is sedation, although tolerance usually develops quickly. Dizziness, EPSs, headache, and anticholinergic effects may occur and may lower seizure threshold. Caution is advised in patients with cardiovascular disease, severe hypertension, respiratory compromise, impaired hepatic function, and epilepsy. Anecdotal evidence suggests that promethazine theoclate (Avomine) is well tolerated and causes less drowsiness than promethazine maleate (Phenergan). Other H_1 antagonists (e.g., diphenhydramine, dimenhydrinate, hydroxyzine, meclizine, cyclizine [not available in the United States]) are mentioned in palliative care guides, and all have similar side effects to promethazine. They vary in their muscarinic activity, and those with more antimuscarinic activity (e.g., cyclizine) may be useful for bowel obstruction.[106] Although prochlorperazine is mainly a dopamine antagonist, it also has some antihistamine activity and may be effective for mild cases of nausea due to a vestibular mechanism.

EVIDENCE FOR ANTIHISTAMINE DRUGS IN NAUSEA OF ADVANCED CANCER

Few data are available. No randomized controlled trials have addressed the role of any of the antihistamines as antiemetics in advanced cancer.[107] In an uncontrolled trial of the mechanistic approach, 5% to 10% of episodes of nausea were treated with cyclizine as the initial drug, apparently all successfully.[33] No other data on its use have been acquired, or for promethazine (maleate or theoclate), diphenhydramine, and dimenhydrinate as antiemetics in advanced cancer.

Other agents
CORTICOSTEROIDS

Steroids have been studied mainly as second-line agents in chemotherapy-induced emesis, in the treatment of nausea and vomiting associated with MBO,[79,108] and in the treatment of symptomatic raised intracranial pressure. They are also used as second-line agents in chronic nausea of advanced cancer.[23] The mechanism of action of steroids as an antiemetic is unknown, but several have been postulated, including depleting gamma-aminobutyric acid (GABA) stores in the medulla, reducing the permeability of the BBB to emetic toxins, and inhibiting brainstem enkephalin release.[103]

Pharmacology of steroids

The effects and toxicities of corticosteroids, including skin, soft tissue, musculoskeletal, renal, cardiovascular, endocrine, psychiatric, gastrointestinal, and hematologic effects, are extensive and have been well described.[109] Caution is needed in diabetic patients and in patients with a psychiatric history, as well as perioperatively. Corticosteroids may be contraindicated in patients on chemotherapy because of the risk of sepsis or masking a fever. If they are to be continued long term, prophylactic cotrimoxazole should be considered. The recommended antiemetic dose is of dexamethasone 4 to 8 mg/day for chronic nausea and up to 16 mg/day for MBO or raised intracranial pressure. In children, the dose is 10 mg/m^2 PO/IV daily (max 20 mg/dose), increasing two- to fourfold for raised intracranial pressure (max daily dose 40 mg). Because treatment may be long term, the lowest possible dose should be used for the briefest period, with withdrawal or reduction considered when maximal effect has been obtained, an adequate trial (approximately 7–10 days) has failed to achieve the desired effect, or side effects occur.

Evidence for steroids in nausea

A meta-analysis found that in bowel obstruction, IV dexamethasone 6 to 16 mg/day showed a nonsignificant trend to hasten resolution of MBO. No impact on survival was seen at 1 month.[8] Only anecdotal evidence reveals the benefit of steroids in chronic nausea due to nonspecific causes in terminal cancer.[103] In the previously mentioned randomized controlled trial of multiple drug combinations,[50] steroid-containing combinations with metoclopramide and chlorpromazine were effective in <20% cases. However, an uncontrolled trial of metoclopramide found that 75% of cases were controlled when steroids were added as second-line agents.[23]

BENZODIAZEPINES

Although short-acting benzodiazepines such as lorazepam and alprazolam are widely administered to nauseated patients,[72] they are only minimally effective as antiemetics. However, they can be particularly useful when anxiety is associated with nausea and vomiting. Their efficacy may be derived from their sedative, anxiolytic, and amnesic properties, which enhance the effectiveness of antiemetic regimens and prevent the development of anticipatory emesis.

NEUROKININ-1 (NK-1) ANTAGONISTS

Substance P and its receptor NK-1 have been implicated in the emetic pathway,[47] and are located in the CTZ and brainstem. Thus NK-1 antagonists represent a new class of antiemetics, with aprepitant being the first one developed.[110] The addition of aprepitant to standard antiemetic therapies for CTIE significantly improves emesis protection in general and, in particular, in the delayed phase.[47] It is effective only when given orally (125 mg/day 1, 80 mg/days 2–3),[111] although its prodrug fosaprepitant now provides an injectable form. It is generally well tolerated, but many potential drug interactions occur through its effects on CYP3A4 and CYP 2C9 metabolism.[111] Other NK-1 antagonists in the pipeline include casopitant,[112] netupitant, and vestipitant. Use of aprepitant for chronic nausea of advanced cancer has not been reported, but neurokinin receptor antagonists may become relevant in palliative care in the future, as substance P and the other tachykinins are also implicated in pain and depression pathways.[113,114]

HYOSCYAMINE

Anticholinergic agents such as hyoscyamine (hyoscine) are used in the medical management of terminal bowel obstruction. By blocking muscarinic receptors, they may reduce gastrointestinal (GI) secretions, thereby relieving nausea and reducing volumes of vomitus. Because they are antispasmodic, they may also relieve colicky pain. The dose of hyoscine butylbromide for this purpose is 80 to 120 mg daily via CSCI (0.5 mg/kg/dose every 6–8 hours PO/SC/IV in children, max 20 mg/dose). The dose of hyoscine hydrobromide is 0.6 to 2.4 mg daily via CSCI or 0.25 to 0.4 mg every 6 hours SC/IV. Toxicities are those of anticholinergic agents.

OCTREOTIDE

This somatostatin analog is used to treat bowel obstruction and may assist with associated nausea and vomiting through a variety of mechanisms, but primarily by reducing the volume of bowel secretions.[115] The dose used is 100 mcg SC 3 times daily or 100 to 600 mcg via CSCI; in pediatrics, the dose is 1 mcg/kg/dose every 8 to 12 hours IV/SC, max 50 mcg/dose. The long-acting depot version may also be used. The most common side effects are local skin reactions (pain, stinging, burning) and gastrointestinal effects. Use with caution in patients with diabetes mellitus, renal failure, and hepatic impairment.

CANNABINOIDS

At a time when more U.S. states are legalizing "medical marijuana," the reality is that little evidence supports the efficacy of cannabinoids in nausea and vomiting. Data are available for their use in CTIE and the anorexia-cachexia syndrome,[116] but no studies have evaluated cannabinoids as antiemetics for the chronic nausea of advanced cancer—only a few case reports have described their use.[117] Short duration of action and side effects are a major problem of current formulations, especially in the elderly, who make up the majority of the supportive care and palliative patient population.

NOVEL PROKINETIC AGENTS

These agents, including ghrelin receptor antagonists, may work in the upper GI tract to improve nausea and vomiting.[118] Activators of CIC-2 chloride channels such as lubiprostone (approved in the United States for idiopathic constipation, but frequently causing nausea as a side effect) and guanate cyclase receptor activators are expected to work only in the lower GI tract.[118]

OTHER MODES OF NAUSEA CONTROL

The application of general measures and specific non-pharmacologic interventions is essential for the good management of cancer pain and cannot be replaced by pharmacologic approaches. Similarly, for nausea, the pharmacologic approaches recommended in this chapter are not meant to be used in isolation and need to be combined with these other approaches for optimal symptom control to be achieved. A range of environmental and psychological factors contribute to the experience of nausea in the terminally ill patient. Although evidence supporting the efficacy of nonpharmacologic approaches in managing nausea is limited, avoidance of environmental stimuli such as sights, sounds, or smells that may initiate nausea has been recommended.[119] It is suggested that fatty, spicy, highly salted food should be avoided, but few published studies have reported on the effectiveness of dietary modification or supplements in reducing nausea. A study of fish oil supplements provided to patients with advanced cancer reported no significant effects on nausea, appetite, or tiredness.[120]

Mixed evidence has been gathered regarding the effect of behavioral approaches, such as relaxation and distraction, on nausea in advanced cancer. Theoretically, these approaches may decrease psychological arousal and distress by refocusing the patient's attention on something else, or they may act as a distracter and increase the patient's feeling of control over symptoms.[121] Relaxation training utilizing progressive muscle relaxation and guided imagery has been successful in reducing nausea and vomiting for patients experiencing chemotherapy-induced emesis and related anxiety in some studies,[122,123] but not in others.[124] Massage has been reported to be effective for nausea and pain in bone marrow transplant patients.[125] Few studies have investigated these therapies in the chronic nausea of advanced cancer unrelated to anticancer treatment. Foot massage was shown to significantly reduce nausea in hospitalized cancer patients.[126]

Similar to behavioral therapies, a systematic review of complementary and alternative medicine (CAM) for symptom management at the end of life found that no large-scale trials have been done in terminally ill patients with nausea and vomiting that is not associated with chemotherapy.[127] Acupuncture and ginger have been shown to be effective for chemotherapy-induced emesis and anticipatory nausea,[128,129] but they have not been evaluated in the nausea of far advanced disease.

NONSURGICAL PROCEDURES IN PALLIATION OF CANCER-RELATED NAUSEA AND VOMITING

Many patients with advanced malignancies, especially those with gastrointestinal cancers, have nausea and vomiting due to GI obstruction but are not candidates for surgery and/or do not respond to pharmacologic measures. Although some patients prefer to die without tubes,[130] palliation of nausea and vomiting in this population may be achieved more quickly and effectively via draining percutaneous gastrostomy tubes, gastrointestinal stents and other endoscopic techniques, and gastric electrical stimulation. Progress in interventional gastroenterology makes these approaches less risky and burdensome than they used to be.

Draining percutaneous endoscopic gastrostomy (PEG) tubes

The first use of PEG tubes for decompression purposes was described in 1987.[131] PEG tubes were initially considered only as a means for enteral feeding and as a substitute for surgical gastrostomy.[132] PEG tube placement is a safe procedure for alleviation of nausea, vomiting, and abdominal distention, as well as pain, in a setting of MBO in a certain subset of patients. Three percent of all advanced cancers lead to MBO. Ovarian cancer is probably the most common (5%–42% of all cases of MBO), followed by colorectal cancer (10%–28%).[133,134] Other malignancies that may be typically complicated by MBO include endometrial, cervical, and primary peritoneal cancer. Some 25% to 50% patients with ovarian cancer will experience at least one episode of MBO.

Nasogastric tubes (NGTs) have been used as an alternative to PEG tubes for decompression. Their major disadvantages are the risk of frequent displacement, poor tolerance, and restrictions in ambulation and daily routine activities. NGTs can cause various complications such as aspiration, hemorrhage, gastric erosion, alar necrosis, and sinusitis or otitis. Placement of NGTs is less invasive, but this modality should not be used over an extended period of time.

Selecting appropriate patients for surgical intervention versus palliative decompressive PEG placement sometimes is difficult. In selected patients (e.g., those with gynecologic malignancies), surgery can prolong life, with median survival being almost 12 months in comparison with less than 4 months for patients who are not surgical candidates.[135] In cases of previous laparotomies, including surgery for prior MBO, diffuse intraperitoneal metastasis with multiple areas of obstruction, and advanced stage of the disease with very short life expectancy, the usual approach is not surgical but rather other palliative measures, such as PEG placement.[136]

The most common approach in the use of gastrostomy tubes is to place them endoscopically, thus the name PEG tubes. It has been reported that in 18% to 35% of placements, sonographic, fluoroscopic, or computed tomography (CT) guidance has been used.[137] In those circumstances, the tubes are technically called percutaneous radiographic gastrostomy (PRG) tubes. Data in the literature regarding which approach has a higher success rate and a lower rate of complications are conflicting. The average procedural time for endoscopic placement of gastrostomy tubes is significantly shorter, equivalent to half the time required for PRG tube placement (24 minutes vs. 53 minutes).[138]

The success rate of PEG placement is very high, ranging from 89% to 100%.[139–142] One of the most comprehensive studies involved 94 patients with MBO in a setting of ovarian cancer.[139] In those cases, 100% of the patients had successful PEG placement, mean age was 56 years, and mean length of time from cancer diagnosis to PEG placement was approximately 3 years. Ninety-one percent reported symptomatic improvement after a mean of 1.7 days before they reported resolution of nausea and vomiting. All patients reported symptomatic relief by day 7 post PEG placement. Additional data from this study showed mean hospital stay after the procedure of 6 days and median overall survival of 8 weeks, and most patients (88%) died at home or in an inpatient hospice facility. Only three patients continued to be unable to tolerate the diet; most patients were able to take sips, liquids, or a soft diet after

PEG placement with and without the tube being clamped. The authors of this study suggested that only the presence of liver metastasis and age older than 55 years were predictors of a shorter life span.

PEG tube maintenance is relatively simple but does require education of the patient and his or her informal caregivers. Initially, the tube is placed to gravity, but within a short time, the patient can be started on an oral diet, which usually consists of liquids or a pureed or soft diet, depending on tolerance. Instructions on frequent water flushes, clamping of the tube, emptying of the bag, and basic wound care are given before the patient is discharged to home. In cases of nausea or vomiting, the PEG tube should stay open to gravity until symptoms resolve. If a PEG tube becomes dislodged, the patient should be brought back to the hospital.

The complication rate of PEG tubes has been summarized in a review of seven studies involving almost 300 patients. The major complication rate was on average 0.33% and included peritonitis (from severe gastric leakage or gastropexy breakdown) and intraperitoneal hemorrhage.[143] In the largest series included in the review, major and minor complications of PEG placement affected 18% of patients, with half of them (9%) complaining of leakage.[139] The prevalence of ascites was high (63%). To prevent possible leakage from a PEG tube, almost a quarter of the patients with ascites underwent preprocedural paracentesis with removal of 2.8 L of ascitic fluid. Other reported complications in this series included peristomal infection, tube obstruction, tube migration, and wound bleeding.

In summary, placement of draining PEG tubes in patients with MBO relieves nausea and vomiting, allows patients to restart and enjoy an oral diet, and presents a safe way of treating patients' distress while facilitating discharge to home or inpatient hospice. In a small study, patients were interviewed using the Symptom Distress Scale before and 7 days after PEG placement. Sixty-four percent of patients reported improvement in nausea, vomiting, intestinal motility, insomnia, weakness, mood, and concentration.[144] This series included only 25 patients; therefore, larger and well-designed studies would be beneficial to document the real degree of quality-of-life improvement after PEG placement.

Gastrointestinal stenting and other endoscopic techniques

Malignant esophageal, gastroduodenal, and colonic partial or complete obstruction is frequently complicated by nausea and vomiting. Blockage of the lumen may occur directly or by extrinsic compression.

Less than 10% of patients with esophageal cancer have a prognosis of 5 years or longer, making palliative management of dysphagia and vomiting a priority in the treatment plan. Some of the endoscopic methods used in treatment of obstructing esophageal cancer include alcohol injection, laser therapy, argon plasma coagulation, photodynamic therapy, and esophageal stent placement.

Injection of alcohol into the cancer tissue is considered a very simple and cost-effective method of de-obstructing the esophageal lumen.[145,146] Laser therapy has a success rate of 75% to 91%.[147,148] A randomized, controlled trial comparing the effectiveness of alcohol injections versus laser therapy found that alcohol injection and laser treatment provided similar durations of relief from dysphagia symptoms (30 days vs. 37 days).[149] The equipment used for delivering laser light is as expensive as stenting, which makes the modality less frequently used nowadays.[150]

Self-expandable metallic stents (SEMSs) can be placed to treat luminal obstruction of the gastrointestinal tract in patients who are not candidates for a surgical intervention (e.g., patients with tumor growth into adjacent organs, distant metastasis, or multiple comorbidities). Multiple studies have shown the advantages of SEMSs compared with rigid plastic stents.[151–155]

Self-expanding plastic stents (SEPSs) have been used in palliation of esophageal obstruction. They have complex composition with polyester monofilaments and silicone, which facilitates food ingestion and prevents stent migration. Their effectiveness has been reported in several studies. Migration rate ranges from 6% to 25%. Repeat interventions were warranted in approximately 25% of cases. This failure of the stent was attributed to tumor overgrowth or stent migration.[156–158]

Gastric outlet obstruction (GOO) can be found in a setting of pancreatic, ampullary, or gastric cancer, as well as cholangiocarcinoma. GOO is associated with vomiting undigested food hours after eating. For treatment of gastric outlet obstruction due to malignancy from all endoscopic modalities, alcohol injection and laser therapy have a role. The most common nonsurgical method by far is enteral stent placement. Enteral stents are very similar to esophageal metal stents. They are permanent devices composed of metal mesh. Some of the complications that may occur after their placement include malfunctioning due to tumor overgrowth in 17% of patients; migration in 5% of cases; and bleeding and perforation in less than 1% of patients.[159] It is important to mention that GOO is frequently associated with biliary tract obstruction. In this scenario, simultaneous placement of a biliary stent and an enteral stent is recommended. Placement of an enteral stent only in such cases would limit access to the papilla and prevent biliary stent placement at a later stage.

Malignant large-bowel obstruction is frequently a life-threatening presentation of very advanced malignancy of the colon or rectum. Patients usually have significant abdominal distention associated with abdominal pain, nausea, and vomiting, including vomiting of feculent material. Nonsurgical methods for palliation include colonic decompression tubes, laser therapy, argon plasma coagulation, and self-expanding metal stents.

Colonic decompression tube placement is often used to provide air (and not necessarily stool) passage in patients who need clinical stabilization before surgery.[160] The stents used for large-bowel obstruction are SEMSs. Studies that compared SEMSs versus surgery have shown that the benefits of SEMS placement include decreased length of hospitalization and reduced costs.[161,162]

Gastric electrical stimulation

Gastroparesis is associated with symptoms and evidence of delayed gastric emptying, in the absence of any mechanical obstruction.[163] Gastroparesis is one of the commonly underdiagnosed conditions in cancer patients, causing chronic nausea and vomiting. The condition is associated with delayed emptying of solids, especially those containing fibers. In those circumstances, the formation of bezoar can lead to mechanical gastric outlet obstruction.[164] The prevalence of malignancy-associated gastroparesis has yet to be established, but it is frequently found among patients with tumors of the upper GI tract. As many as 60% of patients with pancreatic cancer have evidence of gastroparesis.[165] The causes of malignancy-associated gastroparesis are usually mixed. Some of the most common underlying factors include paraneoplastic autonomic dysfunction, tumor-infiltrating celiac plexus or vagal nerve, previous GI surgery, toxic effects of chemotherapy or radiation, and side effects of medications (especially opioids).[166] Usual pharmacologic treatment of gastroparesis involves a combination of prokinetic and antiemetic agents.

Gastric electrical stimulation (GES) is a relatively new treatment for gastroparesis refractory to medical treatment. GES provides series of electrical pulses with a constant current or a constant voltage. Two methods of GES are known: gastric pacing (high-energy/low-frequency stimulation) and neurostimulation (low-energy/high-frequency stimulation). Both methods have been shown to improve the symptoms of gastroparesis.[167] A meta-analysis was performed on 13 studies with data on high-frequency GES (neurostimulator) and showed their substantial benefits.[168] The studied population (265 patients) included diabetic and postsurgical patients. Post-GES measures demonstrated a significant benefit for both nausea and vomiting severity scores. Device removal and/or replacement due to complications was reported in 8.3% of cases. Those complications included infections, erosion through the skin, pain at the implantation site, perforation of the stomach by the stimulation lead, device migration, and small bowel infarction from volvulus around the device wires. Data on the efficacy of gastric neurostimulators are growing. In the United States, this technology has been given human device exemption for patients with diabetic or idiopathic gastroparesis. The FDA has not addressed the use of the device for gastroparesis in a setting of other conditions, including malignancy-associated gastroparesis. Studies on the efficacy of electrical stimulation for gastroparesis secondary to cancer are needed.

CONCLUSION

Nausea and vomiting are common progressive symptoms in patients with advanced cancer receiving supportive care. As with other symptoms, an old school approach to nausea is still advocated by most experts, based on determining the cause and treating it where possible, while using our knowledge of pharmacology to select drugs targeted at the mechanism to ameliorate suffering until treatment of the cause is effective.

Systematic reviews have concluded, however, that the evidence at this time to support the current approach to managing nausea in advanced cancer is weak and contradictory, and much more research is needed on the different drugs and the two approaches to prescribing them. As Perkins et al. concluded in their 2009 Cochrane Review of haloperidol for nausea and vomiting in palliative care:

> *"There is a lack of published evidence for the use of haloperidol for nausea and vomiting in palliative care. No randomized controlled trials of haloperidol in this setting have been published in this setting. Much has been written about methodological challenges when conducting research in palliative medicine. Researchers need to decide whether this is an area where rigorous, high quality research is needed. The alternative is to continue extrapolating from work done in other areas of medicine."[97]*

Work in this area is further complicated by substantial international variations in the armamentarium available and the prescribing practices followed. This is also a changing field, with concerns about safety of traditional agents such as metoclopramide (extrapyramidal syndromes), prochlorperazine (neutropenia), and haloperidol (QTc prolongation); drug interactions in oncology patients on targeted therapies; and the emergence of newer agents that do not fit the conventional emetic pathway. These include mirtazapine, cannabinoids, NK-1 antagonists, erythromycin analogs, and ghrelin analogs. Advances in interventional gastroenterology are creating novel approaches for patients with obstructive symptoms. After many years of challenges, new options for the supportive care of nausea and vomiting are appearing on the horizon.

REFERENCES

1. Pereira J, Bruera E. Chronic nausea. In: Bruera E, Higginson I, eds. *Cachexia-anorexia in cancer patients*. New York: Oxford University Press; 1996:23–27.
2. Baines M. Nausea, vomiting and intestinal obstruction. In: Fallon M, O'Neill WM, eds. *ABC of palliative care*. London: BMJ Books; 1998:16–18.
3. Glare P, Pereira G, Kristjanson LJ, et al. Systematic review of the efficacy of antiemetics in the treatment of nausea in patients with far-advanced cancer. *Support Care Cancer*. 2004;12:432–440.
4. Quigley EM, Hasler WL, Parkman HP. AGA technical review on nausea and vomiting. *Gastroenterology*. 2001;120:263–286.
5. Meineche-Schmidt V, Christensen E. Classification of dyspepsia: identification of independent symptom components in 7270 consecutive, unselected dyspepsia patients from general practice. *Scand J Gastroenterol*. 1998;33:1262–1272.
6. Talley NJ, Phillips SF. Non-ulcer dyspepsia: potential causes and pathophysiology. *Ann Intern Med*. 1988;108:865–879.
7. Bruera E, Belzile M, Neumann C, et al. A double-blind, crossover study of controlled-release metoclopramide and placebo for the chronic nausea and dyspepsia of advanced cancer. *J Pain Symptom Manage*. 2000;19:427–435.
8. Nelson JE, Meier DE, Litke A, et al. The symptom burden of chronic critical illness. *Crit Care Med*. 2004;32:1527–1534.
9. Wolfe J, Grier HE, Klar N, et al. Symptoms and suffering at the end of life in children with cancer. *N Engl J Med*. 2000;342:326–333.
10. Tranmer JE, Heyland D, Dudgeon D, et al. Measuring the symptom experience of seriously ill cancer and noncancer hospitalized patients near the end of life with the memorial symptom assessment scale. *J Pain Symptom Manage*. 2003;25:420–429.
11. Stephenson J, Davies A. An assessment of aetiology-based guidelines for the management of nausea and vomiting in patients with advanced cancer. *Support Care Cancer*. 2006;14:348–353.
12. Ventafridda V, De Conno F, Ripamonti C, et al. Quality-of-life assessment during a palliative care programme. *Ann Oncol*. 1990;1:415–420.
13. Donnelly S, Walsh D, Rybicki L. The symptoms of advanced cancer: identification of clinical and research priorities by assessment of prevalence and severity. *J Palliat Care*. 1995;11:27–32.
14. Vainio A, Auvinen A. Prevalence of symptoms among patients with advanced cancer: an international collaborative study. Symptom Prevalence Group. *J Pain Symptom Manage*. 1996;12:3–10.
15. Reuben DB, Mor V. Nausea and vomiting in terminal cancer patients. *Arch Intern Med*. 1986;146:2021–2023.
16. Coyle N, Adelhardt J, Foley KM, et al. Character of terminal illness in the advanced cancer patient: pain and other symptoms during the last four weeks of life. *J Pain Symptom Manage*. 1990;5:83–93.

17. Fainsinger R, Miller MJ, Bruera E, et al. Symptom control during the last week of life on a palliative care unit. *J Palliat Care.* 1991;7:5–11.

18. Conill C, Verger E, Henriquez I, et al. Symptom prevalence in the last week of life. *J Pain Symptom Manage.* 1997;14:328–331.

19. Power D, Kearney M. Management of the final 24 hours. *Ir Med J.* 1992;85:93–95.

20. Ellershaw JE, Sutcliffe JM, Saunders CM. Dehydration and the dying patient. *J Pain Symptom Manage.* 1995;10:192–197.

21. Lichter I, Hunt E. The last 48 hours of life. *J Palliat Care.* 1990;6:7–15.

22. Radbruch L, Sabatowski R, Loick G, et al. Cognitive impairment and its influence on pain and symptom assessment in a palliative care unit: development of a Minimal Documentation System. *Palliat Med.* 2000;14:266–276.

23. Bruera E, Seifert L, Watanabe S, et al. Chronic nausea in advanced cancer patients: a retrospective assessment of a metoclopramide-based antiemetic regimen. *J Pain Symptom Manage.* 1996;11:147–153.

24. Mercadante S, Casuccio A, Fulfaro F. The course of symptom frequency and intensity in advanced cancer patients followed at home. *J Pain Symptom Manage.* 2000;20:104–112.

25. Chang VT, Hwang SS, Kasimis B, et al. Shorter symptom assessment instruments: the Condensed Memorial Symptom Assessment Scale (CMSAS). *Cancer Invest.* 2004;22:526–536.

26. Bruera E, Neumann C, Brenneis C, et al. Frequency of symptom distress and poor prognostic indicators in palliative cancer patients admitted to a tertiary palliative care unit, hospices, and acute care hospitals. *J Palliat Care.* 2000;16:16–21.

27. Meuser T, Pietruck C, Radbruch L, et al. Symptoms during cancer pain treatment following WHO-guidelines: a longitudinal follow-up study of symptom prevalence, severity and etiology. *Pain.* 2001;93:247–257.

28. Yates P. Clinical and patient perspectives on factors contributing to nausea in advanced cancer. *Oncol Nurs Forum.* 2006;33:468–469.

29. Grossman SA. Undertreatment of cancer pain: barriers and remedies. *Support Care Cancer.* 1993;1:74–78.

30. Reuben D. Nausea and vomiting in terminal cancer patients. *Arch Intern Med.* 1986;146:2021–2023.

31. Greaves J, Glare P, Kristjanson LJ, et al. Undertreatment of nausea and other symptoms in hospitalized cancer patients. *Support Care Cancer.* 2009;17:461–464.

32. Lichter I. Nausea and vomiting in patients with cancer. *Hematol Oncol Clin North Am.* 1996;10:207–220.

33. Bentley A, Boyd K. Use of clinical pictures in the management of nausea and vomiting: a prospective audit. *Palliat Med.* 2001;15:247–253.

34. Walsh D, Donnelly S, Rybicki L. The symptoms of advanced cancer: relationship to age, gender, and performance status in 1,000 patients. *Support Care Cancer.* 2000;8:175–179.

35. Morita T, Tsunoda J, Inoue S, et al. Contributing factors to physical symptoms in terminally-ill cancer patients. *J Pain Symptom Manage.* 1999;18:338–346.

36. Mercadante S, Fulfaro F, Casuccio A. The impact of home palliative care on symptoms in advanced cancer patients. *Support Care Cancer.* 2000;8:307–310.

37. Grossman SA, Sheidler VR, Swedeen K, et al. Correlation of patient and caregiver ratings of cancer pain. *J Pain Symptom Manage.* 1991;6:53–57.

38. Elliott BA, Elliott TE, Murray DM, et al. Patients and family members: the role of knowledge and attitudes in cancer pain. *J Pain Symptom Manage.* 1996;12:209–220.

39. Field L. Are nurses still underestimating patients' pain postoperatively? *Br J Nurs.* 1996;5:778–784.

40. Bruera E, Kuehn N, Miller MJ, et al. The Edmonton Symptom Assessment System (ESAS): a simple method for the assessment of palliative care patients. *J Palliat Care.* 1991;7:6–9.

41. Portenoy RK, Thaler HT, Kornblith AB, et al. The Memorial Symptom Assessment Scale: an instrument for the evaluation of symptom prevalence, characteristics and distress. *Eur J Cancer.* 1994;30A:1326–1336.

42. Melzack R, Rosberger Z, Hollingsworth ML, et al. New approaches to measuring nausea. *CMAJ.* 1985;133:755–758 61.

43. Turner J, Zapart S, Pedersen K, et al. Clinical practice guidelines for the psychosocial care of adults with cancer. *Psychooncology.* 2005;14:159–173.

44. Ward SE, Goldberg N, Miller-McCauley V, et al. Patient-related barriers to management of cancer pain. *Pain.* 1993;52:319–324.

45. Fan G, Filipczak L, Chow E. Symptom clusters in cancer patients: a review of the literature. *Curr Oncol.* 2007;14:173–179.

46. Cheung WY, Le LW, Zimmermann C. Symptom clusters in patients with advanced cancers. *Support Care Cancer.* 2009;17:1223–1230.

47. Hesketh PJ. Chemotherapy-induced nausea and vomiting. *N Engl J Med.* 2008;358:2482–2494.

48. Lichter I. Results of antiemetic management in terminal illness. *J Palliat Care.* 1993;9:19–21.

49. Bruera ED, MacEachern TJ, Spachynski KA, et al. Comparison of the efficacy, safety, and pharmacokinetics of controlled release and immediate release metoclopramide for the management of chronic nausea in patients with advanced cancer. *Cancer.* 1994;74:3204–3211.

50. Mystakidou K, Befon S, Liossi C, et al. Comparison of the efficacy and safety of tropisetron, metoclopramide, and chlorpromazine in the treatment of emesis associated with far advanced cancer. *Cancer.* 1998;83:1214–1223.

51. Cherny N, Ripamonti C, Pereira J, et al. Strategies to manage the adverse effects of oral morphine: an evidence-based report. *J Clin Oncol.* 2001;19:2542–2554.

52. Walkembach J, Bruss M, Urban BW, et al. Interactions of metoclopramide and ergotamine with human 5-HT(3A) receptors and human 5-HT reuptake carriers. *Br J Pharmacol.* 2005;146:543–552.

53. De Maeyer JH, Lefebvre RA, Schuurkes JA. 5-HT4 receptor agonists: similar but not the same. *Neurogastroenterol Motil.* 2008;20:99–112.

54. Cuomo R, Vandaele P, Coulie B, et al. Influence of motilin on gastric fundus tone and on meal-induced satiety in man: role of cholinergic pathways. *Am J Gastroenterol.* 2006;101:804–811.

55. Schuurkes JAJ, Helsen LFM, Ghoos ECR, et al. Stimulation of gastroduodenal motor activity: dopaminergic and cholinergic modulation. *Drug Dev Res.* 1986;8:233–241.

56. Santucci G, Mack JW. Common gastrointestinal symptoms in pediatric palliative care: nausea, vomiting, constipation, anorexia, cachexia. *Pediatr Clin North Am.* 2007;54:673–689.

57. Magueur E, Hagege H, Attali P, et al. Pharmacokinetics of metoclopramide in patients with liver cirrhosis. *Br J Clin Pharmacol.* 1991;31:185–187.

58. Bateman DN, Gokal R, Dodd TR, et al. The pharmacokinetics of single doses of metoclopramide in renal failure. *Eur J Clin Pharmacol.* 1981;19:437–441.

59. Stacher G, Gaupmann G, Steinringer H, et al. Effects of cisapride on postcibal jejunal motor activity. *Dig Dis Sci.* 1989;34:1405–1410.

60. Twycross R, Wilcock A, Charlesworth S, et al. *Palliative care formulary.* 2nd ed. Oxford: Radcliffe Medical Press; 2002.

61. McCallum RW, Prakash C, Campoli-Richards DM, et al. Cisapride: a preliminary review of its pharmacodynamic and pharmacokinetic properties, and therapeutic use as a prokinetic agent in gastrointestinal motility disorders. *Drugs.* 1988;36:652–681.

62. Puisieux FL, Adamantidis MM, Dumotier BM, et al. Cisapride-induced prolongation of cardiac action potential and early afterdepolarizations in rabbit Purkinje fibres. *Br J Pharmacol.* 1996;117:1377–1379.

63. Enger C, Cali C, Walker AM. Serious ventricular arrhythmias among users of cisapride and other QT-prolonging agents in the United States. *Pharmacoepidemiol Drug Saf.* 2002;11:477–486.

64. Barone JA. Domperidone: a peripherally acting dopamine2-receptor antagonist. *Ann Pharmacother.* 1999;33:429–440.

65. Osborne RJ, Slevin ML, Hunter RW, et al. Cardiotoxicity of intravenous domperidone. *Lancet.* 1985;2:385.

66. Corli O, Cozzolino A, Battaiotto L. Effectiveness of levosulpiride versus metoclopramide for nausea and vomiting in advanced cancer patients: a double-blind, randomized, crossover study. *J Pain Symptom Manage.* 1995;10:521–526.

67. Koutsoumbi P, Epanomeritakis E, Tsiaoussis J, et al. The effect of erythromycin on human esophageal motility is mediated by serotonin receptors. *Am J Gastroenterol.* 2000;95:3388–3392.

68. Kim SW, Shin IS, Kim JM, et al. Mirtazapine for severe gastroparesis unresponsive to conventional prokinetic treatment. *Psychosomatics.* 2006;47:440–442.

69. Hardy J, Daly S, McQuade B, et al. A double-blind, randomised, parallel group, multinational, multicentre study comparing a single dose of ondansetron 24 mg p.o. with placebo and metoclopramide 10 mg t.d.s. p.o. in the treatment of opioid-induced nausea and emesis in cancer patients. *Support Care Cancer.* 2002;10:231–236.

70. Abrahamsson H. Treatment options for patients with severe gastroparesis. *Gut.* 2007;56:877–883.

71. Burt M, Scott A, Williard WC, et al. Erythromycin stimulates gastric emptying after esophagectomy with gastric replacement: a randomized clinical trial. *J Thorac Cardiovasc Surg.* 1996;111:649–654.

72. Bonacini M, Quiason S, Reynolds M, et al. Effect of intravenous erythromycin on postoperative ileus. *Am J Gastroenterol.* 1993;88:208–211.

73. Smith AJ, Nissan A, Lanouette NM, et al. Prokinetic effect of erythromycin after colorectal surgery: randomized, placebo-controlled, double-blind study. *Dis Colon Rectum.* 2000;43:333–337.

74. Gregory RE. Ettinger DS. 5-HT3 receptor antagonists for the prevention of chemotherapy-induced nausea and vomiting: a comparison of their pharmacology and clinical efficacy. *Drugs.* 1998;55:173–189.

75. de Bruijn KM. Tropisetron: a review of the clinical experience. *Drugs.* 1992;43(suppl 3):11–22.

76. Lee CR, Plosker GL, McTavish D. Tropisetron: a review of its pharmacodynamic and pharmacokinetic properties, and therapeutic potential as an antiemetic. *Drugs.* 1993;46:925–943.

77. Aapro M. 5-HT(3)-receptor antagonists in the management of nausea and vomiting in cancer and cancer treatment. *Oncology.* 2005;69:97–109.

78. Figg WD, Dukes GE, Pritchard JF, et al. Pharmacokinetics of ondansetron in patients with hepatic insufficiency. *J Clin Pharmacol.* 1996;36:206–215.

79. Gralla RJ, Osoba D, Kris MG, et al. Recommendations for the use of antiemetics: evidence-based, clinical practice guidelines. American Society of Clinical Oncology. *J Clin Oncol.* 1999;17:2971–2994.

80. Currow DC, Coughlan M, Fardell B, et al. Use of ondansetron in palliatve medicine. *J Pain Symptom Manage.* 1997;13:302–307.

81. Currow DC, Coughlan M, Fardell B, et al. Use of ondansetron in palliative medicine. *J Pain Symptom Manage.* 1997;13:302–307.

82. Grunberg SM, Hesketh PJ. Control of chemotherapy-induced emesis. *N Engl J Med.* 1993;329:1790–1796.

83. Richelson E. Pharmacology of neuroleptics in use in the United States. *J Clin Psychiatry.* 1985;46:8–14.

84. Glare PA, Dunwoodie D, Clark K, et al. Treatment of nausea and vomiting in terminally ill cancer patients. *Drugs.* 2008;68:2575–2590.

85. Peroutka SJ, Snyder SH. Antiemetics: neurotransmitter receptor binding predicts therapeutic actions. *Lancet.* 1982;1:658–659.

86. Critchley P, Plach N, Grantham M, et al. Efficacy of haloperidol in the treatment of nausea and vomiting in the palliative patient: a systematic review. *J Pain Symptom Manage.* 2001;22:631–634.

87. Kudo S, Ishizaki T. Pharmacokinetics of haloperidol: an update. *Clin Pharmacokinet.* 1999;37:435–456.

88. Bymaster FP, Calligaro DO, Falcone JF, et al. Radioreceptor binding profile of the atypical antipsychotic olanzapine. *Neuropsychopharmacology.* 1996;14:87–96.

89. Callaghan JT, Bergstrom RF, Ptak LR, et al. Olanzapine: pharmacokinetic and pharmacodynamic profile. *Clin Pharmacokinet.* 1999;37:177–193.

90. Passik SD, Lundberg J, Kirsch KL, et al. A pilot exploration of the antiemetic activity of olanzapine for the relief of nausea in patients with advanced cancer and pain. *J Pain Symp Manage.* 2002;23:526–532.

91. Dineen S, Withrow K, Voronovitch L, et al. QTc prolongation and high-dose olanzapine. *Psychosomatics.* 2003;44:174–175.

92. Meltzer HY, Fibiger C. Olanzapine: a new atypical antipsychotic drug. *Neuropsychopharmacology.* 1996;14:83–85.

93. Bhana N, Foster RH, Olney R, et al. Olanzapine: an updated review of its use in the management of schizophrenia. *Drugs.* 2001;61:111–161.

94. Skinner J, Skinner A. Levomepromazine for nausea and vomiting in advanced cancer. *Hosp Med.* 1999;60:568–570.

95. Patt RB, Proper G, Reddy S. The neuroleptics as adjuvant analgesics. *J Pain Symptom Manage.* 1994;9:446–453.

96. Dahl SG. Pharmacokinetics of methotrimeprazine after single and multiple doses. *Clin Pharmacol Ther.* 1976;19:435–442.

97. Perkins P, Dorman S. Haloperidol for the treatment of nausea and vomiting in palliative care patients. *Cochrane Database Syst Rev.* 2009; CD006271.

98. Buttner M, Walder B, von Elm E, et al. Is low-dose haloperidol a useful antiemetic? A meta-analysis of published and unpublished randomized trials. *Anesthesiology.* 2004;101:1454–1463.

99. Hardy J, Ling J, Mansi J, et al. Pitfalls in placebo-controlled trials in palliative care: dexamethasone for the palliation of malignant bowel obstruction. *Palliat Med.* 1998;12:437–442.

100. Gralla RJ, Itri LM, Pisko SE, et al. Antiemetic efficacy of high-dose metoclopramide: randomized trials with placebo and prochlorperazine in patients with chemotherapy-induced nausea and vomiting. *N Engl J Med.* 1981;305:905–909.

101. Passik SD, Lundberg J, Kirsh KL, et al. A pilot exploration of the antiemetic activity of olanzapine for the relief of nausea in patients with advanced cancer and pain. *J Pain Symptom Manage.* 2002;23:526–532.

102. Twycross R, Bankby G, Hallowood J. The use of low-dose methotrimeprazine (levomepromazine) in the management of nausea and vomiting. *Prog Palliat Care.* 1997;5:49–53.

103. Mannix KA. Palliation of nausea and vomiting. In: Doyle D, Hanks G, Cherny NI, Calman K, eds. *Oxford textbook of palliative medicine.* 3rd ed.Oxford,UK: Oxford University Press; 2004:459–468.

104. Wood CD, Cramer DB, Graybiel A. Antimotion sickness drug efficacy. *Otolaryngol Head Neck Surg.* 1981;89:1041–1044.

105. Twycross R, Wilcock A, Thorp S. PCF1: *palliative care formulary.* Oxon: Radcliffe Medical Press; 1998.

106. Tan LB, Bryant S, Murray RG. Detrimental haemodynamic effects of cyclizine in heart failure. *Lancet.* 1988;1:560–561.

107. Keeley PW. Nausea and vomiting in people with cancer and other chronic diseases. In: *BMJ clinical evidence.* London: BMJ Publishing Group; April 2008.

108. Feuer DJ, Broadley KE. Corticosteroids for the resolution of malignant bowel obstruction in advanced gynaecological and gastrointestinal cancer. *Cochrane Database Syst Rev.* 2000; CD001219.

109. Czock D, Keller F, Rasche FM, et al. Pharmacokinetics and pharmacodynamics of systemically administered glucocorticoids. *Clin Pharmacokinet.* 2005;44:61–98.

110. Jordan K. Neurokinin-1-receptor antagonists: a new approach in antiemetic therapy. *Onkologie.* 2006;29:39–43.

111. Dando TM, Perry CM. Aprepitant: a review of its use in the prevention of chemotherapy-induced nausea and vomiting. *Drugs.* 2004;64:777–794.

112. Arondekar B, Haiderali A, Bandekar R, et al. Single dose oral and 3-day IV/oral regimens of a novel neurokinin-1 (Nk-1) receptor antagonist, casopitant, are effective in reducing the severity of nausea in patients receiving highly emetogenic chemotherapy (HEC). *Support Care Cancer.* 2008;16:629–630.

113. Chahl LA. Tachykinins and neuropsychiatric disorders. *Curr Drug Targets.* 2006;7:993–1003.

114. Chizh BA, Gohring M, Troster A, et al. Effects of oral pregabalin and aprepitant on pain and central sensitization in the electrical hyperalgesia model in human volunteers. *Br J Anaesth.* 2007;98:246–254.

115. Ripamonti C, Twycross R, Baines M, et al. Clinical-practice recommendations for the management of bowel obstruction in patients with end-stage cancer. *Support Care Cancer.* 2001;9:223–233.

116. Bagshaw SM, Hagen NA. Medical efficacy of cannabinoids and marijuana: a comprehensive review of the literature. *J Palliat Care.* 2002;18:111–122.

117. Gonzalez-Rosales F, Walsh D. Intractable nausea and vomiting due to gastrointestinal mucosal metastases relieved by tetrahydrocannabinol (dronabinol). *J Pain Symptom Manage.* 1997;14:311–314.

118. Borman RA, Sanger GJ. Novel approaches and clinical opportunity for gastrointestinal prokinetic drugs. *Drug Discov Today.* 2007;4:165–170.

119. Rhodes VA, McDaniel RW. Nausea, vomiting, and retching: complex problems in palliative care. *CA Cancer J Clin.* 2001;51:232–248 quiz 49–52.

120. Bruera E, Strasser F, Palmer JL, et al. Effect of fish oil on appetite and other symptoms in patients with advanced cancer and anorexia/cachexia: a double-blind, placebo-controlled study. *J Clin Oncol.* 2003;21:129–134.

121. Van Fleet S. Relaxation and imagery for symptom management: improving patient assessment and individualizing treatment. *Oncol Nurs Forum.* 2000;27:501–510.

122. Arakawa S. Relaxation to reduce nausea, vomiting, and anxiety induced by chemotherapy in Japanese patients. *Cancer Nurs.* 1997;20:342–349.

123. Molassiotis A. A pilot study of the use of progressive muscle relaxation training in the management of post-chemotherapy nausea and vomiting. *Eur J Cancer Care (Engl).* 2000;9:230–234.

124. Mundy EA, DuHamel KN, Montgomery GH. The efficacy of behavioral interventions for cancer treatment-related side effects. *Semin Clin Neuropsychiatry.* 2003;8:253–275.

125. Ahles TA, Tope DM, Pinkson B, et al. Massage therapy for patients undergoing autologous bone marrow transplantation. *J Pain Symptom Manage.* 1999;18:157–163.

126. Grealish L, Lomasney A, Whiteman B. Foot massage: a nursing intervention to modify the distressing symptoms of pain and nausea in patients hospitalized with cancer. *Cancer Nurs.* 2000;23:237–243.

127. Pan CX, Morrison RS, Ness J, et al. Complementary and alternative medicine in the management of pain, dyspnea, and nausea and vomiting near the end of life: a systematic review. *J Pain Symptom Manage.* 2000;20:374–387.

128. Ezzo JM, Richardson MA, Vickers A, et al. Acupuncture-point stimulation for chemotherapy-induced nausea or vomiting. *Cochrane Database Syst Rev.* 2006; CD002285.

129. Hickok JT, Roscoe JA, Morrow GR, et al. A phase II/III randomized, placebo-controlled, double-blind clinical trial of ginger (Zingiber officinale) for nausea caused by chemotherapy for cancer: a currently accruing URCC CCOP cancer control study. *Support Cancer Ther.* 2007;4:247–250.

130. Steadman K, Franks A. A woman with malignant bowel obstruction who did not want to die with tubes. *Lancet.* 1996;347:944.

131. Stellato TA, Gauderer MW. Percutaneous endoscopic gastrostomy for gastrointestinal decompression. *Ann Surg.* 1987;205:119–122.

132. Ponsky JL, Gauderer MW. Percutaneous endoscopic gastrostomy: a nonoperative technique for feeding gastrostomy. *Gastrointest Endosc.* 1981;27:9–11.

133. Baines MJ. ABC of palliative care: nausea, vomiting, and intestinal obstruction. *BMJ.* 1997;315:1148–1150.

134. Storey PS. Obstruction of the GI tract. *Am J Hosp Palliat Care.* 1991;8:5.

135. Pothuri B, Vaidya A, Aghajanian C, et al. Palliative surgery for bowel obstruction in recurrent ovarian cancer:an updated series. *Gynecol Oncol.* 2003;89:306–313.

136. Pothuri B, Meyer L, Gerardi M, et al. Reoperation for palliation of recurrent malignant bowel obstruction in ovarian carcinoma. *Gynecol Oncol.* 2004;95:193–195.

137. Levin DC, Matteucci T. "Turf battles" over imaging and interventional procedures in

community hospitals: survey results. *Radiology.* 1990;176:321–324.

138. Hoffer EK, Cosgrove JM, Levin DQ, et al. Radiologic gastrojejunostomy and percutaneous endoscopic gastrostomy: a prospective, randomized comparison. *J Vasc Interv Radiol.* 1999;10:413–420.

139. Pothuri B, Montemarano M, Gerardi M, et al. Percutaneous endoscopic gastrostomy tube placement in patients with malignant bowel obstruction due to ovarian carcinoma. *Gynecol Oncol.* 2005;96:330–334.

140. Cunningham MJ, Bromberg C, Kredentser DC, et al. Percutaneous gastrostomy for decompression in patients with advanced gynecologic malignancies. *Gynecol Oncol.* 1995;59:273–276.

141. Campagnutta E, Cannizzaro R, Gallo A, et al. Palliative treatment of upper intestinal obstruction by gynecological malignancy: the usefulness of percutaneous endoscopic gastrostomy. *Gynecol Oncol.* 1996;62:103–105.

142. Herman LL, Hoskins WJ, Shike M. Percutaneous endoscopic gastrostomy for decompression of the stomach and small bowel. *Gastrointest Endosc.* 1992;38:314–318.

143. Meyer L, Pothuri B. Decompressive percutaneous gastrostomy tube use in gynecologic malignancies. *Curr Treat Options Oncol.* 2006;7:111–120.

144. Campagnutta E, Cannizzaro R. Percutaneous endoscopic gastrostomy (PEG) in palliative treatment of non-operable intestinal obstruction due to gynecologic cancer: a review. *Eur J Gynaecol Oncol.* 2000;21:397–402.

145. Guitron A, Adalid R, Huerta F, et al. [Palliative treatment of esophageal cancer with transendoscopic injection of alcohol]. *Rev Gastroenterol Mex.* 1996;61:208–211.

146. Nwokolo CU, Payne-James JJ, Silk DB, et al. Palliation of malignant dysphagia by ethanol induced tumour necrosis. *Gut.* 1994;35:299–303.

147. Ahlquist DA, Gostout CJ, Viggiano TR, et al. Endoscopic laser palliation of malignant dysphagia: a prospective study. *Mayo Clin Proc.* 1987;62:867–874.

148. Brennan FN, McCarthy JH, Laurence BH. Endoscopic Nd-YAG laser therapy for palliation of upper gastrointestinal malignancy. *Med J Aust.* 1990;153:27–31.

149. Carazzone A, Bonavina L, Segalin A, et al. Endoscopic palliation of oesophageal cancer: results of a prospective comparison of Nd:YAG laser and ethanol injection. *Eur J Surg.* 1999;165:351–356.

150. Dallal HJ, Smith GD, Grieve DC, et al. A randomized trial of thermal ablative therapy versus expandable metal stents in the palliative treatment of patients with esophageal carcinoma. *Gastrointest Endosc.* 2001;54:549–557.

151. De Palma GD, di Matteo E, Romano G, et al. Plastic prosthesis versus expandable metal stents for palliation of inoperable esophageal thoracic carcinoma: a controlled prospective study. *Gastrointest Endosc.* 1996;43:478–482.

152. Mosca F, Consoli A, Stracqualursi A, et al. Portale TR. [Our experience with the use of a plastic prosthesis and self-expanding stents in the palliative treatment of malignant neoplastic stenoses of the esophagus and cardia: comparative analysis of results]. *Chir Ital.* 2002;54:341–350.

153. Knyrim K, Wagner HJ, Bethge N, et al. A controlled trial of an expansile metal stent for palliation of esophageal obstruction due to inoperable cancer. *N Engl J Med.* 1993;329:1302–1307.

154. Mosca F, Consoli A, Stracqualursi A, et al. Comparative retrospective study on the use of plastic prostheses and self-expanding metal stents in the palliative treatment of malignant strictures of the esophagus and cardia. *Dis Esophagus.* 2003;16:119–125.

155. Shimi SM. Self-expanding metallic stents in the management of advanced esophageal cancer: a review. *Semin Laparosc Surg.* 2000;7:9–21.

156. Costamagna G, Shah SK, Tringali A, et al. Prospective evaluation of a new self-expanding plastic stent for inoperable esophageal strictures. *Surg Endosc.* 2003;17:891–895.

157. Dormann AJ, Eisendrath P, Wigginghaus B, et al. Palliation of esophageal carcinoma with a new self-expanding plastic stent. *Endoscopy.* 2003;35:207–211.

158. Decker P, Lippler J, Decker D, et al. Use of the Polyflex stent in the palliative therapy of esophageal carcinoma: results in 14 cases and review of the literature. *Surg Endosc.* 2001;15:1444–1447.

159. Dormann A, Meisner S, Verin N, et al. Self-expanding metal stents for gastroduodenal malignancies: systematic review of their clinical effectiveness. *Endoscopy.* 2004;36:543–550.

160. Lelcuk S, Merhav A, Klausner JM, et al. Rectoscopic decompression of acute recto-sigmoid obstruction. *Endoscopy.* 1987;19:209–210.

161. Xinopoulos D, Dimitroulopoulos D, Theodosopoulos T, et al. Stenting or stoma creation for patients with inoperable malignant colonic obstructions? Results of a study and cost-effectiveness analysis. *Surg Endosc.* 2004;18:421–426.

162. Carne PW, Frye JN, Robertson GM, et al. Stents or open operation for palliation of colorectal cancer: a retrospective, cohort study of perioperative outcome and long-term survival. *Dis Colon Rectum.* 2004;47:1455–1461.

163. Parkman HP, Hasler WL, Fisher RS. American Gastroenterological Association medical position statement: diagnosis and treatment of gastroparesis. *Gastroenterology.* 2004;127:1589–1591.

164. Emerson AP. Foods high in fiber and phytobezoar formation. *J Am Diet Assoc.* 1987;87:1675–1677.

165. Barkin JS, Goldberg RI, Sfakianakis GN, et al. Pancreatic carcinoma is associated with delayed gastric emptying. *Dig Dis Sci.* 1986;31:265–267.

166. Donthireddy KR, Ailawadhi S, Nasser E, et al. Malignant gastroparesis: pathogenesis and management of an underrecognized disorder. *J Support Oncol.* 2007;5:355–363.

167. Cutts TF, Luo J, Starkebaum W, et al. Is gastric electrical stimulation superior to standard pharmacologic therapy in improving GI symptoms, healthcare resources, and long-term health care benefits? *Neurogastroenterol Motil.* 2005;17:35–43.

168. O'Grady G, Egbuji JU, Du P, et al. High-frequency gastric electrical stimulation for the treatment of gastroparesis: a meta-analysis. *World J Surg.* 2009;33:1693–1701.

169. Woodruff R. *Palliative medicine: evidence based symptomatic and supportive care for patients with advanced cancer.* 4th ed. Melbourne: Oxford University Press; 2004.

170. Dahl SG, Strandjord RE. Pharmacokinetics of chlorpromazine after single and chronic dosage. *Clin Pharmacol Ther.* 1977;21:437–448.

171. Griffin DS, Baselt RC. Blood and urine concentrations of cyclizine by nitrogen-phosphorus gas-liquid chromatography. *J Anal Toxicol.* 1984;8:97–99.

172. Heykants J, Hendriks R, Meuldermans W, et al. On the pharmacokinetics of domperidone in animals and man. IV. The pharmacokinetics of intravenous domperidone and its bioavailability in man following intramuscular, oral and rectal administration. *Eur J Drug Metab Pharmacokinet.* 1981;6:61–70.

173. Huang YC, Colaizzi JL, Bierman RH, et al. Pharmacokinetics and dose proportionality of domperidone in healthy volunteers. *J Clin Pharmacol.* 1986;26:628–632.

174. Ebert U, Siepmann M, Oertel R, et al. Pharmacokinetics and pharmacodynamics of scopolamine after subcutaneous administration. *J Clin Pharmacol.* 1998;38:720–726.

175. Bateman DN. Clinical pharmacokinetics of metoclopramide. *Clin Pharmacokinet.* 1983;8:523–529.

176. Kutz K, Nuesch E, Rosenthaler J. Pharmacokinetics of SMS 201–995 in healthy subjects. *Scand J Gastroenterol Suppl.* 1986;119:65–72.

177. Chanson P, Timsit J, Harris AG. Clinical pharmacokinetics of octreotide: therapeutic applications in patients with pituitary tumours. *Clin Pharmacokinet.* 1993;25:375–391.

178. Callaghan JT, Bergstrom RF, Ptak LR, et al. Olanzapine: pharmacokinetic and pharmacodynamic profile. *Clin Pharmacokinet.* 1999;37:177–193.

179. Isah AO, Rawlins MD, Bateman DN. Clinical pharmacology of prochlorperazine in healthy young males. *Br J Clin Pharmacol.* 1991;32:677–684.

180. Taylor WB, Bateman DN. Preliminary studies of the pharmacokinetics and pharmacodynamics of prochlorperazine in healthy volunteers. *Br J Clin Pharmacol.* 1987;23:137–142.

181. Taylor G, Houston JB, Shaffer J, et al. Pharmacokinetics of promethazine and its sulphoxide metabolite after intravenous and oral administration to man. *Br J Clin Pharmacol.* 1983;15:287–293.

182. Paton DM, Webster DR. Clinical pharmacokinetics of H1-receptor antagonists (the antihistamines). *Clin Pharmacokinet.* 1985;10:477–497.

183. Dimmit DC, Choo YS, Martin LA, et al. Intravenous pharmacokinetics and absolute oral bioavailability of dolasetron in healthy volunteers: part 1. *Biopharm Drug Dispos.* 1999;20:29–39.

184. Lerman J, Sims C, Sikich N, et al. Pharmacokinetics of the active metabolite (MDL 74,156) of dolasetron mesylate after oral or intravenous administration to anesthetized children. *Clin Pharmacol Ther.* 1996;60:485–492.

185. Plosker GL, Goa KL. Granisetron: a review of its pharmacological properties and therapeutic use as an antiemetic. *Drugs.* 1991;42:805–824.

186. Roila F, Del Favero A. Ondansetron clinical pharmacokinetics. *Clin Pharmacokinet.* 1995;29:95–109.

187. Simpson KH, Hicks FM. Clinical pharmacokinetics of ondansetron: a review. *J Pharm Pharmacol.* 1996;48:774–781.

188. Wilde MI, Markham A. Ondansetron: a review of its pharmacology and preliminary clinical findings in novel applications. *Drugs.* 1996;52:773–794.

189. Stoltz R, Cyong JC, Shah A, et al. Pharmacokinetic and safety evaluation of palonosetron, a 5-hydroxytryptamine-3 receptor antagonist, in U.S. and Japanese healthy subjects. *J Clin Pharmacol.* 2004;44:520–531.

190. Hunt TL, Gallagher SC, Cullen Jr MT, et al. Evaluation of safety and pharmacokinetics of consecutive multiple-day dosing of palonosetron in healthy subjects. *J Clin Pharmacol.* 2005;45:589–596.

26 Thrombosis in cancer

Laurent Plawny and Mario Dicato

HEMATOLOGY-ONCOLOGY

The correlation between thrombosis and cancer was first described in the 19th century by Trousseau, who observed recurrent superficial thrombophlebitis in a cancer patient. He experienced it himself later in his life when he died of gastric carcinoma.[1] Venous thromboembolism (VTE), consisting essentially of deep vein thrombosis (DVT) and pulmonary embolism (PE), is a frequent complication in cancer patients. It appears in up to 31% of cases and represents the second leading cause of mortality in cancer patients.[2]

This chapter explains some physiopathologic mechanisms of VTE in cancer patients and their diagnostic and prognostic implications. It then focuses on the prevalence of DVT and PE in cancer patients and reviews the different risk factors in favor of VTE.

Finally, questions of thromboprophylaxis and treatment of thrombosis in cancer patients will be addressed.

PATHOPHYSIOLOGY

The classical components of Virchow's triad play a role in the pathophysiology of cancer. Stasis is promoted in the medically ill or surgical patient through bed rest or prolonged immobilization. Vascular injury may result from tumor infiltration or from prolonged central venous catheter insertion.[3,4] A hypercoagulable state or low-grade disseminated intravascular coagulation (DIC) is common in cancer patients. Laboratory results indicate that a process of accelerated fibrin formation and destruction is going on in malignant diseases. The markers of fibrinogen and fibrinolysis can be measured directly (FVIIa, TAT, PF1+2, TF, PAI, plasminogen) or by their products (FDP, D-dimers, fibrin).[2–6] This low-grade DIC may be triggered by a number of factors linked to cancer, such as anticancer therapy, preexisting thrombosis, and compression by a neoplastic mass.[3,4]

PROCOAGULANT ACTIVITY OF TUMOR CELLS

Tumor cells have anticoagulant fibrinolytic and proinflammatory potential, through angiogenic and/or inflammatory cytokine production, or by direct interaction with platelets, leukocytes, and endothelial cells.[2–4,7]

Tissue factor binds to tumor cells, where it activates factor VII, thereby launching fibrin formation (Fig. 26-1). Fibrin is believed to have a central role in tumor progression. The clot's fibrin matrix provides a scaffold where new vessels can proliferate and protects tumor cells against attack by the immune system. The attachment of fibrin to cancer cells will facilitate the attachment of these cells to the endothelium and will facilitate the interaction between circulating tumor cells and endothelial cells. Fibrin has inflammatory properties and stimulates the production of tissue factor by endothelial cells; this allows sustained activation of factor VII by the tumor cells. Fibrin induces the production of pro-angiogenic cytokine interleukin (IL)-8 by endothelial cells.[8]

An in vitro study carried out in 1988 shows that the procoagulant activity of leukemic blasts is partially FVIIa independent.[9] Inhibition of fibrinolysis induced by plasminogen activator inhibitor (PAI), tissue-type plasminogen activator (tPA), and urokinase (uPA) expressed by tumor cells or by endothelial cells under the stimulation of cancer cells may constitute another procoagulant mechanism.[3]

INTERACTION WITH HOST CELLS

Tumor cell–derived cytokines (e.g., IL-1, tumor necrosis factor [TNF]) stimulate the host's neutrophils. Expression of myeloperoxidase and elastase exerts procoagulant activity, and expression of CD11b increases their adhesive properties. Activated monocytes secrete tissue factor, which, in turn, activates coagulation.[6]

P-selectin, secreted by cancer cells, activated endothelial cells, and platelets, plays a major role in tumor-related cell adhesion mechanisms. P-selectins, which are expressed on platelets, and endothelium facilitate the binding of cancer cells to these cells.[2,3,10]

ROLE OF MICROPARTICLES

Tissue factor (TF)-bearing microparticles have been shown to reflect procoagulant activity in breast cancer and in essential thrombocythemia, but also tumor aggressiveness.[1,11,12] Microparticles are shed by the cancer cell as a result of membrane instability. The TF provided by these microparticles triggers coagulation and angiogenesis, as explained previously. Some microparticles also express membrane proteins such as mucin-1 (MUC-1), which allows them to interact with leukocytes or endothelial cells.[1,13] Monocyte-derived microparticles contain the counter-receptor for P-selectin and will enhance platelet aggregation and clot formation.[14]

In 2005, a model explaining the procoagulant properties of tumor cells was proposed. The stimulation of platelets, endothelial cells, and leukocytes by tumor cells localized on the endothelium triggers a localized intravascular coagulation. Monocyte activation will contribute to sustain intravascular

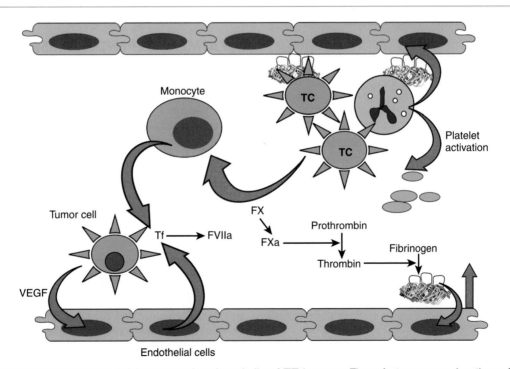

Fig. 26-1 Molecular mechanism underlying venous thromboembolism (VTE) in cancer. Tissue factor expressed on the surface of cancer cells activates factor VII, thereby triggering coagulation. Fibrin enhances angiogenic interleukin (IL)-8 expression by endothelial cells. Endothelial cells further express tissue factor, which will help to maintain activated coagulation. Vascular endothelial growth factor (VEGF) expression by tumor cells (TCs) will favor angiogenesis. Activation of neutrophils by tumor cells will activate the procoagulant and adhesive properties of platelets and endothelial cells. Activation of monocytes by cancer cells induces coagulation through the expression of tissue factor.

coagulation and stabilization of the thrombus by continuous shedding of TF.[6]

PARTICULAR PATHWAYS IN MYELOMA

Besides the previously mentioned pathways, plasmacytes in myeloma patients contribute to thrombosis by secreting pro-angiogenic IL-6. In rare cases, a thrombophilic state can result from the M-component, which exhibits anti–protein S or anti–protein C activity. In other cases, the M- component can act as a lupus anticoagulant.[15]

Acquired protein C resistance has been demonstrated in a small series of newly diagnosed myeloma patients, 50% of whom experienced VTE.[16]

Elevated FVIII and factor von Willebrand (FvW) levels have also been described in myeloma patients suffering from VTE.[15]

EPIDEMIOLOGY AND RISK ASSESSMENT

VTE has been reported in 4% to 31% of patients. The relative risk (RR) of thrombosis in cancer is increased fourfold and rises up to 6.5 in patients under chemotherapy. Venous thromboembolic disease is the second leading cause of death among cancer patients and raises cancer related morality 2 to 8 times.[7,17–19] The rate of VTE in cancer patients has slowly increased over the past 6 years, possibly reflecting the widespread use of new procoagulant drugs.[20]

The occurrence of VTE is variable among cancer patients and depends on a variety of risk factors, some of which are disease-related; others are patient-dependent (Table 26-1).

Table 26-1 Risk factors for cancer-associated thrombosis

Patient-associated	Old age	
	Gender	Females
	Race	Africans>Asians
	Thrombophilic state	
	Past history of VTE	
Cancer-associated	Site of primary cancer	Pancreas>brain> endometrium >GI> ovary>lung>breast
	Stage	
	Period from diagnosis	
Therapy-associated	Hospitalization	
	Surgery	
	Chemotherapy	
	Hormonal therapy	
	ESAs	
	Transfusions	

ESAs, Erythropoiesis-stimulating agents; *GI,* gastrointestinal; *VTE,* venous thromboembolism.

PATIENT-ASSOCIATED RISK FACTORS

Demographic features such as female gender or African race can have a clear impact on the occurrence of VTE. African American patients have a 1.1 odds ratio (OR) of developing DVT or PE, while Asian and Hispanic patients are at lower risk.[20,21] Female cancer patients have a 1.1 times higher risk of developing thrombosis for a reason yet unknown.[20] The presence of preexisting thrombosis increases the risk of DVT or PE in cancer patients. Inherited thrombophilia such as factor V Leiden mutation or prothrombin gene mutations raise the incidence of VTE in cancer patients, but their contribution remains modest.[2,21–23] The impact of antiphospholipids in cancer remains unclear.[2]

CANCER-ASSOCIATED RISK FACTORS

A study by Khorana published in 2007 reviews the occurrence of VTE according to the site of primary cancer. VTE occurs more frequently in pancreatic cancer, complicating 12% of cases. In hematologic malignancies, myeloma is the most potent risk factor of VTE, with a rate of 6%.[20] It is interesting to note that 4% of acute leukemias were complicated by VTE despite thrombocytopenia. A previous in vitro study indeed indicates a rise in procoagulant activity in most myeloid leukemia blasts. This activity is most marked in FAB M3 acute promyelocytic leukemia (AML), reflecting the frequent association between this type of myeloid leukemia and DIC.[9] The 2007 study does not investigate myeloproliferative disorders, although VTE complicates essential thrombocythemia (ET) in 7% to 17% of patients.[24,25]

The stage of disease seems also to play a major role in the occurrence of thrombosis. This is most evident in breast cancer, where the thrombosis rate varies from 0.1% to 45% in stage I patients to 15% to 17% in stage III-IV patients.[26]

TREATMENT-DEPENDENT RISK FACTORS

Surgical treatment is clearly associated with VTE occurrence. The rates of DVT and PE after cancer surgery vary from 22% to 52% and are approximately 3 to 5 times higher than in non-cancer patients.[27–29] For patients presenting with more than one risk factor besides cancer, the overall VTE rate is high: 40% to 80% will present distal DVT, 10% to 20% will present proximal DVT, 4% to 10% will have clinical PE, and 1% to 5% will present fatal PE.[30] Increased risk of postoperative VTE can be assessed for any kind of surgery but is most marked for neurosurgical tumors (Table 26-2).

Chemotherapy markedly increases the relative risk of VTE occurrence. The RR is increased 6 to 8 times in cancer patients undergoing chemotherapy.[2] Blood samples from lymphoma patients display a rise in F1+2 and TAT levels after cyclophosphamide-containing chemotherapy.[31] Cisplatin has been identified as a potent inducer of VTE in lung cancer patients.[32] Asparaginase induces VTE by inducing depletion of antithrombin III (ATIII) and other fibrinolytic and coagulation factors.[7] Levels of ATIII must be carefully monitored, and supplementation must be given if ATIII levels are low when this chemotherapy is used.

Thalidomide has allowed an increase in overall survival and in progression-free survival of myeloma patients. Unfortunately, its use is complicated by a notable increase in VTE, especially when associated with dexamethasone.[33] Antihormone therapy in breast cancer significantly increases the risk of developing VTE. This is especially true for the antiestrogen receptor tamoxifen. Although described, the use of aromatase inhibitors

Table 26-2 Incidence of symptomatic VTE in cancer patients within 91 days of major surgery according to type of surgery

Procedure	VTE (%)
Neurosurgery	2.0–3.6
Head and neck	0.2–1.4
Gastrointestinal	0.9–2.6
Urologic	0.4–3.7
Gynecologic	1.2–2.3
Orthopedic	0.9–3.1

Adapted from White 2003.[29]
VTE, Venous thromboembolism.

less frequently gives rise to VTE.[34] The antiangiogenic drug bevacizumab has also been shown to increase the rates of DVT and PE. A recent meta-analysis shows an increase in VTE in patients receiving bevacizumab in all but one study. The overall RR of developing thrombosis under bevacizumab is estimated at 1.33, with a cumulative incidence of 11%.[35]

The use of erythropoiesis-stimulating agents (ESAs) has also been shown to increase the risk of VTE. The BRAVE study and the BEST study both showed a rise in incidence of DVT and PE (Table 26-3).[36,37] In these studies, however, the target hemoglobin level largely exceeded the normal level of 12 g/dl, which could account for surplus VTE in these patients. However, other studies with a target hemoglobin lower than 12 g/dl also indicate a slight increase in asymptomatic VTE. The RR of developing VTE varies from 1.42 to 1.67, thus indicating a class effect of ESAs, as well as an increased hematocrit.[38]

The use of blood transfusion is also associated with VTE, although to a lesser extent than ESAs.[2]

BIOMARKERS

The prechemotherapy platelet count is shown to be associated with a marked tendency to develop VTE.[39] A prospective cohort study indicates that VTE occurs in 44% of patients presenting high platelets.[10] The incidence increases with higher platelet counts but also with the level of serum P-selectins, which are secreted by the platelets. Another study shows that in patients with a high platelet count, subpopulations can be distinguished according to the presence of TAT complexes. The presence of TAT complexes raises 7.5 times the risk of developing VTE.[40]

In 2009, a prospective study evaluated the value of F1+2 and D-dimers in cancer patients. The hazard ratio (HR) is most elevated in patients presenting both elevated F1+2 and D-dimers, and it is moderately elevated in patients presenting only one of the two markers. This study indicates that D-dimers and F1+2 can be used as prognostic biomarkers for VTE occurrence.[41]

C-reactive protein levels and immunohistochemical tissue factor production are also considered prognostic.[2]

RISK ASSESSMENT

Recently, a risk assessment model based on clinical characteristics and biomarkers has been developed to assess the risk of VTE in cancer patients (Table 26-4). Among the risk factors

Table 26-4 Predictive model for chemotherapy-associated thrombosis

Patient characteristics	Risk score	
Pancreas or stomach cancer	2	
Lung, lymphoma, bladder, gynecologic, testicular	1	
Platelets >350,000/μl	1	
Hemoglobin <10 g/dl or ESAs	1	
Leukocytes >10,000/μl	1	
Body mass index >35	1	
	Low risk	Score 0
	Intermediate risk	Score 1–2
	High risk	Score >3

Adapted from Khorana 2008.[42]
ESAs, Erythropoiesis-stimulating agents.

Table 26-3 Risk of VTE occurrence in major off-label studies on ESAs in cancer-related anemia

Study	Patients (EPO/Transfused)	Target Hb	Tumor	Results
BEST[36] (Leyland-Jones)	448/456	No limit	Breast	HR: 1.37
ENHANCE[83] (Henke)	121/121	No limit	Head and neck	RR: 1.39
EPO-CAN-15[84] (Wright)	52/52	No limit	Small cell lung carcinoma	HR: 1.84
BRAVE[37] (Aapro)	231/232	No limit	Breast	HR: 1.07

EPO, Erythropoietin; *ESAs,* erythropoiesis-stimulating agents; *Hb,* hemoglobin; *HR,* hazard ratio; *RR,* relative risk; *VTE,* venous thromboembolism.

cited, leukocyte counts seem to reflect the inflammatory status of the patient, which could explain the association between leukocytosis and VTE. Anemia is related to VTE for several reasons, the most obvious being ESAs and use of transfusion in anemic cancer patients. Anemia, however, is also related to tumor-induced inflammation. The score allotted to each item allows differentiation of three subpopulations. Low-risk patients have an incidence of VTE of less than 1% in the subsequent 2.5 months; intermediate- and high-risk patients have an incidence of 2% and 7%, respectively, over the same time period.[42]

DIAGNOSIS

The main diagnostic modalities used today for VTE are duplex ultrasound (US) and angio-computed tomography (CT). Duplex US has a weighted mean sensitivity of 97% (95% confidence interval, 96%–98%) for symptomatic proximal DVT, although the yield is far less good for calf vein DVT (sensitivity, 73%) or for asymptomatic distal DVT (sensitivity, 62%).[43] Sensitivity for upper limb DVT is also good. However, duplex US is limited for abdominal thromboses and thrombi residing over the inguinal ligament. In these cases, magnetic resonance imaging (MRI) or CT should be the method of choice.[44]

Angio-CT identifies significantly more PE than ventilation/perfusion scintigraphy. For this reason, it should be reserved for patients with a known allergy to contrast or with renal failure.[44]

Pregnant women should first undergo duplex US. Ventilation/perfusion scintigraphy provides less fetal radiation than angio-CT.[44]

The diagnostic impact of D-dimers is relatively low, given the fact that most cancer patients have positive D-dimers. Negative D-dimers retain a negative predictive value. Currently, the diagnosis should rely essentially on the clinic and on imaging methods, as shown in Figures 26-2 and 26-3.[45]

PREVENTION OF VTE

UNFRACTIONATED HEPARIN

The efficacy of VTE prophylaxis after major surgery has been established since 1975.[46] In a large multicenter trial of 4121 patients, thromboprophylaxis with unfractionated heparin significantly reduced the rate of fatal PE without causing any significant blood loss. However, prophylaxis is associated with slightly increased wound hematomas. Among the 4121 patients, 953 underwent major surgery for cancer. These patients also benefited from unfractionated heparin (UFH) prophylaxis, with a 21% reduction in total surgical mortality, a 68% reduction in fatal PE, and a 67% reduction in asymptomatic DVT.[46]

The concern of major blood loss has been addressed in other studies. A meta-analysis on surgical patients shows a significant reduction in fatal PE (risk reduction, 68%), while bleeding and other causes of mortality are not increased.[47] However, UFH is not devoid of complications; the two most frequent are heparin-induced thrombocytopenia (HIT) and osteoporosis.

LOW-MOLECULAR-WEIGHT HEPARINS

Low-molecular-weight heparins (LMWHs) have been analyzed in cancer patients undergoing major surgery. In 1995, a prospective, randomized, double-blind trial of dalteparin

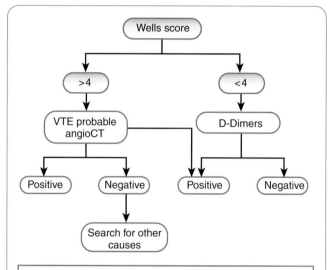

Wells score for PE
Active cancer 1
Surgery or bedridden for 3 days or more during the past 4 weeks 1.5
History of deep venous thrombosis or pulmonary embolism 1.5
Hemoptysis 1
Heart rate > 100 beats per minute 1.5
Pulmonary embolism judged to be most likely diagnosis 3
Clinical signs and symptoms compatible with deep venous thrombosis 3

Fig. 26-2 Algorithm for the diagnosis of pulmonary embolism (PE). If PE is suspected, a score establishing the pretest probability of PE based on clinical and patient-related items should be obtained. High pretest probability should warrant immediate imaging. In cases of low pretest probability, D-dimers can help rule out the diagnosis.

showed a marked reduction in DVT in all analyzed patients.[48] The reduction was proportionate to dalteparin dose administered, but it came at the price of an increase in major bleeding. More recently, the ENOXACANII and FAME studies analyzed the respective effects of enoxaparin 40 mg and dalteparin 5000 U SC versus placebo. Both studies confirmed the reduction in asymptomatic DVT and clinically relevant VTE in cancer patients undergoing surgery without significant bleeding.[49,50] Extended duration of thromboprophylaxis for 21 to 35 days after abdominal or pelvic surgery reduces the risk of fatal PE and DVT without increasing the bleeding risk.[2,49–51]

The MEDENOX and PREVENT studies established the efficacy and safety of LMWHs in medically ill patients who are hospitalized.[52,53]

In the ambulatory care patient, LMWH prophylaxis has been studied in the PROTECHT trial.[54] The PROTECHT trial shows a significant reduction in VTE in cancer, but at the cost of a significant increase in major bleeding. A recent meta-analysis shows that LMWH effectively reduces VTE occurrence in cancer patients, but the risk-benefit ratio seems small.[55] Data show that prevention may be more useful in glioblastoma.[2]

Osteoporosis is infrequent with LMWH. HIT occurs less frequently than with UFH but remains a major concern. Another negative aspect of LMWHs is their accumulation in renal insufficiency. A recent study evaluating adjusted doses of tinzaparin in patients with impaired renal function was complicated by an unacceptable rate of major bleeding.[56]

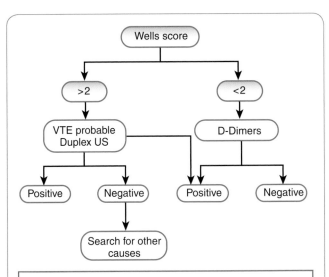

Fig. 26-3 Algorithm for the diagnosis of deep vein thrombosis (DVT). If DVT is suspected, a score establishing the pretest probability of DVT based on clinical and patient-related items should be obtained. High pretest probability should warrant immediate imaging. In cases of low pretest probability, D-dimers can help rule out the diagnosis.

Within the figure:

Wells score

>2 → VTE probable Duplex US → Positive / Negative

<2 → D-Dimers → Positive / Negative

Search for other causes

Wells score for DVT
Active cancer 1
Paralysis, paresis, or recent plaster cast immobilization of the lower extremities 1
Recently bedridden for 3 days or more, or major surgery within the previous 12 weeks requiring general or regional anesthesia 1
Localized tenderness along the distribution of the deep venous system 1
Entire leg swollen 1
Calf swelling at least 3 cm larger than the asymptomatic side (measured 10 cm below the tibial tuberosity) 1
Pitting edema confined to the symptomatic leg 1
Collateral superficial veins (non-varicose) 1
Previously documented deep vein thrombosis 1
Alternative diagnosis at least as likely as deep vein thrombosis –2

FONDAPARINUX

The advantage of fondaparinux over LMWH lies in the few reported cases of HIT. The ARTEMIS study, while analyzing the use of fondaparinux prophylaxis in cancer patients, showed a trend toward risk reduction compared with placebo (47% risk reduction). However, this trend failed to show statistical significance.[57]

VITAMIN K ANTAGONISTS (VKAs)

VKA prophylaxis has been tried with some success in breast cancer patients. The target international normalized ratio (INR) in this study was 1.3 to 1.9. Although VKA effectively reduces the risk of VTE occurrence in ambulatory cancer patients, their use is rendered cumbersome by the need for frequent INR assessment, in which other drugs and some foodstuffs interfere, hence the difficulty of maintaining the target INR in patients undergoing therapy.[58]

NEW MOLECULES

Direct thrombin or factor Xa inhibitors such as dabigatran and rivaroxaban have been used successfully in VTE prophylaxis after orthopedic surgery.[59,60] Dabigatran was superior to warfarin in preventing stroke in atrial fibrillation patients and was not

inferior to VKA in the treatment of VTE.[61,62] Studies with rivaroxaban are ongoing. Although these results seem promising, they have not yet been validated in cancer patients.

MECHANICAL PROPHYLAXIS

Mechanical prophylaxis (intermittent compression device, foot pump, graduated compression stockings [GCS]) achieves a modest risk reduction of VTE.[63] However, its use presents many drawbacks. Compliance with these methods, especially GCS, is not always as good as it should be. Their costs in money and in time are sometimes prohibitive compared with LMWH. Although they were long considered devoid of side effects when compared with LMWH, a recent study of intermittent compression in stroke patients reported higher risks of infection and skin necrosis.[64] Currently, mechanical methods of prophylaxis are recommended only in patients at high risk of developing thrombosis, and in addition to pharmacologic prophylaxis.[2]

RECOMMENDATIONS

According to American College of Chest Physicians (ACCP) 2009, National Comprehensive Cancer Network (NCCN) 2009, American Society of Clinical Oncology (ASCO) 2007, and European Society for Medical Oncology (ESMO) 2009 guidelines, prophylaxis of thrombosis is indicated in cancer patients undergoing surgery or in medically ill cancer patients requiring hospitalization.

According to ESMO 2009, in general, unless there is a contraindication, hospitalized patients with cancer should be considered candidates for VTE prophylaxis with anticoagulants. Routine prophylaxis during outpatient chemotherapy is not indicated in most cases. At the moment evidence as to the safety of VTE prophylaxis in ambulatory cancer patients is insufficient.[65-67] The choice of the prophylactic agent remains at the discretion of the prescriber. However, it should be reminded that VKA prophylaxis is cumbersome and needs frequent laboratory assessment. Furthermore, VKAs interact with many drugs used in chemotherapy or supportive cancer care.

In a recent meta-analysis, LMWH was superior to UFH in terms of VTE reduction, major bleeding, fatal PE, death, wound infection, hematoma, and needed transfusions. LMWH heparin thus remains the first choice in VTE prophylaxis.[68]

American Society of Hematology (ASH) 2009 specifically addressed the problem of myeloma patients. Because myeloma is a great provider of VTE, especially in thalidomide recipients, specific guidelines have been proposed for these patients. Prophylaxis using aspirin can be given to any myeloma patient showing no or one risk factor. Prophylaxis with LMWH can be proposed for any patient showing two or more risk factors, whether patient-related (age, obesity, past history of VTE), myeloma-related (hyperviscosity, high stage), or treatment-related (e.g., thalidomide combined with dexamethasone, polychemotherapy).[69]

TREATMENT OF VTE

INITIAL TREATMENT

In cancer patients, LMWH is preferred to UFH and fondaparinux for the initial treatment of VTE.[66,67] Table 26-5 shows different meta-analyses on studies assessing the effects of

Table 26-5 Results of meta-analysis comparing the outcomes of LMWH treatment vs. UFH treatment for VTE*

	Number of trials	Recurrence of VTE, OR (95% CI)	Major bleeding, OR (95% CI)
Hettiarachi 1998[77]	13	0.77 (0.56–1.04)	0.60 (0.38–0.95)
Gould 1999[85]	11	0.85 (0.63–1.14)	0.57 (0.33–0.99)
Dolovich 2000[86]	13	0.85 (0.65–1.12)	0.63 (0.37–1.05)
Van Dongen 2004[70]	23	0.68 (0.55–0.84)	0.57 (0.39–0.83)

*Show superiority in terms of VTE recurrence and risk reduction of major bleeds with LMWH.
CI, Confidence interval; LMWH, low-molecular-weight heparin; OR, odds ratio; UFH, unfractionated heparin; VTE, venous thromboembolism.

LMWH compared with UFH in terms of VTE recurrence and major bleeding. Although both agents effectively treat thrombosis, the risk of recurrence is reduced by 32% and the bleeding risk is reduced by 43% in LMWH patients compared with UFH recipients. Furthermore, short-term overall survival is better in patients under LMWH compared with UFH.[70]

The MATISSE trial, after analyzing the efficacy and safety of fondaparinux compared with LMWH and UFH, showed no clear-cut advantage in terms of VTE recurrence or major bleeding for any of the three populations in the global population. In the cancer populations, however, the MATISSE study showed an advantage among LMWH patients in terms of VTE recurrence and major bleeding.[71]

LONG-TERM TREATMENT

Recurrence is a major problem in cancer patients, thus stressing the need for long-term VTE treatment. VKAs, which provide first-line long-term treatment for noncancer patients, have an unpredictable response and are complicated by a 21% recurrence rate; the incidence of major bleeding is 12% at 12 months.[72] VKAs are believed to reduce the quality of life in cancer patients as well. Most studies assessing the safety and efficacy of LMWHs compared with VKAs indicate superiority of LMWHs. The CLOT study, an open-label, prospective, randomized controlled trial on cancer patients with symptomatic VTE, compared long-term treatment with warfarin and dalteparin 200 IU/kg daily for 1 month, then 100 mg/kg daily; a clear reduction in symptomatic VTE recurrence was seen in the dalteparin arm (9% vs. 17%, HR 0.48, $P = .002$).[73]

Inferior vena cava filters

The long-term efficacy of inferior vena cava filters is limited, as they do not address the hypercoagulable state seen in cancer patients. Relatively few randomized controlled data are available on their use and on the follow-up of potent side effects. In small trials, they effectively reduce the risk of PE, but their use is complicated by DVT in 4% to 32% of cases. Their use should be restricted to the insertion of retrievable vena cava filters as prophylaxis in patients presenting a transient bleeding risk.[2,23]

RECOMMENDATIONS

ASCO guidelines recommend the use of LMWH for initial treatment of VTE. Long-term treatment with LMWH for at least 6 months is preferred. VKAs are an acceptable option if LMWHs are not available.[65]

ACCP guidelines recommend at least 3 months of LMWH treatment, followed by LMWH treatment or VKA as long as cancer is active.[74]

NCCN recommends LMWHs over VKAs in patients with proximal DVT/PE, or in patients with metastatic disease.[66]

CENTRAL VENOUS CATHETER–RELATED THROMBOSIS

Central venous catheter (CVC) thrombosis is a considerable source of comorbidity, as it may be complicated by fatal PE, catheter-related infection, or septic shock.[2] A recent large multicenter trial on warfarin in CVC patients shows no reduction in VTE in patients receiving warfarin. Furthermore, adjusted-dose warfarin is considered inconvenient because of the need for constant monitoring of INR.[75]

LMWH prophylaxis shows no effect on CVC-related thrombosis.[76] ACCP guidelines recommend against the use of anticoagulants to prevent CVC thrombosis in ambulatory patients.[67]

LMWH AND TUMOR PROGRESSION

Studies showing a gain in survival among LMWH patients compared with UFH patients raised the argument as to the cause of this gain in survival, as the difference could not be explained solely by reductions in fatal PE and in major bleeding.[76,77]

In animal models, the inhibition of formation of fibrinogen is one potential mechanism that could explain the antitumor activity of LMWH. Another possible pathway is the inhibition of P-selectin by heparin and its derivatives. Heparanase is abundant in cancer tissue and may be a marker of bad prognosis. UFH and LMWH have been found to reduce heparanase activity.[78]

A recent randomized trial by Lebeau et al. found an increase in response to chemotherapy in small cell lung carcinoma patients treated with UFH.[79] Two other cohort studies reported similar results with LMWH in prostate or metastatic melanoma.[80,81] Although these results seem encouraging, the previously mentioned studies present some major biases, as they involve inhomogeneous populations and have relatively wide confidence intervals. Currently, available data are considered too scarce to recommend UFH or LMWH in addition to cancer treatment.[78]

ANTICOAGULATION IN THROMBOPENIC PATIENTS

Leukemia and lymphoma patients are at risk for thrombosis. However, this is complicated by therapy-induced or disease-related thrombocytopenia. Anticoagulant therapy poses a major hemostatic challenge in these patients, as it significantly increases bleeding risk. No current guidelines exist as to the use of prophylactic regimens in thrombopenic patients.[82]

The question of treatment of VTE in these patients has not been answered yet in randomized controlled trials.

The American Society of Hematology proposes 50% dose reductions for patients with platelet counts less than 50,000/mm[3] and temporary discontinuation if platelets fall below 20,000/mm[3].[82]

REFERENCES

1. Davizon P, Lopez J. Microparticles and thrombotic disease. *Curr Opin Hematol.* 2009;16:334–341.
2. Sood SL. Cancer-associated thrombosis. *Curr Opin Hematol.* 2009;16:378–385.
3. Rickles FR. *Hemostasis and cancer: hematology education.* Education program for the Annual Congress of the European Hematology Association, Copenhagen, Denmark, June 12-15, 2008:115–119.
4. Falanga A, Rickles FR. The pathogenesis of thrombosis in cancer. *N Oncol Thromb.* 2005;1:9–16.
5. Sud R, Khorana AA. Cancer-associated thrombosis: risk factors, candidate biomarkers and a risk model. *Thromb Res.* 2009;123(suppl 4):S18–S21.
6. Prandoni P, Falanga A, Piccioli A. Cancer and venous thromboembolism. *Lancet Oncol.* 2005;6:401–410.
7. Kwaan HC. *Double hazard of thrombosis and bleeding in malignant hematologic disorders.* Atlanta, GA: American Society of Hematology Program Book; December 8-11, 2007:151–157.
8. Rickles FR, Falanga A. Molecular basis for the relationship between thrombosis and cancer. *Thromb Res.* 2001;102:215–224.
9. Falanga A, Alessio MG, Donati MB, et al. A new procoagulant in acute leukemia. *Blood.* 1998;71:870–875.
10. Ay C, Simanek R, Vormittag R, et al. High plasma levels of soluble P-selectin are predictive of venous thromboembolism in patients with cancer: results from the Vienna Cancer and Thrombosis Study. *Blood.* 2008;112:2703–2708.
11. Toth B, Liebhadt S, Steimig K, et al. Platelet-derived microparticles and coagulation activation in breast cancer patients. *Thromb Haemost.* 2008;100:663–669.
12. Trappenburg MC, van Schilfgaarde M, Narchetti M, et al. Elevated procoagulant microparticles expressing endothelial and platelet markers in essential thrombocythemia. *Haematologica.* 2009;94:911–918.
13. Singhal AK, Orntoft TF, Nudelman E, et al. Profiles of Lewis containing glycoproteins and glycolipids in sera of patients with adenocarcinoma. *Cancer Res.* 1990;50:1375–1380.
14. Pendurthi UR, Rao LV. Role of tissue factor disulfide and lipid rafts in signalling. *Thromb Res.* 2008;122(suppl 1):S14–S18.
15. Eby CS. *Bleeding and thrombosis in plasma cell dyscrasias.* Atlanta, GA: American Society of Hematology Program Book; December 8-11, 2007:158–164.
16. Zangari M, Shaghafifar F, Anaissie E, et al. Activated protein C resistance in the absence of factor V Leiden mutation is a common finding in multiple myeloma and is associated with increased risk of thrombotic complications. *Blood Coagul Fibrinolysis.* 2002;13:187–192.
17. Lee A, Levine M. The thrombophilic state induced by therapeutic agents in cancer patients. *Semin Thromb Hemost.* 1999;25:137–145.
18. Deitcher SR. Cancer and thrombosis: mechanisms and treatment. *J Thromb Thrombolysis.* 2003;16:12–31.

19. Heit JA, Silverstein MD, Mohr DN, et al. Risk factors for deep vein thrombosis and pulmonary embolism: a population based case-control study. *Arch Intern Med.* 2000;160:809–815.
20. Khorana AA, Francis CW, Culakowa E, et al. Frequency, risk factors and trends for venous thromboembolism among hospitalized cancer patients. *Cancer.* 2007;110:2339–2346.
21. Khorana AA, Connolly GC. Assessing risk of venous thromboembolism in the patient with cancer. *J Clin Oncol.* 2009;27:4839–4847.
22. Blom JW, Doggen CJ, Osanto S, et al. Malignancies, prothrombotic mutations and the risk of venous thrombosis. *JAMA.* 2008;293:725–732.
23. Imberti D, Agnelli G, Ageno W, et al. Clinical characteristics and management of cancer-associated acute venous thromboembolism: findings from the MASTER registry. *Haematologica.* 2008;93:273–278.
24. Harrisson CN, Campbell PJ, Buck G, et al. Hydroxyurea compared with anagrelide in high risk essential thrombocythemia. *N Engl J Med.* 2005;353:33–45.
25. Gisslinger H, Gotic M, Holowiecki J, et al. Final results of the ANAHYDRET study: non-inferiority of anagrelide compared to hydroxyurea in newly diagnosed WHO-essential thrombocythemia patients. *Blood.* 2008;112:661.
26. Rickles FR, Levine MN. Epidemiology of thrombosis in cancer. *Acta Haematol.* 2001;106:6–12.
27. Agnelli G, Verso M. *Prophylaxis and treatment of venous thromboembolism in cancer patients: hematology education.* Education program for the Annual Congress of the European Hematology Association, Copenhagen, Denmark, June 12-15. 2008:123–125.
28. Huber O, Bounameaux H, Borst F, et al. Postoperative pulmonary embolism after hospital discharge: an underestimated risk. *Arch Surg.* 1992;127:310–313.
29. White RH, Zhou H, Romano PS. Incidence of symptomatic venous thromboembolism after different elective or urgent surgical procedures. *Thromb Haemost.* 2003;90:446–455.
30. Geerts WH, Bergqvist D, Pineo GF, et al. Prevention of venous thromboembolism: the Seventh ACCP Conference on Antithrombotic and Thrombolytic Therapy. *Chest.* 2004;126(suppl 3):338S–400S.
31. Falanga A, Rickles FR. The pathogenesis of thrombosis in cancer. *N Oncol Thromb.* 2005;1:9–16.
32. Moore RA, Adel NG, Bhutani M, et al. Cisplatin-based chemotherapy is associated with an unacceptably high incidence of thromboembolic events: a large retrospective analysis. *Blood.* 2009;114:456.
33. El Accaoui RN, Shamsheddeen WA, Taher AT. Thalidomide and thrombosis: a meta analysis. *Thromb Haemost.* 2007;97:1031–1036.
34. Fisher B, Constantino JP, Wickerman DL, et al. Tamoxifen for prevention of breast cancer: report of the National Surgical Adjuvant Breast

and Bowel Project P-1 study. *J Natl Cancer Inst.* 1998;90:1371–1388.
35. Nalluri SR, Chu D, Keresztes R, et al. Risk of thromboembolism with the angiogenesis inhibitor bevacizumab in cancer patients: a meta-analysis. *JAMA.* 2008;300:2277–2285.
36. Leyland-Jones B, Semiglazov V, Pawlicki M, et al. Maintaining normal haemoglobin levels with epoetin alfa in mainly non-anemic patients with metastatic breast cancer receiving first-line chemotherapy: a survival study. *J Clin Oncol.* 2005;23:5960–5972.
37. Aapro M, Leonard RC, Barnadas A, et al. Effect of once-weekly epoetin beta on survival in patients with metastatic breast cancer receiving anthracycline- and/or taxane-based chemotherapy: results of the Breast Cancer-Anemia and the Value of Erythropoietin (BRAVE) study. *J Clin Oncol.* 2008;26:592–598.
38. Bohlius J, Wilson J, Seidenfeld J, et al. Recombinant human erythropoietins and cancer patients: updated meta-analysis of 57 studies including 9353 patients. *J Natl Cancer Inst.* 2006;98:708–714.
39. Khorana AA, Francis CW, Colakova E, et al. Risk factors for chemotherapy-associated venous thromboembolism in a prospective observational study. *Cancer.* 2005;104:2822–2829.
40. Falanga A, Ofozu FA, Cortelazzo S, et al. Preliminary study to identify cancer patients at high risk of venous thrombosis following major surgery. *Br J Haematol.* 1993;85:745–750.
41. Ay C, Vormittag R, Dunkler D, et al. D-dimer and prothrombin fragment 1+2 predict venous thromboembolism in patients with cancer: results from the Vienna Cancer and Thrombosis Study. *J Clin Oncol.* 2009;27:4124–4129.
42. Khorana AA, Kuderer NM, Culakowa E, et al. Development and validation of a predictive model for chemotherapy-associated thrombosis. *Blood.* 2008;111:4902–4907.
43. Kearon C, Julian JA, Newman TE, et al. Noninvasive diagnosis of deep venous thrombosis: McMaster diagnostic imaging practice guidelines initiative. *Ann Intern Med.* 1998;128:663–677.
44. Streiff MB. Diagnosis and initial treatment of venous thromboembolism in patients with cancer. *J Clin Oncol.* 2009;27:4889–4894.
45. Carrier M, Lee AY, Bates SM, et al. Accuracy and usefulness of a clinical prediction rule and D-dimer testing in excluding deep vein thrombosis in cancer patients. *Thromb Res.* 2008;123:177–183.
46. Kakkar VV, Corrigan TP, Fossard DP, et al. Prevention of fatal postoperative pulmonary embolism by low doses of heparin: an international multicentre trial. *Lancet.* 1975;2:45–51.
47. Collins R, Scrimgeour A, Yusuf S, et al. Reduction in fatal pulmonary embolism and venous thrombosis by perioperative administration of subcutaneous heparin: overview of results of randomized trials in general, orthopaedic and urologic surgery. *N Engl J Med.* 1988;318:1162–1173.
48. Bergqvist D, Burmark US, Flordal PA, et al. Low molecular weight heparin started before surgery

as prophylaxis against deep vein thrombosis: 2500 vs 5000 XaI units in 2070 patients. *Br J Surg.* 1995;82:496–501.

49. Bergqvist D, Agnelli G, Cohen AT, et al. Duration of prophylaxis against venous thromboembolism with enoxaparin after surgery for cancer. *N Engl J Med.* 2002;346:975–980.

50. Rasmussen MS, Jorgensen LN, Wille Jorgensen P, et al. Prolonged prophylaxis with dalteparin to prevent late thromboembolic complications in patients undergoing major abdominal surgery: a multicenter, randomized open-label study. *J Thromb Haemost.* 2006;4:2384–2390.

51. Bottaro FJ, Elizondo MC, Doti C, et al. Efficacy of extended thromboprophylaxis in major abdominal surgery: what does the evidence show? A meta-analysis. *Thromb Haemost.* 2008;99:1104–1111.

52. Samama MM, Cohen QT, Darmon JY, et al. A comparison of enoxaparin with placebo for the prevention of venous thromboembolism in acutely ill medical patients: prophylaxis in medical patients with enoxaparin study group. *N Engl J Med.* 1999;341:793–800.

53. Leizorovicz A, Cohen AT, Turpie AG, et al. Randomized, placebo controlled trial of dalteparin for the prevention of venous thromboembolism in acutely medically ill patients. *Circulation.* 2004;110:874–879.

54. Agnelli G, Gussoni G, Bianchini C, et al. PROTECHT Investigators. Nadroparin for the prevention of thromboembolic events in ambulatory patients with metastatic or locally advanced solid cancer receiving chemotherapy: a randomised, placebo-controlled double-blind study. *Lancet Oncol.* 2009;10:943–949.

55. Kuderer NM, Ortel TL, Khorana AA, et al. Low molecular weight heparin thromboprophylaxis in ambulatory cancer patients: a systematic review and meta analysis of randomised controlled trials. *Blood.* 2009;114:203.

56. Siguret V, Leizorovicz A, Pautas A, et al. No accumulation of peak anti-Xa activity with tinzaparin in elderly patients with moderate to severe renal impairment: a substudy of IRIS clinical trial. *Blood.* 2009;114:77.

57. Cohen AT, Davison BL, Gallus AS, et al. ARTEMIS Investigators. Efficacy and safety of fondaparinux for the prevention of venous thromboembolism in older acute medical patients: randomised placebo-controlled trial. *BMJ.* 2006;332:325–329.

58. Levine MN, Hirsh J, Gent M, et al. Double-blind randomised trial of very-low-dose warfarin for prevention of thromboembolism in stage IV breast cancer. *Lancet.* 1994;343:886–889.

59. Abrams PJ, Emerson CR. Rivaroxaban, a novel, oral, direct factor Xa inhibitor. *Pharmacotherapy.* 2009;7:552–558.

60. Lassen MR, Ageno W, Borris LC, et al. Rivaroxaban versus enoxaparin for thromboprophylaxis after total knee arthroplasty. *N Engl J Med.* 2008;358:2765–2775.

61. Connolly SJ, Ezekowitz MD, Yusuf S, et al. Dabigatran versus warfarin in atrial fibrillation. *N Engl J Med.* 2009;361:139–151.

62. Schulman S, Eriksson H, Goldhaber S, et al. Dabigatran etexilate versus warfarin in the treatment of venous thromboembolism. *Blood.* 2009;114:3.

63. Roderick P, Ferris G, Wilson K, et al. Towards evidence-based guidelines for the prevention of venous thromboembolism: systematic reviews of mechanical methods, oral anticoagulation, dextran and regional anesthesia as thromboprophylaxis. *Health Technol Assess.* 2005;9:1–78.

64. Blaivas AJ, Dennis M, ACP Journal Club. Graduated compression stockings did not prevent deep venous thrombosis after stroke and increased skin complications. *Lancet.* 2009;373:1958–1965.

65. Lyman GH, Khorana AA, Falanga A, et al. American Society of Clinical Oncology Guideline: recommendations for venous thromboembolism prophylaxis and treatment in patients with cancer. *J Clin Oncol.* 2007;25:5490–5505.

66. National Comprehensive Cancer Network. *Clinical practice guidelines in oncology, version 1.* Available at: http://www.nccn.org. 2009.

67. Geerts WH, Bergqvist D, Pineo GF, et al. Prevention of venous thromboembolism: American College of Chest Physicians evidence-based clinical practice guidelines, ed 8. *Chest.* 2008;133(suppl 6):381S–453S.

68. Mismetti P, Laporte S, Darmon JY, et al. Meta-analysis of low-molecular-weight heparin in the prevention of venous thromboembolism in general surgery. *Br J Surg.* 2001;88:913–930.

69. Palumbo A, Gay F. *How to treat elderly patients with multiple myeloma: combination of therapy or sequencing.* New Orleans, LA: American Society of Hematology Program Book; December 5-8, 2009:566–577.

70. Van Dongen CJ, van den Belt AG, Prins MH, et al. Fixed dose subcutaneous low molecular weight heparins versus adjusted dose unfractionated heparin for venous thromboembolism. *Cochrane Database Syst Rev.* 2004;4: CD001100.

71. Van Dormaal FF, Raskob GE, Davidson BL, et al. Treatment of venous thromboembolism in patients with cancer: subgroup analysis of the Matisse clinical trials. *Thromb Haemost.* 2009;101:762–769.

72. Prandoni P, Lensing AW, Piccioli A, et al. Recurrent venous thromboembolism and bleeding complications during anticoagulant treatment in patients with cancer and venous thrombosis. *Blood.* 2002;100:3484–3488.

73. Lee A, Levine MN, Baker RI, et al. Low-molecular-weight heparin versus a coumarin for the prevention of recurrent venous thromboembolism in patients with cancer. *N Engl J Med.* 2003;349:146–153.

74. Kearon C, Kahn SR, Agnelli G, et al. Antithrombotic therapy for venous thromboembolic disease: American College of Chest Physicians evidence based guidelines, ed 8. *Chest.* 2008;133(suppl 6):454S–545S.

75. Young AM, Billingham LJ, Begum G, et al. Warfarin thromboprophylaxis in cancer patients with central venous catheters (WARP): an open-label randomised trial. *Lancet.* 2009;373:567–574.

76. Niers TM, Di Nisio M, Klerk CP, et al. Prevention of catheter-related venous thrombosis with nadroparin in patients receiving chemotherapy for hematologic malignancies. *J Thromb Haemost.* 2007;5:1578–1582.

77. Hettiarachi RJ, Smorenburg SM, Ginsberg J, et al. Do heparins do more than just treat thrombosis? *Thromb Haemost.* 1999;82:947–952.

78. Prins MH, Beckers NM. *Low molecular weight heparin and cancer progression: hematology education.* Education program for the Annual Congress of the European Hematology Association, Copenhagen, Denmark, June 12-15. 2008:120–122

79. Lebeau B, Chastang C, Brechot JM, et al. Subcutaneous heparin treatment increases survival in small cell lung cancer. *Cancer.* 1994;7:38–45.

80. Gonzalez-Martin A, Fernandez E, Vaz MA, et al. Long-term outcome of a phase II study of weekly docetaxel with a short course of estramustine and enoxaparin in hormone resistant prostate cancer patients. *Clin Transl Oncol.* 2007;9:323–328.

81. Wojtukiewicz MZ, Kozlowski L, Ostrowska K, et al. Low molecular weight heparin treatment for malignant melanoma: a pilot trial. *Thromb Haemost.* 2007;5:729–737.

82. Falanga A, Rickles R. *Management of thrombohemorrhagic syndrome in hematologic malignancies.* Atlanta, GA: American Society of Hematology Program Book; December 8-11, 2007:165–171.

83. Henke M, Laszig R, Rube C, et al. Erythropoietin to treat head and neck cancer patients with anemia undergoing radiotherapy: randomised double-blind, placebo-controlled trial. *Lancet.* 2003;362:1255–1260.

84. Wright JR, Ung YC, Julian JA, et al. Randomized, double-blind, placebo-controlled trial of erythropoietin in non-small-cell lung cancer with disease related anemia. *J Clin Oncol.* 2007;25:1027–1032.

85. Gould MK, Dembitzer AD, Sanders GD, et al. Low-molecular-weight heparins compared with unfractionated heparin for treatment of acute deep venous thrombosis: a cost-effectiveness analysis. *Ann Intern Med.* 1999;130:789–799.

86. Dolovich LR, Ginsberg JS, Douketis JD, et al. A meta-analysis comparing low-molecular-weight heparins with unfractionated heparin in the treatment of venous thromboembolism: examining some unanswered questions regarding location of treatment, product type, and dosing frequency. *Arch Intern Med.* 2000;160:181–188.

Neuromuscular complications

27

Glen H. J. Stevens and Lizbeth Robles

The 5-year relative survival rate for all cancers diagnosed between 1996 and 2004 is 66%, up from 50% between 1975 and 1977. This improvement in survival reflects not only progress in the diagnosis of certain cancers at an earlier stage, but also improvements in therapy.[1] As a result of these advances, the number of late complications from the disease and its treatments has gained increasing importance. Neurologic complications can occur in the central and the peripheral nervous system. Neuromuscular dysfunction can be classified by cause or by anatomic region. Causes may include direct effect of the malignancy through direct compression or infiltration, hematogenous spread, lymphatic spread, meningeal dissemination, or perineural spread; as a paraneoplastic syndrome; or as a complication of cancer treatment.[2]

DIRECT NEUROMUSCULAR EFFECTS OF CANCER

PLEXOPATHIES

Neoplastic plexopathy is usually seen as a late complication of cancer. Brachial and lumbosacral plexopathies are most frequently encountered. Neoplastic plexopathy occurs in approximately 1 of 100 patients with cancer. In cancer patients, the frequency of neoplastic brachial plexopathy is 0.43% and of lumbosacral plexopathy is 0.71%.[3,4]

Brachial plexopathy

Lung and breast carcinomas are the most common associated tumors (Fig. 27-1). Spread occurs via lymphatics to the brachial plexus with predilection for the lower trunk. This predilection is explained by the fact that the lateral group of axillary lymph nodes is in close contact with the lower trunk of the brachial plexus. Less commonly, lymphoma and sarcoma may be involved.[5] Upper plexus involvement suggests epidural disease.[3] Symptoms include paresthesias and pain. Although differentiation between radiation-induced and neoplastic effects may be difficult, shoulder pain radiating down the medial arm and forearm and involving the fourth and fifth digits is a hallmark of metastatic plexopathy. Horner's syndrome secondary to involvement of the stellate ganglion and the sympathetic trunk can be seen in more than half of patients.[3] Electromyogram (EMG) can also help distinguish these two causes of plexopathy. Sixty to seventy percent of patients with radiation-induced plexopathy show myokymia, which spontaneously occurs as grouped action potentials followed by a period of silence, with repetition in a semirhythmic manner.[6,7]

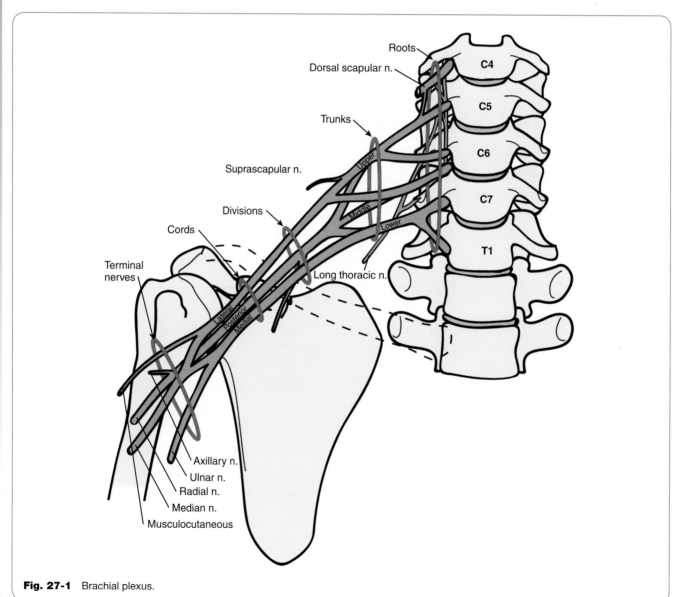

Fig. 27-1 Brachial plexus.

Diagnostic modalities include magnetic resonance imaging (MRI) and positron emission tomography (PET) scans; surgical exploration and biopsy are sometimes required.[7,8] Radiotherapy and chemotherapy may be used as treatment, with radiation relieving pain in only 46% of cases.[3] Regional intra-arterial chemotherapy is used on a limited basis in patients with intractable pain.[9]

Lumbosacral plexopathy

Lumbosacral plexopathy is most commonly caused by direct extension from an intra-abdominal neoplasm (73%).[4,10] Metastatic invasion is less common and is usually associated with breast cancer. Most frequently, colorectal and cervical tumors are involved. Symptoms include low back pain, which progresses to numbness, weakness, paresthesias, and leg edema. Incontinence, impotence, and perineal pain may be present as the result of lower sacral metastases. Bilateral plexopathy can occur in about 25% of patients and is usually related to breast cancer.[7] Diagnostic modalities include MRI and computed tomography (CT). As with neoplastic brachial plexopathy, radiotherapy may be used as treatment.

POLYRADICULOPATHY AND LEPTOMENINGEAL CARCINOMATOSIS

The clinical features of neoplastic polyradiculopathy include radicular pain, weakness, sensory loss, and hyporeflexia. Associated malignancies include breast, lymphoma, lung, gastric, and melanoma.[11,12] Lumbosacral polyradiculopathies commonly present as a cauda equina syndrome with low back pain, bladder and bowel disturbance, weakness, and hyporeflexia. Leptomeningeal metastasis occurs in 3% to 8% of all cancer patients.[13] When leptomeningeal carcinomatosis is suspected, the imaging modality of choice is MRI with gadolinium, which demonstrates leptomeningeal enhancement or compression of the nerve roots and cranial nerves. Cerebrospinal fluid (CSF) analysis is almost always abnormal with increased opening pressure, elevated protein, and pleocytosis.[12] CSF cytology demonstrates malignant cells in less than 50% of cases after an initial lumbar puncture, with the yield increasing to 90% after three specimens are obtained.[14] Prolonged or absent F waves are seen on EMG.[11] Therapy usually involves radiotherapy to symptomatic sites, often followed by intrathecal chemotherapy. Patients with disease from breast, leukemia, and lymphoma tend to respond best.[13] Nonetheless, patients with leptomeningeal carcinomatosis tend to have a poor prognosis, with a median survival of 3 to 6 months with treatment and 4 to 6 weeks without.[15]

PERIPHERAL NEUROPATHY

Mononeuropathies, mononeuropathy multiplex, and a symmetric polyneuropathy may result from direct tumor infiltration of the nerve. Lymphomas and leukemias, particularly chronic lymphocytic leukemia (CLL), have been associated with peripheral neuropathy (PN).[16] The term *neurolymphomatosis* is frequently used to characterize patients with peripheral nervous system (PNS) infiltration as a result of lymphoma. Neurolymphomatosis can mimic inflammatory neuropathies such as acute and chronic inflammatory demyelinating polyneuropathy (AIDP, CIDP) and mononeuritis multiplex.[17,18]

Peripheral neuropathies may also be the result of metastatic compression and invasion. Nerve trunks can be compressed in bony canals as the result of malignancies such as breast, prostate, lung, kidney, and thyroid cancer.[17] Cranial nerve neuropathies secondary to metastasis most commonly affect the third, fifth, sixth, and seventh cranial nerves.[5] The "numb chin syndrome" is due to compression of the inferior alveolar nerve by metastases to the mandible and may be the first presentation of malignancy. Breast cancer is the most common primary site in women, followed by adrenal, colorectal, gynecologic, and thyroid cancers. In men, lung was the most common primary, followed by prostate, kidney, bone, and adrenal cancers.[19] The prognosis for these patients is poor, with a mean survival of 7.3 months from diagnosis of jaw metastasis.[20]

NEUROMUSCULAR EFFECTS OF CANCER TREATMENT

RADIATION-INDUCED BRACHIAL PLEXOPATHY

Radiation-induced brachial plexopathy usually occurs after doses greater than 6000 centigray (cGy) and presents 3 months to 26 years after treatment, with a median of 6 years. Clinical features that allow it to be distinguished from neoplastic plexopathy include involvement of the upper trunk or the entire trunk[21] and lymphedema[9]; pain is less severe and is present in only 15% of patients.[16] As was previously mentioned, myokymic discharge can be seen on EMG.

LUMBOSACRAL PLEXOPATHY

Radiation-induced lumbosacral plexopathy may develop 1 month to 31 years after treatment, most frequently between 12 months and 5 years. Clinical features that allow it to be distinguished from a neoplastic plexopathy include absence of pain, which occurs in only 10% of patients.[22]

RADIATION-INDUCED MYOPATHY

Trismus, which involves the muscles of mastication, may be a result of radiation therapy used for treatment of head and neck cancers. Patient treated for recurrence seem to be at higher risk.[23]

RADIATION-INDUCED NERVE TUMORS

Malignant peripheral nerve sheath tumors (MPNSTs) may appear 16 years after radiation treatment.[24] Malignant transformation from plexiform neurofibromas to MPNSTs has been associated with mutations in the *p53* and *INK4a* genes, with aberrancy signaling in the Notch pathway.[17]

SURGERY RELATED NEUROPATHY

The brachial plexus may be injured during thoracotomy or mastectomy. The spinal accessory muscle is often sacrificed during radical or modified neck dissection for head and neck cancers. The intercostal nerve is frequently damaged during radical or modified radical mastectomy.[2]

STEROID-INDUCED MYOPATHY

Steroids are used in the treatment of acute leukemia in children and in the treatment of lymphoma. They are also used to reduce edema, tumor- or radiation-related, in the brain, spinal cord, and mediastinum. Myopathy, a common complication of steroid therapy, is usually reversible if the drug is withdrawn or the dose reduced.[24]

HEMATOPOIETIC STEM CELL TRANSPLANT

Hematopoietic stem cell transplantation is part of the treatment for hematologic malignancies such as leukemias, lymphoma, and multiple myeloma. Neurologic complications related to bone marrow transplantation (BMT) include drug-related encephalopathies and seizures, septic cerebral infarctions and hemorrhages (most commonly, subdural hematoma), infection by viruses and opportunistic organisms such as herpes zoster, toxoplasmosis, and *Aspergillus,* and neurologic complications of graft-versus-host disease (GVHD).[25] Complications of chronic GVHD in BMT recipients include inflammatory myopathies (polymyositis),[26] myasthenia gravis,[27] and demyelinating polyneuropathies (Guillain-Barré syndrome).[28]

CHEMOTHERAPY-INDUCED NEUROPATHY

Chemotherapy-induced neuropathy is generally characterized by axonal loss. It commonly presents as a subacute, length-dependent polyneuropathy with sensory symptoms greater than motor symptoms (Table 27-1).

VINCA ALKALOIDS

Vinca alkaloids such as vinblastine, vinorelbine, vindesine, and vincristine are used in the treatment of lymphomas, acute lymphocytic leukemia (ALL), and solid tumors. The mechanism of action of vinca alkaloids is to arrest dividing cells in metaphase by binding tubulin and preventing its polymerization into microtubules. This is also the proposed mechanism of causing neuropathy by inhibiting anterograde and retrograde axonal transport, thereby causing axonal degeneration.[29] Toxicity is dose-dependent and is associated with a sensorimotor neuropathy. The initial clinical feature is usually areflexia followed by paresthesias. With further increases in dose, distal weakness of the hands and feet occurs in 25% to 35% of patients.[30] Risk factors for developing vinca alkaloid neuropathy include preceding diabetic neuropathy and Charcot Marie Tooth disease type 1A.[31] Rarely, cranial nerves might be affected. Myopathy is much less frequent and appears after prolonged use.[32] Autonomic neuropathy results in constipation and paralytic ileus.[33]

CISPLATIN AND CARBOPLATIN

Platinum-containing antineoplastic agents are used in the treatment of testicular, ovarian, (small cell lung cancer) SCLC, bladder, and head and neck cancers. The mechanism of action is formation of intra-crosslinks and inter-crosslinks with DNA. In vivo and in vitro cisplatin causes apoptosis in the dorsal root ganglion, resulting in sensory neuronopathy.[34] Symptoms include dysesthesias and sensory ataxia. All sensory modalities are involved, but loss of large fiber function is more significant.[35] Ototoxicity may manifest as tinnitus and high-frequency hearing loss. Its postulated mechanism occurs through reactive oxygen species causing apoptosis of the hair cells.[36] Lhermitte's sign secondary to posterior column demyelination has been described.[32] A coasting phenomenon consisting of worsening neuropathic symptoms despite discontinuation of treatment has been observed.[37] In addition, 60% to 80% of patients develop cold-induced paresthesias consisting of a reversible neuropathy, which occurs within 30 to 60 minutes after infusion and resolves spontaneously.[35]

Oxaliplatin produces acute and chronic forms of neuropathy. The chronic form appears 6 months after treatment. The acute form is more common. Although recent studies support the use of calcium and magnesium salts[38] and supplementation with vitamin E to decrease the incidence and severity of neuropathy,[39] a Cochrane Database Review from 2007

Table 27-1 Chemotherapy-induced neuropathy

Drug	Mechanism	Clinical features	Electrophysiology
Vinca alkaloids	Inhibition of microtubule assembly, inhibiting axonal transport	Symmetric sensorimotor neuropathy, autonomic neuropathy, rarely cranial neuropathy	Axonal sensorimotor polyneuropathy, SNAP and CMAP amplitude reduced
Platinum analogs	Dorsal root ganglia apoptosis	Sensory neuronopathy, Lhermitte's, sensory ataxia, ototoxicity, reversible neuropathy	Axonal neuropathy, SNAP amplitude reduced
Taxanes	Promotion of microtubule assembly, axonal transport	Symmetric sensory neuropathy, autonomic symptoms	Axonal sensorimotor neuropathy, SNAP and CMAP reduced
Surinam	Glycolipid lysosomal inclusion in DRG, inhibition of NGF	Sensorimotor neuropathy, demyelinating neuropathy	Axonal neuropathy, demyelinating neuropathy with conduction blocks
Thalidomide	Inhibition of NGF, antiangiogenesis	Sensory neuropathy, autonomic neuropathy	Axonal sensory neuropathy, SNAP and CMAP reduced
Bortezomib	Proteasome inhibition	Length-dependent neuropathy	Axonal sensory neuropathy involving small fibers

CMAP, Compound muscle action potential; *DRG,* dorsal root ganglia; *NGF,* nerve growth factor; *SNAP,* sensory nerve action potential.

concluded that the evidence is insufficient to recommend the use of any therapy to prevent platinum compound–induced neuropathy.[40]

TAXANES

Paclitaxel is used in the treatment of ovarian, breast, lung, bladder, head and neck cancers, and lymphoma. Docetaxel is a synthetic analog. Both produce a predominantly sensory axonal neuropathy. A proposed mechanism of action involves hyperstabilization of the microtubule assembly, which, in turn, decreases the ability of the cell to reorganize its cytoskeleton and formation of crystal arrays, both of which interfere with axonal transport.[35,41] Also, recent studies have shown that paclitaxel-induced painful sensory neuropathy is related to direct effects in the mitochondria, as evidenced by in vitro studies revealing induction of atypical mitochondrias and mitochondrial swelling after exposure to paclitaxel.[42] These effects have been shown to be related to increases in conductance through the membrane permeability transition pore (mPTP) and cytochrome c release.[42,43] Based on this mechanism, acylcarnitine[44] and, most recently, olexosime[43] have been shown to be effective in vitro in the prevention of paclitaxel-evoked painful neuropathy.

SURAMIN

Suramin is a polysulfonated naphthylurea used for the treatment of refractory malignancies, including adrenal carcinoma. It causes a distal axonal sensorimotor polyneuropathy and a subacute demyelinating polyradiculoneuropathy similar to Guillain-Barré syndrome (GBS).[16,41]

ETOPOSIDE

Etoposide is used for the treatment of lymphoma, leukemia, SCLC, and testicular cancer. It is associated with an axonal distal symmetric sensorimotor polyneuropathy. Autonomic dysfunction can lead to hypotension and gastroparesis.[16,41]

CYTARABINE

Cytarabine is used mainly in the treatment of hematologic malignancies. Although it does not usually cause neuropathy at therapeutic doses, high-dose cytarabine therapy has been associated with a severe sensorimotor neuropathy resembling GBS.[45] High-dose cytarabine has also been associated with an acute irreversible cerebellar syndrome.[46]

IFOSFAMIDE

Ifosfamide is a prodrug alkylating agent. It is used in the treatment of germ cell tumors, sarcomas, and lymphomas. Ten to sixteen percent of patients develop an encephalopathy.[47] Ifosfamide has also been associated with neuropathy occurring in 8% of patients.[35]

THALIDOMIDE

Thalidomide is a glutamic acid derivative that induces production of interferon-γ and interleukin-2 and inhibits tumor necrosis factor-α production and angiogenesis. It is used in patients with multiple myeloma. The neuropathy is mostly sensory. Symptoms include numbness and paresthesias in the hands and feet. Autonomic neuropathy manifesting as constipation affects 56% of patients.[48] Neuropathy develops in 20% to 40% of patients.[35]

BORTEZOMIB

Bortezomib, a proteasome inhibitor used in the treatment of relapsing multiple myeloma and mantle cell lymphoma, has been associated with a peripheral sensory length-dependent distal neuropathy involving small fibers.[49] This neuropathy has been shown to be secondary to reactive oxygen species generation and mitochondrial dysfunction, leading to cytochrome c release and apoptosis.[50] Clinical features include neuropathic pain.

EPITHELONES

Epithelones consist of a group of microtubule-stabilizing agents used in the treatment of metastatic breast cancer. Distal sensory and motor neuropathies have been reported in association with its use.[51] Procarbazine has also been associated with a mild peripheral neuropathy.[52]

Despite the fact that many drugs have been studied as preventive medications for chemotherapy-induced peripheral neuropathy (amifostine, vitamin E, glutamine, glutathione, N- acetylcysteine, acetyl carnitine), evidence is insufficient to recommend the use of any agent.[53]

REMOTE (PARANEOPLASTIC) EFFECTS OF CANCER

Paraneoplastic syndromes are disorders that result from autoimmunity to a common antigen present in the tumor and the neuromuscular system. Tumors commonly involved in paraneoplastic diseases of the CNS include SCLC, neuroblastoma, thymoma, and teratoma. Tumors that produce immunoglobulins (plasma cell dyscrasias, B-cell lymphomas) are commonly involved in paraneoplastic disease of the peripheral nervous system. About 3% to 5% of patients with small cell lung cancer, 15% to 20% with thymomas, and 3% to 10% with B-cell or plasma cell neoplasms develop paraneoplastic disorders (Table 27-2).[54]

PARAEOPLASTIC DISORDERS AFFECTING THE NEUROMUSCULAR JUNCTION
Lambert-Eaton myasthenic syndrome (LEMS)

Lambert-Eaton myasthenic syndrome (LEMS) is a paraneoplastic disorder associated with antibodies against the presynaptic voltage-gated P/Q calcium channels present in more than 85% of patients with LEMS. Binding by the antibody decreases calcium entry into the presynaptic terminal, thereby preventing binding of vesicles to the presynaptic membrane and decreasing acetylcholine release. LEMS is most often associated with small cell lung cancer, although idiopathic presentations are involved in 40% of cases. Symptoms include proximal weakness, areflexia, and autonomic dysfunction. EMG shows small compound muscle action potentials (CMAPs) and facilitation by at least 100% with exercise or 20-Hz repetitive stimulation (Fig. 27-2). Single-fiber EMG

Table 27-2 Paraneoplastic neuromuscular syndromes

Syndrome	Clinical features	Antibody	Tumors	EMG/ QSART	Affected tissues
Sensory neuronopathy	Pain, paresthesias, numbness, asymmetric	Anti-Hu Anti-CRMP-5	SCLC Less commonly: breast, ovarian, adrenal, prostate, neuroblastoma, and Hodgkin's disease	Absent sensory response (asymmetric arms>legs)	Dorsal root ganglia
Sensorimotor polyneuropathy	Weakness, numbness, areflexia	Anti-CRMP-5 Anti-Hu	SCLC, Hodgkin's, osteosclerotic myeloma, leukemia, Waldenström's macroglobu- linemia	Axonal sensorimotor changes	Peripheral nerve
Autonomic neuropathy	Orthostatic hypotension, gastrointestinal dysmotility	Anti-Hu, Anti-CRMP-5, antiacetylcholine ganglionic receptor, anti-PCA-2	SCLC, thymoma	Abnormal QSART	Autonomic ganglia
Vasculitic neuropathy	Mononeuritis multiplex	Anti-Hu	SCLC, lymphoma, renal cell, endometrial, breast	Axonal loss	Peripheral nerve
LEMS	Proximal weakness, areflexia, autonomic dysfunction	P/Q-subtype voltage-gated calcium channel	SCLC	Decreased CMAP with postexercise facilitation	Presynaptic membranes
Myasthenia gravis	Oculobulbar weakness, fatigability	Acetylcholine receptors, anti- striational muscle	Thymoma	Decrement in CMAP after 2 to 3 Hz repetitive stimulation	Postsynaptic membranes
Isaac's syndrome	Muscle stiffness, cramps that persist during sleep	Voltage-gated potassium channel	Thymoma, Hodgkin's, plasmacytoma	Myokymia	Peripheral nerve
Stiff person syndrome	Painful muscle spasms	Anti-GAD, amphiphysin	Hodgkin's, SCLC thymoma, breast	Abnormal exteroceptive reflexes, CMUA	Spinal cord inhibitory neurons
Inflammatory myopathies	Proximal weakness, skin changes	No antibody	Ovarian, lung, pancreatic, stomach, colorectal, Hodgkin's	Myopathic changes, increased abnormal spontaneous activity	Muscle

CMAP, compound muscle action potential; CMUA, continuous motor unit activity; CRMP-5, collapsin response mediated protein-5; EMG, electromyelography; GAD, glutamic acid decarboxylase; LEMS, Lambert-Eaton myasthenic syndrome; PCA-2, Purkinje cell cytoplasmic antibodies; QSART, quantitative sudomotor axon reflex test; SCLC, small cell lung cancer.

shows increased jitter[55] (Fig. 27-3). Patients with idiopathic LEMS should be screened for cancer every 6 months with chest imaging.[55] Symptomatic therapy includes 3,4- diamin-opyridine (DAP) and pyridostigmine. The clinical utility of DAP is limited by seizures, which occur at therapeutic doses.[56]

Myasthenia gravis (MG)

In contrast to LEMS, myasthenia gravis (MG) is a postsynaptic disorder of the neuromuscular junction. The hallmark of MG is fluctuating fatigable weakness with presenting symptoms including bulbar weakness and leg weakness. Approximately 10% of patients with myasthenia gravis are found to have a thymoma, and 30% of patients with thymoma are subsequently found to have myasthenia.[57] Antistriational muscle antibody (also called anti-titin antibody) is found in 80% of patients with MG that is linked to thymoma.[58] EMG shows a decremental motor response in CMAPs with 2 to 3 Hz repetitive stimulation. All patients suspected to have MG should

undergo chest CT to detect a thymoma. Because of the propensity for local invasion, thymectomy is indicated for all patients with thymoma. Approximately 75% of patients with MG benefit from thymectomy.[59] After thymectomy, patients can be followed with CT of the chest and anti-titin (anti-striational) antibody titers.

Many other paraneoplastic conditions have been described in association with thymoma, including thyroiditis, intestinal pseudo-obstruction, pemphigus, stiff person syndrome, and retinopathy.[59]

DISORDERS OF NEUROMUSCULAR HYPERACTIVITY

NEUROMYOTONIA (ISAAC'S SYNDROME)

Isaac's syndrome, or acquired neuromyotonia, is an antibody-mediated channelopathy resulting in hyperexcitability of the motor nerves. Associations with thymoma, Hodgkin's

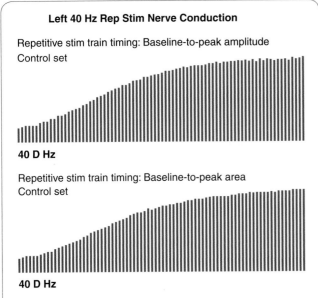

Left 40 Hz Rep Stim Nerve Conduction

Repetitive stim train timing: Baseline-to-peak amplitude
Control set

40 D Hz

Repetitive stim train timing: Baseline-to-peak area
Control set

40 D Hz

Fig. 27-2 Lambert-Eaton myasthenic syndrome (LEMS): facilitation on 40-Hz repetitive stimulation.

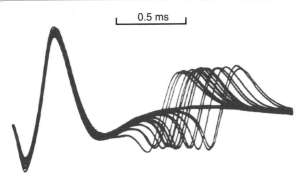

0.5 ms

Fig. 27-3 Single-fiber electromyography (EMG) in neuromuscular junction paraneoplastic disease: jitter.

lymphoma, and plasmacytoma have been reported.[59–62] Antibodies to the voltage-gated potassium channels are associated with the syndrome and are present in 45% of patients. Patients present with muscle twitching (fasciculations and myokymia), which persists during sleep, as well as diffuse muscle stiffness, cramps, and hyperhidrosis. EMG shows spontaneous motor unit activity, including fasciculations, myokymic discharges, and neuromyotonic discharges, as well as voluntary motor unit firing as doublets and triplets.[33] Symptomatic treatment with phenytoin, carbamazepine, and gabapentin has been reported.[63–65]

STIFF PERSON SYNDROME

Stiff person syndrome (SPS) is characterized by painful muscle spasms, often triggered by sudden noise or movement and stiffness that disappears during sleep. Antibodies against glutamic acid decarboxylase are found in up to 60% of patients.[49] Presynaptic anti-amphiphysin antibodies have been found in patients with SPS and breast cancer.[66] SPS has also been reported in association with Hodgkin's lymphoma, SCLC,

and thymoma.[5] EMG shows continuous motor unit activity (CMUA) and abnormal exteroceptive or cutaneomuscular reflexes.[67,68]

MYOPATHIES

Both dermatomyositis and polymyositis have been associated with malignancy. Dermatomyositis is suspected to have a paraneoplastic origin in 30% of patients. Associated malignancies include ovarian, lung, pancreatic, stomach, and colorectal cancers and non-Hodgkin's lymphoma.[69]

PARANEOPLASTIC DISORDERS AFFECTING THE PERIPHERAL NERVOUS SYSTEM

SENSORY NEURONOPATHY

Its onset can be acute or insidiously progressive. There is a female predominance. Pain, paresthesias, and numbness start in the upper extremities in 60% of patients and are asymmetric in 40%; this characteristic helps to distinguish the disorder from a length-dependent sensory neuropathy.[70] The most commonly associated malignancy is SCLC, and the most frequently associated antibody, anti-Hu. Other neoplasms less commonly associated include breast, ovarian, adrenal, prostate, neuroblastoma, and Hodgkin's lymphoma.[5,71] The neuronopathy may precede the diagnosis of neoplasm by up to 2 years.[49] EMG reveals limited changes in small sensory nerve action potentials (SNAPs).[72]

SENSORIMOTOR POLYNEUROPATHY

Use of chemotherapeutic agents, weight loss, malnutrition, and organ failure may predispose and contribute to the development of peripheral neuropathy in cancer patients. Anti–collapsin response-mediated protein-5 (CRMP-5) antibodies have been associated with sensorimotor polyneuropathy and SCLC.[16] EMG reveals an axonal process.

Peripheral neuropathies can also be seen with myelomas. Up to 13% of patients with multiple myeloma have clinically evident peripheral neuropathy, with amyloid deposition as the most common cause.[73] The most frequent monoclonal disorders associated with neuropathy are smoldering myeloma; multiple myeloma; Waldenström's macroglobulinemia; solitary plasmacytoma; systemic immunoglobulin light chain amyloidosis (AL); polyneuropathy, organomegaly, endocrinopathy, monoclonal gammopathy, and skin changes (POEMS); and cryoglobulinemia.[74] In osteosclerotic myeloma, approximately half of patients have an associated polyneuropathy, which is often the presenting symptom.[75] The initial symptoms are pain and paresthesias. Patients can also present with orthostatic hypotension, constipation, or diarrhea, all of which are suggestive of an autonomic dysfunction. Nerve conduction studies reveal an axonal process. Biopsy of abdominal fat pad, rectal mucosa, or sural nerve can reveal amyloid deposition.[74]

VASCULITIC NEUROPATHY

Vasculitic neuropathy as a remote effect of cancer has been reported in association with SCLC, lymphoma, renal cell cancer, adenocarcinoma of the lung, and endometrial, breast, and prostate cancer.[76,77] The usual pattern is a symmetric sensorimotor polyneuropathy, but it may also present as mononeuritis multiplex. EMG findings depend on the stage of the disorder, with axonal loss seen early in the disease.[72]

AUTONOMIC NEUROPATHY

Patients may have symptoms of dysautonomia, including orthostatic hypotension, GI dysmotility, impaired sweating, and impotence. Associated malignancies include thymoma and SCLC, which are present in 15% of patients. Less commonly associated malignancies include non–small cell cancer; cancers of the GI tract, prostate, breast, bladder, kidney, and pancreas; and testicular and ovarian cancer.[71] Antibodies include anti-Hu and antiganglionic acetylcholine receptor (α3-type) binding antibodies,[78] which are detectable in 50% of patients with subacute autoimmune autonomic neuropathy (AAN). Other associated antibodies include Purkinje cell cytoplasmic antibody (PCA-2)[79] and anti-CRMP-5.[80] To assess dysautonomia, autonomic testing includes a quantitative sudomotor axon reflex test (QSART). The acetylcholinesterase inhibitor pyridostigmine is a novel therapy for autonomic failure that acts by enhancing ganglionic synaptic transmission.[81]

INFLAMMATORY DEMYELINATING POLYNEUROPATHY

Hodgkin's lymphoma is the cancer most commonly associated with GBS. Associations with other malignancies, including tongue carcinoma, ovarian dysgerminoma, breast cancer, and non- Hodgkin's lymphoma, are less clear.[82] Chronic inflammatory demyelinating neuropathy has been described in association with pancreatic, colon, and liver cancer.[83]

MOTOR NEURON DISEASE

Many reports have described an association between motor neuron disease and hematologic malignancies. However, whether a true relationship exists is still unclear. True paraneoplastic motor neuron disease is assumed to be rare.[49]

PHYSICAL ACTIVITY

It is likely that much of the functional decline of cancer patients may be improved with exercise.[84] Physical activity capabilities may vary among cancer survivors based on their diagnosis and treatment modalities. For example, patients with significant peripheral neuropathies may benefit from a stationary bicycle, given their possible weakness, loss of balance, and sensory loss.[85] Cancer survivors with a low quality of life may benefit from studies aimed at developing interventions to improve well-being through physical activity.[86]

CONCLUSION

Neuromuscular complications of cancer can occur through a multitude of causes, which include direct compression or infiltration, hematogenous spread, lymphatic spread, meningeal dissemination, and perineurial spread. They can also occur as a paraneoplastic syndrome or as a complication of cancer treatment. Understanding the underlying cause will best help in treatment and alleviation of symptoms.

REFERENCES

1. American Cancer Society. *Cancer facts & figures.* Atlanta, GA: The Society; 2009, p. v.
2. Custodio CM. Neuromuscular complications of cancer and cancer treatments. *Phys Med Rehabil Clin N Am.* 2008;19:27–45.
3. Kori SH, Foley KM, Posner JB. Brachial plexus lesions in patients with cancer: 100 cases. *Neurology.* 1981;31:45–50.
4. Jaeckle KA, Young DF, Foley KM. The natural history of lumbosacral plexopathy in cancer. *Neurology.* 1985;35:8–15.
5. Falah M, Schiff D, Burns TM. Neuromuscular complications of cancer diagnosis and treatment. *J Support Oncol.* 2005;3:271–282.
6. Lederman RJ, Wilbourn AJ. Brachial plexopathy: recurrent cancer or radiation? *Neurology.* 1984;34:1331–1335.
7. Chad DA, Recht LD. Neuromuscular complications of systemic cancer. *Neurol Clin.* 1991;9:901–918.
8. Taylor BV, Kimmel DW, Krecke KN, et al. Magnetic resonance imaging in cancer-related lumbosacral plexopathy. *Mayo Clin Proc.* 1997;72:823–829.
9. Jaeckle KA. Neurological manifestations of neoplastic and radiation-induced plexopathies. *Semin Neurol.* 2004;24:385–393.
10. Evans BA, Stevens JC, Dyck PJ. Lumbosacral plexus neuropathy. *Neurology.* 1981;31:1327–1330.
11. Argov Z, Siegal T. Leptomeningeal metastases: peripheral nerve and root involvement—clinical and electrophysiological study. *Ann Neurol.* 1985;17:593–596.

12. Olson ME, Chernik NL, Posner JB. Infiltration of the leptomeninges by systemic cancer: a clinical and pathologic study. *Arch Neurol.* 1974;30:122–137.
13. DeAngelis LM. Current diagnosis and treatment of leptomeningeal metastasis. *J Neurooncol.* 1998;38:245–252.
14. Wasserstrom WR, Glass JP, Posner JB. Diagnosis and treatment of leptomeningeal metastases from solid tumors: experience with 90 patients. *Cancer.* 1982;49:759–772.
15. Grossman SA, Krabak MJ. Leptomeningeal carcinomatosis. *Cancer Treat Rev.* 1999;25:103–119.
16. Briemberg HR, Amato AA. Neuromuscular complications of cancer. *Neurol Clin.* 2003;21:141–165.
17. Antoine JC, Camdessanche JP. Peripheral nervous system involvement in patients with cancer. *Lancet Neurol.* 2007;6:75–86.
18. Lisak RP, Mitchell M, Zweiman B, et al. Guillain-Barré syndrome and Hodgkin's disease: three cases with immunological studies. *Ann Neurol.* 1977;1:72–78.
19. Evans RW, Kirby S, Purdy RA. Numb chin syndrome. *Headache.* 2008;48:1520–1524.
20. Hirshberg A, Leibovich P, Buchner A. Metastatic tumors to the jawbones: analysis of 390 cases. *J Oral Pathol Med.* 1994;23:337–341.
21. Olsen NK, Pfeiffer P, Mondrup K, et al. Radiation-induced brachial plexus neuropathy in breast cancer patients. *Acta Oncol.* 1990;29:885–890.

22. Thomas JE, Cascino TL, Earle JD. Differential diagnosis between radiation and tumor plexopathy of the pelvis. *Neurology.* 1985;35:1–7.
23. Sciubba JJ, Goldenberg D. Oral complications of radiotherapy. *Lancet Oncol.* 2006;7:175–183.
24. Stubgen JP. Neuromuscular disorders in systemic malignancy and its treatment. *Muscle Nerve.* 1995;18:636–648.
25. Saiz A, Graus F. Neurological complications of hematopoietic cell transplantation. *Semin Neurol.* 2004;24:427–434.
26. Leber B, Walker IR, Rodriguez A, et al. Reinduction of remission of chronic myeloid leukemia by donor leukocyte transfusion following relapse after bone marrow transplantation: recovery complicated by initial pancytopenia and late dermatomyositis. *Bone Marrow Transplant.* 1993;12:405–407.
27. Grau JM, Casademont J, Monforte R, et al. Myasthenia gravis after allogeneic bone marrow transplantation: report of a new case and pathogenetic considerations. *Bone Marrow Transplant.* 1990;5:435–437.
28. Myers SE, Williams SF. Guillain-Barre syndrome after autologous bone marrow transplantation for breast cancer: report of two cases. *Bone Marrow Transplant.* 1994;13:341–344.
29. Paulson JC, McClure WO. Inhibition of axoplasmic transport by colchicine, podophyllotoxin, and vinblastine: an effect on microtubules. *Ann N Y Acad Sci.* 1975;253:517–527.

30. Macdonald DR. Neurologic complications of chemotherapy. *Neurol Clin.* 1991;9:955–967.

31. Graf WD, Chance PF, Lensch MW, et al. Severe vincristine neuropathy in Charcot-Marie-Tooth disease type 1A. *Cancer.* 1996;77:1356–1362.

32. Iniguez C, Larrodé P, Mayordomo JI, et al. Peripheral nervous system neurotoxicity secondary to chemotherapy treatment. *Neurologia.* 2000;15:343–351.

33. Low PA, Vernino S, Suarez G. Autonomic dysfunction in peripheral nerve disease. *Muscle Nerve.* 2003;27:646–661.

34. Gill JS, Windebank AJ. Cisplatin-induced apoptosis in rat dorsal root ganglion neurons is associated with attempted entry into the cell cycle. *J Clin Invest.* 1998;101:2842–2850.

35. Windebank AJ, Grisold W. Chemotherapy-induced neuropathy. *J Peripher Nerv Syst.* 2008;13:27–46.

36. Rybak LP, Whitworth CA, Mukherjea D, et al. Mechanisms of cisplatin-induced ototoxicity and prevention. *Hear Res.* 2007;226:157–167.

37. Behin A, Psimaras D, Hoang-Xuan K, et al. Neuropathies in the context of malignancies. *Curr Opin Neurol.* 2008;21:534–539.

38. Gamelin L, Boisdron-Celle M, Delva R, et al. Prevention of oxaliplatin-related neurotoxicity by calcium and magnesium infusions: a retrospective study of 161 patients receiving oxaliplatin combined with 5-fluorouracil and leucovorin for advanced colorectal cancer. *Clin Cancer Res.* 2004;10:4055–4061.

39. Pace A, Savarese A, Picardo M, et al. Neuroprotective effect of vitamin E supplementation in patients treated with cisplatin chemotherapy. *J Clin Oncol.* 2003;21:927–931.

40. Albers J, Chaudhry C, Cavaletti G, et al. Interventions for preventing neuropathy caused by cisplatin and related compounds. *Cochrane Database Syst Rev.* 2007;(1) CD005228.

41. Peltier AC, Russell JW. Recent advances in drug-induced neuropathies. *Curr Opin Neurol.* 2002;15:633–638.

42. Flatters SJ, Bennett GJ. Studies of peripheral sensory nerves in paclitaxel-induced painful peripheral neuropathy: evidence for mitochondrial dysfunction. *Pain.* 2006;122:245–257.

43. Xiao WH, Zheng FY, Bennett GJ, et al. Olesoxime (cholest-4-en-3-one, oxime): analgesic and neuroprotective effects in a rat model of painful peripheral neuropathy produced by the chemotherapeutic agent, paclitaxel. *Pain.* 2009;147:202–209.

44. Jin HW, Flatters SJ, Xiao WH, et al. Prevention of paclitaxel-evoked painful peripheral neuropathy by acetyl-L-carnitine: effects on axonal mitochondria, sensory nerve fiber terminal arbors, and cutaneous Langerhans cells. *Exp Neurol.* 2008;210:229–237.

45. Openshaw H, Slatkin NE, Stein AS, et al. Acute polyneuropathy after high dose cytosine arabinoside in patients with leukemia. *Cancer.* 1996;78:1899–1905.

46. Gottlieb D, Bradstock K, Koutts J, et al. The neurotoxicity of high-dose cytosine arabinoside is age-related. *Cancer.* 1987;60:1439–1441.

47. Sioka C, Kyritsis AP. Central and peripheral nervous system toxicity of common chemotherapeutic agents. *Cancer Chemother Pharmacol.* 2009;63:761–767.

48. Glasmacher A, Hahn C, Hoffmann F, et al. A systematic review of phase-II trials of thalidomide monotherapy in patients with relapsed or refractory multiple myeloma. *Br J Haematol.* 2006;132:584–593.

49. Richardson PG, Briemberg H, Jagannath H, et al. Frequency, characteristics, and reversibility of peripheral neuropathy during treatment of advanced multiple myeloma with bortezomib. *J Clin Oncol.* 2006;24:3113–3120.

50. Ling YH, Liebes L, Zou Y, et al. Reactive oxygen species generation and mitochondrial dysfunction in the apoptotic response to bortezomib, a novel proteasome inhibitor, in human H460 non-small cell lung cancer cells. *J Biol Chem.* 2003;278:33714–33723.

51. Lee JJ, Swain SM. Peripheral neuropathy induced by microtubule-stabilizing agents. *J Clin Oncol.* 2006;24:1633–1642.

52. Spivack SD. Drugs 5 years later: procarbazine. *Ann Intern Med.* 1974;81:795–800.

53. Kaley TJ, Deangelis LM. Therapy of chemotherapy-induced peripheral neuropathy. *Br J Haematol.* 2009;145:3–14.

54. Dalmau J, Rosenfeld MR. Paraneoplastic syndromes of the CNS. *Lancet Neurol.* 2008;7:327–340.

55. Mareska M, Gutmann L. Lambert-Eaton myasthenic syndrome. *Semin Neurol.* 2004;24:149–153.

56. Kim YI, Goldner MM, Sanders DB. Facilitatory effects of 4-aminopyridine on neuromuscular transmission in disease states. *Muscle Nerve.* 1980;3:112–119.

57. Namba T, Brunner NG, Grob D. Myasthenia gravis in patients with thymoma, with particular reference to onset after thymectomy. *Medicine (Baltimore).* 1978;57:411–433.

58. Yamamoto AM, Gajdos P, Eymard B, et al. Anti-titin antibodies in myasthenia gravis: tight association with thymoma and heterogeneity of nonthymoma patients. *Arch Neurol.* 2001;58:885–890.

59. Tormoehlen LM, Pascuzzi RM. Thymoma, myasthenia gravis, and other paraneoplastic syndromes. *Hematol Oncol Clin North Am.* 2008;22:509–526.

60. Lahrmann H, Albrecht G, Drlicek M, et al. Acquired neuromyotonia and peripheral neuropathy in a patient with Hodgkin's disease. *Muscle Nerve.* 2001;24:834–838.

61. Caress JB, Abend WK, Preston DC, et al. A case of Hodgkin's lymphoma producing neuromyotonia. *Neurology.* 1997;49:258–259.

62. Zifko U, Drlicek M, Michacek E, et al. Syndrome of continuous muscle fiber activity and plasmacytoma with IgM paraproteinemia. *Neurology.* 1994;44:560–561.

63. Dhand UK. Isaacs' syndrome: clinical and electrophysiological response to gabapentin. *Muscle Nerve.* 2006;34:646–650.

64. Serratrice G, Pouget J, Pellissier JF, et al. Carbamazepine-sensitive neuromyotonia and Charcot-Marie-Tooth disease of the neuronal type. *Rev Neurol (Paris).* 1989;145:867–868.

65. Vernino S. Autoimmune and paraneoplastic channelopathies. *Neurotherapeutics.* 2007;4:305–314.

66. Rosin L, DeCamilli P, Butler M, et al. Stiff-man syndrome in a woman with breast cancer: an uncommon central nervous system paraneoplastic syndrome. *Neurology.* 1998;50:94–98.

67. Bartsch T, Herzog J, Baron R, et al. The stiff limb syndrome—a new case and a literature review. *J Neurol.* 2003;250:488–490.

68. Meinck HM, Thompson PD. Stiff man syndrome and related conditions. *Mov Disord.* 2002;17:853–866.

69. Honnorat J, Antoine JC. Paraneoplastic neurological syndromes. *Orphanet J Rare Dis.* 2007;2:22.

70. Chalk CH, Windebank AJ, Kimmel DW, et al. The distinctive clinical features of paraneoplastic sensory neuronopathy. *Can J Neurol Sci.* 1992;19:346–351.

71. Freeman R. Autonomic peripheral neuropathy. *Lancet.* 2005;365:1259–1270.

72. Krarup C, Crone C. Neurophysiological studies in malignant disease with particular reference to involvement of peripheral nerves. *J Neurol.* 2002;249:651–661.

73. Kelly Jr JJ, Kyle RA, Miles JM, et al. The spectrum of peripheral neuropathy in myeloma. *Neurology.* 1981;31:24–31.

74. Hoffman-Snyder C, Smith BE. Neuromuscular disorders associated with paraproteinemia. *Phys Med Rehabil Clin N Am.* 2008;19:61–79, vi.

75. Kelly Jr JJ, Kyle RA, Miles JM, et al. Osteosclerotic myeloma and peripheral neuropathy. *Neurology.* 1983;33:202–210.

76. Oh SJ. Paraneoplastic vasculitis of the peripheral nervous system. *Neurol Clin.* 1997;15:849–863.

77. Kurzrock R, Cohen PR, Markowitz A. Clinical manifestations of vasculitis in patients with solid tumors: a case report and review of the literature. *Arch Intern Med.* 1994;154:334–340.

78. Vernino S, Low PA, Fealey RD, et al. Autoantibodies to ganglionic acetylcholine receptors in autoimmune autonomic neuropathies. *N Engl J Med.* 2000;343:847–855.

79. Vernino S, Lennon VA. New Purkinje cell antibody (PCA-2): marker of lung cancer-related neurological autoimmunity. *Ann Neurol.* 2000;47:297–305.

80. Yu Z, Kryzer TJ, Griesmann GE, et al. CRMP-5 neuronal autoantibody: marker of lung cancer and thymoma-related autoimmunity. *Ann Neurol.* 2001;49:146–154.

81. Singer W, Opfer-Gehrking TL, McPhee BR, et al. Acetylcholinesterase inhibition: a novel approach in the treatment of neurogenic orthostatic hypotension. *J Neurol Neurosurg Psychiatry.* 2003;74:1294–1298.

82. Rudnicki SA, Dalmau J. Paraneoplastic syndromes of the peripheral nerves. *Curr Opin Neurol.* 2005;18:598–603.

83. Antoine JC, Mosnier JF, Absi L, et al. Carcinoma associated paraneoplastic peripheral neuropathies in patients with and without anti-onconeural antibodies. *J Neurol Neurosurg Psychiatry.* 1999;67:7–14.

84. Schwartz AL. Physical activity. *Semin Oncol Nurs.* 2008;24:164–170.

85. Doyle C, Kushi LH, Byers T, et al. Nutrition and physical activity during and after cancer treatment: an American Cancer Society guide for informed choices. *CA Cancer J Clin.* 2006;56:323–353.

86. Irwin ML. Physical activity interventions for cancer survivors. *Br J Sports Med.* 2009;43:32–38.

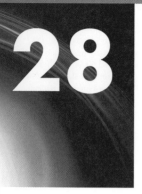

28 Complications of bone metastases—long bone fractures, spinal cord compression, vertebral augmentation

Kathy Pope, Rebecca K. S. Wong, and Isador Lieberman

Recent advances in the diagnosis and treatment of many types of cancers have prolonged and improved the quality of life for cancer patients. Bone metastases remain a common complication of advanced cancer. Occurring most frequently in breast and prostate cancers, bone metastases affect two thirds to three quarters of these patients with advanced disease.[1] Bone metastases can be asymptomatic, but frequently cause pain. Progressive disease can be complicated by soft tissue disease, destruction of bony architecture leading to fractures, spinal deformity, and cord compression. Fracture of weight-bearing bones results in acute painful events, compromise of mobility, and increased risk of medical complications. Other consequences of bone metastases include bone marrow infiltration and hypercalcemia, with significant implications for the patient's morbidity.

In this chapter, we will focus on long bone fractures, spinal cord compression, and their precursors, for which successful therapy has the potential of preventing significant morbidities associated with these complications of bone metastases. The chapter is organized with subsections addressing epidemiology, pathophysiology, clinical features, and risk factors. This is followed by information on management strategies, how to choose between them, and their expected outcomes. In particular, the roles of minimally invasive techniques (including kyphoplasty and vertebroplasty) and stereotactic radiotherapy will be discussed, along with standard radiotherapy and surgery. Bisphosphonates also have a significant role to play in the management of bone metastases depending on the primary site, but this discussion is beyond the scope of this chapter.

EPIDEMIOLOGY

The incidence of fracture and cord compression varies with the primary cancer of origin. Arguably, this is best explored at the population level. Population-based cancer studies involving patients with multiple myeloma or breast or prostate cancer who are on bisphosphonates provide estimates of skeletal complication rates, including fractures and cord compression. Some authors have been able to provide more details by examining institutional cohorts with different clinical characteristics.

LONG BONE AND VERTEBRAL FRACTURES

The risk of sustaining a long bone fracture in cancer patients was examined at the population level by Vestergaard et al., using the Denmark National Hospital Discharge Register.[2] All fractures, including hip, spine, and forearm, were included in this population-based case-control study, which involved a sample of more than 124,600 patients who had sustained a fracture during the year 2000, as well as age- and gender-matched controls that did not. Whether the fractures were pathologic or benign can only be inferred. Twenty percent of this group of patients had at least one cancer diagnosis. The risk of sustaining a fracture was higher than in the general population, with odds ratios (ORs) of 1.3 (95% confidence interval [CI], 1.15–1.47), 1.35 (95% CI, 1.18–1.55), and 1.96 (95% CI, 1.5–2.57) in patients with diagnoses of lung cancer, prostate cancer, and multiple myeloma, respectively. For patients in which "bone metastasis" was the designated cancer diagnosis, the OR was 3.01 (95% CI, 2.34–3.86). Risk of fracture was similar for vertebrae and hips during the first year of diagnosis.

Estimates of pathologic fracture risk for different clinical subgroups have been investigated in greater detail by other investigators. For example, Plunkett et al. retrospectively reviewed more than 800 patients with bone metastases from breast cancer, documenting an incidence of pathologic fracture of 34%. Vertebral fractures were most common, occurring in 20% of patients; long bone fractures occurred in 12%.[3] Similar findings were reported by others.[4] In a study involving 151 hormone-refractory prostate cancer patients from Japan, the bone fracture risk was 14% (15/106).[5] The estimated risk of fracture in lung cancer is more variable. In a cohort of non–small cell lung cancer patients with bone metastases, pathologic fracture was found in 7% (5/70).[6] In another cohort of lung cancer patients with metastatic disease treated with chemotherapy, the incidence of fracture was 2% (5/244).[7] Using a private health insurance claims database to examine the incidence of skeletal complications in 534 patients with lung cancer and bone metastases, Delea et al. reported that the highest incidence of pathologic fracture as inferred from insurance claims was estimated to be 34% (100/295).[8]

The incidence of high-risk bone metastases requiring consideration for treatment to prevent fractures is difficult to establish, but doing so is important for estimating the burden of this complication. In a population-based study by Ristevski et al., prophylactic fixation accounted for 37% of cases among 624 patients who underwent surgical stabilization for femoral metastases.[9] In a separate retrospective report on 116 patients with 152 fractures, 44% were impending fractures (67/152).[10]

SPINAL CORD COMPRESSION

The burden of malignant spinal cord compression (MSCC) was examined by Loblaw et al. using a population-based study design that consisted of 3400 cancer patients from Ontario, Canada. The cumulative probability of MSCC in the 5 years preceding death from cancer was 2.5%.[11] This ranged from 0.2% (pancreas) to 8% (multiple myeloma) for different primary cancer diagnoses. When the prevalence of different cancers is considered, the burden of illness is greatest for lung cancer, representing 23% of all cases of MSCC, followed by breast cancer (20%) and prostate cancer (18%).

Subclinical cord compression (also described as occult or radiologic) can be defined as the presence of radiologic evidence of cord compression without neurologic deficits.[12,13] This is increasingly important in clinical practice, because it represents a window for intervention with potentially the best clinical outcomes. The incidence of subclinical cord compression is difficult to establish, as detection is sensitive to the screening approach and diagnostic tools used. A prospective study by Bayley et al. (n = 68), evaluating prostate cancer patients with known vertebral metastases but without signs or symptoms of cord compression, found that 32% of patients had clinically occult subarachnoid space or spinal cord compression on magnetic resonance imaging (MRI).[12] Similar observations were made by Venkitaraman et al., who reported a 27% incidence of radiologic spinal cord compromise in a cohort of 150 consecutive patients with metastatic prostate cancer, which was detected through MRI in the absence of functional neurologic deficit.[14] The prevalence of occult cord compression in other diseases has not been well characterized.

PATHOPHYSIOLOGY

Bone metastases result in dysregulation of normal bone remodeling. Its effects can be broadly divided into osteolytic (destructive) and osteoblastic (bone-forming) metastases, representing the two ends of the spectrum of bone metabolism dysregulation.[15] This is mediated in part by many growth factors and cytokines, for which activity can be measured through a number of bone turnover markers. Increasing evidence supports the use of these markers to predict impending skeletal-related events, including fracture risk. They also may be useful for monitoring the effects of therapy intended to normalize this process. For example, Coleman et al. demonstrated a strong correlation between skeletal-related events and/or death when n-telopeptide of type I collagen (NTX) values were above 100 nmol/mmol creatinine. A similar relationship has been found in patients with osteoporosis with bone alkaline phosphatase.[16]

Metastatic spinal cord compression (MSCC) is a clinical syndrome caused by invasion of the epidural space by metastatic tumor. It is typically due to mechanical destruction of the vertebral body, compression fracture with or without displacement of bone fragments, or tumor tissue extending into the epidural space. Less commonly, dural-based, leptomeningeal, or intramedullary metastases may cause MSCC. Regardless of the pathology, spinal cord injury typically is associated with disrupted blood flow in both arterial and venous epidural circulations and occlusion of the major spinal arteries. This leads to vasogenic edema and ischemia within the cord.[17] Cytokines and inflammatory mediators such as prostaglandin E_2 (PGE_2) and vascular endothelial growth factor (VEGF), in response to hypoxia, increase vascular permeability and vasogenic edema.[18] Eventually, spinal cord infarction occurs, and this results in permanent neurologic damage.

CLINICAL FEATURES

Patients with bone metastases typically present with escalating pain at or near the site of the bone metastasis. The pain develops over weeks to months and is commonly worse at night or with movement, frequently requiring narcotic analgesia. For pelvic metastases in the ischium or sacrum, pain is often worse with sitting, whereas pubic rami metastases and acetabular and femoral metastases are exacerbated by weight bearing and can cause referral of pain toward the knee. As the degree of mechanical or incident pain increases, so does the risk of fracture. Localized weakness of the proximal lower limbs can occur as a consequence of pain. This can be difficult to distinguish from a presentation of MSCC.

Back pain, the most common presenting symptom of metastatic spinal cord compression, may be sharp, shooting, deep, or burning. The pain can be localized to the back or may radiate in a band-like dermatomal pattern, if tumor compresses the nerve roots in the neural exit foramina. Mechanical back pain is more ominous, as it is associated with spinal instability. Acute exacerbation of back pain on a background of chronic pain suggests recent compression fracture. In addition to pain, other common symptoms of MSCC include motor weakness, sensory changes (paresthesia, loss of sensation), sphincter incontinence, and autonomic dysfunction (hesitancy, urinary retention). At presentation, more patients are paraparetic than paralyzed, and this is often the reason why patients seek medical attention. Patients tend to be less aware of sensory changes than motor weakness. Patients with cauda equina syndrome present differently from those with spinal cord compression, reporting change in or loss of sensation over the buttocks, posterior-superior thighs, and perineal region, in a saddle distribution. Reduced anal tone and urinary retention, with overflow incontinence, are typically present.

ASSESSMENT OF FRACTURE RISK

Assessment of fracture risk is important in identifying patients early to avoid complications and guide management. This is not an exact science, as the risk of fracture involves a complex relationship between extent and location of bone destruction, coupled with the weight-bearing load. Biomechanical models are beginning to provide quantitative insight into the effects of activity on weight-bearing bones and the risk of fracture.[19,20] Clinical and radiologic characteristics remain the main factors used, in clinical practice and research, to obtain estimates of fracture risks. Factors and algorithms that have been developed for the assessment of fracture risk vary according to the anatomic area. This will be discussed for long bone (and acetabulum) and spine.

LONG BONE AND ACETABULAR FRACTURES

For long bone and acetabular metastases, several risk assessment tools have been described. They have common elements, including pain severity, locations of metastases, the nature of bony lesions (lytic, mixed, or blastic), and other radiologic features.[21–23] Mirels' scoring system[24] includes assessment of site of involvement, pain, nature, and size of lesions. Depending on the characteristics of each factor, a total score with a maximum of 12 can be calculated. Scores of 7 or more were found to be predictive for increasing risk of pathologic fracture. This was best validated subsequently in the assessment of fracture risk in long bones[19,25] and is widely adopted as a research and, to a certain extent, clinical tool for assessing fracture risk (Table 28-1). A simpler system

Table 28-1   Mirels' score[24]

Feature	1	2	3
Site	Upper limb	Lower limb	Peritrochanteric
Pain (0–10)	Mild (1–4)	Moderate (5–6)	Severe (7–10)
Lesion	Blastic	Mixed	Lytic
Size (circumference)	<⅓	⅓ to ⅔	>⅔

Circle one for each feature. Total score max = 12.
Scores >7 typically are used for significant risk of pathologic fracture.

Chance of pathological fracture vs. Mirels' score

described by van der Linden et al.[22] is based on a cohort of 102 patients (14 subsequently developed fractures) with femoral metastases treated within a dose fractionation radiotherapy trial. Degree of axial cortical involvement >30 mm was found to have a strong negative predictive value (97%) for subsequent fracture despite radiotherapy. For patients with acetabular involvement, Harrington described a classification based on the degree of acetabular wall involvement[26] (Table 28-2). The utility of the system in guiding the choice of surgical approach can be observed. In broad terms, the more extensive the periacetabular defect, the larger is the construct that will be necessary to successfully reinforce the deficit and distribute weight from the lower extremity to the remaining pelvis and spine.[27] Variations of this system have also been described.[27,28]

VERTEBRAL FRACTURE RISK

To estimate vertebral fracture risk, investigators have applied the concept of dividing the vertebra into adjacent cubes or cells.[29,30] Based on a sample of 113 fractured vertebrae from 67 patients, Shah et al. described a fourfold increase (hazard ratio [HR], 4.6; 95% CI, 1.7–12.7) in fracture risk when the vertebrae were >80% involved according to MRI assessment (Fig. 28-1). A greater risk of fracture was described for the upper lumbar spine when compared with cervical and thoracic vertebrae. Symmetric fractures with fragments were found to have the greatest risk of epidural compression. For clinical decision making, a simpler system using the concept

of different "zones" of involvement to predict fracture risk is frequently used.[30,31] Its application is further discussed in the section on complications of vertebral metastases—spinal cord compression: surgery.

MANAGEMENT

The optimal management strategy for individual patients with impending, established fractures or cord compression involves a complex decision-making process. It requires due consideration for multiple factors such as the patient's general condition, natural history and prognosis related to the underlying cancer, the effectiveness of different management strategies, and the goals of treatment.

In the field of supportive oncology, outcomes are almost always multidimensional and can be measured and quantitatively analyzed in many ways. For example, dose fractionation trials for painful bone metastases focus on the probability of pain relief, while spinal cord compression trials focus on response rates at 1 month post treatment, and the single trial comparing surgery and radiotherapy versus radiotherapy alone for cord compression used availability to walk after treatment as the primary endpoint (Table 28-3). In the following sections, treatment options and ways to choose between them are discussed under the headings of impending fractures of long bones, vertebral compression fracture, and spinal cord compression. Equivalent outcomes are presented wherever possible to facilitate contrast between different treatment options.

Table 28-2 Harrington classification of periacetabular metastatic destruction[26]

Class	
I	Sufficient bone to permit conventional arthroplasty
II	Medial wall defect
III	Acetabular dome defect
IV	Isolated lesion that could be resected in an attempted curative procedure

IMPENDING FRACTURES OF LONG BONES

Patients with impending fractures of the long bones may present with escalating pain but could be asymptomatic, having been identified through investigations such as plain films, bone scans, or computed tomography (CT) scans performed as part of patients' metastatic workup. Active treatment options include best supportive care, radiotherapy, prophylactic surgery, or a combined approach. Decision making regarding these approaches is based on multidisciplinary assessment of fracture risk, severity of symptoms, type of surgery required, surgical risk, life expectancy, and patient preference.[27]

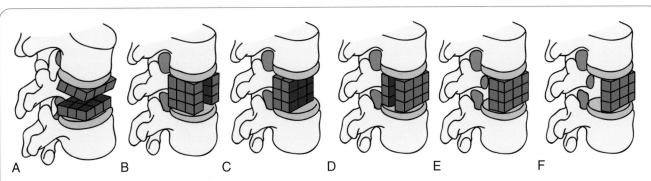

Fig. 28-1 Extent of vertebral involvement and compression fracture risk.[31] Tumor infiltration or damage to portions of the cube. **A,** Destruction of the middle third of the axial plane results in gross instability. **B,** Destruction of the middle third of the sagittal plane may not be associated with significant destabilization. **C,** A lesion in the ventral portion of the vertebral body in the coronal plane affects stability to a greater extent than a lesion in the middle **(D)** or dorsal **(E and F)** portion.

Table 28-3 Outcomes reported for different randomized trials

	RCT on dose fractionation for painful bone metastases[35]	RCT on radiotherapy dose fractionation for spinal cord compression[72,76]	RCT on radiotherapy vs. surgery and radiotherapy cord compression[74]
Pain relief—probability	√ (primary endpoint)	√	
Pain relief—duration	√		
Narcotic use			√
Response rate—mobility			√ (primary endpoint)
Duration of ambulation preservation			√
Response rate—for pain, motor function, sphincter dysfunction		√ (primary endpoint)	
Risk of cord compression	√		
Risk of fracture	√		
In-field recurrences		√	
Retreatment probability	√		
Acute toxicity	√	√	
Late toxicity			
Survival		√	√

RCT, Randomized controlled trial.

RADIOTHERAPY

The efficacy of radiotherapy for pain relief from bone metastases has been well established, supporting the choice of a single fraction for an equivalent likelihood of achieving pain relief when compared with more protracted fractionation schedules.[32–35] In contrast, its efficacy in preventing or deferring fractures in patients who are at high risk for fracture is not well established. The observation that remineralization occurs following radiotherapy is well recognized. However, this process can take several months, and the strength of the remineralized bone is uncertain.[36,37] Although dose fractionation randomized trials comparing lower versus higher doses demonstrated no significant difference in fracture risk,[34] patients who entered into these trials were not at high risk for fracture; therefore the power of inference of the analysis was severely limited. In general terms, for patients with impending fractures of the long bones, prophylactic surgery followed by radiotherapy is usually preferred, and radiotherapy alone is reserved for patients with relative contraindications to surgery. A higher biological dose (e.g., 20 Gy in 5 fractions, 30 Gy in 10 fractions) is generally favored,[36] although high-level evidence to support this practice is lacking.

For patients for whom prophylactic surgery is recommended, postoperative radiotherapy is generally considered following surgical fixation. The efficacy of postoperative radiotherapy is supported by retrospective data only. Townsend et al. described the outcomes of 60 consecutive patients undergoing surgery with or without surgery for femoral metastases. The estimated probability of achieving normal use of the extremity was 12% for surgery alone and 53% for surgery and radiotherapy. The need for a second orthopedic procedure was greater with surgery alone, occurring in 15% of patients, in contrast to 3% when radiotherapy was added.[38] Contemporary series and a comparative trial are needed.

The longer term goals of reducing the risk of tumor progression, the instability of the hardware, and the need for repeat surgery or instrumentation are common reasons for offering postoperative radiotherapy. Although pain secondary to mechanical instability is typically improved following prophylactic surgery, incremental pain relief can often be gained from postoperative radiotherapy through its effect on the residual tumor, providing a further clinical rationale for postoperative radiotherapy. For patients in whom extensive surgery has been performed, a delay in postoperative radiotherapy is frequently recommended (e.g., 3 weeks) to allow adequate soft tissue healing. When surgery is limited (e.g., prophylactic pinning), early radiotherapy (e.g., within a few days) can be administered safely. It is generally recommended that cutaneous surgical sites be excluded from the radiotherapy high dose volume. Following prophylactic pinning, the entire traversed marrow space is generally included in the target volume to prevent tumor seeding along the track. Fractionated courses of treatment are commonly recommended (e.g., 20 Gy in 5 fractions), although single fractions also merit consideration.

PROPHYLACTIC SURGERY

For patients at high risk of fracture, prophylactic fixation is generally advocated to avoid a higher risk of delayed union or nonunion, longer rehabilitation, and the technical complexity associated with postfracture fixation.[39,40] This also avoids the morbidity and distress typically experienced by the patient in an acute fracture event. Contemporary prosthetic devices available today provide a wide range of options, from replacement to reinforcement and repair, depending on the patients' circumstances. Replacement may be favored when the metastasis involves articular and periarticular areas, or when simpler techniques are not feasible. Repair and reinforcement procedures, particularly for long bones, may involve the use of intramedullary nailing techniques, plates, and screws[41] (Figs. 28-2 and 28-3). The use of a combination of plates and poly methyl methacrylate could provide superior biomechanical properties and is preferred for patients with a better prognosis.[42]

Only two prospective surgical series focusing on lesions of the pelvis and lower extremities have quantitatively addressed functional outcomes following surgery for impending or frank pathologic fractures.[43,44] Functional improvement was observed at 6 weeks[43,44] and 3 months.[44] With the use of commonly used limb function scales, including Musculoskeletal Tumor Society (MSTS)-87,[45] MSTS-93,[46] and Toronto Extremity Salvage Score (TESS),[47] improvement was observed as follows when preoperative versus postoperative scores were compared: MSTS 1987: 14.1 ± 7.4 vs. 19.1 ± 6.4; MSTS 1993: 7.9 ± 7.5 vs. 14.4 ± 5.8; and TESS: 39.7 ± 22.1 vs. 53.8 ± 23.7, respectively. Further improvement in functional scores was observed at 3 months.[44] Longer term outcomes were not available, given the relatively short life expectancies and high attrition rates characteristic of patients with advanced malignancies.

COMPLICATIONS OF VERTEBRAL METASTASES—COMPRESSION FRACTURES

Metastases involving the spine complicated by compression fracture can result in pain and kyphosis. The presence of soft tissue disease or bony fragments following compression fracture can result in nerve root, cauda equina, or cord compression. For patients who are at high risk (Fig. 28-4) or who have established compression fractures, especially when symptomatic with pain, local management options include radiotherapy, and minimally invasive techniques such as vertebral augmentation can be considered. Surgery is typically reserved for exceptional cases. Stereotactic spinal radiotherapy provides an additional treatment option for selected patients.

VERTEBRAL AUGMENTATION

Multiple authors have demonstrated the safety of vertebral augmentation—vertebroplasty and kyphoplasty techniques (Fig. 28-5)—in the treatment of spinal metastases.[48–52] Indications for considering vertebral augmentation include osteolytic lesions involving large portions of the weight-bearing vertebral body, osteolytic collapse, painful metastases, and intravertebral reinforcement for screws if a formal reconstruction is required. Commonly cited contraindications to vertebral augmentation are systemic pathology such as sepsis, prolonged

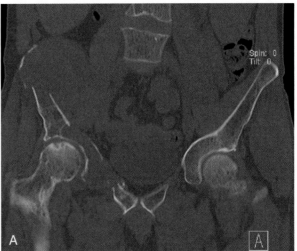

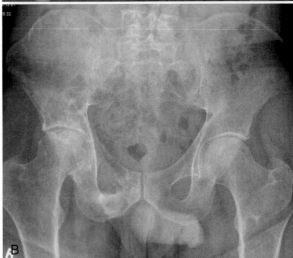

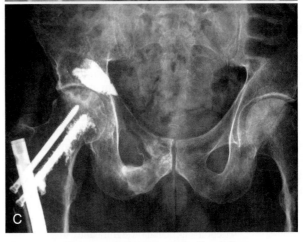

Fig. 28-2 Right acetabular metastasis. Coexisting metastases in right neck of femur. Preoperative and postoperative images. **A,** Preoperative coronal computed tomography (CT) image of patient with right acetabular (including soft tissue mass) and right neck of femur lytic metastases. **B** and **C,** Preoperative X-ray image of the same patient with right acetabular and right neck of femur metastases.

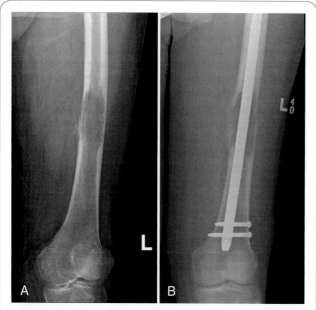

Fig. 28-3 Femoral metastasis at high risk of fracture, before and after prophylactic pinning. **A,** Patient with multiple myeloma. Mid shaft left femur, lytic lesion 8 cm in length with destruction of cortex. Mirels' score = 11. **B,** Same patient after prophylactic intramedullary pinning.

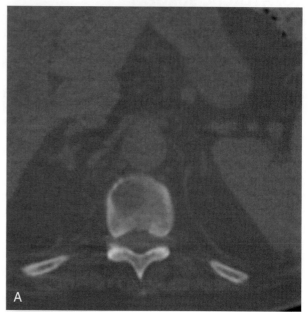

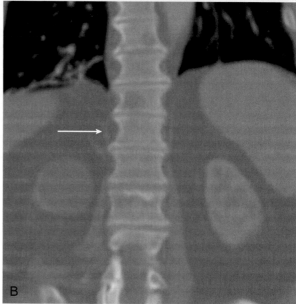

Fig. 28-4 Lytic metastasis within vertebra at risk of collapse. **A,** Patient with metastatic non–small cell lung cancer. Axial computed tomography (CT) image through T12 vertebra shows large lytic metastasis. **B,** Coronal CT image through thoracolumbar spine shows the same lytic metastasis almost filling the height of the T12 vertebra.

bleeding times, and cardiopulmonary pathology, which would preclude safe completion of the procedure. Other contraindications include neurologic signs or symptoms, nonosteolytic infiltrative spinal metastases, vertebral height collapse of more than 60%, burst fractures, and vertebral bodies with deficient posterior cortices.[53,54] Control of local disease and potential dissemination of disease are concerns and serve as potential limitations of these vertebral augmentation techniques.

Complications associated with vertebral augmentation are rare and, when they do occur, are usually related to cement extravasation. Pulmonary embolism of cement material, the most serious complication, has been reported to occur in 1.7% to 3.4% of patients.[48,51] Local clinical complications reported include transitory radiculopathy, permanent radiculopathy, cauda equina syndrome, hemothorax, and hematoma.

The efficacy of vertebral augmentation in patients with metastatic osteolytic fractures has been well demonstrated, with one study showing equivalent statistically significant improvements with regard to functional outcome between osteoporotic compression fractures and those secondary to multiple myeloma.[50] Furthermore, in patients with compression fracture secondary to multiple myeloma, vertebral augmentation with kyphoplasty demonstrated restoration and stabilization of height of the vertebral body at 1-year follow-up.[55,56] Vertebral augmentation significantly improved many patients' global quality-of-life scores and function by markedly decreasing their back pain and reducing their intake of pain medications.[52] Anselmetti et al. reported that age, underlying pathology, and length of follow-up did not seem to influence the outcome.[57] Hentschel et al. demonstrated that vertebral augmentation was safe and effective in patients with severe back pain caused by vertebral body fracture that is unresponsive to other therapies, even in the presence of relative contraindications to the procedure.[58]

In a study undertaken to assess the safety and efficacy of percutaneous vertebroplasty in 64 patients with osteolytic lesions

due to multiple myeloma, Masala et al. showed excellent postoperative pain reduction; however, no difference in pain levels at 1 and 6 months was reported, and no procedure-related complications were observed.[59] Lee et al. reviewed their experience with percutaneous vertebroplasty in 19 patients with spinal metastasis from solid organs. The authors found percutaneous vertebroplasty to be an effective palliative procedure in patients with compression fractures secondary to metastatic solid malignancy; its use can be successfully combined with other treatment modalities such as radiotherapy and chemotherapy.[60] Tseng treated 57 patients (78 vertebrae) with spinal metastatic tumor

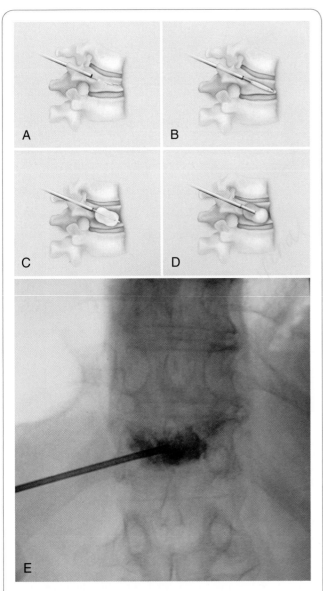

Fig. 28-5 Kyphoplasty.[103] Steps in the kyphoplasty procedure: **A,** cannulation of the vertebral body; **B,** placement of the inflatable bone tamp (IBT); **C,** inflation of the IBT and restoration of vertebral body height; and **D,** resultant cavity and cement fill. **E,** Anteroposterior (AP) fluoroscopy image of vertebroplasty procedure (T12 vertebral body).

Pflugmacher et al. prospectively assessed the long-term efficacy and safety of balloon kyphoplasty in treating thoracic and lumbar spinal metastatic fractures that resulted in pain or instability in 65 patients. The authors found that mean pain VAS and Oswestry Disability Index significantly improved from pretreatment to posttreatment ($P < .0001$); this improvement was sustained for up to 24 months. A gain in height restoration and a reduction in the postoperative kyphotic angle were seen postoperatively and at 3 months, although these radiographic outcomes returned to preoperative levels at 12 months. Balloon kyphoplasty was associated with rates of cement leakage and subsequent vertebral fracture of 12% and 8%, respectively. No symptomatic cement leaks or serious adverse events were seen during 24 months of follow-up.[63]

Vertebral augmentation can be performed as an open procedure in patients in need of neural decompression and stabilization of the vertebral column. Fuentes et al. demonstrated good pain control and neurologic improvement in their series.[64] In selected patients, vertebral augmentation can be used in combination with other minimally invasive techniques (e.g., percutaneous pedicle screw stabilization, limited open tumor evacuation) to provide symptom relief and spine stabilization while avoiding the perioperative morbidity associated with open procedures (Fig. 28-6).

SURGERY

In the absence of spinal cord compression and with the availability of vertebral augmentation and contemporary radiotherapy and chemotherapy, the role of open surgery for impending and actual vertebral compression fractures is limited. An open excisional biopsy may be needed in those cases where percutaneous biopsy is unsuccessful, or in those cases where a solitary metastasis is identified and presumptive cure can be obtained. These circumstances are exceptionally rare and are debated on a case-by-case basis.

RADIATION THERAPY

In patients with a longer life expectancy, with vertebral metastases displaying features at high risk of compression fracture, the desire to prevent progression and avoid a painful fracture is a common goal of therapy. As in dose fractionation consideration in the treatment of impending fractures of the long bones, evidence to guide the best choice of therapy is weak. The additional factor to consider is the intimate relationship between vertebral metastases and the spinal cord. The desire to avoid the need for retreatment over the spinal cord frequently motivates radiation oncologists to recommend fractionated treatments. Pattern-of-practice surveys confirm that multiple fractions, which allow a higher biological dose to be delivered, are considered appropriate treatment options (e.g., 20 Gy in 5 fractions) and are commonly recommended according to the treatment intent.[65] Additional studies are required.

STEREOTACTIC SPINAL RADIOTHERAPY

For patients who have had prior radiotherapy to the spine, residual spinal cord tolerance limits the amount or dose of radiotherapy that can be delivered safely. Generally, spinal cord tolerance expressed as biological equivalent dose (BED) is considered to be on the order of BED 100 Gy_{10}. This means for patients who had received prior radiotherapy doses of 8

using percutaneous vertebroplasty. The authors found marked pain reduction and a significant reduction in the quantity of narcotic and nonnarcotic analgesics required.[61] McDonald performed a retrospective review of clinical outcome data from 67 multiple myeloma patients treated with percutaneous vertebroplasty. Outcome measures, including Roland Morris Disability Questionnaire, a visual analog scale (VAS), and VAS with rest and activity improved by 11.0 (48%; $P < .0001$), 2.7 (25%; $P < .001$), and 5.3 (48%; $P < .0001$) points, respectively, with persistent improvement noted at 1 year ($P < .01$; $P < .03$; $P < .001$). Eighty-two percent and 89% of patients experienced a significant improvement in subjective rest pain and activity pain, respectively. Subjective scores achieved durable improvements, with 65% of patients requiring fewer narcotics after vertebroplasty and 70% having improved mobility.[62]

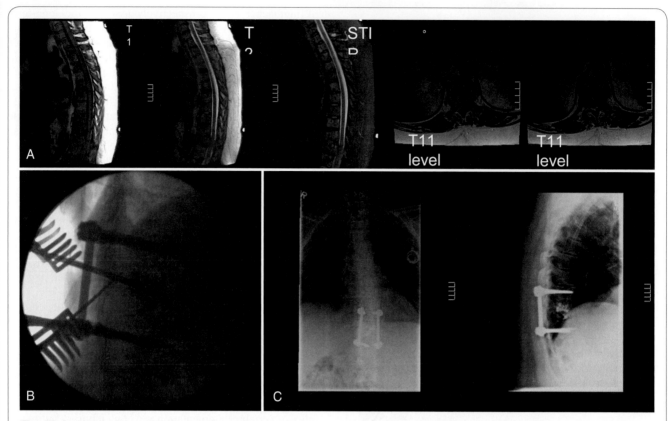

Fig. 28-6 Vertebral augmentation used in combination with other minimally invasive techniques. **A,** Patient with metastatic breast cancer. Magnetic resonance imaging (MRI; sagittal and axial) shows multiple levels of spinal metastases and epidural disease causing early cord compression at T11. **B,** Intraoperative fluoroscopic image demonstrates the use of combination minimally invasive procedures, including percutaneous pedicle screw stabilization, limited open tumor evacuation, and percutaneous vertebral cement augmentation. **C,** Plain radiograph (anteroposterior and lateral views) illustrates good alignment of the spine 6 months post treatment.

Gy in 1 fraction or 20 Gy in 5 fractions, a maximum additional dose on the order of 20 Gy in 8 fractions can be safely delivered. Beyond this, risk of radiation myelitis escalates, and this in turn can result in paraplegia, typically occurring approximately 6 months following radiotherapy.

Stereotactic spinal radiation allows radiotherapy to be given to the vertebral body while sparing the spinal cord, in some instances allowing treatment to those who would have been denied treatment on the basis of cord tolerance limits. Although the technical aspects of stereotactic radiotherapy are now well established, allowing radiation doses on the order of 8 to 24 Gy in 1 fraction, 4 to 6 Gy × 5 fractions, and 8 to 9 Gy × 3 fractions (BEDs of 43 to 82 Gy_{10}) to be safely delivered, evidence to guide the optimal use of this approach is still evolving but is mounting.[66]

In current practice, the typical reason for recommending stereotactic radiotherapy is progressive spinal disease in a patient who has had previous radiotherapy,[67] or highly selected cases such as solitary bone metastases in which maximal tumoricidal doses are intended to provide local control. In addition, tumors previously considered radioresistant (i.e., renal cell metastases) may now be treated with higher targeted doses. The planning and treatment delivery process is demanding, compared with conventional radiotherapy, and is not suitable for patients with poorly managed pain or acute cord compression. Advantages of stereotactic radiotherapy hinge on the ability to create a steep dose gradient between tumor and

adjacent spinal cord within a distance of a few millimeters (Fig. 28-7). High-quality imaging, including diagnostic and planning MRI and CT scans, is needed for treatment decision making and radiotherapy planning. To ensure reproducibility of the treatment plan, rigid immobilization is required. Together with the need for robust quality image guidance to ensure that radiation is being delivered to exactly where it was intended, the radiotherapy planning process can take several days. Each fraction of radiotherapy typically requires an hour of delivery time while the patient remains immobilized on the treatment couch. All of these requirements can be demanding for some and can preclude the use of this approach in others. Nevertheless it can be a powerful tool for patients with progressive spinal disease or occult cord compression, for whom other options are suboptimal. In selected patients with small volume solitary metastasis, the high doses achievable with this technique can offer the potential for tumor eradication.

COMPLICATIONS OF VERTEBRAL METASTASES—SPINAL CORD COMPRESSION

For patients with signs and symptoms suggestive of cord compression, rapid diagnosis and management are essential for optimal preservation of function. Much of the literature presented in the following section addresses patients with

with a median life expectancy of 3 months.[11] However, there exist subgroups of patients who are expected to have a more favorable prognosis where a more aggressive approach is warranted. Finally, there is the subgroup of patients with subclinical cord compression (i.e., those with radiologic evidence of cord compression in the absence of neurologic symptoms). Treatment options for the management of spinal cord compression include surgery, radiotherapy, or combination surgery and radiotherapy. Whether more aggressive treatments such as combination surgery and radiotherapy should be generalized to these patients requires further definition. Noninvasive treatment options such as conventional radiotherapy and stereotactic radiotherapy may have a bigger role to play, although randomized controlled trials in this setting are lacking.

SURGERY

Surgery is the only method that leads to immediate relief of spinal compression and direct mechanical stabilization of disease and the weakened vertebral column.[18] Key indications for surgical intervention include bony fragments causing cord compression, spinal instability, preferably single-level disease with good bone stock above and below (Fig. 28-8, *A* and *B*), and good performance status (i.e., patient with expected survival of greater than 3 months). Other reasons for surgical management include the need for tissue diagnosis, progression of symptoms during or after radiotherapy, and prior radiotherapy precluding further treatment.[68–70] If the tumor is known to be highly vascular (e.g., renal cell carcinoma), embolization 24 hours before surgery should be considered. For primary tumor histologies that are highly responsive to radiotherapy and/or chemotherapy, such as lymphoma, small cell lung cancer, and germ cell tumor, the demand for surgical intervention is less.

The type of surgery that is appropriate depends on the extent of tumor involvement. Weinstein described the division of the vertebral body into four zones to guide surgical planning (Fig. 28-9). The recommendation for Zones I and II includes a posterior or posterolateral approach with stabilization; for Zone III, an anterior approach with reconstruction using plates or poly methyl methacrylate implants; and for Zone IV, a combined anterior and posterior approach with reconstruction.[31] The approach of performing a posterior decompressive laminectomy for patients with an anterior lesion may translate into spinal instability, kyphosis, and pain, and generally is best avoided.

RADIOTHERAPY

Radiotherapy is one of the most common recommendations for the management of spinal cord compression. It can be used alone or in combination with surgery. Combined results from prospective nonrandomized studies of radiotherapy for malignant cord compression suggest that ambulation can be preserved in 94% of those who were ambulatory before treatment. It can be restored in 63% of those who needed assistance with ambulation, 38% who were paraparetic, and 13% of those who were paraplegic before treatment.[71] Complete relief of back pain is reported in 54% to 59% of patients.[72,73]

Radiotherapy used alone is usually indicated when patients have multiple vertebral levels (see Fig. 28-8, *C*), poor performance status, limited life expectancy, or medical contraindications to surgery or radiosensitive tumors. Typically, radiotherapy is designed to include areas of gross

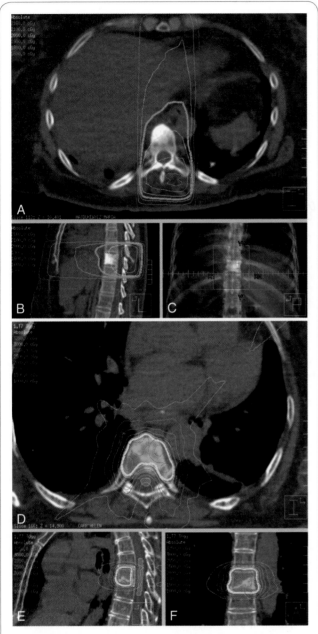

Fig. 28-7 Comparison of three-dimensional (3D) conformal external beam radiation therapy (RT) plan for painful spinal metastasis versus stereotactic spinal RT plan. **A through C,** 3D conformal RT plan for patient with sclerotic metastasis in T9 vertebra due to metastatic colorectal cancer. Prescription is 20 Gy in 5 fractions with 95% isodose (19 Gy = bright green line) covering T8-T10 vertebrae using a weighted parallel pair. **A,** Axial view. **B,** Sagittal view. **C,** Field placed to cover T8-T10 inclusive. **D through F,** Stereotactic spinal RT plan for patient with metastatic non–small cell lung cancer. Previously treated with 20 Gy in 5 fractions. Prescription is 30 Gy in 4 fractions. **D,** Axial view of dosimetry (9 co-planar beams) demonstrating improved conformity compared with 3D conformal plan sparing spinal cord. (30 Gy = bright yellow line, T7 vertebra; PTV = shaded red area; spinal cord = shaded green area). **E,** Sagittal view. **F,** Coronal view.

clinical spinal cord compression (i.e., those presenting with escalating pain and neurologic features leading to subsequent radiologic confirmation of the diagnosis). The diagnosis of spinal cord compression in general implies a poor prognosis

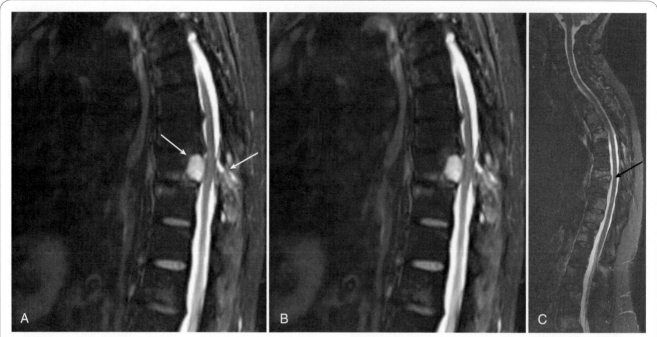

Fig. 28-8 Spinal cord compression (**A** and **B**, single level; **C**, multiple levels). **A**, Sagittal magnetic resonance imaging (MRI; T2 weighted, postgadolinium) shows a solitary metastasis at the T9 vertebral level, causing malignant spinal cord compression from non–small cell lung cancer. *Arrows* show anterior and posterior masses causing malignant spinal cord compression (MSCC). **B**, The same patient. Axial MRI (T1 weighted, fluid-attenuated inversion recovery [FLAIR]) through the T9 vertebra at the level of cord compression. **C**, Different patient with metastatic breast cancer. Sagittal MRI (short tau inversion recovery [STIR]) of whole spine showing multiple levels of vertebrae involved with metastatic disease. *Arrow* indicates impending MSCC at the T5 vertebral level.

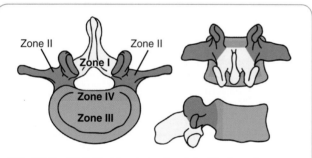

Fig. 28-9 Four discrete zones of vertebral body and suggested guide to surgical approaches.[31] Recommended surgical approaches: Zones I and II: Posterior or posterolateral stabilization. Zone III: Anterior with reconstruction using plates or poly methyl methacrylate implants. Zone IV: Combined anterior and posterior approach.

disease (as seen on MRI) with a margin of 2 cm, or 1 to 2 vertebral bodies, above and below the level of involvement. High-dose dexamethasone (e.g., 4 mg 4 times daily) is frequently recommended to reduce edema. In patients with complete paraplegia lasting >72 hours, radiotherapy has a very low likelihood of restoring neurologic function. Rapid commencement of therapy is critical for best functional outcomes.

COMBINED RADIOTHERAPY AND SURGERY

Use of radiotherapy alone has several limitations. In patients with spinal instability, although radiation can provide effective tumor shrinkage, pain relief, and neurologic improvement, the weakened vertebrae remain without any structural support. The effect of radiotherapy is not immediate. The time to reduction in mass effect and pressure relief on the spinal cord is delayed, compared with surgery. For rapidly progressing cord compression, this may be of critical importance. In patients in whom initial radiation is ineffective and progressive deficits are observed, the use of salvage surgery within a few weeks of receiving radiotherapy is associated with increased wound complications and is best avoided.

A single randomized trial examined the role of direct decompressive surgery (maximal debulking) with stabilization and postoperative radiotherapy (3 Gy × 10 fractions) versus radiotherapy alone.[74] Patients were eligible if they had a single area of extradural cord compression, paraplegia for less than 48 hours, and life expectancy greater than 3 months, and were able to undergo surgery and irradiation. Patients with spinal instability or the presence of bony compression were also eligible. Patients with radiosensitive tumors, multiple discrete compressive lesions, prior radiotherapy precluding the study radiotherapy, and preexisting neurologic problems were excluded. High-dose dexamethasone (96 mg/day) was given to both groups. Treatment in both groups started within 24 hours of the spinal cord compression diagnosis by MRI.

One hundred one patients were included (of a planned sample of 200). The study was stopped early because of a predetermined early stopping rule based on efficacy. Significantly more patients in the surgery group (S; 84%) than in the radiotherapy group (RT; 57%) were able to walk after treatment (*P* = .001). Patients treated with surgery retained the ability to walk and preserve sphincter control significantly longer than those with radiotherapy alone. Lower analgesic requirements and a longer life expectancy (126 days S + RT vs. 100 days RT) were also noted in the surgical arm. The results of this study were practice changing, supporting the use of combined modality for eligible patients with spinal cord compression (Table 28-4).

Following surgery, postoperative RT should be recommended and is typically commenced within 2 to 3 weeks after surgery, depending on the extent of surgery and wound healing (Fig. 28-10). The radiotherapy dose used in the Patchell study[74] was 30 Gy in 10 fractions, although the regimen of 20 Gy in 5 fractions is frequently used in clinical practice.

RADIOTHERAPY DOSE FRACTIONATION FOR SPINAL CORD COMPRESSION

Although radiotherapy is the most common modality for the management of spinal cord compression, the optimal dose and treatment regimen remain controversial.[75] Fractionated regimens such as 30 Gy in 10 fractions and 20 Gy in 5 fractions are frequently given clinically. Single-fraction radiotherapy tends to be reserved for patients with shorter life expectancies.

Two randomized controlled trials have examined the effects of different dose fractionation regimens.[72,76] Before these studies were conducted, only retrospective study results were available.[71] In the first study, patients were randomized to 16 Gy in 2 fractions (6 days apart) or 30 Gy in 8 fractions (5 Gy × 3, 4-day rest, then 3 Gy × 5). Study designs of the two trials were similar. Patients with MSCC and a shorter life expectancy (defined as ≤6 months) were included. Those with spinal instability, bony compression of the spinal cord, or previous radiation to the target area were excluded. The primary end-

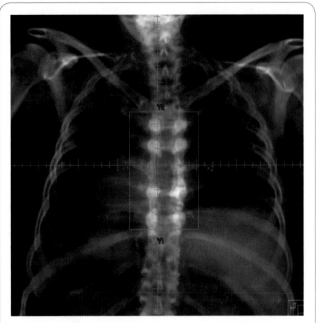

Fig. 28-10 Postoperative radiation therapy (RT) field covering surgical hardware. The patient developed cord compression from multiple myeloma and underwent decompression and instrumentation. This digitally reconstructed radiograph from a computed tomography (CT) simulation image shows the posterior RT field covering the surgical hardware (vertebral levels T5-T9 included).

point consisted of "response rate" for pain relief, motor function, and sphincter function. Both studies were designed as equivalence trials. Sample sizes for both studies were similar, at 276 and 303, respectively.

Neurologic status at study entry was similar to that of patients enrolled in the combined modality trial,[74] where the proportions of patients who were ambulatory at study entry were 67%[72] and 65%,[76] and normal sphincter control was noted in 89%[72] and 86%,[76] respectively. Patients were older, with median ages of 68 years[72] and 67 years.[76] Those with indications for surgery, including unstable spines, were excluded. This study was intended to apply to patients with "shorter" life expectancies; the median survival was 4 months—similar to results reported in the Patchell study.[74]

No significant difference in response (back pain, ambulation, and bladder function), duration of response, survival, or toxicity was found between the two arms; measurements were taken at 1 month post treatment[72,76] (Table 28-5). Both studies showed no difference in the incidence of in-field recurrent cord compression, although a trend favored higher doses. Taken together, these trials would support a single 8 Gy to be equivalent to 16 Gy in 2 fractions[76]; this in turn was equivalent to 30 Gy in 8 fractions[72] for patients with spinal cord compression who had a short life expectancy and no indications for surgery.

The biological equivalent doses (BEDs) of 8 Gy in 1 fraction, 16 Gy in 2 fractions, and 30 Gy in 8 fractions are estimated to be 19 Gy_{10}, 28 Gy_{10}, and 44 Gy_{10}, respectively. The question of whether higher BEDs (e.g., 30 Gy in 10 fractions with BED of 60 Gy_{10}) would provide superior outcomes remains unanswered. Clinical judgment alone has

Table 28-4 Summary of outcomes of RCT comparing surgery versus RT and surgery

Outcomes	RT and surgery for cord compression RCT		
	RT	S + RT	P
Pain response: mean daily morphine equivalent	4.8 mg	0.4 mg	.002
Mobility response:			
Proportion ambulatory post treatment	29/51 (57%)	42/50 (84%)	.001
Maintenance of ASIA score	72 days	566 days	.001
Maintenance of Frankel score	72 days	566 days	.0006
Duration able to ambulate (median)	13 days	122 days	.0017
Maintenance of sphincter control	17 days	156 days	.016
Survival (median)	100 days	126 days	.033

Adapted from Patchell.[74]
ASIA, American Spinal Injury Association; *RCT,* randomized controlled trial; *RT,* radiation therapy.

Table 28-5 Summary of outcomes of two RCTs on dose fractionation comparison for spinal cord compression

	2005	
Outcomes*	16 Gy in 2 French	30 Gy in 8 French[72]
Pain relief	56%	59%
"Responders"[†] in ambulation	68%	71%
Duration of improvement (median)	3.5 mo	3.5 mo
Responders[†] in sphincter control	90%	89%
Survival (median)	4 mo	4 mo
	2009	
Outcomes*	8 Gy in 1 French	16 Gy in 2 French
Pain relief	52%	53%
"Responders"[†] in ambulation	62%	69%
Duration of improvement (median)	5 mo	5 mo
Responders[†] in sphincter control	85%	87%
Survival (median)	4 mo	4 mo

Adapted from Marazano 2005.[72]
Adapted from Marazano 2009.[76]
*Outcomes measured at 1 month cessation of RT.
[†]"Responders" included patients who maintained or regained ability to walk and/or sphincter control and patients without pain or with pain responsive to minor analgesics after treatment.
RCT, Randomized controlled trial.

COMBINATION SURGERY AND RADIOTHERAPY OR RADIOTHERAPY ALONE?

The decision of whether to recommend combination surgery and radiotherapy or radiotherapy alone is based on a complex interaction between clinical and radiologic factors. How do we decide between combined modality and radiotherapy alone?

In a prospective database of patients, including those with radiologic evidence of cord compression with or without neurologic symptoms, within a clinical environment where combined modality therapy is readily available, combined modality was recommended in only 35% of patients.[81] The characteristics of patients accrued into the Patchell study[74] would shed some light on the types of patients to which the study results can best be generalized. In this study, 69% were walking and 62% had preservation of sphincter function at study entry. Patients with bony fragments or instability represented 38% of study patients.[82] Secondary analysis suggests a significant interaction of age and treatment outcome. The best estimate for the age at which surgery is no longer superior to radiation alone was calculated to be between 60 and 70 years.[83]

Until further robust evidence is available to refine the types of radiologic and patient characteristics that would be best suited for combined modality in patients with clinical evidence of cord compression (at least one sign or symptom of cord compression), a single level of cord compression, a favorable life expectancy (e.g., >3 months), and younger age (e.g., <70 years), combined modality therapy should be considered. In addition, patients who had prior radiotherapy to the target area and those with unstable spine or bony fragments contributing to cord compression are expected to have poor outcomes from radiotherapy alone and should also be considered for surgery. For patients at the two extremes of prognosis, those with radiologic evidence of cord compression only, and those with dense neurologic deficits and poor life expectancy or surgical risks, radiotherapy is likely the ideal management strategy.

PREDICTING OUTCOMES IN PATIENTS WITH SPINAL CORD COMPRESSION

Many different factors have been examined in an effort to predict both survival[78] and ambulation[79,84] following treatment of spinal cord compression. Rades et al.[78] evaluated one of the largest clinical cohorts, including 1852 patients with spinal cord compression treated with radiotherapy. Thirteen disease factors, radiologic characteristics of cord compression, adjacent bony architecture, and treatment factors were examined. Based on multivariate analysis, six disease factors were found to be significantly predictive of overall survival: favorable tumor type (myeloma, lymphoma, and breast), interval between cancer diagnosis and spinal cord compression of greater than 15 months, time to develop motor deficits of greater than 7 days, preradiotherapy ambulatory status, absence of visceral metastases, and presence of other bone metastases. Bony destruction at the level of cord compression and in adjacent areas was not studied in detail. However, cases of one or two involved vertebrae were associated with

been shown to be inadequate when survival predictions are made in patients with advanced cancer.[77] The inaccuracies in prognosis prediction and the devastating effect of progressive cord compression frequently formed the basis in practice for radiation oncologists in their quest to pursue more durable effects with higher BEDs.

Retrospective trials[78,79] and a recent prospective non-randomized study (Spinal Cord cOmpression Recurrence Evaluation [SCORE-1]) comparing different radiation schedules provide tantalizing evidence to suggest potential advantages of higher doses (e.g., 30 Gy in 10 fractions, 37 Gy in 15 fractions, 40 Gy in 20 fractions) compared with lower doses (8 Gy in 1 fraction, 20 Gy in 5 fractions) with respect to local control.[80]

For patients with a poor prognosis, 8 Gy in 1 fraction provides an equivalent likelihood of preserving ambulatory function. For patients with a favorable prognosis, combined modality therapy provides superior neurologic outcomes and survival and should be recommended. For patients between the two extremes, the optimal choice of dose fractionation is unclear.

a favorable survival outcome. From a treatment perspective, patients receiving long-course radiotherapy (e.g., 30 Gy in 10 fractions, 37.5 Gy in 15 fractions, and 40 Gy in 20 fractions), with a favorable response to radiotherapy were found to have a more favorable survival outcome.

The authors provided a method of integrating these factors for the purpose of prognostication, yielding a "First Score"[85] (Table 28-6 and Fig. 28-11). Six key prognostic factors, including tumor type, interval between tumor diagnosis and metastatic spinal cord compression, bone, or visceral metastases, ambulatory status, and duration of motor deficits, were incorporated. Different subgroups were given different weighting to arrive at an overall maximum score of 40. Overall 6-month

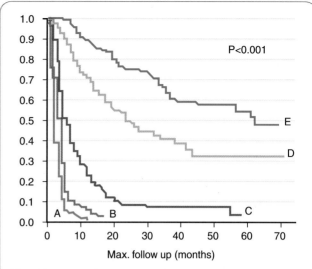

Fig. 28-11 Kaplan-Meier survival curves for the five groups. Group A: 21 to 25 points; Group B: 26 to 30 points; Group C: 31 to 35 points; Group D: 36 to 40 points; and Group E: 41 to 45 points.

Table 28-6 Rades first score: total score from each of the six categories (max 45)[85]

	Survival at 6 months, %	Score
Type of primary tumor		
Breast cancer	78	8
Prostate cancer	66	7
Myeloma/lymphoma	85	9
Lung cancer	25	3
Other tumors	40	4
Other bone metastases at the time of RT		
Yes	48	5
No	65	7
Visceral metastases at the time of RT		
Yes	17	2
No	80	8
Interval from tumor diagnosis to MSCC		
< 15 mo	41	4
>15 mo	71	7
Ambulatory status before RT		
Ambulatory	71	7
Nonambulatory	31	3
Time to develop motor deficits before RT		
1–7 days	26	3
8–14 days	55	6
>14 days	78	8

MSCC, Metastatic spinal cord compression; *RT*, radiotherapy.

survival rates were 4% for patients with a score of 20 to 25, 11% with scores of 26 to 30, 48% with scores of 31 to 35, 87% with scores of 36 to 40, and 99% for scores measuring 41 to 45. As an example, a patient with lung cancer, other bone metastases, visceral metastases, ≤15 months from tumor diagnosis to MSCC, nonambulatory status, and time to development of motor deficit before radiotherapy of <7 days receives a score of 20. Although the system is perhaps too complex for routine clinical use, the relative importance of the clinical factors is noteworthy and is deserving of further validation and investigation. Similar models have been described for patients treated by surgery.[86–90]

Leithner et al.[91] compared seven preoperative prognostic systems for spinal metastases (n = 69 patients) and found the Bauer score[89] to have the best correlation with survival. Three factors, including presence or absence of visceral metastases, primary site (lung vs. others), and number of bone metastases (solitary vs. multiple), were included in this system.

Predicting functional outcome after treatment allows the clinician to advise the patient and caregivers about the probability of meaningful recovery, so they can start planning for future care needs, and helps guide management decisions by evaluating potential benefits against risks. Large prospective series exploring predictive factors are uncommon. Hessler et al.[92] described a 16 times higher likelihood of recovery in patients (194 with neurologic deficit) undergoing surgery who presented with neurologic symptoms for less than a day before operative decompression, compared with greater than 15 days. Furstenberg[93] described recovery in 71% of 35 patients with a neurologic deficit who were operated on within 48 hours compared with recovery in only 29% of those who were operated on after 48 hours. Chaichana[94] (in 78 patients) described that preoperative ability to walk, the presence of pathologic fracture at presentation, the presence of symptoms for less than 48 hours, and postoperative radiotherapy all predicted an increased likelihood of regaining ambulation.

OTHER SUPPORTIVE MEASURES

Regardless of the treatment option chosen, dexamethasone is a useful supportive measure once the diagnosis has been made. The action of dexamethasone is mediated through antiinflammatory and antiedema effects. Three small randomized trials[95–97] were reviewed in the 2008 Cochrane meta-analysis[98] that examined interventions for the treatment of MSCC; none showed significant benefit for high-dose corticosteroids (96 to 100 mg/day) over moderate-dose corticosteroids (10 to 16 mg/day). Given the potentially significant side effects of high-dose dexamethasone, including gastrointestinal bleeding and metabolic disturbances, a dose of 16 mg over 24 hours in 2 to 4 divided doses is usually prescribed. Dexamethasone is continued during radiotherapy and is tapered upon completion of treatment.

FACILITATING MULTIDISCIPLINARY OPINION FOR THE MANAGEMENT OF CORD COMPRESSION

The strongest prognostic factor for overall survival and ability to ambulate after treatment is pretreatment neurologic status, specifically, motor function.[99] Prompt MRI to assess the whole spine in patients with known or suspected cancer who present with new symptoms (e.g., neurologic compromise, escalating neuropathic pain) is of utmost importance to minimize neurologic decline before treatment.[100] Once the diagnosis has been made, prompt assessment by surgical oncology or radiation oncology is needed to confirm the best treatment option.

A telephone rapid referral service or "hotline"[101] has been described as a simple, affordable, and practical approach to help triage patients obtain urgent MRI. A virtual consult process has been tested to facilitate multidisciplinary opinions from specialists that are geographically separate. This process hinges on a priori agreement between radiation and surgical oncology on the type of clinical information that is critical in clinical decision making, and on common access to electronic imaging and the willingness to respond urgently (often within minutes to hours depending on the clinical urgency) on the part of both disciplines. The process allows accurate multidisciplinary opinion to be rendered while limiting patient transfers to patients who are candidates for surgery after discussion.[102] Finally, the importance of continued education of the healthcare team and of patients at high risk for cord compression cannot be overemphasized for early diagnosis, rapid decision making, and treatment delivery for patients with malignant spinal cord compression.

SUMMARY

Progressive bone metastases can lead to disruption of bony architecture, mechanical instability, fractures, and spinal cord compression. Treatment goals range from pain relief to restoration of stability and preservation of function. Radiotherapy, minimally invasive procedures such as vertebral augmentation procedures, stereotactic radiotherapy, surgery, and combination approaches are all considered to formulate an optimal strategy, depending on the clinical circumstances. Treatment decision making requires due consideration of treatment effectiveness, life expectancy, treatment-related morbidity, and patient values and preferences. Although expeditious diagnosis, multidisciplinary discussion, and prompt treatment are the hallmark of excellent care, nowhere are these principles as critical as in the management of spinal cord compression.

REFERENCES

1. Coleman RE. Clinical features of metastatic bone disease and risk of skeletal morbidity. *Clin Cancer Res*. 2006;12:6243s–6249s.
2. Vestergaard P, Rejnmark L, Mosekilde L, et al. Fracture risk in patients with different types of cancer. *Acta Oncol*. 2009;48:105–115.
3. Plunkett TA, Smith P, Rubens RD. Risk of complications from bone metastases in breast cancer: implications for management. *Eur J Cancer*. 2000;36:476–482.
4. Domchek SM, Younger J, Finkelstein DM, et al. Predictors of skeletal complications in patients with metastatic breast carcinoma. *Cancer*. 2000;89:363–368.
5. Inoue T, Segawa T, Kamba T, et al. Prevalence of skeletal complications and their impact on survival of hormone refractory prostate cancer patients in Japan. *Urology*. 2009;73:1104–1109.
6. Tsuya A, Kurata T, Tamura K, et al. Skeletal metastases in non-small cell lung cancer: a retrospective study. [see comment]. *Lung Cancer*. 2007;57:229–232.
7. Sekine I, Nokihara H, Yamamoto N, et al. Risk factors for skeletal-related events in patients with non-small cell lung cancer treated by chemotherapy. *Lung Cancer*. 2009;65: 219–222.
8. Delea T, Langer C, McKiernan J, et al. The cost of treatment of skeletal-related events in patients with bone metastases from lung cancer. *Oncology*. 2004;67:390–396.
9. Rietevski B, Finkelstein JA, Stephen DJ, et al. Mortality and complications following stabilization of femoral metastatic lesions: a population-based study of regional variation and outcome. *J Can Chir*. 2009;52:302–308.
10. Van Geffen E, Wobbes T, Veth RP, et al. Operative management of impending pathological fractures: a critical analysis of therapy. *J Surg Oncol*. 1997;64:190–194.
11. Loblaw DA, Laperriere NJ, Mackillop WJ. A population-based study of malignant spinal cord compression in Ontario. *Clin Oncol (R Coll Radiol)*. 2003;15:211–217.
12. Bayley A, Milosevic M, Blend R, et al. A prospective study of factors predicting clinically occult spinal cord compression in patients with metastatic prostate carcinoma. *Cancer*. 2001;92:303–310.
13. Venkitaraman R, Barbachano Y, Dearnaley DP, et al. Outcome of early detection and radiotherapy for occult spinal cord compression. *Radiother Oncol*. 2007;85:469–472.
14. Venkitaraman R, Sohaib SA, Barbachano Y, et al. Detection of occult spinal cord compression with magnetic resonance imaging of the spine. *Clin Oncol (R Coll Radiol)*. 2007;19:528–531.
15. Roodman GD. Mechanisms of bone metastasis. *N Engl J Med*. 2004;350:1655–1664.
16. Bergmann P, Body JJ, Boonen S, et al. Evidence-based guidelines for the use of biochemical markers of bone turnover in the selection and monitoring of bisphosphonate treatment in osteoporosis: a consensus document of the Belgian Bone Club. *Int J Clin Pract*. 2009;63:19–26.
17. Abrahm JL. Assessment and treatment of patients with malignant spinal cord compression. *J Support Oncol*. 2004;2:377.
18. Prasad D, Schiff D. Malignant spinal-cord compression. [see comment]. *Lancet Oncol*. 2005;6:15–24.
19. Damron TA, Ward WG, Damron TA, et al. Risk of pathologic fracture: assessment. *Clin Orthop Relat Res*. 2003;(suppl 415):S208–S211.
20. Tschirhart CE, Finkelstein JA, Whyne CM, et al. Biomechanics of vertebral level, geometry, and transcortical tumors in the metastatic spine. *J Biomech*. 2007;40:46–54.
21. Harrington KD. Impending pathologic fractures from metastatic malignancy: evaluation and management. *Instr Course Lect*. 1986;35:357–381.
22. van der Linden YM, Kroon HM, Dijkstra SP, et al. Simple radiographic parameter predicts fracturing in metastatic femoral bone lesions: results from a randomised trial. *Radiother Oncol*. 2003;69:21–31.
23. Keyak JH, Kaneko TS, Rossi SA, et al. Predicting the strength of femoral shafts with and without metastatic lesions. *Clin Orthop Relat Res*. 2005;439:161–170.
24. Mirels H. Metastatic disease in long bones: a proposed scoring system for diagnosing impending pathologic fractures. *Clin Orthop Relat Res*. 1989;249:256–264.

25. Evans AR, Bottros J, Grant W, et al. Mirels' rating for humerus lesions is both reproducible and valid. *Clin Orthop Relat Res*. 2008;466:1279–1284.

26. Harrington KD. The management of acetabular insufficiency secondary to metastatic malignant disease. *J Bone Joint Surg Am*. 1981;63:653–664.

27. Biermann JS, Holt GE, Lewis VO, et al. Metastatic bone disease: diagnosis, evaluation, and treatment. *J Bone Joint Surg Am*. 2009;91:1518–1530.

28. Ghert M, Alsaleh K, Farrokhyar F, et al. Outcomes of an anatomically based approach to metastatic disease of the acetabulum. *Clin Orthop Relat Res*. 2007;459:122–127.

29. Krishnaney AA, Steinmetz MP, Benzel EC. Biomechanics of metastatic spine cancer. *Neurosurg Clin N Am*. 2004;15:375–380.

30. Shah AN, Pietrobon R, Richardson WJ, et al. Patterns of tumor spread and risk of fracture and epidural impingement in metastatic vertebrae. *J Spinal Disord Tech*. 2003;16:83–89.

31. Georgy BA. Metastatic spinal lesions: state-of-the-art treatment options and future trends. *Am J Neuroradiol*. 2008;29:1605–1611.

32. Wu JS, Wong R, Johnston M, et al. Meta-analysis of dose-fractionation radiotherapy trials for the palliation of painful bone metastases. [see comment]. *Int J Radiat Oncol Biol Phys*. 2003;55:594–605.

33. Falkmer U, Jarhult J, Wersall P, et al. A systematic overview of radiation therapy effects in skeletal metastases. *Acta Oncol*. 2003;42:620–633.

34. Chow E, Harris K, Fan G, et al. Palliative radiotherapy trials for bone metastases: a systematic review. *J Clin Oncol*. 2007;25:1423–1436.

35. Sze WM, Shelley M, Held I, et al. Palliation of metastatic bone pain: single fraction versus multifraction radiotherapy a systematic review of the randomised trials. *Cochrane Database Syst Rev*. 2004; CD004721.

36. Koswig S, Budach V. Remineralization and pain relief in bone metastases after after different radiotherapy fractions (10 times 3 Gy vs. 1 time 8 Gy): a prospective study. *Strahlenther Onkol*. 1999;175:500–508.

37. Ural AU, Avcu F, Baran Y, et al. Bisphosphonate treatment and radiotherapy in metastatic breast cancer. *Med Oncol*. 2008;25:350–355.

38. Townsend PW, Rosenthal HG, Smalley SR, et al. Impact of postoperative radiation therapy and other perioperative factors on outcome after orthopedic stabilization of impending or pathologic fractures due to metastatic disease. [see comment]. *J Clin Oncol*. 1994;12:2345–2350.

39. Coleman RE. Metastatic bone disease: clinical features, pathophysiology and treatment strategies. *Cancer Treat Rev*. 2001;27:165–176.

40. Jacofsky DJ, Haidukewych GJ, Jacofsky DJ, et al. Management of pathologic fractures of the proximal femur: state of the art. *J Orthop Trauma*. 2004;18:459–469.

41. Ogilvie CM, Fox EJ, Lackman RD, et al. Current surgical management of bone metastases in the extremities and pelvis. *Semin Oncol*. 2008;35:118–128.

42. Sarahrudi K, Wolf H, Funovics P, et al. Surgical treatment of pathological fractures of the shaft of the humerus. *J Trauma*. 2009;66:789–794.

43. Clohisy DR, Le CT, Cheng EY, et al. Evaluation of the feasibility of and results of measuring health-status changes in patients undergoing surgical treatment for skeletal metastases. *J Orthop Res*. 2000;18:1–9.

44. Talbot M, Turcotte RE, Isler M, et al. Function and health status in surgically treated bone metastases. *Clin Orthop Relat Res*. 2005;438:215–220.

45. Enneking WF. Modification of the system for functional evaluation of surgical management of musculoskeletal tumors. In: Enneking WF, ed. *Limb salvage in musculoskeletal oncology*. New York: Churchill-Livinstone; 1987:626.

46. Enneking WF, Dunham W, Gebhardt MC, et al. A system for the functional evaluation of reconstructive procedures after surgical treatment of tumors of the musculoskeletal system. *Clin Orthop Relat Res*. 1993;286:241–246.

47. Davis AM, Wright JG, Williams JI, et al. Development of a measure of physical function for patients with bone and soft tissue sarcoma. *Qual Life Res*. 1996;5:508–516.

48. Khanna AJ, Togawa D. *Functional outcomes of kyphoplasty for the treatment of spinal metastases*. Presented at: 72th Annual Meeting of American Academy Orthopaedic Surgeons, Washington DC; 2005.

49. Barragan-Campos HM, Vallee JN, Lo D, et al. Percutaneous vertebroplasty for spinal metastases: complications. *Radiology*. 2006;238:354–362.

50. Khanna AJ, Reinhardt MK, Togawa D, et al. Functional outcomes of kyphoplasty for the treatment of osteoporotic and osteolytic vertebral compression fractures. *Osteoporos Int*. 2006;17:817–826.

51. Calmels V, Vallee JN, Rose M, et al. Osteoblastic and mixed spinal metastases: evaluation of the analgesic efficacy of percutaneous vertebroplasty. *Am J Neuroradiol*. 2007;28:570–574.

52. Cheung G, Chow E, Holden L, et al. Percutaneous vertebroplasty in patients with intractable pain from osteoporotic or metastatic fractures: a prospective study using quality-of-life assessment. *Can Assoc Radiol J*. 2006;57:13–21.

53. Bai B, Jazrawi LM, Kummer FJ, et al. The use of an injectable, biodegradable calcium phosphate bone substitute for the prophylactic augmentation of osteoporotic vertebrae and the management of vertebral compression fractures. *Spine*. 1999;24:1521–1526.

54. Cotten A, Boutry N, Cortet B, et al. Percutaneous vertebroplasty: state of the art. *Radiographics*. 1998;18:311–320 discussion 313–20.

55. Pflugmacher R, Kandziora F, Schroeder RJ, et al. Percutaneous balloon kyphoplasty in the treatment of pathological vertebral body fracture and deformity in multiple myeloma: a one-year follow-up. [see comment]. *Acta Radiol*. 2006;47:369–376.

56. Pflugmacher R, Beth P, Schroeder RJ, et al. Balloon kyphoplasty for the treatment of pathological fractures in the thoracic and lumbar spine caused by metastasis: one-year follow-up. *Acta Radiol*. 2007;48:89–95.

57. Anselmetti GC, Corrao G, Monica PD, et al. Pain relief following percutaneous vertebroplasty: results of a series of 283 consecutive patients treated in a single institution. *Cardiovasc Intervent Radiol*. 2007;30:441–447.

58. Hentschel SJ, Burton AW, Fourney DR, et al. Percutaneous vertebroplasty and kyphoplasty performed at a cancer center: refuting proposed contraindications. *J Neurosurg Spine*. 2005;2:436–440.

59. Masala S, Anselmetti GC, Marcia S, et al. Percutaneous vertebroplasty in multiple myeloma vertebral involvement. *J Spinal Disord Tech*. 2008;21:344–348.

60. Lee B, Franklin I, Lewis JS, et al. The efficacy of percutaneous vertebroplasty for vertebral metastases associated with solid malignancies. *Eur J Cancer*. 2009;45:1597–1602.

61. Tseng YY, Lo YL, Chen LH, et al. Percutaneous polymethylmethacrylate vertebroplasty in the treatment of pain induced by metastatic spine tumor. *Surg Neurol*. 2008;70(suppl 1):S178–S183 discussion S183–4.

62. McDonald RJ, Trout AT, Gray LA, et al. Vertebroplasty in multiple myeloma: outcomes in a large patient series. *Am J Neuroradiol*. 2008;29:642–648.

63. Pflugmacher R, Taylor R, Agarwal A, et al. Balloon kyphoplasty in the treatment of metastatic disease of the spine: a 2-year prospective evaluation. *Eur Spine J*. 2008;17:1042–1048.

64. Fuentes S, Metellus P, Pech-Gourg G, et al. Open kyphoplasty for management of metastatic and severe osteoporotic spinal fracture: technical note. *J Neurosurg Spine*. 2007;6:284–288.

65. Janjan N, Lutz ST, Bedwinek JM, et al. Therapeutic guidelines for the treatment of bone metastasis: a report from the American College of Radiology Appropriateness Criteria Expert Panel on Radiation Oncology. *J Palliat Med*. 2009;12:417–426.

66. Sahgal A, Larson DA, Chang EL, et al. Stereotactic body radiosurgery for spinal metastases: a critical review. *Int J Radiat Oncol Biol Phys*. 2008;71:652–665.

67. Sahgal A, Ames C, Chou D, et al. Stereotactic body radiotherapy is effective salvage therapy for patients with prior radiation of spinal metastases. *Int J Radiat Oncol Biol Phys*. 2009;74:723–731.

68. Quinn JA, DeAngelis LM. Neurologic emergencies in the cancer patient. *Semin Oncol*. 2000;27:311–321.

69. Loblaw DA, Laperriere NJ. Emergency treatment of malignant extradural spinal cord compression: an evidence-based guideline. *J Clin Oncol*. 1998;16:1613–1624.

70. Sundaresan N, Sachdev VP, Holland JF, et al. Surgical treatment of spinal cord compression from epidural metastasis. *J Clin Oncol*. 1995;13:2330–2335.

71. Loblaw DA, Perry J, Chambers A, et al. Systematic review of the diagnosis and management of malignant extradural spinal cord compression: the Cancer Care Ontario Practice Guidelines Initiative's Neuro-Oncology Disease Site Group. [see comment]. *J Clin Oncol*. 2005;23:2028–2037.

72. Maranzano E, Bellavita R, Rossi R, et al. Short-course versus split-course radiotherapy in metastatic spinal cord compression: results of a phase III, randomized, multicenter trial. *J Clin Oncol*. 2005;23:3358–3365.

73. Maranzano E, Latini P. Effectiveness of radiation therapy without surgery in metastatic spinal cord compression: final results from a prospective trial. *Int J Radiat Oncol Biol Phys*. 1995;32:959–967.

74. Patchell RA, Tibbs PA, Regine WF, et al. Direct decompressive surgical resection in the treatment of spinal cord compression caused by metastatic cancer: a randomised trial. *Lancet*. 2005;366:643–648.

75. Cole JS, Patchell RA. Metastatic epidural spinal cord compression. *Lancet Neurol*. 2008;7:459–466.

76. Maranzano E, Trippa F, Casale M, et al. 8 Gy single-dose radiotherapy is effective in metastatic spinal cord compression: results of a phase III randomized multicentre Italian trial. *Radiother Oncol*. 2009;93:174–179.

77. Christakis NA, Lamont EB. Extent and determinants of error in doctors' prognoses in terminally ill patients: prospective cohort study. [see comment]. *BMJ*. 2000;320:469–472.

78. Rades D, Fehlauer F, Schulte R, et al. Prognostic factors for local control and survival after radiotherapy of metastatic spinal cord compression. *J Clin Oncol*. 2006;24:3388–3393.

79. Rades D, Stalpers LJ, Veninga T, et al. Evaluation of five radiation schedules and prognostic factors

for metastatic spinal cord compression. *J Clin Oncol.* 2005;23:3366–3375.

80. Rades D, Lange M, Veninga T, et al. Preliminary results of spinal cord compression recurrence evaluation (score-1) study comparing short-course versus long-course radiotherapy for local control of malignant epidural spinal cord compression. *Int J Radiat Oncol Biol Phys.* 2009;73:228–234.

81. Grabarz D, Rampersaud R, Fehlings M, et al. *The virtual consultation project—enhancing multidisciplinary care for patients with malignant spinal cord compression (SCC).* Presented at: 11th World Congress on Internet in Medicine, Toronto. Available at: http://www.mednetcongress.org/fullpapers/MEDNET-54_GrabarzDanielA_e.pdf; 2006.

82. Loblaw D. Does surgery provide better outcomes in malignant spinal cord compression? Commentary. *Support Oncol.* 2004;2:391–393.

83. Chi JH, Gokaslan Z, McCormick P, et al. Selecting treatment for patients with malignant epidural spinal cord compression—does age matter? Results from a randomized clinical trial. *Spine.* 2009;34:431–435.

84. Helweg-Larsen S, Sorensen PS, Kreiner S. Prognostic factors in metastatic spinal cord compression: a prospective study using multivariate analysis of variables influencing survival and gait function in 153 patients. *Int J Radiat Oncol Biol Phys.* 2000;46:1163–1169.

85. Rades D, Dunst J, Schild SE. The first score predicting overall survival in patients with metastatic spinal cord compression. *Cancer.* 2008;112:157–161.

86. Tokuhashi Y, Matsuzaki H, Toriyama S, et al. Scoring system for the preoperative evaluation of metastatic spine tumor prognosis. *Spine.* 1990;15:1110–1113.

87. Tokuhashi Y, Ajiro Y, Umezawa N, et al. Outcome of treatment for spinal metastases using scoring system for preoperative evaluation of prognosis. *Spine.* 2009;34:69–73.

88. Tomita K, Kawahara N, Kobayashi T, et al. Surgical strategy for spinal metastases. *Spine.* 2001;26:298–306.

89. Bauer HC, Wedin R. Survival after surgery for spinal and extremity metastases: prognostication in 241 patients. *Acta Orthop Scand.* 1995;66:143–146.

90. Sioutos PJ, Arbit E, Meshulam CF, et al. Spinal metastases from solid tumors: analysis of factors affecting survival. *Cancer.* 1995;76:1453–1459.

91. Leithner A, Radl R, Gruber G, et al. Predictive value of seven preoperative prognostic scoring systems for spinal metastases. [see comment]. *Eur Spine J.* 2008;17:1488–1495.

92. Hessler C, Burkhardt T, Raimund F, et al. Dynamics of neurological deficit after surgical decompression of symptomatic vertebral metastases. *Spine.* 2009;34:566–571.

93. Furstenberg CH, Wiedenhofer B, Gerner HJ, et al. The effect of early surgical treatment on recovery in patients with metastatic compression of the spinal cord. *J Bone Joint Surg Br.* 2009;91:240–244.

94. Chaichana KL, Woodworth GF, Sciubba DM, et al. Predictors of ambulatory function after decompressive surgery for metastatic epidural spinal cord compression. *Neurosurgery.* 2008;62:683–692.

95. Graham PH, Capp A, Delaney G, et al. A pilot randomised comparison of dexamethasone 96 mg vs 16 mg per day for malignant spinal-cord compression treated by radiotherapy: TROG 01.05 Superdex study. *Clin Oncol (R Coll Radiol).* 2006;18:70–76.

96. Sorensen S, Helweg-Larsen S, Mouridsen H, et al. Effect of high-dose dexamethasone in carcinomatous metastatic spinal cord compression treated with radiotherapy: a randomised trial. *Eur J Cancer.* 1994;30A:22–27.

97. Vecht CJ, Haaxma-Reiche H, van Putten WL, et al. Initial bolus of conventional versus high-dose dexamethasone in metastatic spinal cord compression. *Neurology.* 1989;39:1255–1257.

98. George R, Jeba J, Ramkumar G, et al. Interventions for the treatment of metastatic extradural spinal cord compression in adults. *Cochrane Database Syst Rev.* 2008;(4) CD006716.

99. Talcott JA, Stomper PC, Drislane FW, et al. Assessing suspected spinal cord compression: a multidisciplinary outcomes analysis of 342 episodes. *Support Care Cancer.* 1999;7:31–38.

100. Husband DJ. Malignant spinal cord compression: prospective study of delays in referral and treatment. *BMJ.* 1998;317:18–21.

101. Allan L, Baker L, Dewar J, et al. Suspected malignant cord compression—improving time to diagnosis via a 'hotline': a prospective audit. *Br J Cancer.* 2009;100:1867–1872.

102. Hashimoto S, Shirato H, Kaneko K, et al. Clinical efficacy of telemedicine in emergency radiotherapy for malignant spinal cord compression. *J Digit Imaging.* 2001;14:124–130.

29

Pulmonary complications of cancer therapy and central airway obstruction

Ai-Ping Chua, Jose Fernando Santacruz, and Thomas R. Gildea

In this chapter we will review several of the more common pulmonary conditions that occur in the context of cancer therapy. Lung injury as a result of cancer therapy and central airway obstruction due to cancer in the thorax are just simple groupings that do not capture the wide array of cancer-related illnesses that cause dyspnea, cough, pain, or death. Each of these is commonly seen in pulmonary practice.

CHEMOTHERAPY-RELATED LUNG TOXICITY

Chemotherapy can cause pulmonary toxicity and lung injury, giving rise to new respiratory symptoms and radiographic abnormalities. This may be further aggravated if the oncologic patient already has underlying concurrent cardiopulmonary disease. The incidence of pneumotoxicity from anticancer therapies is less common than radiation-induced lung injury and ranges anywhere from less than 1% to 30%. Nonspecific interstitial pneumonitis/fibrosis, hypersensitivity pneumonitis syndrome, and noncardiogenic pulmonary edema are the common clinical manifestations. The number of antineoplastic agents causing parenchymal lung diseases is expected to steadily increase, leading to a rise in the incidence of lung toxicity as more new pharmacotherapeutic options are made available. Lung toxicity may carry a higher mortality risk than radiation pneumonitis.

Several mechanisms of lung toxicity have been postulated. One of the proposed pathogenic processes involves direct injury to the alveolar epithelial and endothelial cells, leading to activation of the inflammatory cascade and release of various active immunologic mediators, including cytokines (i.e., prostaglandins and leukotrienes), causing capillary leak. Growth factors are also released as by-products that stimulate myofibroblasts and their proliferation with resultant pathologic expansion of the extracellular matrix and increased fibrosis. The other common mechanism is the production of reactive oxygen species by activated neutrophils (e.g., hydrogen peroxide, superoxide anions, and hydroxyl radicals), which can cause direct pulmonary toxicity via redox reactions and fatty acid oxidation, or in turn can trigger the activation of other inflammatory metabolites.[1–3]

Cytotoxic drugs can cause pulmonopathy by creating a homeostatic imbalance in collagen synthesis and cellular immunity, causing tissue damage.[4].

Diagnosis of drug-related lung injury is often challenging because of the paucity of specific and distinct features that are apparent clinically and radiographically. However, one should always maintain a high index of suspicion when these medications are used. Integrating a thorough history and physical examination with changes on physiologic testing and radiographic imaging is essential in diagnosing chemotherapy-induced lung toxicity. Dyspnea and hypoxia are the most common clinical manifestations caused by impaired gas exchange. Other symptoms may include dry cough and constitutional symptoms of fever, fatigue, and malaise. Physical findings are often normal. Bibasilar velcro-like end-inspiratory crepitations may be heard on lung auscultation when significant pulmonary fibrosis is present. In the absence of pathognomonic findings, clinical investigation is directed to rule out other concomitant and alternative diagnoses such as infection, thromboembolic disease, and tumor recurrence. Radiographic changes are nonspecific. Plain chest radiographs oftentimes are normal, even in the presence of active histologic changes.[4].

Radiographic patterns commonly seen on high-resolution computed tomography (HRCT) scans are interstitial and include reticular thickening, nonspecific diffuse ground-glass infiltrates, fibrosis, and nodules. Pleural effusion is uncommon. Hilar adenopathy and cavitating nodules are exceedingly rare.[4]

Bronchoscopy with bronchoalveolar lavage is used primarily to evaluate for opportunistic infections, although the preponderant type of inflammatory cells may help to differentiate the toxicity of one drug from another. Cytologic examination of the bronchoalveolar lavage of patients with bleomycin lung injury showed abundant neutrophilic infiltrates versus a lymphocytic predominance in methotrexate-induced toxicity. Because the primary finding in acute infection is also neutrophilic, this alone is insufficient, and additional modalities may be required.[5–7]

Surgical biopsies and transbronchial or surgical lung biopsy may be necessary to establish a firm diagnosis by distinguishing between scarring, viable residual, or progressive cancer versus drug-induced pneumopathy. The tissue histology of drug-induced lung toxicity is nonspecific and is not unique to any of the cytotoxic agents. Histopathologic features are characterized by damage and desquamation of type I pneumocytes, proliferation of type II pneumocytes, infiltration by predominantly mononuclear cells, and abundant fibroblasts with increased fibrosis. Swelling and destruction of endothelial cells are noted, along with interstitial and alveolar edema. Eosinophilic inflammation and granuloma formation are seen in hypersensitivity reactions caused by procarbazine, methotrexate, and bleomycin.[4,6,8]

Spirometry and diffusion lung capacity for carbon monoxide (DLCO) are useful in screening and assessing for drug toxicity. Because the pathology involves mainly the interstitium, giving rise to impairment in gas exchange, restrictive ventilatory limitation and reduced DLCO are the most common spirometric findings. It had been recommended that screening pulmonary function tests given at baseline and periodically may predict the risk of developing lung toxicity in patients receiving cytotoxic drugs, and that they may help in early detection while clinical symptoms and signs are monitored closely, but this has not been well established.[9]

Once the diagnosis is suspected, the alleged causative drug should be stopped. High-dose steroids are an effective mainstay treatment for interstitial and parenchymal lung diseases caused by these systemic agents when administered in the early disease state. This is gradually tapered off very slowly once a response is established. Prophylaxis against peptic ulcer, infection, and osteoporosis should be administered if steroid treatment is going to be prolonged. Oxygen may be necessary to relieve hypoxia. Bronchodilators, antibiotics, diuretics, and anticoagulation may be indicated for coexisting cardiorespiratory comorbidities. In rare circumstances, lung transplantation has been offered to long-term survivors with permanent lung injury. Rates of resolution of lung injury are variable and are based on the agent and the underlying condition of the lung.

BLEOMYCIN

Among the many chemotherapeutic drugs that can lead to lung damage, bleomycin is by far the most notorious and deserves special mention. Others include methotrexate, mitomycin, nitrosoureas, specifically, carmustine, and cytosine arabinoside. Bleomycin is most commonly associated with lung injury, with reported incidence ranging from 3% to 40%.[10,11]

Because bleomycin is the most extensively studied drug, the pathogenesis of lung damage is the best understood, and various mechanisms of pulmonary damage have been defined. By complexion with Fe^{3+}, bleomycin releases oxygen free radicals, causing injury to the pulmonary capillary endothelial cells and type I alveolar epithelial cells; this further activates the inflammatory cascade and promotes cellular injury and scarring.[12,13]

In vitro studies have demonstrated reduction in fibrosis in the lungs of mice treated with iron chelators.[13]

Bleomycin enhances the synthesis and deposition of collagen and promotes the release of pro-fibrotic cytokines (e.g., transforming growth factor-β [TGF-β], macrophage inflammatory protein-1, interleukin-1, monocyte chemoattractant protein-1) through increased genetic transcription.[1,4,14–16]

In addition, bleomycin enhances pulmonary proteolytic enzyme activity and fibrin deposition.[4] The synergistic effects of thoracic radiation and oxygen administration on the pulmonary toxicity of bleomycin lend further support to this pathogenesis.

The risk of lung toxicity is dose related, and pneumopathy increases in incidence at a total cumulative dose of 300 to 400 units.[10,17] However, toxicity had been reported to occur at a much lower cumulative dose of less than 50 mg at a rate of less than 5%.[5]

The most frequent clinical presentation is still dyspnea, although dry cough, fever, and bibasilar crepitations are not uncommon. Interstitial and reticular-nodular infiltrates on computed tomography (CT) scans can be localized to the lung bases or subpleural region, but may progress to be diffuse.[18] Rarely, lung toxicity can produce a unique acute chest pain syndrome[8,19] and may present with cavitating nodules, mimicking metastatic lesions.[4]

Reduced DLCO, which is common, is the earliest indicator of an adverse effect. This should prompt the clinician to consider stopping the drug, although cessation of the drug immediately, upon documentation of a decrease in DLCO, may not prevent a further decline in pulmonary function. It is recommended that DLCO readings should be obtained before bleomycin treatment is initiated and at regular intervals, as long as the treatment lasts. Currently, no agreement has been reached on what constitutes a clinically significant decline in DLCO, although most oncologists are using a cutoff of 20% before advising their patients to discontinue the drug.[20]

It had been suggested that a decline in total lung capacity correlates better with radiographic changes than does diffusing capacity.[21,22]

Besides dose, age and the presence of concomitant renal disease are other risk factors for bleomycin-induced lung toxicity.[10,17]

Older age has also been found to be predictive of death from bleomycin pneumopathy.[23]

The concurrent administration of oxygen, radiation, and other cytotoxic agents (e.g., cisplatin, gemcitabine) and granulocyte-colony stimulating factor (G-CSF) has been shown to be predictive in the development of bleomycin-induced lung injury.[4,24]

Bleomycin is metabolized mainly by the kidneys. Cisplatin is known to cause renal impairment, which can lead to reduced bleomycin clearance. The risk of lung toxicity is increased by accumulation of bleomycin in the body.[24]

Fatality may result from severe bleomycin-induced lung injury with the use of granulocyte-colony stimulating factor and a bleomycin-containing regimen. It is thought that the underlying pathogenesis consists of increased alveolar neutrophil recruitment and inflammation, which causes further endothelial damage.[25,26]

Bleomycin is converted to inactive metabolites by the enzyme, bleomycin hydrolase, of which concentration is lowest in skin and lungs—the two organs most frequently involved in bleomycin toxicity.[8] It has been postulated that genetically determined levels of bleomycin hydrolase could account for one's inherent predisposition to bleomycin-induced lung toxicity.[7,27]

Bleomycin-dependent electron transport is dependent on O_2. Worsening of lung injury from bleomycin, including severe acute respiratory distress syndrome, had been demonstrated in rats given higher oxygen concentrations during operative anesthesia.[4,28-30]

The dose or duration of oxygen supplementation at which lung toxicity does occur with bleomycin is unknown; therefore, it is prudent to minimize the use of oxygen supplementation to maintain adequate tissue oxygenation.[31]

Most patients eventually recover from the insult, with complete or near-complete response of lung function to withdrawal of the drug and/or steroid administration. The fatality rate is low at an estimated incidence of 3%; severe life-threatening and fatal toxicity had been rarely reported at a much lower cumulative dose.[23]

Figure 29-1 shows the chest CT of a 57-year-old man taken at the time of presentation with exertional dyspnea, dry cough, low-grade fever, restrictive ventilatory defect, and 50% reduction in DLCO following 6 months of bleomycin therapy (total dose, 276 units) for stage IIIB classical Hodgkin's lymphoma. Bronchial lavage was negative for microorganisms, and histopathologic examination of a transbronchial lung biopsy specimen showed organizing acute lung injury. The patient

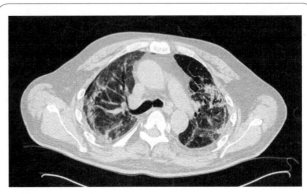

Fig. 29-1 Chest computed tomography (CT) scan shows bleomycin-induced pneumonitis.

was treated with 60 mg prednisone tapered over 3 months and responded, but with incomplete resolution of his symptoms and moderate radiographic improvement in infiltrates. He no longer requires oxygen but does have persistent exercise limitations.

ANTIMETABOLITES

Similar to bleomycin, methotrexate can cause interstitial pneumonitis.[32-35]

Hypersensitivity reaction in the lungs is likely the mechanism[6]; it often is apparent radiographically with bilateral nodular or alveolar infiltrates, which resolve rapidly.[4]

In some instances, pleural effusion may be present, and mediastinal lymphadenopathy has been reported.[4] A favorable response to steroids is often seen. Lymphocytic alveolitis with an increased CD4/CD8 ratio in bronchial fluid is uniformly noted in methotrexate pneumonitis, supporting an immunologically mediated injury. This resolves and the ratio normalizes when the lungs recover.[6]

Gemcitabine is used increasingly for the treatment of solid tumors. Gemcitabine used in isolation as an antineoplastic agent usually is not associated with significant lung toxicity. However, rarely, severe adult respiratory distress syndrome can result from capillary leak.[36] On the other hand, gemcitabine has been shown to increase the risk of lung injury caused by other cytotoxic agents when used in combination, particularly with taxanes.[37,38]

Fludarabine is another fairly well tolerated antimetabolite drug used commonly in the treatment of hematologic malignancy. It has been reported to cause interstitial pneumonitis associated with fever in 8% of cases, which appeared to be fairly steroid responsive.[39,40]

NITROSOUREAS AND ALKYLATORS

Nitrosoureas and alkylators, which are commonly used in bone marrow transplant (BMT) at high doses, had an additive effect on pulmonary insult that is separate from direct toxicity resulting from BMT itself.

Carmustine commonly causes lung injury when used as adjuvant therapy in breast cancer and lymphoma. Patients who had received previous irradiation may develop toxicity at a lower dose of 600 mg/m² and may demonstrate a poor treatment response to steroids.[41]

The risk of chronic pulmonary fibrosis is related to dose and age, and the condition is poorly responsive to steroids.[42–45]

The risk of pulmonary fibrosis increases at a higher cumulative total dose of 1400 mg/m².[46] Focal upper lobe fibrosis that is poorly responsive to steroids has been reported after 2 decades of carmustine treatment.[43]

When used in non-BMT patients, cyclophosphamide, melphalan, and ifosfamide are alkylators that have been known to cause interstitial pneumonitis, which may be reversible with steroids, as well as progressive pulmonary fibrosis decades after cessation of treatment.[47,48]

Cyclophosphamide may contribute to lung toxicity when used in combination with other cytotoxic agents, but rarely causes pneumopathy by itself. It may promote proteolysis in the lungs by ameliorating the effects of the antiprotease system and intensifying the effects of proteolytic enzymes.[4]

A higher incidence of interstitial pneumonitis with delayed pulmonary toxic syndrome was found when high-dose chemotherapy regimens comprising cyclophosphamide/cisplatin and carmustine were used followed by autologous bone marrow transplant in patients with breast malignancy.[32]

ANTHRACYCLINES

Mitomycin can cause pneumopathy, especially when combined with cisplatin and vinca alkaloids as neoadjuvant treatment for advanced non–small cell lung cancer. Acute dyspnea from bronchospasm, pleural effusion, and noncardiogenic pulmonary edema with diffuse interstitial infiltrate and hypoxemia had been reported shortly after an infusion of vinca alkaloid when used with mitomycin for non–small lung cancer.[49,50]

The mechanism of injury is thought to be secondary to initial vascular insult, leading to capillary leak. The risk of pneumopathy is not clearly related to dose; it occurs in approximately 5% of patients receiving the drug.[51] Clinical improvement has been demonstrated in most symptomatic patients after a trial of steroid treatment.[52,53]

Anthracyclines such as doxorubicin commonly cause cardiotoxicity but are rarely associated with lung injury. However, when these agents are combined with intensive thoracic radiation therapy, the resultant pneumopathy can be highly fatal, especially in susceptible patients with lung cancer.[54,55]

TAXANES

Weekly use of docetaxel is associated with increased risk of pulmonary toxicity when compared with 3-weekly dosing.[56] Docetaxel has been shown to potentiate radiation-induced pneumonitis in lung cancer patients,[57] as well as high risk of lung injury when added to gemcitabine treatment in patients with underlying pulmonary disease.[58]

Because of the high incidence of pneumonitis, it is not advisable to use weekly paclitaxel with concurrent thoracic radiation therapy following adjuvant anthracycline-based chemotherapy for early-stage breast cancer.[59]

BIOLOGIC MODIFIERS AND TARGET-SPECIFIC AGENTS

Biological agents such as interleukins and interferons, through which antineoplastic mechanisms act via immune modulation, can cause interstitial pneumonitis and noncardiogenic pulmonary edema, which is generally steroid responsive. Recombinant β-interferon, when added to conventional chemotherapeutic regimen therapy, has been shown to be implicated in increased risk of lung toxicity.[60,61]

Rare reports of interstitial pneumonitis and pulmonary hemorrhage have emerged with the use of new targeted therapies. These include the oral tyrosine kinase inhibitors, which act on specific signal transduction pathways (e.g., gefitinib, erlotinib, imatinib), the anti-CD 20 antibody rituximab, and the antiangiogenic agent, bevacizumab (anti–vascular endothelial growth factor [VEGF]). Data have yet to emerge regarding their exact pulmonary toxicity profiles and mechanisms.[62–66]

Chemotherapy-induced pulmonary toxicity represents a broad spectrum of disease and often poses a diagnostic challenge. Early diagnosis and discontinuation of drug with or without steroid use are essential to achieve a favorable outcome. Further data on means of predicting who is at risk for this complication and preventive strategies are necessary to maximize the therapeutic potential of these agents.

MALIGNANT CENTRAL AIRWAY OBSTRUCTION

The malignant process that causes mechanical obstruction of the major airways—the trachea and the main bronchi—is known as malignant central airway obstruction. Malignant central airway obstruction is not infrequently seen in clinical practice, especially in advanced or metastatic malignancies. It causes significant morbidity and mortality with a major negative impact on quality of life.[67,68]

Obstruction of the major airways by malignant tumors is usually a late complication, and unfortunately most patients have a limited life expectancy. Malignant central airway obstruction causes significant psychological and physical distress.[69] Furthermore, in those patients presenting with severe malignant central airway obstruction and impending arrest from suffocation, modalities such as chemotherapy or external beam radiation are ineffective for the acute management and restoration of oxygenation and ventilation in symptomatic patients.

Multiple interventional pulmonology techniques are now available and, in fact, are highly effective in the palliative management of malignant central airway obstruction.

EPIDEMIOLOGY

The precise incidence and prevalence of malignant airway obstruction are not known; however, it is estimated that approximately one third of patients with lung cancer will have complications related to obstruction of major airways, such as dyspnea, postobstructive pneumonia, atelectasis, hypoxemia, bleeding, or respiratory distress.[67,70] Also, around 40% of patients with lung cancer eventually die as the result of a complication of advanced locoregional disease (e.g., hemoptysis, respiratory infection, asphyxia).[67,71]

The central airways become obstructed by direct extension with airway invasion from an adjacent tumor; by the growth of a primary endobronchial malignancy; by metastatic endobronchial disease; or by compression from a contiguous tumor or cancer-related lymphadenopathy.

Malignant central airway obstruction is classified a intrinsic (purely intraluminal obstruction), extrinsic (purely extraluminal compression), or a combination of both, known as mixed obstruction (Figs. 29-2 through 29-4).

ETIOLOGY

Lung cancer is the second most common diagnosed malignancy and the most common cause of cancer-related death in the United States.[72,73] As such, it represents the most frequently reported cause of malignant central airway obstruction.[74] Non–small cell lung carcinoma (NSCLC) is the most common cause of malignant central airway obstruction.[75,76] Among histologic cell types, squamous cell carcinoma accounts for more than half of central airway–related obstructions, followed by adenocarcinoma.[70] Lung cancer commonly obstructs airways by direct extension with or without external compression. Other malignancies that generally obstruct the airways by direct extension are esophageal, laryngeal, and thyroid tumors.[67,76]

Primary large airway malignancies are rare. Among tracheal tumors, squamous cell carcinoma and adenoid cystic carcinoma represent the two most common cell types.[67,77] Carcinoid tumors are the most frequent primary airway tumors in the bronchi, distal to the main carina.[67,78] Other less common primary endobronchial tumors include mucoepidermoid and salivary gland–type tumors.[77]

Malignant central airway obstruction due to endobronchial metastatic extrathoracic disease is uncommon. The incidence ranges from 2% to 50% of extrathoracic malignancies have endobronchial metastases.[79,80] This discrepancy may be related to the definition. Some studies have reported only endobronchial metastases; others have reported general intrathoracic metastatic disease, with or without an endobronchial component. Tumors that frequently metastasize to the airways are breast, renal cell, colorectal, and thyroid carcinomas.[67]

Mediastinal malignancies, such as lymphomas, thymomas, thymic carcinomas or germ cell tumors, and cancer-related lymphadenopathy, cause major airway obstruction by external compression or mixed obstruction.

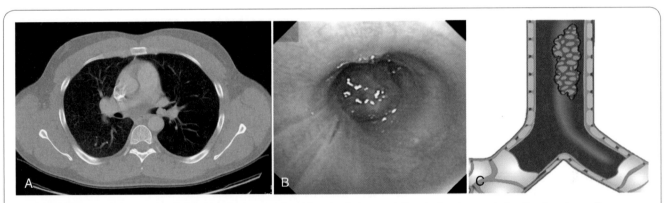

Fig. 29-2 Intrinsic obstruction. **A,** Computed tomography of the chest shows a left mainstem tumor obstructing the airway. **B,** Bronchoscopic image of the left mainstem tumor causes an almost complete endobronchial obstruction. After bronchoscopic resection, the pathologic diagnosis was an endobronchial carcinoid tumor. **C,** Graphic illustration of pure intraluminal obstruction.

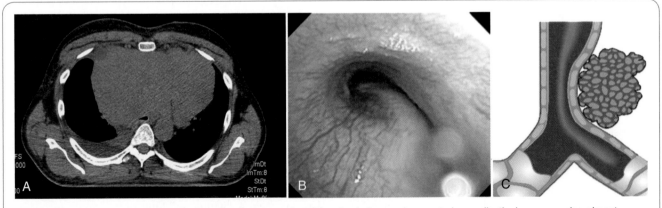

Fig. 29-3 Extrinsic compression. **A,** Computed tomography of the chest shows a large anterior mediastinal mass causing almost complete compression of the lower mid trachea. **B,** Bronchoscopic image at the lower third of the trachea shows significant external compression causing almost complete occlusion, especially at the right mainstem take-off. The pathologic diagnosis of an anterior mediastinal mass was consistent with lymphoma. **C,** Graphic illustration of a pure extraluminal compression.

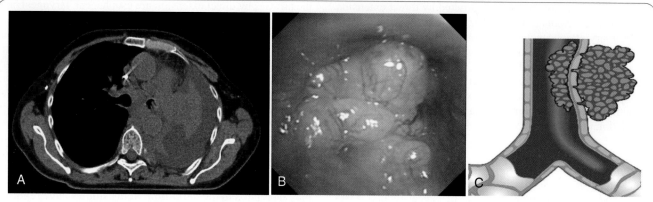

Fig. 29-4 Mixed obstruction. **A,** Computed tomography of the chest shows a large left mass causing encasement of the left mainstem and endobronchial tumor. **B,** Bronchoscopic image of the left mainstem tumor with significant endobronchial obstruction and airway wall involvement. Bronchogenic carcinoma was the final pathologic diagnosis. **C,** Graphic illustration of a mixed airway obstruction.

DIAGNOSIS

The presentation of central airway obstruction is variable. Symptoms may be mild with a chronic persistent cough; subacute, with progressive shortness of breath; or acute, in an asphyxiating patient with imminent suffocation and respiratory collapse.

The diagnosis of malignant central airway obstruction is challenging. It is based on the combination of patient history; signs and symptoms; and imaging, and endoscopic studies. Ultimately, the diagnosis is made by visualization of the tracheobronchial tree by bronchoscopy.

A detail clinical history is invaluable in making a prompt diagnosis. Risk factors such as smoking and personal or familial history of malignancy should be assessed.

SYMPTOMS

Commonly reported symptoms include cough, shortness of breath, hemoptysis, hoarseness, chest discomfort, orthopnea, and dysphagia.[75,81–83] The cough is usually chronic and dry; however, if associated with an infectious process (e.g., obstructive pneumonia), it may be productive and accompanied by systemic symptoms such as malaise and fever. Dyspnea appears late in the course of the disease. Dyspnea on exertion emerges once the trachea is <8 mm in diameter. When the airway lumen is <5 mm in diameter, dyspnea will occur at rest.[67,69,83] Patients with preexisting lung disease (e.g., chronic obstructive pulmonary disease [COPD]) may become dyspneic with lesser degrees of airway obstruction. Also, mild endoluminal obstructions may become symptomatic during episodes of respiratory infection, because of edema and accumulation of secretions that further narrow the already compromised airway. Patients with large tumors will complain of orthopnea due to airway compression when assuming a recumbent position. Hemoptysis is frequently seen with endobronchial lesions. It may be mild with blood-streaked sputum, or be massive. Dysphagia is seen as esophageal tumors extend into or compression airways, or when large bronchogenic or mediastinal tumors secondarily compress the esophageal. Cough provoked by eating or expectoration of food particles should raise suspicion of a aerodigestive fistula.

The type, intensity, response to treatment, and duration of symptoms are crucial to know, not only for diagnosis but also for therapeutic options. For example, if a malignant tumor causes a lung to collapse; it would be important to know the exact length of time the lung has been collapsed when making management decisions, because the longer the time of collapse, the less likely it is that the lung may recover despite airway clearance.

PHYSICAL EXAMINATION

Chest auscultation on physical examination, may be normal despite central airway collapse or may be associated with stridor, wheezing, localized crackles, frank consolidation, or complete absence of air movement.

Stridor points to severe subglottic or tracheal occlusion, and indicates that the airway lumen is <5 mm in diameter.[84,85] Stridor may be inspiratory, expiratory, or biphasic, and is best heard over the neck. Wheezing may be inspiratory or expiratory and may be heard over the trachea or the lung fields and does not usually conform to the area of obstruction.[85] On occasion, wheezing may be confined to one hemithorax, indicating an obstruction distal to the main carina. In fact, the finding of unilateral monophonic wheezing should always prompt further investigation to rule out a central airway obstruction.

In more severe obstructions, patients may present with signs and symptoms of impending respiratory arrest, such as anxiety, agitation, tachycardia, tachypnea, hypoxemia, and accessory muscle use.

IMAGING
Chest X-ray

A chest radiograph (CXR) should be obtained in patients suspected to have malignant central airway obstruction,[67] despite its low sensitivity in detecting abnormalities in major airways, especially the trachea. It is rarely diagnostic; however, findings associated with malignant central airway obstruction may be easily recognized and appropriate studies obtained.[86] For example, obstructive or recurrent pneumonia, atelectasis, and lobar or complete lung collapse is seen. A "white-out" lung is commonly recognized, and differs to the findings in a massive pleural effusion. Malignant central airway obstruction is associated with an elevated hemidiaphragm, ipsilateral mediastinal shift and volume loss (Fig. 29-5, *A*). Also, a pared inhalation and exhalation CXR demonstrates unilateral air trapping due to, tumor–induced check-valve obstruction.[87] Moreover, the classic "golden S-sign," indicative of an obstructive mass, has been reported in the literature[87] (Fig. 29-6).

Computed tomography (CT) scan of the chest

Conventional computed tomography (CT) or high-resolution computed tomography (HRCT) of the chest is the imaging modality of choice in diagnosing malignant central airway obstruction. HRCT has a sensitivity of 97% to detect anomalies in the trachea and main bronchi.[87] Considerable technologic advances in the last few years have significantly improved airway imaging. With the introduction of multidetector computed tomography (MDCT), high-quality reconstruction techniques are available, including multiplanar reconstructions (MPRs), external representations with three-dimensional (3D) shaded surface displays, and volumetric representations with internal rendering, the so-called virtual bronchoscopy (VB).[88,89]

In clinical practice, chest CT is extremely helpful not only in the diagnosis of malignant central airway obstruction but also in management, it is particularly important in planning interventional bronchoscopic procedures. HRCT of the chest allows recognition of the size and length of the tumor, and whether the obstruction is intrinsic, extrinsic, or mixed. Furthermore, careful examination of the CT scan helps to verify whether a viable airway is present distal to the obstruction. With the addition of intravenous (IV) contrast, CT of the chest will evaluate the relationship of the obstructive process to nearby structures, such as major vessels.

Magnetic resonance imaging (MRI) of the chest is useful in evaluating the mediastinum and vascular structures.

Endoscopy

Bronchoscopy, whether rigid or flexible, is the gold standard in the diagnosis of malignant central airway obstruction.[67,75,77] Endoscopy will allow biopsies to be taken if needed. Also, by endoscopic direct visualization, the physician will most accurately evaluate the lesion location, size, length, morphology, and degree of intraluminal and extraluminal disease, as well as the presence or absence of distal airways. However, endoscopy has some limitations, for example, the degree of extrinsic compression may be difficult to estimate without the help of HRCT of the chest; in the same way, to evaluate distal airways, other interventional bronchoscopic

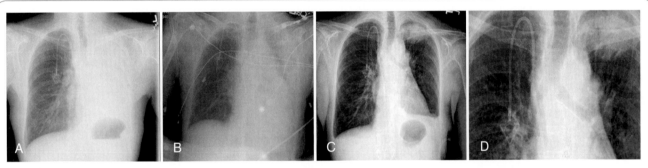

Fig. 29-5 Chest X-ray image (CXR) of a left upper lobe tumor. **A,** CXR shows a left "white-out" lung, with complete lung collapse and mild ipsilateral mediastinal and diaphragmatic shift. The patient underwent therapeutic rigid bronchoscopy with left mainstem self-expanding hybrid stent placement. **B,** Immediately after airway stenting, improvement is noted with greater aeration of the left upper lobe. **C,** Two weeks later, follow-up CXR shows significant improvement with resolution of lung collapse and good entry of air into the left hemithorax. **D,** Close-up image of the major airways shows the left mainstem metallic airway stent in place.

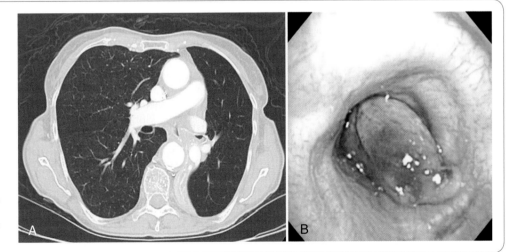

Fig. 29-6 The "golden-S or reverse-S sign." **A,** Essentially, when a lobe collapses around a large central mass, the peripheral lung tissue collapses, and the central portion of the lung is prevented from collapsing by the presence of the mass. The involved lung fissure is concave toward the lung peripherally and convex centrally, resembling a reverse S. **B,** Endoscopic image of metastatic colon cancer in the left mainstem bronchi.

procedures (e.g., laser) may be needed to "find a lumen" distal to the obstruction.

Although in general, flexible bronchoscopy (FB) represents a safe procedure, occasionally in the patient with severe malignant central airway obstruction presenting as impeding respiratory failure, it becomes a potentially dangerous procedure.[90] The narrow lumen may be further compromised by the flexible bronchoscope itself, or by accumulation of secretions and/or bleeding. Also, moderate sedation may impair ventilation and muscle performance, creating an unstable emergent airway. For these reasons, a team with expertise in the management of complex airway diseases should be present when diagnostic FB is to be done in such patients. Because of these factors, a two-step endoscopic approach is commonly planned: first, a diagnostic flexible bronchoscopy; second, a therapeutic one, which may be rigid or flexible. This procedure is usually performed by the interventional bronchoscopist in the operating theater with the patient under general anesthesia.

Pulmonary function tests (PFTs)

Whenever possible, especially if the acuity of the clinical presentation allows, a pulmonary function survey should be obtained.

Spirometry is not sensitive or specific for chronic airway obstruction (CAO), and usually the airway orifice is severely reduced ($\leq 6\,mm$ in diameter) before detection of significant changes in forced expiratory volume (FEV_1).[91] However, other parameters are useful. For instance, if the peak expiratory flow rate (PEFR) is disproportionately reduced in comparison with the reduction in FEV_1, an obstruction of the upper airway should be suspected.[91] Also, if the maximal voluntary ventilation (MMV) is reduced in association with a normal FEV_1, the possibility of an upper airway obstruction should be considered.[91]

The most important step when PFTs are used to assess a major airway obstruction is to look at the tracings. "Classic patterns" in the flow-volume loop (FVL) spirogram have been described for obstructions of the trachea. Although not sensitive, they may appear before changes in the FEV_1. The diameter of the trachea is around 8 to 10 mm to show FVL abnormalities.[84]

These changes have been classically divided into three patterns of upper airway obstruction (UAO)[84]:

1. Dynamic (nonfixed or variable) extrathoracic UAO: A flattened inspiratory limb is seen in the extrathoracic part of the trachea (above the suprasternal notch) as the result of an accentuated folding of the trachea with slower airflow during forced inspiration. This pattern may be seen with neck malignancies causing external compression of the upper one third of the trachea, or in subglottic endoluminal tumors.
2. Dynamic (nonfixed or variable) intrathoracic UAO: A flattened expiratory limb is seen in the intrathoracic part of the trachea (two thirds below the suprasternal notch) as the result of an accentuated folding of the airway with slower airflow during forced exhalation. This pattern may be seen in endoluminal tracheal tumors or in tracheobronchial compression due to malignant processes.

3. Fixed UAO: Flattened inspiratory and expiratory limbs are seen as the result of a fixed lesion in the upper airways that does not change in response to transmural pressure alterations during the respiratory cycle. This pattern may be seen in malignant tumors that cause encasement of the upper airway.

When assessing the FVL, keep in mind that the configuration of the loops is not sensitive, nor is it specific, and that preexisting diseases (e.g., COPD) may alter the configuration, as well as a suboptimal effort, during the forced expiratory maneuver.

Differential diagnosis

Diagnosis of malignant airway obstruction is not uncommonly delayed, and the condition may be misdiagnosed as progression of COPD, a COPD exacerbation, or a "difficult to treat asthma." Because the common signs and symptoms of malignant central airway obstruction (i.e., progressive dyspnea, chronic cough, and wheezing) are very nonspecific and are shared with many other more common diseases, the clinician must have a high index of suspicion when dealing with an appropriate set of patients at risk. Obviously, malignant central airway obstruction symptoms do not respond to pharmacotherapy, such as antibiotics, corticosteroids, or bronchodilators. Moreover, malignant central airway obstruction symptoms are persistent, instead of episodic, and ultimately are progressive. The quote "All that wheezes is not asthma" applies to malignant central airway obstruction; in addition, wheezing related to obstruction of the central airways is frequently unilateral. A nonresolving or recurrent pneumonia should alert the physician to the possibility of tracheobronchial obstruction.

MANAGEMENT

The management of malignant central airway obstruction is challenging and requires a multidisciplinary team approach that may include the pulmonologist, medical and radiation oncologists, thoracic surgeons, the anesthesiologist, and interventional bronchoscopists.

In general, the treatment largely depends on the clinical presentation. In the stable patient without impending respiratory failure, a step-wise approach may be taken. Initially, detailed preprocedural studies (e.g., HRCT, diagnostic flexible bronchoscopy) are performed; these are followed by a planned intervention (e.g., rigid debulking, laser photoresection). On the other hand, in the patient with severe malignant central airway obstruction (i.e., complete lung collapse and respiratory distress), the first priority is to secure the airway; then, urgent recanalization of the tracheobronchial obstruction is needed to maintain ventilation and/or oxygenation and to improve survival by avoiding death from suffocation.

Surgery is the best therapy for malignant central airway obstruction. Unfortunately, in most instances, patients present with advanced malignancies that are not curable by surgical resection. In those rare cases where malignant central airway obstruction is localized in a medically operable patient, every effort must be made to offer a radical surgical approach to improve the chance of cure. In addition, it is important to note that in some patients with localized, nonmetastatic malignant central airway obstruction and impending respiratory failure, interventional bronchoscopic procedures may improve patient status and function as a "bridge" to a definitive surgical resection.[92]

Nonetheless, as stated previously, most patients present with locally advanced or metastatic disease, with failed prior therapies (e.g., chemoradiation), or with multiple medical comorbidities; therefore, palliative management is frequently offered. Historically, external beam radiation (EBR) with or without chemotherapy has been the modality of choice. However, nowadays, interventional bronchoscopic procedures should be offered as the initial treatment of choice for palliative management of malignant central airway obstruction.

The literature has classically divided the management of malignant central airway obstruction into two main interventions: airway or initial stabilization and endoscopic therapy.[86]

A detailed description of airway stabilization/management in malignant central airway obstruction is beyond the purpose of this chapter; however, excellent reviews have been published elsewhere.[83,93] Briefly, the mandatory priority in malignant central airway obstruction management is to have a secure airway. This may be accomplished most frequently by endotracheal intubation or rigid bronchoscopy; however, in some instances a surgical tracheotomy may be needed. The support of an anesthesiologist with some expertise in major airways obstruction is of invaluable help.

Once the airway has been secured, endoscopic management of malignant central airway obstruction may be provided by flexible or rigid bronchoscopy (RB). Over the past decade, the field of interventional pulmonology and the armamentarium for dealing with malignant central airway obstruction have dramatically improved, and several different modalities may be used. These modalities can be encompassed in three categories: (1) thermal therapies, (2) nonthermal therapies, and (3) radiation therapies. Many times, these modalities are actually complementary and are used in conjunction, tailored to patient necessities (Fig. 29-7). Most of these techniques may be used with the flexible or the rigid bronchoscope. Some argue that FB should be done whenever possible, given that it is readily available and does not require general anesthesia or an operating theater. However, RB is the procedure of choice when severe CAO has been diagnosed, or when the stability of the airway is in doubt.[67]

Rigid bronchoscopy is a safe and effective way to secure the airway.[94] It allows ventilation and oxygenation, while the rigid bronchoscope barrel itself may be used to "core-out" lesions and dilate stenosis.[95] Through the rigid scope, several large instruments may be passed (e.g., laser, suction catheters), as may the flexible bronchoscope. It does requires general anesthesia and must be performed in the operating room. Contraindications to RB are those related to the anesthesia

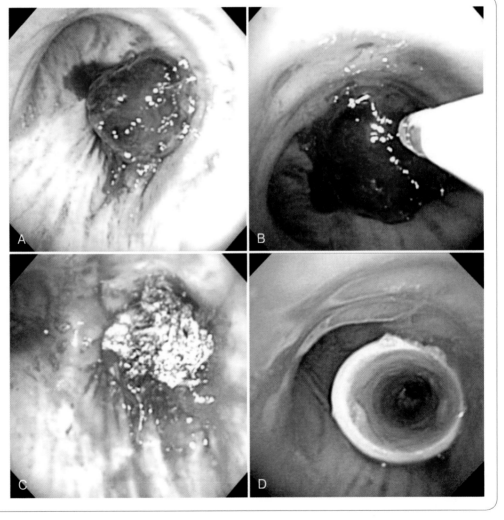

Fig. 29-7 Combination of bronchoscopic techniques in the management of malignant central airway occlusion (MCAO). **A,** Bronchoscopic image of a large friable tumor obstructing the right mainstem bronchus. **B,** Different techniques may be used to ablate the tumor and regain passage to the obstructed airways. In this image, the electrocautery probe is seen. **C,** The right mainstem mass shows the effects of electrofulguration of the tumoral tissue; here, significant necrosis is seen. **D,** After tumor destruction and debulking, a silicone stent was placed to maintain airway patency.

and to the patient's neck and jaw anatomy. Common complications include gum and tooth injuries, tracheal or bronchial tears, and bleeding. The overall complication rate related to the procedure itself is <0.1% in experienced hands.[96]

In general, the physician needs to determine the following points before choosing the optimal procedure for malignant central airway obstruction palliation:

- Is the obstruction intrinsic, extrinsic, or mixed?
- Is the location amenable to intervention?
- Does the patient's medical condition allow safe intervention to be performed?
- Will the intervention improve the patient's current status and quality of life?
- Is a viable airway present distal to the obstruction?

Here, we present a brief description of various interventional pulmonology therapies used in the management of malignant central airway obstruction.

Thermal therapies: laser, electrocautery, argon plasma coagulation, and cryotherapy

LASER*

Laser (*l*ight *a*mplification of *s*timulated *e*mission of *r*adiation) photoresection refers to the application of laser energy to cause thermal, photodynamic, and electromagnetic changes in living tissues.

The first report of the use of the laser to ablate endobronchial malignant tumors dates back to the mid-70s; since that time, multiple reports have documented its safety and efficacy.

Multiple types of lasers are available. The *neodymium: yttrium-aluminum-garnet* (Nd:YAG) laser is currently the most commonly used by interventional pulmonologists.

The Nd:YAG laser may be used through the flexible or rigid bronchoscope. It has a wavelength of 1064 nm, and contact and noncontact probes are available. The depth of tissue penetration by the Nd:YAG laser ranges from 3 to 5 mm, depending on the settings. However, the depth of tissue destruction is not immediately evident, so extreme caution must be used to direct the laser parallel to the airway to avoid complications.

Laser photoresection is indicated in the therapy of major airway obstruction by malignant tumors. Because of its immediate effect, it may be used in the management of acute malignant central airway obstruction with respiratory compromise, in cases where a rapid recanalization technique is needed. Multiple studies have documented excellent results with use of the laser in endobronchial tumor debulking and lumen restoration, with success rates from 83% to 93%. Also, a rate of up to 94% in symptom relief has been historically described. Furthermore, retrospective studies using historical controls have documented improved survival and quality of life in patients with malignant central airway obstruction treated with laser photoresection.

Laser endoscopy is a safe procedure when performed by experienced hands. A complication rate of <3% has been described. Complications include airway perforation, pneumothorax, hypoxia, bleeding, arrhythmias, myocardial infarction, gas embolism, and airway ignition. To avoid airway fires, the fraction of inspired oxygen (FiO_2) must be

rigorously kept below 40% during laser firing. To minimize risks and avoid complications with laser bronchoscopy, the "Mehta's rule of four" has been published.

The only absolute contraindication for laser photoresection is purely extrabronchial compression. Major drawbacks to laser endoscopy include its high cost and the fact that it is not available at most institutions.

ELECTROCAUTERY*

Electrocautery or electrosurgery refers to the use an electrical current to heat and destroy tissue. Often referred to as "the poor man's laser," it provides laser-like tissue effects at a lower cost.

It was in 1926 when the first report of using energy to destroy an endobronchial tumor was published. In that case, a music wire introduced through the rigid bronchoscope was used.

In electrosurgery, a high-frequency, alternating electrical current is used to generate heat, which is proportionally related to tissue resistance, and inversely related to tissue vascularity and moisture content. The current leaves the body through a grounding plate. Its effect ultimately depends on the power used, the application time, the surface in contact, and the tissue type.

Electrocautery may be performed by flexible or rigid bronchoscopy. It is usually a contact mode of therapy. Different types of probes are available for different purposes. Probes commonly used are the blunt-tip probe, the electrocautery knife, the wire snare, and the forceps. In general, three settings are commonly used: a pure cut mode (high current, low voltage), a coagulate mode (low current, high voltage), and a blend mode that allows cutting and coagulation simultaneously.

Electrocautery has the same indications as laser photoresection. It also achieves rapid tumor debulking and may be used in cases of severe, acute malignant central airway obstruction for which rapid recanalization is indicated. Electrocautery is particularly useful in polypoid endobronchial lesions that are attached to the airway by a stalk (Fig. 29-8). With the use of the wire snare, the pedunculated lesion may be removed by cauterizing the stalk and leaving the rest of the tissue undestroyed for pathologic review, if needed. Several studies have documented the efficacy of electrocautery in treating malignant central airway obstruction. A reported rate of 89% of lumen restoration has been described. Also, up to 97% of symptom relief may be achieved.

Bronchoscopic electrosurgery has an excellent safety profile. Reported complications include bleeding, hypoxemia, airway perforation, endobronchial ignition, and electrical shock to the operator if not adequately grounded. As with laser photoresection, the FiO_2 must be kept at <40%; the procedure is contraindicated in purely external airway compression.

A major drawback to electrocautery is the fact that because it is a contact mode, frequent cleaning of the probe may be needed. Also, the electrical current may loss efficacy in cases of bleeding as the result of diffusion across a larger surface area. In addition, in patients with pacemakers or automatic implantable cardioverter/defibrillators (AICDs), the risk of creating an arrhythmia or a device malfunction is present.

*References 67, 69, 74, 75, 90, 94, 95, 97.

*References 67, 69, 74, 75, 90, 94, 95, 97–100.

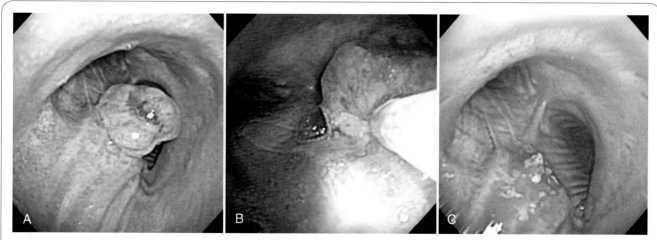

Fig. 29-8 Polypoid lesion at the main carina. **A,** A polypoid malignant tumor is seen close to the main carina. The pedunculated lesion shows an attachment to the posterior airway wall. **B,** In this image, with use of the electrocautery snare, the lesion is removed by cauterization at the stalk. **C,** The polypoid lesion has been removed, leaving minimal bleeding at the posterior airway wall.

ARGON PLASMA COAGULATION (APC)*

Argon plasma coagulation (APC) is a form of noncontact electro-coagulation that uses ionized argon gas to conduct an electrical current between the delivery catheter probe and the target tissue. With the use of a high-voltage electrical field created at the tip of the probe, argon gas is ionized, creating a monopolar current that makes an "arc" conducted by the argon plasma to the nearest grounded tissue, producing coagulation necrosis. The flow of argon plasma from the probe to the tissue creates a noncontact diathermy that is homogeneous and superficial (2 to 3 mm in depth).

APC is conducted by a flexible catheter through the rigid or flexible bronchoscope. It is a noncontact type of procedure with a superficial effect. Energy released from the probe may be applied in an axial, radial, or retrograde manner, providing the important advantage of treating tumors laterally to the probe, or at sharp angles from the probe tip. This is a significant quality of APC when compared with laser or electrocautery. Also, APC is an excellent tool for hemostasis.

APC is indicated in the management of malignant central airway obstruction, and its use has increased recently, as part of a multimodality approach or instead of laser or electrosurgery. Nonetheless, unlike electrocautery and Nd:YAG photoresection, APC does not vaporize tissue, so other debulking modalities may be needed to resect a large tumor. Also, because of its low penetration depth, increased time may be needed when APC is used as a debulking tool. A luminal restoration rate of 91% has been reported with APC.

APC is a safe procedure with an overall complication rate of <1%. Complications include airway perforation, hemorrhage, airway fire, and systemic gas embolism. As with laser and electrocautery, the FiO_2 must be kept at <40%. APC is contraindicated in pure external airway compression. As with electrocautery, APC should not be used in patients with a pacemaker or AICD.

CRYOTHERAPY†

Cryotherapy refers to the application of extreme cold to create a hypothermic destruction of tissue. Three different cooling agents exist: liquid nitrogen, nitrous oxide, and carbon dioxide. Currently, nitrous oxide is the cryogen that is most commonly used.

It was in the mid-60s when the first report was published describing the use of endobronchial cryotherapy to treat an endobronchial carcinoma obstructing a large airway.

The effects of cryotherapy are multiple. When extracellular ice crystals form, extracellular space tonicity significantly increases, leading to cell membrane destruction by dehydration. Also, intracellular ice crystals form, damaging organelles. Furthermore, freezing causes vasoconstriction and formation of microthrombi.

The cryotherapy probe may be used by the flexible or rigid bronchoscope. The cryogen passes through the catheter probe, cooling the metal tip; then under direct visualization, the tip is applied parallel to the lesion. This is a contact mode of therapy. Cryotherapy effect basically depends on the number of freezing-thawing cycles, the temperature reached (below −40° C), and the type of tissue being treated. Maximal cellular damage occurs with repetitive rapid freezing–slow thawing cycles. Cryosensitive tissues include skin, nerve, endothelium, granulation tissue, and mucous membranes. Cryoresistant tissues consist of connective and fibrous tissues, as well as cartilage and fat.

The use of cryotherapy may be indicated in malignant central airway obstruction when the presentation is not acute with impending respiratory failure. Because cryotherapy effects are delayed as opposed to those of laser or electrocautery, it is not used when rapid recanalization of the airway is needed. However, it is very useful in the removal of polypoid lesions, blood clots, and foreign materials, and in the treatment of vascular tumors.

The main advantages of cryotherapy are its excellent safety profile, low cost, low risk for airway perforation, and lack of risk for airway ignition. Complications may include airway sloughing and the need to follow "cleaning bronchoscopies" and postprocedure fever. Furthermore, unlike other thermal therapies, cryotherapy with high FiO_2 concentrations may be used.

PHOTODYNAMIC THERAPY*

Photodynamic therapy (PDT) refers to the method of activating a chemical compound with a nonthermal laser light to

---

*References 67, 69, 75, 90, 94, 95, 97, 99, 101, 102.
†References 67, 69, 75, 94, 95, 97, 100, 101, 103.

*References 67, 69, 75, 94, 95, 97, 101.

produce a phototoxic reaction, leading to cellular death. PDT is used in malignant central airway obstruction as a delayed tumor destruction method.

It was in the early 1980s when the use of PDT to treat early lung cancer was first described. Since that time, it has evolved into a complex interventional technique.

In PDT, the patient receives a local or systemic injection of a photosensitizing drug; this is preferentially retained in malignant cells, but also in the skin, liver, and spleen. Then, about 24 to 72 hours after the drug injection, a laser light of specific wavelength is applied by flexible bronchoscopy to activate the chemical compound. The phototoxic reaction causes tumor destruction by oxygen radical species generation, direct cell damage, indirect ischemic effects, apoptosis, and inflammatory reactions. Subsequently, immediately and 48 hours after the procedure, bronchoscopic cleaning and debulking of the area are performed to clean debris and establish airway patency. The most common photosensitizer compound used is dihematoporphyrin ether (DHE).

PDT is indicated in the palliative treatment of malignant endobronchial obstruction presenting with no acute dyspnea. Also, in patients who are not surgical candidates or have contraindications to external beam radiation, PDT may be used in treating early lung cancer without extension beyond the airway wall. The literature has described an 80% success rate in malignant airway obstruction palliation.

Complications of PDT include skin photosensitivity for 4 to 6 weeks after the procedure, local airway edema, airway strictures, bleeding, and formation of fistulas. Major drawbacks to PDT are the need for repetitive procedures and the inconvenience for the patient regarding severe skin photosensitivity and its delayed tumor destructive effect.

Nonthermal therapies: rigid debulking, balloon dilatation, the microdebrider, and airway stents

RIGID BRONCHOSCOPIC DEBULKING[69,75,96]

Rigid bronchoscopy is a safe and effective way of securing the airway and, at the same time, allowing therapeutic interventions. In emergent cases, the bronchoscope itself may be used for rapid tumor debulking and stenosis dilatation.

The distal end of the bronchoscope is beveled and is ideal for "coring out" through large endobronchial tumors. At the same time, the barrel of the scope is used to tamponade bleeding while debulking malignancies. Its large internal diameter allows multiple instruments to be passed through (e.g., large suction catheters, forceps, flexible bronchoscopes) if needed. Also, at the proximal end, it has several ports that allow ventilation (positive pressure or jet ventilation). In general, debulking of tumors is a multimodality approach. Coring out lesions with the scope has the risk of damaging the airway; however, mechanical core-out is still commonly performed to treat malignant central airway obstruction.

BALLOON DILATATION (BALLOON TRACHEOPLASTY/BRONCHOPLASTY)[67,75,97,104,105]

With the use of special balloons of various lengths and diameters, the airway may be dilated. Balloon tracheoplasty (dilatation of the trachea) or bronchoplasty (dilatation of the bronchi) allows gentler airway dilatation, as compared with the rigid scope, with less mucosal trauma. It is commonly performed in the management of malignant central airway obstruction, usually in combination with other modalities.

Balloon dilatation may be performed by rigid or flexible bronchoscopy. The balloons are filled with saline until full deployment is reached, with the help of a pressure-measuring syringe. A prespecified pressure unit diameter is obtained and commonly is maintained for seconds up to a few minutes. Then, the procedure may be repeated several times, or, if needed, larger balloons may be used subsequently.

It has a reported immediate effect of 79% in malignant obstruction; however, its effect typically is not long sustained. Because of its common short-lived effect, balloon dilatation is performed in combination with other procedures such as laser endoscopy, or before airway stenting.

Airway balloon dilatation is a relatively safe procedure. Complications include airway tear or rupture, pneumothorax, pneumomediastinum, pain, and bleeding. The exact incidence of complications after airway balloon dilatation is unknown. Minimal airway tears are universally expected after dilatation; however, a vast majority of them do not cause additional problems. In a report of 126 balloon dilatations for malignant airway disease, 41 minor bleeds without the need for specific therapy were seen.[104] In that report, one fatal bleed occurred that was related to a laceration of a branch of the pulmonary artery surrounded by malignant tumor.

THE MICRODEBRIDER[106,107]

The endobronchial microdebrider is a relatively new addition to the tools used in interventional pulmonology.

It is a metallic instrument that may be inserted through the rigid scope and has at the tip a powered rotating blade coupled with suction for the rapid debridement of endobronchial tumors. Because it has instantaneous suction capacity, in theory a clean field that allows visual maintenance is achieved.

Two different lengths are available to treat lesions at the trachea and at the main bronchi. Few studies have been published; however, the microdebrider represents a practical tool that may be useful in the management of malignant central airway obstruction.

AIRWAY STENTS*

Airway stents are endoluminal prostheses made from various materials that support and maintain patency of the hollow tubular airway structure.

In the 1960s, the Montgomery T-tube was introduced to treat subglottic stenosis. Then, in the early 90s, the Dumon silicone stent was conceived, which in fact was the first dedicated airway stent. Since that time, multiple prototypes of stents made from different materials have been produced in attempts to find the ideal stent.

In general, three different types of stents exist: silicone, metallic, and hybrid stents.

Silicone stents are made of synthetic silicone elastomers. They are available in different shapes (i.e., straight or Y-shaped), lengths, and diameters, and can be easily customized to the airway anatomy before deployment (Fig. 29-9). Rigid bronchoscopy is required for their insertion. Once deployed, these stents can be repositioned and removed effortlessly. Also, they are relatively inexpensive. Disadvantages of silicone stents include a higher migration rate, the induction of

---

*References 67, 69, 71, 74, 75, 90, 94, 95, 97, 101, 108–114.

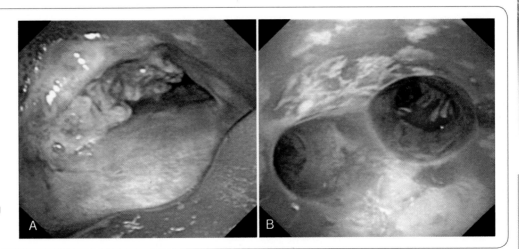

Fig. 29-9 Silicone Y-stent at the main carina. **A,** A friable irregular mass is seen at the main carina, causing almost complete occlusion of the left mainstem and partial obstruction of the right main bronchi. **B,** After tumor debulking, a Dumon silicone "Y-stent" was placed, keeping the main carina and both mainstem bronchi patent.

granulation tissue at stent edges, accumulation of secretions, and the need for general anesthesia and rigid bronchoscopy for placement.

Metallic stents are made from different metal alloys (e.g., nitinol:titanium, nickel). They are available in different lengths and diameters. Uncovered and covered (hybrid) versions can be found in the market. Most of the new-generation metallic stents are self-expandable once deployed. Metallic stents are easily deployed by flexible bronchoscopy under moderate sedation or by rigid bronchoscopy (Fig. 29-10). They have a minimal migration rate, resist extrinsic compression, may conform to tortuous airways, and may allow ventilation across lobar orifices. One of the major disadvantages of metallic stents is the difficulty in their repositioning and removal once epithelialized. Other complications attributed to metallic stents include granulation tissue formation at the edges and through the metallic mesh, tumor in-growth across the metallic orifices, metal fracture or rupture, and risk for airway or vascular perforation (Fig. 29-11). In the management of malignant central airway obstruction, uncovered metallic stents currently have minimal or no indication for placement.

The use of airway stents is indicated in malignant airway obstruction in cases of extrinsic compression or intrinsic or mixed obstruction, if, after tumor debulking, the airway lumen remains with >50% intraluminal occlusion. In the appropriate setting, stenting of malignant airway obstruction provides rapid palliation of symptoms (up to 94% symptom relief), enhanced quality of life, and possibly improved survival. Also, silicone and metallic covered stents have been used in the palliative management of malignant tracheoesophageal fistula. Tumor debulking and stenting in many instances are complementary procedures, depending on case complexity. Furthermore, interventional procedures, such as airway stenting, may be complementary to chemotherapy and/or radiation therapy. For instance, relieving a central airway obstruction by stenting may allow a patient to have the necessary respiratory reserve to continue with oncologic therapy, such as external beam radiation.

In summary, stent indications in malignant processes include a rapidly growing tumor, >50% endobronchial obstruction, tracheoesophageal fistula (TEF), tumor refractory to other therapies, airway obstruction with an anticipated slow response to other therapies, and external compression of the airways.

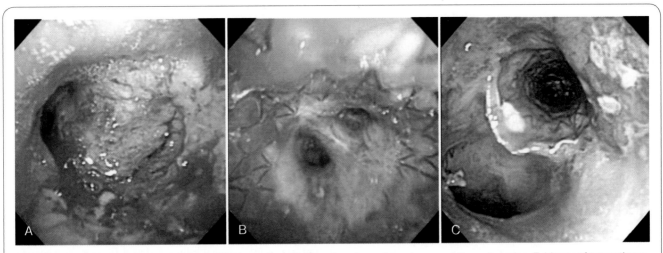

Fig. 29-10 Self-expanding covered metallic stents. **A,** A friable, edematous airway is seen at the main carina. Evidence of tumor tissue is seen endobronchially and involving the airway walls. **B,** After tumor debulking and dilatation, two covered metallic stents were placed. Here, evidence of patent airways distal to the left mainstem is seen after stenting. **C,** Two fully covered metallic stents were placed, keeping the airways patent.

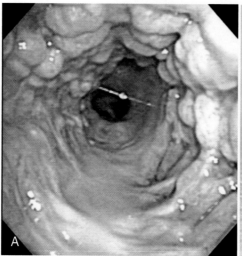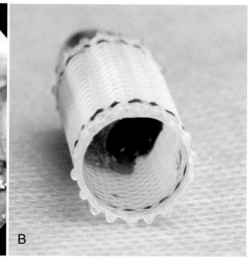

Fig. 29-11 Stent complications. Images **A** and **B** show two of the most common and feared stents complications. Image **A** shows a metallic stent with significant neoepithelialization, making its removal extremely difficult and potentially dangerous. Image **B** shows a hybrid silicone stent after removal, with a mucous plug. As can be seen in the image, the mucous plug caused complete occlusion of the stent, placing the patient at risk of suffocation.

Radiation therapies: brachytherapy
BRACHYTHERAPY*

Brachytherapy involves the delivery of radioactivity endo-bronchially. By flexible bronchoscopy under fluoroscopic guidance, a polyurethane afterloading catheter is placed into the airway tumor or in close proximity. Then, the catheter is secured and the radioactive source, usually iridium-192, is placed within or very close to the tumor. Brachytherapy may be given as a low-dose rate (LDR) or as a high-dose rate endo-bronchial (HDR) method. High-dose rate brachytherapy is preferred because higher radiation doses are given with less time on each fraction, given that treatment may be administered on an outpatient basis.

Brachytherapy is indicated for the palliation of symptoms related to malignant central airway obstruction. Its effects are not due to direct tissue destruction, but are related to DNA alteration, including cell apoptosis. The effects are delayed and, depending on dosage per fraction, may take up to 3 weeks. In consequence, brachytherapy is not indicated in the management of acute malignant central airway obstruction. Nevertheless, it has a long-lasting effect and may be used combined with other techniques, as is laser photoresection or external beam radiation. A 78% to 85% rate of airway lumen recanalization has been described, with a 69% to 93% rate of symptom improvement. Another advantage of brachytherapy is the short-distance radiation, with subsequent protection of surrounding normal tissue.

Complications of brachytherapy include hemorrhage, fistulas, arrhythmias, hypotension, bronchospasm, bronchial stenosis or necrosis, and radiation bronchitis. A 0% to 32% fatal hemorrhage incidence has been described. However, it is not clear if the complication was related to the radiation itself, or if it was due to tumor progression. It is interesting to note that a higher incidence of hemoptysis has been found in tumors located in the right and left upper lobes; probability is related to proximity to the great vessels.

Outcome

Unfortunately, the evidence-based literature in interventional bronchoscopy is limited. Most reported studies are retrospective and usually descriptive, and have included heterogeneous populations and diseases. However, the immediate benefit of central airway de-obstruction is seen in significant improvements in dyspnea, performance indexes, and quality-of-life measurements. Also, a retrospective study has shown that patients presenting with malignant central obstruction treated with interventional bronchoscopic procedures plus chemotherapy or radiation therapy have the same life expectancy as those without central airway obstruction treated with the same adjunctive therapies.[70]

In the vast majority of malignant central airway obstruction patients, the disease is not curable; therefore, patients and family members must be aware of the palliative nature of the interventions.

Given the common dramatic presentation of malignant central airway obstruction and the dramatic symptom improvement observed after airway recanalization, a randomized controlled trial of intervention versus nonintervention to assess mortality benefits is unethical. Anyway, because of high efficiency in symptom relief, interventional bronchoscopy should be offered to every patient presenting with malignant central airway obstruction.

RADIATION-INDUCED LUNG INJURY

A significant proportion of lung cancer patients at some point during their disease course will receive lung radiotherapy.[115] Furthermore, other thoracic or chest wall malignancies, such as lymphoma, breast, or esophageal cancer, will also be managed with thoracic irradiation.[116] Unfortunately, radiation will kill cancer cells and will provoke severe damage to normal parenchymal cells. Thus, because of concerns regarding normal tissue damage, high-dose radiation is limited.

Two radiation-induced lung injury (RILI) entities have been well described: acute radiation pneumonitis and chronic radiation fibrosis.[117] Although lung-induced fibrosis may represent a continuum from acute pneumonitis, the two conditions might be unrelated. The pathophysiology of RILI is beyond the scope of this chapter; however, the generation of oxygen free radicals, as well as cytotoxic cell damage, has been implicated.[118]

*References 67, 69, 81, 94, 95, 97, 100.

No method of predicting lung injury following radiation is highly accurate. Some risk factors have been described, and the volume of tissue treated, the dose of therapy delivered, and the sizes of fractions given are important issues to consider.[116,117,119] In the same way, concurrent treatment with chemotherapy enhances lung injury. Doxorubicin, bleomycin, gemcitabine, and docetaxel, among other chemotherapy agents, are some of the most potent radiation sensitizers.[117,119,120] Other reported factors include smoking, pretherapy performance status, pretherapy lung function, prior thoracic radiation, and glucocorticoid withdrawal during radiotherapy.[117,120] The dose of radiation is very important in predicting the possibility of lung injury. The mean radiation dose may be a predictor of the risk of radiation pneumonitis, with an estimated 5% risk at a mean dose of 20 Gy.[119]

Acute radiation pneumonitis, typically presents within 4 to 12 weeks after therapy. Common symptoms include nonproductive cough, dyspnea, pneumonia-like symptoms, and low-grade fever.[116-119] Chest radiography may show diffuse haziness in the treatment field.[117] CT of the chest is more sensitive and may show ground-glass opacities or consolidations. In many instances, a discrepancy between symptoms and imaging is noted. Pulmonary function tests may show decreased FEV_1 and DLCO.[116,119] Bronchoscopic alveolar lavage may reveal an increased lymphocyte count but is not specific. No randomized trials regarding its treatment are under way, and recommendations are based on expert opinion.[116] Steroids given at high doses with a slow taper course represent the mainstay of treatment.[118] An 80% response rate has been described.[117,119] Fortunately, most cases are mild, and no therapy is required.[119]

Chronic radiation fibrosis may present within 6 to 24 months after radiotherapy.[117,119] Typical symptoms include a nonproductive cough associated with shortness of breath. Chest X-ray may show opacifications, volume loss, or pleural thickening. Often, a sharp demarcation delineating the radiation field is evident, more commonly in CT imaging. This so-called "nonanatomic margination" represents a straight-line effect that corresponds not with anatomic landmarks, but rather with the radiation field.[118] These findings are almost diagnostic. A restrictive pattern with reduced DLCO is seen on pulmonary function surveys. Unfortunately, no treatment exists, and supportive and palliative management is usually offered.[118,119]

REFERENCES

1. Sakanashi Y, Takeya M, Yoshimura T, et al. Kinetics of macrophage subpopulations and expression of monocyte chemoattractant protein-1 (MCP-1) in bleomycin-induced lung injury of rats studied by a novel monoclonal antibody against rat MCP-1. *J Leukoc Biol.* 1994;56:741–750.

2. Lewis RA, Austen KF. The biologically active leukotrienes. biosynthesis, metabolism, receptors, functions, and pharmacology. *J Clin Invest.* 1984;73:889–897.

3. Freeman BA, Crapo JD. Biology of disease: free radicals and tissue injury. *Lab Invest.* 1982;47:412–426.

4. Cooper Jr JA, White DA, Matthay RA. Drug-induced pulmonary disease, part 1: cytotoxic drugs. *Am Rev Respir Dis.* 1986;133:321–340.

5. White DA, Kris MG, Stover DE. Bronchoalveolar lavage cell populations in bleomycin lung toxicity. *Thorax.* 1987;42:551–552.

6. White DA, Rankin JA, Stover DE, et al. Methotrexate pneumonitis: bronchoalveolar lavage findings suggest an immunologic disorder. *Am Rev Respir Dis.* 1989;139:18–21.

7. Nuver J, Lutke Holzik MF, van Zweeden M, et al. Genetic variation in the bleomycin hydrolase gene and bleomycin-induced pulmonary toxicity in germ cell cancer patients. *Pharmacogenet Genomics.* 2005;15:399–405.

8. Jules-Elysee K, White DA. Bleomycin-induced pulmonary toxicity. *Clin Chest Med.* 1990;11:1–20.

9. Ignoffo RJ, Viele CS, Damon LE, Venook A. *Cancer chemotherapy pocket guide.* Baltimore, MD: Lippincott-Raven; 1998.

10. Sleijfer S. Bleomycin-induced pneumonitis. *Chest.* 2001;120:617–624.

11. Saxman SB, Nichols CR, Einhorn LH. Pulmonary toxicity in patients with advanced-stage germ cell tumors receiving bleomycin with and without granulocyte colony stimulating factor. *Chest.* 1997;111:657–660.

12. McCullough B, Collins JF, Johanson Jr WG, Grover FL. Bleomycin-induced diffuse interstitial pulmonary fibrosis in baboons. *J Clin Invest.* 1978;61:79–88.

13. Herman EH, Hasinoff BB, Zhang J, et al. Morphologic and morphometric evaluation of the effect of ICRF-187 on bleomycin-induced pulmonary toxicity. *Toxicology.* 1995;98:163–175.

14. Khalil N, Whitman C, Zuo L, et al. Regulation of alveolar macrophage transforming growth factor-beta secretion by corticosteroids in bleomycin-induced pulmonary inflammation in the rat. *J Clin Invest.* 1993;92:1812–1818.

15. King SL, Lichtler AC, Rowe DW, et al. Bleomycin stimulates pro-alpha 1 (I) collagen promoter through transforming growth factor beta response element by intracellular and extracellular signaling. *J Biol Chem.* 1994;269:13156–13161.

16. Chandler DB. Possible mechanisms of bleomycin-induced fibrosis. *Clin Chest Med.* 1990;11:21–30.

17. O'Sullivan JM, Huddart RA, Norman AR, et al. Predicting the risk of bleomycin lung toxicity in patients with germ-cell tumours. *Ann Oncol.* 2003;14:91–96.

18. Rimmer MJ, Dixon AK, Flower CD, et al. Bleomycin lung: computed tomographic observations. *Br J Radiol.* 1985;58:1041–1045.

19. White DA, Schwartzberg LS, Kris MG, et al. Acute chest pain syndrome during bleomycin infusions. *Cancer.* 1987;59:1582–1585.

20. Straus DJ, Portlock CS, Qin J, et al. Results of a prospective randomized clinical trial of doxorubicin, bleomycin, vinblastine, and dacarbazine (ABVD) followed by radiation therapy (RT) versus ABVD alone for stages I, II, and IIIA nonbulky Hodgkin disease. *Blood.* 2004;104:3483–3489 Epub 2004 Aug 17.

21. Wolkowicz J, Sturgeon J, Rawji M, et al. Bleomycin-induced pulmonary function abnormalities. *Chest.* 1992;101:97–101.

22. Rossi SE, Erasmus JJ, McAdams HP, et al. Pulmonary drug toxicity: radiologic and pathologic manifestations. *Radiographics.* 2000;20:1245–1259.

23. Simpson AB, Paul J, Graham J, et al. Fatal bleomycin pulmonary toxicity in the West of Scotland 1991–95: a review of patients with germ cell tumours. *Br J Cancer.* 1998;78:1061–1066.

24. Rabinowits M, Souhami L, Gil RA, et al. Increased pulmonary toxicity with bleomycin and cisplatin chemotherapy combinations. *Am J Clin Oncol.* 1990;13:132–138.

25. Azoulay E, Herigault S, Levame M, et al. Effect of granulocyte colony-stimulating factor on bleomycin-induced acute lung injury and pulmonary fibrosis. *Crit Care Med.* 2003;31:1442–1448.

26. Lei KI, Leung WT, Johnson PJ. Serious pulmonary complications in patients receiving recombinant granulocyte colony-stimulating factor during BACOP chemotherapy for aggressive non-Hodgkin's lymphoma. *Br J Cancer.* 1994;70:1009–1013.

27. Haston CK, Wang M, Dejournett RE, et al. Bleomycin hydrolase and a genetic locus within the MHC affect risk for pulmonary fibrosis in mice. *Hum Mol Genet.* 2002;11:1855–1863.

28. Blom-Muilwijk MC, Vriesendorp R, Veninga TS, et al. Pulmonary toxicity after treatment with bleomycin alone or in combination with hyperoxia: studies in the rat. *Br J Anaesth.* 1988;60:91–97.

29. Gilson AJ, Sahn SA. Reactivation of bleomycin lung toxicity following oxygen administration: a second response to corticosteroids. *Chest.* 1985;88:304–306.

30. Ingrassia 3rd TS, Ryu JH, Trastek VF, et al. Oxygen-exacerbated bleomycin pulmonary toxicity. *Mayo Clin Proc.* 1991;66:173–178.

31. Mathes DD. Bleomycin and hyperoxia exposure in the operating room. *Anesth Analg.* 1995;81:624–629.

32. Wilczynski SW, Erasmus JJ, Petros WP, et al. Delayed pulmonary toxicity syndrome following high-dose chemotherapy and bone marrow transplantation for breast cancer. *Am J Respir Crit Care Med.* 1998;157:565–573.

33. Cannon GW. Methotrexate pulmonary toxicity. *Rheum Dis Clin North Am.* 1997;23:917–937.

34. Imokawa S, Colby TV, Leslie KO, et al. Methotrexate pneumonitis: review of the literature and histopathological findings in nine patients. *Eur Respir J.* 2000;15:373–381.

35. Chap L, Shpiner R, Levine M, et al. Pulmonary toxicity of high-dose chemotherapy for breast cancer: a non-invasive approach to diagnosis and treatment. *Bone Marrow Transplant.* 1997;20:1063–1067.

36. Vansteenkiste JF, Vandebroek JE, Nackaerts KL, et al. Clinical-benefit response in advanced non-small-cell lung cancer: a multicentre prospective randomised phase III study of single agent gemcitabine versus cisplatin-vindesine. *Ann Oncol.* 2001;12:1221–1230.

37. Kouroussis C, Mavroudis D, Kakolyris S, et al. High incidence of pulmonary toxicity of weekly docetaxel and gemcitabine in patients with non-small cell lung cancer: results of a dose-finding study. *Lung Cancer.* 2004;44:363–368.

38. Belknap SM, Kuzel TM, Yarnold PR, et al. Clinical features and correlates of gemcitabine-associated lung injury: findings from the RADAR project. *Cancer.* 2006;106:2051–2057.

39. Stoica GS, Greenberg HE, Rossoff LJ. Corticosteroid responsive fludarabine pulmonary toxicity. *Am J Clin Oncol.* 2002;25:340–341.

40. Helman Jr DL, Byrd JC, Ales NC, et al. Fludarabine-related pulmonary toxicity: a distinct clinical entity in chronic lymphoproliferative syndromes. *Chest.* 2002;122:785–790.

41. Weaver CH, Appelbaum FR, Petersen FB, et al. High-dose cyclophosphamide, carmustine, and etoposide followed by autologous bone marrow transplantation in patients with lymphoid malignancies who have received dose-limiting radiation therapy. *J Clin Oncol.* 1993;11:1329–1335.

42. O'Driscoll BR, Kalra S, Gattamaneni HR, et al. Late carmustine lung fibrosis: age at treatment may influence severity and survival. *Chest.* 1995;107:1355–1357.

43. O'Driscoll BR, Hasleton PS, Taylor PM, et al. Active lung fibrosis up to 17 years after chemotherapy with carmustine (BCNU) in childhood. *N Engl J Med.* 1990;323:378–382.

44. Block M, Lachowiez RM, Rios C, et al. Pulmonary fibrosis associated with low-dose adjuvant methyl-CCNU. *Med Pediatr Oncol.* 1990;18:256–260.

45. Nelson DF, Diener-West M, Weinstein AS, et al. A randomized comparison of misonidazole sensitized radiotherapy plus BCNU and radiotherapy plus BCNU for treatment of malignant glioma after surgery: final report of an RTOG study. *Int J Radiat Oncol Biol Phys.* 1986;12:1793–1800.

46. Twohig KJ, Matthay RA. Pulmonary effects of cytotoxic agents other than bleomycin. *Clin Chest Med.* 1990;11:31–54.

47. Malik SW, Myers JL, DeRemee RA, et al. Lung toxicity associated with cyclophosphamide use: two distinct patterns. *Am J Respir Crit Care Med.* 1996;154:1851–1856.

48. Spector JI, Zimbler H, Ross JS. Early-onset cyclophosphamide-induced interstitial pneumonitis. *JAMA.* 1979;242:2852–2854.

49. Kris MG, Pablo D, Gralla RJ, et al. Dyspnea following vinblastine or vindesine administration in patients receiving mitomycin plus vinca alkaloid combination therapy. *Cancer Treat Rep.* 1984;68:1029–1031.

50. Rivera MP, Kris MG, Gralla RJ, et al. Syndrome of acute dyspnea related to combined mitomycin plus vinca alkaloid chemotherapy. *Am J Clin Oncol.* 1995;18:245–250.

51. Castro M, Veeder MH, Mailliard JA, et al. A prospective study of pulmonary function in patients receiving mitomycin. *Chest.* 1996;109:939–944.

52. Stover DE, Kaner RJ. Pulmonary complications in cancer patients. *CA Cancer J Clin.* 1996;46:303–320.

53. Chang AY, Kuebler JP, Pandya KJ, et al. Pulmonary toxicity induced by mitomycin C is highly responsive to glucocorticoids. *Cancer.* 1986;57:2285–2290.

54. Maurer LH, Herndon 2nd JE, Hollis DR, et al. Randomized trial of chemotherapy and radiation therapy with or without warfarin for limited-stage small-cell lung cancer: a cancer and leukemia group B study. *J Clin Oncol.* 1997;15:3378–3387.

55. Lebeau B, Urban T, Brechot JM, et al. A randomized clinical trial comparing concurrent and alternating thoracic irradiation for patients with limited small cell lung carcinoma: "petites cellules" group. *Cancer.* 1999;86:1480–1487.

56. Chen YM, Shih JF, Perng RP, et al. A randomized trial of different docetaxel schedules in non-small cell lung cancer patients who failed previous platinum-based chemotherapy. *Chest.* 2006;129:1031–1038.

57. Dincbas FO, Atalar B, Koca S. Two-dimensional radiotherapy and docetaxel in treatment of stage III non-small cell lung carcinoma: no good survival due to radiation pneumonitis. *Lung Cancer.* 2004;43:241–242.

58. Friedlander PA, Bansal R, Schwartz L, et al. Gemcitabine-related radiation recall preferentially involves internal tissue and organs. *Cancer.* 2004;100:1793–1799.

59. Burstein HJ, Bellon JR, Galper S, et al. Prospective evaluation of concurrent paclitaxel and radiation therapy after adjuvant doxorubicin and cyclophosphamide chemotherapy for stage II or III breast cancer. *Int J Radiat Oncol Biol Phys.* 2006;64:496–504. Epub 2005 Oct 21.

60. van Zandwijk N, Groen HJ, Postmus PE, et al. Role of recombinant interferon-gamma maintenance in responding patients with small cell lung cancer: a randomised phase III study of the EORTC Lung Cancer Cooperative Group. *Eur J Cancer.* 1997;33:1759–1766.

61. Bradley JD, Scott CB, Paris KJ, et al. A phase III comparison of radiation therapy with or without recombinant beta-interferon for poor-risk patients with locally advanced non-small-cell lung cancer (RTOG 93–04). *Int J Radiat Oncol Biol Phys.* 2002;52:1173–1179.

62. Onozawa M, Hashino S, Sogabe S, et al. Side effects and good effects from new chemotherapeutic agents, case 2: thalidomide-induced interstitial pneumonitis. *J Clin Oncol.* 2005;23:2425–2426.

63. Lin JT, Yeh KT, Fang HY, et al. Fulminant, but reversible interstitial pneumonitis associated with imatinib mesylate. *Leuk Lymphoma.* 2006;47:1693–1695.

64. Endo M, Johkoh T, Kimura K, et al. Imaging of gefitinib-related interstitial lung disease: multi-institutional analysis by the West Japan Thoracic Oncology Group. *Lung Cancer.* 2006;52:135–140. Epub 2006 Mar 29.

65. Leon RJ, Gonsalvo A, Salas R, et al. Rituximab-induced acute pulmonary fibrosis. *Mayo Clin Proc.* 2004;79:949, 953.

66. Herbst RS. Toxicities of antiangiogenic therapy in non-small-cell lung cancer. *Clin Lung Cancer.* 2006;8(suppl 1):S23–S30.

67. Ernst A, Feller-Kopman D, Becker HD, et al. Central airway obstruction. *Am J Respir Crit Care Med.* 2004;169:1278–1297.

68. Rafanan AL, Mehta AC. Role of bronchoscopy in lung cancer. *Semin Respir Crit Care Med.* 2000;21:405–420.

69. Wahidi MM, Herth FJ, Ernst A. State of the art: interventional pulmonology. *Chest.* 2007;131:261–274.

70. Chhajed PN, Baty F, Pless M, et al. Outcome of treated advanced non-small cell lung cancer with and without central airway obstruction. *Chest.* 2006;130:1803–1807.

71. Miyazawa T, Miyazu Y, Iwamoto Y, et al. Stenting at the flow-limiting segment in tracheobronchial stenosis due to lung cancer. *Am J Respir Crit Care Med.* 2004;169:1096–1102.

72. Dubey S, Powell CA. Update in lung cancer 2008. *Am J Respir Crit Care Med.* 2009;179:860–868.

73. *Common cancer types. [homepage on the Internet].* Available at: http://www.cancer.gov/cancertopics/commoncancers; May, 7. 2009.

74. Beamis Jr JF. Interventional pulmonology techniques for treating malignant large airway obstruction: an update. *Curr Opin Pulm Med.* 2005;11:292–295.

75. Seijo LM, Sterman DH. Interventional pulmonology. *N Engl J Med.* 2001;344:740–749.

76. Jeon K, Kim H, Yu CM, et al. Rigid bronchoscopic intervention in patients with respiratory failure caused by malignant central airway obstruction. *J Thorac Oncol.* 2006;1:319–323.

77. Gaissert HA, Grillo HC, Shadmehr MB, et al. Uncommon primary tracheal tumors. *Ann Thorac Surg.* 2006;82:268–272; discussion 272–3.

78. Wood DE. Management of malignant tracheobronchial obstruction. *Surg Clin North Am.* 2002;82:621–642.

79. Kiryu T, Hoshi H, Matsui E, et al. Endotracheal/endobronchial metastases: clinicopathologic study with special reference to developmental modes. *Chest.* 2001;119:768–775.

80. Shepherd MP. Endobronchial metastatic disease. *Thorax.* 1982;37:362–365.

81. Lee P, Kupeli E, Mehta AC. Therapeutic bronchoscopy in lung cancer: laser therapy, electrocautery, brachytherapy, stents, and photodynamic therapy. *Clin Chest Med.* 2002;23:241–256.

82. Dutau H, Toutblanc B, Lamb C, et al. Use of the Dumon Y-stent in the management of malignant disease involving the carina: a retrospective review of 86 patients. *Chest.* 2004;126:951–958.

83. Brodsky JB. Bronchoscopic procedures for central airway obstruction. *J Cardiothorac Vasc Anesth.* 2003;17:638–646.

84. Aboussouan LS, Stoller JK. Diagnosis and management of upper airway obstruction. *Clin Chest Med.* 1994;15:35–53.

85. Hollingsworth HM. Wheezing and stridor. *Clin Chest Med.* 1987;8:231–240.

86. Simoff MJ, Sterman DH, Ernst A, ed. *Thoracic endoscopy: advances in interventional pulmonology.* 1st ed. Malden, MA: Blackwell Publishing; 2006.

87. Collins J, Stern EJ. *Chest radiology: the essentials.* 2nd ed. Philadelphia, PA: Wolters Kluwer, Lippincott Williams & Wilkins; 2008.

88. Boiselle PM. Imaging of the large airways. *Clin Chest Med.* 2008;29:181–193.

89. Naidich DP, Webb WR, Muller NL, et al. *Computed tomography and magnetic resonance of the thorax.* 4th ed. Philadelphia, PA: Wolters Kluwer, Lippincott Williams & Wilkins; 2007.

90. Bolliger CT, Sutedja TG, Strausz J, et al. Therapeutic bronchoscopy with immediate effect: laser, electrocautery, argon plasma coagulation and stents. *Eur Respir J.* 2006;27:1258–1271.

91. Fishman AP, Elias JA, Fishman JA, et al. *Fishman's pulmonary diseases and disorders.* 4th ed. New York: The McGraw-Hill Companies; 2008.

92. Chhajed PN, Eberhardt R, Dienemann H, et al. Therapeutic bronchoscopy interventions before surgical resection of lung cancer. *Ann Thorac Surg.* 2006;81:1839–1843.

93. Finlayson GN, Brodsky JB. Anesthetic considerations for airway stenting in adult patients. *Anesthesiol Clin.* 2008;26:281–291, vi.

94. Bolliger CT, Mathur PN, Beamis JF, et al. ERS/ATS statement on interventional pulmonology. European Respiratory Society. *Eur Respir J.* 2002;19:356–373.

95. Ernst A, Silvestri GA, Johnstone D. Interventional pulmonary procedures: guidelines from the American College of Chest Physicians. *Chest.* 2003;123:1693–1717.

96. Ayers ML, Beamis Jr JF. Rigid bronchoscopy in the twenty-first century. *Clin Chest Med.* 2001;22:355–364.

97. Folch E, Mehta AC. Airway interventions in the tracheobronchial tree. *Semin Respir Crit Care Med.* 2008;29:441–452.

98. Coulter TD, Mehta AC. The heat is on: impact of endobronchial electrosurgery on the need for Nd-YAG laser photoresection. *Chest.* 2000;118:516–521.

99. Sheski FD, Mathur PN. Endobronchial electrosurgery: argon plasma coagulation and electrocautery. *Semin Respir Crit Care Med.* 2004;25:367–374.

100. Sheski FD, Mathur PN. Cryotherapy, electrocautery, and brachytherapy. *Clin Chest Med.* 1999;20:123–138.

101. Wang K-P, Mehta AC, Turner J. *Flexible bronchoscopy.* 2nd ed. Malden, MA: Blackwell Publishing; 2004.

102. Morice RC, Ece T, Ece F, Keus L. Endobronchial argon plasma coagulation for treatment of hemoptysis and neoplastic airway obstruction. *Chest.* 2001;119:781–787.

103. Mathur PN, Wolf KM, Busk MF, et al. Fiberoptic bronchoscopic cryotherapy in the management of tracheobronchial obstruction. *Chest.* 1996;110:718–723.

104. Hautmann H, Gamarra F, Pfeifer KJ, et al. Fiberoptic bronchoscopic balloon dilatation in malignant tracheobronchial disease: indications and results. *Chest.* 2001;120:43–49.

105. McArdle JR, Gildea TR, Mehta AC. Balloon bronchoplasty: its indications, benefits, and complications. *J Bronchol.* 2005;12:123–127.

106. Kennedy MP, Morice RC, Jimenez CA, et al. Treatment of bronchial airway obstruction using a rotating tip microdebrider: a case report. *J Cardiothorac Surg.* 2007;2:16.

107. Lunn WM, Bagherzadegan NM, Munjampalli SK. Initial experience with a rotating airway microdebrider. *J Bronchol.* 2008;15:91–94.

108. Colt HG, Dumon JF. Airway stents. present and future. *Clin Chest Med.* 1995;16:465–478.

109. Dumon JF. A dedicated tracheobronchial stent. *Chest.* 1990;97:328–332.

110. Dumon J, Cavaliere S, Diaz-Jimenez J, et al. Seven year experience with the Dumon prosthesis. *J Bronchol.* 1996;3:6–10.

111. Lund ME, Garland R, Ernst A. Airway stenting: applications and practice management considerations. *Chest.* 2007;131:579–587.

112. Makris D, Marquette CH. Tracheobronchial stenting and central airway replacement. *Curr Opin Pulm Med.* 2007;13:278–283.

113. Mehta AC, Dasgupta A. Airway stents. *Clin Chest Med.* 1999;20:139–151.

114. Santacruz JF, Folch E, Mehta AC. Silicone and metallic stents in interventional pulmonology. *Minerva Pneumol.* 2009;48:243–259.

115. Tyldesley S, Boyd C, Schulze K, et al. Estimating the need for radiotherapy for lung cancer: an evidence-based, epidemiologic approach. *Int J Radiat Oncol Biol Phys.* 2001;49:973–985.

116. Abratt RP, Morgan GW, Silvestri G, et al. Pulmonary complications of radiation therapy. *Clin Chest Med.* 2004;25:167–177.

117. Movsas B, Raffin TA, Epstein AH, et al. Pulmonary radiation injury. *Chest.* 1997;111:1061–1076.

118. Ghafoori P, Marks LB, Vujaskovic Z, et al. Radiation-induced lung injury: assessment, management, and prevention. *Oncology (Williston Park).* 2008;22:37–47.

119. Spiro SG, Douse J, Read C, et al. Complications of lung cancer treatment. *Semin Respir Crit Care Med.* 2008;29:302–317.

120. Yahalom J, Portlock CS. Long-term cardiac and pulmonary complications of cancer therapy. *Hematol Oncol Clin North Am.* 2008;22:305–318.

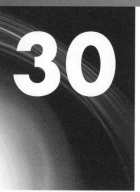

30 Malignant bowel obstruction

Raimundo Correa, Carla I. Ripamonti,
Jason E. Dodge, and Alexandra M. Easson

Malignant bowel obstruction (MBO) represents a frequent complication for patients with advanced intra-abdominal malignancy. Overall, the frequency of MBO is as high as 51%[1-4] in patients with ovarian cancer, compared with 28% with colorectal malignancies.[3] This condition can also occur as the result of intra-abdominal metastatic disease due to non–intra-abdominal primaries such as melanoma and breast and lung cancer.[5]

The term *malignant bowel obstruction* can refer to any bowel obstruction caused by malignancy, and can be categorized from its time of onset as follows:

1. At the time of diagnosis of the malignancy.
2. As part of recurrent disease, sometimes associated with an end-of-life state.

The approach to management of the patient with MBO is unique to each patient. Although MBO is usually associated with advanced-stage disease when it occurs at the time of initial diagnosis, regardless of the primary site of malignancy, management generally proceeds with curative intent, and each patient should be managed according to appropriate principles/guidelines for the underlying malignancy. On the other hand, MBO as part of recurrent disease is often managed with palliative intent; in this context, different factors that will be discussed later should be considered to determine the most appropriate treatment.

For patients with recurrent disease, MBO generally occurs in a chronic and slow fashion that results in narrowing of the diameter of the small or large bowel (or both simultaneously). The obstruction can be single or may be seen at multiple levels. In autopsies performed on patients who had died secondary to ovarian malignancy, obstruction was usually found at multiple levels and in both the small and large bowel. When only one portion of bowel was affected, the small bowel was affected more often than the large bowel.[2]

The clinical presentation of MBO differs according to the primary origin of the malignancy. Colorectal cancer can present with obstructive symptoms, especially arising from the left colon; these patients are treated with curative intent in the absence of metastatic disease and are not the focus of this paper. In ovarian cancer, although bowel obstruction can be present at initial diagnosis, MBO most often represents recurrent and noncurable disease. This is also the case in advanced colorectal cancer and other intraabdominal malignancies that are discussed in this book. This occurs in patients with colorectal cancer.[6-8]

Intraperitoneal carcinomatosis represents the presence of multiple implants of metastatic disease throughout the serosal surfaces along the peritoneal cavity. This finding is frequently observed in patients with recurrent disease who present with MBO. For patients with metastatic colorectal disease, disseminated intraperitoneal carcinomatosis has a very ominous prognosis because of the lack of effective curative systemic treatment, although this may change with new chemotherapy regimens now available for this condition. For patients with recurrent ovarian cancer and carcinomatosis, the likelihood of responding to chemotherapy is greater, especially when the patient has received only one or two previous lines of chemotherapy, and the progression-free survival is at least 6 months between lines of chemotherapy. Although it is often not possible to accurately predict life expectancy in this clinical scenario, survival for these patients has been reported to be less than 6 months in the absence of anticancer therapy.[6,9] Moreover, some authors have stated that life expectancy is very poor, estimated at less than 3 months.[10,11] Patients with low-grade tumors who have pseudomyxoma peritoneii will have a longer life expectancy.[12,13] Management of patients with MBO is challenging because the clinical presentation and management options vary according to the characteristics of the underlying malignancy, which can vary widely for an individual patient.

It is important to emphasize that benign conditions such as adhesions or hernias can be responsible for intestinal obstruction, even in patients with known advanced intra-abdominal malignancy. Benign causes of obstruction need to be considered in the workup and management of patients with apparent MBO. In certain series of patients, benign causes account for 50% of obstructions in patients with known malignancy.[14–16] Benign conditions are more likely to occur in patients with colorectal malignancies than in those with gynecologic cancer.[17] However, in one study of women with gynecologic cancer who presented with intestinal obstruction, 34% had a benign condition that caused the obstruction.[18] Intussusceptions of the bowel are uncommonly seen in adults, accounting for only 1% to 5% of intestinal obstructions. Among patients older than 18 years of age, a mass at the lead point, benign or malignant, usually accounted for the intussusceptions.[19] Recent series have found 50% to 65% of malignant tumors to be the cause of intestinal intussusceptions.[20,21] Computed tomography (CT) or magnetic resonance imaging (MRI) can help identify the lead point. Surgery is necessary only if the patient has symptoms of bowel obstruction; asymptomatic intussusceptions seen incidentally on high-resolution CT imaging are more frequent than clinically apparent and do not require intervention.

This chapter reviews the pathophysiology of MBO for healthcare practitioners who manage cancer patients at risk for developing an MBO during their disease course. We discuss therapeutic options in the management of patients with MBO, including medical and surgical therapies. Finally, we conclude with a brief summary of colorectal and ovarian cancer to highlight the differences between these diseases and to explain why patients are often managed in a different manner, even though bowel obstruction may present in a similar apparent clinical manner.

DEFINITION

A multidisciplinary committee of experts met in 2004 to discuss MBO with the aim of developing randomized trials.[22] First of all, the panel included only patients with obstructions located distal to the ligament of Treitz because gastric and esophageal obstructions can generally be managed with endoscopic stenting or surgical bypass. Also, the panel included only patients with noncurable cancers presenting with MBO. The experts justified this decision based on the fact that patients with potentially curable cancer would not be suitable candidates for a clinical trial that would include randomization to noncurative treatment.[23] This chapter focuses on management of MBO in the setting of advanced metastatic recurrent disease; thus, we use the same definitions proposed by the group of experts.

MBO is defined as follows[23]:

1. Clinical evidence of a bowel obstruction (history, physical, and radiographic examination).
2. Bowel obstruction beyond the ligament of Treitz.
3. Intra-abdominal primary cancer with incurable disease; or
4. Non–intra-abdominal primary cancer with intraperitoneal disease.

PATHOPHYSIOLOGY

Bowel obstruction secondary to any malignancy usually results from insidious narrowing of the lumen of the bowel due to different mechanisms.

Traditionally, bowel obstruction is classified as mechanical or functional (Fig. 30-1). Mechanical obstructions are due to progressive narrowing of the lumen of the bowel by a tumor, either extrinsically or intrinsically. Functional obstruction results from tumor infiltration within the bowel wall involving enteric nerves, as occurs with peritoneal carcinomatosis, extensive pelvic encasement with colon cancer, or malignant involvement of the celiac plexus, which interferes with normal peristalsis. Such patients have no physical blockage of the lumen with tumor; rather, intestinal contents cannot be propelled forward because of impaired peristalsis. Patients with lung cancer may have a paraneoplastic neuropathy that causes chronic intestinal pseudo-obstruction.[24–26]

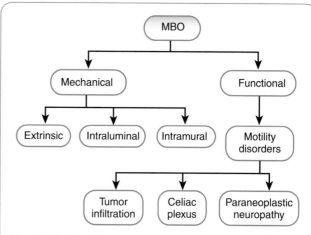

Fig. 30-1 Classification of the causes of malignant bowel obstruction.

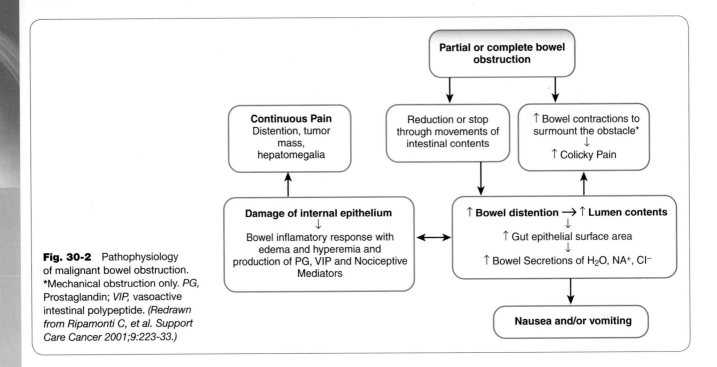

Fig. 30-2 Pathophysiology of malignant bowel obstruction. *Mechanical obstruction only. PG, Prostaglandin; VIP, vasoactive intestinal polypeptide. (Redrawn from Ripamonti C, et al. Support Care Cancer 2001;9:223-33.)*

Regardless of the initial mechanism leading to the obstruction, as soon as any portion of bowel becomes critically narrowed, diverse consequences may occur[18] (Fig. 30-2):

1. Excessive accumulation of bowel contents due to:
   a. Excessive secretion of water and sodium into the intestinal lumen (which, in turn, worsens the degree of obstruction).
   b. Decreased absorption of water and sodium from the intestinal lumen.
2. Accumulation of three types of gastrointestinal secretions (gastric, pancreatic, and biliary) within the bowel lumen, which serves as a stimulus for additional secretions proximal to the level of obstruction.
3. Bowel wall edema proximal to the level of obstruction secondary to an inflammatory response.

All these consequences worsen the degree of obstruction. This phenomenon is summarized as distention-secretion-motor activity, which results in a vicious circle of events.[24]

CLINICAL MANIFESTATIONS

MBO is initially partial rather than complete obstruction. For this reason, symptoms occur gradually and worsen slowly instead of acutely. To gain a better understanding of the symptoms related to MBO, it is very important to understand the mechanisms that contribute to obstruction.[27]

Patient history is characterized by abnormal bowel movements in terms of the physical characteristics of stools (i.e., diarrhea, loose stools, or small solid fragments) and decreasing frequency of evacuation. As soon as the bowel becomes critically narrowed, but not necessarily completely obstructed, bowel movements become irregular, and the patient experiences abdominal pain (persistent or colicky in nature), abdominal distention, nausea, and vomiting.[27] At the same time, the affected bowel segment becomes progressively distended secondary to accumulation of intestinal contents resulting from mechanical obstruction and related to irregularity in bowel peristalsis, which itself may lead to colicky abdominal pain.

As the bowel wall becomes edematous, patients feel persistent nausea. The severity of this feeling varies with the level of obstruction and the amount of fluid retained. Vomiting occurs upon buildup of fluids within the stomach.

Table 30-1 compares the symptoms typically experienced with small and large MBO.[18,28]

Table 30-1 Clinical symptoms that suggest the site of the malignant bowel obstruction (MBO)

Symptom	Small-bowel obstruction (SBO)	Large-bowel obstruction (LBO)
Vomiting		
Amount	Frequent	Infrequent
Character	Watery, bilious	Malodorous, feculent
Timing	May be feculent if longstanding	Later, usually hours after oral intake
	Early, usually within an hour after oral intake	
Pain		
Timing	Early onset	Late onset
Location	Periumbilical	Localized
Character	Cramps occasionally	Cramps frequently
Abdominal distention	Occasional	Frequent
Anorexia	Frequent	Occasional

DIAGNOSIS

HISTORY AND PHYSICAL EXAMINATION

A complete history and a thorough physical examination are mandatory before any radiographic investigation is ordered. Table 30-2 summarizes key questions in the assessment.

Investigations

A diagnosis usually is suspected clinically and is confirmed using various imaging modalities.

Plain X-rays of the abdomen are the easiest and cheapest way to confirm the diagnosis and are readily available. Radiographs show the presence or absence of dilated bowel loops, air fluid levels, gas in the rectum, and free air (if a perforation is suspected). However, plain abdominal radiographs do not distinguish an ileus from a bowel obstruction with any degree of sensitivity, and they cannot determine the exact location of the obstruction or whether multiple levels of obstruction coexist (Fig. 30-3).

Computed tomography (CT) scans are more useful and better demonstrate the site, severity, and number of obstructions; the extent of cancer; and whether or not the patient has ascites (Fig. 30-4, *A* through *F*). The sensitivity of CT scans in the diagnosis of small-bowel obstruction is between 81% and 94%, and specificity is 94%.[29–32] Diagnostic accuracy is greater with a complete obstruction, in which often a definite transition point is visualized, proximal bowel loops are dilated, and distal bowel is collapsed.[33]

Magnetic resonance imaging (MRI) has also been used to image the abdomen.[34] Gadolinium-enhanced MRI is useful in distinguishing benign from malignant bowel obstruction in a patient with a previous history of malignancy.[35] One prospective study compared the accuracy of MRI and helical CT scans for determining the cause of bowel obstruction (benign vs. malignant). Sensitivity and specificity reported for MRI were 95% and 100%, respectively, compared with 71% and 71% for CT scans.[36] In general practice, however, MRI is not the usual imaging modality for these patients.

Table 30-2 Key questions as part of the clinical history at the time of assessment in a patient who presents with diagnosis suggestive of malignant bowel obstruction (MBO)

Symptoms

A. Pain: location, intensity, nature (colicky vs. continuous), previous use of pain medications.

B. Nausea/vomiting: aspect (watery, bilious, malodor), quantity, duration/progression, timing of onset since last intake.

C. Anorexia: history of weight loss, appetite.

D. Other: concurrent use of opioids (r/o constipation); previous history of MBO.

Signs

A. Vital signs: Are they acutely ill?

B. Abdominal examination: distention, peritonitis, hernias, scars, bowel sounds.

Disease characteristics

A. Determine primary origin and histology of tumor.

B. Determine time between diagnosis and presentation of the obstruction.

Treatment

A. History of previous treatments, including numbers and types of previous surgeries, lines of chemotherapy and drugs used in each line, previous radiation and the location if any.

B. Ask what the patient understands about estimated life expectancy and further anticancer therapy.

C. Elicit patient goals.

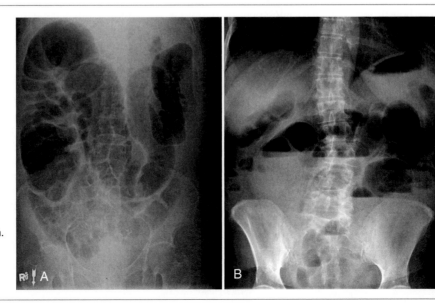

Fig. 30-3 Plain film of the abdomen. **A,** Dilated loops of small and large bowel are clearly evident, suggesting that the bowel is obstructed. **B,** Air-fluids levels.

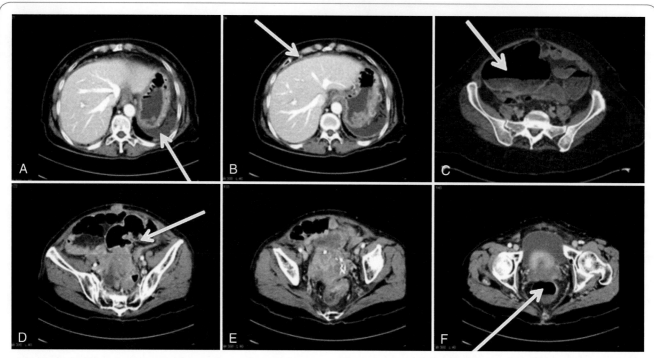

Fig. 30-4   Computed tomography (CT) scan of the abdomen and pelvis in a 50-year-old woman who had a history of metastatic ovarian cancer and presented with malignant large-bowel obstruction. **A,** Ascites. **B,** Signs of intraperitoneal carcinomatosis. **C,** Diameter of the cecum. **D** through **F,** Different planes where the obstruction was located: dilated proximal segment **(D)**, transition point does not show the presence of gas **(E)**, distal segment with the presence of gas and normal bowel wall appearance **(F)**. Usually, obstruction is partial; therefore, gas can often be seen in the distal colon.

Contrast-enhanced studies can be done transorally or per rectum and may distinguish between functional (dysmotility) and mechanical causes of obstruction (intrinsic lesion/extrinsic compression). They also determine the length of the affected bowel segment and the luminal characteristics of the lesion. Water-soluble contrast, such as gastrografin (diatrizoate meglumine), is preferable to barium because of its lower risk for impaction and association with reduced luminal edema compared with barium.[27] Barium is associated with higher risk of complications with aspiration and may be retained longer within the bowel, thus delaying endoscopic or fluoroscopic procedures.[18] Transrectal contrast imaging is critical when a distant large-bowel obstruction is suspected and a colorectal stent is being considered. Also, when the role of surgery in the management of small-bowel obstruction (SBO) is considered, transrectal investigations rule out distal concurrent large-bowel obstruction (LBO), thus perhaps avoiding an unsuccessful procedure. However, high-quality CT imaging, usually with oral and/or transrectal contrast, will provide the same information without the need for these tests.[37]

Figure 30-5 shows different radiologic procedures for the diagnosis and treatment of malignant large-bowel obstruction (MLBO).

TREATMENT

One problem when most previous reports regarding the treatment of MBO are considered is the fact that multiple definitions of success may be used, including survival,[38–45] ability to tolerate oral intake,[9,46–52] or rate of reobstruction.[39,40,44,50,53–55] Infrequently is quality of life and/or quality of death included in outcomes.[28] One article addressed quality of life in patients with MBO.[56] Selby et al. used the Edmonton Symptom Assessment Scale (ESAS) (an assessment tool validated in many languages)[57] and the Rochester Symptom Checklist (RSCL)[58] to assess the impact of treatment. This study evaluated symptoms at the time of diagnosis and 1 week, 1 month, and 3 months after initial assessment. Although this study has some limitations (such as the fact that treatment was not uniform among patients, patients with gynecologic malignancies were not included, only fluent English speakers were allowed to take part in the study, and not all patients were able to answer the questionnaire at the time of admission because of severe symptoms), it is the first study to evaluate quality-of-life issues prospectively in patients with MBO. The authors concluded that therapy had a positive outcome in the following areas: physical, psychological, and quality of life, 1 week and 1 month after initiation of treatment. However, at 3 months, the psychological component was not improved because of patient anxiety about the future. As per the authors, physical activity was not improved because the disease continued in its course, resulting in a progressive decline despite successful management of the MBO.[56]

CONSERVATIVE (BEST SUPPORTIVE CARE)

Historically, surgery was the treatment of choice for patients with MBO. If surgical intervention was not feasible, the patient's last days of life were spent in bed with a nasogastric

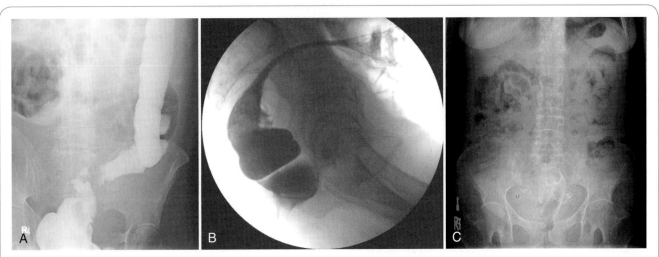

Fig. 30-5 Different radiologic techniques for the diagnosis and management of malignant large-bowel obstruction. **A,** Water-soluble contrast enema shows an obstruction at the level of the rectosigmoid junction. **B,** Fluoroscopic-guidance insertion of a colorectal stent demonstrating the passage of contrast through the stent. **C,** Plain radiography of the abdomen in a patient with metastatic ovarian cancer who presented with MBO and underwent colorectal stent insertion. Stent has deployed adequately and is located in the correct position.

(NG) tube in place. In 1985, a seminal report involving 40 patients described an effective but aggressive medical management approach to MBO as an alternative to surgery for patients who were not fit enough for surgery. Only 2 of 40 patients were managed using a surgical approach. For the remaining 38 patients, a combination of medications, including morphine, loperamide, atropine, hyoscine, prochlorperazine, chlorpromazine, and haloperidol was used as an alternative to surgery; this combination successfully relieved symptoms without the need for an NG tube.[10] Since that time, literature reports have supported the successful medical management of symptoms in MBO.[24,59–63]

Because MBO generally presents in chronic or subacute fashion rather than in an acute situation, and with partial rather than complete obstruction, when these patients require admission into a hospital and do not require emergency surgery (e.g., clinical and laboratory signs of peritonitis, acute onset of symptoms, cecum diameter ≥8 cm), they usually can be managed first by supportive care focused on symptom management.[27] If after 48 to 72 hours, a patient does not improve, then the individual should be reassessed, and a decision made as to whether surgery or a fluoroscopic/endoscopic procedure is feasible and appropriate. Supportive care includes both nonpharmacologic and pharmacologic therapies (Table 30-3, Boxes 30-1 and 30-2).

NONPHARMACOLOGIC TREATMENT

Fluid restriction, intravenous or subcutaneous hydration, and the use of gastric and proximal small-bowel decompression with an NG tube are the most common interventions.

Oral intake restriction

Because most patients are intolerant of oral intake and have been vomiting before they were hospitalized, it is imperative to address fluid and electrolyte imbalances and fluid resuscitation with appropriate volume and electrolytes given intravenously or subcutaneously. Fluid administration should be monitored carefully because overhydration increases bowel secretions and subsequently worsens symptoms.

Nasogastric tubes

NG suction is most useful for patients who have a small-bowel obstruction and are vomiting profusely and persistently. NG tubes were first described in 1978 for diagnostic and therapeutic purposes, as a means of decompressing the bowel and/or stomach perioperatively, or in the setting of an inoperable intestinal obstruction.[64] Unfortunately, when NG tubes are used for long periods of time, patients experience significant complications and discomfort as the result of restricted physical activity and poor tolerance. Long-term NG tube use is associated with aspiration, alar necrosis, hemorrhage, erosion, and respiratory infection.[65] Therefore, these tubes should be used transiently and selectively in appropriate patients with MBO.

Nutritional considerations

Malignancy will influence patients' nutritional status[66] as the result of the disease or cancer-related treatments. Nutritional status is further impaired in MBO by decreased oral intake, which adversely affects the course of disease[67] and the prognosis.[68–70]

Cachexia is a catabolic metabolic state commonly seen in advanced cancer; cachectic patients are unable to benefit from nutrition and continue to catabolize muscle, protein, and fat. Cachexia is associated with a state of inflammation as measured by increased C-reactive protein, hypercatabolism, and hormonal alterations (high cortisol). Specific cytokines produced by the patient and the tumor are responsible for cachexia. No universal consensus is evident in the literature regarding how best to diagnose cachexia. However, it is important to try to distinguish cachexia from malnutrition due to inadequate oral intake from MBO. Cachexia is not reversed by supplementing nutritional intake and represents an irreversible process; therefore interventions to improve oral intake

Table 30-3   **Steps in the assessment and management of a patient presenting with malignant bowel obstruction**

INITIAL assessment by healthcare provider (ideally a multidisciplinary team).

INVESTIGATIONS:

1. Plain films of the abdomen and/or CT scan/MRI of the abdomen and pelvis within the first 24 hours of admission to confirm the diagnosis and determine the site(s) of obstruction. If malignant LBO suspected, rectal contrast might be considered.

2. CBC, electrolytes, and albumin to determine the acuity of illness: evidence of peritonitis, electrolyte imbalance due to vomiting, and nutritional status.

DURING THE FIRST 48 TO 72 HOURS:

BEST SUPPORTIVE CARE
MEDICAL MANAGEMENT
A. Nonpharmacologic treatment

   1. NPO and intravenous hydration, with correction of electrolyte abnormalities.

   2. Nasogastric tube only if patient is vomiting significantly and/or with severe abdominal distention.

B. Pharmacologic treatment

Pain Medications

   1. *Pain management according to WHO ladder recommendations.[13,14]

Antisecretory Drugs

   1. *Octreotide 0.1 to 0.9 mg/day SC every 8 hours or intravenous infusion.

   2. *Dexamethasone 4 to 8 mg SC/IV every 24 hours.[15]

Antiemetic Drugs

   1. *Metoclopramide 10 mg IV every 6 hours if partial obstruction and no colicky pain.

   2. Prochlorperazine 25 mg per rectum every 8 hours.

   3. *Haloperidol 5 to 15 mg/day SC/IV (every 4 hours), especially in the context of complete bowel obstruction.

   4. Methotrimeprazine 6.25 to 50 mg/day SC (every 8 hours).

   5. Chlorpromazine 50 to 100 mg every 8 hours per rectum/IM.

Anticholinergic Drugs

   1. Hyoscine butylbromide 40 to 120 mg/day SC/IV (every 6 hours).

   2. Hyoscine hydrobromide 0.8 to 2.0 mg/day SC (every 4 hours).

   3. Glycopyrrolate 0.1 to 0.2 mg 3 times daily SC/IV (every 4 hours).

Antihistaminic Drugs

   1. Cyclizine 100 to 150 mg/day SC (every 8 hours) or 50 mg every 8 hours per rectum.

   2. Dimenhydrinate 50 to 100 mg SC as needed.

ASSESS THE FEASIBILITY OF AN INTERVENTIONAL PROCEDURE (SURGICAL vs. FLUOROSCOPIC/ENDOSCOPIC)

1. Surgical decision making:

   a. Identify the site and location of the obstruction (single vs. multiple, partial vs. complete).

   b. Determine whether an intervention will relieve the obstruction in the context of the patient's illness.

     i. Endoscopic/fluoroscopic procedures.

     ii. Open laparotomy.

     iii. Risk of complications.

   c. Formulate recommendations: no obligation to offer futile treatments.

2. Patient factors:

   a. Age: biological/physiological.

   b. Performance status.

   c. Stage of the cancer: previous treatments, available anticancer treatments if unobstructed.

   d. Malnutrition/cachexia.

   e. Concurrent illness.

   f. Ascites.

   g. Patient values and preferences.

3. Decision making with patient and family:

   a. What do they understand of their disease?

   b. What do they expect from the intervention?

   c. Are the risks worth the potential benefits?

   d. Does this procedure fit with the patient's goals of care?

If no interventional/surgical procedure is performed, continue with aggressive medical management with the goal of removing the nasogastric tube as soon as possible.

*Medications most commonly used.

will not be helpful. In advanced cancer patients, cachexia, MBO, and poor nutritional status are often seen together.[71]

The European Society for Clinical Nutrition and Metabolism (ESPEN) has defined severe malnutrition as the presence of at least one of the following risk factors: weight loss ≥10% to 15% within 7 months; body mass index (BMI) ≤18 kg/m^2, and serum albumin ≤30 g/L (without evidence of renal and/or liver dysfunction).[72]

The use of parenteral nutrition (PN) in advanced cancer remains controversial. Recent guidelines put forth by ESPEN were published for patients with cancer who will undergo surgery[72] and for patients with cancer who will not undergo a surgical intervention.[73] For those who meet the ESPEN definition of severe malnutrition or undernourished (BMI <18.5 to 22 kg/m^2, depending on age), in whom surgery is planned, and who cannot be fed enterally, the Society recommended starting PN 7 to 10 days preoperatively to decrease the rate of postoperative infection, length of stay in hospital, and postoperative mortality. Postoperative PN is indicated for malnourished patients who require emergency surgery.[72]

For those patients with advanced cancer and poor nutritional status who do not require surgery, PN is ineffective if the cause of the poor nutritional status does not reside in the gastrointestinal tract. Also, PN does not have a role as a supplement for patients who are receiving chemotherapy, radiation treatment, or both, or for those who are able to take oral or enteral nutrition adequately.[73]

One recently published study evaluated the effectiveness of a home PN program in 38 patients with advanced malignant disease. The most common indication for home PN in this group was MBO. Patients on PN with a Karnofsky performance status ≥50 had longer survival compared with patients who had a score of <50 at the time of PN.[74] Therefore, PN may have a role in selected patients with MBO for whom some improvement in quality of life and extension of life may be expected.

PHARMACOLOGIC TREATMENT

Although it is not possible to predict an individual patient's response, early and aggressive pharmacologic management focused on controlling symptoms benefits most patients.[75,76] Table 30-3 summarizes various drugs that are effective in the management of MBO.[24]

Pain management

The most accepted approach for optimal treatment of pain is to follow the World Health Organization (WHO) pain ladder.[77–79] In most patients with MBO, the use of opioids is necessary to control continuous and/or colicky pain. Intravenous, subcutaneous, and transdermal routes are preferred. If pain is not well controlled with adequate opioids, anticholinergics such as scopolamine can be added,[17] particularly for patients with severe colicky pain.

Nausea and vomiting

Nausea and vomiting are managed by drugs that decrease gastrointestinal (GI) secretions (antisecretory drugs, anticholinergics, and steroids) or that act at the level of the central nervous system (dopamine antagonists).[24,27]

OCTREOTIDE

Octreotide, a synthetic somatostatin-analog, has been widely used in patients with MBO.[63,75,80,81] Octreotide is administered through a continuous (subcutaneous or intravenous) infusion or by subcutaneous boluses. First described in the management of MBO in 1993,[80] this drug acts within the intestinal epithelium to decrease the secretion of sodium, water, and chloride and, at the same time, to increase the absorption of water and electrolytes. It also decreases splanchnic blood flow.[81]

Octreotide has been used successfully for patients with MBO. In a recent case report, for example, a 60-year-old man with MBO secondary to disseminated pancreatic cancer was treated with octreotide. Multiple levels of small bowel were obstructed on CT scan on admission to hospital associated with small-bowel edema. Ten days later, the edema had disappeared completely on repeat imaging. Clinically, he had very mild pain (2/10) and no nausea and/or vomiting.[82] Shima et al. recently demonstrated that octreotide (300 µg/day SC) decreased the amount of vomiting and improved quality of life in terminally ill patients with MBO. The overall response rate was 44% in their study.[83] Three randomized trials have compared octreotide versus hyoscine butylbromide (HB).[61,84,85] In all trials, octreotide was superior in terms of control of symptoms. Indeed, in one study, patients on octreotide had decreased gastrointestinal secretions by days 2 and 3.[61] Other authors have confirmed rapid response with treatment[86] consisting of a significant decrease in nausea and vomiting and overall symptoms in the majority of patients.[87]

Two studies involving 25 patients in total have examined the use of long-acting octreotide in patients with advanced cancer and MBO.[88,89] These studies show an acceptable response and tolerance to the drug, as well as no grade III-IV toxicities. It would be of interest to investigate low-acting octreotide in the management of MBO in the outpatient, ambulatory setting.

ANTICHOLINERGICS

Anticholinergic drugs, such as hyoscine butylbromide, hyoscine hydrobromide, and glycopyrrolate, alter neural transmission at the level of the bowel wall by inhibiting muscarinic receptors in the smooth muscle and in enteric neurons. This leads to decreased peristalsis and decreased segmental contractions.[62]

ANTIEMETICS AND PROKINETICS

Antiemetics and prokinetics are usually prescribed as part of a multidrug multimodal strategy rather than as single drugs.[6,10,60,76] Metoclopramide is the antiemetic and prokinetic drug of choice for symptomatic partial bowel obstruction. It acts at the level of acetylcholine and dopamine receptors, stimulating peristalsis. It is contraindicated in patients with complete bowel obstruction and in those with significant colic.[17,27,90]

Antiemetics such as prochlorperazine and chlorpromazine, part of the phenothiazine family, are used in MBO to reduce nausea and vomiting.[10] They act centrally as dopamine antagonists. Prochlorperazine is less sedative but has more extrapyramidal effects compared with chlorpromazine. Another dopamine antagonist, haloperidol, is commonly used and is a good option when obstruction is complete.[27] This drug serves as a potent suppressor of chemoreceptor trigger zone activation by blocking the D_2 (dopamine) receptor family.

Serotonin (5-HT$_3$) receptors play a role in chemotherapy-induced nausea and vomiting. They are present in the chemotherapy trigger zone and distally at the level of the peripheral afferent vagal neurons. Ondansetron and granisetron are widely used to prevent nausea and vomiting in patients receiving chemotherapy.[91] Constipation is a side effect with 5-HT$_3$ receptor antagonists, especially when used for prolonged periods of time; in fact, one study reported 2 episodes of bowel obstruction in a patient who took ondansetron 8 mg daily over 14 and 5 days, respectively.[92] The authors do not recommend the routine use of 5-HT$_3$ antagonists for patients with MBO.

CORTICOSTEROIDS

Corticosteroids are used for their antiinflammatory effects. No consensus has been reached as to which corticosteroid is most effective; dexamethasone and methylprednisolone are most commonly used. A systematic review found a trend toward reduction in symptoms in the steroid-treated group compared with placebo. No differences in mortality were observed between those treated with steroids and those not treated. Of note, all patients who participated in these trials were considered inoperable before entry into the study and received steroids for a short period of time—no longer than 5 days.[93]

Laval et al. described a three-step protocol for the treatment of MBO in those deemed inoperable.[60] Patients initially received symptomatic management for 5 days, including IV fluids, antisecretory drugs, antiemetics, corticosteroids, and analgesics ± NG tube, excluding octreotide (step I). If symptoms persisted, corticosteroids were discontinued and octreotide was added (step II). If after 3 additional days, patients were still vomiting, octreotide was stopped and the decision was made to proceed with a definitive procedure (surgical or fluoroscopic/endoscopic stenting or PEC) (step III). Using this simple scheme, the authors were able to relieve symptoms in 67% with use of step I only. Although this protocol is easy to follow, controversy continues regarding whether or not octreotide should be included as part of step I. The authors commented that the cost/benefit ratio of routinely using octreotide needs to be assessed.[60] It is the opinion of the authors that because the goal of treatment is to improve quality of life in patients with a short life expectancy, and because evidence indicates that early use of octreotide provides significant symptom benefit, octreotide should be part of the initial medical management despite its cost.

OTHER DRUGS

Proton pump inhibitors (PPIs) and histamine receptor antagonists have also been reported in the management of MBO. A recent meta-analysis, based on seven randomized controlled trials involving 445 patients, compared the effectiveness of histamine-2 receptor antagonists and PPIs in reducing gastric secretions in MBO.[94] Both classes of drugs were able to reduce gastric secretions, and between them, ranitidine appeared to be the most potent.[94] Based on this report, we cannot make recommendations, but our findings may provide another means to manage MBO symptoms and may reveal something that needs further investigation.

INTERVENTIONAL PROCEDURES

If significant clinical improvement is seen after 72 hours of medical management for MBO, patients can often be managed by continuing and potentially tapering the medicines, including octreotide. On the other hand, if patients have not improved after this period of time, the option to decompress the bowel should be considered.

Historically, surgery has been the modality of choice to manage the symptoms of MBO. Surgical options include diversion (ileostomy or colostomy), bowel resection with primary anastomoses, or intestinal bypass. Table 30-4 lists different factors related to the underlying disease and to the individual patient, which will have an impact in a positive or negative way on the course of the disease. It is imperative to consider the options before making a final decision with regard to surgical management. When it is considered that patients with MBO are in the late stages of their illness, and when it is noted that surgery is associated with high morbidity and mortality, it is extremely important to evaluate carefully each patient and to consider her or his wishes before making a decision for the individual patient for the purpose of achieving an adequate quality of

Table 30-4 Important factors to consider when selecting an interventional procedure for a patient with malignant bowel obstruction (MBO)

Related to the patient	Related to the disease
• Age	• Time from first diagnosis
• Nutritional status	• Primary cancer (histology)
• Performance status	• Ascites
• Comorbidities	• Distribution of disease
• Patient values and wishes	• Characteristics of obstruction
	• # of previous treatments and other options
	• Previous surgery for MBO

life. Some authors have tried to develop surgical algorithms/guidelines/recommendations for patients with MBO,[26,95,96] but there remains consensus only on the approach that management should be tailored to each individual's needs, meaning that the wishes of the patient and the goals of care for improving his or her quality of life are critically important.

Fluoroscopic/endoscopic procedures

"VENTING" GASTROSTOMY TUBES

A venting gastrostomy is a surgically placed tube that decompresses the stomach and exits through the anterior abdominal wall. Initially used to feed patients,[97–102] it is now more often used in advanced cancer patients to decompress an obstructed bowel as an alternative to abdominal surgery for patients whose symptoms require NG decompression.

This procedure is generally done under endoscopic or fluoroscopic visualization, requires intravenous conscious sedation, takes a few minutes to be done,[103] and is associated with a low complication rate. Patients are still able to take in small amounts orally; they cover the tube with their clothing. The venting gastrostomy does not carry the risk of aspiration and nasal damage of the NG tube. Because of high output in some, and to avoid electrolyte disturbance in this setting, an aggressive oral intake (fluids) has been recommended.[104] Patients (1) with significant nausea and vomiting who have a proximal small bowel or multilevel obstruction, (2) who are very ill or malnourished, and (3) who do not have anticancer treatment options or have a short life expectancy are generally considered ideal candidates for venting gastrostomy.

One study compared the endoscopic versus the fluoroscopic approach to tube placement. Endoscopy was quicker but had a lower success rate and a higher complication rate compared with fluoroscopic guidance.[105]

Extensive ascites is a relative contraindication for a venting gastrostomy tube because of leakage of ascitic fluid around the tube, which results in skin excoriations. One study in patients with severe ascites used paracentesis before insertion of the gastrostomy; this reduced the leakage.[106] However, further research involving this approach is needed to confirm the benefits.

Complications of venting gastrostomy include cutaneous infection, cellulitis, and, in a small number of individuals, necrotizing fasciitis. Drainage around the tube may be an indication of a tube lumen obstruction. Imaging the location of the tube by using contrast injected into the venting gastrostomy tube will clarify the location of the tube and will confirm whether the tube is obstructed. Replacement of the venting gastrostomy and repositioning can be done under fluoroscopy.

Table 30-5 summarizes the experiences of different authors with this technique used in the setting of MBO.

Venting jejunostomy tubes are an alternative for those patients who develop bowel obstructions.[107–109]

COLORECTAL STENTS

The use of colorectal expandable metallic stents was first described in 1991.[110] Since that time, multiple investigators have reported colorectal stent in benign and malignant disease. Most reports involve patients with colorectal cancer (Table 30-6).

Malignant large-bowel obstruction normally occurs distal to the splenic flexure, at the level of the descending colon, sigmoid colon, or rectum.[111] Patients with underlying gynecologic malignancies can have large-bowel obstruction, but this is less common than small-bowel obstruction and frequently occurs in both places at the same time. In this group, colorectal stents are used less often than in patients with colorectal malignancy.

Because of the anatomic location of colorectal cancer and the increasing availability of colonoscopy throughout the world, stenting has been used more frequently during the last few years.

It is possible to place stents endoscopically or under fluoroscopy. Although no studies have compared these techniques, success with either technique reportedly has been very high. Although having both options seems preferable,[18,112] unfortunately only a few centers have the capability of doing both.

Colonoscopy has the capability of reaching the obstructing lesion with greater ease compared with fluoroscopy, but it has the disadvantage of being unable to see the proximal end of the obstructed segment. Fluoroscopy, when the obstruction is located in the sigmoid colon or rectum, has the advantage of visualizing the obstruction completely during insertion. If the procedure is successful, patients will note passing gas and bowel movements soon afterward. Although not used routinely, some recommend a plain abdominal X-ray 1 day after the procedure to confirm whether the stent is deployed properly, and to rule out stent migration (Fig. 30-6).

Colorectal stents are used in two clinical situations. The first involves patients who present with an acute left-sided colonic obstruction at the time of initial diagnosis. We will not discuss this scenario because it goes beyond the scope of this chapter on MBO in patients with recurrent (i.e., incurable) disease. This approach, however, allows relief of obstruction and time to prepare the patient for surgery without the need to do emergency surgery. A one-stage rather than two-stage surgical approach is possible in this situation if decompression is successful.

The second approach is to stent the bowel obstruction late in the course of disease, after multiple lines of chemotherapy and radiation treatment, and when surgery is not an option. This situation is very common in women with gynecologic malignancies. Three reports have been published on women with ovarian cancer[113–115]; 37 patients in total were included. The biggest series involved 35 patients and reported a technical success rate of 78%.[113] These were highly selected individuals, and so the response rate may be biased and inflated.

Although not well documented, extrinsic lesions seem to be more difficult to stent compared with intrinsic lesions. Obstructions due to colonic primary malignancies are concentric and more localized, whereas obstructions secondary to other malignancies are often eccentric, and tumor infiltrations are usually associated with torsion. In this context, one study reported that technical success was significantly higher in patients with colorectal malignancies than in those with noncolorectal cancer.[116] This study is retrospective in nature and included only 34 patients with colorectal cancer and 25 with other malignancies. This finding has not been confirmed by other reports, for example, in patients with obstruction secondary to gynecologic cancer, as described previously.[113–115]

Complications of stenting include pain, bowel perforation, stent migration, and reobstruction.[117,118] In the biggest review reported to date, morbidity and mortality rates were 4% and 1%, respectively.[119]

Table 30-5 A review of the use of venting gastrostomy tubes in the setting of malignant bowel obstruction due to gynecologic and nongynecologic malignancies

Author	N	Technical success	Outcome	Comments
Campagnutta et al.[1]	34	32/34 (94.1%)	Symptomatic relief 84%. Median hospital stay: 7 days. No complications reported. Median survival 74 days.	25% of patients received chemotherapy after the tube was placed.
Cunningham et al.[2]	20	20/20 (100%)	Symptomatic relief 100%. Hospital stay not reported. No complications reported. Median survival 53 days.	7 patients required tube replacement for different reasons.
Pothuri et al.[3]	94	94/94 (100%)	Symptomatic relief 91%. Median hospital stay: 6 days. Complication rate 19.1%. Median survival 56 days.	29 patients received chemotherapy. Four of the 29 underwent tube removal.
Brooksbank et al.[4]	49	47/49 (95.9%)	Symptomatic relief 92%. Hospital stay not reported. No complications reported. Median survival 17 days.	Authors included 4 extra patients. They were excluded from this summary because they did undergo an open laparotomy for insertion of the gastrostomy tube.
Scheidbach et al.[5]	24	24/24 (100%)	Symptomatic relief 92%. Median hospital stay 6 days. Complication rate 25%. Median survival 147 days.	One patient presented with spontaneous tube dislodgment.
Cannizzaro et al.[6]	22	21/22 (95%)	Symptomatic relief 100%. No morbidity associated with the procedure was reported.	This study randomized patients to receive a 15 French or a 20 French tube size. No differences were seen.
Herman et al.[7]	46	41/46 (89%)	Symptomatic relief 88%. Complications 4%.	This study utilized a 28 French tube size.

[1]Campagnutta E, et al. Palliative treatment of upper intestinal obstruction by gynecological malignancy: the usefulness of percutaneous endoscopic gastrostomy. *Gynecol Oncol.* 1996;62:103–105.
[2]Cunningham MJ, et al. Percutaneous gastrostomy for decompression in patients with advanced gynecologic malignancies. *Gynecol Oncol.* 1995;59:273–276.
[3]Pothuri B, et al. Percutaneous endoscopic gastrostomy tube placement in patients with malignant bowel obstruction due to ovarian carcinoma. *Gynecol Oncol.* 2005;96:330–334.
[4]Brooksbank MA, Game PA, Ashby MA. Palliative venting gastrostomy in malignant intestinal obstruction. *Palliat Med.* 2002;16:520–526.
[5]Scheidbach H, et al. Percutaneous endoscopic gastrostomy/jejunostomy (PEG/PEJ) for decompression in the upper gastrointestinal tract: initial experience with palliative treatment of gastrointestinal obstruction in terminally ill patients with advanced carcinomas. *Surg Endosc.* 1999;13:1103–1105.
[6]Cannizzaro R, et al. Percutaneous endoscopic gastrostomy as a decompressive technique in bowel obstruction due to abdominal carcinomatosis. *Endoscopy.* 1995;27:317–320.
[7]Herman LL, Hoskins WJ, Shike M. Percutaneous endoscopic gastrostomy for decompression of the stomach and small bowel. *Gastrointest Endosc.* 1992;38:314–318.

Location of the obstruction is reported as an important factor to consider. Patients who present with lesions localized within the distal 5 cm above the anal verge usually complain of pressure sensation and persistent pain with stenting. To our knowledge, no definitive studies have supported this contention. On the other hand, lesions located proximal to the splenic flexure are more difficult to stent and are not reported as frequently as distant colon stenting.[117] A recent study reported the experience of stenting proximal obstructions over 5 years; 97 stenting procedures were performed, 16 proximal to the splenic flexure. Technical and clinical success rates were 94% and 87.5%, respectively.[119] Although scant data are available, the authors do not consider obstructions located proximal to the splenic flexure a contraindication per se for stenting.

One randomized, prospective trial compared colostomy versus colorectal stent in patients with unresectable obstructions or with distant metastases. Eleven patients were included in each group, and all of them had primary colorectal cancer.

No difference in mortality or morbidity was seen, although the stented group had a shorter procedure time and hospital stay compared with the surgical group. Survival and quality of life were not reported in either group.[120]

Two systematic reviews[117,118] have reviewed the evidence for stents placed as palliation or as a bridge to surgery. Technical and clinical success and mortality, migration, perforation, and reobstruction rates were similar in both groups.[117,118] In terms of clinical success, both trials reported improved outcomes in 88%. These outcomes are not comparable with those achieved by the largest gynecologic series (78%) because definitions of success differed between reports.[115,117,118]

CECOSTOMY TUBES

Cecostomy tubes have the same basic purpose as gastrostomy tubes in the management of MBO; the difference is that cecostomies are used only for decompression, not for feeding.[121] The

Table 30-6 A review of the use of colorectal stents in the setting of malignant bowel obstruction due to gynecologic and nongynecologic malignancies

Author	N	Technical success clinical success	Outcomes	Comments
Jung et al.[8]	39	39/39 (100%) 34/39 (87.5%)	Complication rate 10.2%. Median survival 11 days. Median event-free survival time 83 days.	Stents shorter than 10 cm and lesions located distal to the splenic flexure had better long-term outcomes.
Suh et al.[9]	55	54/55 (98.2%) 52/55 (94.4%)	Mean stent patency period 184 days. Complication rate 30.9%.	Stent expansion ≤70% during the first 48 hours was associated with an increase in stent occlusion.
Watson et al.[10]	107	100/107 (93%) 97/100 (97%)	Median survival time after stenting 42 days. Complication rate 9%.	All 3 patients in whom stent did not deploy had ovarian cancer. Mortality related to the procedure 1% (bowel perforation).
Caceres et al.[11]	35	27/35 (77%) 27/35 (77%)	Median survival time post procedure 7.7 months. Median hospital stay: 15 days. This long stay is explained by the fact that many of these patients received chemotherapy after the procedure was done.	Largest series including only patients with gynecologic malignancies. Median survival time for patients with unsuccessful procedure 1.9 months.
Dronamraju et al.[12]	16	15/16 (94%) 14/16 (88%)	Median survival time 9 months (subgroup for palliation). No morbidity/mortality related to the procedure was reported. Hospital stay post procedure was 1.6 days.	This trial included lesions located proximal to the splenic flexure. Five patients had the stent placed as a bridge to surgery.

[8]Jung MK, et al. Factors associated with the long-term outcome of a self-expandable colon stent used for palliation of malignant colorectal obstruction. *Surg Endosc.* 2010;24:525–530.

[9]Suh JP, et al. Effectiveness of stent placement for palliative treatment in malignant colorectal obstruction and predictive factors for stent occlusion. *Surg Endosc.* 2010;24:400–406.

[10]Watson AJ, et al. Outcomes after placement of colorectal stents. *Colorectal Dis.* 2005;7:70–73.

[11]Caceres A, et al. Colorectal stents for palliation of large-bowel obstructions in recurrent gynecologic cancer: an updated series. *Gynecol Oncol.* 2008;108:482–485.

[12]Dronamraju SS, et al. Role of self-expanding metallic stents in the management of malignant obstruction of the proximal colon. *Dis Colon Rectum.* 2009;52:1657–1661.

evidence of benefit in MBO is limited, however. Cecostomy decompresses the large bowel, but cecostomy tubes often leak and are difficult to take care of at home; they should be used only if colostomy cannot be done for technical reasons. It is common to place these tubes at the time of the laparotomy when diversion, resection, or colostomy cannot be done.

SURGICAL PROCEDURES

Surgery is an option for these patients but has high morbidity and mortality rates,* and reobstruction rates are significant.[39,50,53-55,122] Some authors believe that surgery should be considered only for patients with a life expectancy ≥2 months.[18,96,123]

Some studies reported better survival for patients who have successful surgical decompression compared with those who undergo exploration only, or who did not have surgery at all or underwent endoscopic/fluoroscopic procedures.[38,52,124,125] These studies may, however, represent less than optimal patient selection and noncomparable cohorts with different clinical and tumor characteristics. The challenge is to carefully select those patients who will truly benefit from a surgical procedure.

In 1983, Krebs and Goplerud developed a prognostic scoring system based on the following factors: age, nutritional status, tumor status (palpable masses and liver metastases), ascites, and previous radiation and/or chemotherapy treatments. These authors selected six parameters (age, nutritional status, tumor status, ascites, previous chemotherapy, and prior radiation treatment) and numerically scored each (0-1-2). They reported that 20% of patients with a total score ≥7 showed improvement of their obstruction and survived at least 8 weeks postoperatively, compared with 84% of those with a total score ≤6.[44] Performance status is another prognostic factor.[126]

The decision whether to proceed with surgery or not will depend on the extent of disease seen on imaging studies. Other factors will play a role in the decision as well. For those patients who undergo a surgical procedure, it is at the time of the laparotomy that the definite procedure will be decided.

The most common procedures are intestinal resection, intestinal bypass and creation of diverting stomas (either ileostomy or colostomy), insertion of gastric tubes, and a combination of these modalities. Based on intraoperative exploration, the surgeon will decide the most appropriate approach. In this sense, the experience of the surgeon in managing an MBO becomes critical.

*References 9, 14, 39, 41, 42, 44, 45, 47, 49, 50, 53, 54.

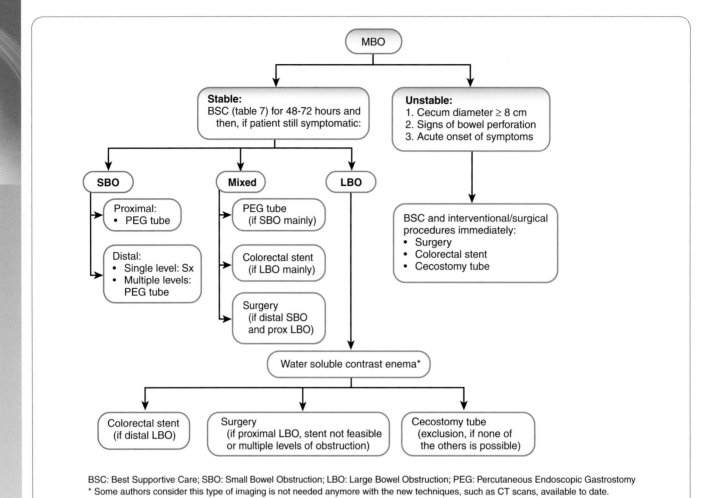

Fig. 30-6 Options for surgical vs. endoscopic/fluoroscopic treatment of malignant bowel obstruction. *BSC,* Best supportive care; *LBO,* large-bowel obstruction; *PEG,* percutaneous endoscopic gastrostomy; *SBO,* small-bowel obstruction. *Some authors believe that this type of imaging is not needed anymore with new techniques, such as computed tomography (CT) scans, available to date. *(Adapted from information in Stevenson G. Can Assoc Radiol J 2008;59:174–182.)*

Another important aspect to consider before planning surgery is the goals of care as expressed by patients. Treatment is largely palliative rather than curative, and surgeons need to consider this because colostomy/ileostomy/cecostomy affects quality of life.[127–129]

Most reports are retrospective and methods differ considerably. A systematic review to evaluate the role of surgery in management found no randomized studies; thus the evidence for benefit relies on cohort, case series, and individual patient reports. Data are inadequate to reveal in which situation(s) surgery is indicated or contraindicated. Better standardization of outcomes in prospective studies would be helpful to the clinician in determining the best approach.[11]

One prospective study involving patients with ovarian cancer included only 26 patients. The authors used no criteria. Ninety days following any intervention, half of the patients had died or had another episode of obstruction. Survival was significantly longer in the surgical group than in the endoscopic group (191 vs. 78 days).[38] This may be to the result of a selection bias. Individuals undergoing surgery may have had lower tumor burden or were better nutritionally. The small numbers also could represent a sample bias.

The role of repeat surgery in patients who have undergone prior surgery for MBO has been studied as well. Two studies, both in gynecologic cancer, involved only 19 patients in total. In both studies, successful palliation was accomplished in 30%, procedure-related morbidity was high, and overall survival was not improved.[124,126] The authors believe that in this group of patients, surgery rarely is a good option. Patients should generally be managed by endoscopic/fluoroscopic procedures whenever possible.

FURTHER RESEARCH

Many unanswered questions remain as to the diagnosis and the best management of MBO. Further research is clearly needed to elucidate answers to these questions with the objective of improving care.

In terms of diagnosis, multidetector computed tomography (MDCT) has been reported in evaluation of the whole bowel over the past few years.[130,131] One report of MDCT in patients with bowel obstruction secondary to benign or malignant conditions concluded that a combination of axial and coronal views gives optimal images.[132] If a repeat study confirms these findings, MDCT might replace contrast enemas.[133]

Regarding treatment, one of the most important issues to address is the appropriate outcomes to study for this condition. Investigators have used survival, reobstruction rates, and ability to tolerate oral intake as main outcomes. We believe that quality of life should be included as an outcome, and studies in the future must include this as part of the study outcomes.

High-quality evidence requires prospective clinical trials. Randomized trials are difficult to perform in these patients, especially in those with advanced disease for whom surgery may not be feasible.

The development of less invasive procedures using endoscopic/fluoroscopic techniques and, over time, additional improvements in technology are to be expected. Recently, spiral enteroscopy in the placement of stents for obstructions located in the small bowel distal to the ligament of Treitz has been reported.[134] This is preliminary, as only two patients were treated. If further experience demonstrates effectiveness of this procedure, it may serve as an alternative to venting gastrostomy tubes.

Chemotherapy is a potential treatment for patients with MBO as well. Available evidence for the treatment of MBO using chemotherapy is small and retrospective in nature. Chemotherapy is most effective in patients with platinum-sensitive disease.[135] Conversely, patients who have been previously treated with chemotherapy are not usually benefited by salvage chemotherapy.[136] A prospective trial using new chemotherapy regimens for colorectal and ovarian cancer might prove beneficial as an alternative to surgery, or for those patients who are not considered surgical candidates.

CONCLUSION

Malignant bowel obstruction remains a very challenging clinical complication of cancer. The primary goals are to make a correct diagnosis and to offer the more appropriate treatment to patients who, unfortunately, most of the time are facing the end of their lives, and for whom the treatment is palliative rather than curative. This is a difficult task because most of the evidence available to date is retrospective and involves only small numbers of patients with no standardized outcomes measures.

Although little evidence supports or refutes its clinical utility, we believe that a multidisciplinary assessment should be considered first in the management of each patient who presents with MBO in the setting of recurrent/incurable disease, before any attempt at surgical intervention is made (unless in emergency conditions).

Because this condition rarely presents as an emergency, there is no reason to define definitive treatment at the time of diagnosis. Best supportive care represents the first step in the management of patients with MBO for at least 48 to 72 hours (see Table 30-3). For patients who do not respond to supportive care alone, consider surgical management or fluoroscopic/endoscopic decompression, if appropriate. Choices are dependent on the likelihood of successful palliation and improved quality of life, as well as the goals of the patient and multidisciplinary care team.

Ideally, an algorithm of optimal sequences in the management of MBO would facilitate care of these patients. Because of numerous factors influencing these decisions and the lack of currently available good evidence, no single algorithm has been universally accepted.

The authors of this chapter have developed a simple algorithm that might facilitate optimal decision making regarding the role of definitive surgical or fluoroscopic/endoscopic management (see Table 30-3 and Fig. 30-6).

It is extremely important that further research be done in this area to improve management of patients with MBO, and ultimately quality of life. The fact is that most patients are facing the end of their lives, and this condition creates a lot of anxiety for patients, families, and caregivers alike. A multidisciplinary approach that includes psychosocial and spiritual care is important.

ACKNOWLEDGMENTS

Dr. Correa would like to thank Drs. Joan Murphy, Camilla Zimmermann, Gary Rodin, and Amit Oza, and the other chapter authors, for their invaluable assistance, recommendations, and clinical advice.

REFERENCES

1. Dvoretsky PM, et al. Survival time, causes of death, and tumor/treatment-related morbidity in 100 women with ovarian cancer. *Hum Pathol.* 1988;19:1273–1279.
2. Dvoretsky PM, et al. Distribution of disease at autopsy in 100 women with ovarian cancer. *Hum Pathol.* 1988;19:57–63.
3. Ripamonti C, et al. Management of bowel obstruction in advanced and terminal cancer patients. *Ann Oncol.* 1993;4:15–21.
4. Rose PG, et al. Metastatic patterns in histologic variants of ovarian cancer: an autopsy study. *Cancer.* 1989;64:1508–1513.
5. Idelevich E, et al. Small bowel obstruction caused by secondary tumors. *Surg Oncol.* 2006;15:29–32.
6. Randall TC, Rubin SC. Management of intestinal obstruction in the patient with ovarian cancer.

Oncology (Williston Park). 2000;14:1159–1163: discussion 1167–8, 1171–5.
7. Deans GT, Krukowski ZH, Irwin ST. Malignant obstruction of the left colon. *Br J Surg.* 1994;81:1270–1276.
8. Fielding LP, et al. Prediction of outcome after curative resection for large bowel cancer. *Lancet.* 1986;2:904–907.
9. Pecorelli S, Sartori E, Santin A. Follow-up after primary therapy: management of the symptomatic patient-surgery. *Gynecol Oncol.* 1994;55:S138–S142.
10. Baines M, Oliver DJ, Carter RL. Medical management of intestinal obstruction in patients with advanced malignant disease: a clinical and pathological study. *Lancet.* 1985;2:990–993.
11. Feuer DJ, et al. Systematic review of surgery in malignant bowel obstruction in advanced gynecological and gastrointestinal cancer. The

Systematic Review Steering Committee. *Gynecol Oncol.* 1999;75:313–322.
12. Krouse RS, et al. When the sun can set on an unoperated bowel obstruction: management of malignant bowel obstruction. *J Am Coll Surg.* 2002;195:117–128.
13. Averbach AM, Sugarbaker PH. Recurrent intraabdominal cancer with intestinal obstruction. *Int Surg.* 1995;80:141–146.
14. Spears H, et al. Treatment of bowel obstruction after operation for colorectal carcinoma. *Am J Surg.* 1988;155:383–386.
15. Butler JA, et al. Small bowel obstruction in patients with a prior history of cancer. *Am J Surg.* 1991;162:624–628.
16. Edna TH, Bjerkeset T. Small bowel obstruction in patients previously operated on for colorectal cancer. *Eur J Surg.* 1998;164:587–592.

17. Ripamonti C, Bruera E. Palliative management of malignant bowel obstruction. *Int J Gynecol Cancer*. 2002;12:135–143.

18. Roeland E, von Gunten CF. Current concepts in malignant bowel obstruction management. *Curr Oncol Rep*. 2009;11:298–303.

19. Marinis A, et al. Intussusception of the bowel in adults: a review. *World J Gastroenterol*. 2009;15:407–411.

20. Hanan B, et al. Intussusception in adults: a retrospective study. *Colorectal Dis*. 2010;12:574–578.

21. Wang N, et al. Adult intussusception: a retrospective review of 41 cases. *World J Gastroenterol*. 2009;15:3303–3308.

22. Krouse RS. The international conference on malignant bowel obstruction: a meeting of the minds to advance palliative care research. *J Pain Symptom Manage*. 2007;34(suppl 1):S1–S6.

23. Anthony T, et al. Report of the clinical protocol committee: development of randomized trials for malignant bowel obstruction. *J Pain Symptom Manage*. 2007;34(suppl 1):S49–S59.

24. Ripamonti C, et al. Clinical-practice recommendations for the management of bowel obstruction in patients with end-stage cancer. *Support Care Cancer*. 2001;9:223–233.

25. Roberts PF, Stebbings WS, Kennedy HJ. Granulomatous visceral neuropathy of the colon with non-small cell lung carcinoma. *Histopathology*. 1997;30:588–591.

26. Sodhi N, et al. Autonomic function and motility in intestinal pseudoobstruction caused by paraneoplastic syndrome. *Dig Dis Sci*. 1989;34:1937–1942.

27. Ripamonti CI, Easson EM, Gerdes H. Management of malignant bowel obstruction. *Eur J Cancer*. 2008;44:1105–1115.

28. Helyer L, Easson AM. Surgical approaches to malignant bowel obstruction. *J Support Oncol*. 2008;6:105–113.

29. Burkill GJ, Bell JR, Healy JC. The utility of computed tomography in acute small bowel obstruction. *Clin Radiol*. 2001;56:350–359.

30. Maglinte DD, et al. Obstruction of the small intestine: accuracy and role of CT in diagnosis. *Radiology*. 1993;188:61–64.

31. Maglinte DD, et al. Reliability and role of plain film radiography and CT in the diagnosis of small-bowel obstruction. *AJR Am J Roentgenol*. 1996;167:1451–1455.

32. Megibow AJ, et al. Bowel obstruction: evaluation with CT. *Radiology*. 1991;180:313–318.

33. Furukawa A, et al. Helical CT in the diagnosis of small bowel obstruction. *Radiographics*. 2001;21:341–355.

34. Martin DR, et al. Magnetic resonance imaging of the gastrointestinal tract. *Top Magn Reson Imaging*. 2005;16:77–98.

35. Low RN, Chen SC, Barone R. Distinguishing benign from malignant bowel obstruction in patients with malignancy: findings at MR imaging. *Radiology*. 2003;228:157–165.

36. Beall DP, et al. Imaging bowel obstruction: a comparison between fast magnetic resonance imaging and helical computed tomography. *Clin Radiol*. 2002;57:719–724.

37. Stevenson G. Colon imaging in radiology departments in 2008: goodbye to the routine double contrast barium enema. *Can Assoc Radiol J*. 2008;59:174–182.

38. Chi DS, et al. A prospective outcomes analysis of palliative procedures performed for malignant intestinal obstruction due to recurrent ovarian cancer. *Oncologist*. 2009;14:835–839.

39. Pothuri B, et al. Reoperation for palliation of recurrent malignant bowel obstruction in ovarian carcinoma. *Gynecol Oncol*. 2004;95:193–195.

40. Soo KC, et al. Intestinal obstruction in patients with gynaecological malignancies. *Ann Acad Med Singapore*. 1988;17:72–75.

41. Bais JM, et al. Intestinal obstruction in patients with advanced ovarian cancer. *Int J Gynecol Cancer*. 1995;5:346–350.

42. Castaldo TW, et al. Intestinal operations in patients with ovarian carcinoma. *Am J Obstet Gynecol*. 1981;139:80–84.

43. Jong P, Sturgeon J, Jamieson CJ. Benefit of palliative surgery for bowel obstruction in advanced ovarian cancer. *Can J Surg*. 1995;38:454–457.

44. Krebs HB, Goplerud DR. Surgical management of bowel obstruction in advanced ovarian carcinoma. *Obstet Gynecol*. 1983;61:327–330.

45. Redman CW, et al. Survival following intestinal obstruction in ovarian cancer. *Eur J Surg Oncol*. 1988;14:383–386.

46. Ely CA, Arregui ME. The use of enteral stents in colonic and gastric outlet obstruction. *Surg Endosc*. 2003;17:89–94.

47. Ellis CN, et al. Small bowel obstruction after colon resection for benign and malignant diseases. *Dis Colon Rectum*. 1991;34:367–371.

48. Katz LB, et al. Ovarian carcinoma complicated by gastric outlet obstruction. *J Surg Oncol*. 1981;18:261–264.

49. Larson JE, et al. Bowel obstruction in patients with ovarian carcinoma: analysis of prognostic factors. *Gynecol Oncol*. 1989;35:61–65.

50. Lo NN, Kee SG, Nambiar R. Palliative gastrojejunostomy for advanced carcinoma of the stomach. *Ann Acad Med Singapore*. 1991;20:356–358.

51. Nakane Y, et al. Management of intestinal obstruction after gastrectomy for carcinoma. *Br J Surg*. 1996;83:113.

52. Rubin SC, et al. Palliative surgery for intestinal obstruction in advanced ovarian cancer. *Gynecol Oncol*. 1989;34:16–19.

53. Lau PW, Lorentz TG. Results of surgery for malignant bowel obstruction in advanced, unresectable, recurrent colorectal cancer. *Dis Colon Rectum*. 1993;36:61–64.

54. Lund B, et al. Intestinal obstruction in patients with advanced carcinoma of the ovaries treated with combination chemotherapy. *Surg Gynecol Obstet*. 1989;169:213–218.

55. Solomon HJ, et al. Bowel complications in the management of ovarian cancer. *Aust N Z J Obstet Gynaecol*. 1983;23:65–68.

56. Selby D, et al. Room for improvement? A quality of life assessment in patients with malignant bowel obstruction. *Palliat Med*. 2010;24:38–45.

57. Bruera E, et al. The Edmonton Symptom Assessment System (ESAS): a simple method for the assessment of palliative care patients. *J Palliat Care*. 1991;7:6–9.

58. de Haes JC, van Knippenberg FC, Neijt JP. Measuring psychological and physical distress in cancer patients: structure and application of the Rotterdam Symptom Checklist. *Br J Cancer*. 1990;62:1034–1038.

59. Feuer DJ, Broadley KE. Corticosteroids for the resolution of malignant bowel obstruction in advanced gynaecological and gastrointestinal cancer. *Cochrane Database Syst Rev*. 2000;(2): CD001219.

60. Laval G, et al. Protocol for the treatment of malignant inoperable bowel obstruction: a prospective study of 80 cases at Grenoble University Hospital Center. *J Pain Symptom Manage*. 2006;31:502–512.

61. Ripamonti C, et al. Role of octreotide, scopolamine butylbromide, and hydration in symptom control of patients with inoperable bowel obstruction and nasogastric tubes: a prospective randomized trial. *J Pain Symptom Manage*. 2000;19:23–34.

62. Mercadante S, Casuccio A, Mangione S. Medical treatment for inoperable malignant bowel obstruction: a qualitative systematic review. *J Pain Symptom Manage*. 2007;33:217–223.

63. Mercadante S, et al. Aggressive pharmacological treatment for reversing malignant bowel obstruction. *J Pain Symptom Manage*. 2004;28:412–416.

64. Hodge J. The clinical use of the naso-gastric duodenal mercury tip sump tube in abdominal surgery and in the management of intestinal obstruction. *Ann Surg*. 1978;187:100–102.

65. Meyer L, Pothuri B. Decompressive percutaneous gastrostomy tube use in gynecologic malignancies. *Curr Treat Option Oncol*. 2006;7:111–120.

66. Dewys WD, et al. Prognostic effect of weight loss prior to chemotherapy in cancer patients. Eastern Cooperative Oncology Group. *Am J Med*. 1980;69:491–497.

67. Bozzetti F, et al. Impact of cancer, type, site, stage and treatment on the nutritional status of patients. *Ann Surg*. 1982;196:170–179.

68. Andreyev HJ, et al. Why do patients with weight loss have a worse outcome when undergoing chemotherapy for gastrointestinal malignancies? *Eur J Cancer*. 1998;34:503–509.

69. Kadar L, et al. The prognostic value of body protein in patients with lung cancer. *Ann N Y Acad Sci*. 2000;904:584–591.

70. Aviles A, et al. Malnutrition as an adverse prognostic factor in patients with diffuse large cell lymphoma. *Arch Med Res*. 1995;26:31–34.

71. Blum D, Omlin A, Fearon K, et al. Evolving classification systems for cancer cachexia: ready for clinical practice? *Support Care Cancer*. 2010;18:273–279.

72. Braga M, et al. ESPEN guidelines on parenteral nutrition: surgery. *Clin Nutr*. 2009;28:378–386.

73. Bozzetti F, et al. ESPEN guidelines on parenteral nutrition: non-surgical oncology. *Clin Nutr*. 2009;28:445–454.

74. Soo I, Gramlich L. Use of parenteral nutrition in patients with advanced cancer. *Appl Physiol Nutr Metab*. 2008;33:102–106.

75. The challenge of treating malignant bowel obstruction. *J Support Oncol*. 2006;4:83–84.

76. Weber C, Zulian GB. Malignant irreversible intestinal obstruction: the powerful association of octreotide to corticosteroids, antiemetics, and analgesics. *Am J Hosp Palliat Care*. 2009;26:84–88.

77. WHO. *Cancer pain relief*. Geneva, Switzerland: World Health Organization; 1986.

78. WHO. *Cancer pain relief*. 2nd ed. Geneva, Switzerland: World Health Organization; 1996.

79. Miguel R. Interventional treatment of cancer pain: the fourth step in the World Health Organization analgesic ladder? *Cancer Control*. 2000;7:149–156.

80. Mercadante S, et al. Octreotide in relieving gastrointestinal symptoms due to bowel obstruction. *Palliat Med*. 1993;7:295–299.

81. Ripamonti C, Mercadante S. How to use octreotide for malignant bowel obstruction. *J Support Oncol*. 2004;2:357–364.

82. Shinjo T, Kagami R. Radiological imaging change in a malignant bowel obstruction patient treated with octreotide. *Support Care Cancer*. 2009;17:753–755.

83. Shima Y, et al. Clinical efficacy and safety of octreotide (SMS201–995) in terminally ill Japanese cancer patients with malignant bowel obstruction. *Jpn J Clin Oncol*. 2008;38:354–359.

84. Mercadante S, et al. Comparison of octreotide and hyoscine butylbromide in controlling

gastrointestinal symptoms due to malignant inoperable bowel obstruction. *Support Care Cancer*. 2000;8:188–191.

85. Mystakidou K, et al. Comparison of octreotide administration vs conservative treatment in the management of inoperable bowel obstruction in patients with far advanced cancer: a randomized, double-blind, controlled clinical trial. *Anticancer Res*. 2002;22:1187–1192.

86. Khoo D, et al. Palliation of malignant intestinal obstruction using octreotide. *Eur J Cancer*. 1994;30A:28–30.

87. Mangili G, et al. Octreotide in the management of bowel obstruction in terminal ovarian cancer. *Gynecol Oncol*. 1996;61:345–348.

88. Massacesi C, Galeazzi G. Sustained release octreotide may have a role in the treatment of malignant bowel obstruction. *Palliat Med*. 2006;20:715–716.

89. Matulonis UA, et al. Long-acting octreotide for the treatment and symptomatic relief of bowel obstruction in advanced ovarian cancer. *J Pain Symptom Manage*. 2005;30:563–569.

90. Jatoi A, et al. Pathophysiology and palliation of inoperable bowel obstruction in patients with ovarian cancer. *J Support Oncol*. 2004;2:323–334; discussion 334–7.

91. Morrow G, Hickok J, Rosenthal S. Progress in reducing nausea and emesis. *Cancer*. 1995;76:343–357.

92. Lebrun C, et al. Recurrent bowel occlusion with oral ondasentron with no side effects of the intravenous route: a previously unknown adverse event. *Ann Oncol*. 1997;8:919–920.

93. Feuer DJ, Broadley KE. Systematic review and meta-analysis of corticosteroids for the resolution of malignant bowel obstruction in advanced gynaecological and gastrointestinal cancers. Systematic Review Steering Committee. *Ann Oncol*. 1999;10:1035–1041.

94. Clark K, Lam L, Currow D. Reducing gastric secretions—a role for histamine 2 antagonists or proton pump inhibitors in malignant bowel obstruction? *Support Care Cancer*. 2009;17:1463–1468.

95. Finan PJ, et al. The management of malignant large bowel obstruction: ACPGBI position statement. *Colorectal Dis*. 2007;9(suppl 4):1–17.

96. Krouse RS. Surgical palliation of bowel obstruction. *Gastroenterol Clin North Am*. 2006;35:143–151.

97. Gauderer MW, Ponsky JL, Izant RJ. Gastrostomy without laparotomy: a percutaneous endoscopic technique. *J Pediatr Surg*. 1980;15:872–875.

98. Ponsky JL, Gauderer MW. Percutaneous endoscopic gastrostomy: a nonoperative technique for feeding gastrostomy. *Gastrointest Endosc*. 1981;27:9–11.

99. Abuksis G, et al. Percutaneous endoscopic gastrostomy: high mortality rates in hospitalized patients. *Am J Gastroenterol*. 2000;95:128–132.

100. Chowdhury MA, Batey R. Complications and outcome of percutaneous endoscopic gastrostomy in different patient groups. *J Gastroenterol Hepatol*. 1996;11:835–839.

101. Cunliffe DR, et al. Percutaneous endoscopic gastrostomy at the time of tumour resection in advanced oral cancer. *Oral Oncol*. 2000;36:471–473.

102. Zera RT, Nava HR, Fischer JI. Percutaneous endoscopic gastrostomy (PEG) in cancer patients. *Surg Endosc*. 1993;7:304–307.

103. Gutt CN, et al. Experiences with percutaneous endoscopic gastrostomy. *World J Surg*. 1996;20:1006–1008 discussion; 1108–9.

104. Gemlo B, et al. Home support of patients with end-stage malignant bowel obstruction using hydration and venting gastrostomy. *Am J Surg*. 1986;152:100–104.

105. Hoffer EK, et al. Radiologic gastrojejunostomy and percutaneous endoscopic gastrostomy: a prospective, randomized comparison. *J Vasc Interv Radiol*. 1999;10:413–420.

106. Lee MJ, et al. Malignant small bowel obstruction and ascites: not a contraindication to percutaneous gastrostomy. *Clin Radiol*. 1991;44:332–334.

107. Freeman C, Delegge MH. Small bowel endoscopic enteral access. *Curr Opin Gastroenterol*. 2009;25:155–159.

108. Maple JT, et al. Direct percutaneous endoscopic jejunostomy: outcomes in 307 consecutive attempts. *Am J Gastroenterol*. 2005;100:2681–2688.

109. Piccinni G, et al. Venting direct percutaneous jejunostomy (DPEJ) for drainage of malignant bowel obstruction in patients operated on for gastric cancer. *Support Care Cancer*. 2005;13:535–539.

110. Dohmoto M. Endoscopic implantation of rectal stents in palliative treatment of malignant stenosis (in Japanese). *Endosc Dig*. 1991;3:1507–1512.

111. Mainar A, et al. Colorectal obstruction: treatment with metallic stents. *Radiology*. 1996;198:761–764.

112. DeBernardo R. Surgical management of malignant bowel obstruction: strategies toward palliation of patients with advanced cancer. *Curr Oncol Rep*. 2009;11:287–292.

113. Caceres A, et al. Colorectal stents for palliation of large-bowel obstructions in recurrent gynecologic cancer: an updated series. *Gynecol Oncol*. 2008;108:482–485.

114. Carter J, et al. Management of large bowel obstruction in advanced ovarian cancer with intraluminal stents. *Gynecol Oncol*. 2002;84:176–179.

115. Pothuri B, et al. The use of colorectal stents for palliation of large-bowel obstruction due to recurrent gynecologic cancer. *Gynecol Oncol*. 2004;95:513–517.

116. Keswani RN, et al. Stenting for malignant colonic obstruction: a comparison of efficacy and complications in colonic versus extracolonic malignancy. *Gastrointest Endosc*. 2009;69:675–680.

117. Khot UP, et al. Systematic review of the efficacy and safety of colorectal stents. *Br J Surg*. 2002;89:1096–1102.

118. Sebastian S, et al. Pooled analysis of the efficacy and safety of self-expanding metal stenting in malignant colorectal obstruction. *Am J Gastroenterol*. 2004;99:2051–2057.

119. Dronamraju SS, et al. Role of self-expanding metallic stents in the management of malignant obstruction of the proximal colon. *Dis Colon Rectum*. 2009;52:1657–1661.

120. Fiori E, et al. Palliative management of malignant rectosigmoidal obstruction: colostomy vs.

endoscopic stenting. A randomized prospective trial. *Anticancer Res*. 2004;24:265–268.

121. Holm AN, Baron TH. Palliative use of percutaneous endoscopic gastrostomy and percutaneous endoscopic cecostomy tubes. *Gastrointest Endosc Clin N Am*. 2007;17:795–803.

122. Caprotti R, et al. Palliative surgery for recurrent bowel obstruction due to advanced ovarian cancer. *Minerva Gynecol*. 2006;58:239–244.

123. Ripamonti C. Management of bowel obstruction in advanced cancer patients. *J Pain Symptom Manage*. 1994;9:193–200.

124. Pothuri B, et al. Palliative surgery for bowel obstruction in recurrent ovarian cancer: an updated series. *Gynecol Oncol*. 2003;89:306–313.

125. Tunca JC, et al. The management of ovarian-cancer-caused bowel obstruction. *Gynecol Oncol*. 1981;12:186–192.

126. Mangili G, et al. Palliative care for intestinal obstruction in recurrent ovarian cancer: a multivariate analysis. *Int J Gynecol Cancer*. 2005;15:830–835.

127. Rubin GP, Devlin HB. The quality of life with a stoma. *Br J Hosp Med*. 1987;38:300–303 306.

128. Smith DM, et al. Happily hopeless: adaptation to a permanent, but not to a temporary, disability. *Health Psychol*. 2009;28:787–791.

129. Yau T, et al. Longitudinal assessment of quality of life in rectal cancer patients with or without stomas following primary resection. *Dis Colon Rectum*. 2009;52:669–677.

130. Sinha R, Verma R. Multidetector row computed tomography in bowel obstruction, part 2: large bowel obstruction. *Clin Radiol*. 2005;60:1068–1075.

131. Sinha R, Verma R. Multidetector row computed tomography in bowel obstruction, part 1: small bowel obstruction. *Clin Radiol*. 2005;60:1058–1067.

132. Filippone A, Cianci R, Storto ML. Bowel obstruction: comparison between multidetector-row CT axial and coronal planes. *Abdom Imaging*. 2007;32:310–316.

133. Jacob SE, Lee SH, Hill J. The demise of the instant/unprepared contrast enema in large bowel obstruction. *Colorectal Dis*. 2008;10:729–731.

134. Lennon AM, et al. Spiral-enteroscopy-assisted enteral stent placement for palliation of malignant small-bowel obstruction (with video). *Gastrointest Endosc*. 2010;71:422–427.

135. Bryan DN, Radbod R, Berek JS. An analysis of surgical versus chemotherapeutic intervention for the management of intestinal obstruction in advanced ovarian cancer. *Int J Gynecol Cancer*. 2006;16:125–134.

136. Abu-Rustum NR, et al. Chemotherapy and total parenteral nutrition for advanced ovarian cancer with bowel obstruction. *Gynecol Oncol*. 1997;64:493–495.

137. Ozols RF, et al. Phase III trial of carboplatin and paclitaxel compared with cisplatin and paclitaxel in patients with optimally resected stage III ovarian cancer: a Gynecologic Oncology Group study. *J Clin Oncol*. 2003;21:3194–3200.

138. Wasserberg N, Kaufman HS. Palliation of colorectal cancer. *Surg Oncol*. 2007;16:299–310.

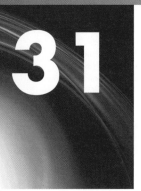

31 Management of malignant wounds and pressure ulcers

Vincent Maida

The cutaneous system (integument) is the largest organ in the body.[1] It includes the skin, mucous membranes, hair, and nails.[1] Cutaneous manifestations of systemic disease are numerous and, metaphorically, represent windows into a patient's overall health. Wounds represent a breach in the intactness of the skin and mucous membranes and occur in many forms and have varied causes.[1] Wounds may be acute or chronic.[1-4] Acute wounds are induced by trauma or are acquired through surgical interventions. Unlike acute wounds, chronic wounds are associated with significant systemic illness and generally fail to heal in an orderly and timely manner.[1-4] Cancer patients are at high risk for the development of multiple wound issues

resulting from disease-related complications, failing performance status, and iatrogenic factors like chemotherapy, radiotherapy, and the use of corticosteroids and immunosuppressive drugs.[1-3] A recent prevalence and incidence study involving advanced cancer patients catalogued 43 different wound types grouped into 9 distinct classes.[5] The two most common wound classes that afflict advanced cancer patients are pressure ulcers and malignant wounds.[5,6]

Chronic wounds are increasingly recognized as an emerging epidemic within health care. In addition, pressure ulcers are becoming an increasing concern from a medico-legal perspective.[7,8] As such, wounds represent a major threat to public health and the economy.[9,10] On any given day, 27% to 50% of acute hospital beds are occupied by patients with wounds.[11] A 2005 point prevalence study at a 754-bed academic hospital in Paris identified 327 patients (52% of 624 evaluated patients) with 933 wounds.[12] These concerns will only increase as the population in developed countries ages. In the United States, chronic wounds afflict more than 6.5 million people.[9] It is estimated that the United States spends more than $25 billion annually on the management of chronic wounds, and it is projected that annual costs for wound management products alone will exceed $15.3 billion by 2010.[9] The net annual cost for the management of pressure ulcers in the United States is approximately $11 billion.[8,13] Wound infections are associated with numerous potential complications[14] that may add to the economic burden. The key to stemming this looming economic crisis is to optimize overall wound prevention while minimizing wound-related complications like those induced by infection. In addition, more research is needed to adopt a truly "evidence-based" approach to wound management.

The human costs of wounds are staggering. Wounds are capable of generating significant multidimensional suffering to the patient that encompasses physical, social, spiritual, psychological, and existential domains with resultant decreased quality of life.[15-17] They may be associated with a number of physical symptoms such as pain, exudation, odor, pruritus, bleeding, edema, and physical mass effect.[18-22] In addition, patients with wounds may have psychosocial problems such as changes in body image (due to unsightly and unnecessarily exuding, malodorous, painful wounds), emotional responses (anger, embarrassment, anxiety, depression, guilt, disgust, shame, and denial), withdrawal and social isolation (relationship problems due to uncontrolled wound symptoms and altered body image), and social restrictions (as a result of frequent dressing changes and poorly controlled symptoms).[19,23–25] Wounds may lead to lowered self-esteem and loss of control as well.[20,23–25]

Wound management is an all-encompassing term that includes the complete spectrum of holistic clinical measures, methods, and interventions in the care of patients with wounds. Wound management, operating in tandem with wound prevention (primary prevention and secondary prevention), comprises multiple goals and objectives including wound healing, wound maintenance (stabilization), and wound palliation, and fulfillment of "patient-centered concerns."[26,27] Wound palliation is synonymous with "wound pain and symptom management" and "palliative wound care."[28,29] Goals of care need to be negotiated with the patient once clinical details and prognostic data have been disclosed to patients. This is vital, as most wounds in the setting of advanced cancer are not healable. However, goals of care and their ranking are not necessarily static or fixed and may change as the natural history of the patient's underlying illness evolves. Goals of care are not mutually exclusive, as attempts at wound healing may improve wound palliation and vice versa.[30] Successful wound management is predicated on the ability to relieve suffering, improve the patient's quality of life, and potentially elevate functional status and independence.

WOUND ASSESSMENT

Objective clinical assessment is one of the keys to successful outcomes in all domains of health care. In addition, assessment is foundational in conducting clinical audits and research. Comprehensive assessments must be conducted in systematic fashion and should incorporate both quantitative and qualitative methods. In addition, there must be an interprofessional commitment to carrying out systematic assessments at baseline and serially. The assessment of wounds should not be limited to the wound ("the hole in the patient") alone but must include an overall assessment of the "whole patient."[31] Ideally, it must also include assessment of all patient-centered concerns.[26,27] A thorough assessment of the patient and the wound will facilitate appropriate goal setting.

A prime requisite for systematic assessment is the use of standardized instruments, questionnaires, or tools. Ideally, they should be validated and reliable and should demonstrate ease of application. Tools that are excessively complex or onerous to the patient or clinicians are destined to fail. Examples of tools include classification systems for wounds. The National Pressure Ulcer Advisory Panel (NPUAP) has recently updated its classification system for pressure ulcers in collaboration with the European Pressure Ulcer Advisory Panel (EPUAP).[32–34] The NPUAP classification places pressure ulcers into six categories (formerly known as grades or stages): suspected deep tissue injury, category I through IV, and unstageable (Table 31-1). This updated system acknowledges that pressure ulcers do not necessarily evolve, in orderly fashion, from one stage or grade to another. The European system (EPUAP) classifies suspected deep tissue injury with category 4. The Pressure Ulcer Scale for Healing (PUSH) score has been in use since 1997 and is recommended by the NPUAP.[32] The PUSH instrument assesses wound length and width, amount of exudate (none, light, moderate, heavy), and tissue type (closed, epithe-

lial tissue, granulation tissue, slough, necrotic tissue). However, PUSH does not include wound depth. A number of classification systems have been proposed for malignant wounds, but none have attained general consensus.

Another vital aspect of wound assessment is patient-rated scoring of wound-related symptoms and overall distress. This can be facilitated through the use of the Toronto Symptom Assessment System for Wounds (TSAS-W).[21] TSAS-W (Fig. 31-1) is a concise tool. It is applicable to all wound classes. TSAS-W uses 10 numeric rating scales, each ranging between 0 and 10, which allow for scoring of the most common wound-related symptoms. The summation of all ten scales equates to the Global Wound Distress Score (GWDS), which may be used to monitor efficacy of therapies. TSAS-W may also be useful in evaluating wound palliation through clinical audits and research.[21]

Even the most thorough of clinical assessments cannot translate into better outcomes if its documentation is not in a format that is standardized, accessible, and legible. Electronic medical records (EMRs) are part of the overall trend of Electronic Health Informatics, commonly referred to as "ehealth."[35] Studies demonstrate that adoption of EMRs translates into improvements in the quality of health care, increased patient safety, and reduced costs.[36] In addition, EMRs are capable of improving communication within the interprofessional team and of enabling evidence-based practice. EMRs also have the potential to facilitate clinical research.[35,36] Over the past decade, electronic records have been increasingly used in wound management. Such records contain all pertinent health data and include all classification systems and assessment tools in digital format. Digital wound photography is an intrinsic component of such wound electronic medical records (WEMRs).[37] Digital photography of wounds promotes increased accuracy in the documentation of wound morphology, geometry, and dimensions.[37] Examples of two-dimensional digital protocols include VERG and VISITRAK.[38] These digital methods demonstrate increased accuracy over manual two-dimensional documentation of wounds. The use of stereophotographic technology and protocols has the potential to document wounds in three dimensions, hence allowing estimation of wound volumes. Examples of three-dimensional digital protocols include ATOS II and MAVIS.[38] High-quality clinical wound assessment and documentation combined with appropriate goal setting and communication with patients and their families translates into improved quality of care.

MALIGNANT WOUNDS

EPIDEMIOLOGY AND PATHOPHYSIOLOGY

Malignant wounds (Fig. 31-2), also referred to as malignant cutaneous wounds or malignant cutaneous lesions, occur in up to 15% of patients with advanced cancer and had an incidence rate of 3.9 new wounds per month per 100 patients in one study.[5] Malignant wounds are extremely varied and may represent primary disease, local recurrence, or metastatic disease. Examples of primary cutaneous malignancies include melanoma, basal cell carcinoma, squamous cell carcinoma, Kaposi's sarcoma, angiosarcoma, and cutaneous T-cell lymphoma (mycosis fungoides).[3,6,16,19,20] Local and

Table 31-1 2007 National pressure ulcer advisory panel pressure ulcer stages

Category	Morphology	Further Description
Suspected Deep Tissue Injury (DTI)	Purple or maroon localized area of discolored intact skin or blood-filled blister due to damage of underlying soft tissue from pressure and/or shear. The area may be preceded by tissue that is painful, firm, mushy, boggy, warmer or cooler compared to adjacent tissue.	Deep tissue injury may be difficult to detect in individuals with dark skin tones. Evolution may include a thin blister over a dark wound bed. The wound may further evolve and become covered by thin eschar. Evolution may be rapid exposing additional layers of tissue even with optimal treatment.
Stage I	Intact skin with nonblanchable redness of a localized area usually over a bony prominence. Darkly pigmented skin may not have visible blanching; its color may differ from the surrounding area.	The area may be painful, firm, soft, warmer or cooler as compared to adjacent tissue. Stage I may be difficult to detect in individuals with dark skin tones. May indicate "at risk" persons (a heralding sign of risk).
Stage II	Partial thickness loss of dermis presenting as a shallow open ulcer with a red-pink wound bed, without slough. May also present as an intact or open/ruptured serum-filled blister.	Presents as a shiny or dry shallow ulcer without slough or bruising.* This stage should not be used to describe skin tears, tape burns, perineal dermatitis, maceration, or excoriation.
Stage III	Full-thickness tissue loss. Subcutaneous fat may be visible, but bone, tendon, or muscle is not exposed. Slough may be present but does not obscure the depth of tissue loss. May include undermining and tunneling.	The depth of a stage III pressure ulcer varies by anatomic location. The bridge of the nose, ear, occiput, and malleolus do not have subcutaneous tissue and stage III ulcers can be shallow. In contrast, areas of significant adiposity can develop extremely deep stage III pressure ulcers. Bone/tendon is not visible or directly palpable.
Stage IV	Full-thickness tissue loss with exposed bone, tendon, or muscle. Slough or eschar may be present on some parts of the wound bed. Often include undermining and tunneling.	The depth of a stage IV pressure ulcer varies by anatomic location. The bridge of the nose, ear, occiput, and malleolus do not have subcutaneous tissue and these ulcers can be shallow. Stage IV ulcers can extend into muscle and/or supporting structures (e.g., fascia, tendon, or joint capsule) making osteomyelitis possible. Exposed bone/tendon is visible or directly palpable.
Unstageable (US)	Full-thickness tissue loss in which the base of the ulcer is covered by slough (yellow, tan, gray, green, or brown) and/or eschar (tan, brown, or black) in the wound bed.	Until enough slough and/or eschar is removed to expose the base of the wound, the true depth, and therefore stage, cannot be determined. Stable (dry, adherent, intact without erythema or fluctance) eschar on the heels serves as "the body's natural (biological) cover" and should not be removed.

Adapted from NPUAP. Permission obtained on December 18, 2009. http://www.npuap.org.
* Bruising indicates suspected deep tissue injury.

regional recurring malignancies most commonly arise from primary skin cancers but may also be associated with breast cancers and head and neck cancers; they are thought to be due to residual microscopic disease or intraoperative wound contamination.[39] Thus, they propagate through contiguous spread. Truly metastatic cutaneous lesions arise through hematogenous or lymphogenous spread from remote primary cancers.[3,6,16,19,20] Malignant wounds may occasionally develop within a chronic wound such as a pressure ulcer, in the case of Marjolin's ulcer, a form of squamous cell carcinoma.[40] In advanced cancer patients, the malignancies with the highest point prevalence of malignant wounds were primary skin cancers (53.8%), breast cancer (48.3%), and head and neck cancers (46.2%).[18] Morphologically, they may be complex. Several common morphologic types are known: exophytic (fungating), ulcerative, nodular, indurated, and zosteriform (Table 31-2). Malignant wounds seldom manifest singular morphologic features and usually contain multiple morphologic elements (see Table 31-2). For this reason, it is challenging to develop a universally accepted classification system. In one study of advanced cancer patients, 60%

of the malignant wounds had a predominance of fungating (exophytic) morphology.[5] The most common anatomic sites for malignant wounds are the chest/breast and head/neck areas.[5] Malignant wounds may evolve complications like superficial infections (critical colonization), deep infections (cellulitis, abscess, lymphangitis), or systemic infections (osteomyelitis, peritonitis, pleuritis, septicemia).[41] Malignant wounds also have a propensity to develop into fistulas if located in anatomic proximity of the gastrointestinal or genitourinary system.[16–20] In addition, owing to the invasion and obstruction of local lymphatic channels, they may produce lymphedema.[39] Aside from the obvious physical effects, malignant wounds are associated with significant psychosocial morbidity, as the cutaneous disfigurement is a constant and visible reminder of the cancer and its progression.[16–20] These factors lead to disturbances of body image, decreased feelings of self-worth, and affective disorders, all resulting in reduced quality of life.[16] Research studies using Heideggerian hermeneutic phenomenologic approaches are elucidating the patient's perspective on living with a malignant wound.[23]

Toronto Symptom Assessment System for Wounds (TSAS-W)

Patient's Name: _____   **Date:** ___ ____ _____   **Time:** _____
          dd   mm   yyyy

Study ID: _____   **Wound ID:** _____   **Wound assessment number:** _____

Wound Location:
1☐ **Face/Head/Neck**   5☐ **Upper Extremity**   9☐ **Sacrum/Coccyx**
2☐ **Chest/Breast**   6☐ **Lower Extremity**   10☐ **Foot (excluding heel)**
3☐ **Abdomen/Flank**   7☐ **Pelvis/Hips**   11☐ **Heel**
4☐ **Upper/Lower Back**   8☐ **Perineum/Genitalia**

Side: 1☐**Left** 2☐**Right** 3☐**Center**   Describe location further if needed: _____

Wound Class:
1☐ **Malignant**   4☐ **Diabetic Foot ulcer**   7☐ **Iatrogenic**
2☐ **Pressure Ulcer**   5☐ **Venous ulcer**   8☐ **Infection/Inflammatory**
3☐ **Traumatic**   6☐ **Arterial ulcer**   9☐ **Ostomy**
Stage: _____   Size: _____ (cm^2)   10☐ **Other**

*Please circle the number that best describes your **wound-related symptoms** over the past 24 hours:*

No Pain **with** dressings and/or debridement	0 1 2 3 4 5 6 7 8 9 10	Most severe Pain **with** dressings and/or debridement
No Pain **between** dressings and/or debridement	0 1 2 3 4 5 6 7 8 9 10	Most severe Pain **between** dressings and/or debridement
No Drainage or Exudation	0 1 2 3 4 5 6 7 8 9 10	Most severe and/or continuous Drainage or Exudation
No Odor	0 1 2 3 4 5 6 7 8 9 10	Most severe Odor
No Itching	0 1 2 3 4 5 6 7 8 9 10	Most severe Itching
No Bleeding	0 1 2 3 4 5 6 7 8 9 10	Most severe and/or continuous Bleeding
No Cosmetic or Aesthetic concern and/or distress	0 1 2 3 4 5 6 7 8 9 10	Most severe Cosmetic or Aesthetic concern and/or distress
No Swelling or Edema **around** wound	0 1 2 3 4 5 6 7 8 9 10	Most severe Swelling or Edema **around** wound
No Bulk or Mass effect from **wound**	0 1 2 3 4 5 6 7 8 9 10	Most severe Bulk or Mass effect from **wound**
No Bulk or Mass effect from **dressings**	0 1 2 3 4 5 6 7 8 9 10	Most severe Bulk or Mass effect from **dressings**

Completed by: 1☐**Patient**   2☐**Patient assisted by caregiver**   3☐**Caregiver**

☐ Dr. Vincent Maida 2008

Fig. 31-1 Toronto Symptom Assessment System for Wounds.

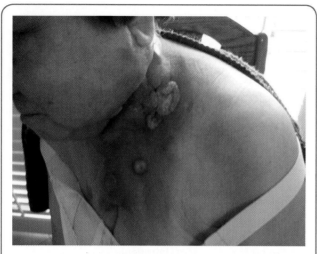

Fig. 31-2 A complex malignant wound that possesses elements of fungating, ulcerative, nodular, and induration.

Table 31-2 Elements of malignant wounds

Common nomenclature	Morphologic features
Fungating	Exophytic
Ulcerative	Cavitating
Subcutaneous nodules	Hard nodules beneath intact skin
Carcinoma erysipeloid	Indurated skin that is flat but erythematous having the appearance of cellulitis but does not respond to antibiotics
Carcinoma en cuirasse	Indurated skin that is flat
Elephantiasic	Indurated skin that is raised, thick, and lymphedematous; hyperkeratosis and papillomatosis are often present
Schirrous (morphea)	Scleroderma-like tightness due to dermal reaction; May be localized or multifocal
Carcinoma telangiectoides	Red patches with telangiectasia
Zosteriform	Pustular appearance similar to herpes zoster; often in a peripheral nerve or dermatomal distribution because of perineural propagation

PREVENTION

Several preventive strategies aimed at reducing the occurrence of malignant wounds are currently being used. Early excision of primary cutaneous malignancies may decrease the risk of recurrence.[42] In the case of primary cutaneous melanomas, a recent systematic review and meta-analysis has provided more evidence to support a 2-cm margin rather than a 1-cm margin as the minimum margin for surgical excision; this was associated with the best overall disease-free survival and the lowest rate of locoregional recurrence.[43] Adjuvant radiotherapy and chemotherapy in the setting of women with breast cancer, following a modified radical mastectomy, have been associated with improved survival and reduced rates of cutaneous recurrence in both premenopausal and postmenopausal women who presented with nodal disease.[44] Methods targeting intraoperative wound contamination and residual microscopic tumor at surgical sites are being studied. A xenograft model with human hypopharyngeal squamous cell carcinoma demonstrated lower rates of locoregional recurrence in both treatment groups that were irrigated with gemcitabine or saline.[45]

MANAGEMENT

Given that most malignant wounds occur in the setting of advanced cancer,[5] the probability of healing is marginal.[46] Therefore, in large part, the management of malignant wounds consists of wound palliation.[3,6,16–20],[29] Nonetheless, there remains a significant role for optimized systemic and disease-modulating therapies, such as chemotherapy and hormonal therapies, because they may be effective in the stabilization/maintenance of existing wounds as well as in reducing the incidence of new lesions.[39] Moreover, novel chemotherapeutic classes such as the monoclonal antibodies, trastuzumab and bevacizumab, are demonstrating significant potential.[47] Intra-arterial infusion of chemotherapy also may be effective for larger fungating lesions.[48] Topical chemotherapeutic agents have demonstrated efficacy. Topical 6% miltefosine, a cytotoxic agent, was associated with delayed tumor progression in a randomized controlled study involving women with malignant wounds.[49] Photodynamic therapy may have some efficacy in smaller malignant wounds in the setting of breast cancer and mycosis fungoides.[50] In selected cases, surgical excision, in conjunction with lymph node resection or debulking of fungating lesions, may be indicated.[39] Radiotherapy may play a significant role in the management of malignant wounds. The degree of responsiveness of a tumor to radiation, however, is dictated by its cell type, level of differentiation, and size.[51] The most radiosensitive tumors are lymphomas, myelomas, seminomas, and small cell cancers, followed by breast, gastrointestinal, prostate, and lung cancers.[51] The least radiosensitive tumors are melanomas, sarcomas, and renal cancers.[51] Radiotherapy may help to relieve pain and control bleeding from malignant wounds. A low dose of 800 cGy in 1 fraction is often sufficient to control bleeding within a few days, whereas it may take a few weeks to achieve analgesia.[51]

Malignant wounds, like all chronic wounds that are colonized polymicrobially, may develop signs and symptoms of infection.[41] Targeted topical or systemic antimicrobial therapy, guided by accurate wound cultures, is indicated.[41] Prevention of infection may be achieved with wound cleansing using topical antiseptic agents such as chlorhexidine and povidone-iodine.[41] Both agents possess broad-spectrum coverage and relatively low tissue toxicity.[41] Topical acetic acid may be used in cases colonized with *Pseudomonas* species.[52] Finally, given the profound psychosocial impact of malignant wounds, other nonpharmacologic treatments and psychotherapy may also be indicated.[23–25]

WOUND PALLIATION

Malignant wounds are associated with the highest burden of pain and other symptoms relative to other wound classes.[21] Wound palliation aims to improve quality of life through the relief of physical symptoms.[16,28,29] This is achieved mostly through local wound measures such as specialized wound products and dressings (Table 31-3). The choice of dressings should be consistent with patient-centered concerns and should offer the greatest efficacy and convenience while minimizing dressing changes and being cosmetically and economically favorable.[16–20]

Pain

Pain is the most common symptom associated with malignant wounds, as it is reported by almost one third of patients.[18,21] The morphologic type most associated with pain is the malignant ulcer.[39] It must be acknowledged that cancer pain, as originally described by Dame Cicely Saunders, is a multifactorial construct that includes not only the physical, but also the psychological, social, and spiritual/existential dimensions.[53] Local wound factors contribute to the patient's wound-related pain perspective.[54] Pain associated with malignant wounds may occur within the wound itself or in the peri-wound skin, or it may be regional. Pain may be caused by tumor-induced damage to nerve fibers, blood vessels, and dermal nerve endings.[6,22] This may be exacerbated by edema, fibrosis, and infection. Pain associated with malignant wounds is complex. Generally speaking, patients experience constant or background (baseline) pain that is persistent, as well as episodic pain that may be spontaneous or provoked by contact, movement, or dressing changes. The latter is termed "incident pain," a subset of "breakthrough pain."[55,56]

Although malignant wound pain results from a combination of inflammatory and neuropathic mechanisms, most chronic pain syndromes invariably become secondarily neuropathic through mechanisms such as N-methyl-d-aspartate (NMDA) activation, sensitization (peripheral and central),

Table 31-3. Common Local Wound Management Products

Wound Product Primary Objective	Product Category	Sample Product	Collateral benefits
Absorbent	Foam	Biatain IBU	Topical analgesic
Absorbent	Hydrofiber	Aquacel Ag	Topical antimicrobial
Absorbent	Alginate	Katostat™	Topical hemostatic
Absorbent	Alginate with ethylene methylacrylate contact layer	Silvercel nonadherent	Topical antimicrobial Non-adherent
Absorbent	Cellulose pulp with polypropylene contact layer	Mesorb	Nonadherent + protects clothing
Absorbent	Textile with silver complex	InterDryAg	Skin fold management to treat & prevent moisture lesions
Hydrating agent	Hydrocolloid	NU-DERM Hydrocolloid	Autolytic debridement
Hydrating agent	Hydrogel	Purilon Gel	Autolytic debridement
Protease modulator	ORC/Collagen	Promogran	Topical hemostatic
Protease modulator	ORC/Collagen	Prisma	Topical antimicrobial Topical hemostatic
Topical antimicrobial	Nanocrystalline silver	Acticoat	Absorbent
Topical antimicrobial	Ionic silver + hydrogel	Silvasorb Gel	Hydrating agent + topical antimicrobial
Topical antimicrobial	Cadexomer iodine	Iodosorb	Absorbent
Topical antimicrobial	10% povidone iodine	Inadine	Nonadherent
Anti-odor	Metronidazole	Metrogel	Topical antimicrobial
Anti-odor	Charcoal	Actisorb Silver 220	Absorbent
Nonadherent wound contact layer	Cotton + polyethylene contact layer	Telfa	Allows moisture vapour exchange
Nonadherent wound contact layer	Polyamide net covered with Silicone	Mepetel	Flexible & conforms to contours
Protect Peri-wound skin	Barrier cream	Cavilon	Hypoallergenic

and neuroplasticity.[57] Optimal analgesia may be achieved using a combination of systemic and topical agents. As no one analgesic is a panacea, combination therapy is indicated as described by the World Health Organization (WHO) pain ladder and Twycross' approach of "broad-spectrum" analgesia.[58] Generally speaking, combinations of opioids and adjuvants such as the gabapentinoids, tricyclic antidepressants, serotonin-norepinephrine reuptake inhibitors (SNRIs), selective serotonin reuptake inhibitors (SSRIs), and cannabinoids, as outlined in the Canadian Pain Society's guidelines for chronic neuropathic pain, are effective in most cases.[59] Topical analgesia may be achieved through the use of lidocaine-prilocaine (eutectic mixture of local anesthetics [EMLA]),[60] opioids such as morphine sulfate[61,62] or methadone[63] compounded with hydrogels, or Biatain IBU, a novel foam dressing that elutes ibuprofen.[64] The degree and frequency of "incident pain" may be reduced, but not necessarily eliminated, with optimal management of baseline pain. It may be exacerbated by removal of dressing materials that have become adherent to dry wound beds. This may be obviated by application of hydrating agents such as Nu-Derm gel or other hydrogels and/or the use of non-adherent wound contact layers such as Telfa or Mepetel.[19,20]

For incident pain associated with dressing changes, rapid-onset and short-acting agents such as the fentanyl series of opioids may be used IV, or transmucosally (orobuccal or nasal), in preemptive fashion, 5 to 10 minutes before the procedure.[65] Nitrous oxide gas (Entonox) may also be beneficial in anticipated cases of severe incident pain.[66] Patients with wound-related pain may have concomitant anxiety and depression that tend to further exacerbate their pain, hence indicating the need for a multimodal and interprofessional approach.[16,17,23–25]

Drainage

Drainage or exudation from malignant wounds is the second most common symptom, experienced by 28.6% of patients with malignant wounds.[18,21] Optimal control of drainage helps to reduce complications involving peri-wound tissues. Extravasation of chemotherapy through wound exudation may be associated with peri-wound sequelae that range from minor skin irritation to necrosis.[67] Protection of peri-wound skin may also be achieved through the use of barrier ointments (zinc oxide ointment, petrolatum) or windowed hydrocolloid dressings or film-forming liquid acrylates.[6,19,20] Numerous dressing products may be used singularly or in combination to absorb drainage and contain it within the dressing system to prevent leakage and soiling of clothing. Examples of absorbent dressings include foams, alginates, and hydrofibers. Multilayer dressings such as Mesorb combine the capacity for high exudate absorption with high retention. In malignant wounds that have developed into fistulas, application of ostomy dressings may be indicated to collect high-volume effluents.[6,19,20]

Odor

Approximately 10% of patients report malodor emanating from their malignant wound.[18,21] Patients experience a wide range of feelings associated with malodor, including embarrassment, disgust, guilt, and shame, which can lead to social isolation and relationship problems.[16,17,19,20] Wound-related odor may be due to infection, stagnant exudates, saturated dressings, or necrotic tissue. Necrotic tissue is heavily colonized with anaerobic bacteria

that generate volatile fatty acid end products such as cadaverine (1,5-diaminopentane) and putrescine (1,4-diaminopentane) that cause foul wound odors. Debridement of necrotic material within malignant wounds may be helpful but must be carried out with great scrutiny because vascular structures are difficult to identify and resultant bleeding may be difficult to control. Metronidazole, effective against anaerobic bacteria, has demonstrated efficacy in reducing odor from malignant wounds through randomized trials with topical and systemic administration.[68] Other interventions to reduce odor include wound cleansing, antisepsis, and treatment of infection, if present. The use of outer dressing layers containing activated charcoal as filters to adsorb malodorous volatile chemicals emanating from the wound may be effective, but only if the overall dressing is airtight.[19,20] Environmental methods such as the use of aromatherapy oils and odor adsorbents such as charcoal briquettes and pet litter materials may also be considered.

Itching

Pruritus has many possible causes and aggravating factors. It is increasingly being regarded as a neuropathic phenomenon.[69] Dryness of the skin is frequently a precipitating or exacerbating factor; therefore moisturizers are beneficial.[69] Several systemic agents may be useful in the symptomatic relief of pruritus, including antihistamines, tricyclic antidepressants, particularly doxepin, anticonvulsants, and cannabinoids.[69] Recent studies demonstrated 95% resolution of pruritus associated with lymphedema using Olivamine-based skin care products,[70] and topical cannabinoid agonists caused an average 86.4% reduction in pruritus.[71]

Bleeding

Bleeding is reported by about 5% of patients with malignant wounds.[18,21] It may be spontaneous or induced by minor trauma or dressing changes. Minor bleeding may be abated with a number of topical agents, including Kaltostat, a calcium alginate, topical thromboplastin (100 u/ml), and silver nitrate (0.5%–1%).[72] For more severe cases, interventional methods such as arterial embolization may be considered. Antifibrinolytic agents such as tranexamic acid, given orally or intravenously, may also be effective in controlling persistent bleeding.[19] A recent study has demonstrated the use of a chemical hemostatic treatment for bleeding breast cancer fungating wounds using zinc chloride paste (Mohs paste).[73]

Cosmetic/esthetic concerns

Concerns regarding the cosmetic/esthetic appearance of malignant wounds are reported by 17.9% of patients.[18,21] Strategies to mask or cloak the wound, while maintaining body contour, symmetry, and concealment beneath clothing, should be used.[72] Bulky dressings that impede body movement or other activities should be avoided. Given the importance of this issue, the ultimate goal is to restore and enhance a patient's self-image, self-confidence, and self-esteem.[72]

PROGNOSIS

The survival of patients with malignant wounds has been increasing over the past four decades.[74,75] Data published in 1966 demonstrate that patients survived an average of only 3 months after the development of cutaneous metastases.[74]

Data published in 1993 demonstrate that patients survived an average of 11.27 months after the development of cutaneous metastases, with patients diagnosed with cancers of the lung, ovary, and foregut faring the worst.[75] A recent prospective study has revealed that malignant wounds are not associated with decreased survival[76]; after controlling for the co-occurrence of all other wounds, age, sex, Charlson Comorbidity Index (CCI), and Palliative Performance Scale version 2 (PPSv2), malignant wounds did not demonstrate statistically significant associations with decreased survival, with a hazard ratio (HR) of 1.17 (95% confidence interval [CI], 0.88–1.56; $P = .285$).[76] A Canadian study[77] published in 2000 and a Hong Kong–based study[78] published in 2007 also demonstrated that malignant wounds were not associated with decreased survival in advanced cancer patients. These positive trends are clearly the result of advancements in oncologic therapeutics over the past few decades, especially in breast cancer. Thus the presence of a malignant wound should not be automatically regarded as a disqualifying criterion for additional attempts at disease-modulating therapies.

PRESSURE ULCERS

EPIDEMIOLOGY AND PATHOPHYSIOLOGY

Pressure ulcers (Fig. 31-3), also referred to as decubitus, decubitus ulcers, pressure sores, or "bed-sores," are the most common wound class in patients with advanced cancer, occurring in 22.4% of patients, and having an incidence rate of 22.4 new wounds per month per 100 patients.[5] In addition, their prevalence and incidence increase with age.[5] The most common sites for pressure ulcer development in cancer patients are the sacrococcygeal area and the posterior heel.[5] Pressure ulcers develop over bony prominences and represent an ischemic necrosis of skin and underlying tissues resulting from arterial, venous, and lymphatic dysfunction and stasis induced by prolonged unrelieved pressure, as well as repetitive friction and shearing forces.[3,6,8,79] Cancer-induced anorexia-cachexia is a major causative factor in the development of pressure ulcers because it is associated with loss of muscle and subcutaneous fat interposed between bony prominences and skin; such loss also makes the skin looser, thereby allowing for a greater shearing

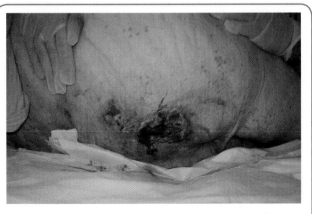

Fig. 31-3 A complex pressure ulcer that possesses elements of suspected deep tissue injury stage I, stage II, and Unstageable.

effect.[3,6,8,79] Extremes in the level of skin hydration also predispose to pressure ulcers.[80,81] Excessively dry skin is less elastic and more likely to fissure; wet skin, possibly exacerbated by incontinence, may become macerated, which reduces tensile strength and predisposes to invasion by bacteria and fungi.[80,81]

Poor overall pain management may also promote decreased mobility and recumbence, thereby predisposing to increased pressure, friction, and shearing effects. Moreover, pain may cause vasoconstriction of small arterial channels that further increases risk for the development of pressure ulcers and reduces their probability of healing.[82] Other risk factors for the development of pressure ulcers in advanced cancer patients include corticosteroid usage, paralysis, spinal cord compression, orthopedic deformities (flexion contractures, kyphoscoliosis), fractures, peripheral vascular disease, diabetes mellitus, and sensory neuropathy.[3,6,8,79] Pressure ulcers may become complicated by infections such as abscesses, cellulitis, osteomyelitis, septic arthropathies, gangrene, and septicemia. Chemotherapy may cause neutropenia and thrombocytopenia; this decreases the availability of inflammatory cells such as neutrophils and platelets for skin repair.[3] These deficits also render the patient more susceptible to infection. Chronic pressure ulcers also predispose to the development of malignant transformation (Marjolin's ulcer)[40] and amyloidosis.[83]

PREVENTION

Although many pressure ulcers may be preventable, some remain unavoidable. Langemo et al, in 2003, postulated the concept of "skin failure" to explain the often inevitable development of pressure ulcers in patients with advanced illness.[79] Thus skin failure needs to be acknowledged and accepted as part of the natural history and context of disease, much like heart failure and renal failure.[79] Three main themes are evident in the prevention of pressure ulcers:

1. **Risk assessment:** The key to prevention is the identification and stratification of risk through the use of risk assessment tools. Of course, appropriate actions must follow the risk assessment. A number of risk assessment tools are described in the healthcare literature. The tool with the highest level of acceptance in a wide range of healthcare settings is the Braden Scale (BS) because it provides the best balance between sensitivity and specificity.[84] A recent study demonstrated a strong correlation between PPSv2[85] and BS ($r = 0.885$, $P < .001$).[86] Therefore PPSv2 may be used as a proxy for the assessment of pressure ulcer risk in cancer patients.[86] The use of infrared thermometry may provide additional data in assessing risk for pressure ulcer development.[87] Although a 2008 *Cochrane Systematic Review* found no evidence to recommend a specific risk assessment tool, it did not stratify according to clinical setting.[88]

2. **Skin care:** Skin integrity may be promoted by daily skin inspection, gentle cleaning, cleansing after incontinence, containment of drainage, avoidance of massage over bony prominences, and use of moisturizers for dry skin.[6,80] All are essential for those patients with wounds and for those at high risk for their development. Prevention of infection may be achieved with wound cleansing using topical antiseptic agents such as chlorhexidine and povidone-iodine.[41] Both agents possess broad-spectrum coverage and low toxicity. Topical acetic acid may be used in cases colonized with *Pseudomonas* species.[52]

3. **Mechanical loading and support surfaces:** Pressure redistribution, commonly referred to as "off-loading," is imperative for preventing new lesions, potentially healing existing pressure ulcers, or allowing their stabilization/maintenance. Traditionally, frequent repositioning of bed-bound patients was the original method for pressure redistribution. A recent Cochrane meta-analysis concluded that patients at high risk for pressure ulcer development should be offered higher-specification foam mattresses rather than standard hospital foam mattresses, and dynamic low–air-loss mattresses and alternating–air pressure mattresses may be more cost effective than static alternating pressure overlays.[89] Avoidance of shearing and friction forces may be achieved with the use of lift sheets and mechanical trapeze lift devices.

Although it seems intuitive that nutritional support is useful to prevent and treat pressure ulcers, a recent Cochrane meta-analysis did not find enough data to support routine hyper-alimentation to prevent or treat pressure ulcers.[90] This is not surprising in that the weight loss and nutritional depletion seen in advanced cancer patients are mostly related to primary cancer-related cachexia rather than to cachexia due to anorexia. Nutritional supplementation is of greatest value in patients with nonmalignant disease who are not terminally ill.

MANAGEMENT

Less than 10% of pressure ulcers are healable in the advanced cancer setting.[46] Therefore the goals of care involve wound stabilization (maintenance), wound prevention, and wound palliation, while maintaining respect for patient-centered concerns. Management of pressure ulcers may be guided by the wound bed preparation paradigm (Fig. 31-4) (forwarded by Sibbald et al) that is enabled by the "DIME" mnemonic[91]:

1. **Debridement:** Eradication of necrotic tissue, through debridement, may serve to reduce bacterial burden, odor, and exudation.[92] The most rapid methods are sharp and surgical debridement; their utility may be limited by pain or hemostatic issues. Alternative modes of debridement may include autolytic (hydrogels), enzymatic (collagenase), and mechanical (wound lavage) methods. Medical larvae (maggots) may also be considered because they consume both necrotic material and bacteria.[92] Heel ulcers in the setting of severe peripheral vascular disease (ankle-brachial index <0.5) represent a contraindication for debridement and constitute an exception to the paradigm of moist-wound healing forwarded by Winter in 1963.[93]
2. **Infection/Inflammation:** Pressure ulcers are usually colonized by a mixture of aerobic (gram-positive and gram-negative) and anaerobic bacteria.[41] Treatment of infection

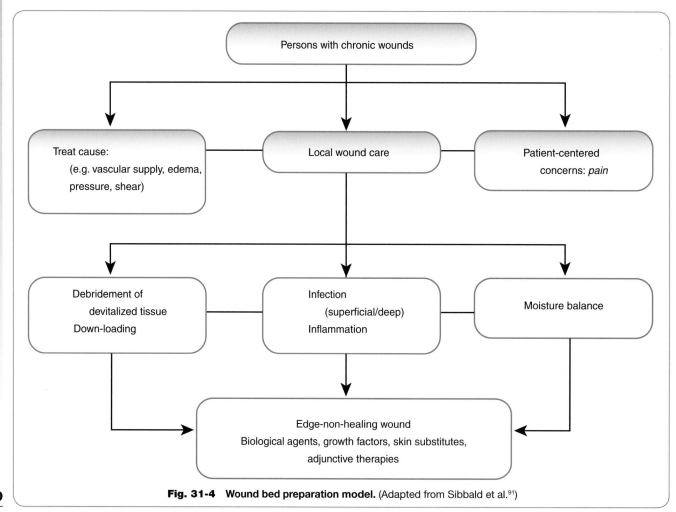

Fig. 31-4 Wound bed preparation model. (Adapted from Sibbald et al.[91])

is important because it may lead to rapid deterioration of ulcers and exacerbation of symptoms such as pain, exudation, and odor.[41] However, if the patient is imminently dying, treatment of infection may not be appropriate. The clinical diagnosis of wound infection may be guided by mnemonic enablers created by Sibbald et al[41]: **NERDS:** N = Nonhealing wounds, E = Exudative wounds, R = Red and bleeding wound surface granulation tissue, D = Debris (yellow or black necrotic tissue) on the wound surface, S = Smell or unpleasant odor from the wound. **STONES:** S = Size is bigger, T = Temperature increased, O = Os (probe to or exposed bone), N = New or satellite areas of breakdown, E = Exudate, Erythema, Edema, S = Smell. The presence of a majority of the NERDS criteria supports the presence of superficial infection (critical colonization) and indicates the need for topical antimicrobials such as ionic silver or povidone-based dressings.[41] The presence of a majority of the STONES criteria supports the presence of deep infection and indicates the need for systemic antimicrobials.[41] Targeted antimicrobial therapy should be guided by the use of semiqualitative swabs and cultures and should follow established guidelines, such as the 39th Edition, *The Sanford Guide to Antimicrobial Therapy 2009,* based on microbial sensitivities.[94] In addition to the inflammatory reactions generated in response to microbial exotoxins and endotoxins, another cause of inflammation within wounds derives from excessive levels of proteases, especially the matrix metalloproteases (MMPs). Levels of MMPs may be normalized through the use of modulating agents such as Promogran or Prisma.[41]

3. **Moisture balance:** In general, wounds with the potential to heal require a moist wound environment, and nonhealable and maintenance wounds are best managed in a dryer state.[81] Therefore the choice of dressings is dependent on the goals of care. In general, foams, hydrofibers, and alginates are the most absorptive; hydrocolloids and hydrogels are the most hydrating dressings.[81] In cases where exudation is extreme, negative-pressure wound therapy (NPWT) may be considered; NPWT also has the capacity to reduce periwound edema, stimulate granulation tissue, stimulate neovascularization, and reduce bacterial burden.[95]

4. **Edge effect:** This refers to the failure of epithelium to migrate across a granulating wound base.[95] Assuming that the goal of care is wound healing, the following adjunctive therapies have demonstrated some efficacy and may be considered: biological agents (honey, spruce resin[96]), growth factor therapy, hyperbaric oxygen therapy, NPWT, and electrotherapy. In selected cases, where the patient is thought to have a longer survival, surgical methods such as musculocutaneous flaps and skin grafts may also be considered.[95]

PROGNOSIS

Although controversy looms over the link between pressure ulcers and increased mortality, consensus is growing that they are mostly predictors of impending death rather than a direct cause of death.[97] In patients with advanced noncancer illness, a controlled prospective study has demonstrated an HR of 2.42 (95% CI, 1.34–4.38; $P = .003$) among patients with pressure ulcers.[98] A case-matched retrospective cohort study of 33 cancer patients demonstrated a 39% mortality rate; patients who died did so within a mean of 3 weeks after developing pressure ulcers.[99] A prospective study involving a sequential case series of 418 advanced cancer patients demonstrated univariate HR of 2.07 (95% CI, 1.60–2.67; $P < .001$) for patients with pressure ulcers.[76] After controlling for the co-occurrence of all other wounds, age, sex, CCI, and PPSv2, a large sex–mortality differential was demonstrated, with women affected by pressure ulcers having worse survival than men with pressure ulcers, by a factor of 1.85 ($P = .020$).[76] The preservation of statistical significance for women affected with pressure ulcers supports the conclusion that they represent an independent risk factor for decreased survival among patients with advanced cancer.[76]

REFERENCES

1. Burns DA, Breathnach SM, eds. *Rook's textbook of dermatology*. Malden, MA: Blackwell Science; 2004.
2. Bruera E. Medical and psychosocial implications of skin disorders. In: Portenoy RK, Bruera E, eds. *Topics in palliative care, vol 3, section IV*. New York: Oxford University Press; 2002:231–283.
3. Gerlach MA. Wound care issues in the patient with cancer. *Nurs Clin N Am*. 2005;40:295–323.
4. Lazarus GS, Cooper DM, Knighton DR, et al. Definitions and guidelines for assessment of wounds and evaluation of healing. *Arch Dermatol*. 1994;130:489–493.
5. Maida V, Corbo M, Irani S, et al. Wounds in advanced illness: a prevalence and incidence study based on a prospective case series. *Int Wound J*. 2008;5:305–314.
6. MacDonald A, Lesage P. Palliative management of pressure ulcers and malignant wounds in patients with advanced illness. *J Palliat Med*. 2006;9:285–295.
7. Ayello EA, Capitulo KL, Fife CE, et al. Legal issues in the care of pressure ulcer patients: key concepts for health care providers. A consensus paper from the international expert wound care advisory panel. *J Palliat Med*. 2009;12:995–1008.
8. Reddy M, Gill SS, Rochon PA. Preventing pressure ulcers: a systematic review. *JAMA*. 2006;296:974–984.
9. Sen CK, Gordillo GM, Roy S, et al. Human skin wounds: a major and snowballing threat to public health and the economy. *Wound Repair Regen*. 2009;17:763–771.
10. Posnett J, Franks PJ. The burden of chronic wounds in the UK. *Nurs Times*. 2008;104:44–45.
11. Posnett J, Gottrup F, Lundgren H, et al. The resource impact of wounds on health-care providers in Europe. *J Wound Care*. 2009;18:154–161.
12. Mahe E, Langlois G, Baron G, et al. Results of a comprehensive hospital based wound survey. *J Wound Care*. 2006;15:381–384.
13. Gordon MD, Gottschlisch MM, Helvig EI, et al. Review of evidence-based practice for the prevention of pressure sores in burn patients. *J Burn Care Rehabil*. 2004;25:388–410.
14. Bjarnsholt T, Kirketerp-Moller K, Madsen KG, et al. Why chronic wounds will not heal: a novel hypothesis. *Wound Repair Regen*. 2008;16:2–10.
15. Brown GC, Brown JM, Nelson EA, et al. Impact of pressure ulcers on quality of life in older patients: a systematic review. *J Am Geriatr Soc*. 2009;57:1175–1183.
16. Grocott P, Browne N, Cowley S. Quality of life: assessing the impact and benefits of care to patients with fungating wounds. *Wounds*. 2005;17:8–15.
17. Alexander S. Malignant fungating wounds: key symptoms and psychosocial issues. *J Wound Care*. 2009;18:325–329.
18. Maida V, Ennis M, Kuziemsky C, Trozzolo L. Symptoms associated with malignant wounds: a prospective case series. *J Pain Symptom Manage*. 2009;37:206–211.
19. Naylor WA. A guide to wound management in palliative care. *Int J Palliat Nurs*. 2005;11:572–579.
20. Hatsfield-Wolfe ME, Rund C. Malignant cutaneous wounds: a management protocol. *Ostomy Wound Manage*. 1997;43:56–66.
21. Maida V, Ennis M, Kuziemsky C. The Toronto Symptom Assessment System for Wounds (TSAS-W): a new clinical and research tool. *Adv Skin Wound Care*. 2009;22:468–474.

22. Reddy M, Kohr R, Queen D, et al. Practical treatment of wound pain and trauma: a patient-centered approach. An overview. *Ostomy Wound Manage.* 2003;49(suppl 4A):2–15.

23. Piggin C, Jones V. Malignant fungating wounds: an analysis of the lived experience. *J Wound Care.* 2009;18:57–64.

24. Lund-Nielsen B, Muller K, Adamsen L. Malignant wounds in women with breast cancer: Feminine and sexual perspectives. *J Clin Nurs.* 2005;14:56–64.

25. Lo SF, Hu WY, Hayter M, et al. Experiences of living with a malignant fungating wound: a qualitative study. *J Clin Nurs.* 2008;17:2699–2708.

26. Picker Institute. *Patient-centered care 2015: Scenarios, vision, goals and next steps.* 2004. Available at: http://www.pickerinstitute.org. Accessed December 31, 2009.

27. Lin GA, Dudley RA. Patient-centered care: what is the best measuring stick? *Arch Intern Med.* 2009;169:1551–1553.

28. Ferris FD, Al Khateib AA, Fromantin I, et al. Palliative wound care: managing chronic wounds across life's continuum: a consensus statement from the International Palliative Wound Care Initiative. *J Palliat Med.* 2007;10:37–39.

29. Alvarez OM, Kalinski C, Nusbaum J, et al. Incorporating wound healing strategies to improve palliation (symptom management) in patients with chronic wounds. *J Palliat Med.* 2007;10:1161–1189.

30. Liao S, Arnold RM. Wound care in advanced illness: application of palliative care principles. *J Palliat Med.* 2007;10:1159–1160.

31. Sibbald RG, Williamson D, Orsted HL, et al. Preparing the wound bed: debridement, bacterial balance, and moisture balance. *Ostomy Wound Manage.* 2000;46:14–22.

32. National Pressure Ulcer Advisory Panel. Available at: http://www.npuap.org. Accessed December 31, 2009.

33. European Pressure Ulcer Advisory Panel. Available at: http://www.epuap.org. Accessed December 31, 2009.

34. Dealey C. A joint collaboration: international pressure ulcer guidelines. *J Wound Care.* 2009;18:368–372.

35. Oh H, Rizo C, Enkin M, et al. What is eHealth: a systematic review of published definitions. *J Med Internet Res.* 2005;7:e1.

36. Poissant L, Pereira J, Tamblyn R, Kawasumi Y. The impact of electronic health records on time efficiency of physicians and nurses: a systematic review. *J Am Med Informatics Assoc.* 2005;12:505–516.

37. Rennert R, Golinko M, Kaplan D, et al. Standardization of wound photography using the wound electronic medical record. *Adv Skin Wound Care.* 2009;22:32–38.

38. Ahn C, Salcido R. Advances in wound photography and assessment methods. *Adv Skin Wound Care.* 2008;21:85–95.

39. Schulz VN. Cutaneous metastases and malignant wounds. In: Nabholtz JM, ed. *Breast cancer management.* 2nd ed. Philadelphia: Lippincott Williams & Wilkins; 2003:475–488.

40. Esther RJ, Lamps L, Schwartz HS. Marjolin ulcers: secondary carcinomas in chronic wounds. *J South Orthop Assoc.* 1999;8:181–187.

41. Sibbald RG, Woo K, Ayello EA. Increased bacterial burden and infection: the story of NERDS and STONES. *Adv Skin Wound Care.* 2006;19:447–461.

42. Sladden MJ, Balch C, Barzilai DA, et al. Surgical excision margins for primary cutaneous melanoma. *Cochrane Database Syst Rev.* 2009;4:CD004835.

43. Haigh PI, DiFronzo LA, McCready DR. Optimal excision margins for primary cutaneous melanoma: a systematic review and meta-analysis. *Can J Surg.* 2003;46:419–426.

44. Rutqvist LE, Johansson H. Long-term follow-up of the Stockholm randomized trials of postoperative radiation therapy versus adjuvant chemotherapy among "high risk" pre- and postmenopausal breast cancer patients. *Acta Oncol.* 2006;45:517–527.

45. Allegretto M, Selkaly H, Mackey JR. Intraoperative saline and gemcitabine irrigation improves tumour control in human squamous cell carcinoma-contaminated surgical wounds. *J Otolaryngol.* 2001;30:121–125.

46. Maida V. *Healing rates of wounds in patients with advanced illness.* Poster presented at: 16th International Congress on Palliative Care, Montreal, Canada; 2006.

47. Harmer V. Breast cancer. Part 2: Present and future treatment modalities. *Brit J Nurs.* 2008;17:1028–1035.

48. Murakami M, Kuroda Y, Sano A, et al. Validity of local treatment including intraarterial infusion chemotherapy and radiotherapy for fungating adenocarcinoma of the breast. *Am J Clin Oncol.* 2001;24:388–391.

49. Leonard R, Hardy J, van Tienhoven G, et al. Randomized, double-blind, placebo-controlled, multicenter trial of 6% miltefosine solution, a topical chemotherapy in cutaneous metastases from breast cancer. *J Clin Oncol.* 2001;19:4150–4159.

50. Wang X, Zhang W, Xu Z, et al. Sonodynamic and photodynamic therapy in advanced breast carcinoma: a report of 3 cases. *Integr Cancer Ther.* 2009;8:283–287.

51. Ferris FD, Bezjak A, Rosenthal SG. The palliative uses of radiation therapy in surgical oncology patients. *Surg Oncol Clin N Am.* 2001;10:185–201.

52. Ryssel H, Kloeters O, Germann G, et al. The antimicrobial effect of acetic acid—an alternative to common local antiseptics? *Burns.* 2009;35:695–700.

53. Saunders C. The treatment of intractable pain in terminal cancer. *Proc Royal Soc Med.* 1963;56:195–197.

54. Woo KY, Sibbald RG. Chronic wound pain: a conceptual model. *Adv Skin Wound Care.* 2008;21:175–188.

55. Portenoy RK, Hagen NA. Breakthrough pain: definition, prevalence and characteristics. *Pain.* 1990;41:273–281.

56. Payne R. Recognition and diagnosis of breakthrough pain. *Pain Med.* 2007;8(suppl 1):S3–S7.

57. Jarvis MF, Boyce-Rustay JM. Neuropathic pain: models and mechanisms. *Curr Pharm Des.* 2009;15:1711–1716.

58. Twycross R. *Introducing palliative care.* 3rd ed. Oxford: Radcliffe Medical Press; 1999.

59. Moulin DE, Clark AJ, Gilron I, et al. Pharmacological management of chronic neuropathic pain—Consensus statement. *Pain Res Manage.* 2007;12:13–21.

60. Vanscheidt W, Sadjadl Z, Lilliborg S. EMLA anaesthetic cream for sharp leg ulcer debridement: a review of the clinical evidence for analgesic efficacy and tolerability. *Eur J Dermatol.* 2001;11:90–96.

61. Twillman RK, Long TD, Cathers TA, et al. Treatment of painful skin ulcers with topical opioids. *J Pain Symptom Manage.* 1999;17:288–292.

62. Zeppetella G, Paul J, Ribeiro MD. Analgesic efficacy of morphine applied topically to painful ulcers. *J Pain Symptom Manage.* 2003;25:555–558.

63. Gallagher RE, Arndt DR, Hunt KL. Analgesic effects of topical methadone: a report of four cases. *Clin J Pain.* 2005;21:190–192.

64. Coutts P, Woo KY. Bourque. Treating patients with painful chronic wounds. *Nurs Stand.* 2008;23:42–46.

65. Casuccio A, Mercadante S, Fulfaro F. Treatment strategies for cancer patients with breakthrough pain. *Expert Opin Pharmacother.* 2009;10:947–953.

66. Parlow JL, Milne B, Tod DA, et al. Self-administered nitrous oxide for the management of incident pain in terminally ill patients: a blinded case series. *Palliat Med.* 2005;19:3–8.

67. Wyatt AJ, Leonard GD, Sachs DL. Cutaneous reactions to chemotherapy and their management. *Am J Clin Dermatol.* 2006;7:45–63.

68. Bale S, Tebble N, Price P. A topical metronidazole gel used to treat malodorous wounds. *Brit J Nurs.* 2004;13:S4–S11.

69. Pogatzi-Zahn E, Marziniak M, Schneider G, et al. Chronic pruritus: targets, mechanisms and future therapies. *Drug News Perspect.* 2008;21:541–551.

70. McCord D, Fore J. Using Olivamine-containing products to reduce pruritic symptoms associated with localized lymphedema. *Adv Skin Wound Care.* 2007;20:441–444.

71. Stander S, Reinhardt HW, Luger TA. Topical cannabinoid agonists: an effective new possibility for treating chronic pruritus. *Hautarzt.* 2006;57:801–807.

72. Barton P, Parslow N. Malignant wound management: a patient centered approach. In: Krasner D, ed. *Chronic wound care: a clinical source book for health care professionals.* 4th ed. Malvern, PA: HMP Communications; 2007:715–725 [chapter 70].

73. Kakimoto M, Tokita H, Okamura T, Yoshino K. A chemical hemostatic technique for bleeding from malignant wounds. *J Palliat Med.* 2009;12:1–3.

74. Reingold IM. Cutaneous metastases from internal carcinoma. *Cancer.* 1966;19:162–168.

75. Lookingbill DP, Spangler N, Helm KF. Cutaneous metastases in patients with metastatic carcinoma: a retrospective study of 4020 patients. *J Am Acad Dermatol.* 1993;29:228–236.

76. Maida V, Ennis M, Kuziemsky C, Corban J. Wounds and survival in cancer patients. *Eur J Cancer.* 2009;45:3237–3244.

77. Vigano A, Bruera E, Jhandri GS, et al. Clinical survival predictors in patients with advanced cancer. *Arch Intern Med.* 2000;160:861–868.

78. Lam PT, Leung MW, Tse CY. Identifying prognostic factors for survival in advanced cancer patients: a prospective study. *Hong Kong Med J.* 2007;13:453–459.

79. Langemo DK. When the goal is palliative care. *Adv Skin Wound Care.* 2006;19:148–154.

80. Sibbald RG, Norton L, Woo KY. Optimized skin care can prevent pressure ulcers. *Adv Skin Wound Care.* 2009;22:392.

81. Okan D, Woo K, Ayello EA, Sibbald G. The role of moisture balance in wound healing. *Adv Skin Wound Care.* 2007;20:39–53.

82. Ueno C, Hunt TK, Hopf HW. Using physiology to improve surgical wound outcomes. *Plast Reconstr Surg.* 2006;117(suppl 7):59S–71S.

83. Silver JR. Pressure ulcer and amyloidosis. *Spinal Cord.* 1998;36:293.

84. Pancorbo PL, Garcia-Fernandez FP, Lopez-Medina IM, et al. Risk assessment scales for pressure ulcer prevention: a systematic review. *J Adv Nurs.* 2006;54:94–110.

85. Anderson F, Downing GM, Hill J, et al. Palliative performance scale (PPS): a new tool. *J Palliat Care.* 1996;12:5–11.

86. Maida V, Lau F, Downing M, Yang J. Correlation between Braden Scale and Palliative Performance Scale in advanced illness. *Int Wound J.* 2008;5:585–590.

87. Rapp MP, Bergstrom N, Padhye NS. Contribution of skin temperature regularity to the risk of developing pressure ulcers in nursing facility residents. *Adv Skin Wound Care.* 2009;22:506–513.

88. Moore ZEH, Cowman S. Risk assessment tools for the prevention of pressure ulcers. *Cochrane Database Syst Rev.* 2008;(3): CD006471.

89. McInnes E, Cullum NA, Bell-Syer SEM, et al. Support surfaces for pressure ulcer prevention. *Cochrane Database Syst Rev.* 2008;(4): CD001735.

90. Langer G, Knerr A, Kuss O, et al. Nutritional interventions for preventing and treating pressure ulcers. *Cochrane Database Syst Rev.* 2003;(4): CD003216.

91. Sibbald RG, Orsted HL, Coutts PM, et al. Best practice recommendations for preparing the wound bed: update 2006. *Adv Skin Wound Care.* 2007;20:390–405.

92. Kirshen C, Woo K, Ayello EA, Sibbald RG. Debridement: a vital component of wound bed preparation. *Adv Skin Wound Care.* 2006;19: 506–517.

93. Winter GD, Scales JT. Effect of air drying and dressings on the surface of the wound. *Nature.* 1963;197:91–92.

94. Gilbert DN, Moellering Jr RC, Eliopoulos GM, et al, eds. *The Sanford guide to antimicrobial therapy.* 39th ed. Sperryville, VA: Antimicrobial Therapy; 2009.

95. Woo K, Ayello EA, Sibbald RG. The edge effect: current therapeutic options to advance the wound edge. *Adv Skin Wound Care.* 2007;20:99–117.

96. Sipponen A, Jokinen JJ, Sipponen P, et al. Beneficial effect of resin salve in treatment of severe pressure ulcers: a prospective, randomized and controlled multicentre trial. *Brit J Dermatol.* 2008;158:1055–1062.

97. Thomas DR, Goode PS, Tarquine PH, Allman RM. Hospital-acquired pressure ulcers and risk of death. *J Am Geriatr Soc.* 1996;44:1435–1440.

98. Maida V, Ennis M, Kuziemsky C, Corban J. Wounds and survival in non-cancer patients. *J Palliat Med.* 2010;13:453–459.

99. Waltman NL, Bergstrom N, Armstrong N, et al. Nutritional status, pressure sores, and mortality in elderly patients with cancer. *Oncol Nurs Forum.* 1991;18:867–873.

32 Pleural and pericardial effusions

Ani Balmanoukian and Julie R. Brahmer

Common complications of advanced malignancy are pleural effusions and pericardial effusions. Under most circumstances, these fluid accumulations occur secondary to advanced disease and may be refractory to multiple therapeutic regimens. Oftentimes, they are the initial presentation of a malignancy. Clinically, patients present with various symptoms and severity, ranging from asymptomatic to significant degrees of discomfort and end-organ damage. Physicians are often faced with choosing from a menu of various therapeutic options and need to take into consideration the patient's underlying medical condition, the tolerability of the procedure, and life expectancy. Management of pleural and pericardial effusions and ascites will be discussed in this chapter.

MALIGNANT PLEURAL EFFUSIONS

One of the most common complications of advanced malignancy is the development of pleural effusion. The estimated annual incidence is 150,000 patients.[1,2] In most instances, the presence of a pleural effusion is indicative of advanced disease and of unresponsiveness to systemic therapy; however, pleural effusions are caused by a variety of diseases and complications, including pneumonia, congestive heart failure, pulmonary embolus, and atelectasis (Table 32-1). Careful workup of the underlying cause is necessary before any decisions regarding therapy are made. The development of malignant pleural effusion for most malignancies, including those of lung and gastrointestinal cancers, portends a poor prognosis with a usual median survival ranging from 3 to 12 months[3,4]; however, complete remission and even cure are possible, despite the presence of pleural effusions with germ cell tumors and certain types of lymphomas.[5]

PATHOPHYSIOLOGY

The pleural space lies between the visceral pleura, which covers the lung; interlobar fissures; and the parietal pleura, which covers the chest wall, diaphragm, and mediastinum. The origin of malignant pleural effusions is complex and multifactorial. Effusions result from both increased entry and decreased exit of fluid within the pleural space. Impaired lymphatic drainage causes fluid to accumulate[6] by direct tumor invasion of the pleurae or by lymph node involvement. Under most circumstances, tumor has spread to the parietal and visceral pleurae, leading to fluid accumulation. Seeding of the pleurae with tumor cells increases pleural fluid formation, leading to increased fluid in the pleural space.[7]

CLINICAL MANIFESTATIONS

Patients present with various symptoms, including dyspnea, chest pain, cough, or orthopnea. Hemoptysis is rare. A pleural effusion may also be a purely incidental finding on imaging

Table 32-1 Causes of pleural effusions

Transudative pleural effusions

Heart failure
Nephrotic syndrome
Hepatic hydrothorax
Hypoalbuminemia
Atelectasis
Constrictive pericarditis

Exudative pleural effusions

Bacterial pneumonia
Atpical pneumonias
Carcinoma
Lymphoma
Mesothelioma
Leukemia
Chylothorax
Pulmonary embolism
Radiation therapy
Sarcoidosis
Esophageal perforation
Hemothorax

with no discomfort to the patient. Dyspnea is due to loss of functional lung volume caused by compressive atelectasis, reduced chest wall compliance, depression of the ipsilateral hemidiaphragm, or mediastinal shift.[8]

A thorough physical examination is necessary for patients who present with any of the suspected symptoms of a pleural effusion. The chest has dullness to percussion, decreased or absent breath sounds, and absence of fremitus on the involved side. Depending on the cause of the effusion, the physician should pay attention to other clinical findings such as bilateral decreased breath sounds, elevated jugular venous pressure due to congestive heart failure, or any signs of infection.

DIAGNOSIS AND EVALUATION

Workup should initially include a chest X-ray, which is the quickest test for an evaluation. Pleural effusions are apparent on X-ray when at least 200 ml of fluid is present.[9] An effusion that has reached the fourth rib indicates a volume of about 1000 ml. Decubitus films are obtained to ensure that the fluid is free flowing and to exclude a loculated effusion. An effusion that is thicker than 1 cm on a decubitus film can be reached by thoracentesis.[10] Chest computed tomography (CT) is more accurate in detecting small effusions and in identifying loculated effusions. An ultrasound can also detect loculated effusions, as well as effusions as small as 5 ml.[11]

For those patients with advanced malignancy in which a pleural effusion provides obvious evidence of their disease progression, a thorough evaluation is not warranted if the patient is asymptomatic. Observation with the intent to

intervene therapeutically if the patient develops symptoms is a reasonable approach. The effusion can be used as a marker of response if salvage systemic chemotherapy or hormone therapy is initiated by the oncologist. In patients for whom a pleural effusion is not clearly explained by their malignancy, a thorough workup is essential to rule out other causes.

MANAGEMENT
Thoracentesis

The initial approach to a malignant pleural effusion is a thoracentesis, which is both diagnostic and therapeutic. Even though a thoracentesis provides relief of acute symptoms, the chance of reaccumulation of a malignant pleural effusion is high after the procedure.[12,13]

Before the patient undergoes a thoracentesis, the chest X-ray or CT scan should be reviewed to evaluate for any possibility of loculated fluid, which would require ultrasound-guided drainage.[14,15] Relative contraindications to a thoracentesis include bleeding disorders, anticoagulation, elevated international normalized ratio (INR), platelets <20,000, infections of the chest wall, pneumothorax, hemothorax, and pain.[16,17] Caution should be taken with patients who are on mechanical ventilation with a high positive end-expiratory pressure (PEEP). Even though thoracentesis is not contraindicated under these circumstances, the possibility of developing a tension pneumothorax is high if a complication does occur. Risks involved with a thoracentesis include pneumothorax, bleeding, infection, pain, and possible liver or spleen laceration.

A thoracentesis is done to evaluate for an exudative or transudative process. Depending on the rapidity of fluid reaccumulation, a thoracentesis may or may not be repeated, and the physician may opt to pursue other therapeutic options. If pleural fluid reaccumulates slowly, repeat thoracentesis as needed to alleviate symptoms may be all that is required. For most patients with a malignant effusion, fluid accumulates quickly, making other therapeutic options more appealing.

DIAGNOSTIC CRITERIA

Light's criteria are most frequently used to differentiate between a transudate and an exudate. In 1972, Richard Light published his criteria,[18] and they have since become the standard by which medical practitioners evaluate pleural fluid. His criteria use ratios of effusion to serum lactate dehydrogenase (LDH) and protein to classify an exudate by the following three criteria:

1. Pleural fluid protein-to-serum protein ratio of greater than 0.5
2. Pleural fluid LDH greater than two thirds of upper limit of normal for serum
3. Pleural fluid LDH-to-serum LDH ratio of greater than 0.6

Other tests should include cell count and differential, albumin, pH, glucose, amylase, gram stain, culture, and cytology. Cholesterol and triglyceride are obtained on the pleural fluid if a chylothorax is suspected, and fungal culture should be ordered depending on the clinical scenario. Even though cell count is frequently obtained on pleural fluid, it is usually not helpful unless a high number (>50,000 per milliliter) of nucleated cell counts are present, which indicates a complicated parapneumonic effusion or empyema.[19] Pleural fluid cytology provides the most definitive criteria for diagnosing a malignant effusion, whereas tumor markers are not generally helpful. The sensitivity of cytology ranges from 62% to 90%,[20] depending on the malignancy and the expertise of the cytopathologist. A positive cytology of malignant effusion is predictive of poor survival.

The pH of the pleural fluid should always be measured. Normal pH for pleural fluid is between 7.60 and 7.64. Transudates have a pH between 7.40 and 7.55, whereas exudates have a pH between 7.30 and 7.45.[21] A low pleural fluid pH has diagnostic and prognostic implications. Those patients with pleural effusions with a pH <7.30 have a shorter survival and a worse outcome with pleurodesis.[22–24] A parapneumonic effusion with a low pleural pH (<7.15) will likely require placement of a pleural tube drain.[25,26]

Pleurodesis

For those patients who symptomatically respond to thoracentesis, pleurodesis is considered a good therapeutic option. Pleurodesis is the closing of the pleural space by fusion through chemical or mechanical irritation.[27] Obliteration of the pleural space prevents fluid reaccumulation.[28] Patients have to demonstrate improvement with a thoracentesis to clarify that the effusion is the predominant cause of symptoms—not lung metastases, pulmonary embolism, or pulmonary fibrosis. Reexpansion with thoracentesis is necessary to ensure that the lung is not trapped.[29] Pleurodesis requires an inflammatory reaction, local activation of coagulation with fibrin deposition, and collagen deposition for fusion of both pleural surfaces.[30–32]

Chemical pleurodesis is performed more often than mechanical pleurodesis because it is usually more effective and minimally invasive.[33,34] Chemical pleurodesis requires placement of a chest tube to drain the pleural fluid, followed by instillation of a chemical sclerosant into the pleural space. The chest tube is clamped for 1 to 4 hours following sclerosis to prevent backflow of the sclerosant into the chest tube. The chest tube is then unclamped and is left to drain until output is less than 150 ml. At this point, a radiographic image is obtained to confirm that the effusion has resolved, and that apposition of the two pleural surfaces has occurred. Once these criteria are met, the chest tube is removed.[35–37] This procedure usually requires hospitalization for 3 to 7 days. A few reports describe the use of small-caliber catheters connected to a plastic drainage system to prevent a pneumothorax. These catheters can be placed on an outpatient basis.[38,39] If drainage continues to measure >250 ml despite pleurodesis, a second pleurodesis and use of another sclerosing agent may be needed.

Multiple agents have been used for pleurodesis; however, no ideal agent has been found. Some of the most frequently used agents include talc slurry, tetracycline class compounds such as doxycycline, and bleomycin. Talc is currently the most widely used and the best studied agent. It is also substantially less expensive than other agents. Several studies[34,40–42] have demonstrated the relative superiority of talc over other sclerosing agents for recurrent malignant effusions. A meta-analysis[34] of 10 randomized trials included 308 patients and

found talc superior to other sclerosants such as bleomycin, tetracycline, and mustine in preventing reaccumulation of pleural fluid. Tetracycline derivatives such as doxycycline are the next best option.[43]

Video-assisted thoracic surgery (VATS) with talc insufflation is another method of pleurodesis performed under general anesthesia with single-lung ventilation. The choice between talc slurry by chest tube versus VATS depends on the clinical scenario. VATS has the advantage of allowing complete fluid drainage, lysis of adhesions, and equal distribution of talc during insufflation. For those patients with a poor performance status, talc slurry via a chest tube is preferred because it is less invasive. Talc slurry via VATS or chest tube has similar efficacy in achieving palliation.[44]

The most common complications of talc slurry are pain and fever. Empyema is also a possibility. Pulmonary complications include acute respiratory distress syndrome (ARDS), pneumonitis, and respiratory failure.[45,46]

Thoracoscopic mechanical pleurodesis is a means of creating apposition between parietal and visceral pleurae by abrasion to the parietal pleura, which causes inflammation and adhesion of the pleura during the healing process. An injury to the visceral pleura is usually avoided to limit the risk of lung parenchymal damage leading to air leak. Thoracoscopic mechanical pleurodesis and talc pleurodesis were studied in a series of breast cancer patients.[47] The two procedures had a similar success rate (92% and 91%, respectively, in patients with pleural effusions with pH >7.3); however, mechanical pleurodesis was better in effusions with pH <7.3. For the most part, chemical pleurodesis has been reported to be more effective.[33,34]

INTRAPLEURAL THERAPY

Therapy applied directly to the pleural space has had variable results over the years. Agents that have been used include 5-fluorouracil (5-FU),[48] cisplatin,[48–51] doxorubicin,[52] cytarabine,[49] mitomycin,[50] and docetaxel.[53] Shoji et al.[48] reported the use of intrapleural chemotherapy using an implantable access system with biweekly 5-FU and cisplatin in 22 patients with malignant pleural effusion. No systemic toxicity was observed with the use of intrapleural chemotherapy. Intraoperative intrapleural hypotonic cisplatin treatment has been shown to suppress the development of malignant pleural effusion, but with no significant effect on overall survival.[51] Jones et al.[53] recently reported findings of a phase I trial using intrapleural docetaxel administered through an implantable catheter in patients with malignant pleural effusion. All 15 patients tolerated therapy well, and most had a complete radiographic response.

More randomized trials are needed until intrapleural chemotherapeutic agents are used routinely. Currently, the chance of systemic absorption and the cost of intrapleural chemotherapy make the use of talc and other such agents more favorable.

Indwelling catheter

The most frequently used approach to control symptoms of recurrent malignant pleural effusion is a PleurX catheter, which is an indwelling tunneled catheter. The FDA approved it in 1997 for use with pleural effusions. The PleurX is a 15.5 French silicone catheter that is soft and relatively comfortable, with side holes and a polyester cuff that induces fibrosis along the catheter tunnel. Tunnel fibrosis decreases the risks of leakage, dislodgment, and infection.[54] A proximal hub prevents air entry and fluid leakage. A cap is placed over the hub when the tube is not used.

The ideal candidate for a PleurX catheter has a free-flowing recurrent effusion or a large locule. A trapped lung is another indication for a PleurX catheter.[55] Again, for a PleurX to be used, the patient should have shown signs of improvement after a prior thoracentesis. The catheter can be placed at the bedside with local or conscious sedation rather than in the operating room or the procedure room. No more than 1500 ml is drained initially to avoid reexpansion pulmonary edema. The catheter is drained every other day afterwards by the patient, a family member, or a designated caretaker. The schedule for drainage will depend on the size of the effusion and the patient's symptoms. The catheter can be removed if three consecutive drainages yield low output, and imaging shows resolution of the fluid. The PleurX catheter may induce spontaneous pleurodesis. A patient series published by Musani reported spontaneous pleurodesis in 58% of patients.[56]

The major advantages of a PleurX catheter include improvement in dyspnea in about 70% to 80% of patients,[57] low cost as compared with pleurodesis,[58] and improvement in quality of life and in the ability of patients to be out of the hospital. Complications associated with a PleurX catheter include poor drainage requiring replacement, tumor migration along the catheter, and infection.

Pleurectomy

Pleurectomy is an alternative approach to the treatment of recurrent malignant pleural effusions. Pleurectomy is a palliative debulking procedure that includes resection of visceral and parietal pleurae and decortication by removal of fibrous pleural rind. It has been used as a primary therapeutic approach in patients with malignant pleural mesothelioma.[59] It can also be used as a palliative approach in patients with other malignant pleural effusions. Pleurectomy is effective in obliterating the pleural space and controlling recurrent malignant pleural effusions.

An ideal candidate for this procedure is a patient with a good performance status and a reasonably long expected survival, given that this is a major surgical procedure. The procedure itself is well tolerated and has a low mortality rate (1.5%–5%).[60] Complications include bronchopleural fistula, hemorrhage, pneumonia, subcutaneous emphysema, empyema, and, rarely, vocal cord paralysis.[61-63]

Shunt

Pleuroperitoneal shunting is an option that is rarely used with recurrent malignant pleural effusions. Patients need to be under general anesthesia, and the procedure itself involves a shunt catheter placement, with one end inserted into the pleural cavity and the other into the peritoneum through a tunnel. The shunt pumping chamber is placed in a subcutaneous pocket overlying the costal margin.[64]

Shunt complications occur in about 15% of patients,[65] with risk of occlusion and infection as the major associated problems. Tumor seeding into the chest wall at the site of shunt insertion has been reported. Palliation is achieved in 73% to 90% of patients.[65,66]

PERICARDIAL EFFUSION

Malignant pericardial effusions do not occur as frequently as pleural effusions and are rarely the initial presentation of a malignancy.[67] Similar to pleural effusions, pericardial effusions occur as a result of various systemic diseases or disorders (Table 32-2). Malignant pericardial effusions are common in patients with lung cancer, breast cancer, lymphoma, leukemia, or melanoma. The prognosis of patients with malignant pericardial effusions depends on the extent of the underlying malignancy. Survival may be as long as 10 to 13 months in some patients with breast cancer[68,69] and less than 6 months in those with other cancers.[70,71]

PATHOPHYSIOLOGY

The pericardium consists of two layers: a visceral pericardium, which adheres to the external surface of the heart, and a parietal pericardium, in which a fibrous layer is formed by the visceral pericardium reflecting back on itself. The potential space between these two layers is called the pericardial cavity. This space normally contains 15 to 50 ml of serous fluid,[72] which serves as a lubricant to reduce friction and as a barrier against infection.

Malignant involvement of the pericardium can result from primary tumors of the pericardium,[73,74] but more frequently from other malignancies such as breast or lung. Malignant cells gain access to the pericardial space by direct invasion from adjacent tumor in the lung or mediastinum, or by hematogenous or lymphatic spread. Alternative causes of pericardial effusion are lymphatic and/or venous obstruction by a malignancy.

CLINICAL MANIFESTATIONS

The potential space in the pericardial cavity is less than that of the pleural space. Cardiac chamber capacity is reduced by the accumulation of pericardial effusion, limiting venous return and decreasing cardiac output leading to cardiac tamponade. Reduced compliance of the pericardium and acuity of fluid collection causes patients to develop symptoms rapidly. Rapid accumulation of fluid in the pericardial space is poorly tolerated, whereas slow accumulation may allow large amounts of

---

Table 32-2 Causes/types of pericardial effusion

Malignancy

Myocardial infarction (Dressler's syndrome)

Myxedema

Trauma

Acute idiopathic

Drug induced

Radiation induced

Collagen vascular disease

Viral (coxsackievirus, human immunodeficiency virus, mumps, adenovirus)

Tuberculosis

Fungal (histoplasmosis, coccidiomycosis)

Bacterial (*Pneumococcus, Streptococcus, Staphylococcus*)

pericardial fluid to collect and pericardium to accommodate to the volume without producing symptoms. Filling pressures in all chambers of the heart are elevated as fluid accumulates. The clinical features typically result from decreased cardiac output and elevated venous pressure.

The most common clinical manifestations of symptomatic pericardial effusion are dyspnea, cough, chest pain, palpitations, tachypnea, tachycardia, and edema. Ewart's sign refers to subscapular dullness with percussion due to compression of the left lung by a massively enlarged heart. Physical signs of low cardiac output include cool extremities, jugular venous distention, distant heart sounds, narrowed pulse pressure, pericardial friction rub, and pulsus paradoxus. Electrocardiography (ECG) has low-voltage complexes across all leads and electrical alternans.

DIAGNOSIS AND EVALUATION

Pericardial effusion is caused by a variety of mechanisms, and a search as to the cause is warranted. Exposure to radiation and certain medications may cause a pericardial effusion, which may falsely be assumed to be due to a malignancy.

The initial workup includes a chest X-ray, which may show cardiomegaly or the characteristic water-bottle heart or triangular heart with smoothed-out cardiac borders. Echocardiography (ECHO) is both specific and sensitive for detecting pericardial effusions and assesses the hemodynamic significance of the effusion. It is the most important study performed for the diagnosis and quantification of an effusion. The 2003 American College of Cardiology/American Heart Association/American Society of Echocardiography (ACC/AHA/ASE) guidelines encourage and recommend the use of echocardiography in all patients with suspected pericardial disease.[75] An echocardiogram should be done emergently if a tamponade physiology is suspected clinically. Echocardiograms detect as little as 15 ml fluid. When tamponade physiology is present, the ECHO shows a compressed right side of the heart, increased respiratory variation of the mitral and tricuspid inflow velocity, and right atrial and ventricular collapse during diastole. A diagnosis of tamponade is based on both clinical and echocardiographic findings.

Other radiographic procedures for assessing a pericardial effusion include a chest CT scan, which is sensitive, detects 50 ml of pericardial fluid, and allows visualization of intrapericardial metastasis.[76] Chest magnetic resonance imaging (MRI) is an alternative radiographic modality for directly visualization of the epicardium.[77] An MRI is more sensitive in differentiating between malignant and benign lesions.

MANAGEMENT

Not all pericardial effusions need to be treated; patients who are asymptomatic do not need pericardiocentesis. Under most circumstances, a malignancy causes rapid accumulation of fluid with symptoms that require drainage.

Pericardiocentesis

Pericardiocentesis can be done semi-electively, but often it must be performed on an emergent basis with impending cardiac collapse due to cardiac tamponade.

Pericardiocentesis is usually performed with local anesthesia using a 16- to 22-gauge needle attached to a syringe, with the patient elevated at a 45-degree angle. The subxiphoid approach is usually used, with the needle inserted into the angle formed between the left costal arch and the xiphoid process and directed approximately 15 degrees posterior to the head or either shoulder.[72] Echocardiographically guided pericardiocentesis is one approach to visualize the space where the needle is being placed. The procedure is simple, safe, and effective for primary treatment of clinically significant postoperative pericardial effusion.[78] In one patient series, 132 consecutive pericardiocenteses were performed under ECHO guidance, with a procedural morbidity of 4% and mortality of 0%.[79] Nowadays, a more frequent approach is to perform the pericardiocentesis under direct visualization in the cardiac catheterization laboratory.

Among patients who are clinically unstable with hypotension and impending cardiac collapse due to cardiac tamponade, aggressive fluid resuscitation is necessary with emergent pericardiocentesis at the bedside.

Major complications are ventricular perforation, arrhythmias, hemopericardium, and pneumothorax. The complication rate ranges from 5% to 20%. Echocardiography reduces the complication rate.[80]

The recurrence rate of pericardial fluid after initial drainage is as high as 50%.[81] With recurrence, an indwelling pigtail drainage catheter (6–8 French) is introduced over a guidewire during pericardiocentesis. Kopecky et al. reported use of the pigtail catheter, which allowed drainage without obstruction and without significant risk of infection when maintained for 72 hours.[82] A drainage catheter does carry a significant complication risk, including greater morbidity observed with acute cardiac tamponade.[83] The use of ECHO reduces the risk of complications.[84]

Evaluation of pericardial fluid

Unlike what has been observed with pleural effusions, no diagnostic criteria can be used to differentiate a transudate from an exudate for pericardial effusions. Fluid should be evaluated for cell count and differential, culture, LDH, glucose, protein, and cytology. The sensitivity of cytology ranges from 50% to 90%.[85,86] A negative cytology does not exclude malignancy. In a study by Monte et al., only 10 of 47 pericardial fluids were positive for malignancy.[87] By the same token, other causes for pericardial effusion such as radiation-induced pericardial effusion should be considered if the cytology is negative. The history is an important component in the overall evaluation when one is trying to determine the cause of a pericardial effusion.

Surgical approaches

Surgical intervention is a safe and reliable method for treating chronic pericardial effusions. It also provides pericardial tissue for diagnosis of the underlying cause. The three most common surgical approaches are subxiphoid pericardial window, thoracostomy with creation of a pericardial window, and thoracotomy with pericardiectomy.

The subxiphoid pericardial window is the most common surgical procedure and can be performed under local anesthesia with the pericardium isolated under direct visualization through the xiphoid process. A 4- to 6-cm window is created; then a catheter is inserted into the pericardial cavity and is left in place until drainage decreases over a few days. The catheter can be used for sclerosis.[84,88,89] Complications of the procedure include wound dehiscence and pneumothorax.[90,91]

Alternative surgical techniques such as thoracostomy with pericardial window or pericardiectomy carry a higher risk of complications compared with the subxiphoid approach. Park et al.[90] compared the subxiphoid window to the lateral thoracotomy approach with or without pericardiectomy and found that the latter group had a 50% incidence of major complications and a 44% occurrence of early mortality compared with no complications and 10% mortality with the subxiphoid group. Selection bias might have played a role in the differences in morbidity and mortality between the two groups. Nevertheless, Vaitkus et al.[92] also reported a decreased number of pericardial complications with subxiphoid pericardiostomies compared with open pericardiectomies. For those patients in whom a subxiphoid pericardiostomy is not contraindicated (such as those with acute substernal angles, associated gross ascites, or adhesions due to previous procedures), this procedure should be the first selected when surgical options are considered.

Sclerosing therapy and chemotherapy

Pericardiocentesis with instillation of sclerosants or chemotherapy is another option for treating pericardial effusions. The most common sclerosing agents are tetracycline[93,94] and bleomycin.[95,96] Mitomycin C,[97] OK-432,[98] carboplatin,[99] cisplatin,[100,101] and interferon[102] are chemotherapy agents that have also been used successfully. The technique entails draining the pericardial fluid and injecting the sclerosing agent into the pericardial space, followed by clamping the catheter for 10 minutes to 4 hours. The most common side effects are nonseptic fever up to 38° C and chest pain. Chest pain is reduced with the use of bleomycin.[95] Long-term success ranges from 70% to 100% with bleomycin[95,96] and from 68% to 91% with tetracycline.[93,94] Mitomycin C has a success rate of 70%,[97] and OK-432 100%.[98] Cisplatin is the best studied chemotherapy agent directly instilled into the pericardial space, with success rates of 67% to 87%.[100] It has been reported by Moriya et al.[99] that use of carboplatin leads to complete resolution of effusion in 8 out of 10 patients with non–small cell lung cancer. Sclerosing therapy is not associated with constrictive pericarditis or any significant mortality. Despite this evidence, sclerosing chemotherapy is infrequently used, given the complexity and time commitment of the therapy, because it must be done several times for it to be effective.

PERCUTANEOUS BALLOON PERICARDIOTOMY

Percutaneous balloon pericardiotomy is a safe nonsurgical method used to relieve symptoms of pericardial effusion. It is typically performed in a cardiac catheterization laboratory under fluoroscopic guidance with the use of local lidocaine. It is an extension of the procedure used to place a percutaneous pigtail catheter with the addition of a balloon-dilating catheter (20 mm diameter, 3 cm long) that is exchanged over a guidewire and inserted into the pericardial space.[72] The pericardial drainage catheter is left in place until drainage is less than 100 ml/day.[103] This technique is particularly helpful for relieving symptoms with minimal morbidity and discomfort for patients with a short life expectancy.[104]

CONCLUSION

Pleural effusions and pericardial effusions represent a common complication of advanced malignancy. In patients with these complications, an evaluation to exclude causes other than malignancy is important in the initial workup; however, under most circumstances, malignancy is usually found to be the cause. Any decision regarding further therapy should take into consideration the patient's underlying co-morbid medical conditions and overall life expectancy, as well as complications of the procedure. Ultimately, the intention with any therapy is to provide maximum relief and the best quality of life to achieve adequate palliation for patients.

REFERENCES

1. Neragi-Miandoab S. Malignant pleural effusion, current and evolving approaches for its diagnosis and management. *Lung Cancer.* 2006;54:1–9.
2. American Thoracic Society. Management of malignant pleural effusions. *Am J Respir Crit Care Med.* 2000;162:1987–2001.
3. Sears D, Hajdu SI. The cytologic diagnosis of malignant neoplasm in pleural and peritoneal effusions. *Acta Cytol.* 1987;31:85–97.
4. Van de Molengraft FJ, Voojis GP. Survival of patients with malignancy-associated effusions. *Acta Cytol.* 1989;33:911–916.
5. Weick JK, Keily JM, Harrison Jr EG, et al. Pleural effusion in lymphoma. *Cancer.* 1973;31:848.
6. Sahn SA. State of the art: the pleura. *Am Rev Respir Dis.* 1988;138:184–234.
7. Lynch Jr TJ. Management of malignant pleural effusions. *Chest.* 1993;103(4 suppl):385S–389S.
8. Judson MA, Sahn SA. Pulmonary physiologic abnormalities caused by pleural disease. *Semin Respir Crit Care Med.* 1995;16:346–353.
9. Collins JD, Burwell D, Furmaski S, et al. Minimal detectable pleural effusions: a roentgen pathology model. *Radiology.* 1972;105:51–53.
10. Stark P. The pleura. In: Taveras J, Ferucci C, ed. *Radiology: diagnosis, imaging, intervention.* Philadelphia: Lippincott; 2003:454–460.
11. Grogan DR, Irwin RS, Channick R, et al. Complications associated with thoracentesis: a prospective, randomized study comparing three different methods. *Arch Intern Med.* 1990;150:873–877.
12. Sorensen PG, Svendsen TL, Enk B. Treatment of malignant pleural effusion with drainage, with and without instillation of talc. *Eur J Respir Dis.* 1984;65:131–135.
13. Groth G, Gatzemeier U, Haussingen K, et al. Intrapleural palliative treatment of malignant pleural effusions with mitoxantrone versus placebo(pleural tube alone). *Ann Oncol.* 1991;2:213–215.
14. Lipscomb DJ, Flower CD, Hadfield JW. Ultrasound of the pleura: an assessment of its clinical value. *Clin Radiol.* 1981;32:289–290.
15. Grogan DR, Irwin RS, Channick R, et al. Complications associated with thoracentesis: a prospective, randomized study comparing three different methods. *Arch Intern Med.* 1990;150:873–877.
16. Sahn SA. Pleural diagnostic techniques. *Curr Opin Pulm Med.* 1995;1:324–330.
17. McVay PA, Toy PT. Lack of increased bleeding after paracentesis and thoracentesis in patients with mild coagulation abnormalities. *Transfusion.* 1991;31:164–171.
18. Light RW, Macgregor MI, Luchsinger PC, et al. Pleural effusions: the diagnostic separation of transudates and exudates. *Ann Intern Med.* 1972;77:507–513.
19. Sahn SA. State of the art: the pleura. *Am Rev Respir Dis.* 1988;138:184–234.
20. Starr RL, Sherman ME. The value of multiple preparations in the diagnosis of malignant pleural effusions: a cost-benefit analysis. *Acta Cytol.* 1991;35:533–537.
21. Sahn SA. Pleural fluid pH in the normal state and in disease effecting the pleural space. In: Chestian J,

Bignon J, Hirsch A, ed. *The pleura in health and disease*. New York: Marcel Dekker; 1985:253.

22. Burrows CM, Mathews WC, Colt HG. Predicting survival in patients with recurrent symptomatic malignant pleural effusions: an assessment of the prognostic values of physiologic, morphologic, and quality of life measures of extent of disease. *Chest*. 2000;117:73.

23. Heffner JE, Nietert PJ, Barbieri C. Pleural fluid pH as predictor of survival for patients with malignant pleural effusions. *Chest*. 2000;117:79.

24. Heffner JE, Nietert PJ, Barbieri C. Pleural fluid pH as a predictor of pleurodesis failure: analysis of primary data. *Chest*. 2000;117:87.

25. Heffner JE, Heffner JN, Brown LK. Multilevel and continuous pleural fluid pH likelihood ratios for draining parapneumonic effusions. *Respiration*. 2005;72:351.

26. Jimenez Castro D, Diaz Nuevo G, Sueiro A, et al. Pleural fluid parameters identifying complicated parapneumonic effusions. *Respiration*. 2005;72:357.

27. Neragi S. Malignant pleural effusion, current and evolving approaches for its diagnosis and management. *Lung Cancer*. 2006;54:1–9.

28. Ukale V, Bone D, Hillerdal G, et al. The impact of pleurodesis in malignant effusion on respiratory function. *Respir Med*. 1999;93:898–902.

29. Perpina M, Benlloch E, Marco V, et al. Effect of thoracentesis on pulmonary gas exchange. *Thorax*. 1983;38:747–750.

30. Bouros D, Froudarakis M, Siafakas NM. Pleurodesis: everything flows. *Chest*. 2000;118:577–579.

31. Kroegel C, Antony VB. Immunobiology of pleural inflammation: potential implications for pathogenesis, diagnosis and therapy. *Eur Respir J*. 1997;10:2411–2418.

32. Antony VB. Pathogenesis of malignant pleural effusions and talc pleurodesis. *Pneumologie*. 1999;53:493–498.

33. Dresler CM, Olak J, Herndon JE, et al. Phase III intergroup study of talc poudrage vs. talc slurry sclerosis for malignant pleural effusion. *Chest*. 2005;127:909.

34. Shaw P, Agarwal R. Pleurodesis for malignant pleural effusions. *Cochrane Database Syst Rev*. 2004;(1): CD002916.

35. Sahn SA. Management of malignant pleural effusions. *Monaldi Arch Chest Dis*. 2001;56:394–399.

36. Lorch DG, Gordon L, Wooten S, et al. Effect of patient positioning on distribution of tetracycline in the pleural space during pleurodesis. *Chest*. 1988;93:527–529.

37. Yim AP, Chung SS, Lee TW, et al. Thoracoscopic management of malignant pleural effusions. *Chest*. 1996;109:1234–1238.

38. Hewitt JB, Janssen W. A management strategy for malignancy-induced pleural effusion: long-term thoracostomy drainage. *Oncol Nurs Forum*. 1987;14:17–22.

39. Patz EF, McAdams HP, Goodman PC, et al. Ambulatory sclerotherapy for malignant pleural effusions. *Radiology*. 1996;199:133–135.

40. Tan C, Sedrakyan A, Brown J, et al. The evidence on the effectiveness of management for malignant pleural: a systematic review. *Eur J Cardiothorac Surg*. 2006;29:829.

41. Cardillo G, Facciolo F, Carbone L, et al. Long-term follow-up of video-assisted talc pleurodesis in malignant recurrent pleural effusions. *Eur J Cardiothorac Surg*. 2002;21:302.

42. Steger V, Mika U, Toomes H, et al. Who gains most? A 10-year experience with 611 thoracoscopic talc pleurodeses. *Ann Thorac Surg*. 2007;83:1940.

43. Robinson LA, Fleming WH, Galbraith TA. Intrapleural doxycycline control of malignant pleural effusions. *Ann Thorac Surg*. 1993;55:1115.

44. Erickson KV, Yost M, Bynoe R, et al. Primary treatment of malignant pleural effusions: video-assisted thoracoscopic surgery poudrage versus tube thoracostomy. *Am Surg*. 2002;68:955–959.

45. De Campos JR, Vargas FS, de Campos WE, et al. Thoracoscopy talc poudrage: a 15-year experience. *Chest*. 2001;119:801–806.

46. Campos JR, Werebe EC, Vargas FS, et al. Respiratory failure due to insufflated talc. *Lancet*. 1997;349:251–252.

47. Hausheer FH, Yarbro JW. Diagnosis and treatment of malignant pleural effusion. *Semin Oncol*. 1985;12:54–75.

48. Shoji T, Tanaka F, Yanagihara K, et al. Phase II study of repeated intrapleural chemotherapy using implantable access system for management of malignant pleural effusion. *Chest*. 2002;121:821–824.

49. Moon YW, Choi ST, Cho BC, et al. A case of successful intrapleural chemotherapy with cisplatin plus cytarabine for intractable malignant pleural effusion. *Yonsei Med J*. 2007;48:1035–1038.

50. Rusch VW, Niedzwiecki D, Tao Y, et al. Intrapleural cisplatin and mitomycin for malignant mesothelioma following pleurectomy: pharmacokinetic studies. *J Clin Oncol*. 1992;10:1001–1006.

51. Ichinose Y, Tsuchiya R, Koike T, et al. A prematurely terminated phase III trial of intraoperative intrapleural hypotonic cisplatin treatment in patients with resected non-small cell lung cancer with positive pleural lavage cytology: the incidence of carcinomatous pleuritis after surgical intervention. *J Thorac Cardiovasc Surg*. 2002;123:695–699.

52. Ike O, Shimizu Y, Hitomi S, et al. Treatment of malignant pleural effusions with doxorubicin hydrochloride-containing poly(L-lactic acid) microspheres. *Chest*. 1991;99:911–915.

53. Jones DR, Taylor MD, Petroni GR, et al. Phase I trial of intrapleural docetaxel administered through an implantable catheter in subjects with a malignant pleural effusion. *J Thorac Oncol*. 2010;5:75–81.

54. Pollack JS. Malignant pleural effusions: treatment with tunneled long-term drainage catheters. *Curr Opin Pulm Med*. 2002;8:302–307.

55. Putnam Jr JB, Light RW, Rodriguez RM, et al. A randomized comparison of indwelling pleural catheter and doxycycline pleurodesis in the management of malignant pleural effusions. *Cancer*. 1999;86:1992–1999.

56. Musani AI, Haas AR, Seijo L, et al. Outpatient management of malignant pleural effusions with small-bore, tunneled pleural catheters. *Respiration*. 2004;71:559–566.

57. Van den Toorn LM, Schaap E, Surmont VF, et al. Management of recurrent malignant pleural effusions with a chronic indwelling pleural catheter. *Lung Cancer*. 2005;50:123–127.

58. Putnam JB, Walsh GL, Swisher SG, et al. Outpatient management of malignant pleural effusion by a chronic indwelling pleural catheter. *Ann Thorac Surg*. 2000;69:369–375.

59. Flores RM, Pass HI, Seshan VE, et al. Extrapleural pneumonectomy versus pleurectomy/decortications in the surgical management of malignant pleural mesothelioma: results in 663 patients. *J Thorac Cardiovasc Surg*. 2008;135:620.

60. Rusch VW. Pleurectomy/decortications in the setting of multimodality treatment for diffuse malignant pleural mesothelioma. *Semin Thorac Cardiovasc Surg*. 1997;9:367–372.

61. Pass HI, Pogrebniak HW. Malignant pleural mesothelioma. *Curr Probl Surg*. 1997;30:921–1012.

62. Pass HI, Temeck BK, Kranda K, et al. Preoperative tumor volume is associated with outcome in malignant pleural mesothelioma. *J Thorac Cardiovasc Surg*. 1998;115:310–317.

63. Brancatisano RP, Joseph MG, McCaughan BC. Pleurectomy for mesothelioma. *Med J Aust*. 1991;154:455–457, 460.

64. Tsang V, Fernando HC, Goldstraw P. Pleuroperitoneal shunt for recurrent malignant pleural effusions. *Thorax*. 1990;45:369.

65. Genc O, Petrou M, Ladas G, et al. The long-term morbidity of pleuroperitoneal shunts in the management of recurrent malignant effusions. *Eur J Cardiothorac Surg*. 2000;18:143.

66. Little AG, Ferguson MK, Golomg HM, et al. Pleuroperitoneal shunting for malignant effusions. *Cancer*. 1986;58:2740.

67. Permanyer-Miralda G, Sagrista-Sauleda J, Soler-Soler J. Primary acute pericardial disease: a prospective series of 231 consecutive patients. *Am J Cardiol*. 1985;56:623–630.

68. Buck M, Ingle JN, Guiliani ER, et al. Pericardial effusion in women with breast cancer. *Cancer*. 1987;60:263–269.

69. Woll PJ, Knight RK, Rubens RD. Pericardial effusion complicating breast cancer. *J R Soc Med*. 1987;80:490–491.

70. Celermajer DS, Boyer MJ, Bailey BP, et al. Pericardiocentesis for symptomatic malignant pericardial effusion. *Med J Aust*. 1991;154:19–22.

71. Markiewicz W, Borovik R, Ecker S. Cardiac tamponade in medical patients. *Am Heart J*. 1986;111:1138–1142.

72. Karam N, Patel P, deFilippi C. Diagnosis and management of chronic pericardial effusions. *Am J Med Sci*. 2001;322:79–87.

73. Thomazon R, Schlegel W, Lucca M, et al. Primary malignant mesothelioma of the pericardium: case report and literature review. *Tex Heart Inst J*. 1994;21:170–174.

74. Holtan SG, Allen RD, Henkel DM, et al. Angiosarcoma of the pericardium presenting as hemorrhagic pleuropericarditis, cardiac tamponade, and thromboembolic phenomena. *Int J Cardiol*. 2007;115:e8–9.

75. Cheitlin MD, Armstrong WF, Aurigemma GP, et al. *ACC/AHA/ASE 2003 guideline for the clinical application of echocardiography* Available at: www.acc.org/qualityandscience/clinical/statement.htm.

76. Chong HH, Plotnick GD. Pericardial effusion and tamponade: evaluation, imaging modalities, and management. *Compr Ther*. 1995;21:378–385.

77. Sechtem U, Tscholakoff D, Higgins CB. MRI of the abnormal pericardium. *Am J Roentgenol*. 1986;147:245–252.

78. Tsang T, Barnes M, Hayes S, et al. Clinical and echocardiographic characteristics of significant pericardial effusions following cardiothoracic surgery and outcome of echo-guided pericardiocentesis for management. *Chest*. 1999;116:322–331.

79. Callahan J, Seward J, Nishimura R, et al. Two dimensional echocardiographic guided pericardiocentesis: experience in 117 consecutive patients. *Am J Cardiol*. 1985;55:476–479.

80. Hall JB, Schmidt LD. Emergencies in critical care. In: Hall JB, Schmidt GA, Wood LD, Crinc PF, ed. *Principles of critical care*. New York: McGraw Hill; 1997:1405–1410.

81. Markiewicz W, Borovik R, Ecker S. Cardiac tamponade in medical patients: treatment and prognosis in the echocardiographic era. *Am Heart J*. 1998;111:1138–1142.

82. Kopecky S, Callahan J, Tajik A, et al. Percutaneous pericardial catheter drainage: report of 42 consecutive cases. *Am J Cardiol.* 1986;58:633–635.

83. Wong B, Murphy H, Chang C, et al. The risk of pericardiocentesis. *Am J Cardiol.* 1979;44:1110–1114.

84. Susini G, Pepi M, Sisillo E, et al. Percutaneous pericardiocentesis versus subxiphoid pericardiotomy in cardiac tamponade due to postoperative pericardial effusion. *J Cardiothorac Vasc Anesth.* 1993;7:178–183.

85. Wilkes JD, Fidias P, Vaickus L, et al. Malignancy-related pericardial effusion: 127 cases from the Roswell Park Cancer Institute. *Cancer.* 1995;76:1277–1387.

86. Porte HL, Jaceki-Delebecq TJ, Finzi L, et al. Pericardioscopy for primary management of pericardial effusion in cancer patients. *Eur J Cardiothorac Surg.* 1999;16:287–291.

87. Monte SA, Ehya H, Lang W. Positive effusion cytology as the initial presentation of malignancy. *Acta Cytol.* 1987;31:448–452.

88. Piehler J, Pluth J, Schaff H, et al. Surgical management of effective pericardial disease: influence of extent of pericardial resection on clinical course. *J Thorac Cardiovasc Surg.* 1985;90:506–516.

89. Okamoto H, Shinkai T, Yamakido M, et al. Cardiac tamponade caused by primary lung cancer and the management of pericardial effusion. *Cancer.* 1993;71:93–98.

90. Park J, Rentschler R, Wilbur D. Surgical management of pericardial effusions in patients with malignancies. *Cancer.* 1991;67:76–80.

91. Lema L, McHara O. Subxiphoid pericardiostomy in the management of pericardial effusions. *Cent Afr J Med.* 1991;37:265–268.

92. Vaitkus PT, Herrmann HC, LeWinter MM. Treatment of malignant pericardial effusion. *JAMA.* 1995;272:59–64.

93. Shepard F, Ginsberg J, Evans W, et al. Tetracycline sclerosis in the management of malignancy pericardial effusion. *J Clin Oncol.* 1985;3:1678–1682.

94. Davis S, Rambotti P, Grignani F. Intrapericardial tetracycline sclerosis in the treatment of malignant pericardial effusion: an analysis of 33 cases. *J Clin Oncol.* 1984;2:631–638.

95. Van Belle S, Volckaert A, Taeymans Y, et al. Treatment of malignant pericardial tamponade with sclerosis induced by instillation of bleomycin. *Int J Cardiol.* 1987;16:155–160.

96. Van Der Gaast A, Kok T, Van Der Linden N, et al. Intrapericardial instillation of bleomycin in the management of malignant pericardial effusion. *Eur J Cancer Clin Oncol.* 1989;25:1505–1506.

97. Lee L, Yang P, Chang D, et al. Ultrasound guided pericardial drainage and intrapericardial instillation of mitomycin C for malignant pericardial effusion. *Thorax.* 1994;49:594–595.

98. Inamura T, Tamura K, Takenago M, et al. Intrapericardial OK-432 instillation for the management of malignant pericardial effusion. *Cancer.* 1991;68:259–263.

99. Moriya T, Takiguchi Y, Tabeta H, et al. Controlling malignant pericardial effusion by intrapericardial carboplatin administration in patients with primary non-small-cell lung cancer. *Br J Cancer.* 2000;83:858–862.

100. Florentino M, Daniele O, Morandi P, et al. Intrapericardial instillation of platin in malignant pericardial effusion. *Cancer.* 1988;62:1904–1906.

101. Tomkowski W, Szturmowicz M, Fijalkowska A, et al. Intrapericardial cisplatin for the management of patients with large malignant pericardial effusion. *J Cancer Res Clin Oncol.* 1994;120:434–436.

102. Wilkins H, Cacioppo J, Connoly M, et al. Intrapericardial interferon in the management of malignant pericardial effusion. *Chest.* 1998;114:330–331.

103. Ziskind A, Pearce A, Lemmon C, et al. Percutaneous balloon pericardiotomy for the treatment of cardiac tamponade and large pericardial effusions: description of technique and report of the first 50 cases. *J Am Coll Cardiol.* 1993;21:1–5.

104. Jackson G, Keane E, Mishra B. Percutaneous balloon pericardiotomy in the management of recurrent malignant pericardial effusions. *Br Heart J.* 1992;159:1704–1708.

33 Ascites

Gerhild Becker

Ascites is defined as pathologic accumulation of protein-rich fluid in the peritoneal cavity. The word *ascites* is derived from the Greek term ασκός (Gr. sack, wineskin), meaning "a leather bag or sheepskin used to carry wine, water, or oil." Ascites is the most common complication of cirrhosis and is associated with poor quality of life, increased risk of infection, renal failure, and poor long-term outcomes.[1,2] Already in the 4th century BCE , Hippocrates stated, "When the liver is filled with water and bursts into the epiplöon (the omentum), in this case the belly is filled with water and the patient dies."[3] In addition to cirrhosis of the liver, ascites occurs in heart failure, tuberculosis, and malignancy.

PREVALENCE AND PATHOPHYSIOLOGY

Malignant ascites accounts for ≈10% of all cases of ascites and occurs in association with a variety of neoplasms. Malignant effusion is the escape of fluid from the blood or vessels into tissues or cavities; it is a common problem in patients with cancer. All types of cancer can metastasize to any of the body's serous cavities, resulting in malignant effusion. In the Western world, the most common cause of malignant ascites is ovarian cancer. Other common primary sites are the pancreas, stomach, and uterus, with breast, lung, and lymphoma representing the most common extra-abdominal sites.[4] Up to 20% of all patients with malignant ascites have cancer of unknown primary origin.[5] Except in breast and ovarian cancer, the presence of malignant ascites in patients with neoplastic disease frequently signals the terminal phase of cancer. The mean survival time for ovarian cancer is 30 to 35 weeks, and for tumors of lymphatic origin 58 to 78 weeks, whereas for cancers of the gastrointestinal tract, mean survival is only 12 to 20 weeks. In patients with carcinoma of unknown primary (CUP), the median survival shows great variability, ranging from 1 week to 3 months in different series.

Fluid accumulation in the peritoneal cavity is dependent on the amount of fluid generated and the rate at which it leaves the abdominal cavity. When fluid production exceeds its clearance, free transudate will accumulate. Under physiologic conditions, transudation of plasma through capillary membranes of the peritoneal serosa continuously produces free fluid to lubricate the serosal surfaces. This fluid production is under the influence of portal pressure, plasma oncotic pressure, sodium and water retention, hepatic lymph production, and microvascular permeability for macromolecules. Under physiologic conditions, at least two thirds of the peritoneal fluid reabsorbs into open-ended lymphatic channels of the diaphragm and is propelled cephalad by negative intrathoracic pressure. This fluid proceeds through mediastinal lymph channels into the right thoracic duct and empties into the right subclavian vein. The ability of the healthy subject to resorb fluid is much greater than the fluid generated, with the result that normally only a small volume of fluid is present in the peritoneal cavity. Healthy men have little or no intraperitoneal fluid, but women may normally have as much as 50 ml, depending on the phase of the menstrual cycle.

Ascites as an abnormal accumulation of fluid in the peritoneal cavity can be induced by several causes. In principle, four types can be identified: (1) ascites due to raised hydrostatic pressure, caused by cirrhosis, congestive heart failure, inferior vena cava obstruction, or hepatic vein occlusion; (2) ascites due to decreased osmotic pressure, caused by protein depletion (e.g., nephrotic syndrome), reduced protein intake (malnutrition), or reduced protein production (cirrhosis of the liver); (3) ascites due to fluid production exceeding resorptive capacity, caused by infection or malignancy; and (4) chylous ascites, caused by obstruction and leakage of the lymph channels draining the gut.

The pathophysiology of malignant ascites is multifactorial and is insufficiently understood. Ascites may result from obstruction of lymphatic drainage by tumor cells that prevent absorption of intraperitoneal fluid and protein,[6] as is often seen in lymphoma and breast cancer.[7] Because the ascites of many patients with malignant ascites has a high protein content, alterations in vascular permeability have been implicated in the pathogenesis of ascites production.[8] The tumor induces increasing production of peritoneal fluid caused by increased microvascular permeability of the tumor vasculature; the amount of ascites production correlates with the extent of neovascularization. Aside from mechanical obstruction and cytokines, the pathophysiology of malignant ascites also involves hormonal mechanisms. Because of decreased removal of fluid as a consequence of obstructed lymphatics, the circulating blood volume is reduced, thus activating the renin-angiotensin-aldosterone system, which leads to sodium retention. Therefore, reduced sodium intake together with diuretics is often used to treat malignant ascites, but no consensus on effectiveness has been reached.

DIAGNOSIS

In most cases, ascites can be diagnosed by performing a careful physical examination and taking a detailed history. The main clinical symptoms of ascites include abdominal distention, ankle edema, continuous abdominal discomfort or pain, nausea, vomiting, shortness of breath, and decreased mobility. Greater quantities of ascites cause abdominal distention, bulging flanks that are dull to percussion, shifting dullness, and a fluid wave. Ultrasound is able to detect free peritoneal fluid if its volume is greater than 100 ml. Computed tomography (CT) and magnetic resonance imaging (MRI) are also able to detect small quantities of ascites. Malignancy is indistinguishable by physical examination from ascites caused by nonmalignant conditions. Ascites detected by ultrasound, CT, or MRI in the presence of typical imaging features of a malignant tumor is strongly suggestive of malignant ascites. Diagnosis is confirmed by positive cytology of malignant cells in the fluid. A positive cytology result has a specificity of nearly 100%, but it is not very sensitive, with only about 60% of malignant aspirates cytologic positive.[4,9,10] Immunohistochemical staining combined with conventional cytologic examination increases diagnostic sensitivity. Tumor markers, especially carcinoembryonic antigen (CEA) and cancer antigen (CA)-125, can be useful in diagnosing malignant ascites, although they lack specificity.[11] Compared with ascites caused by cirrhosis, malignant ascites usually contains more white blood cells and a higher level of lactate dehydrogenase. Exudative or transudative ascites on the basis of total protein content (>2.5 or <2.5 g/dl) shows a large overlap between malignant and nonmalignant ascites. Up to 25% of patients with cirrhosis (mostly those with cardiac cirrhosis) can have high protein levels in ascites, and 18% of malignant ascites will be low in protein levels by nature.[12]

Fibronectin, cholesterol, lactate dehydrogenase, sialic acid, proteases, and antiproteases have been studied, with fibronectin performing best in differentiating malignant and nonmalignant ascites in most series, although the origin of fibronectin is unclear. However, at present, no single test is available that routinely differentiates between malignant and nonmalignant ascites. Table 33-1 shows the specificity and sensitivity of different diagnostic variables. In case of doubt, abdominal paracentesis with chemical and cytologic analysis of the ascitic fluid should be used. The cell count provides immediate information about the potential for bacterial infection. Samples with at least 250 neutrophils per cubic millimeter of ascitic fluid are suggestive of infection. Gram stains and culture for bacterial, fungal, and acid-fast organisms are mandatory. Spontaneous bacterial peritonitis (SBP) is characterized by the spontaneous infection of ascitic fluid in the absence of an intra-abdominal source for infection. SBP involves the translocation of bacteria from the intestinal lumen to the lymph nodes, with subsequent bacteremia and infection of ascitic fluid. Third-generation cephalosporins are the treatment of choice for SBP. Ascitic fluid amylase content helps to detect pancreatitis associated ascites and gut perforation.

Eighty percent of all cases of ascites are caused by cirrhosis of the liver. The chief factor contributing to ascites in cirrhosis is portal hypertension. Patients with ascites caused by liver disease usually have a serum-ascites albumin concentration gradient (SAAG; calculated by subtracting the albumin concentration of the ascitic fluid from the albumin concentration of a serum specimen obtained on the same day) >1.1 g/dl. A serum albumin:ascites albumin gradient of >1.1 g/dl indicates with 97% accuracy[13] that the patient has portal hypertension

Table 33-1 Diagnostic parameter for malignant ascites

Parameter	Discrimination	Specificity, %	Sensitivity, %
Total protein concentration in ascitic fluid	>2.5 g/dl	≈70	≈75
Concentration of cholesterol in ascitic fluid	>45 mg/dl	≈70	≈80
Ascites/serum lactate dehydrogenase	>1.0	≈75	≈60
Cytology	Positive	≈100	≈80
Tumor marker (e.g., CEA)	Positive (>2.5 ng/ml)	≈100	≈45

Modified from Wiest.[11]
CEA, Carcinoembryonic antigen.

resulting from liver cirrhosis, massive hepatic metastasis, congestive heart failure, constrictive pericarditis, or Budd-Chiari syndrome.[14] If the gradient is less than 1.1 g/dl, portal hypertension can be essentially excluded. The SAAG need not be repeated after the initial measurement is taken.

TREATMENT

The onset and progression of malignant ascites are associated with deterioration in quality of life and portend a poor prognosis. Symptoms include abdominal distention, nausea, vomiting, early satiety, dyspnea, reduced mobility, weight gain, and problems with body image. It has been estimated that treatment for ascites accounts for 6% of hospice admissions.[15] Different approaches to the treatment of malignant ascites may be used, ranging from symptomatic relief with simple drainage procedures to chemotherapy and debulking surgery aimed at treating the underlying cancer. Paracentesis and diuretics are the most commonly used approaches to management of malignant ascites, followed by peritoneovenous shunts or permanent drains, diet measures, and other modalities such as systemic or intraperitoneal chemotherapy. In general, the management of malignant ascites seems to be guided by evidence derived by managing nonmalignant ascites, especially ascites caused by liver disease. Malignant ascites accounts for approximately 10% of all ascites, whereas more than 80% of cases are clues to chronic liver disease. In contrast to treatment of the underlying cancer, no gold standard to guide the management of malignant ascites is generally accepted.

PHARMACOLOGIC MANAGEMENT

DIET

When ascites is caused by cirrhosis, the most important treatments are restriction of sodium intake and use of oral diuretics; patients with liver cirrhosis retain sodium and water as a result of activation of the renin-angiotensin-aldosterone pathway. Therefore, reduced sodium intake together with diuretics is often used to treat malignant ascites, but no consensus has been reached on effectiveness.[16] Malignant ascites is often highly resistant to salt restriction. However, selected patients with portal hypertension due to hepatic metastases are more likely to respond to salt restriction.[17] Treatment has to be tailored to the illness situation, the life expectancy, and the wishes and needs of the patient.

DIURETIC THERAPY

In liver disease, good evidence for combined therapy with the diuretics spironolactone and furosemide is supported by several randomized controlled trials. No randomized trials have assessed the efficacy of diuretic therapy in malignant ascites. Available data are controversial, and no clear predictors are available to identify patients who would benefit. Therefore, the use of diuretics should be considered in all patients with malignant ascites but must be evaluated individually. Phase II data suggest that patients with malignant ascites due to massive hepatic metastasis are more likely to respond to diuretics than those with malig-

nant ascites caused by peritoneal carcinomatosis or chylous ascites.[18] The SAAG gradient could serve as a guideline for a trial of diuretic therapy. The choice of diuretics is not evidence based. However, available data suggest that efficacy in malignant ascites depends on elevated plasma renin/aldosterone concentrations; aldosterone antagonists such as spironolactone are logical choices, given alone or in combination with a loop diuretic.

CHEMOTHERAPY

For patients suffering from ascites secondary to a primary tumor of known origin, systemic chemotherapy is indicated if the primary has known chemosensibility. This applies, for example, to patients suffering from ovarian carcinoma with malignant ascites,[19] who have a comparatively long median survival of almost 2 years.[20] Systemic chemotherapy may also be considered in patients with symptoms secondary to visceral metastases. However, the benefit of systemic chemotherapy must be balanced against the risk of its toxicity, especially in a palliative treatment situation.

Chemotherapeutic agents can be delivered intraperitoneally immediately after ascites is removed. Through this treatment, high cytotoxic concentrations of active agents can be reached in the abdominal cavity, preventing the recurrence of malignant ascites by destroying cancer at the peritoneal surface and inducing a fibrotic reaction, thereby preventing the formation of peritoneal fluid. Treatment seems to be more effective when the tumor has been responsive to earlier systemic chemotherapy.[8] Debulking of ovarian cancer followed by intraperitoneal chemotherapy improves survival over standard therapy but requires special expertise to deliver the therapy. A significant barrier to effective therapy is drug penetration into bulky, large-volume tumors. The choice of intraperitoneal drug given should be guided by tumor type, prior chemotherapy, drug toxicity profile, and patient's performance status. Intraperitoneal tested drugs include bleomycin, cisplatin plus 5-fluorouracil, cisplatin plus mitomycin, mechlorethamine, thiotepa, and modified FOLFOX (fluorouracil, leucovorin, and oxaliplatin).[21]

Laparoscopic hyperthermic intraperitoneal preoperative chemotherapy (HIPEC) was introduced as a new approach to improve tissue penetration and enhance the cytotoxicity of certain chemotherapeutic agents.[21] Drugs used with HIPEC include cisplatin and etoposide, mitomycin C, paclitaxel, gemcitabine, and 5-fluorouracil.[21,22] Debulking surgery for disseminated intraperitoneal tumors has conflicting reported outcomes. To improve efficacy, a combined approach consisting of optimal debulking surgery immediately followed by HIPEC was investigated in several studies. Data show that cytoreductive surgery in combination with hyperthermic chemotherapy may prolong survival and reduce recurrence of ascites in selected patients with low-grade metastatic gastrointestinal (GI) cancers limited to the peritoneum.[21]

INTRAPERITONEAL RADIOTHERAPY

The instillation of radioactive gold or phosphorous isotopes (Au-198, P-32), which was commonly used in the 1960s, is rarely used now. Even though remissions of 30% are seen with yttrium-90, it is rarely used because of the complex logistics involved in delivery.

IMMUNOTHERAPY

Several immunomodulators have been investigated in the treatment of malignant ascites. These agents work not directly as cytotoxics, but by inducing the immune system to destroy malignant cells. Cytokines such as alpha- and beta-interferon, interleukin-2, and tumor necrosis factor (TNF)-α have been investigated in several studies.[21] In tumors associated with increased activity of vascular endothelial growth factor (VEGF), as is seen in ovarian, gastric, colon, and pancreatic carcinomas, and omental or hepatic metastatic malignancies, biologicals may reduce the production of ascites by inhibiting neovascularization and VEGF through anti–VEGF-receptor antibodies. This concept is comparatively new and is based on small studies. Recent evidence suggests that targeting VEGF through intraperitoneal application of the anti-VEGF antibody bevacizumab (Avastin), which is already in use as an intravenous therapeutic drug for a variety of tumors, might have the potential to suspend the ascites production resulting from peritoneal metastases. However, this therapeutic approach has been studied only in small, single-arm patient series, with 9 patients included in the largest study.[23] An overview of the preclinical and clinical data on bevacizumab for the treatment of malignant effusions was recently published.[24] Bevacizumab might present a new approach for the therapy of malignant ascites, but the first clinical data have to be confirmed in daily clinical practice.

Another new group of active agents for intraperitoneal immunotherapy of malignant ascites is the so-called trifunctional antibodies. The trifunctional antibody catumaxomab has been designed to specifically adhere to the epithelial cell adhesion molecule (EpCAM) of carcinoma cells with one binding arm, with the second binding arm to CD3 receptors of T cells, and with its Fc portion to the Fcγ receptors of accessory cells such as macrophages and natural killer cells, to induce a complex immune response. EpCAM is an antigen that is expressed on many carcinomas, such as breast, lung, colorectal, gastric, prostate, head and neck, pancreatic, and ovarian cancers. The European Medicines Agency (EMEA) recently approved catumaxomab (Removab) for the treatment of malignant ascites in patients with EpCAM-positive tumors for whom no standard therapy is available. Trifunctional antibodies may become an option for the treatment of malignant ascites in selected patients, but the high cost of this therapy has to be considered.

OTHER PHARMACOLOGIC APPROACHES

Infectious agents in nonpathogenic (invasive) form have been utilized as co-stimulatory immunotherapy. Administration of agents such as *Corynebacterium parvum* or OK-432 (a penicillin- and heat-treated powder of Su-strain *Streptococcus pyogenes* A3) into the peritoneal cavity has been investigated in several studies, with responses ranging from 55% to 100% in GI cancer.[21] These studies suggest that this type of therapy may have a role in the management of malignant ascites. Another interesting approach is the inhibition of matrix metalloproteinases (MMPs). MMPs are a family of enzymes present within normal healthy individuals, but produced in high concentrations by a variety of tumors. They are involved in angiogenesis, tumor invasion, and metastasis. Inhibition of these enzymes plays a role in targeting tumor spread. MMP inhibitors such as Batimastat (BB94) are cytostatics but are

synergistic when combined with chemotherapy. Octreotide, a somatostatin analog known to decrease the secretion of fluid by the intestinal mucosa, and to increase water and electrolyte reabsorption, has been used in the symptomatic management of bowel obstruction and uncontrolled diarrhea. It was used successfully in case reports on managing malignant ascites[25]; its efficacy is currently being evaluated in a randomized, placebo-controlled trial.[26] The corticosteroid triamcinolone hexacetanide has been used for hemodialysis patients who develop ascites refractory to salt restriction and diuretic therapy.[27] In ascites associated with cancer, it prolonged the mean time to the need for paracentesis from 2.5 to 17.5 days in 15 patients. It was postulated that the therapeutic effect was mediated by inhibition of VEGF-induced capillary leakage.[28] A phase II study found that repeated instillation of Iscador M (viscum album extract) into the peritoneal cavity reduced malignant ascites accumulation and the need for repeated paracentesis.[29] However, all of these investigational therapies have been studied in small, single-arm patient series only. Randomized controlled studies and comparative trials are lacking.

NONPHARMACOLOGIC MANAGEMENT

Patients with cirrhosis whose ascites is resistant to standard diuretics are treated by paracentesis, peritoneovenous shunting, transjugular portosystemic stenting, and extracorporeal ultrafiltration of ascitic fluid with reinfusion or liver transplantation. Whereas transjugular portosystemic stenting, extracorporeal ultrafiltration, and liver transplantation are specific to liver disease, abdominal paracentesis and peritoneovenous shunting are often used in managing malignant ascites.

THERAPEUTIC PARACENTESIS

Paracentesis provides temporary relief of symptoms related to fluid in about 90% of patients. No consensus has been reached on the amount or rate of fluid withdrawal. The timing of paracentesis varies from 30 to 90 minutes[30] to 24 hours.[31] Complications include peritonitis, pulmonary emboli, and hypotension.[32] Repeated large-volume paracentesis without plasma volume expansion is associated with a significantly higher incidence of hypotension and renal impairment. Several studies have explored this topic in the context of benign ascites due to liver disease,[4] but in the context of malignant ascites, only limited evidence is available. Fischer reported about 300 individuals undergoing abdominal paracentesis for malignant ascites. Dextrose 5% was infused intravenously simultaneously, and no episodes of severe hypotension were reported.[33] Patients with benign ascites who undergo large-volume paracentesis benefit from intravenous albumin, which is superior to other plasma expanders in preventing circulatory dysfunction.[34] However, randomized studies show no significant difference in survival between patients receiving albumin and those treated with other plasma expanders.[34] With malignant ascites, no trials of concurrent intravenous albumin infusions have been reported. In the context of liver disease, up to 5 L can be removed quickly without the risk of adversely affecting plasma volume or renal function.[35–37]

Stephenson and Gilbert retrospectively analyzed 30 cases of paracentesis in 12 patients with malignant ascites after implementing a guideline that allowed up to 5 L of fluid to drain without clamping, and intravenous fluids only when specifically indicated. Intravenous fluids or blood products were given during six procedures, and no instances of symptomatic hypotension occurred.[38] McNamara conducted a prospective study in patients. Significant improvement in symptoms of abdominal pressure was noted with the removal of a few liters (range, 0.8–15 L; mean, 5.3 L; median, 4.9 L). Severe adverse effects were not seen. It was assumed that patients did not receive intravenous fluids, plasma expanders, or blood products, although this was not explicitly stated.[39] No randomized trials have been undertaken to compare paracentesis versus the use of diuretics in the management of malignant ascites.

PERITONEOVENOUS SHUNTS

Although paracentesis is an effective modality to relieve symptomatic ascites, recurrence is an issue, and many patients require multiple paracenteses. Patients need to return repeatedly for the procedure, and each puncture is associated with a small but existing risk of bleeding and/or infection. Concerns have been expressed regarding loss of protein from the ascitic fluid, which would worsen hypoalbuminemia. For patients with longer life expectancies who need repeated large-volume paracentesis, peritoneovenous shunting is another option. Originally, the peritoneovenous shunt was developed for patients with intractable ascites from cirrhosis,[8] but it subsequently became a popular procedure for managing malignant ascites.[16] Two main types of shunts are available for use: the LeVeen shunt[40] and the Denver shunt.[41] The LeVeen shunt drains ascitic fluid into the superior vena cava through a one-way valve, which opens with a pressure of 3 cm of H_2O. The Denver shunt works on the same principle. The valves open at a positive pressure gradient of about 1 cm H_2O; this is one way of preventing detectable reflux. No prospective randomized studies have compared the patency rates of the two systems in malignant ascites.

The objective of using shunts is to achieve symptom relief and prevent the need for repeat paracentesis and resulting protein and fluid depletion. Hemorrhagic ascites and ascitic fluid protein content greater than 4.5 g/L are considered contraindications for shunting because of the high risk of shunt occlusion.[8] Loculated ascites, portal hypertension, coagulation disorders, and advanced cardiac or renal failure are also contraindications.[8] Although the shunt drains fluid with malignant cells from the peritoneal space to the venous system, clinical observations and findings at necropsy do not reveal clinically important hematogenous metastases.[18] However, postmortem examinations are not performed routinely, and this complication may be underreported. Median survival of patients with malignant ascites and shunting varies between 52 and 266 days, reflecting better patient selection than is seen with repeat paracentesis.[8] In all reported studies, patients with ovarian and breast cancer who undergo peritoneovenous shunting have the best response rate (≥50%), whereas the response rate in patients with GI cancers is far worse (10%–15%).[8] Because of poor prognosis and response, it is agreed by most investigators that shunt insertion is contraindicated in patients with malignant ascites due to gastrointestinal cancer.[8,32]

Shunts are associated with potentially fatal side effects and are costly in terms of time and money. Patients need to be monitored closely for at least 24 hours after operation with a central venous pressure line to monitor fluid balance. Therefore, a shunt should be used only when other treatment options, such as diuretics, have failed, and when life expectancy is long enough to derive benefit. No consensus has been reached on expected survival; some investigators advocate longer than 1 month, and others suggest an expected survival of at least 3 months.[18] The use of shunts has to be balanced by potential risks of this procedure. A review of 27 studies and 634 patients treated with LeVeen or Denver shunts found that major complications such as disseminated intravascular coagulation, infection, pulmonary edema, or pulmonary emboli are to be expected in 6% of patients.[18]

PERMANENT DRAINS

Patients with limited life expectancy should have permanent drains when management requires serial paracentesis. Two types of exteriorized drainage catheters are used. One type is tunneled under the skin (e.g., Tenckhoff catheter,[42] peritoneal Port-A-Cath,[43] PleurX catheter[44]); the other type is an external pigtail catheter. At Freiburg University Hospital, we use the PleurX catheter, a system that is approved by the FDA for the treatment of malignant ascites (original manufacturer: Denver Biomedical, Golden, CO; current manufacturer: Care Fusion, San Diego, CA). The PleurX catheter is a silicone catheter with an airtight valve in the hub, which allows the catheter to remain in place indefinitely and can be accessed by the patient or caregiver for intermittent drainage using a vacuum bottle (Fig. 33-1). Tunneled catheter systems have two potential advantages over nontunneled (pigtail) catheters: lower infection rates and greater stability.[45] Recently published data support the use of permanent drains to provide symptom relief for most patients with comparatively few side effects.[45,46] Complications include infection, malfunction or occlusion, dislodgment, and protein loss. Permanent drains are generally managed by patients and their families; therefore, families need to be educated about the care and use of permanent catheters. The catheters are placed under local anesthesia with ultrasonographic guidance. With appropriate patient and family education, these catheters can be placed on an outpatient basis, and intermittent drainage can be performed by the patient or caregiver at home.

Life expectancy in patients with advanced cancer and malignant ascites is limited, and placement of permanent drains maximizes time spent out of hospital. On the other hand, permanent catheters can adversely influence psychosocial function and produce physical constraints associated with exteriorized drains. These catheters require patient cooperation in terms of the ability to live with and care for the catheter system.

MANAGEMENT OF SYMPTOMATIC MALIGNANT ASCITES

Although abdominal paracentesis, diuretics, peritoneovenous shunting, and insertion of permanent drains are commonly used procedures in managing malignant ascites, randomized controlled trials evaluating the efficacy and safety of these therapies are lacking.

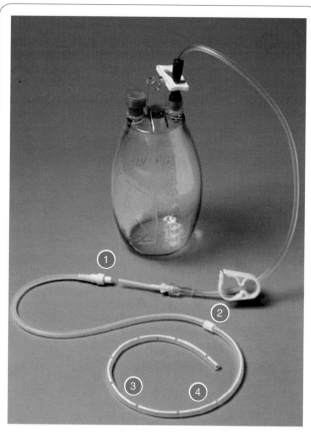

Fig. 33-1 PleurX catheter.
1. **Safety valve:** Helps prevent inadvertent passage of air or fluid through the catheter.
2. **Polyester cuff:** Promotes tissue in-growth to help reduce infection risk and hold the catheter securely in place.
3. **15.5 French silicone catheter:** Conforms to the peritoneal space and minimizes insertion site discomfort.
4. **Fenestrated length 26 cm:** Fenestrations with beveled edges promote drainage and help avoid plugging.

Based on a systematic review critically summarizing available evidence on the effectiveness of diuretics, abdominal paracentesis, and peritoneovenous shunting,[18] on a literature overview of indwelling peritoneal catheters,[45,46] and on data on the use of catumaxomab,[47] the following recommendations from the revised grading system prepared by the Scottish Intercollegiate Guidelines Network (SIGN) are given:

1. Paracentesis is indicated for those patients who have symptoms of increasing intra-abdominal pressure. The strength of evidence is good, although only temporary relief of symptoms occurs in most patients. Discomfort, dyspnea, nausea, and vomiting are relieved by draining up to 5 L of fluid. (Grade of Recommendation: D)
2. When up to 5 L of fluid is removed, intravenous fluids are not routinely required. (Grade of Recommendation: D)
3. When patients are hypotensive or dehydrated or are known to have severe renal impairment and paracentesis is indicated, intravenous hydration should be considered. Infusion therapy has not been sufficiently studied to support the practice. The only therapy reported in malignant ascites is infusion of dextrose 5%. No evidence is available to support the practice of concurrent albumin infusions in patients with malignant ascites. (Grade of Recommendation: D)
4. When patients have a long life expectancy, peritoneovenous shunting should be considered to avoid repeated paracentesis. Major complications (pulmonary edema, pulmonary emboli, clinically relevant disseminated intravascular coagulation, and infection) are expected in 6% of patients. (Grade of Recommendation: D)
5. In patients with limited life expectancy, insertion of indwelling intraperitoneal (IP) catheters may be considered when fluid control cannot be achieved by paracentesis. Indwelling IP catheters are an effective and safe palliative strategy for managing refractory malignant ascites. Major complications include catheter-related infection, leakage from the catheter site, catheter occlusion, and fatal hypotension. Independent of the catheter type, the risk of peritonitis seems to be lower with tunneled IP catheters than with nontunneled systems. (Grade of Recommendation: D)
6. No randomized controlled trials have been undertaken to assess the efficacy of diuretic therapy in malignant ascites. The evidence is controversial, and no clear predictors can identify which patients would benefit from diuretics. The use of diuretics should be considered in all patients but has to be evaluated individually. Patients with malignant ascites due to massive hepatic metastasis are more likely to respond to diuretics than are patients with malignant ascites caused by peritoneal carcinomatosis or chylous ascites. (Grade of Recommendation: D)
7. The choice of diuretics is not evidence based. Efficacy in malignant ascites depends on plasma renin/aldosterone concentration. It is reasonable to consider aldosterone antagonists such as spironolactone given alone or in combination with a loop diuretic. (Grade of Recommendation: D)
8. Doses and schedules of diuretics have not been evaluated in patients with malignant ascites. There is no reason to diverge from standard clinical practice in treating ascites from cirrhosis. Dosage and schedule should be selected according to the manufacturer's instructions and package inserts. (Grade of Recommendation: D)
9. In patients with EpCAM-positive tumors, refractory ascites, and adequate life expectancy, treatment with the trifunctional antibody catumaxomab (Removab) may be considered. Randomized controlled trials in patients with ovarian cancer and malignant ascites demonstrate that patients receiving catumaxomab have a fourfold increased puncture-free survival over those treated with paracentesis alone. The European Medicines Agency (EMEA) has approved this agent for the treatment of malignant ascites in patients with EpCAM-positive tumors for whom no standard therapy is available. (Grade of Recommendation: B)

REFERENCES

1. Ginès P, Quintero E, Arroyo V, et al. Compensated cirrhosis: natural history and prognostic factors. *Hepatology.* 1987;7:122–128.
2. Ginès P, Fernández-Esparrach G. Prognosis of cirrhosis with ascites. In: Arroyo V, Ginès P, Rodés J, Schrier RW, ed. *Ascites and renal dysfunction in liver disease: pathogenesis, diagnosis and treatment.* Malden, MA: Blackwell Science; 1999:431–441.
3. Adams F. Trans. *The genuine works of Hippocrates.* [Translated from the Greek with a preliminary discourse and annotations.] Volume II, Aphorisms, Section VII, 55. London: The Syndenham Society London; 1949:770.
4. Runyon BA. Care of patients with ascites. *N Engl J Med.* 1994;330:337–342.
5. Ringenberg QS, Doll DC, Loy TS, et al. Malignant ascites of unknown origin. *Cancer.* 1989;64:753–755.
6. Garrison RN, Galloway RH, Heuser LS. Mechanisms of malignant ascites production. *J Surg Res.* 1987;42:126–132.
7. Olopade OI, Ultmann JE. Malignant effusions. *CA Cancer J Clin.* 1991;41:166–179.
8. Adam RA, Adam YG. Malignant ascites: past, present, and future. *J Am Coll Surg.* 2004;198:999–1011.
9. Castaldo G, Oriani G, Cimino L, et al. Total discrimination of peritoneal malignant ascites form cirrhosis and hepatocarcinoma-associated ascites by assays of ascetic cholesterol and lactate dehydrogenase. *Clin Chem.* 1994;40:478–483.
10. Runyon BA, Hoefs JC, Morgan TR. Ascitic fluid analysis in malignancy related ascites. *Hepatology.* 1988;8:1104–1109.
11. Wiest R, Schölmerich J. Diagnosis and therapy of ascites. *Dtsch Ärztebl.* 2006;103:1972–1981.
12. Siddiqui RA, Kochhar R, Singh V, et al. Evaluation of fibronectin as a marker of malignant ascites. *J Gastroenterol Hepatol.* 1992;7:161–164.
13. Aslam N, Marino CR. Malignant ascites: new concepts in pathophysiology, diagnosis, and management. *Arch Intern Med.* 2001;161:2733–2737.
14. Saif MW, Siddiqui IAP, Sohail MA. Management of ascites due to gastrointestinal malignancy. *Ann Saudi Med.* 2009;29:369–377.
15. Regnard C, Mainx K. Management of ascites in advanced cancer—a flow diagram. *Palliat Med.* 1989;4:45–47.
16. Lee CW, Bociek G, Faught W. A survey of practice in management of malignant ascites. *J Pain Symptom Manage.* 1998;16:96–101.
17. Parsons SL, Lang MW, Steele RJ. Malignant ascites: a 2-year review from a teaching hospital. *Eur J Surg Oncol.* 1996;22:237–239.

18. Becker G, Galandi D, Blum HE. Malignant ascites: systematic review and guideline for treatment. *Eur J Cancer.* 2006;42:589–597.
19. Du Bois A, Lück HJ, Meier W, et al. A randomized clinical trial of cisplatin/paclitaxel versus carboplatin/paclitaxel as first-line treatment of ovarian cancer. *J Natl Cancer Inst.* 2003;95:1320–1329.
20. Ayantunde AA, Parsons SL. Pattern and prognostic factors in patients with malignant ascites: a retrospective study. *Ann Oncol.* 2007;18:945–949.
21. Chung M, Kozuch P. Treatment of malignant ascites: current treatment options in oncology. *Curr Treat Options Oncol.* 2008;9:215–233.
22. Valle M, Van der Speeten K, Garofalo A. Laparoscopic hyperthermic intraperitoneal preoperative chemotherapy (HIPEC) in the management of refractory malignant ascites: a multi-institutional retrospective analysis in 52 patients. *J Surg Oncol.* 2009;100:331–334.
23. El-Shami K, Elsaid A, El-Kem Y. Open label safety and efficacy pilot trial of intraperitoneal bevacizumab as palliative treatment in refractory malignant ascites. ASCO Abstract. *J Clin Oncol.* 2007;25(18 suppl):9043.
24. Kobold S, Hegewisch-Becker S, Oechsle K, et al. Intraperitoneal VEGF inhibition using bevacizumab: a potential approach for the symptomatic treatment of malignant ascites? *Oncologist.* 2009;14:1242–1251.
25. Cairns W, Malone R. Octreotide as an agent for the relief of malignant ascites in palliative care patients. *Palliat Med.* 1999;13:429–430.
26. National Cancer Institute. *Phase III randomized study of octreotide in patients with cancer-related symptomatic malignant ascites.* Protocol summary at: http://www.cancer.gov/clinicaltrials/NCCTG-N04C2; Accessed 29.01.20.
27. Diaz-Buxo JA, Chandler JT, Farmer CD, et al. Intraperitoneal infusion of non-absorbable steroids in the treatment of ascites and sterile peritonitis. *J Dial.* 1980;4:43–50.
28. Mackey JR, Wood L, Nabholtz JM, et al. A phase II trial of triamcinolone hexacetanide for symptomatic recurrent malignant ascites. *J Pain Symptom Manage.* 2000;19:193–199.
29. Bar-Sela G, Goldberg H, Beck D, et al. Reducing malignant ascites accumulation by repeated intraperitoneal administrations of a Viscum album extract. *Anticancer Res.* 2006;26:709–713.
30. Gotlieb WH, Feldman B, Feldman-Moran O, et al. Intraperitoneal pressures and clinical parameters of total paracentesis for palliation of symptomatic ascites in ovarian cancer. *Gynecol Oncol.* 1998;71:381–385.
31. Appelqvist P, Silvo J, Salmela L, et al. On the treatment and prognosis of malignant ascites:

is the survival time determined when the abdominal paracentesis is needed? *J Surg Oncol.* 1982;20:238–242.
32. Parsons SL, Watson SA, Steele RJC. Malignant ascites. *Br J Surg.* 1996;83:6–14.
33. Fischer DS. Abdominal paracentesis of malignant ascites. *Arch Intern Med.* 1979;139:235.
34. Gines P, Cardenas A, Arroyo V, et al. Management of cirrhosis and ascites. *N Engl J Med.* 2004;350:1646–1654.
35. Kao HW, Rakov NE, Savage E, et al. The effect of large volume paracentesis on plasma volume—a cause of hypovolemia? *Hepatology.* 1985;5:403–407.
36. Kellerman PS, Linas SL. Large volume paracentesis in treatment of ascites. *Ann Intern Med.* 1990;112:889–891.
37. Reynolds TB. Renaissance of paracentesis in the treatment of ascites. *Adv Intern Med.* 1990;112:365–374.
38. Stephenson J, Gilbert J. The development of clinical guidelines on paracentesis for ascites related to malignancy. *Palliat Med.* 2002;16:213–218.
39. McNamara P. Paracentesis—an effective method of symptom control in the palliative care setting? *Palliat Med.* 2000;14:62–64.
40. LeVeen HH, Cristoudias G, Ip M, et al. Peritoneovenous shunting for ascites. *Ann Surg.* 1974;180:580–590.
41. Lund RH, Newkirk JB. Peritoneovenous shunting system for surgical management of ascites. *Contemp Surg.* 1979;14:31–45.
42. Barnett TD, Rubins J. Placement of a permanent tunneled peritoneal drainage catheter for palliation of malignant ascites: a simplified percutaneous approach. *J Vasc Interv Radiol.* 2002;13:379–383.
43. Ozkan O, Akinci D, Gocmen R, et al. Percutaenous placement of peritoneal port-catheter in patients with malignant ascites. *Cardiovasc Intervent Radiol.* 2007;30:232–236.
44. Iyengar TD, Herzog TJ. Management of symptomatic ascites in recurrent ovarian cancer patients using an intra-abdominal semi-permanent catheter. *Am J Hosp Palliat Care.* 2002;19:35–38.
45. Flemming ND, Alvarez-Secord A, Fleming ND, et al. Indwelling catheters for the management of refractory malignant ascites: a systematic literature overview and retrospective chart review. *J Pain Symptom Manage.* 2009;38:341–349.
46. Rosenberg S, Courtney A, Nemcek AAJ, et al. Comparison of percutaneous management techniques for recurrent malignant ascites. *J Vasc Interv Radiol.* 2004;15:1129–1131.
47. Sebastian M, Kuemmel A, Schmidt M, et al. Catumaxomab: a bispecific trifunctional antibody. *Drugs Today.* 2009;45:589–597.

Venous access systems, port catheters, and central lines

34

Hans-Heinrich Wolf, Karin Jordan, and Christof Kramm

Central venous catheters (CVCs) are widely used to provide safe venous access for hemodialysis, administration of cytotoxic drugs and antimicrobial therapies, parenteral nutrition, balanced electrolyte infusion treatment, and support of blood components, but also for diagnostic reasons such as cardiovascular management. Especially in children and intensive care patients, CVCs are useful for collecting venous blood samples for analysis. Therefore, physicians should be aware of specific advantages and typical complications of different catheter systems.

Infections are the most common complications related to CVCs; these include exit site infections, endoluminal infections, and catheter-associated septicemia. However, mechanical complications also can be seen in daily practice. Because most of these complications can be prevented or attenuated by proper handling, strategies should be established for insertion and management of CVCs in every department. To develop a special standard of care in every hospital, complication rates and a survey of catheter-associated infections should be registered.[1] Documentation of catheter days and parameters such as flushing, patient diaries, types of permanent catheters, date of insertion, and flushing technique, as well as management programs for healthcare professionals and patients, are useful. Totally implantable venous access ports are valuable for long-term intravenous treatment, especially when chemotherapy is administered. This chapter provides an overview of typical complications associated with central venous lines (CVLs) with a focus on port devices. Infectious complications are the most frequent; however, thromboembolic and mechanical complications such as extravasation, the pinch-off syndrome, catheter dislocation, occlusion, and leakage are also discussed.

MECHANICAL COMPLICATIONS

Individuals performing venous and arterial puncture routinely use assisted sonography for catheter placement to avoid bleeding complications, especially in thrombocytopenic patients.[2] In some pediatric hospitals, patients are examined even more carefully to avoid incorrect or arterial CVC placement with radiographic, echocardiographic, and blood oxygenation assessments. Before a CVL is used for chemotherapy, a blood sample should be aspirated; this should be followed by injection of saline, then drug infusion should be started.[3] Local discomfort or swelling should be assessed. After chemotherapy administration, the device should be flushed with at least 25 ml saline. Compatibility of cytotoxic drugs and central venous devices needs to be considered to avoid chemical interactions.

This chapter does not focus on surgical problems following the implantation of catheters and ports; however, complication rates depend on perioperative conditions, surgical experience, technique of catheter placement used, the product that is being administered, and postoperative care. They are also influenced by the patient's condition, age, and performance status. The port should be sutured in the fascia, preferably with nonabsorbable sutures to prevent distortion and possible catheter retraction. Port catheter retraction is a rare complication. A safe connection between catheter and port chamber should be assured by the surgeon. Any use of clamps has to be avoided. Radiographs are performed postoperatively and after extraction to ensure placement.

Implantation of port catheters is intended to provide safe venous access. However, extravasation injuries can still range up to 6%. Irritant drugs cause inflammation and pain at the site of an extravasation; vesicant drugs may induce severe soft tissue necrosis or persistent ulceration, which will require surgical treatment. Extravasation may occur as the result of leakage or needle dislocation during infusion: The puncture may have been made outside the reservoir, or the needle may have become dislodged from the port membrane. Correct placement and proper infusion rate control are important to avoid needle dislocation. Correct placement requires the catheter tip to be in the distal superior caval vein; this should be documented by radiography. Radiography should also be performed if malfunction of the port system, port occlusion, or venous thrombosis is suspected. Spontaneous migration of the catheter tip can cause pain in the neck and shoulder, phlebitis, or ascending thrombosis of cervical and cerebral veins, with an incidence of 0.9% to 1.8%. Catheters should be replaced interventionally by experienced radiologists.

Catheter disconnection is a rare complication (incidence, 0.1%–2 %). Several patient-related reasons for catheter disconnection are known, such as extensive arm movements during sports and the use of backpacking equipment. Increased intraluminal pressure, especially with catheter flushing, increases the risk of disconnection or will cause damage to the port reservoirs. To avoid excessive intraluminal peak pressures, the syringe used for injections should hold at least 10 ml; in very small children (body weight less than 10 kg), even less volume (5-ml syringes) and reduced injection time (at least 1 minute) should be provided for flushing. Port chamber defects are related to flaws in the port material or construction port defects; the device should be disposed of immediately.

Other mechanical complications include the pinch-off syndrome (Fig. 34-1),[4] catheter fragmentation, rupture or embolization, catheter disconnection, port chamber defects (Fig. 34-2),[4] and port catheter retraction, respectively. Mechanical compression of the CVL between the clavicle and the upper rib is referred to as the pinch-off syndrome and is observed in up to 5% of ports. Compression causes transient obstruction of the catheter and possibly catheter fragmentation. Impaired reflux and reduced flow may be warning signs.

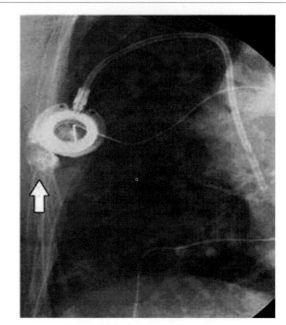

Fig. 34-2 Port chamber defect.

The incidence of pinch-off syndrome rises with medial and infraclavicular catheter insertions. The syndrome is prevented by introducing the catheter into the internal jugular vein or by inserting it into the subclavian vein at a more lateral position between clavicle and rib. If chest radiography reveals the pinch-off syndrome, the catheter should be replaced. Catheter embolization can induce ventricular tachycardia, mechanical irritation of the myocardium, thrombosis, and endocarditis. Embolized catheters should be removed transvenously by an interventional radiologist.

THROMBOTIC COMPLICATIONS

The frequency of symptomatic venous thrombosis ranges up to16%. Catheter-related thrombus may occur at the catheter tip (ball valve clot), intraluminally (fibrin sheath), or intravascularly. The cause of thrombosis is often multifactorial.[5] Vascular insertion or mechanical irritation causes endothelial damage and local activation of the coagulation system. Chemotherapeutic agents or electrolyte infusions can induce endothelial damage, leading to thrombosis.

Clinically suspected venous thrombosis should be confirmed sonographically. No significant risk of pulmonary embolism is associated with catheter-related thrombosis of the subclavian veins. Thrombosis should be treated with low-molecular-weight heparin (LMWH) or fondaparinux in case of heparin-induced thrombocytopenia type II (HIT II). Progressive thrombosis during heparin therapy should give reason for consideration of HIT II and initiation of tests.

A close correlation has been noted between catheter-related thrombosis and catheter-related infection. Colonization of the CVC by microorganisms without clinical signs of infection is a major risk factor for subsequent catheter-related thrombosis. Therefore, strict antiseptic handling of catheters is crucial to avoid both thrombosis and infection.

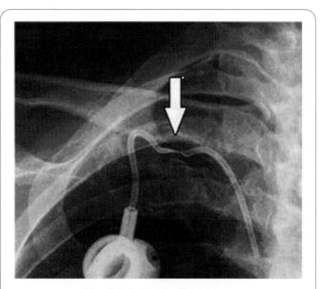

Fig. 34-1 Pinch-off syndrome.

Up to 25% of CVCs will occlude. Prophylactic heparin instillation (500 IU unfractionated heparin/ml) into the catheter does not reduce the risk of catheter occlusion. In cases of recent occlusion of permanent catheters (e.g., Hickman, Broviac), thrombolysis by instillation of low-dose urokinase may be helpful, even if no clear recommendation can be found in the literature. Thrombus embolization caused by bolus injection must be avoided. In summary, in case of obstruction of the permanent catheter, any further need for CVC should be evaluated critically, and extraction should be preferred if new placement of another CVC seems possible.

No clear evidence of benefit has been found for prophylactic anticoagulation in adults with CVLs; no type or dosage of anticoagulant and no duration of treatment have been effective. Neither low-dose warfarin nor LMWH prophylaxis clearly reduces the risk of catheter-related thrombosis in every subgroup of cancer patients. Furthermore, anticoagulant prophylaxis increases bleeding complications in thrombocytopenic patients. Because low-dose heparin increases the risk of HIT II, hematologists prefer to flush without heparin.

Children with cancer and endogenous plasminogen activator inhibitor type 1 (PAI-1) polymorphism, gene mutations in methylenetetrahydrofolate reductase (MTHFR), or coagulation factor II or V genes are at increased risk for catheter-related thrombosis. In adults, however, the incidence of catheter-related thrombosis is related to factors other than genetic risk, including tumor type and growth, venous compression, and vessel obstruction. Administration of procoagulant drugs or drugs that favor procoagulant to fibrinolytic factors such as asparaginase increases thrombotic risk. For patients who present with one of these risk factors, the implantation of a permanent port catheter should be evaluated carefully.[5a]

INFECTIOUS COMPLICATIONS

The diagnosis of catheter-related infection (CRI) is based on clinical symptoms (redness, swelling, pain, purulent exudate) along the subcutaneous tunnel of the CVC or around the port systems. Local signs of inflammation may be absent in neutropenic patients.

Bacterial colonization at the insertion site is a major risk factor for occlusion, infection, or septicemia. Skin lesions secondary to chemotherapy or graft-versus-host disease increase the risk of infection. To avoid extraluminal spread of bacteria along the central venous tunnel, the lines should be changed routinely. Catheter hubs, infusion solutions, and connecting branches to the CVL should be changed under sterile conditions. Inside the endoluminal lining of the inner surface of catheters, a so-called biofilm develops within 24 hours after insertion. This biofilm is composed of polysaccharides, fibrin, fibronectin, or lamina and appears to be important in the pathogenesis of CRI. Microorganisms are embedded and protected from host defense mechanisms and antimicrobial drugs. After colonization, microorganisms proliferate within the biofilm, and this may lead to systemic infection.[6–8]

Catheter colonization is believed to occur when microorganisms are detected on the catheter surface, even if clinical signs of infection are absent. Microorganism adherence depends on the physical properties of the catheter material and the biofilm electric charge. Hydrophobic staphylococci and *Candida* spp. seem to colonize polyvinylchloride and silicone catheters more frequently than polyurethane catheters.

EPIDEMIOLOGY OF CENTRAL VENOUS CATHETER–RELATED INFECTIONS

Data concerning the incidence of CRI are difficult to compare because of inconsistent definitions, the heterogeneity of patient populations (e.g., different predisposition in surgical patients, patients with burn injuries, cancer or HIV patients, bone marrow transplant recipients, neonates), the use of different types of catheters, and the selection of different local strategies to prevent infection.[9] To specify CRI rates, most authors refer to the number of catheter-related infections per 1000 days of catheter placement (CRI/1000 days CVC).

The lowest infection rates (0.1 infection/1000 CVC days) are reported in oncology patients with port systems. Tunneled catheters are preferred for use in high-risk patients (e.g., allogeneic bone marrow transplant recipients) and are associated with an infection rate of 5 to 6 per 1000 catheter days. Tunneled catheters are at increased risk for CRI during neutropenic periods of time compared with non-neutropenic periods. Nontunneled CVCs are associated with a substantially higher rate of infection. No difference is seen in infection rates between peripherally and directly inserted CVCs.

RISK FACTORS FOR CRI

Catheter time frame, frequency of manipulation (e.g., blood samplings, injections), site of insertion, and administration of (high-caloric) parenteral nutrition are identified risk factors for CRI. Two studies in hemato-oncologic patients suggest that even subclinical thrombosis of the catheterized vein, as detected by ultrasound, is an important risk factor for subsequent CRI.[11] Colonization of CVC by microorganisms is a major risk factor for subsequent catheter-related thrombosis. Most reviews stress that CRI is a significant risk factor for disease-related mortality. The risk of septic complications is correlated with duration of neutropenia.

PATHOGENS

A broad spectrum of pathogens may cause catheter-related infections, but gram-positive bacteria predominate. A U.S. surveillance study analyzing all pathogens isolated from blood cultures in cancer patients with or without CVCs found that gram-positive organisms accounted for more than 70% of all nosocomial bloodstream infections. Coagulase-negative staphylococci (CoNS) are the most common isolates in catheter-related bacteremia. *Staphylococcus aureus, Corynebacteria, Enterococci,* gram-negative bacteria *(Pseudomonas aeruginosa, Stenotrophomonas maltophilia, Acinetobacter baumannii),* and *Candida* spp. are also seen commonly.[12]

Diagnosis of catheter-related bacteremia or fungemia is confirmed by detection of the identified organism in blood and catheter cultures. In clinical practice, identified isolated organisms are assumed to be the cause of CRI when results of in vitro susceptibility testing are identical. However, a recent study evaluating infection due to coagulase-negative staphylococci demonstrated genetically different organisms by DNA fingerprinting in one quarter of infections, despite in vitro susceptibility testing. According to the Centers for Disease Control and Prevention (CDC) definition, a diagnosis of nosocomial bloodstream infection (laboratory-confirmed bloodstream infection) is confirmed in patients with indwelling intravascular devices treated with appropriate antimicrobial therapy through detection of "skin contaminants" in at least one blood culture.

DIAGNOSIS

Diagnostic procedures are initiated quickly to avoid a concomitant systemic infection. Clinical signs of infection may include local induration or tenderness (within 2 cm of the venipuncture), fever, and/or sepsis, or a combination of these. If tunnel infection is suspected, ultrasound should be performed along the catheter. Physical examinations, chest X-ray, and microbiological tests (blood cultures) are recommended. Additional diagnostic procedures depend on clinical symptoms because no gold standard has been established for the diagnosis of CRI.

Skin swabs of purulent secretions at the exit site may be misleading if a difference between colonizing and pathogenic organisms is detected. Therefore, "targeted" antimicrobial therapy based on swab cultures is not sufficient in every case of catheter-related systemic infection.

Most countries have recommendations for empirical antibiotic and antimycotic treatment for neutropenic patients with suspected CRI.[13–16]

Blood cultures

At least two pairs of blood cultures with adequate volume (≥20 ml in adults) must be obtained: one from a peripheral vein, the other from every single-catheter lumen, as colonization may occur within one lumen only. Differential time to positivity (DTTP) is a useful diagnostic indicator; it refers to the time interval to positive microbiological results of blood cultures taken from the CVC and peripheral vein. This method does not require any additional resources because information is provided by timed automated blood culture incubation. Studies involving hematopoietic stem cell transplant neutropenic and cancer patients with short-interval or long-interval catheter implants reveal that DTTP >2 hours is a sensitive and specific predictor in diagnosing catheter-related bacteremia. Only one study in critically ill patients did not reproduce the findings using this method. To determine DTTP, blood cultures have to arrive at the microbiological laboratory within a 12-hour time interval.[17] Quantitative blood cultures improve specificity. Blood cultures taken from catheters usually demonstrate higher bacterial concentrations than those taken from peripheral veins in the case of CRI. A ratio of hub colony-forming unit (CFU)-to-peripheral CFU >10 is indicative of catheter-related infection. However, special transport bottles, immediate sample processing, and significant resources in staff and materials are needed. By meta-analysis, this was found to be the most accurate test.

Quantitative detection of bacterial 16S ribosomal DNA in catheter-derived blood samples has not yet become standard clinical practice. Cytospin slide preparations are stained with gram/acridine orange stains to provide high sensitivity and specificity rates (96% and 92%, respectively) for detecting CRI. Endoluminal brushing of the CVC remains useful in cases of obturation. Some authors collect swab cultures from catheter hubs routinely for early diagnosis of CRI. This method is controversial in terms of sensitivity and specificity and is not recommended. In summary, DTTP is recommended for routine diagnostic purposes; quantitative blood cultures or DNA testing is not yet standard, despite validation in scientific studies.

Microbiological diagnosis after catheter removal

If catheter removal is clinically indicated, the catheter tip should be cut to a length of 5 cm and placed into a sterile and dry container for transport. Catheter tips should be processed within 12 hours. If immediate transport to the laboratory cannot be arranged, the catheter tip should be refrigerated at 4° C to 8° C. Immersing the catheter tip in culture broth is not recommended because this method is associated with a high rate of false positivity. The role plate method with semiquantitative cultures is standard for microbiological diagnosis of CRI after catheter removal. Only bacteria adhering to the outer surface of the catheter are captured by this method. Growth of at least 15 CFUs on the plate is interpreted as evidence of CRI. In a prospective trial involving intensive care unit (ICU) patients, the quantitative method was not shown to be superior to the role plate technique. Several methods have been tested to improve sensitivity and specificity, including quantitative cultures obtained from the interior surface of the catheter using vortex and ultrasound methods to remove catheter material and disengage adhesive bacteria. The Brun-Buisson method is based on quantitative analysis after vortexing of the catheter. A cutoff limit of 103 CFUs is interpreted as positive.

All methods used for catheter tip processing have not been validated for catheters coated with antibiotics or antiseptics.[18,19]

MANAGEMENT

After CRI has been diagnosed, decisions must be made regarding catheter removal and the choice and duration of antimicrobial therapy.

For complicated CRI, catheter removal is required. The definition of a complicated CRI includes positive blood cultures despite 48 hours of antibiotic therapy combined with the development of endocarditis, osteomyelitis, septic thrombosis or embolism, or abscess formation. These conditions require intensified antimicrobial therapy and consideration of surgical intervention in some cases. In some hospitals Taurolidine/Citrate is used for CVC blocking.[19a]

Uncomplicated CRI occurs as a response of bacteremia to antibiotic therapy (i.e., defervescence, negative blood culture) within 48 hours of initiation of antimicrobial treatment.

Catheter removal is recommended in clinically unstable patients (e.g., severe sepsis, septic shock), patients with persistent fever, and patients with breakthrough fever after discontinuation of antimicrobial therapy. Catheter removal is required if *Staphylococcus aureus* organisms are isolated from blood cultures: Remission rates as low as 20% are associated with a high risk of secondary complications such as endocarditis and osteomyelitis. Catheter removal is also recommended in patients with CRI due to *Candida* spp. and *Bacillus* spp. if appropriate antibiotics are provided and patients do not present with clinical signs of sepsis. Preservation of the CVC could be attempted in patients with coagulase-negative staphylococci, *Corynebacterium jeikeium*, *Acinetobacter baumannii*, *Stenotrophomonas maltophilia*, *Pseudomonas aeruginosa*, and *Bacillus* spp. receiving appropriate antibiotics if the patients' conditions are stable without developing clinical signs of sepsis. Special arrangements should be made for neutropenic patients.

Catheter exit site infections usually respond to local procedures and antibiotics. However, patients with tunnel or pocket infection require catheter explantation. Management of CRI in neutropenic patients is based on the same principles as treatment of fever of unknown origin (FUO). However, preemptive antimicrobial treatment should take into account the institution's commonly isolated microorganisms.

Initial empirical treatment with glycopeptides is not standard. Therapy with penicillinase-resistant penicillin is as effective and therefore is preferable to the use of glycopeptide antibiotics in patients without methicillin-resistant *Staphylococcus aureus* (MRSA) infection.

Glycopeptides are indicated in patients who are intolerant to penicillin or who have methicillin-resistant staphylococci cultures. Newer drugs active against multiresistant gram-positive bacteria (e.g., linezolid, quinupristin/dalfopristin) are reserved for patients who are intolerant to glycopeptides or are infected by organisms resistant to glycopeptide antibiotics.

Before pathogen-specific antimicrobial therapy is initiated, the significance of cultured pathogens should be reviewed critically. For coagulase-negative staphylococci and *Corynebacterium* spp., significance is indicated by detection of the same pattern of antibiotic sensitivity in at least two separate blood cultures. In regard to microbial culture results and in vitro susceptibility testing, antimicrobial treatment should be modified.

Independent risk factors for hematogenous complications resulting from catheter-related *S. aureus* bacteremia include duration of clinical signs and symptoms of infection, hemodialysis, the presence of a long-term intravascular catheter or noncatheter device, and infection with MRSA. Therefore, sufficient time is needed for intravenous antimicrobial treatment if complications are to be avoided. In immunosuppressed patients, the duration of treatment with appropriate systemic antibiotics is at least 2 weeks.

Instillation of antibiotics (e.g., vancomycin, gentamicin) within the catheter lock, in addition to parenteral antibiotic therapy, was shown to reduce CRI relapse rates in a small randomized study involving non-neutropenic patients.

PROPHYLAXIS

Stringent sterile management criteria for CVC systems are necessary. Strict compliance with antiseptic principles during insertion (i.e., hand hygiene, standardized puncture techniques, use of sterile covers, gloves and clothing including mask and cap) prevents infection.

Ultrasound-guided placement is helpful to further reduce CRI rates. Qualified and experienced teams specializing in CVC insertion and management are a major factor in preventing CRI. Educational programs for nurses and physicians that focus on catheter management reduce CRI rates.[20,21]

A single-lumen catheter is preferred. A nonpermanent CVC placed via the subclavian vein is preferred to the internal jugular vein approach in terms of infection prevention, but the risk of other complications such as severe hemorrhage (particularly in thrombocytopenic patients) or pneumothorax should be taken into account.

Use of the femoral vein should be avoided because of the high microbial colonization rate and the greater risk of deep venous thrombosis.

Chlorhexidine solutions are used in preference to aqueous povidone-iodine solutions for catheter insertion. Alcoholic chlorhexidine solutions, alcoholic povidone-iodine solutions, and 70% propranolol are alternatives. One randomized controlled study demonstrated that serial combinations of alcoholic chlorhexidine solutions and aqueous povidone-iodine were superior to single preparations.[22]

Catheter replacement without clinically proven infection does not reduce infection rates. Systemic prophylactic antibiotic treatment before insertion of the catheter does not reduce CRI.

Sterile gauze or transparent film may be used to cover the CVC insertion site. Sterile gauze is changed every 2 days, unless local contamination, signs of inflammation, or detachment occurs.[23] More frequent replacement does not reduce the incidence of infection.

Infusion tubing for systems for lipid emulsions is changed every 24 hours. Impregnation of CVCs with antiseptics (chlorhexidine/silver sulfadiazine) or antibiotics (minocycline/rifampicin) lowers the incidence of catheter colonization, but the clinical implications have not yet been determined. Therefore, use of impregnated catheters generally is not recommended.[24]

REFERENCES

1. Harbarth S, Sax H, Gastmeier P. The preventable proportion of nosocomial infections: an overview of published reports. *J Hosp Infect.* 2003;54:258–266.

2. Hind D, Calvert N, McWilliams R, et al. Ultrasonic locating devices for central venous cannulation: meta-analysis. *BMJ.* 2003;327:361–368.

3. Johansson E, Björkholm M, Björvell H. Totally implantable subcutaneous port system versus central venous catheter placed before induction chemotherapy in patients with acute leukemia—a randomized study. *Support Care Cancer.* 2004;12:99–105.

4. Jordan K, Behlendorf T, Surov A, et al. Venous access ports: frequency and management of complications in oncology patients. *Oncology.* 2008;31:404–410.

5. Joynt GM, Kew J, Gomersall CD, et al. Deep venous thrombosis caused by femoral venous catheters in critically ill adult patients. *Chest.* 2000;117:178–183.

5a. Nowak-Göttl U, Heinecke A, von Kries R, et al. Thrombotic events revisited in children with acute lymphoblastic leukemia: impact of concomitant Escherichia coli asparaginase/prednisone administration. *Thromb Res.* 2001;103:165–172.

6. Kuhn DM, Ghannoum MA. Candida biofilms: antifungal resistance and emerging therapeutic options. *Curr Opin Investig Drugs.* 2004;5:186–197.

7. Pierce GE. *Pseudomonas aeruginosa, Candida albicans,* and device-related nosocomial infections: implications, trends, and potential approaches for control. *J Indian Micobiol Biotechnol.* 2005;32:309–318.

8. Schinabeck MK, Long A, Hossain MA. Rabbit model of *Candida albicans* biofilm infection: liposomal amphotericin B antifungal lock therapy. *Antimicrob Agents Chemother.* 2004;48:1727–1732.

9. Wisplinghoff H, Seifert H, Wenzel RP, et al. Current trends in the epidemiology of nosocomial bloodstream infections in patients with hematological malignancies and solid neoplasms in hospitals in the United States. *Clin Infect Dis.* 2003;36:1103–1110.

10. Reference deleted in proofs.

11. Safdar N, Maki DG. Risk of catheter-related bloodstream infection with peripherally inserted central venous catheters used in hospitalized patients. *Chest.* 2005;128:489–495.

12. Kojic EM, Darouiche RO. Candida infections of medical devices. *Clin Microbiol Rev.* 2004;17:255–267.

13. Mermel LA, Barry MF, Sherertz RJ, et al. Guidelines for the management of intravascular catheter related infections. *Clin Infect Dis.* 2001;32:1249–1272.

14. Wolf H-H, Leithäuser M, Maschmeyer G, et al. Central venous catheter-related infections in hematology and oncology: guidelines of the Infectious Diseases Working Party (AGIHO) of the German Society of Hematology and Oncology (DGHO). *Ann Hematol.* 2008;87:863–876.

15. O'Grady NP, Alexander M, Dellinger EP, et al. Guidelines for the prevention of intravascular catheter-related infections. *Infect Control Hosp Epidemiol*. 2002;23:759–769.

16. Raad II, Hanna HA, Boktour M, et al. Management of central venous catheters in patients with cancer and candidemia. *Clin Infect Dis*. 2004;38:1119–1127.

17. Abdelkefi A, Achour W, Ben Othman T, et al. Difference in time to positivity is useful for the diagnosis of catheter-related bloodstream infection in hematopoietic stem cell transplant recipients. *Bone Marrow Transplant*. 2005;35:397–401.

18. Dobbins BM, Kite P, Catton JA, et al. In situ endoluminal brushing: a safe technique for the diagnosis of catheter-related bloodstream infection. *J Hosp Infect*. 2004;58:233–237.

19. Brun-Buisson C, Abrouk F, Legrand P, et al. Diagnosis of central venous catheter-related sepsis: critical level of quantitative tip cultures. *Arch Intern Med*. 1987;147:873–877.

19a. Simon A, Ammann RA, Wiszniewsky G, et al. Taurolidine-citrate lock solution (TauroLock) significantly reduces CVAD-associated grampositive infections in pediatric cancer patients. *BMC Infect Dis*. 2008;8:102.

20. Coopersmith CM, Rebmann TL, Zack JE, et al. Effect of an education program on decreasing catheter-related bloodstream infections in the surgical intensive care unit. *Crit Care Med*. 2002;30:59–64.

21. Berenholtz SM, Pronovost PJ, Lipsett PA, et al. Eliminating catheter-related bloodstream infections in the intensive care unit. *Crit Care Med*. 2004;32:2014–2020.

22. Tietz A, Frei R, Dangel M, et al. Octenidine hydrochloride for the care of central venous catheter insertion sites in severely immunocompromised patients. *Infect Control Hosp Epidemiol*. 2005;26:703–707.

23. Gillies D, O'Riordan L, Carr D, et al. Gauze and transparent polyurethane dressings for central venous catheters. Review. *Cochrane Database Syst Rev*. 2003;(4) CD003827.

24. Brun-Buisson C, Doyon F, Sollet JP, et al. Prevention of intravascular catheter-related infection with newer chlorhexidine-silver sulfadiazine-coated catheters: a randomized controlled trial. *Intensive Care Med*. 2004;30:837–843.

Stents for palliative treatment of digestive cancer

35

César V. Lopes, Júlio C. Pereira-Lima, and Marc Giovannini

In oncologic practice, advanced gastrointestinal cancers often lead to obstructive symptoms, either by direct blockage or by extrinsic compression. The endoscopic placement of stents, especially self-expandable metal stents (SEMS), in patients with malignant esophageal, gastroduodenal, biliary, and colonic obstruction has made possible the reestablishment of luminal continuity and improvement in the quality of life. Because palliation is the goal of care for most malignant strictures and fistulas of the gastrointestinal tract, stents are a well-accepted alternative for palliation as first-line therapy in patients not suitable for surgery.[1–5]

In this chapter, we introduce the reader to the most important aspects of endoscopic placement of stents for palliative treatment of malignant obstruction of the gastrointestinal tract.

ESOPHAGEAL CANCER

Esophageal cancer is an important cause of cancer-related death worldwide. Despite advances in therapy, more than 50% of esophageal cancers are incurable at presentation, and the 5-year survival rate is below 10%.[6]

A large number of options are available for the treatment of unresectable esophageal cancer, but the results of treatment in relation to costs, complications, quality of life, and survival are not better than those obtained by stenting.[1,7,8] Furthermore, to reinforce the value of SEMS for treatment in these cases, a new stent loaded with ^{125}I seeds for intraluminal brachytherapy has recently been reported to produce significantly longer relief of dysphagia, as well as better survival, when compared with conventional stents[9]—a result that to date has not been achieved by any other palliative therapy for malignant dysphagia.

Esophageal stents are usually placed successfully in all patients (Fig. 35-1). Procedure-related and life-threatening complications are rare.[4,10,11] The rate of late complications (i.e., those occurring more than 2 weeks after the procedure) ranges from 14% to 64%, especially obstruction due to tumor overgrowth–in-growth and stent migration, whether for covered or bare stents.[4,10–12] In an attempt to prevent obstruction due to tumor in-growth, which can affect up to 36% of individuals treated with uncovered stents,[10,13] the routine use of covered stents for any individual with esophageal advanced cancer seems to be the best choice. Dislodgment and migration of covered stents range from 4.5% to 15%.[4,10,12] Overall, reintervention rates are lower for covered stents than for noncovered ones.[14,15] Fortunately, most of these complications are within the control of the endoscopist and can be managed conservatively by inserting a second stent or by repositioning the migrated stent.

Stent complications are related to the level of obstruction. Stents deployed in the proximal third of the esophagus are more hazardous than those placed more distally. In the experience of Verschuur et al.,[16] SEMS were effective for palliation of dysphagia in 104 patients with malignant stricture close to the upper esophageal sphincter, and although major complications (e.g., aspiration pneumonia, hemorrhage, fistula, perforation) occurred in 21% of the patients, no procedure-related mortality was reported. In a comparative study, bleeding occurred in 14% of patients whose stents were placed in the proximal third of the esophagus, but in none with stents placed more distally.[12]

Self-expandable metal stents are used to seal off esophageal fistulas and can offer a chance for survival, even in severely ill patients. Recovery with complete healing of the fistula is seen in 57% to 89% of patients.[17,18]

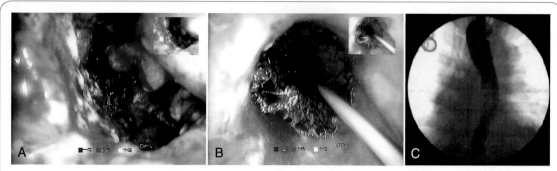

Fig. 35-1 **A,** Endoscopic view of an obstructing esophageal adenocarcinoma. **B,** Covered metal stent guaranteeing luminal patency. **C,** Fluoroscopic image demonstrating free passage of contrast.

To date, the safety of placing SEMS for patients with inoperable esophageal cancer who are undergoing chemotherapy and/or radiotherapy before or after stent placement remains controversial. Sumiyoshi et al.[19] evaluated morbidity and mortality in patients with esophageal cancer and stent placement after chemoradiotherapy. Most individuals with tumor invasion of the aorta died of massive hemorrhage. Conversely, in the experience of Raijman et al.,[20] among patients with no previous chemotherapy or radiotherapy, the occurrence of complications was only 9.5%. In contradiction, among patients who received radiotherapy, chemotherapy, or both, life-threatening complications occurred in 8% of cases. Another study compared complications in 116 patients who had undergone chemotherapy and radiation versus those who had not. The study involved 116 individuals. Early and late complications were more frequent in patients who had undergone chemotherapy or radiation (23% vs. 3.3%, $P < .002$; and 21.6% vs. 5%, $P < .02$, respectively).[21] To clarify this finding, a study of 200 patients followed prospectively found that stent placement after radiation was safe and prior treatment was not a contradiction. Retrosternal pain after stent placement occurred more often in patients undergoing treatment; this pain needs to be adequately treated because it compromises quality of life in these patients.[22]

GASTRIC OUTLET OBSTRUCTION

Patients with malignant gastric outlet obstruction (GOO) typically have advanced primary malignancies arising from the stomach, pancreas, ampulla, and biliary tree.[23] Two clues to suggest that malignant GOO is present are a history of vomiting undigested food hours after eating and the absence of bile from the vomitus.

Endoscopic enteral stenting, in addition to being safe and effective in the management of GOO, averts surgical morbidity from laparotomy, promptly restores oral intake, and shortens hospital stay compared with palliative gastrojejunostomy.[24,25] Enteral stenting is successful in more than 95% of individuals, and for most only one stent is needed to maintain oral intake until death (Fig. 35-2). Life-threatening complications are rare. Stent obstruction and migration, whether procedure related or as a late complication, are found in 16% to 32% of patients.[2,4,24,26]

Biliary obstruction is found frequently in patients with malignant GOO. Enteral stents will make it difficult or even impossible to place stents endoscopically in the major papilla. For this reason, it is recommended to place a prophylactic biliary metal stent before duodenal stenting. In situations where biliary obstruction occurs after enteral stent placement, percutaneous or echoendoscopically guided stenting can allow biliary drainage.[23,27]

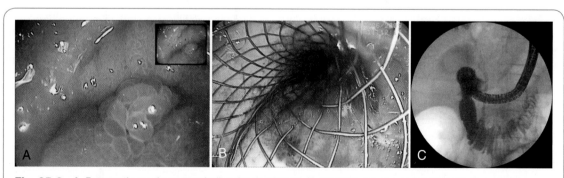

Fig. 35-2 **A,** Pancreatic carcinoma occluding the duodenum. **B,** Deployment of a metal stent. **C,** Fluoroscopy demonstrating free passage of contrast. Note the biliary metal stent in place.

MALIGNANT BILE DUCT OBSTRUCTION

Endoscopic biliary stenting is the treatment of choice for unresectable malignant jaundice and is preferred over percutaneous approaches, except when complex intrahepatic biliary strictures are present, when the papilla cannot be reached with a duodenoscope because of prior surgery, or when hospitals have expert interventional radiologists and no endoscopists.[5,28] Metal and plastic stents are available for the endoscopic approach to malignant strictures of the biliary tree for distal or proximal obstruction, as well as for endoscopic ultrasound–guided access to the biliary tree when the papilla is not accessible with the use of duodenoscopes. Management of these individuals is discussed in the following sections.

DISTAL OBSTRUCTION

In a population-based study evaluating 32,348 individuals with pancreatic cancer, curative surgery was feasible in less than 15% with malignant distal strictures.[29]

Endoscopic retrograde cholangiopancreatography (ERCP) with stent placement is the preferred treatment for 75% of patients with malignant distal bile duct obstruction. In a Cochrane Review of 21 trials involving 1454 individuals, endoscopic stenting with plastic endoprostheses was associated with fewer complications and reduced 30-day mortality compared with surgical bypass. However, endoscopic stents were associated with a higher risk of recurrent biliary obstruction.[5] Stent occlusion can be resolved with stent changing, either plastic or SEMS. Self-expandable metal stents can reach a 30 French diameter after insertion and can remain open longer than 10 French/11.5 French plastic stents in randomized controlled trials. This guarantees fewer reinterventions and better quality of life (Fig. 35-3).[5,28]

Prognostic factors associated with shorter survival (e.g., liver metastases, tumor size >3 cm, anemia, pain, carcinoembryonic antigen [CEA]/cancer antigen [CA] 19-9 levels) should be used to select patients for metal or plastic stents. In general, plastic stents are inserted in patients with a survival expectancy of less than 4 months, and metal stents are inserted in those with a better prognosis.[5,28]

Early complications from biliary stent insertion can be related to ERCP or to stenting. Pancreatitis, sphincterotomy-related bleeding, or perforation occurs in up to 7% and is related to difficulties in biliary cannulation, pre-cut papillotomy, sphincterotomy before insertion, previous cholangitis, and coagulopathy.[30,31]

Long-term complications of plastic biliary stents consist of occlusion and migration. The cause of obstruction is biliary sludge deposition. Plastic stents typically last from 3 to 4 months.[32] Conversely, metal stents are superior to plastic stents in terms of patency and patient quality of life,[5] and in clinical practice, there is some indication that metal stents improve survival.[33,34] Occlusion of uncovered metal stents and recurrent jaundice happen in up to 20% of patients and are usually caused by tumor in-growth–overgrowth. They are rarely due to sludge deposition or migration,[35] and they usually occur between 5 and 9 months after insertion. To overcome these problems and reestablish stent patency, several techniques have been used, including tissue ablation with thermal probes, mechanical cleaning with basket and balloon, and insertion of a new stent. The introduction of a plastic prosthesis through an occluded metal stent is the easiest and most cost-effective measure to reestablish patency.[35–39] Covered metal stents can also fail as the result of tumor overgrowth, epithelial hyperplasia, sludge occlusion, or stent migration. To resolve these complications, the same methods are used as for uncovered metal stents.[36]

Plastic or covered metal biliary stents can cause cholecystitis through cystic duct occlusion. Cholangitis may be noted after plastic stent insertion for an obstructed SEMS. Covered metal biliary stents may also cause pancreatitis as the result of pancreatic duct occlusion. Covered stents can minimize the problem of tumor in-growth and actually confer higher patency during the midterm compared with noncovered metal stents; early complications, particularly cholecystitis and pancreatitis, are more frequent.[37,39] It should be kept in mind that these patients have a limited life expectancy, so the fewer the complications and the more time they spend outside the hospital, the better. Covered stents should never be inserted into hilar tumors because they will obstruct small intrahepatic bile

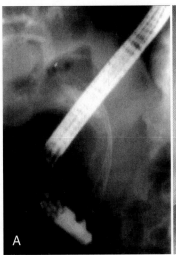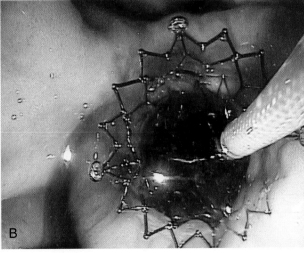

Fig. 35-3 A, Pancreatic cancer with a metal stent inserted into the bile duct. **B,** Metal stent viewed from the duodenum.

ducts. Covered metal stents are a good initial option only in patients with a previous cholecystectomy and malignant lower bile duct obstruction.

PROXIMAL BILIARY OBSTRUCTION

Malignant proximal duct strictures are caused most often by hilar tumors. Primary hilar tumors have a better prognosis than pancreatic cancer; however, most are unresectable because of vessel invasion, hepatic metastasis, or spread through the biliary tree.[27,28]

Drainage of malignant distal bile duct obstruction is undoubtedly safer and more effective by endoscopy than by percutaneous intubation. However, in malignant proximal bile duct strictures, there is a serious question about the best approach: percutaneous or endoscopic. In clinical practice, whether patients undergo endoscopic or radiologic biliary drainage with metal stents depends on patient selection and local expertise. Two randomized trials before the advent of SEMS demonstrated that inserting plastic stents through the papilla was safer and more efficient (fewer sessions).[40,41] In a retrospective review, percutaneously inserted stents were more successful than (92% vs. 77%) and as safe as endoscopic stenting.[40] Endoscopic stenting is usually recommended for Bismuth type II/III Klatskin tumors (Fig. 35-4), and percutaneous stenting is recommended for type III/IV lesions (as determined by magnetic resonance cholangiopancreatography). Unfortunately, both methods are suboptimal, and reintervention will be necessary in up to 10% of cases.[41]

The introduction of one (draining just one lobe) or two stents (draining both liver lobes) produces similar clinical results in trials.[42] Moreover, the placement of two stents is associated with a higher risk of early complications and a longer procedure time.[43] Some authors[43,44] advocate selective drainage with one stent placed in the dominant duct, as determined by magnetic resonance cholangiopancreatography. On the other hand, De Palma et al.[45] demonstrated that draining

the duct, which can be reached easily by guidewire with a single stent, yields the same clinical results. Indeed, given that 25% of volume drainage is enough to normalize liver function, the benefits of draining the left and right lobe are clinically similar.[46]

An essential goal in stenting hilar cancers is to drain the ducts. Nondraining opacified ducts are associated with higher morbidity and mortality.[47]

ECHOENDOSCOPICALLY GUIDED HEPATICOGASTROSTOMY FOR BILIARY DRAINAGE

ERCP is the procedure of choice for establishing biliary decompression for malignant jaundice; success rates exceed 90% at academic centers.[28] However, in certain situations, bile ducts are not endoscopically accessible because of surgical diversion, anatomic variation, periampullary diverticula, or tumor invasion. In such cases, percutaneous transhepatic biliary drainage (PTBD) is the standard method at most institutions.[48] The complication rate is 10% to 30%, and complications include cholangitis, bile leak, bleeding, fistulas, peritonitis, and stent occlusion.[27]

In an attempt to overcome the drawbacks of external biliary drainage, echoendoscopically guided hepaticogastrostomy has been recommended as an alternative. Because endoscopic ultrasound provides excellent imaging of the left lobe of the liver, a transgastric approach to the dilated left biliary system, in the absence of ascites or coagulopathy, is a good option, resulting in internal biliary drainage into the stomach (Fig. 35-5). To date, the clinical success rate of the procedure is reported to be 75% to 100%. Complications include stent migration, bile leaks, and cholangitis.[48,49]

Additional clinical trials comparing echoendoscopically guided hepaticogastrostomy and PTBD are needed to identify the best treatment option for managing malignant biliary obstruction after failure of ERCP.[48]

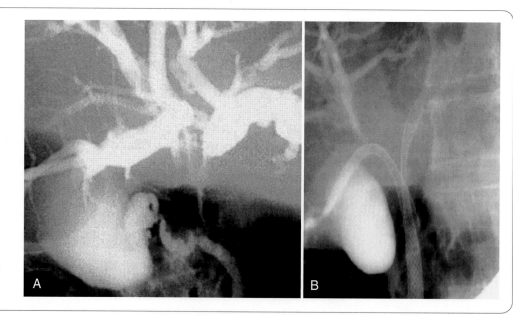

Fig. 35-4 A, Bismuth type III cholangiocarcinoma. **B,** Bilateral metal stents.

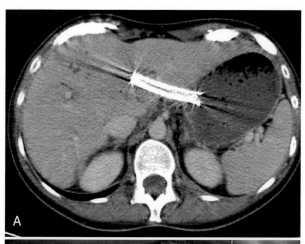

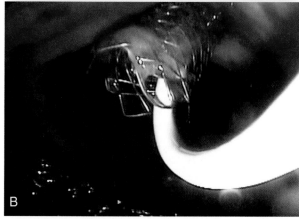

Fig. 35-5 Malignant stricture of the duodenum with dilated left biliary tree. **A,** Tomographic image demonstrating a transgastric metal stent after echoendoscopically guided hepaticogastrostomy. **B,** Endoscopic image of a transgastric metal stent.

COLORECTAL OBSTRUCTION

Colorectal cancer is one of the most common neoplastic diseases throughout the world. Patients with malignant large-bowel obstruction usually have advanced disease and frequently are poor candidates for surgical decompression. Individuals undergoing palliative procedures for relief of large-bowel

obstruction have a surgical mortality rate that can exceed 10%.[50] Furthermore, colostomy considerably worsens the quality of life of these patients. Colorectal stents, on the other hand, decompress the colon and lead to prompt restoration of colonic transit (Fig. 35-6). SEMS for colorectal cancer are used in two settings: as definitive palliation for malignant colorectal obstruction in patients not suitable for surgery and as a bridge to surgery.

Sebastian et al.[3] analyzed 54 studies reporting the use of stents in a total of 1198 patients. The technical success rate was 94%. Major early complications included stent migration (11.8%), obstruction (7.3%), and perforation (3.8%). Overall, late complications occurred in 27%; most were non–life threatening and were easily managed by replacing the stent.[4,51,52] Few randomized studies have compared colonic SEMS with surgery. Although SEMS do not improve survival, fewer complications, shorter hospital stays, lower costs, and a better quality of life have been reported with stents.[53–55]

Patients with acute malignant colorectal obstruction commonly present with an unprepared and dilated colon, which makes surgery in these patients a high-risk procedure.[52] SEMS is a minimally invasive and cost-effective procedure that allows definitive elective one-stage surgery for most after stenting, which does not happen necessarily for those who do not undergo stenting but only a temporary colostomy. A temporary colostomy and a second definitive en bloc resection are required. Stenting is associated with fewer complications and a shorter length of stay.[3,56]

Malignant colonic obstruction may also arise from extracolonic tumors causing extrinsic compression or invading the lumen. Palliative surgery in this situation is associated with significant morbidity.[57,58] A minimally invasive approach would be desirable. Colorectal stenting might be a reasonable alternative in treating extrinsic colonic obstruction and avoiding a colostomy, but so far, effectiveness for extracolonic malignancy is not well established. In a study by Keswani et al.,[58] stenting of colonic obstruction due to malignant extrinsic compression was less successful (20% vs. 94%, $P < .0001$) and was associated with a higher rate of complications (33% vs. 9%, $P = .046$) when compared with treatment for obstructive colorectal cancer. On the other hand, in a series of 39 patients, most of whom had peritoneal carcinomatosis, the technical success rate was 87% and the complication rate was 38.6%, which accounted for stent obstruction and migration.[59] In another case series involving 36 patients suffering from colonic obstruction managed by SEMS, 9 had extracolonic malignancy and peritoneal carcinomatosis. No differences in

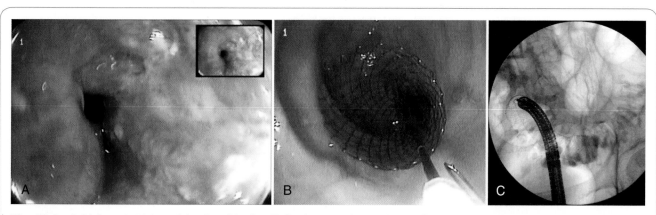

Fig. 35-6 **A,** Malignant stricture of the sigmoid colon. **B,** Deployment of a metal stent. **C,** Fluoroscopy confirming luminal patency.

complications were noted after stenting in comparison with cases without neoplastic ascites (22% vs. 44%, P = .430).[4] Clinical trials on this evolving approach should be undertaken to clarify the value of endoscopic stenting for this particular group of patients who were not suitable for cytoreductive surgery and hyperthermic intraperitoneal chemotherapy.[60,61]

CONCLUSION

Endoscopic stenting is an important tool for palliation and restoration of the luminal continuity of malignant advanced gastrointestinal cancers not suitable for surgery. Stents are usually placed successfully in all patients. Procedure-related and life-threatening complications are rare. Late complications can occur, especially stent obstruction and migration, but they can be managed conservatively. The endoscopic insertion of stents for advanced gastrointestinal cancers leads to fewer complications, shorter hospital stays, lower costs, and a better quality of life than palliative surgical interventions.

REFERENCES

1. Xinopoulos D, Dimitroulopoulos D, Moschandrea I, et al. Natural course of inoperable esophageal cancer treated with metallic expandable stents: quality of life and cost-effectiveness analysis. *J Gastroenterol Hepatol.* 2004;19:1397–1402.

2. Kim JH, Song HY, Shin JH, et al. Metallic stent placement in the palliative treatment of malignant gastroduodenal obstructions: prospective evaluation of results and factors influencing outcome in 213 patients. *Gastrointest Endosc.* 2007;66:256–264.

3. Sebastian S, Johnston S, Geoghegan T, et al. Pooled analysis of the efficacy and safety of self-expanding metal stenting in malignant colorectal obstruction. *Am J Gastroenterol.* 2004;99:2051–2057.

4. Lopes CV, Pesenti C, Bories E, et al. Self-expandable metallic stents for palliative treatment of digestive cancer. *J Clin Gastroenterol.* 2008;42:991–996.

5. Moss AC, Morris E, MacMathuna P. Palliative biliary stents for obstructing pancreatic carcinoma. *Cochrane Database Syst Rev.* 2006;(19): CD004200.

6. Stein HJ, Siewert JR. Improved prognosis of resected esophageal cancer. *World J Surg.* 2004;28:520–525.

7. Wenger U, Johnsson E, Bergquist H, et al. Health economic evaluation of stent or endoluminal brachytherapy as a palliative strategy in patients with incurable cancer of the oesophagus or gastro-oesophageal junction: results of a randomized clinical trial. *Eur J Gastroenterol Hepatol.* 2005;17:1369–1377.

8. Eroglu A, Turkyilmaz A, Subasi M, et al. The use of self-expandable metallic stents for palliative treatment of inoperable esophageal cancer. *Dis Esophagus.* 2010;23:64–70.

9. Guo JH, Teng GJ, Zhu GY, et al. Self-expandable esophageal stent loaded with ^{125}I seeds: initial experience in patients with advanced esophageal cancer. *Radiology.* 2008;247:574–581.

10. Homann N, Noftz MR, Klingenberg-Noftz RD, et al. Delayed complications after placement of self-expanding stents in malignant esophageal obstruction: treatment strategies and survival rate. *Dig Dis Sci.* 2008;53:334–340.

11. White RE, Parker RK, Fitzwater JW, et al. Stents as sole therapy for oesophageal cancer: a prospective analysis of outcomes after placement. *Lancet Oncol.* 2009;10:240–246.

12. Wang MQ, Sze DY, Wang ZP, et al. Delayed complications after esophageal stent placement for treatment of malignant esophageal obstructions and esophagorespiratory fistulas. *J Vasc Interv Radiol.* 2001;12:465–474.

13. Acunas B, Rozanes I, Akpinar S, et al. Palliation of malignant esophageal strictures with self-expanding nitinol stents: drawbacks and complications. *Radiology.* 1996;199:648–652.

14. Vakil N, Morris AI, Marcon N, et al. A prospective, randomized, controlled trial of covered expandable metal stents in the palliation of malignant esophageal obstruction at the gastroesophageal junction. *Am J Gastroenterol.* 2001;96:1791–1796.

15. Hills KS, Chopra KB, Pal A, et al. Self-expanding metal oesophageal endoprostheses, covered and uncovered: a review of 30 cases. *Eur J Gastroenterol Hepatol.* 1998;10:371–374.

16. Verschuur EM, Kuipers EJ, Siersema PD. Esophageal stents for malignant strictures close to the upper esophageal sphincter. *Gastrointest Endosc.* 2007;66:1082–1090.

17. Johnsson E, Lundell L, Liedman B. Sealing of esophageal perforation or ruptures with expandable metallic stents: a prospective controlled study on treatment efficacy and limitations. *Dis Esophagus.* 2005;18:262–266.

18. Ross WA, Lee JH. Endoscopic approach to tracheoesophageal fistulas in adults. *Tech Gastrointest Endosc.* 2008;10:155–163.

19. Sumiyoshi T, Gotoda T, Muro K, et al. Morbidity and mortality after self-expandable metallic stent placement in patients with progressive or recurrent esophageal cancer after chemoradiotherapy. *Gastrointest Endosc.* 2003;57:882–885.

20. Raijman I, Siddique I, Lynch P. Does chemoradiation therapy increase the incidence of complications with self-expanding coated stents in the management of malignant esophageal strictures? *Am J Gastroenterol.* 1997;92:2192–2196.

21. Lecleire S, Di Fiore F, Ben-Soussan E, et al. Prior chemoradiotherapy is associated with a higher life-threatening complication rate after palliative insertion of metal stents in patients with oesophageal cancer. *Aliment Pharmacol Ther.* 2006;23:1693–1702.

22. Homs MY, Hansen BE, van Blankenstein M, et al. Prior radiation and/or chemotherapy has no effect on the outcome of metal stent placement for esophagogastric carcinoma. *Eur J Gastroenterol Hepatol.* 2004;16:163–170.

23. Adler DG, Merwat SN. Endoscopic approaches for palliation of luminal gastrointestinal obstruction. *Gastroenterol Clin North Am.* 2006;35:65–82.

24. Jeurnink SM, Steyerberg EW, Hof G, et al. Gastrojejunostomy versus stent placement in patients with malignant gastric outlet obstruction: a comparison in 95 patients. *J Surg Oncol.* 2007;96:389–396.

25. Espinel J, Sanz O, Vivas S, et al. Malignant gastrointestinal obstruction: endoscopic stenting versus surgical palliation. *Surg Endosc.* 2006;20:1083–1087.

26. Kim GH, Kang DH, Lee DH, et al. Which types of stent, uncovered or covered, should be used in gastric outlet obstructions? *Scand J Gastroenterol.* 2004;39:1010–1014.

27. van Delden OM, Lameris JS. Percutaneous drainage and stenting for palliation of malignant bile duct obstruction. *Eur Radiol.* 2008;18:448–456.

28. Jakobs R, Weickert U, Hartmann D, et al. Interventional endoscopy for benign and malignant bile duct strictures. *Z Gastroenterol.* 2005;43:295–303.

29. Shaib Y, Davila J, Naumann C, et al. The impact of curative intent surgery on the survival of pancreatic cancer patients: a U.S. Population-based study. *Am J Gastroenterol.* 2007;102:1377–1382.

30. Ryan ME. ERCP complication rates: how low can we go? *Gastrointest Endosc.* 2009;70:89–91.

31. Cotton PB, Garrow DA, Gallagher J, et al. Risk factors for complications after ERCP: a multivariate analysis of 11,497 procedures over 12 years. *Gastrointest Endosc.* 2009;70:80–88.

32. Pereira-Lima JC, Jakobs R, Maier M, et al. Endoscopic biliary stenting for the palliation of pancreatic cancer: results, survival predictive factors, and comparison of 10-French with 11.5-French gauge stents. *Am J Gastroenterol.* 1996;91:2179–2184.

33. Weber A, Mittermeyer T, Wagenpfeil S, et al. Self-expanding metal stents versus polyethylene stents for palliative treatment in patients with advanced pancreatic cancer. *Pancreas.* 2009;38:7–12.

34. Schmassmann A, von Gunten E, Knuchel J, et al. Wallstents versus plastic stents in malignant biliary obstruction: effects of stent patency of the first and second stent on patient compliance and survival. *Am J Gastroenterol.* 1996;91:654–659.

35. Carr-Locke DL. Metal stents for distal biliary malignancy: have we got you covered? *Gastrointest Endosc.* 2005;61:534–536.

36. Rogart JN, Boghos A, Rossi F, et al. Analysis of endoscopic management of occluded metal biliary stents at a single tertiary care center. *Gastrointest Endosc.* 2008;68:676–682.

37. Yoon WJ, Lee JK, Lee KH, et al. A comparison of covered and uncovered wallstents for the management of distal malignant biliary obstruction. *Gastrointest Endosc.* 2006;63:996–1000.

38. Bueno JT, Gerdes H, Kurtz RC. Endoscopic management of occluded biliary wallstents: a

cancer center experience. *Gastrointest Endosc.* 2003;58:879–884.

39. Isayama H, Komatsu Y, Tsujino T, et al. A prospective randomised study of covered versus uncovered diamond stents for the management of distal malignant biliary obstruction. *Gut.* 2004;53:729–734.

40. Paik WH, Park YS, Hwang JH, et al. Palliative treatment with self-expandable metallic stents in patients with advanced type III or IV hilar cholangiocarcinoma: a percutaneous versus endoscopic approach. *Gastrointest Endosc.* 2009;69:55–62.

41. Geller A. Klatskin tumor—palliative therapy: the jury is still out or may be not yet in. *Gastrointest Endosc.* 2009;69:63–65.

42. De Palma GD, Galloro G, Siciliano S, et al. Unilateral versus bilateral endoscopic hepatic duct drainage in patients with malignant hilar biliary obstruction: results of a prospective, randomized, and controlled study. *Gastrointest Endosc.* 2001;53:681–684.

43. Freeman ML, Overby C. Selective MRCP and CT-target drainage of malignant hilar biliary obstruction with self-expanding metallic stents. *Gastrointest Endosc.* 2003;58:41–49.

44. Hintze RE, Abou-Rebyeh H, Adler A, et al. Magnetic resonance cholangiopancreaticography-guided unilateral endoscopic stent placement for Klatskin tumors. *Gastrointest Endosc.* 2001;53:40–46.

45. De Palma GD, Pezzullo A, Rega M, et al. Unilateral placement of metallic stents for malignant hilar obstruction: a prospective study. *Gastrointest Endosc.* 2003;58:50–53.

46. Polydorou AA, Chisholm EM, Romanos AA, et al. A comparison of right versus left hepatic duct endoprosthesis insertion in malignant hilar biliary obstruction. *Endoscopy.* 1989;21:266–271.

47. Chang WH, Kortan P, Haber GB. Outcomes in patients with bifurcation tumors who undergo unilateral versus bilateral hepatic duct drainage. *Gastrointest Endosc.* 1998;47:354–362.

48. Savides TJ, Varadarajulu S, Palazzo L. EUS 2008 Working Group document: evaluation of EUS-guided hepaticogastrostomy. *Gastrointest Endosc.* 2009;69(2 suppl):S3–S7.

49. Bories E, Pesenti C, Caillol F, et al. Transgastric endoscopic ultrasonography-guided biliary drainage: results of a pilot study. *Endoscopy.* 2007;39:287–291.

50. Deans GT, Krukowski ZH, Irwin ST. Malignant obstruction of the left colon. *Br J Surg.* 1994;81:1270–1276.

51. Law WL, Choi HK, Lee YM, et al. Palliation for advanced malignant colorectal obstruction by self-expanding metallic stents: prospective evaluation of outcomes. *Dis Colon Rectum.* 2004;47:39–43.

52. Regimbeau JM, Yzet T, Brazier F, et al. Self expanding metallic stent in the management of malignant colonic obstruction. *Ann Chir.* 2004;129:203–210.

53. Carne PW, Frye JN, Robertson GM, et al. Stents or open operation for palliation of colorectal cancer: a retrospective, cohort study of perioperative outcome and long-term survival. *Dis Colon Rectum.* 2004;47:1455–1461.

54. Xinopoulos D, Dimitroulopoulos D, Theodosopoulos T, et al. Stenting or stoma creation for patients with inoperable malignant colonic obstructions? Results of a study and cost-effectiveness analysis. *Surg Endosc.* 2004;18:421–426.

55. Tilney HS, Lovegrove RE, Purkayastha S, et al. Comparison of colonic stenting and open surgery for malignant large bowel obstruction. *Surg Endosc.* 2007;21:225–233.

56. Khot UP, Lang AW, Murali K, et al. Systematic review of the efficacy and safety of colorectal stents. *Br J Surg.* 2002;89:1096–1102.

57. Bedirli A, Mentes BB, Onan A, et al. Colorectal intervention as part of surgery for patients with gynaecological malignancy. *Colorectal Dis.* 2005;7:228–231.

58. Keswani RN, Azar RR, Edmundowicz SA, et al. Stenting for malignant colonic obstruction: a comparison of efficacy and complications in colonic versus extracolonic malignancy. *Gastrointest Endosc.* 2009;69(3 suppl):675–680.

59. Shin SJ, Kim TI, Kim BC, et al. Clinical application of self-expandable metallic stent for treatment of colorectal obstruction caused by extrinsic invasive tumors. *Dis Colon Rectum.* 2008;51:578–583.

60. Koppe MJ, Boerman OC, Oyen WJ, et al. Peritoneal carcinomatosis of colorectal origin: incidence and current treatment strategies. *Ann Surg.* 2006;243:212–222.

61. Elias D, Raynard B, Farkhondeh F, et al. Peritoneal carcinomatosis of colorectal origin: long-term results of intraperitoneal chemohyperthermia with oxaliplatin following complete cytoreductive surgery. *Gastroenterol Clin Biol.* 2006;30:1200–1204.

36 Interventional approaches to treatment in supportive oncology

Abraham Levitin, Matthew Tam,
Karunakaravel Karuppasamy, and Raghid Kikano

Interventional radiology plays an ever expanding role in the supportive and palliative care of cancer patients. These procedures range from placement of catheters to decompress an obstructed system to direct local or regional tumor destruction, with the goal of symptom relief and, in many cases, improved survival. This chapter will focus on the role of interventional radiology in symptom management and improved quality of life. The chapter is organized by organ systems and their associated cancer-related symptoms and includes discussion of both vascular and nonvascular techniques of symptom relief.

CHEST

Supportive interventions in the chest may be provided to palliate important clinical problems such as hemoptysis, airway obstruction, superior vena cava syndrome, and recurrent pleural effusions. Palliative ablative therapy for lung carcinoma is increasingly useful.

HEMOPTYSIS

Massive hemoptysis is a life-threatening medical emergency. Although the major causes of massive hemoptysis are related to inflammatory lung disease, malignancy can also be a cause. In 90% of cases, bleeding occurs from the bronchial arteries. Selective catheterization of the bronchial arteries (typically arising from the proximal descending thoracic aorta) allows the bronchial arteries to be occluded by embolization with microscopic particles (Fig. 36-1). The success rate of bronchial artery embolization for hemoptysis due to primary lung cancer in terms of complete cessation of bleeding at 30 days has been reported at 62%, with a significant decrease in hemoptysis in 79%.[1]

Transient postembolization chest pain and dysphagia from nontargeted embolization of the chest wall and esophageal branches, respectively, are the most common complications of bronchial artery embolization.[2] One serious complication, spinal cord ischemia, is reported to occur in about 1% of patients and can be avoided with careful attention to technique. Preembolization contrast-enhanced computed tomography (CT) and bronchoscopy are useful for localizing the area of bleeding to a specific lobe.

SUPERIOR VENA CAVA SYNDROME

Stenting for malignant superior vena cava (SVC) obstruction produces rapid and dramatic improvement in patients' symptoms. Patients can present with severe headache and breathlessness exacerbated by position; facial and upper limb edema and pain; altered consciousness; blurred vision; retro-orbital pressure; and dilated collateral chest wall veins. This distressing syndrome can be rapidly reversed. The obstruction may

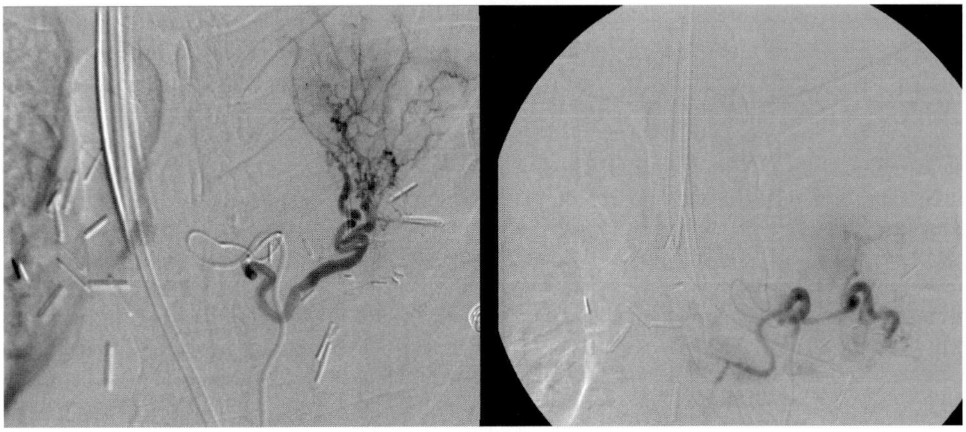

Fig. 36-1 Bronchial artery embolization for massive hemoptysis. Patient with a left upper lobe lesion and massive hemoptysis. Pre-embolization and post-embolization angiographic images demonstrate successful embolization with cessation of bleeding.

result from direct extension of cancer, but more likely may be due to extrinsic compression by enlarged mediastinal lymph nodes.

When symptoms are not severe, standard management consists of radiotherapy (RT), chemotherapy, or both. Stenting is an important primary treatment if the patient is extremely symptomatic and cannot wait for or tolerate standard treatments, or if chemoradiation treatment fails to relieve symptoms. SVC obstruction is approached from jugular, femoral, or upper limb venous access points, and commonly, a self-expanding metallic stent is deployed (Fig. 36-2). If associated thrombus is seen around the obstruction, this is managed with mechanical or infusion thrombolytic therapy. Mechanical thrombectomy can reduce the burden of clot sufficiently to allow stent deployment. Infusion thrombolysis may be contraindicated by the presence of concurrent brain metastases or hemoptysis. In one series, 52 patients reported symptomatic relief within 24 to 72 hours, and most patients improved within 24 hours.[3] An associated procedural mortality of 2% has been reported.[4] Pulmonary embolus, pericardial tamponade, and SVC or cardiac rupture are serious complications related to stent expansion or migration.

LUNG CANCER

Pain in lung cancer patients is typically due to osseous metastases, Pancoast (superior sulcus) tumor, and chest wall involvement.[5] Standard treatment consists of RT and combined modality therapy (CMT). When these treatments fail to relieve symptoms, alternative treatments such as embolization of bone tumor or image-guided tumor ablation should be considered.

Applications of image-guided tumor ablation have technically improved and are becoming part of standard practice for renal cell carcinoma, primary and metastatic lung lesions, and liver and bone lesions. Methods of image-guided ablation include radiofrequency ablation (RFA), cryoablation, microwave, and focused ultrasound and laser technologies. RFA is a useful palliative option for the treatment of lung lesions, particularly if patients have poor pulmonary reserve. Pain relief and improved quality of life have been demonstrated for patients with advanced inoperable lung cancer treated with RFA.[6] Greico and colleagues reported 100% response among patients who received RT within 90 days before RFA, suggesting a synergistic effect when both modalities are used.[7] The main complication associated with

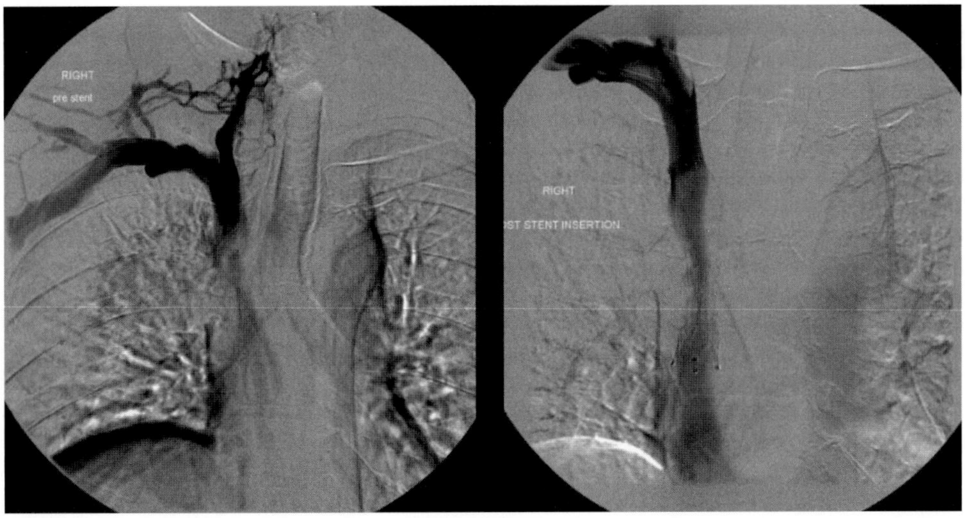

Fig. 36-2 Angiographic images before and after superior vena cava (SVC) stenting. The patient presented with symptoms and signs of SVC obstruction. An SVC stent resulted in dramatic and rapid resolution of symptoms.

RFA is pneumothorax (up to 12% of patients require chest tube placement). Some experience periprocedural pain.[8]

AIRWAY OBSTRUCTION

Airway obstruction presents with symptoms such as shortness of breath that worsens with exertion or lying flat, or with a nonproductive cough. With more severe airway obstruction, stridor will be present. Malignancy will cause airway problems via compression of airways or airway infiltration. Radiotherapy may cause focal stenosis and tracheobronchomalacia.

The trachea and bronchi (as far as second-order divisions) can be stented via a flexible bronchoscope. Complications include stent migration, tumor in-growth around the stent, formation of granulation tissue, mucous retention, infection, and hemorrhage. Metallic stents are used increasingly for palliation of symptoms associated with inoperable malignant tracheobronchial obstruction. Retrievable metallic stents are safe and effective as a temporizing measure for managing malignant tracheobronchial strictures, followed by CMT or RT.[9]

PLEURAL DISEASE

Pleural effusions occur in up to 50% of patients with metastatic malignancy and are most frequently encountered in those with breast cancer or non–small cell lung cancer. Guidelines for treatment of pleural effusions involve thoracentesis as the first step. If this results in symptomatic improvement and lung reexpansion, pleurodesis is next if the effusion recurs. Options for persistent/recurrent malignant pleural effusions include thoracoscopy, creation of a pleuroperitoneal shunt, and placement of a PleurX catheter.[10]

Chemical pleurodesis is an established palliative therapy for recurrent, symptomatic malignant pleural effusions. Talc is the most effective agent. A long-term tunneled pleural catheter (PleurX, Cardinal Health, Twinsburg, OH) is another effective alternative option for symptomatic relief of malignant pleural effusions.[11] This is a tunneled multi-sidehole drainage catheter that can be drained continuously or intermittently as needed on an outpatient basis.

ASCITES

Malignant refractory ascites is associated with a poor prognosis in cancer and is a marker of advanced stage. Patients present with increasing abdominal girth, abdominal pain, bloating, early satiety, and respiratory insufficiency. The median survival is less than 6 months, except with untreated ovarian cancer; efforts are aimed at reducing morbidity and minimizing hospitalization.[12] Several management options are available, including use of diuretics, paracentesis, intracavitary chemotherapy, hyperthermic chemotherapy, intracavitary biological agents (such as immunomodulators and radioimmunotherapy), intracavitary radioisotopes, and surgical shunting.[13] Paracentesis is a low-risk drainage procedure that is usually performed at the patient's bedside. When it is complicated by loculated ascites or failed bedside blinded paracentesis, interventional radiology (IR) and image-guided paracentesis can be done for both diagnostic and therapeutic purposes. In most cases, immediate relief is good; unfortunately, rapid reaccumulation may require repeated paracentesis.[14] To minimize the need for repeated paracentesis, a multi-sidehole catheter (PleurX, Denver Biomaterials, Golden, CO) is placed percutaneously with image guidance into the ascites; ultrasound or fluoroscopic modalities are used as outpatient procedures with the patient under conscious sedation. These drainage catheters have a polyester cuff and are tunneled, which reduces the risk of sepsis, as is seen with tunneled central venous catheters.[15] Drainage may be continuous or intermittent as required, thereby negating the need for repeated paracentesis and limiting hospitalization.

Rosenberg and colleagues reported more effective palliation and acceptable complication rates when PleurX catheters were placed during a single hospital visit compared with repeated large-volume outpatient clinical paracentesis that required frequent hospital trips. The PleurX catheter can become clogged and may require replacement.[16]

HEPATOBILIARY CANCER

Interventional radiology procedures for primary and secondary hepatic and biliary cancers are used primarily for cytoreduction or drainage techniques to relieve symptoms from tumor bulk and/or to relieve obstructive symptoms. The most common symptoms are pain, fatigue, anorexia, weight loss, jaundice, and pruritus. Locoregional treatments are indicated for relief of local symptoms (pruritus, pain, or signs of jaundice) in inoperable patients whose cancers are not responding well to CMT or who are unable to tolerate CMT. These treatments are used in conjunction with medical treatment of liver failure symptoms. Treatment options to cytoreduce tumor include image-guided percutaneous thermal or chemical ablation, transarterial chemoembolization (TACE), transarterial bland embolization (TAE), and selective internal radiation therapy (SIRT). Treatment options for relief of biliary obstructive symptoms include percutaneous transhepatic biliary drainage and biliary stenting. The most common tumors are hepatocellular carcinoma (HCC), cholangiocarcinoma (CC), metastatic colorectal carcinoma (mCRC), metastatic neuroendocrine tumor (mNET), and pancreatic cancer.

CYTOREDUCTION

Image-guided ablative therapies include chemical or thermal ablation. In either case, the treatment is performed (percutaneously) by placing a needle or probe into the lesion. Ablation can be done for tumors up to 3 to 5 cm in diameter.[17] Although larger tumors are treated with ablation as well, this typically requires multiple overlapping ablation procedures. Treatment of larger lesions with this technique is not likely to completely obliterate the targeted metastases but may be sufficient for symptom relief. Larger lesions are more typically treated with transarterial ablative embolization therapy or a combination of percutaneous and transarterial techniques.

Percutaneous treatment can involve ethanol injection (PEI), RFA, cryoablation, microwave ablation, and laser ablation. Typically, RFA is used if the goal is complete tumor necrosis and curative intent; however, it can be utilized for symptom palliation as well. In a randomized controlled trial that compared PEI with RFA for patients with HCC, RFA was more effective with fewer treatments than PEI, albeit with a slightly higher incidence of nonserious complications.[18] Another trial demonstrated improved survival with RFA in patients with HCC compared with PEI (64% vs. 54%), along with a similar rate of adverse events.[19] Additionally, in a mixed group of patients with HCC and mCRC,[20] individuals who underwent RFA had a lower recurrence rate than those treated with PEI (2% vs. 14%) and had a significantly lower complication rate (3% vs. 41%). PEI is typically completed in several treatment sessions, and RFA is typically done in a single treatment session. Because of these advantages, RFA is the most popular ablative technique used in the United States.

Cholangiocarcinomas are typically perihilar in location and ablative techniques are rarely of benefit (because of the risk of biliary duct injury); only a minority of those with intrahepatic cholangiocarcinoma can undergo ablative procedures with some expectation of benefit.[21] In contrast, RFA is very valuable for palliating symptoms of patients with metastatic neuroendocrine tumor. In a large series of patients, RFA provided at least some relief of symptoms in 95% of patients.[22]

For large, more extensive hepatic tumors, intra-arterial therapies provide relief of symptoms. These treatments involve transarterial hepatic chemoembolization, bland embolization, or yttrium-90 (Y^{90}) microsphere selective internal radiation therapy/radioembolization. Patient selection for any of these transarterial methods is important, as functional liver reserve, portal vein patency, and anatomy need to be considered.

TACE is ideally suited for highly vascularized tumors. TACE involves intra-arterial treatment using CMT (typically cisplatin, doxorubicin, and mitomycin C) combined with ethiodol (iodized poppy seed oil) and small (typically 300 to 500 micron sized) inert embolic particles delivered subselectively into the hepatic artery. This results in a very high concentration of CMT within the tumor (10 to 25 times that obtained with intra-arterial infusion alone), prolonged CMT dwell time within the hepatic metastases, increased CMT uptake by tumor cells, and ischemic necrosis of the tumor with decreased systematic toxicity. In a recent systematic review of cohort and randomized trials using TACE, Marelli

et al. reported an overall objective response rate of 40% ± 20% and 1-, 2-, and 3-year survival rates of 62% ± 20%, 42% ± 17%, and 30% ± 15%, respectively; mean survival time was 18 ± 9 months.[23] Some studies suggest that bland embolization (TAE) performs as well as TACE.[23]

The value of TACE and/or TAE in the treatment of mNET is seen in rapid progression of liver metastases, symptoms related to tumor bulk, and symptoms related to hormonal excess. mNET frequently results in "carcinoid syndrome," which consists of variable degrees of diarrhea, facial flushing/rash, hypertension, and electrolyte disorders. Only a small percentage of patients with mNET are candidates for surgical resection and/or percutaneous ablation. TACE or TAE is effective at cytoreduction and symptom control of carcinoid syndrome, as well as pain due to enlarging metastases, with an average response rate in multiple case series publications ranging from 32% to 56%.[24]

Drug-eluting beads (DEBs) have emerged as a chemoembolization method for treating HCC and liver metastases. These beads are loaded with chemotherapeutic agents such as doxorubicin and irinotecan. Potential advantages include higher tumor levels and lower systemic concentrations of the drug, thus reducing the risk of systemic side effects such as myelosuppression. Currently, however, only limited data on this technique have been published. A recently published prospective randomized trial compared DEB with TACE and demonstrated a statistically significant improved objective response to DEB compared with TACE, and a trend toward higher response rates and greater disease control overall in those with more advanced metastatic disease.[25]

Intra-arterial selective internal radioembolization therapy using yttrium-90 (Y^{90}) microspheres in multiple clinical trials has provided effective palliation for those with primary HCC and for individuals with liver metastases (predominantly colorectal cancer) (Fig. 36-3). Survival times were 21.6 to 24.4 months for patients with Okuda I disease, and 10 to 12.5 months for those with Okuda II stage HCC.[26,27] In cases of radioembolization metastatic (predominantly colorectal) cancer in which standard therapy had failed, standard of care systemic chemotherapy resulted in a median survival of 457 days for patients with CRC and 776 days for those with mNET.[28]

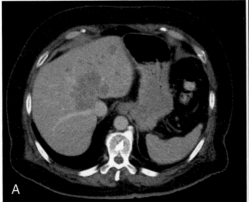 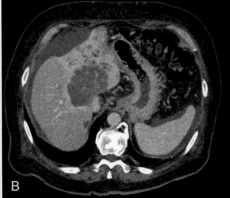

Fig. 36-3 Patient with unresectable central hepatic cholangiocarcinoma treated with yttrium-90 (Y^{90}) radioembolization of the entire liver in two sessions separated by 6 weeks. Pretreatment computed tomography (CT) scan demonstrates a central, low-density, enhancing mass. An additional low-density lesion in the left lobe represents left hepatic biliary dilatation resulting from obstruction. At 6 months following treatment, CT scan demonstrates necrosis of the mass. Treatment resulted in left hepatic atrophy and ascites. Persistent left biliary dilatation is evident.

OBSTRUCTION

Most patients with advanced cancer of the pancreas and extrahepatic biliary ducts develop symptomatic biliary obstruction. Goals of palliation involve relief from jaundice, pruritus, and gastrointestinal symptoms in the hope of improving quality of life.[29] Percutaneous transhepatic biliary drainage is indicated when endoscopic management fails to relieve biliary obstruction or is contraindicated, or when intrahepatic obstruction is not amenable to endoscopic decompression. Frequently, initial management consists of endoscopic placement of biliary drainage catheter(s). However, the usual plastic catheters have a high occlusion rate, requiring replacement every 2 to 3 months. They also are uncomfortable and inconvenient for patients, and their use may lead to recurrent cholangitis. Internalized metallic stents have a median patency of 6 to 7 months[30] and are preferred whenever possible. About 10% to 30% of metallic stents will require reintervention for recurrent jaundice.[31]

PANCREATIC CANCER PAIN

Approximately 75% of patients with pancreatic cancer have pain at diagnosis, as do 90% with advanced stages.[32] As symptoms worsen, standard treatment with escalating doses of opioids[33] is utilized with increased risk of opioid-related adverse effects and toxicities. The use of neurolytic celiac plexus block (NCPB) for pancreatic cancer pain has been extensively documented. NCPB involved needles placed percutaneously under image guidance and injection of 50% ethanol into the region of the celiac plexus to destroy sensory nerve tissue. Yan et al., in a systemic review and meta-analysis of several randomized controlled trials, concluded that NCPB improved pain control and reduced opioid narcotic usage and constipation compared with standard systematic analgesic treatment.[32]

GASTROINTESTINAL OBSTRUCTION AND MALNUTRITION TREATED BY ENTERAL TUBE PLACEMENT

Gastrostomy (G), gastrojejunostomy (GJ), and jejunostomy (J) tubes are used for nutritional support. When a patient is unable to eat for longer than a couple of weeks with a functional gut, G, GI, or J enteral feeding is preferred over prolonged nasogastric tube feeding. In patients with mechanical bowel obstruction, decompression of the bowel to alleviate associated symptoms is accomplished through a venting enterogastrostomy. The method of access depends on the underlying pathologic process. A G tube may be used for gastric feeding in patients with an inoperable malignant esophageal obstruction following failed stent placement, or with bowel obstruction for venting with malignant bowel obstruction and decompression. GJ tubes are placed for duodenal carcinoma, and the gastrostomy port decompresses a distended stomach, while the jejunal port threaded across the duodenal obstruction enables enteral nutrition to occur in the jejunum. J-tube placement enables enteral nutrition following gastrectomy.

G and GJ tubes are placed endoscopically or radiologically under conscious sedation, whereas J tubes are placed surgically following transfixation of a jejunal loop to the abdominal wall. If the jejunal tube is dislodged, or if it malfunctions, it is replaced under fluoroscopic guidance by an interventional radiologist, thus reducing the need for reoperation.

In a large meta-analysis involving G-tube placement, Wollman and colleagues reported that major complications and 30-day procedure-related mortality following percutaneous radiologic gastrostomy (PRG) were significantly less compared with percutaneous endoscopic gastrostomy (PEG) or surgical placement. The risk of wound-related problems (e.g., major infection, septicemia, dehiscence) was 0.8% for PRG versus 3.3% for PEG.[34]

Fortunately, major procedure-related complications with PRG or PEG (inadvertent injury to neighboring structures such as colon, liver, and spleen) are rare and manifest shortly after the procedure. Other complications include tube site pain, infection, leakage, herniation, bleeding, ulceration, tumor seeding, gastric outlet obstruction, gastroparesis, volvulus, tube dislodgment, clogging, and aspiration.[35] In a recent retrospective review, PEG (n = 30) and PRG (n = 44) were equally safe; however, PRG was significantly costlier than PRG in spite of the older age of the PRG group. On average, the PEG group had a longer hospital stay and a greater amount of medical care.[36] Results from a retrospective analysis involving children (n = 98) who had undergone one of the three methods (PEG, PRG, or surgery) revealed that PRG may be more economical than PEG or surgery.[37]

GASTROINTESTINAL OBSTRUCTION: ENTERAL STENT PLACEMENT

Intrinsic esophageal tumors or extrinsic compression commonly caused by lung cancer can result in dysphagia and/or tracheoesophageal fistula. Less than 7% of individuals with a symptomatic malignant obstruction survive beyond 1 year following stent placement. The main role of stent placement in inoperable patients is to relieve dysphagia and improve quality of life.[38,39] Stent migration, tumor in-growth, and reflux are some of the common complications that occur following successful stenting. Specialized stents have been developed to deal with each.[40–42] For patients whose nutritional status fails to improve because of reduced intake, whose fistula fails to heal, or in whom dysphagia persists despite a patent esophagus after stenting, a percutaneous gastrostomy should be considered.

Current management options for malignant gastroduodenal obstruction include surgical bypass and placement of GJ or J tubes. However, several studies have shown the usefulness of metal stents, which is similar to that of esophageal stents. Endoscopists and interventional radiologists can place these stents. In a systematic review of 32 studies, Dormann and colleagues reported successful stenting in 97%, with nearly 90% experiencing resolution of symptoms and able to take soft solids or a full diet for 4 days. However, as with esophageal stents, migration and tumor in-growth can occur.[43]

Jeurnink and colleagues reported from their systematic review 44 studies on the use of GJ and stent placements. Technical success (>95%) and complication rates (<20%) were similar among these studies. Stents provided rapid clinical symptom improvement and shorter hospital stays. However, recurrence of symptoms was common with stents. The authors concluded that for patients with a relatively short life expectancy, stents should be considered as the first option and GJ tubes should be reserved for patients with prospects of longer survival.[44]

Current indications for colonic stenting include temporary stenting as a "bridge to surgery" and palliation in patients unsuitable for surgery.[45] Left-sided colonic stent placement without endoscopic guidance is feasible. However, more proximal colonic lesions require endoscopic guidance with or without fluoroscopic assistance. In a meta-analysis of 10 studies, Tilney and colleagues reported that stent placement for malignant colonic obstruction offered a good alternative to emergency surgery that uniformly resulted in stoma formation and colostomy. Primary stent placement was highly successful (93%) and less risky; this procedure was associated with fewer complications than surgery and did not adversely affect patients' survival. It also reduced the longitudinal need for colostomy.[46]

Perforation, the most feared complication of stent placement, occurs in about 2.5%, as determined by a literature review of 27 studies. Other complications include stent migration (4.4%), pain and tenesmus (2.2%), stent occlusion (<1%), and rectovesical fistula (<1%).[47] Current covered stents, which theoretically could delay tumor in-growth and stent obstruction, are not effective and are prone to more complications when compared with uncovered metal stents.[48]

HYDRONEPHROSIS

Patients with malignant urinary obstruction present with hydronephrosis as an incidental finding on imaging studies, or they present with symptoms, with findings of renal insufficiency, urosepsis, or flank pain. Malignant unilateral ureteral obstruction is due to intrinsic tumors such as ureteral transitional cell carcinoma, invasive bladder tumor, or an extrinsic tumor compressing the ureter, as occurs with gynecologic malignancies, colorectal carcinomas, and soft tissue sarcomas. Distal obstruction can result from locally extensive bladder, prostate, cervical, or rectal carcinomas.

Urinary drainage preserves renal function and treats infection. Management depends on the level of obstruction and the potential for urinary diversion. For bladder outlet obstruction, the interventional radiologist can do an image-guided suprapubic catheter placement or bilateral nephrostomy for continuous drainage. For ureteral obstruction, cystoscopic cannulation with placement of a ureteral stent is typically the first option. Infiltrating large bladder tumors or severe ureteral strictures may prevent this approach. Percutaneous nephrostomy (PCN) by IR is an alternative, and is the first line of management with urosepsis. PCN also provides a means to subsequent ureteral stricture dilatation and placement of stents. These can then be exchanged transurethrally by the urologist on a regular basis through cystoscopic guidance. Patients who cannot have indwelling ureteral stents because of small irritable bladders or bladder obstruction tumors, and those who have had a cystectomy without a functioning diverting pouch or neobladder, will need continuous, externally accessible nephrostomy tubes, and will require exchange every 2 to 3 months to prevent encrustation and clogging of the catheters. Externally accessible nephroureteral catheters, which also require periodic exchanges, are an alternative.

Patients who have had a curative radical cystectomy and ileal conduit may experience recurrent malignancy, benign strictures, chronic infection, and stone formation. Strictures usually occur at the distal ureter and, if benign, may be amenable to balloon ureteroplasty or serial catheter dilatation, performed by an interventionalist via an antegrade percutaneous transrenal approach.[49] A subset of ileal loop strictures requires surgical revision.[50] Patients with ileal conduits and long-term ureteral catheters should have them converted to retrograde trans-stoma catheters and eliminate the transcutaneous catheter. These are then exchanged periodically (usually every 2–3 months) to prevent obstruction with encrustation. This is a safe and effective alternative to surgery.[51]

GENITOURINARY HEMORRHAGE

Bleeding secondary to genitourinary malignancy can be massive and life threatening. Morbidity and associated increased resource utilization may be due to repeat admissions and transfusions.

Renal cancer is typically managed surgically with radical or partial nephrectomy. For patients who are poor surgical candidates because of comorbidities such as solitary kidney, renal insufficiency, and multiple tumors, percutaneous ablative or cryoablation techniques such as RFA should be considered.[52] Peripheral lesions and lesions smaller than 4 cm are best suited to image-guided ablation.[53] Although RFA has been used as palliative therapy to treat intractable hematuria, embolotherapy is more frequently used for inoperable renal cancers. Palliative embolization of renal tumors involves the transarterial subselective injection of ethanol or biodegradable particles into the renal artery under conscious sedation. This technique has significant benefit for most patients who require transfusion because of gross hematuria and flank pain,[54] with less than 5% risk of complications from the procedure.[55] Although most patients develop a post-infarction syndrome, it is usually mild and self-limiting. The role of preoperative embolization in facilitating surgical nephrectomy has been a subject of debate in the medical literature. After an extensive review of the literature, Kalman and Vanhorst concluded that this technique is most beneficial for patients with large vein-invading tumors; the material of choice for embolization is ethanol, as it causes microvascular occlusion and necrosis of perivascular tissue, and the optimal delay between embolization and nephrectomy is 1 day.[56]

Hemorrhage from pelvic genitourinary neoplasm can be treated successfully by transarterial subselective iliac artery embolization. Liguori and colleagues reported control of bleeding in 36 of 44 patients who experienced intractable hematuria secondary to advanced pelvic malignancies due to bladder invasion when bilateral selective internal iliac artery embolization was performed. Five patients underwent a second embolization, which was successful in two. The conclusion of this study is that bilateral internal iliac artery embolization should be considered as the treatment of choice before surgery because of the fact that embolization decreases costs, operating time, and blood loss in operable patients.[57]

BONE METASTASES

Bone metastases resulting from a primary or a nonosseous primary are the most common causes of pain in cancer. Patients present with chronic pain and incident pain due to instability and pathologic fracture. Depending on functional deficits and location and extent of disease, patients should be managed surgically. Pain is controlled by high doses of opiates and by radiotherapy and/or chemotherapy. For many for whom anticancer therapy provides little benefit, the interventional radiologist is able to play an active role in pain management and in improvement of quality of life through efficient imaging-guided techniques. The interventional radiologist may also play an important role by performing preoperative embolization to facilitate surgical correction.

Spinal metastases can be treated by percutaneous vertebral augmentation techniques such as vertebroplasty and kyphoplasty. These procedures are sometimes used in conjunction with ablative therapies. Peripheral bone pain can be managed by thermal ablation techniques, namely, radiofrequency and cryoablation, sometimes in conjunction with cement injection (cementoplasty), particularly in weight-bearing bones such as the acetabulum.

Conventional vertebroplasty involves the introduction of a large-bore needle into the vertebral body through the pedicles, as well as injection of radiopaque cement under direct fluoroscopic guidance. Careful attention to technique is necessary to prevent complications that may arise from cement extravasation into the spinal canal, the epidural venous plexus, or the intervertebral disk. Significant pain relief is expected in more than 70% of patients with vertebral metastasis and multiple myeloma treated with vertebroplasty.[58,59] In a large retrospective study of vertebroplasty conducted by Gangi and colleagues, pain relief was obtained in 83% of patients with vertebral tumors; analgesic effects were experienced within 6 to 48 hours after the procedure.[60]

Acetabulum cementoplasty is performed in the same way; a large-bore needle is positioned in the metastasis under CT guidance or fluoroscopy, and ablation is followed by injection of cement under fluoroscopy to avoid leakage into the joint or soft tissues. Placement of additional needles is sometimes necessary for good filling of the metastatic cavity within the bone.[61]

Kyphoplasty involves introducing a balloon device similar to those used for angioplasty into the compressed vertebral body and inflating it to create a cavity. This cavity is filled with radiopaque cement under fluoroscopic guidance following removal of the balloon. Vertebroplasty and kyphoplasty are safe and are similarly effective in relieving pain and improving quality of life.[62]

Percutaneous RF ablation is effective for painful soft tissue and osteolytic metastatic lesions (Fig. 36-4). Callstrom

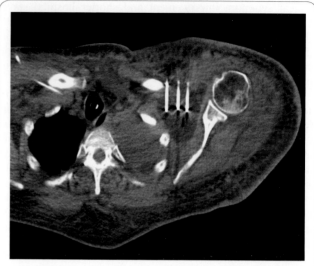

Fig. 36-4 Cryoablation of the left brachial plexus. The patient had severe left upper extremity pain from recurrent breast carcinoma with extensive axillary invasion. Post ablation, the patient's pain levels were significantly reduced. Computed tomography (CT) scan demonstrates three probes in the left axilla. The low-density region surrounding the probes is the "ice ball," or ablation zone.

and colleagues (2002) reported on the use of RFA to treat 12 patients with a single painful osteolytic metastasis ranging from 1 to 11 cm in diameter. Chemotherapy and radiation therapy had failed to relieve pain. A decrease in mean pain score from 6.5 to 1.8 (out of 10) was achieved within 4 weeks after treatment without complications and with reduced consumption of analgesics.[63] Several additional reports have described the successful application of cryoablation in the treatment of primary and metastatic bone cancers.[64,65]

Many metastatic bone lesions, most notably renal cell carcinoma and primary bone cancers, are highly vascular and may benefit from preoperative or palliative transarterial embolization. Preoperative embolization results in significantly reduced perioperative blood loss and reduced tumor volume and provides a safer, easier, more complete resection.[66] Palliative embolization has been shown to be effective in controlling pain[66]; it reduces the size of metastases to facilitate the benefits of other therapies such as radioiodine therapy, radiation therapy, and ablative therapy.

In conclusion, interventional radiology plays an important role in symptom management, quality of life, and survival for cancer patients suffering from a wide range of potentially debilitating tumors.

REFERENCES

1. Park HS, Kim YI, Kim HY, et al. Bronchial artery and systemic artery embolization in the management of primary lung cancer patients with hemoptysis. *Cardiovasc Intervent Radiol.* 2007;30:638–643.
2. Yoon W, Kim JK, Kim YH, et al. Bronchial and non-bronchial systemic artery embolization for life-threatening hemoptysis: a comprehensive review. *Radiographics.* 2002;22:1395–1409.
3. Lanciego C, Chacon JL, Julian A, et al. Stenting as first option for endovascular treatment of

malignant superior vena cava syndrome. *AJR Am J Roentgenol.* 2001;177:585–593.
4. Nguyen NP, Borok TL, Welsh J, et al. Safety and effectiveness of vascular endoprostheses for malignant superior vena cava syndrome. *Thorax.* 2009;64:174–178.
5. Watson PN, Evans RJ. Intractable pain with lung cancer. *Pain.* 1987;29:163–173.
6. Van Sonnenberg E, Shankar S, Morrison PR, et al. Radiofrequency ablation of thoracic lesions: part 2, initial clinical experience—technical and

multidisciplinary considerations in 30 patients. *AJR Am J Roentgenol.* 2005;184:381–390.
7. Greico CA, Simon CJ, Mayo-Smith WW, et al. Percutaneous image-guided thermal ablation and radiation therapy: outcomes of combined treatment for 41 patients with inoperable stage I/II non-small-cell lung cancer. *J Vasc Interv Radiol.* 2006;17:1117–1124.
8. de Baere T, Palussiere J, Auperin A, et al. Midterm local efficacy and survival after radiofrequency ablation of lung tumors with minimum follow-up

of 1 year: prospective evaluation. *Radiology.* 2006;240:587–596.

9. Kim JH, Shin JH, Song HY, et al. Palliative treatment of inoperable malignant tracheobronchial obstruction: temporary stenting combined with radiation therapy and/or chemotherapy. *AJR Am J Roentgenol.* 2009;193:W38–W42.

10. Antony VB, Loddenkemper R, Astoul P, et al. Management of malignant pleural effusions. *Eur Respir J.* 2001;18:402–419.

11. Courtney A, Nemcek Jr AA, Rosenberg S, et al. Prospective evaluation of the PleurX catheter when used to treat recurrent ascites associated with malignancy. *J Vasc Interv Radiol.* 2008;19:1723–1731.

12. Ayantunde AA, Parsons SL. Pattern and prognostic factors in patients with malignant ascites: a retrospective study. *Ann Oncol.* 2007;18:945–949. Epub 2007 Feb 13.

13. Adam RA, Adam YG. Malignant ascites: past, present, and future. *J Am Coll Surg.* 2004;198:999–1011.

14. Lee CW, Bociek G, Faught W. A survey of practice in management of malignant ascites. *J Pain Symptom Manage.* 1998;16:96–101.

15. Richard HM, Coldwell DM, Boyd-Kranis RL, et al. PleurX tunneled catheter in the management of malignant ascites. *J Vasc Interv Radiol.* 2001;12:373–375.

16. Rosenberg S, Courtney AL, Nemcek AA, et al. Comparison of percutaneous management techniques for recurrent malignant ascites. *J Vasc Interv Radiol.* 2004;15:1129–1131.

17. Cormier JN, Thomas KT, Chari RS, et al. Management of hepatocellular carcinoma. *J Gastrointest Surg.* 2006;10:761–780.

18. Livraghi T, Goldberg SN, Lazzaroni S, et al. Small hepatocellular carcinoma: treatment with radio-frequency ablation versus ethanol injection. *Radiology.* 1999;210:655–661.

19. Shiina S, Teratani T, Obi S, et al. A randomized controlled trial of radiofrequency ablation with ethanol injection for small hepatocellular carcinoma. *Gastroenterology.* 2005;129:122–130.

20. Pearson AS, Izzo F, Fleming RY, et al. Intraoperative radiofrequency ablation or cryoablation for hepatic malignancies. *Am J Surg.* 1999;178:592–596.

21. Ustundag Y, Bayraktar Y. Cholangiocarcinoma: a compact review of the literature. *World J Gastroenterol.* 2008;14:6458–6466.

22. Gillams A, Cassoni A, Conway G, et al. Radiofrequency ablation of neuroendocrine liver metastases: the Middlesex experience. *Abdom Imaging.* 2005;30:435–441.

23. Marelli L, Stigliano R, Triantos C, et al. Transarterial therapy for hepatocellular carcinoma: which technique is more effective? A systematic review of cohort and randomized studies. *Cardiovasc Interv Radiol.* 2007;30:6–25.

24. Madoff DC, Gupta S, Ahrar K, et al. Update on the management of neuroendocrine hepatic metastases. *J Vasc Interv Radiol.* 2006;17:1235–1250.

25. Lammer J, Malagari K, Vogl T, et al. Prospective randomized study of doxorubicin-eluting-bead embolization in the treatment of hepatocellular carcinoma: results of the PRECISION V study. *Cardiovasc Interv Radiol.* 2010;33:41–52.

26. Salem R, Lewandowski RJ, Atassi B, et al. Treatment of unresectable hepatocellular carcinoma with use of 90Y microspheres (TheraSphere): safety, tumor response, and survival. *J Vasc Interv Radiol.* 2005;16:1627–1639.

27. Carr BI. Hepatic arterial 90Yttrium glass microspheres (Therasphere) for unresectable hepatocellular carcinoma: interim safety and survival data on 65 patients. *Liver Transpl.* 2004;10:S107–S110.

28. Sato KT, Lewandowski RJ, Mulcathy MF, et al. Unresectable chemo-refratory liver metastases: radioembolization with 90Y microspheres—safety, efficacy, and survival. *Radiology.* 2008;247:507–515.

29. Nakakura EK, Warren RS. Palliative care for patients with advanced pancreatic and biliary cancers. *Surg Oncol.* 2007;16:293–297.

30. Garcea G, Ong SL, Dennison AR, et al. Palliation of malignant obstructive jaundice. *Dig Dis Sci.* 2009;54:1184–1198.

31. van Delden OM, Lameris JS. Percutaneous drainage and stenting for palliation of malignant bile duct obstruction. *Eur Radiol.* 2008;18:448–456.

32. Yan BM, Myers RP. Neurolytic celiac plexus block for pain control in unresectable pancreatic cancer. *Am J Gastroenterol.* 2007;102:430–438.

33. Carr DB, Goudas LC, Balk EM, et al. Evidence report on the treatment of pain in cancer patients. *J Natl Cancer Inst Monogr.* 2004;32:23–31.

34. Wollman B, D'Agostino HB, Walus-Wigle JR, et al. Radiologic, endoscopic, and surgical gastrostomy: an institutional evaluation and meta-analysis of the literature. *Radiology.* 1995;197:699–704.

35. Schrag SP, Sharma R, Jaik NP, et al. Complications related to percutaneous endoscopic gastrostomy (PEG) tubes: a comprehensive clinical review. *J Gastrointest Liver Dis.* 2007;16:407–418.

36. Galaski A, Peng WW, Ellis M, et al. Gastrostomy tube placement by radiological versus endoscopic methods in an acute care setting: a retrospective review of frequency, indications, complications and outcomes. *Can J Gastroenterol.* 2009;23:109–114.

37. Goretsky MF, Johnson N, Farrell M, et al. Alternative techniques of feeding gastrostomy in children: a critical analysis. *J Am Coll Surg.* 1996;182:233–240.

38. Johnson E, Enden T, Noreng HJ, et al. Survival and complications after insertion of self-expandable metal stents for malignant oesophageal stenosis. *Scand J Gastroenterol.* 2006;41:252–256.

39. Maroju NK, Anbalagan P, Kate V, et al. Improvement in dysphagia and quality of life with self-expanding metallic stents in malignant esophageal strictures. *Indian J Gastroenterol.* 2006;25:62–65.

40. Verschuur EM, Repici A, Kuipers EJ, et al. New design esophageal stents for the palliation of dysphagia from esophageal or gastric cardiac cancer: a randomized trial. *Am J Gastroenterol.* 2008;103:304–312. Epub 2007 Sep 25.

41. Vakil N, Morris AI, Marcon N, et al. A prospective, randomized, controlled trial of covered expandable metal stents in the palliation of malignant esophageal obstruction at the gastroesophageal junction. *Am J Gastroenterol.* 2001;96:1791–1796.

42. Laasch HU, Marriott A, Wilbraham L, et al. Effectiveness of open versus antireflux stents for palliation of distal esophageal carcinoma and prevention of symptomatic gastroesophageal reflux. *Radiology.* 2002;225:359–365.

43. Dormann A, Meisner S, Verin N, et al. Self-expanding metal stents for gastroduodenal malignancies: systematic review of their clinical effectiveness. *Endoscopy.* 2004;36:543–550.

44. Jeurnink SM, van Eijck CH, Steyerberg EW, et al. Stent versus gastrojejunostomy for the palliation of gastric outlet obstruction: a systematic review. *BMC Gastroenterol.* 2007;7:18.

45. Homs MY, Siersema PD. Stents in the GI tract. *Expert Rev Med Devices.* 2007;4:741–752.

46. Tilney HS, Lovegrove RE, Purkayastha S, et al. Comparison of colonic stenting and open surgery for malignant large bowel obstruction. *Surg Endosc.* 2007;21:225–233.

47. Dionigi G, Villa F, Rovera F, et al. Colonic stenting for malignant disease: review of literature. *Surg Oncol.* 2007;16(suppl 1):S153–S155. Epub 2007 Nov 26.

48. Lee KM, Shin SJ, Hwang JC, et al. Comparison of uncovered stent with covered stent for treatment of malignant colorectal obstruction. *Gastrointest Endosc.* 2007;66:931–936.

49. Martin EC, Fankuchen EI, Casarella WJ. Percutaneous dilatation of ureteroenteric strictures or occlusions in ileal conduits. *Urol Radiol.* 1982;4:19–21.

50. Hildell J. Balloon dilatation of stricture of the ileal loop after ileal conduit diversion. *AJR Am J Roentgenol.* 1987;149:993–994.

51. Tal R, Bachar GN, Baniel J, et al. External-internal nephro-uretero-ileal stents in patients with an ileal conduit: long-term results. *Urology.* 2004;63:438–441.

52. Uppot RN, Silverman SG, Zagoria RJ, et al. Imaging-guided percutaneous ablation of renal cell carcinoma: a primer of how we do it. *AJR Am J Roentgenol.* 2009;192:1558–1570.

53. Gervais DA, McGovern FJ, Arellano RS, et al. Radiofrequency ablation of renal cell carcinoma, part 1: indications, results, and role in patient management over a 6-year period and ablation of 100 tumors. *AJR Am J Roentgenol.* 2005;185:64–71.

54. Maxwell NJ, Saleem Amer N, Rogers E, et al. Renal artery embolisation in the palliative treatment of renal carcinoma. *Br J Radiol.* 2007;80:96–102.

55. Schwartz MJ, Smith EB, Trost DW, et al. Renal artery embolization: clinical indications and experience from over 100 cases. *BJU Int.* 2007;99:881–886.

56. Kalman D, Varenhorst E. The role of arterial embolization in renal cell carcinoma. *Scand J Urol Nephrol.* 1999;33:162–170.

57. Liguori G, Amodeo A, Mucelli FP, et al. Intractable haematuria: long-term results after selective embolization of the internal iliac arteries. *BJU Int.* 2010;106:500–503.

58. McDonald RJ, Trout AT, Gray LA, et al. Vertebroplasty in multiple myeloma: outcomes in a large patient series. *AJNR Am J Neuroradiol.* 2008;29:642–648.

59. Cortet B, Cotten A, Boutry N, et al. Percutaneous vertebroplasty in patients with osteolytic metastases or multiple myeloma. *Rev Rheum Engl Ed.* 1997;64:177–183.

60. Gangi A, Guth S, Imbert JP, et al. Percutaneous vertebroplasty: indications, technique, and results. *Radiographics.* 2003;23:e10.

61. Kelekis A, Lovblad KO, Mehdizade A, et al: Pelvic osteoplasty in osteolytic metastases: technical approach under fluoroscopic guidance and early clinical results. *J Vasc Interv Radiol* 2005;16:81–88.

62. Mathis JM. Percutaneous vertebroplasty or kyphoplasty: which one do I choose? *Skeletal Radiol.* 2006;35:629–631.

63. Callstrom MR, Charboneau JW, Goetz MP, et al. Painful metastases involving bone: feasibility of percutaneous CT- and US-guided radiofrequency ablation. *Radiology.* 2002;224:87–97.

64. Beland MD, Dupuy DE, Mayo-Smith WW. Percutaneous cryoablation of symptomatic extra abdominal metastatic disease: preliminary results. *AJR Am J Roentgenol.* 2005;184:926–930.

65. Callstrom MR, Atwell TD, Charboneau JW, et al. Painful metastases involving bone: percutaneous image-guided cryoablation—prospective trial interim analysis. *Radiology.* 2006;241:572–580.

66. Owen RJT. Embolization of musculoskeletal tumors. *Radiol Clin N Am.* 2008;46:535–543.

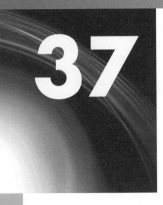

37 Palliative care and surgery

Geoffrey P. Dunn, Daniel B. Hinshaw,
and Timothy M. Pawlik

Palliative surgery enjoys a rich and ancient tradition, although contemporary surgeons remain surprisingly ambivalent about it. Most surgeons now associate palliative surgery with advanced and incurable oncologic disease. However, before the antibiotic era and well into it, palliative surgery was widely practiced beyond the specialty of oncology, as when treating complications of chronic orthopedic and pulmonary conditions resulting from tuberculous and staphylococcal infection. Indirect and direct surgical treatments for symptomatic coronary occlusive disease and mitral commissurotomy for overwhelmingly symptomatic congestive heart failure were accepted treatments before any improvement in survival was demonstrated with these interventions. As surgical cure for all types of disease became more frequent, the appeal of palliative surgery lessened because it became mistakenly synonymous with noncurative surgery. This has created a sense of cognitive dissonance for surgeons attempting to reconcile the need for intervention for distressing symptoms with the increasingly common perception that palliative surgery represents "failure." The previous framework of surgical oncology, structured as it has been upon the disease-based model, has not had the scope or depth to rescue the negative perceptions

about palliative surgery from a death-denying profession and public. This has created the need for a new framework to provide a meaningful and appropriate context for palliative surgery. Palliative surgery for the patient with oncologic illness is best appreciated in the greater context of *surgical palliative care,* which is the treatment of suffering and the promotion of quality of life for seriously or terminally ill patients under surgical care.[1]

Through the perspective of palliative care, a practical, appealing, and evidence-based interdisciplinary approach to patient care for serious or advanced illness, the opportunity now exists for a more consistent and affirmative redefinition of palliative surgery. This transition has been guided by increased emphasis on determining personal relevance for symptom relief ("patient-centered"), minimizing morbidity, improving nonphysical domains, and expanding the durability of symptom relief. A series of position statements (Table 37-1),[2] certification requirements,[3] and educational initiatives[4] suggest that the field of surgery is accommodating itself to this transformation from the hopelessness stemming from failure to cure toward the hopefulness that accompanies our role in mitigating suffering and redefining meaning in our patients' lives. To quote a current authority on palliative surgery, "Almost ironically, a palliative surgical procedure can be an oncologic failure (tumor left behind, margins positive) but a palliative success, achieving relief of an intestinal obstruction in the face of diffuse carcinomatosis."[5]

PALLIATIVE SURGERY DEFINED

Palliative surgery was not consistently defined in the surgical literature until recently. One traditional definition of palliative surgery, surprising now given the primacy of symptom control for palliative care, describes it as surgery resulting in residual microscopic or gross disease at the end of the procedure. Another definition based squarely on the disease-centered model of treatment without any reference to symptom control or quality-of-life outcomes, defined palliative surgery as a resection for recurrent or persistent disease after primary treatment failure.[6] These definitions undoubtedly reflect and contribute

Table 37-1 Statement of principles of palliative care

- Respect the dignity and autonomy of patients and patients' surrogates and caregivers.
- Honor the right of the competent patient or surrogate to choose among treatments, including those that may or may not prolong life.
- Communicate effectively and empathically with patients, their families, and their caregivers.
- Identify the primary goals of care from the patient's perspective, and address how the surgeon's care can achieve the patient's objectives.
- Strive to alleviate pain and other burdensome physical and nonphysical symptoms.
- Recognize, assess, discuss, and offer access to services for psychological, social, and spiritual issues.
- Provide access to therapeutic support, encompassing the spectrum from life-prolonging treatments through hospice care, when they can realistically be expected to improve the quality of life as perceived by the patient.
- Recognize the physician's responsibility to discourage treatments that are unlikely to achieve the patient's goals, and encourage patients and families to consider hospice care when the prognosis for survival is likely to be less than a half-year.
- Arrange for continuity of care by the patient's primary and/or specialist physician, alleviating the sense of abandonment that patients may feel when "curative" therapies are no longer useful.
- Maintain a collegial and supportive attitude toward others entrusted with care of the patient.

From the Bulletin of the American College of Surgeons 2005;90:34-5.

general surgeons in palliative care is limited.[10] In fact, 95% of surgeons reported receiving 10 or fewer hours of palliative care content in medical school, 79% reported 10 or fewer hours in residency or fellowship, and 74% reported 10 or fewer hours of continuing education in palliative care since completing their training. Galante et al.[10] postulated that the lack of postgraduate palliative care training for surgeons accounted for the striking inconsistency in surgical management of symptomatic patients with advanced cancer.

A pioneer of surgical palliative care philosophy, Blake Cady, summarized the intellectual and psychological difficulty confronting surgeons as they contemplate palliative surgery: "One of the basic principles of palliation is that it is easier to make day-to-day surgical decisions in the framework of some overall surgical philosophy. Certainly if you have a mature surgical philosophy that understands the vicissitudes of life, you're better equipped to deal with some of these situations than a surgeon who thinks that "I can cure all problems."[11] Previously, the framework for surgical decision making has been centered on the disease process itself, not on the personhood of the patient or the symptomatic expression of illness. Surgeons have traditionally not "staged" pain, dyspnea, or nausea, nor have many been comfortable with the "patient centering" of care by making concessions to the quirks and uniqueness of each individual, especially in the environment of accountability for mortality and morbidity that follows operative procedures.

PRINCIPLES AND PATIENT ASSESSMENT FOR PALLIATIVE SURGERY

The principles of palliative surgery are derived from the general principles of palliative care and include honest and clear communication, individual acknowledgement of the relevance of the symptom to be treated and the goals of treatment, and the moral and ethical legitimacy of treatment that is noncurative in intent (Table 37-2). Primary considerations for selecting a palliative procedure include the patient's symptoms and personal expectations, the expected

to the persistence of the disease-focused model of treatment as the prevailing approach to treatment for advanced and incurable disease, even when symptom control remains the only achievable clinical objective. It was not until the 1980s that quality of life (QoL) following cancer surgery was acknowledged in the surgical literature as equally important to survival outcomes.[7] Even after another decade had passed, few good studies had been undertaken to address QoL outcomes of oncologic surgical procedures. It was only recently that a more consistent and clinically practical definition of palliative surgery began to emerge. Broad-based advocacy for patient comfort and dignity at the end of life during the 1980s and 1990s in the United States and elsewhere now appears to be influencing the field of surgical oncology. The current consensus definition of palliative surgery that has emerged is well expressed by Miner: "Surgical palliation for cancer is defined best as a procedure used with the primary intention of improving QoL or relieving symptoms caused by the advanced malignancy. The effectiveness of a palliative intervention should be judged by the presence and durability of patient-acknowledged symptom resolution."[8]

IS SURGERY READY FOR PALLIATIVE SURGERY?

A landmark survey[9] of oncologic surgeons showed that palliative surgery is a significant part of many surgeons' practice, with a fifth of cancer operations described as palliative in nature. Data have shown, however, that education among

Table 37-2 Principles of palliative surgery

- Palliation is not the opposite of cure; it has its own distinct indications and goals and should be evaluated independently.
- Asymptomatic patients cannot be palliated.
- Palliative surgery is as morally and ethically legitimate as surgery for curative intent.
- Day-to-day surgical decisions are best made in the framework of ethical, scientific, and technical principles.
- The patient or surrogate must acknowledge the personal relevance of the symptom to be treated.
- Meaningful survival expectations should exist before surgical palliation is offered.
- Goals must be clearly and honestly defined to patient and family, yourself, the surgical team, and other members of the healthcare team.

From Dunn GP, Martensen R, Weissman D, editor. Surgical palliative care: a resident's guide. Chicago, IL: American College of Surgeons; 2009, p. 136.

impact of the procedure on function and the disease trajectory, and the likely prognosis or projected survival, with the expectations for functional decline independent of the effect of surgical intervention. Secondary considerations include the skill and temperament of the surgeon, adjunctive measures to be taken (e.g., radiation following pathologic fracture fixation), reconstructive and rehabilitation requirements, and psychological, social, and economic impact (e.g., days spent in hospital in the face of progressive life-limiting illness). Major operative complications dramatically worsen the prospects of achieving durable symptom relief up to the time of death. The principles and interventions useful for the palliation of malignant disease can be applied to non-neoplastic disorders frequently encountered, such as regional pain syndromes, cardiomyopathy, intestinal failure, and chronic liver failure.

Currently, no consensus has been reached about the estimated life expectancy that would preclude palliative surgery, perhaps because prognostication itself has been so inconsistent. However, in general, any patient with a projected survival based on an Eastern Cooperative Oncology Group (ECOG) performance status of 3 or greater with likely survival measured in days to weeks usually should not be offered a major operative intervention (e.g., general anesthesia with laparotomy/thoracotomy). Less invasive surgical interventions (e.g., endoscopic stenting) may be appropriate even in very late stages of illness, albeit with appropriate informed consent and clear articulation of the increased risks of performing these procedures in very ill patients. In some instances, intractable symptoms rather than progression of disease account for the decline in function. In calculating the impact of surgery, transient loss of function due to the immediate postoperative state must also be considered. The window for tallying postoperative mortality and morbidity is 30 days, making this amount of time a likely minimal prerequisite for operation for many surgeons. One large study[9] of palliative surgery outcomes found that all patients who had relief of the symptom for which treatment was targeted demonstrated this improvement within 6 weeks. For highly burdensome symptoms, such as a pathologic fracture, which would respond dramatically and rapidly to surgical treatment, a more modest expectation for survival (weeks) should not rule out surgery.

The patient assessment for palliative surgery is fundamentally the same as assessments for nonsurgical treatment: Do the patient and family understand the nature and prognosis of the underlying illness? Does the patient comprehend the risks and benefits? Because of its invasive nature, patients and families may have unrealistic expectations about the impact of surgery, including actual cure, even in the face of disseminated disease. Does the patient have an advance directive and a surrogate decision maker? Will the patient and family tolerate the physical, psychological, social, and economic consequences of the proposed procedure?

The prospect of palliative surgery offers the surgeon and other interdisciplinary team members a unique opportunity to explore the patient's broader experience of illness with all of the opportunities for redefining a "good outcome" that can result. Surgeons will increasingly contribute to palliative care through their operative skills and in their clinical decisions as they become more comfortable with the redefinition of success that has occurred in the nonsurgical palliative disciplines during the past 30 years.

Although "cure" is usually the goal of most surgical interventions to treat malignancies, the aim of any procedure must be framed within the context of the broader personal goals of the patient. These goals often include palliation of symptoms through the appropriate use of surgery to palliate bleeding, obstruction, perforation, or pain. Although cure and palliation may be mutual goals in some patients, in other instances the sole intent of the surgical intervention will be palliative. Ultimately, the goal of any invasive intervention should be to improve the individual patient's life.

Surgery has a long tradition of palliating patients through the use of surgical procedures. In the past, many surgical procedures often involved lengthy operations with potential morbidity and mortality. More recently, however, perioperative morbidity has decreased, and, perhaps more important, significant advances have been made in the fields of laparoscopy and endoscopy.[12] Given this, procedures aimed at palliation have become increasingly able to achieve the goals of symptom relief and improved QoL with a reduction in the surgical burden. Surgeons therefore need to be aware of when a palliative surgical procedure may be indicated and must be knowledgeable about nonsurgical and minimally invasive surgical approaches that may benefit the patient in need of palliation.

Two of the more common general surgical indications for palliative surgical intervention involve patients with gastrointestinal malignancies. For example, given that colon cancer is the second leading cause of cancer-related death in the United States,[13] the surgeon is not infrequently confronted with a patient who may have incurable metastatic disease with an intact primary. Data suggest that the primary tumor will be asymptomatic in many patients, but up to 15% to 20% of patients will have obstruction, and another 10% may have significant hemorrhage from the primary colorectal lesion.[14,15] Although significant symptoms may dictate surgical management, the treatment of asymptomatic patients is more controversial. Data[16,17] suggest that most patients with incurable stage IV colorectal cancer and an intact primary can be managed safely without primary tumor resection. When patients are symptomatic, management has traditionally consisted of open resection or diversion. Recently, the use of laparoscopic diversion has been suggested as a better option that can be performed safely while diminishing recovery time and improving overall QoL.[18] Another option for patients with symptomatic rectal obstruction may be the use of self-expanding metallic stents.[19] The placement of rectal stents is generally well tolerated and can be performed on an outpatient basis. These stents have been shown to be effective, with some series showing that the use of rectal stents may avoid surgical intervention in many patients.

Pancreatic cancer is another disease process that surgeons frequently struggle with in terms of how best to palliate. Pancreatic cancer is associated with high case mortality and short overall survival. As such, effective palliation of this disease with minimal associated morbidity is important to ensure the highest QoL in this group of patients with limited survival. Open "double bypass" (e.g., hepaticojejunostomy plus gastrojejunostomy) has been advocated in the past as an effective method of palliation for patients with advanced pancreatic cancer. Although it is still indicated in a subset of patients, several noninvasive or minimally invasive techniques designed to palliate patients with advanced pancreatic cancer have emerged recently. Specifically, nonoperative biliary decompression by an endoscopic or percutaneous approach may be a better alternative in some patients.[20,21] Stent placement is associated with less morbidity and a shorter hospital stay. In addition, metallic stents that have longer patency rates and require fewer repeat procedures can be placed. Gastric outlet obstruction can often be dealt with by using endoscopic techniques. Duodenal stent placement is successful in up to 90% of patients and has a median duration of 6 months.[22]

Management of pleural effusions and peritoneal ascites presents another set of clinical problems that general surgeons are often asked to help with in the palliative setting. Pleural effusions can be a significant source of morbidity and can have an adverse impact on patient QoL. Pleural effusions can lead to progressive dyspnea and an impaired ability to carry out normal activities of daily living. Several malignancies, including breast, ovarian, and lung, may be associated with the formation of malignant pleural effusions. Although thoracentesis may be helpful initially, its role in the ongoing management of malignant effusions is frequently much more limited. Given this, palliative procedures such as chemical pleurodesis via tube thoracostomy or open video-assisted thoracoscopic surgery (VATS) may be required. Some studies have reported that closed pleurodesis via a small-bore chest tube can be efficacious.[23,24] However, other studies have suggested that VATS may be used as primary treatment, because its use may result in shorter hospital stays, less time with the chest tube, and better overall results.[25] Peritoneal ascites can be a challenging clinical problem in patients with advanced malignant disease. Ascites can cause restricted mobility, pain, and respiratory difficulty. Malignancies commonly associated with ascites include breast, pancreas, stomach, and ovarian. Although diuretic therapy may help control ascites, it usually does not provide a durable solution for patients with malignant ascites. Peritoneovenous shunts were popular in the past for managing malignant ascites, but they have recently fallen out of favor because of risks and associated costs. Large-volume paracentesis can be effective in dealing with malignant ascites; however, the need for repeat procedures can be cumbersome to patients. Given this, the use of indwelling catheters may be preferable to repeated large-volume paracentesis in patients who are in need of ascites management.[26]

In general, palliative surgical procedures should be discussed openly between patients and physicians. Any decision to proceed with a surgical intervention must be placed within the larger context of the patient's physical, psychological, and social well-being. The terms and goals of the procedure need to be clearly delineated. Whenever possible, minimally invasive or nonoperative approaches to palliation should be explored, as these approaches often can provide the best option for improving a patient's quality of life.

MEASUREMENT OF SURGICAL OUTCOMES AND PALLIATIVE SURGERY

Traditionally, assessment of outcomes in surgical oncology has focused on perioperative morbidity and mortality, and whether or not the underlying neoplasm was cured by the surgical intervention. Recent decades have seen a growing recognition that although these outcomes are certainly important, they do not adequately reflect the patient's experience of the disease and its treatment. They may not identify key

differences in otherwise equally efficacious treatment options with respect to cure that would be more consistent with patient preferences and goals of care. Such measures may have even less utility for patients who will not be cured of their underlying cancer.

Considerable efforts have been made over the past three decades to develop measures of health-related quality of life (HRQoL). QoL has been defined as "a multidimensional patient-centered outcome."[27] A schematic depicting some of the many health-related factors and dimensions that define QoL is presented in Figure 37-1.[28] A number of health-related and non–health-related factors have been identified as contributing to QoL. Non–health-related elements of QoL include financial status, location of residence, and time for leisure activities. Three main domains of HRQoL have been identified: physical, social, and psychological.[29] Elements reflective of the physical domain of HRQoL include pain, other forms of physical distress, and functional ability. The social domain relates to the ability to perform one's duties in society, and the psychological domain includes one's emotional and cognitive state.[29] In recognition of the importance of a patient's subjective experience of serious illness and the impact of associated distress, disability, and treatment-related morbidity, several instruments have been developed to measure HRQoL. These instruments have been created to provide more objective reproducible means of measuring the subjective patient experience, especially in the context of clinical trials of different therapies. Instruments used to measure HRQoL have typically been designed for general (generic instruments), disease-specific, or symptom-specific assessment of HRQoL (Table 37-3).[29] Generic instruments are

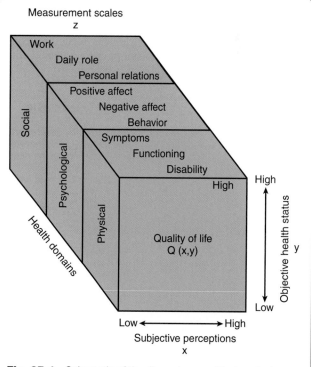

Fig. 37-1 Schematic of the dimensions and factors that make up quality of life. *(Redrawn from Testa MA, Simonson DC. Assessment of quality of life outcomes. N Engl J Med 1996;334:835–840.)*

Table 37-3 Types of quality-of-life instruments

Type of instrument	Application	Examples
Generic instrument	Comparisons across health conditions and interventions	Short Form 36-item Health Survey, Sickness Impact Profile, Nottingham Health Profile
Disease-specific instrument	Specific diagnostic groups and patient populations	Functional Living Index, Rotterdam Symptom Checklist, Cancer Rehabilitation Evaluation System, EORTC QLQ-C30, FACT-G
Symptom-specific instrument	Symptoms of a certain disease process (e.g., pain)	Gastrointestinal Symptom Rating Scale, McGill Pain Questionnaire

From Langenhoff BS, Krabbe PFM, Wobbes T, et al. Quality of life as an outcome measure in surgical oncology. Br J Surg 2001;88:643-52.

designed to facilitate comparisons across broad categories of illnesses, and because of this, they may have limited utility in the assessment of a specific disease that has its own unique set of issues such as cancer. The Short Form 36 (SF-36) is an example of a generic instrument. Disease-specific instruments have been developed to assess HRQoL within various patient populations carrying specific diagnoses. Examples of disease-specific instruments for patients with cancer include the European Organization for Research and Treatment of Cancer Quality of Life Questionnaire (EORTC QLQ-C30) and the Functional Assessment of Cancer Therapy–General (FACT-G). Symptom-specific instruments focus on detailed measurement and assessment of symptoms associated with a

disease process. Their usefulness may be limited to the extent that symptoms alone adequately reflect QoL. The McGill Pain Questionnaire is an example of a symptom-specific instrument that is commonly used in the assessment of cancer-related pain. Recently, the palliative surgery outcome score (PSOS) has been developed to help define QoL-related outcomes in patients undergoing surgical interventions in the setting of advanced cancer.[30] The remainder of this section will focus on a more detailed discussion and comparison between the EORTC QLQ-C30 (and its variants) and the FACT-G. Use of the PSOS as an adjunct to these instruments in further evaluation of the impact of surgical intervention on HRQoL in patients with advanced cancer will also be reviewed.

The EORTC QLQ-C30 represents a modular approach that consists of a core questionnaire to which a cancer-specific module is added as a supplement. The core questionnaire comprises 30 items for patient self-report, which include scales addressing a patient's functional role on physical, cognitive, emotional, and social levels. It also assesses specific symptoms such as pain, fatigue, nausea, vomiting, anorexia, diarrhea, constipation, dyspnea, and insomnia. Other scales assess global health, HRQoL, and the patient's perception of the financial impact of the disease. To address the unique impact of a given type of cancer, supplemental modules have been developed to facilitate comparisons within specific cancer populations (e.g., EORTC QLQ-PAN26 for patients with pancreatic cancer,[31] EORTC QLQ-OES18 for patients with esophageal cancer[32]). The esophageal cancer module from EORTC QLQ-OES18 is presented in Figure 37-2 to illustrate the detailed and focused character of the questions asked in the EORTC cancer-specific modules.

The FACT-G is essentially the U.S. equivalent to the EORTC QLQ-C30 and is similar in many ways to the European instrument. It also uses a modular approach consisting of a generic core questionnaire that is supplemented with disease-specific modules (e.g., FACT-B specific for breast cancer). The generic version (FACT-G) consists of 28 items that broadly

---

EORTC QLQ – QES18

Patients sometimes report that they have the following symptoms or problems. Please indicate the extent to which you have experienced these symptoms or problems during the past week. Please answer by circling the number that best applies to you.

During the past week:	Not at all	A little	Quite a bit	Very much
1. Could you eat solid foods?	1	2	3	4
2. Could you eat liquidized or soft foods?	1	2	3	4
3. Could you drink liquids?	1	2	3	4
4. Have you had trouble swallowing your saliva?	1	2	3	4
5. Have you choked when swallowing?	1	2	3	4
6. Have you had trouble enjoying your meals?	1	2	3	4
7. Have you felt full too quickly?	1	2	3	4
8. Have you had trouble with eating?	1	2	3	4
9. Have you had trouble with eating in front of other people?	1	2	3	4
10. Have you had a dry mouth?	1	2	3	4
11. Have you had problems with your sense of taste?	1	2	3	4
12. Have you had trouble with coughing?	1	2	3	4
13. Have you had trouble with talking?	1	2	3	4
14. Have you had acid indigestion or heartburn?	1	2	3	4
15. Have you had trouble with acid or bile coming into your mouth?	1	2	3	4
16. Have you had pain when you eat?	1	2	3	4
17. Have you had pain in your chest?	1	2	3	4
18. Have you had pain in your stomach?	1	2	3	4

Fig. 37-2 Esophageal cancer module from the European Organization for Research and Treatment of Cancer Quality of Life Questionnaire (EORTC QLQ-OES18). *(Redrawn and adapted from the European Organisation for the Research and Treatment of Cancer.)*

address physical, emotional, and social health issues of cancer patients. A structural difference between the two instruments is that the EORTC QLQ-C30 uses a question format for the generic items, whereas the FACT-G uses statements.[29] When the two instruments have been compared directly in the assessment of patients with breast cancer or Hodgkin's disease, it has been demonstrated that even though substantial overlap may be noted between the two instruments, each instrument measures different elements of QoL and cannot be used interchangeably or compared directly in clinical studies.[33] In addition to differences between the two instruments in phrasing of the items, the FACT-G has unique items that focus on patients' relationships with their doctors, whereas the EORTC QLQ-C30 includes unique items that address cognitive function, the financial impact of the illness, and global QoL.[33]

Both instruments should be effective in providing a detailed portrait of the impact of cancer and cancer treatment on a patient's QoL, and both have limitations for assessing HRQoL outcomes specific to a patient with advanced cancer who is undergoing a palliative surgical intervention. Because survival after a palliative surgical intervention is uncertain and sometimes may be measured in days or weeks at best, potential outcomes in terms of HRQoL must be sufficiently compelling to justify the procedure. Miner et al. used the FACT-G (QoL), the Karnofsky Scale (functional status), and the Memorial Pain Assessment Card (pain) to study outcomes of palliative surgical procedures requiring a general anesthetic in patients with advanced cancer.[34] A critical component of this study was that study personnel asked the patient and a trusted family member (as well as the surgeon) to define the single-most important problem/symptom that she/he wanted to have palliated by the procedure. Of 26 patients participating in the study, 15 patients had undergone operations for gastrointestinal obstruction, 3 for biliary obstruction, 3 for pleural effusion, 3 for management of fungating, malodorous lesions, and 2 for abdominal pain. Twelve of the 26 patients (46%) were noted to have clinical improvement after the palliative operation (based on at least a 25% improvement in one of the parameters measured in the study). The benefits seen in patients with clinical improvement were short-lived (median, only 3.4 months). This study highlights several important observations related to assessing the outcomes of palliative surgical procedures:

1. It is likely that only a minority of patients will have significant improvement in overall QoL, functional status, and pain relief following a palliative surgical procedure, emphasizing the need for careful patient selection.
2. The durability of such benefits may be short-lived.
3. The value of acknowledging the patient's and the family's priorities in a shared decision-making process between surgeon, patient, and family cannot be underestimated, particularly in a context where the potential benefits are often limited and of short duration.

Attempts have been made to better assess the relative therapeutic benefit of palliative surgery for symptomatic patients in the context of advanced cancer. These attempts have led to the development of the PSOS,[30] which is expressed as the percentage of postoperative days during the first 6 months after the operation on which a patient does not require hospitalization, is relieved of the symptom treated by the operation, and has not experienced a major surgical complication.[30] If the patient dies within 6 months after the operation, the remaining days of life after the operation are used as the denominator for the calculation. Using this approach, McCahill et al. identified a PSOS >70% as a good outcome.[30] The authors noted that accurate estimation of patient prognosis by the surgical oncologist is critical to the process of identifying candidates for palliative surgical intervention who will be more likely to achieve a PSOS >70%. In fact, the authors noted that patients were much less likely to have a good PSOS (only 36%)—just 4 of 11 symptomatic patients—if they had <6 months survival time after palliative surgery.[30]

FUTURE OF OUTCOMES ASSESSMENT IN PALLIATIVE SURGERY

Four areas that have been neglected or that require further development are awaiting major advances to yield significant improvements in palliative surgical practice:

1. Recognition that the quality of dying for surgical patients is of equal importance to their QoL
2. Extension of the PSOS concept to surgical oncology patients who will be free of their disease after surgical intervention but maimed by the treatment with a new chronic symptom burden or persistent and unrelieved preoperative symptoms (i.e., recognition that cure accompanied by the sequelae of unrelieved symptoms and potentially chronic suffering represent an ongoing responsibility of the surgeon to provide palliative care)
3. Additional refinements (including better education of surgeons in prognostication) are greatly needed to enhance the accuracy of prognostication in advanced illness.
4. Awareness of the existential/spiritual needs of surgical oncology patients (neglected or underemphasized by most HRQoL instruments) and their crucial importance in any discussion regarding surgical intervention late in an advanced illness.[35]

A study by Steinhauser et al. in which a random national survey of patients, bereaved family members, nurses, social workers, chaplains, physicians, and hospice volunteers explored the perceived attributes of a "good death" demonstrated some remarkable differences in physician attitudes compared with all other individuals surveyed.[36] Patients and most of the other individuals surveyed felt that the following attributes were very important elements of a "good death":

1. To be mentally aware
2. To be at peace with God
3. To not be a burden to one's family
4. To be able to help others
5. To be able to pray
6. To have funeral arrangements planned
7. To not be a burden to society
8. To feel one's life is complete

Unfortunately, physicians who were surveyed did not perceive any of these attributes of a "good death" to be important ($P < .001$).[36] Quantitative survival has been so ingrained into the surgical consciousness as the major surgical outcome that these "soft" outcomes may naturally be viewed as of less importance to many surgeons as well. However, spiritual and existential issues will often weigh the most on the minds of patients with a poor prognosis when they consider additional medical or surgical interventions near the end of life.[35] Surgeons must be open to having discussions with their patients and families about their spiritual concerns, especially when the outcome of any proposed surgical intervention may adversely affect the patient's ability to pursue a good death.

PALLIATIVE CARE, SURGERY, AND ETHICAL CONSIDERATIONS

The ethics of palliative care involves many dimensions of patient care, including consent, truth telling, decisional capacity, and withholding/withdrawing life-sustaining therapy.[37] A comprehensive review of these topics is beyond the scope of this review; however, we herein highlight issues of decisional capacity and withholding/withdrawing life-sustaining therapy.

The principle of autonomy recognizes self-determination as independently and inherently valuable. Each person has the fundamental right to control his or her own body and be protected from unwanted intrusions. As such, physicians need to respect the capacity of individuals to make their own decisions regarding palliative therapy, or end-of-life decision making. When a decision is made to begin the shift from life-sustaining therapies to palliative care, the patient always should be involved directly in all discussions and decision-making processes. Discussions with the patient need to be rooted in an accurate and truthful, yet sensitive, accounting of the medical and prognostic details. Although medical information might not always be perfect, accurate data on the clinical situation are mandatory for patients and families to make informed decisions. Unfortunately, many seriously ill patients are unable to speak for themselves when discussions regarding palliative care/end-of-life treatment are begun.[38] Physicians need to be aware of this and should engage patients early on in the therapeutic relationship, so that palliative and end-of-life decisions can be addressed when patients have full decision-making capacity. For those patients who do not have independent decision-making capacity, physicians need to be aware of substituted judgment. In this situation, a surrogate determines what is best for the patient with decreased or loss of decision-making capacity or the incompetent or incapacitated patient based on the surrogate's understanding of the patient's wishes. Often a proxy decision maker is a family member or close friend who has been chosen because he or she has the best perception of the patient's values and interests. The physician should work with the proxy decision maker to improve the patient's decision-making capacity when possible, and when not possible, should work with the proxy to ensure best understanding of the anticipated wishes of the patient.

Other principles that have implications for palliative care ethics include nonmaleficence and beneficence. Nonmaleficence implies an obligation not to inflict harm intentionally on another; beneficence refers to the duty to contribute proactively to the welfare of others. These principles have been cited commonly in the ethical discussion surrounding the foregoing of life-sustaining therapy, specifically, withholding versus withdrawing life-sustaining therapy.[39] Not uncommonly, physicians are confronted by such issues

near the end of life. However, traditionally, they have found it easier to limit or withhold certain therapeutic efforts (e.g., chest compressions) rather than withdraw already instituted life-sustaining treatments (e.g., stopping mechanical ventilation, nutrition).[40] Most ethicists, however, have concluded that the distinction between withholding and withdrawing life-sustaining therapy is morally irrelevant. Treatment can always be permissibly withdrawn if it can be permissibly withheld.[37,39] As such, physicians, patients, and proxy decision makers are permitted to withdraw life-sustaining therapies if these interventions prove not to have the expected physiologic effect or to be commensurate with the patient's personal goals.

Frequently, an appropriate candidate for palliative surgery will have a preexisting Do-Not-Resuscitate (DNR) order. Surgeons and anesthesiologists may inappropriately invoke the presence of a DNR order as a reason to refuse surgery. Basing their respective positions on the principle of patient autonomy, the American College of Surgeons, the Association of Operating Room Nurses, and the American Society of Anesthesiologists have condemned policies requiring automatic cancellation of existing DNR orders for patients undergoing anesthesia. All organizations recommend preoperative discussion ("required reconsideration") during which the patient or surrogate confirms the patient's treatment goals and limits of care, including revision or implementation of a DNR order; risks of a patient's care plan; and recommendations of the anesthesiologist and the surgeon. During this discussion, the anesthesiologist and the patient can set the parameters for resuscitation for the procedure itself and for time in the recovery room. Two suggested approaches for setting resuscitation parameters include (1) procedures permitted or proscribed may be listed, as in a list of medical directives (e.g., "No chest compressions, but cardioversion and vasopressors permitted") or, (2) the surgeon and the anesthesiologist may be given discretion on the scope of interventions.

SUMMARY

A major advance for surgical oncology in the future will be the recognition within the specialty that dichotomous thinking with respect to palliation is no longer necessary. Palliation as relief of suffering and restoration of function and QoL should be a primary goal of surgical oncologic intervention. When cure of the underlying cause of the patient's suffering is achieved by surgical intervention, the goals of cure and palliation are fully united in the same act. This should become the gold standard for surgical oncologic outcomes: holistic relief of suffering coupled with surgical extirpation of the underlying cancer. When surgical intervention with curative intent causes new or additional suffering that is not accompanied by effective palliative care, this should be seen as a failure (or at least as an unacceptable outcome), even if the underlying cancer is cured by the surgical procedure. When surgical cure is not attainable, excellent attention given from the beginning of surgical care to palliation of suffering can support good QoL for the life remaining and can help ensure a "good death."

REFERENCES

1. Dunn GP. Surgical palliative care. In: Cameron JL, ed. *Current surgical therapy*. Philadelphia: Mosby; 2007:1179–1187.
2. Task Force on Surgical Palliative Care; Committee on Ethics. Statement of principles of palliative care. *Bull Am Coll Surg*. 2005;90:34–35.
3. The American Board of Surgery, Inc. *Booklet of information—surgery*. Philadelphia: American Board of Surgery; 2009, p 8.
4. Dunn GP, Martensen R, Weissman D. *Surgical palliative care: a resident's guide*. Chicago, IL: American College of Surgeons; 2009.
5. Wagman LD. Progress in palliative surgery—is it a subspecialty? *J Surg Oncol*. 2007;96:449–450.
6. Finlayson CA, Eisenberg BL. Palliative pelvic exenteration: patient selection and results. *Oncology*. 1996;10:313–322.
7. Sugarbaker PH, Barofsky I, Rosenberg SA, et al. Quality of life assessment of patients in extremity sarcoma clinical trials. *Surgery*. 1982;91:17–23.
8. Miner TJ. Palliative surgery for advanced cancer: lessons learned in patient selection and outcome assessment. *Am J Clin Oncol*. 2005;28:411–414.
9. McCahill LE, Krouse R, Chu D, et al. Indications and use of palliative surgery—results of Society of Surgical Oncology survey. *Ann Surg Oncol*. 2002;9:104–112.
10. Galante JM, Bowles TL, Khatri VP, et al. Experience and attitudes of surgeons toward palliation in cancer. *Arch Surg*. 2005;140:873–878 discussion 78–80.
11. Cady B, Easson A, Aboulafia AJ, et al. Part 1: Surgical palliation of advanced illness—what's new, what's helpful. *J Am Coll Surg*. 2005;200:115–127.
12. Augustine MM, Pawlik TM. Palliation of advanced gastrointestinal malignancies using minimally invasive strategies. *Prog Palliat Care*. 2009;17:250–260.
13. Jemal A, Siegel R, Ward E, et al. Cancer statistics, 2008. *CA Cancer J Clin*. 2008;58:71–96.
14. McGregor JR, O'Dwyer PJ. The surgical management of obstruction and perforation of the left colon. *Surg Gynecol Obstet*. 1993;177:203–208.
15. Serpell JW, McDermott FT, Katrivessis H, et al. Obstructing carcinomas of the colon. *Br J Surg*. 1989;76:965–969.
16. Scoggins CR, Meszoely IM, Blanke CD, et al. Nonoperative management of primary colorectal cancer in patients with stage IV disease. *Ann Surg Oncol*. 1999;6:651–657.

17. Scheer MG, Sloots CE, van der Wilt GJ, et al. Management of patients with asymptomatic colorectal cancer and synchronous irresectable metastases. *Ann Oncol*. 2008;19:1829–1835.
18. Ludwig KA, Milsom JW, Garcia-Ruiz A, et al. Laparoscopic techniques for fecal diversion. *Dis Colon Rectum*. 1996;39:285–288.
19. Watt AM, Faragher IG, Griffin TT, et al. Self-expanding metallic stents for relieving malignant colorectal obstruction: a systematic review. *Ann Surg*. 2007;246:24–30.
20. Smith AC, Dowsett JF, Russell RC, et al. Randomised trial of endoscopic stenting versus surgical bypass in malignant low bile duct obstruction. *Lancet*. 1994;344:1655–1660.
21. Artifon EL, Sakai P, Cunha JE, et al. Surgery or endoscopy for palliation of biliary obstruction due to metastatic pancreatic cancer. *Am J Gastroenterol*. 2006;101:2031–2037.
22. Nassif T, Prat F, Meduri B, et al. Endoscopic palliation of malignant gastric outlet obstruction using self-expandable metallic stents: results of a multicenter study. *Endoscopy*. 2003;35:483–489.
23. Parker LA, Charnock GC, Delany DJ. Small bore catheter drainage and sclerotherapy for malignant pleural effusions. *Cancer*. 1989;64:1218–1221.
24. Clementsen P, Evald T, Grode G, et al. Treatment of malignant pleural effusion: pleurodesis using a small percutaneous catheter: a prospective randomized study. *Respir Med*. 1998;92:593–596.
25. Erickson KV, Yost M, Bynoe R, et al. Primary treatment of malignant pleural effusions: video-assisted thoracoscopic surgery poudrage versus tube thoracostomy. *Am Surg*. 2002;68:955–959 discussion 59–60.
26. Barnett TD, Rubins J. Placement of a permanent tunneled peritoneal drainage catheter for palliation of malignant ascites: a simplified percutaneous approach. *J Vasc Interv Radiol*. 2002;13:379–383.
27. Temple L, Fuzesi S, Patil S. The importance of determining quality of life in clinical trials. *Surgery*. 2009;145:622–626.
28. Testa MA, Simonson DC. Assessment of quality-of-life outcomes. *N Engl J Med*. 1996;334:835–840.
29. Langenhoff BS, Krabbe PF, Wobbes T, et al. Quality of life as an outcome measure in surgical oncology. *Br J Surg*. 2001;88:643–652.
30. McCahill LE, Smith DD, Borneman T, et al. A prospective evaluation of palliative outcomes for surgery of advanced malignancies. *Ann Surg Oncol*. 2003;10:654–663.

31. Fitzsimmons D, Johnson CD, George S, et al. Development of a disease specific quality of life (QoL) questionnaire module to supplement the EORTC core cancer QoL questionnaire, the QLQ-C30 in patients with pancreatic cancer. EORTC Study Group on Quality of Life. *Eur J Cancer*. 1999;35:939–941.
32. Blazeby JM, Conroy T, Hammerlid E, et al. Clinical and psychometric validation of an EORTC questionnaire module, the EORTC QLQ-OES18, to assess quality of life in patients with oesophageal cancer. *Eur J Cancer*. 2003;39:1384–1394.
33. Kemmler G, Holzner B, Kopp M, et al. Comparison of two quality-of-life instruments for cancer patients: the functional assessment of cancer therapy-general and the European Organization for Research and Treatment of Cancer Quality of Life Questionnaire-C30. *J Clin Oncol*. 1999;17:2932–2940.
34. Miner TJ, Jaques DP, Shriver CD. A prospective evaluation of patients undergoing surgery for the palliation of an advanced malignancy. *Ann Surg Oncol*. 2002;9:696–703.
35. Woll ML, Hinshaw DB, Pawlik TM. Spirituality and religion in the care of surgical oncology patients with life-threatening or advanced illnesses. *Ann Surg Oncol*. 2008;15:3048–3057.
36. Steinhauser KE, Christakis NA, Clipp EC, et al. Factors considered important at the end of life by patients, family, physicians, and other care providers. *JAMA*. 2000;284:2476–2482.
37. Hinshaw DB, Pawlik T, Mosenthal AC, et al. When do we stop, and how do we do it? Medical futility and withdrawal of care. *J Am Coll Surg*. 2003;196:621–651.
38. Nyman DJ, Sprung CL. End-of-life decision making in the intensive care unit. *Intensive Care Med*. 2000;26:1414–1420.
39. Pawlik TM. Withholding and withdrawing life-sustaining treatment: a surgeon's perspective. *J Am Coll Surg*. 2006;202:990–994.
40. Dowdy MD, Robertson C, Bander JA. A study of proactive ethics consultation for critically and terminally ill patients with extended lengths of stay. *Crit Care Med*. 1998;26:252–259.

38 Symptom management in the last days of life

S. Lawrence Librach and Janet R. Hardy

As a cancer illness progresses, the patient and family will face many different challenges and many different sources of distress. Multiple symptoms—physical, psychological, social, and spiritual—produce suffering that should be addressed by an interprofessional team. At the end of life,

care must be comprehensive, responsive, humane, and systematic to address and prevent unnecessary distress for both patient and family.

SETTING THE STAGE

To come to terms with the last days of life, the patient and family must be prepared to address the issues surrounding dying and death. This task requires the following:

1. *Delineation of the goals of care all along the illness spectrum.* Most advanced solid tumors remain incurable, and the mode of dying from specific malignancies is often predictable. Patients with cancer are usually aware of dying as a possibility, but initially, the goals of care are focused on cure or disease control. As the disease progresses, conversations with patient and family must include a change of emphasis toward the goals of care that will ensure a "good death." Lack of acknowledgment of an imminent death places the patient at risk of "unfinished business," unnecessary investigations and interventions, and increased suffering. Care pathways for end-of-life care provide a model for the change in emphasis of care and goals to be met to optimize that care.[1] These goals are shown in Table 38-1.
2. *Advance care planning.* Advance care planning describes the type of care a person would want (or not want) if he or she were unable to make healthcare decisions. It is a process of conversation between healthcare providers, patients, and their families and is not just a document or a decision about resuscitation. It allows a substitute decision maker to be nominated, documents a person's preferred setting of death, and specifies what interventions are acceptable or not acceptable at the very end of life. Few patients and families understand complex medical technologies and their effectiveness or lack thereof. Many are not aware of the care they can expect when dying at home, or in a nursing home, palliative care unit, acute care hospital, or other facility. Advance care planning is the responsibility of all members of the oncology care team. The Preferred Priorities for Care program within the U.K. End of Life strategy and a national education

Table 38-1 Goals of care for patients in the dying phase[1]

Comfort measures

- Assessment of current medication and discontinuation of nonessentials
- As required subcutaneous drugs written up according to protocol (pain, agitation, respiratory tract secretions, nausea, vomiting)
- Discontinuation of inappropriate interventions (blood tests, antibiotics, intravenous fluids or drugs, turning regimens, vital signs); documentation that patient is not for cardiopulmonary resuscitation

Psychological and insight issue

- Insight into condition assessed

Religious and spiritual support

- Religious and spiritual needs assessed with patient and family

Communication with family and others

- Information on how family or other people involved are to be informed of patient's impending death
- Relevant information given to family or other people involved regarding the care setting and how to contact care providers

Communication with primary healthcare team

- Primary care physician is aware of patient's condition.
- Plan of care is explained and discussed with patient and family.
- Family or other people involved express understanding of the plan of care.

Care after death

- Primary care physician informed
- Procedure for laying out explained
- Procedure following death discussed
- Family given information regarding procedures
- Policy regarding valuables explained
- Necessary documentation given to family
- Bereavement literature given

program in Canada have been designed to help both patients and health professionals address these issues.[2,3]

3. *Communication.* None of the issues discussed above can be addressed without the patient's full knowledge of the status of his or her disease and the likely prognosis. Full and open discussion regarding the inevitability of death and the change in focus of care should be encouraged between patients, their families and carers, and health professionals. Guidelines have been published to help healthcare professionals undertake these difficult discussions.[4]

4. *Delineation of rites and rituals that patient and family desire at the end of life.* This might include cultural issues (e.g., requirements for dressing and burial following death) or acknowledging a patient's wish as to who should or should not be present at the time of death.

5. *Careful documentation* of all of the above in the medical record is essential, as is disclosure to other health professionals who have been involved in the patient's care, especially the primary health practitioner.

6. *An interprofessional team approach* to address the diverse physical, psychological, social, functional, and spiritual needs of patients and families during the last days of life.

7. *24-Hour access (if possible)* to an interprofessional team experienced in providing care at the very end of life.

8. *Care provider acceptance of dying and death.* Death may be seen as failure by oncology professionals, leaving them with feelings of powerlessness and helplessness.[5] Healthcare professionals facing a patient's death may develop practice avoidance, may disengage emotionally, may withdraw from the care of the patient, or may advocate "just one more treatment" as an alternative to addressing issues surrounding death. It is important that all members of the interprofessional team are open and consistent in their approach to care of the patient and family.

HOW TO DETERMINE WHEN SOMEONE IS ENTERING THE LAST FEW DAYS OF LIFE

Symptoms and signs that indicate that a patient is entering the last few days or hours of life include the following:

- *Rapidly increasing weakness and fatigue.* Patients with advanced cancer often complain about fatigue and generalized weakness. Patients nearing death will report daily changes in these symptoms. For example, getting out of bed or sitting up becomes increasingly difficult. Ultimately, they will become bedridden and require full assistance in all activities.

- *Rapid decline in oral intake.* Patients will become less and less interested in consuming food and fluids and will rarely complain of hunger or thirst. Oral intake declines to sips of fluids as tolerated because of difficulty swallowing. This is accompanied by decreasing urine output and often a decrease in peripheral edema or ascites.

- *Decreasing level of consciousness.* Patients will spend more time sleeping. They lose interest in their surroundings and have decreased response to tactile or verbal stimuli. Eventually, they will be completely unresponsive.

- *Decreased communication.* Patients will have little interest in communicating beyond a few words. Their ability to concentrate on conversations will decrease. Eventually, communication is reduced to single words or head nods.

- *Tachycardia.* Patients often will develop a sinus tachycardia in the week or two before their death. This is not usually symptomatic.

- *Pain.* Families often fear that pain will increase at the end of life. In reality, pain may increase, decrease, or stay the same.[6] The use of breakthrough medication may decrease because patients are less active, and the subjective sense of pain decreases as awareness decreases.

Later signs and symptoms include the following:

- *Respiratory changes.* Up to 50% to 70% of terminally ill cancer patients experience dyspnea in the last 6 weeks of life.[7] Dyspnea can be extremely distressing for both patient and family and is an independent predictor of near death.[8] A variety of changes in respiratory rate are seen in patients, often without respiratory compromise. The most frequent sign is apneic spells that gradually lengthen in duration as death approaches. Patients who become acidotic may develop the typical deep, regular breathing pattern that is typically seen in patients with renal failure.

- *Loss of ability to swallow.* As death nears, patients lose the ability to swallow and often will choke or aspirate when food and fluids are administered. A formal review by an appropriate health professional is indicated if oral intake is considered unsafe, as relatives may be loathe to stop offering sustenance to their loved ones.

- *Retained respiratory secretions.* As death approaches, patients are not able to swallow secretions and may develop noisy breathing or gurgling, commonly referred to as a "death rattle." The airway may be narrowed by relaxation of the muscles of the tongue and pharynx, allowing the tongue to fall posteriorly in the pharynx. This may be misinterpreted as pneumonia and is often very distressing for relatives, care providers, and other patients in the room.

- *Moaning.* Toward the end of life, patients may moan on expiration. This can result from the vibration of vocal cords and pharyngeal muscles and does not necessarily mean that the patient is in pain.

- *Cardiovascular changes.* Blood pressure may be decreased for weeks as the patient's status deteriorates. In the last hours of life, peripheral mottling, cyanosis, and cooling may occur as blood flow to the extremities is decreased to maintain central blood flow.

- *Eye changes.* Patients at the very end of life will blink much less often and will rest with eyelids partially open.

- *Skin changes.* Patients' peripheries become cold and their skin mottled. Pressure areas are common and can contribute significantly to patient morbidity and care provider burden.

- *Loss of sphincter control.* This is variable, but incontinence of bowel and bladder must be dealt with effectively to avoid extra burden on the family and care providers.

- *Delirium.* Progressive cognitive dysfunction with confusion, agitation, hallucinations, and moaning complicates care at the end of life. Delirium is a frequent multifactorial complication of advanced cancer.[9]

Although these signs and symptoms indicate that death is near, they are not absolutely prognostic as far as time remaining is concerned, except for very late cardiovascular and respiratory changes.

CRISES AT THE END OF LIFE

Crises in the terminal phase are rare but should be anticipated so that appropriate prophylactic measures can be put in place.

1. *Exsanguination.* This is occasionally seen in patients with hematologic malignancies or in those with tumors encroaching upon major blood vessels. Appropriate doses of analgesia and anxiolytics should be charted in advance for use if a catastrophic hemorrhagic event is anticipated. Practical measures such as the use of dark towels can reduce the visual distress.

2. *Large airway obstruction aspiration and asphyxia.* This should be managed with appropriate doses of opioids and benzodiazepines or other major sedatives.

3. *Status epilepticus* in patients with brain tumors or brain metastases, as discussed later.

4. *Severe pain* (e.g., a pathologic fracture, bleeding into the capsule of an organ such as liver or spleen, peritonitis from bowel perforation) can complicate the terminal phase.

MANAGING THE SYMPTOMS OF THE LAST DAYS OR HOURS OF LIFE

GENERAL APPROACHES

1. Educate the family and other care providers about the significance of the symptoms and signs described above. Clarify the goals of care and the revised care plan. This information may have to be delivered several times because family anxiety may inhibit the ability to listen and learn, and because changes are progressive. Providing a document that outlines the approach to the last hours can be helpful.

2. Discuss with the family issues surrounding communication with the dying patient. Explain that the apparent withdrawal of the dying person is normal. Encourage family and friends to talk with the dying person but not to expect a response. Help them understand that even the patient who seems unconscious may still be hearing. Share updates and bad news away from the bedside.

3. Encourage the family to surround the patient with people, objects, and activities that were part of his or her life. Music may be important. Encourage children to be present, and teach their parents and caregivers what to say to allow children to understand dying in an age-appropriate fashion and to grieve appropriately. Encourage expressions of intimacy.

4. Maintain privacy and confidentiality, particularly in hospitals. Try to move dying patients to private rooms.

5. Stop monitoring of vital signs but ensure regular observation for symptom control.

6. Stop all unnecessary tests and investigations.

7. Ensure ongoing support from care team members. Ensure that all team members are aware of resuscitation discussions.

8. Discuss what will happen when the patient dies. Deal with common fears and misconceptions about dead bodies, the lack of need to involve emergency personnel, and regulatory issues around certifying death and transfer to funeral homes. Ensure that relatives of patients in hospital have all needed practical information (e.g., where to park, eat, toilet).

9. Discuss all ethical issues (e.g., those surrounding parenteral feeding, antibiotics, do-not-resuscitate orders).

10. Ensure that all patients have access to pastoral care and spiritual support if this is their wish.

MANAGING SYMPTOMS

See Table 38-2.

REVIEWING MEDICATIONS

1. Stop all unnecessary medications (e.g., drugs for hypertension, cardiac disease, hyperlipidemia, anticoagulation, and other chronic diseases).

Table 38-2 Essential medications and equipment for use at end of life

Symptom	Drug	Comments
Pain	Parenteral opioids	For intermittent administration or by constant subcutaneous infusion
	Transmucosal fentanyl, buprenorphine	Provides an alternate route of drug delivery
Dyspnea	Opioids Benzodiazepines Oxygen, if necessary	If on opioids, increase the dose by 10% to 25%, but watch for possible toxicity
Nausea	Parenteral metoclopramide, haloperidol, dimenhydrinate, methotrimeprazine	Methotrimeprazine is particularly useful if sedation is desirable
Terminal agitation	Parenteral haloperidol, methotrimeprazine, chlorpromazine, midazolam, clonazepam Sublingual lorazepam, midazolam	See text
Noisy respirations	Parenteral hyoscine hydrobromide, hyoscine butylbromide, glycopyrrolate, ipratropium bromide	Reposition first, suctioning occasionally needed
Oral care	Saline solution or peppermint water Oral swabs Sponge-tipped swabs	Avoid lemon-glycerin swabs
Incontinence	Urinary catheters Adult diapers Incontinence pads	

2. Ensure ongoing prescription of truly essential drugs such as analgesics, anxiolytics, and antiemetics, and make sure they are available by parenteral formulation should this be required.
3. It may be appropriate to continue other medications such as antibiotics, anticonvulsants, and insulin if the patient is likely to become symptomatic without them. Insulin dosages should be adjusted to an "as required" schedule because oral caloric intake is diminished.
4. Ensure that all drugs are prescribed for delivery by an appropriate route (e.g., subcutaneous, intravenous) as dying patients will be unable to take oral medications.
5. Ensure that all "as required" medications are charted, along with regular medications.

PAIN AT THE END OF LIFE

At the time of death, most cancer patients will be receiving opioid analgesia,[6] especially if they are in a hospital or a specialist palliative care unit.[10]

Opioids must be delivered by an appropriate route, that is, parenterally (by subcutaneous or intravenous infusion), transdermally (e.g., fetanyl or buprenorphine patch), sublingually, or rectally. Continuous infusion of opioids by the parenteral route is considered ideal in many countries, in that it allows the dose to be increased or decreased quickly according to response, toxicity, or the number of extra or breakthrough doses required. In other settings, especially in the home, setting up a continuous infusion may introduce complex technology and care complexity at this time and has been criticized as "over-medicalization" of death.[11]

Short-acting opioids must always be available to be given concurrently with baseline opioids for breakthrough pain. Many co-analgesics or adjuvants can be given only orally and must be discontinued in the terminal phase, with some exceptions (e.g., nonsteroidal antiinflammatory drugs, steroids, benzodiazepines). Carefully assess the necessity of these drugs at the very end of life.

Renal impairment is an inevitable consequence of decreased oral intake and dehydration as death approaches. This can lead to retention of active metabolites of some opioids (e.g., morphine, hydromorphone), potentially causing toxicity and delirium. Some have advocated the use of intravenous fluids during the terminal phase to prevent opioid toxicity.[12] Others prefer to monitor the patient closely for signs of toxicity and to reduce the dose accordingly. Another option is to use opioids that are not dependent on renal function for clearance (e.g., fentanyl, methadone).[13] However, changing opioids in the last few days requires careful monitoring, as dosage equivalencies are not exact. Not only is great interindividual variation seen in the opioid dose required at the end of life,[6] variation in the pattern of prescribing is also evident. Most published series show an increase in opioid dose in the 48 hours before death, but a significant number of patients have a stable or decreased dose.[6,10] Palliative care units in a number of different countries have attempted to benchmark the use of opioids at the end of life.[10,14,15] Contrary to common concern, no series has shown an association between opioid dose or rate of opioid increase and survival.[16]

RESPIRATORY SYMPTOMS

The changing pattern of respiration in the terminal phase can be misinterpreted by family members as hypoxia or impending suffocation requiring oxygen. Oxygen has been shown to be no better than air for alleviating dyspnea except in patients with documented hypoxia.[7] Relatives can be reassured of this and encouraged to use nonpharmacologic means of relieving the distress, for example, a fan or cold facecloth on the forehead. Nurse-led interventions based on breathing techniques with a focus on the emotional experience can improve breathlessness.[7]

Evidence of the benefit of opioids in reducing the subjective sensation of refractory breathlessness is increasing.[7] Common practice is to increase the baseline opioid dose by about 10% if the aim is to palliate dyspnea, as well as pain. The sedative effect of benzodiazepines can be used to advantage in this scenario. One trial has demonstrated that the addition of midazolam to morphine was significantly more effective than morphine alone in palliating dyspnea without additional adverse events.[17]

Pneumonia is common in the terminal phase. Discussions with the patient and family at this stage should center on whether antibiotics are likely to reduce secretions and improve symptoms or serve only to prolong an inevitable death.

At the very last few minutes or hours of life, deep but infrequent agonal respirations may be seen. Careful support and education of family members as to the meaning of these is important, as they can be distressing to watch. The patient by this time will usually be comatose. The family should be reassured that the unresponsive patient will not be distressed by breathlessness, and that oxygen will not be of benefit.

RETAINED RESPIRATORY SECRETIONS

This can sometimes be managed by repositioning the patient on his or her side with the head down or semiprone, supported by pillows in both positions. This will allow the tongue to come forward and open the airway. Secretions will accumulate at the side of the mouth and can be removed by swabs or by gentle suctioning.

Anticholinergic drugs (e.g., hyoscine hydrobromide, hyoscine butylbromide [Buscopan], glycopyrrolate, ipratropium bromide [Atropine]) are commonly used in this situation in an attempt to dry secretions (Table 38-3). No evidence indicates that any one drug is better than another.[18] Transdermal scopolamine is available in some countries but takes a number of hours to take effect. If the transdermal patch is to be used, it should be preceded by a loading dose given by injection.

ORAL CARE

Careful attention to oral care is imperative during the terminal phase, as the oral mucosa can become dry and caked with secretions unless frequent, careful mouth care is performed. Avoid lemon-glycerin swabs and use soft-cotton or sponge-tipped swabs moistened with a solution of water, salt, and baking soda; lubricating jelly and water; or peppermint water. Swabbing should be directed particularly at the gingival mucosa, tongue, and palate. Swabbing can be done every half hour to 1 hour (or less often if water trickling down the throat causes distress), and family members can be taught to perform this simple comfort measure. If the patient has dentures, ask the family (and patient, if possible) if they would like them left in place or taken out for comfort. If they wish to keep them in, gently remove and rinse with warm water and brush off debris. Moisten the lips with lip balm, but avoid petroleum jelly, as this tends to harden in lip folds, has an unpleasant taste, and can damage plastic tubing.

SKIN CARE

Some degree of impairment or compromise of skin integrity is almost inevitable in a bed-bound patient. During the terminal phase, the frequency of turning and repositioning of patients should be reduced to every 6 or 8 hours to minimize shearing forces on the skin, especially over the sacrum. Ensure that the bed surface is smooth and supportive without potential pressure areas. Minimize the quantity of bedclothes and sheets that may cause skin friction. If a patient wishes to be sat up in bed, then ensure that the end of the bed is elevated or pillows are placed under the thighs to prevent the patient from slipping down the bed, causing friction or shearing to sacral skin. A light sheet, an incontinence pad, and a hospital gown are often all that is required. Ensure that the patient's skin is clean and dry. Check the heels, elbows, and ears for redness. If incontinence pads are indicated, change frequently to avoid skin maceration and to eliminate odors. Gentle moisturizing of the skin may provide some comfort and can be a useful task for family members.

EYE CARE

Artificial tear preparations, solutions, or ointments will provide corneal hydration for the patient who is not blinking or is lying with eyes half open.

BOWEL AND BLADDER PROBLEMS

The problem encountered most commonly is urinary incontinence. Most patients will agree to the insertion of a Silastic urinary catheter when the effort required in toileting becomes too great. Others prefer incontinence pads, although the perceived loss of dignity and the expense incurred (especially for patients who are being managed at home) may be off-putting. Stool incontinence can be minimized if laxatives are discontinued. Frequent stool incontinence or diarrhea may necessitate the use of incontinence pads.

SEIZURES

If frequent seizures have been a problem, phenytoin can be given once daily if the patient has intravenous access in situ. Alternatively, benzodiazepines can be delivered subcutaneously or sublingually (midazolam, clonazepam) or rectally (diazepam). Clonazepam has a longer half-life and is therefore probably preferable in this context. Phenobarbitone and

Table 38-3	Medications for excessive secretions	
Drug	**Dose**	**Special Issues**
Scopolamine (hyoscine hydrobromide)	0.4–0.6 mg SC, IV, q4–6h to maintain, or transdermal patch 1–3 every 3 days,	Can increase delirium
Buscopan (hyoscine hydrobromide)	20 mg SC q4h	
Ipratropium bromide (Atropine)	0.4–0.6 mg SC q4–6h	Caution, potential cardiac toxicity
Glycopyrrolate	0.2–0.4 mg SC q2–4h	As does not cross blood-brain barrier, can be given to conscious patients

propofol given intravenously are recommended only when other measures have failed. Both require close monitoring and should not be used in the community setting.

TERMINAL AGITATION

Lucidity at the end of life has been identified by patients and their families as very important.[19] Unfortunately, a state of unease, restlessness, and agitation is common at the end of life and is not always possible to avoid. This condition is multifactorial (Table 38-4) and sometimes can be reversed by simple measures, such as insertion of a urinary catheter to relieve retention, adequate pain relief, and careful management of opioids and other drugs to reduce drug toxicity. In other instances, agitation may be the result of metabolic factors such as hypercalcemia or organ failure, and treatment for these may be impossible or inappropriate.

Antipsychotics are considered by most clinicians as first-line pharmacotherapeutic agents for terminal agitation,[20] with anxiolytics (e.g., benzodiazepines) used second line. However, very little evidence supports the use of any of these agents over another, or the use of supportive drug therapy over supportive care alone (e.g., transfer to a familiar environment, the presence of relatives, good lighting, soothing music).

In the absence of evidence, most clinicians will use antipsychotics such as haloperidol, methotrimeprazine, or chlorpromazine in an attempt to improve cognitive function and will use benzodiazepines for sedation (Table 38-5). Most of these drugs can be delivered parenterally and are compatible, so they can be used concurrently with other drugs used in the terminal phase.

FOOD AND FLUID INTAKE

One of the more difficult and controversial issues to deal with at the very end of life is the issue of fluid and food intake.[21] The issue of withdrawal of food and fluids should be discussed with the patient and family as part of the advance care planning process. A common fear on the part of family members is that the person will die of starvation and dehydration if not given food or fluid supplements. Repeated education about this issue is required, and most families will allow the gradual withdrawal of fluids and food, especially when informed that enteral feeding tubes or parenteral feed-

Table 38-5 Medications for terminal agitation

Drug	Dose	Special Issues
Lorazepam	1–2 mg buccal mucosal, PR, SL, SC, IV q1h to titrate, then q4h to maintain sedation	Can cause paradoxical agitation
Midazolam	2.5–5 mg SC q1h until settled 0.5–1 mg IV q30min until settled, and then prn 10–30 mg/24 hr continuous subcutaneous infusion	Can cause paradoxical agitation. Duration of action, 15 min to several hours
Chlorpromazine Methotrimeprazine	25–50 mg q2h IM until settled, and then q6h prn 6.25–50 mg/24 hr by SC infusion or in divided dose	Can be given SC, but injections may be painful and absorption less certain
Haloperidol	0.5–5 mg SC, IV q6h titrate to effect, then q6h to maintain	Be aware of potential adverse effects (e.g., extrapyramidal movements)

ing does not improve morbidity or prolong survival in terminally ill patients.[22,23] Relatives should be cautioned against trying to give food or fluids to a patient who has difficulty swallowing, as this may lead to aspiration. Declining intake of food and fluid can be explained as part of the natural process of dying.

The issue of dehydration must be explored and its limited impact on the dying process explained. The fact that the patient is unlikely to complain of thirst reinforces this. Emphasizing oral care as a way of maintaining moist oral membranes may help family members understand that dehydration need not be distressing. Moreover, hydration can necessitate frequent toileting, can exacerbate ascites, edema, and bronchial secretions, and can cause fluid overload. Every case should be considered individually, and the cultural and spiritual beliefs of the patient and relatives should be considered at all times.

SEDATION AT THE END OF LIFE

Low-dose sedation has a useful role in the management of anxiety, pain, dyspnea, and distress. In cases in which agitation is difficult to control, pain is resistant to analgesia, dyspnea is distressing, and/or physical distress is overwhelming, higher-dose sedation may be indicated. This should be delivered in a carefully titrated manner to achieve the desired effect with the lowest possible dose. Sedation at the end of life is a controversial issue that demands experienced providers and patient and family education and consent.[6] Guidelines should be followed, and these can be institutional, national, or international in scope.[24,25]

Table 38-4 Causes of terminal agitation

Drugs	Opioids, anticholinergic drugs, corticosteroids, and corticosteroid withdrawal
Disease factors	Brain metastases, infection, paraneoplastic syndromes
Metabolic	Renal failure, liver failure, hypercalcemia
Uncontrolled symptoms	Urinary retention, severe constipation, pain, dyspnea
Psychosocial and spiritual distress	Anxiety, fear

WHEN A PATIENT DIES

Respect the spirituality around the experience of death. Teach family members to spend some time with the deceased and to engage in rites and rituals. Tears are very appropriate. With good preparation for the event of dying and death, family members are often at peace. There is no rush to move the deceased to a funeral home. Children can also be brought to the bedside to observe adult grief, to express their own grief, and to observe rituals.

It is also important for care providers to be able to say their goodbyes to patient and family. There should be no inordinate rush in an institution to clear the bed for another patient. Palliative care units may move the patient to a chapel, so that other patients and staff can pay their respects.

This is also a time for initial grief counseling, especially around funerals, the early stages of bereavement, and the availability of grief counseling should family members require it. Recognize those at risk for abnormal grief,[26] and provide appropriate follow-up and counseling.

CONCLUSION

The last hours or days of life are an extremely important time of providing care to patient and family. A systematic and comprehensive approach can minimize symptoms and can prepare a family effectively for death.

REFERENCES

1. Ellershaw J, Wilkinson S, eds. *Care of the dying—a pathway to excellence.* New York: Oxford University Press; 2003.
2. National End of Life Care Programme. *Care Pathway Step 5: Last Days of Life:* http://www.endoflifecareforadults.nhs.uk/care-pathway/5-lastdays. Accessed November 21, 2010.
3. Librach SL, Hanvey L, et al. from the Educating Future Physicians in Palliative and End of Life Care Project. Facilitating advance care planning: an interprofessional education program. Ottawa, Ontario, Canada: Association of Faculties of Medicine of Canada; 2007.
4. Clayton JM, Hancock KM, Butow PN, et al. Clinical practice guidelines for communicating prognosis and end-of-life issues with adults in the advanced stages of life-limiting illness, and their caregivers. *Med J Aust.* 2007;186:S77–S108.
5. Meier DE, Back AL, Morrison RS. The inner life of physicians and care of the seriously ill. *JAMA.* 2001;286:3007–3014.
6. Sykes N, Thorns A. The use of opioids and sedatives at the end of life. *Lancet Oncol.* 2003;4:312–318.
7. Ben-Aharon I, Gafter-Gvili A, Paul M, et al. Interventions for alleviating cancer-related dyspnoea: a systematic review. *J Clin Oncol.* 2008;26:2396–2404.
8. Glare P, Sinclair C, Downing M, et al. Predicting survival in patients with advanced disease. *Eur J Cancer.* 2008;44:1146–1156.
9. Lawlor PG, Bruera ED. Delirium in patients with advanced cancer. *Hematol Oncol Clin North Am.* 2002;163:701–714.
10. Wilcock A, Chauhan A. Benchmarking the use of opioids in the last days of life. *J Pain Symptom Manage.* 2007;34:1–3.
11. O'Neil W. Subcutaneous infusions—a medical last rite. *Palliat Med.* 1994;8:91–93.
12. Bruera E, Sala R, Rico MA, et al. Effects of parenteral hydration in terminally ill cancer patients: a preliminary study. *J Clin Oncol.* 2005;23:2366–2371.
13. White C, Hardy J, Boyd A, et al. Subcutaneous sufentanil for palliative care patients in a hospital setting. *Palliat Med.* 2008;22:89–90.
14. Good PD, Ravenscroft PJ, Cavenagh J. Effects of opioids and sedatives on survival in an Australian inpatient palliative care population. *Intern Med J.* 2005;35:512–517.
15. Bilsen J, Norup M, Deliens L, et al. Drugs used to alleviate symptoms with life shortening as a possible side effect: end-of-life care in six European countries. *J Pain Symptom Manage.* 2006;31:111–121.
16. Hardy J. Opioids in the terminal phase. In: Davis M, Glare P, Hardy J, et al., eds. *Opioids in cancer pain.* 2nd ed. New York: Oxford University Press; 2009:453–459.
17. Navigante AH, Cerchietti LC, Castro MA, et al. Midazolam as an adjunct therapy to morphine in the alleviation of severe dyspnoea perception in patients with advanced cancer. *J Pain Symptom Manage.* 2006;31:38–47.
18. Wee B, Hillier R. Interventions for noisy breathing in patients near to death. *Cochrane Database Syst Rev.* 2008;(1) CD005177.
19. Steinhauser K, Christakis N, Clipp E, et al. Factors considered important at the end of life by patients, family, physicians and other care providers. *JAMA.* 2000;284:2476–2482.
20. Boettger S, Breitbart W. Atypical antipsychotics in the management of delirium: a review of the empirical literature. *Palliat Support Care.* 2005;3:227–237.
21. Viola RA, Wells GA, Peterson J. The effects of fluid status and fluid therapy on the dying: a systematic review. Review. *J Palliat Care.* 1997;13:41–52.
22. Lipman TO. Clinical trials of nutritional support in cancer: parenteral and enteral therapy. *Hematol Oncol Clin North Am.* 1991;5:91–102.
23. Winter SM. Terminal nutrition: framing the debate for the withdrawal of nutritional support in terminally ill patients. Review. *Am J Med.* 2000;109:723–726.
24. De Graeff A, Dean M. Palliative sedation therapy in the last weeks of life: a literature review and recommendations for standards. *J Palliat Med.* 2007;10:67–85.
25. Royal Dutch Medical Association. National guideline for palliative sedation. Utrecht. The Netherlands: Royal Dutch Medical Association; 2005.
26. Kristjanson LJ, Cousins K, Smith J, et al. Evaluation of the Bereavement Risk Index (BRI): a community hospice care protocol. *Int J Palliat Nurs.* 2005;11:612–618.

REHABILITATION AND SURVIVORSHIP

SECTION OUTLINE

39 Cancer rehabilitation

Lisa Ruppert, Juliet Hou, Lynn Jedlicka,
Michael D. Stubblefield, and Vernon W. H. Lin

PRINCIPLES OF CANCER REHABILITATION

Physical medicine and rehabilitation is the medical specialty concerned with restoring and maintaining the highest possible level of function, independence, and quality of life. This relatively new specialty has evolved into a number of subspecialties to meet the needs of patients from all age groups whose primary medical issues may be neurologic, cardiac, pulmonary, amputation, sports injury, orthopedic, or pain, among others. Cancer rehabilitation is a rapidly emerging subspecialty of rehabilitation medicine whose primary focus is the evaluation and treatment of functional disorders in cancer patients and survivors. These disorders can result directly or indirectly from cancer, or from cancer treatments such as surgery, chemotherapy, and radiation. Disorders commonly addressed by the cancer rehabilitation specialist include neuromuscular and musculoskeletal pain, spasticity, stroke, myopathy, neuropathy, spinal cord injury, bowel and bladder dysfunction, amputation, fatigue, lymphedema, abnormalities of gait, and so forth. Lehmann et al.[1] assessed 805 hospitalized cancer patients and identified that 54% had a physical medicine problem (Fig. 39-1). These problems occurred with all tumor types; among those with central nervous system, breast, lung, or head and neck tumors, rehabilitation

needs were identified in more than 70%. Psychological problems were found in 42% of patients. A large gap was noted between identified rehabilitation needs and services actually delivered to this population. This gap improved dramatically after initiation of a program for patient education, automatic screening of patients for their rehabilitation needs, and the inclusion of a physiatrist as a member of the clinical oncology team.

REHABILITATION TEAM

Rehabilitation efforts for cancer patients and survivors require a comprehensive treatment approach to address their unique and often multidimensional problems. The optimal cancer rehabilitation team includes physiatry, nursing, physical and occupational therapy, speech and language pathology, recreational therapy, nutritionists, social workers, psychologists, orthotists, and prosthetists, among others. Chaplains, vocational counselors, hospice liaisons, home care agencies, support groups, and educational outreach programs may play an important role. The patient and family members are also a vital part of the rehabilitation team.[2,3] Medical and radiation oncologists, as well as oncologic surgeons, are instrumental in maximizing the function and quality of life of cancer patients and survivors, and a close working relationship with these practitioners is imperative for the overall success of rehabilitation efforts.

The physiatrist (or rehabilitation medicine specialist) is a neuromuscular and musculoskeletal physician trained to assess functional disability, biomechanics, and human movement. Physiatrists who specialize in cancer rehabilitation should also be expert in understanding and incorporating their knowledge of medical comorbidities, such as cardiac, pulmonary, and rheumatologic disease, into optimal patient care. They should possess an intimate knowledge of oncology and various oncologic treatments, as this knowledge will heavily influence their ability to safely and effectively restore function and quality of life to cancer patients. The ability to appropriately prescribe medications, modalities, and orthotic, prosthetic, and assistive devices in a way that accounts for all competing medical and psychosocial issues faced by

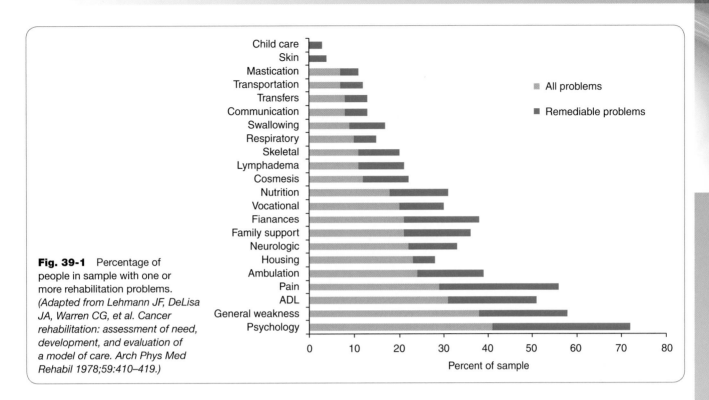

Fig. 39-1 Percentage of people in sample with one or more rehabilitation problems. *(Adapted from Lehmann JF, DeLisa JA, Warren CG, et al. Cancer rehabilitation: assessment of need, development, and evaluation of a model of care. Arch Phys Med Rehabil 1978;59:410–419.)*

the patient is key to the success of a cancer rehabilitation specialist. The physiatrist serves as the link between the clinical oncology team and the multidisciplinary rehabilitation team to coordinate rehabilitation services. He or she prepares a comprehensive plan for treatment and follows up to enhance function, reduce pain, and prevent disability.[2]

Successful rehabilitation of the cancer patient or survivor is dependent on a team of specialists with unique skills. Consistent communication between members of the oncology team and rehabilitation team and patient and family members is essential. This is especially vital during periods when the patient's clinical status, prognosis, and treatment strategies are changing. This communication ensures that realistic expectations for rehabilitation can be set.[3]

The physical therapist generally concentrates on the patient's gross motor function and mobility and trains the patient in the use of orthotics and gait aids. The physical therapist may also prove invaluable in the management of disorders such as pain or swelling from lymphedema. The occupational therapist focuses on the restoration of activities of daily living (ADLs) that emphasize fine motor function, self-care, adapted equipment, home safety, and cognitive function. Speech and language pathologists specialize in the evaluation and treatment of dysphagia and communication. Prosthetists and orthotists assist the physiatrist and therapist in evaluating gait and functional deficits, and then in helping to design, construct, and fit braces and limb prostheses to aid mobility and function. The recreational therapist provides leisure activities and community reintegration to facilitate independence in school, work, and other social settings. Recreational activities benefit people both physically and emotionally through enjoyment, exercise, competition, and meeting other people.[4] Vocational rehabilitation involvement allows persons with physical disabilities to engage in gainful employment. The roles of

psychologist, social worker, and nutritionist are described in other chapters.

BASIC REHABILITATION PRINCIPLES

Morbidity and decreased functional status and disability are significant concerns during the various stages of cancer and its treatment.[5] These concerns must be acknowledged when realistic rehabilitation goals are formulated.

In 1947, Dr. J. Herbert Dietz introduced several cancer rehabilitation approaches that are still in use today.[2] When establishing realistic rehabilitation goals, it is important to consider which Dietz rehabilitation approach would be most appropriate for the patient.

1. Preventive rehabilitation is the approach indicated when the disability can be predicted; it focuses on reducing the severity and duration of the disability's effect. For instance, preoperative instruction in ambulation with an appropriate assistive device both on level ground and on stairs will improve function, increase confidence, and enhance the speed of postoperative gait training in a prospective amputee patient.[6]
2. Restorative rehabilitation attempts to restore pre-morbid function in a patient when permanent impairment is not expected.[6] Physical and occupational therapy measures focusing on upper extremity strengthening and range of motion can improve upper extremity function and independence in a patient with shoulder impairment secondary to breast cancer treatment.
3. Supportive rehabilitation focuses on maximizing function when a permanent impairment exists. For example, providing a Becker knee extension orthosis, a Townsend

knee immobilizer, or a hip flexion assist orthosis to a patient with a femoral neuropathy can reduce the risk of falls, increase ambulation distances, and improve confidence.[7]

4. Palliative rehabilitation provides comfort and support and reduces complications that may develop when increasing disability is expected from disease progression.[6] Bed mobility and proper positioning can decrease the incidence of skin breakdown in patients requiring prolonged bed rest. Providing resting hand splints may prevent contractures, allowing improved hand hygiene and decreasing the incidence of skin breakdown.

A primary role of the cancer rehabilitation specialist is patient assessment. Assessment of functional limitations is of limited utility if an accurate diagnosis of the specific cause or causes of these limitations is not ascertained. Specificity in diagnosis is imperative, so that treatment can be targeted to provide maximal benefit to the patient while minimizing potential complications of treatment. Functional assessment is often qualitative and geared toward specific limitations of concern to the patient, such as steadiness of gait, difficulty with ADLs, or pain. Several functional assessment tools, including the Karnofsky Performance Scale, the Functional Assessment of Cancer Therapy–General Scale, and the Functional Independence Measure, have utility in the cancer rehabilitation setting. Accuracy in diagnosing the cause of a specific complaint starts with a comprehensive clinical evaluation. Key components of such an assessment are the history and physical examination. Physiatrists have extensive training in the use of physical examination to diagnose a multitude of neuromuscular and musculoskeletal disorders. Imaging often plays a critical role in evaluation of pain and functional deficits in the cancer setting. Such imaging may include X-rays, computed tomography (CT), and magnetic resonance imaging (MRI). Imaging, although often invaluable, can be misleading in the accurate diagnosis of a given disorder. The clinician should always strive to demonstrate congruence between the patient's clinical situation, physical examination, and imaging.[2] Electrodiagnostic testing can be an extremely valuable diagnostic and prognostic tool in the cancer population for evaluation and treatment of neuromuscular and musculoskeletal disorders. A well-designed study can help clarify the origin of a patient's symptoms, localize peripheral nerve lesions, exclude competing diagnostic possibilities, predict neurologic prognosis, and assist in chemotherapeutic decision making.[3]

NEUROMUSCULAR COMPLICATIONS OF CANCER

Neuromuscular complications are common in cancer patients and can be directly or indirectly related to the malignancy or may result from its treatment.[8] Neurologic complications occur in about 15% to 20% of cancer patients and are a frequent reason for hospital admissions.[9] Any segment of the neuromuscular system, including the brain, spinal cord, nerve roots, plexus, peripheral nerve, neuromuscular junction, and muscle, can be affected.

Brain metastases are common in patients with systemic cancer and occur much more frequently than primary brain tumors. Manifestations of both primary and metastatic brain tumors include headaches, mental status changes, focal weakness such as hemiparesis, cognitive decline, sensory loss, seizures, speech impairment, dysphagia, gait abnormalities, visual disturbances, and nausea/emesis.[10–13] Signs and symptoms of brain tumors depend largely on their location, size, and number, and they are often symptomatic. Suspected brain metastasis can be confirmed by CT or MRI.

Spinal metastases and spinal cord or nerve root compression occur in 5% to 10% of patients with systemic cancer, with potentially devastating consequences for function. Most tumors that affect the spinal axis are metastatic. Tumor can occur in the epidural, intramedullary, or leptomeningeal space (Fig. 39-2). Epidural tumor is most common and can cause spinal cord compression by progressing from the vertebrae or epidural space, through the neural foramen, to surround and compress the spinal cord within the thecal sac. The first manifestation of spinal cord compression is usually axial spinal pain, which may precede weakness by hours or months. Weakness usually precedes sensory deficits and ataxia. Once weakness develops, it can progress rapidly to paraplegia or quadriplegia. Spinal cord compression resulting from epidural tumor usually requires emergent medical (steroids or chemotherapy), surgical, or radiotherapeutic intervention to prevent progressive neurologic deficits.[14,15] Intramedullary and leptomeningeal tumors are less common but can be every bit as devastating to function. Intramedullary tumor describes disease within the parenchyma of the spinal cord that may manifest as spasticity, paraplegia, pain, ataxia, bowel and bladder dysfunction, and so forth. Leptomeningeal tumor is disease that is present within the thecal sac but outside the parenchyma of the spinal cord (i.e., within the leptomeningeal space where the cerebrospinal fluid flows). Leptomeningeal disease can cause frank spinal cord compression but more commonly presents as monoradiculopathy or polyradiculopa-

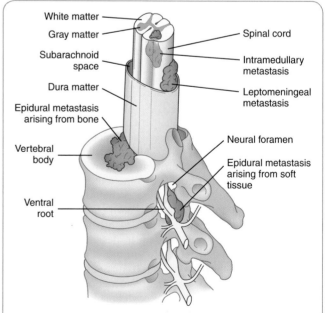

Fig. 39-2 Tumor affecting the spinal axis can be epidural, intramedullary, or leptomeningeal. (*Redrawn from Stubblefield MD, O'Dell MW. Cancer rehabilitation: principles and practice. New York: Demos Medical Publishing; 2009.*)

thy or cauda equina syndrome. Contrast MRI is the gold standard for excluding epidural or intramedullary tumor. Serial lumbar punctures may be required to diagnose leptomeningeal disease suspected but not visualized on MRI.

Radiation myelopathy may develop immediately following radiation or months to years later and may progress to complete plegia. Damage to the spinal cord can also occur from radiation, regardless of whether it is used with intent to cure (e.g., head and neck cancer, lymphoma) or palliatively (e.g., metastatic breast or prostate cancer). Acute myelopathy may be due to transient demyelination and typically resolves in 1 to 9 months.[16] Delayed myelopathy, however, is irreversible, with an incidence of 1% to 12%[17] and typical onset within 9 to 18 months after treatment; the latency period decreases as the dose of radiation increases.[18] The prototypical symptom pattern consists of lower extremity sensory changes, bowel/bladder dysfunction, and weakness, but it can also present as a Brown-Séquard–type pattern of hemisensory changes and motor deficits on the contralateral side below the level of involvement. Central pain (funicular pain) can occur in up to 20% with a history of radiation-associated myelopathy and likely results from ectopic activity in the ascending spinothalamic tracts.

Plexopathy can occur from tumor infiltration (breast, lung, lymphoma) and/or as a result of radiation therapy. Signs and symptoms of radiation plexopathy can present from 1 month to 15 years or longer following radiation therapy.[19] Chemotherapy can further amplify the effects of radiation plexopathy and decrease the time to onset of symptoms.[20] Pain is usually more common and severe in plexopathy resulting from tumor invasion; however, radiation and tumor-associated plexopathy can be present together.[21] Radiation can cause radiation-induced sarcomas and other secondary malignancies. This phenomenon is commonly seen in survivors of Hodgkin's lymphoma treated with radiation. Electrodiagnostic testing can help confirm the presence of plexopathy and can clarify the cause, extent, and severity of plexopathy. Myokymia, if present, suggests a radiation component of plexopathy; however, imaging with contrast MRI should always be the final arbiter when tumor is excluded.[22] Lumbosacral plexopathies can be caused by local invasion from pelvic and gastrointestinal tumors or by radiation for such tumors. They are generally less common than brachial plexopathies.[23] Neurotoxic chemotherapies such as platinum analogs, taxanes, and vinca alkaloids can contribute to or worsen plexopathy and are well known to be associated with polyneuropathy.[24]

Neuropathy is very common in the cancer setting. The pattern of nerve involvement can be seen as mononeuropathy, mononeuropathy multiplex, or polyneuropathy. Mononeuropathy can result from several causes, including direction invasion by tumor (e.g., sciatic neuropathy, extremity sarcoma), surgery, radiation therapy, weight loss (e.g., peroneal neuropathy), and compression from immobility. Mononeuropathy multiplex often implicates a vasculitic component of neuropathy; it can be seen to result from paraprotein disorders, amyloid deposition, and vasculitis or graft-versus-host disease, and can progress to a polyneuropathy. Polyneuropathy is the most commonly seen pattern of neuropathy in the cancer setting; it can result from a paraneoplastic process (anti-Hu antibody syndrome), advanced paraprotein disorders, or amyloid deposition, or can be vasculitic from lymphoma, multiple myeloma, and so forth. Preexisting neuropathy from diabetes and other nononcologic causes of neuropathy can predispose patients to demonstrating worse signs and symptoms of neuropathy when challenged with neurotoxic chemotherapy or another cancer-related cause of neuropathy.[25] Numerous chemotherapeutic agents, including taxanes, vinca alkaloids, platinum agents, bortezomib, and thalidomide, are causative of neuropathy. Clinical manifestations of neuropathy caused by various agents differ somewhat and largely depend on the mechanism of damage associated with the particular agent. For instance, the vinca alkaloids and taxanes are tubulin inhibitors and generally cause sensory more than motor axonal polyneuropathy in a length-dependent distribution. Dysfunction resulting from these agents may improve over time. However, platinum agents damage the DNA of axons in the cell body that is located at the dorsal root ganglion for sensory nerves and in the anterior horn of the spinal cord for motor nerves. This produces a potentially severe non–length-dependent sensory neuropathy with little effect on the motor nerves, which are sequestered behind the blood-brain barrier. Pain, sensory ataxia, and diminished ADLs are common. Because DNA dysfunction is the primary cause of pathology, symptoms can progress for months (coasting effect) following treatment and in some cases may not improve significantly over time.

Treatment of neuropathy depends on the clinical manifestations. Weakness, ataxia, and gait abnormalities are treated with physical and/or occupational therapy and gait aids/orthotics as necessary. Pain is generally treated with nerve stabilizers (pregabalin, gabapentin, duloxetine). More than one agent may be required. For instance, nerve stabilizers of differing mechanisms and opioids are commonly used in combination to treat refractory pain.

The Lambert-Eaton myasthenic syndrome (LEMS) is a rare paraneoplastic presynaptic neuromuscular junction disorder associated with small cell lung and other cancers. It is caused by immunoglobulin (Ig)G antibodies against voltage-gated calcium channels and may lead to weakness that is worst proximally; it may affect ocular and bulbar muscles and may cause fatigue and autonomic symptoms.

Myopathy is common in the cancer setting as a result of high-dose and prolonged steroid use or following critical illness. Weakness is usually worse proximally, but in severe cases, it may cause frank quadriplegia. Weakness of the cervical and/or thoracic paraspinal muscles with subsequent neck extensor weakness and wasting can be seen in patients treated with local radiation (head and neck cancer, Hodgkin's lymphoma). Myopathy can also result from exposure to toxins such as vincristine or zidovudine, or from amyloid infiltration of muscle or paraneoplastic disorders.

Cancer-related fatigue (CRF) occurs in a majority of cancer survivors and is a major factor in their diminished quality of life. Although the significance of this symptom has been recognized, the pathophysiology and site of origin of CRF remain largely unknown. Studies were carried out to determine the effects of motor activity–induced fatigue on subjective and objective fatigue ratings, motor performance, and physiologic measurements to address central and peripheral neuromuscular function adaptations in advanced cancer patients.[26,27] Patients (n = 29) who had advanced solid tumors and age-, gender-, and body mass index (BMI)-matched healthy controls (n = 16) participated completed a Brief Fatigue Inventory (BFI). BFI scores, motor performance, central drive, neuromuscular junction propagation (NMJP) function, electromyographic (EMG) and electroencephalographic (EEG) signals, EEG-EMG signal coupling (coherence), and force-generating capability (FGC) of the muscle were evaluated before and after a fatigue task that required participants to sustain a low-intensity muscle contraction to exhaustion. Compared with healthy controls, CRF patients exhibited greater BFI score, reduced motor performance (shorter time to exhaustion or fatigue), greater central fatigue and less significant muscle fatigue, impaired NMJP function, abnormal EEG signal, and reduced EEG-EMG signal coupling. In summary, patients with CRF *feel* significantly more fatigued (BFI scores), which limits their motor performance (feel exhausted sooner), but their level of muscle fatigue (physiologic fatigue) is lower. The fatigue induced by motor performance in cancer survivors with CRF is more of central origin and may be contributed to, at least in part, by abnormal brain function, impaired functional corticomuscular coupling, and diminished NMJP function.

MUSCULOSKELETAL COMPLICATIONS OF CANCER

Musculoskeletal disorders are common in the cancer setting and often keep company with neurologic or neuromuscular complications. Bone metastases, for instance, may cause severe pain, pathologic fractures, and/or deformity. Bony fracture can cause compression of the spinal cord, cauda equina, nerve roots, plexus, or peripheral nerves. Impending pathologic fractures are a significant potential barrier to functional recovery and should be addressed appropriately with radiation therapy or surgery before rehabilitation is initiated.[28]

Cancer patients are often at higher risk for fractures secondary to osteoporosis. Accelerated bone loss leading to osteoporosis results from the high incidence of steroid use, treatment-related hormone deprivation, and debility from the primary disorder.[29,30] Medical intervention with hormonal therapy, chemotherapy, radiation, or surgical removal of testicles/ovaries can have direct or indirect consequences on bone, leading to loss of bone mass and strength. The typical method of measuring bone mineral density is the dual-energy X-ray absorptiometry (DEXA) scan. Normal is defined as being within one standard deviation (SD) of the young adult's mean peak bone mass. Osteopenia is defined as being between −1 and −2.5 SD, and osteoporosis as being −2.5 SD or less than the mean peak bone mass of the young adult.[31] The risk for fracture doubles for every SD the affected patient is below the young adult's mean peak bone mass.[32,33] Treatments for osteopenia and osteoporosis in the cancer setting are the same as for non–cancer-related bone loss and include bisphosphonates, diet, exercise, supplementation with vitamin D and calcium, and weight-bearing exercise,[34] as well as cessation of smoking[35-37] and decreased alcohol ingestion. Hormone replacement therapy is absolutely contraindicated in breast and prostate cancers.

Radiation treatment can have significant direct and indirect effects on the musculoskeletal system. Direct effects can result from progressive fibrosis of muscle, joint, ligaments, and other supportive tissues. Indirect effects of radiation commonly result from damage to the neural innervation of muscles. For instance, damage to the upper cervical nerve roots or the upper brachial plexus in patients with head and neck cancer treated with radiation can result in weakness of the rotator cuff muscles and shoulder dysfunction, including rotator cuff tendonitis and adhesive capsulitis.[38] These disorders can benefit greatly from therapeutic intervention to improve range of motion, posture, and body mechanics, and to strengthen and condition supporting and affected muscles.

LYMPHEDEMA

Lymphedema is the abnormal accumulation of lymph in an extremity or on the trunk or face. Left untreated, accumulations of protein-rich lymphatic fluid eventually result in fibrotic deposition with progressive sclerosis and potentially elephantiasis.[39] Primary lymphedema is due to aplastic or hypoplastic development of the lymphatics, whereas secondary lymphedema is usually the result of infection, tumor, or lymphatic injury. Lymphedema in and of itself does not cause pain, but can cause a feeling of extremity heaviness or constriction and may cause associated traction on the neck and shoulder due to altered biomechanics from a larger limb.[38]

Lymphedema is most commonly seen in breast cancer patients following axillary dissection, radiation, or tumor recurrence, but it can be seen in any malignancy in which the lymphatics are affected by tumor, surgery, or radiation. Reports on the incidence of lymphedema vary greatly depending on the type of surgery, the extent of axillary dissection, the amount of radiation given, and the method of measurement used.[40] Swelling may occur immediately after surgery and may resolve spontaneously. Postoperative swelling may be due to axillary cording (superficial thrombophlebitis) and may not necessarily prognosticate the future development of lymphedema. Lymphedema that presents longer than 2 years following primary treatment should prompt suspicion for tumor recurrence. Imaging is generally indicated and should include a contrast MRI to exclude tumor recurrence and a duplex ultrasound to evaluate for deep venous thrombosis.[39] Screening CT scans of the chest, abdomen, and pelvis commonly used by the primary oncologist will likely miss an axillary recurrence. Positron emission tomography (PET) alone or with CT is very sensitive for recurrence but is not generally preferred over MRI.

Cancer and related treatments are not the only causes of edema, thus there is a need to differentiate lymphedema from other causes of edema. Typical lower extremity lymphedema will involve the dorsal foot but will spare the metatarsal-phalangeal joints and will not involve peripheral vascular disease; stigmata of overt vasculature and ulceration are rare. Studies such as lymphoscintigraphy, which evaluates lymphatic transport and abnormalities, can clarify the origin of venous edema from mixed or lymphatic edema. Lymphoscintigraphy is rarely done, however, as it is highly dependent on the skill of the examiner and carries considerable morbidity without providing significant information to contribute to a comprehensive clinical evaluation. Impedance plethysmography is a noninvasive technique that uses small changes in electrical resistance to evaluate and follow lymphedema. Impedance plethysmography is becoming more clinically relevant as the technology improves, its price falls, and research validating the study becomes available.

The focus of treatment for lymphedema should be on patient education, prevention, early treatment, and avoidance of infection. Goals of intervention should include maintenance of skin and soft tissues, decreased risk of lymphangitis, reduction in and later maintenance of limb volume, and avoidance of contractures and secondary musculoskeletal abnormalities. Early treatment decreases the risk of chronic sequelae of lymphatic damage and late-stage progression of lymphedema changes.

Conventional interventions for lymphedema require close collaboration between the physiatrist and the physical or occupational therapist with specialized training in lymphedema. Therapy includes manual lymphatic drainage (MLD), elevation, wrapping, compressive garments, and occasionally pumps. MLD is a specialized massage technique that progresses from proximal to distal and can be very effective in improving lymphatic flow. Elevation can be used to assist lymph movement. MLD is often followed by or used in combination with compressive wrapping. Compressive wrapping involves the application of layers of special low-elasticity fabric under the direction of a skilled lymphedema therapist. Properly applied wrapping uses the body's own muscle to gently pump the lymphatic fluid out of an extremity. Once the volume reduction goal is reached, compression garments are used, typically with a 30 to 40 or a 40 to 50 mm Hg gradient, to help prevent reaccumulation of lymph fluid.[39] Pneumatic pumping may be instituted for patient populations unable to use MLD or wrapping techniques. Such patients may not have the manual dexterity, strength, flexibility, or cognitive capacity to safely or effectively use MLD or wrapping. Pumping is generally not preferred for fear that it may damage the lymphatics and ultimately worsen lymphedema. Newer multichamber pumps may mitigate this issue, but more research is needed. Optimal management of lymphedema requires meticulous skin hygiene to minimize the risk of infection. Skin should be kept clean, with special care given to protection from injury and avoidance of needle sticks, blood pressure cuffs, or IV lines in the involved limb. If superficial cellulitis does occur, antibiotic intervention should be instituted without delay.

Several treatments are used less commonly for lymphedema. Benzyopyrones, a type of flavonoid, can decrease the amount of high-protein edema fluid by promoting proteolysis and thus the risk of lymphedema formation, but they are not available in the United States, and their efficacy is unclear.[41] Diuretics may be used for temporary effect for overall loss of volume from the interstitium, but they will not affect the protein-rich fluids of the extravascular space.[42] Surgical intervention is uncommon and often is a treatment of last resort. Procedures of resection are aimed at tissue volume reduction, whereas lymphatic reanastomoses are technically difficult and often unsuccessful.

MEDICAL COMPLICATIONS AND REHABILITATION

The nature of cancer and its treatment is such that medical derangements are common and can severely affect the safety and efficacy of rehabilitation efforts. Physiatrists should routinely check for such conditions and consider appropriate changes to their rehabilitation plans, which may include alteration, delay, or even halting of therapy, depending on the clinical scenario.[43] Common conditions that should prompt reconsideration of rehabilitation efforts include the following:

1. Hematologic profile: hemoglobin <8.0 g/dl, platelets <20,000/mm³, white blood cell count <5,000/mm³ if accompanied by fever.
2. Metastatic bone disease with involvement of long bones (femur, tibia, humerus) such that more than 50% of the cortex is involved, intramedullary lesions have a greater than 50% to 60% cross-sectional diameter, or the diameter of the lesion femur measures more than 2.5 cm.

3. Compression of a hollow viscus (bowel, bladder, or ureter), vessel, or spinal cord.
4. Fluid accumulation in the pleura, pericardium, abdomen, or retroperitoneum associated with persistent pain, dyspnea, or problems with mobility.
5. Central nervous system depression or coma, or increased intracranial pressure.
6. Hypokalemia/hyperkalemia, hyponatremia, or hypocalcemia/hypercalcemia.
7. Orthostatic hypotension or hypertension with blood pressure in excess of 160/100 mm Hg.
8. Heart rate in excess of 110 beats/min, or ventricular arrhythmia.
9. Fever greater than 101° Fahrenheit.

Hematologic and cardiovascular abnormalities secondary to cancer treatments, such as anemia, thrombocytopenia, and neutropenia, are common in this population and may present a limitation to rehabilitation efforts.[28] Neutropenia and thrombocytopenia can be detected as early as the ninth day following administration of certain chemotherapeutics. The nadir of blood counts generally occurs between days 14 and 18, and recovery begins by day 21.[39] Neutropenia, with white blood cell counts below 1500/ml of blood, has been associated with increased risk of infection. Physical and occupational therapy is generally provided when white blood cell counts fall below 5000/ml of blood if the patient is febrile.[28] Thrombocytopenia from chemotherapy can result in bleeding from the nasal and oral mucosae, the gastrointestinal tract, and the urinary tract. Platelet counts less than 20,000/ml blood can result in bleeding. Therapy is usually provided when platelet counts are below 20,000/ml.[28] Patients with thrombocytopenia should avoid medications that affect platelet function, such as ibuprofen, aspirin, and naproxen. Patients with anemia or thrombocytopenia may require transfusions of packed red blood cells or single-donor platelets. Several causes of anemia, including hemorrhage, hemolysis, nutritional deficiencies, bone marrow infiltration, chemotherapy or radiation therapy, and anemia of chronic disease, are recognized in cancer patients.[44] Therapy is often provided when hematocrit levels fall below 25%, or hemoglobin below 8 g/dl.[28] It should be noted that the hematologic guidelines for withholding therapy are not strict rules. The decision to continue patients on therapy when their laboratory values fall below the recommended minimum is a risk-benefit assessment that should include key members of the oncologic and rehabilitation teams.

Patients with cancer are predisposed to venous thromboembolism secondary to prolonged bed rest, along with immobilization. They may have tumors that obstruct or slow blood flow, or indwelling venous catheters that predispose to clotting. Clotting may also be promoted by the release of procoagulants from tumor cells. Nearly 15% of patients who develop deep venous thrombosis or pulmonary embolism have a diagnosis of cancer.[45] The guidelines used at the Memorial Sloan-Kettering Cancer Center for decision making with regard to physical, occupational, and lymphedema therapy in patients with venous thromboembolism are presented in Table 39-1.

PAIN

Pain is often one of the most significant barriers affecting successful rehabilitation. Pain can be nociceptive, somatic, neuropathic, or visceral in origin. Multiple competing causes

Table 39-1   Guidelines for physical, occupational, and lymphedema therapy in patients with venous thromboembolism

Lower extremities	1. For patients with acute lower extremity deep vein thrombosis (DVT), with or without pulmonary embolism (PE), and no inferior vena cava (IVC) filter, therapy (including physical, occupational, and lymphedema with bandaging and manual lymphatic drainage [MLD]) can be initiated once they are therapeutic on an anticoagulant. Resistive exercises generally should be deferred for 48 to 72 hours.	• Definition of therapeutic anticoagulation by modality: • Low-molecular-weight heparin (LMWH) preparations are preferred, as they are therapeutic immediately following the first injection. Monitoring is not required. Common preparations include enoxaparin (Lovenox), dalteparin (Fragmin), and tinzaparin (Innohep). • Unfractionated heparin may take 1 to 2 days to become therapeutic and is more prone to bleeding complications than LMWH. The adjusted partial thromboplastin time (APTT) should be monitored, and therapy can begin when it is between 50 and 70. • Warfarin (Coumadin) may take several days to become therapeutic. The international normalized ratio (INR) should be monitored, and therapy can begin when it is between 2 and 3.
	2. For patients with acute lower extremity DVT (with or without PE) and an IVC filter, therapy can be initiated immediately, regardless of their anticoagulation status.	
	3. For patients with acute lower extremity DVT who cannot be anticoagulated and in whom an IVC filter cannot be placed, therapy can be started immediately but should be functional in nature (ambulation, balance, activities of daily living [ADL] training) and should avoid resistive and repetitive exercise. Such patients are at very high risk for PE and death. Therapists are advised to discuss therapy interventions with the patient's primary attending or the rehabilitation medicine attending, so that the relative risks and benefits of therapy can be better delineated.	
Upper extremities	1. Upper extremity DVT carries the same risk for PE and death as lower extremity DVT. IVC filters are not protective. For patients with acute upper extremity DVT with or without PE, therapy (including physical, occupational, and lymphedema with bandaging and manual lymphatic drainage [MLD]) can be initiated once they are therapeutic on an anticoagulant. Resistive exercises should generally be deferred for 48 to 72 hours. (See anticoagulation guidelines above.)	
	2. For patients with acute upper extremity DVT who cannot be anticoagulated, therapy should be functional in nature (ambulation, balance, ADL training) and should avoid resistive and repetitive exercise. Such patients are at very high risk for PE and death. Therapists are advised to discuss therapeutic interventions with the patient.	

are common in the cancer setting. A thorough clinical assessment is critical in the accurate assessment of pain, so that treatments can be targeted to provide maximum therapeutic impact while minimizing side effects. Successful treatment of pain often requires a multimodal approach that may include nonsteroidal antiinflammatory drugs (NSAIDs), opioids, nerve-stabilizing agents, injections, physical or occupational therapy, radiation therapy, surgery, or changes in chemotherapy. A comprehensive discussion of pain management in the cancer setting is beyond the scope of this chapter but is provided elsewhere in this book.

RADIATION-RELATED INJURIES

Radiation can damage any tissue in the body, including all levels of the nervous system and muscle. Effects of radiation can be classified as acute, subacute, or late. Late effects of radiation therapy result from progressive fibrosis of the microvasculature of affected tissue with local fibrin formation both within the blood vessels and in the extracellular matrix. The clinical manifestations of this progressive fibrosis are termed radiation fibrosis syndrome (RFS). RFS is common in patients with Hodgkin's lymphoma treated with mantle filed radiation, head and neck cancers, and extremity sarcomas. Common clinical manifestations include radiation-induced cervical dystonia, trismus, and dropped head syndrome.[46] Trismus may result from pathologic spasm of the muscles of mastication and from progressive fibrosis of the supporting tissues of the jaw and oropharynx. Trismus can significantly affect eating, oral hygiene, and speech.[47] Dropped head syndrome is a late complication of RFS commonly seen in Hodgkin's lymphoma and head and neck cancer survivors treated with radiation. The neck extensor weakness of dropped head syndrome results from local myopathy of radiated cervical and thoracic muscles, as well as from damage to their neural innervations.[3]

Radiation-related dysfunction of the neuromuscular, musculoskeletal, and other systems such as the cardiac and pulmonary systems should be anticipated and recognized by physiatrists.

Although the underlying pathophysiology of progressive fibrosis that causes RFS cannot be affected, many of the neuromuscular, musculoskeletal, cardiac, pulmonary, and other complications that result can be effectively treated. Cervical dystonia from radiation to the head and neck has been successfully treated with botulinum toxin injections.[46] Botulinum toxin has also been used in the management of trismus. Use of a prescribed Dynasplint trismus system and collaboration with therapists have proved beneficial. The Dynasplint trismus system provides low-load, prolonged duration stretch to reduce contractures.[47] Range of motion, strengthening exercises, manual fibrous tissue release techniques, postural correction, and compression garments are utilized in the treatment of dropped head syndrome.[39] Cervical collars can assist with energy conservation in upright head posturing for these patients.

REFERENCES

1. Lehmann JF, DeLisa JA, Warren CG, et al. Cancer rehabilitation: assessment of need, development, and evaluation of a model of care. *Arch Phys Med Rehabil.* 1978;59:410–419.
2. DeLisa JA. A history of cancer rehabilitation. *Cancer.* 2001;92:970–974.
3. Stubblefield MD, Custodio CM, Franklin DJ. Cardiopulmonary rehabilitation and cancer rehabilitation. 3. Cancer rehabilitation. *Arch Phys Med Rehabil.* 2006;87:S65–S71.
4. Bundy AC. Assessment of play and leisure: delineation of the problem. *Am J Occup Ther.* 1993;47:217–222.
5. Aziz NM. Cancer survivorship research: state of knowledge, challenges and opportunities. *Acta Oncol.* 2007;46:417–432.
6. Dietz JH. *Rehabilitation oncology.* 99th ed. New York: John Wiley & Sons Inc; 1981.
7. Jones VA, Stubblefield MD. The role of knee immobilizers in cancer patients with femoral neuropathy. *Arch Phys Med Rehabil.* 2004;85:303–307.
8. Newton HB. Neurologic complications of systemic cancer. *Am Fam Physician.* 1999;59:878–886.
9. Clouston PD, DeAngelis LM, Posner JB. The spectrum of neurological disease in patients with systemic cancer. *Ann Neurol.* 1992;31:268–273.
10. O'Neill BP, Buckner JC, Coffey RJ, et al. Brain metastatic lesions. *Mayo Clin Proc.* 1994;69:1062–1068.
11. Patchell RA. The treatment of brain metastases. *Cancer Invest.* 1996;14:169–177.
12. Nussbaum ES, Djalilian HR, Cho KH, et al. Brain metastases: histology, multiplicity, surgery, and survival. *Cancer.* 1996;78:1781–1788.
13. Patchell RA, Tibbs PA, Walsh JW, et al. A randomized trial of surgery in the treatment of single metastases to the brain. *N Engl J Med.* 1990;322:494–500.
14. Sioutos PJ, Arbit E, Meshulam CF, et al. Spinal metastases from solid tumors: analysis of factors affecting survival. *Cancer.* 1995;76:1453–1459.
15. Klein SL, Sanford RA, Muhlbauer MS. Pediatric spinal epidural metastases. *J Neurosurg.* 1991;74:70–75.
16. Dropcho EJ. Central nervous system injury by therapeutic irradiation. *Neurol Clin.* 1991;9:969–988.
17. Schultheiss T, El-Jahdi A. *Statistical analysis of two hundred radiation myelopathy cases.* Presented at: Seventh International Congress of Radiation Research, Amsterdam, The Netherlands, July 8; 1983:3–41.
18. Liebel S, Guten P, Avis R. Tolerance of the brain and spinal cord. In: Guten P, ed. *Radiation injury to the nervous system.* New York: Raven Press; 1991:239–256.
19. Louton RB, Terranova WA. The use of suction curettage as adjunct to the management of lymphedema. *Ann Plast Surg.* 1989;22:354–357.
20. Olsen NK, Pfeiffer P, Mondrup K, et al. Radiation-induced brachial plexus neuropathy in breast cancer patients. *Acta Oncol.* 1990;29:885–890.
21. Lederman RJ, Wilbourn AJ. Brachial plexopathy: recurrent cancer or radiation? *Neurology.* 1984;34:1331–1335.
22. Harper Jr CM, Thomas JE, Cascino TL, et al. Distinction between neoplastic and radiation-induced brachial plexopathy, with emphasis on the role of EMG. *Neurology.* 1989;39:502–506.
23. Numata K, Ito M, Uchiyama S, et al. A case of delayed radiation lumbo-sacral plexopathy. *No To Shinkei.* 1990;42:629–633.
24. Forman A. Peripheral neuropathy in cancer patients: clinical types, etiology, and presentation, part 2. *Oncology (Williston Park).* 1990;4:85–89.
25. Stubblefield MD, Slovin S, MacGregor-Cortelli B, et al. An electrodiagnostic evaluation of the effect of pre-existing peripheral nervous system disorders in patients treated with the novel proteasome inhibitor bortezomib. *Clin Oncol.* 2006;18:410–418.
26. Khoshknabi DS, Davis MP, Ranganathan VK, et al. Combining objective and subjective outcomes in cancer-related fatigue: illustrations from a single case report. *J Palliat Med.* 2008;11:829–833.
27. Yavuzsen T, Davis MP, Ranganathan VK, et al. Cancer-related fatigue: central or peripheral? *J Pain Symptom Manage.* 2009;38:587–596.
28. Stubblefield MD, Bilsky MH. Barriers to rehabilitation of the neurosurgical spine cancer patient. *J Surg Oncol.* 2007;95:419–426.
29. Kerr D, Ackland T, Maslen B, et al. Resistance training over 2 years increases bone mass in calcium-replete postmenopausal women. *J Bone Miner Res.* 2001;16:175–181.
30. Sheth P. Osteoporosis and exercise: a review. *Mt Sinai J Med.* 1999;66:197–200.
31. World Health Organization. *Prevention and management of osteoporosis, WHO Technical Report Series.* Geneva, Switzerland: WHO; 2003:N921.
32. Chien AJ, Goss PE. Aromatase inhibitors and bone health in women with breast cancer. *J Clin Oncol.* 2006;24:5305–5312.
33. Kaste SC, Chesney RW, Hudson MM, et al. Bone mineral status during and after therapy of childhood cancer: an increasing population with multiple risk factors for impaired bone health. *J Bone Miner Res.* 1999;14:2010–2014.
34. Aksnes LH, Bruland OS. Some musculo-skeletal sequelae in cancer survivors. *Acta Oncol.* 2007;46:490–496.
35. Bae DC, Stein BS. The diagnosis and treatment of osteoporosis in men on androgen deprivation therapy for advanced carcinoma of the prostate. *J Urol.* 2004;172:2137–2144.
36. Conde FA, Aronson WJ. Risk factors for male osteoporosis. *Urol Oncol.* 2003;21:380–383.
37. Hawkins R. Osteoporosis. *Cancer Nurs.* 2006;29:78–82.
38. Stubblefield MD, Custodio CM. Upper-extremity pain disorders in breast cancer. *Arch Phys Med Rehabil.* 2006;87:S96–S99.
39. Braddom RL, ed. *Physical medicine and rehabilitation.* 3rd ed. Philadelphia, PA: WB Saunders; 2007.
40. Brennan MJ. Lymphedema following the surgical-treatment of breast-cancer: a review of pathophysiology and treatment. *J Pain Symptom Manage.* 1992;7:110–116.
41. Tubiana-Hulin M. Incidence, prevalence and distribution of bone metastases. *Bone.* 1991;12(suppl 1):S9–S10.
42. DeVita J, Hellman S, Rosenberg S. *Cancer: principles and practice of oncology.* 3rd ed. Philadelphia, PA: JB Lippincott; 1989:2231.
43. Delisa J. *Physical medicine and rehabilitation.* 4th ed. Philadelphia, PA: Lippincott Williams & Wilkins; 2005.
44. Sood A, Moynihan TJ. Cancer-related fatigue: an update. *Curr Oncol Rep.* 2005;7:277–282.
45. Kasper DL, Braunwald E, Fauci AS, et al. *Harrison's principles of internal medicine.* 16th ed. New York: McGraw-Hill Medical Publishing; 2005.
46. Harti DM, Cohen M, Julieron M, et al. Botulinum toxin for radiation-induced facial pain and trismus. *Otolaryngol Head Neck Surg.* 2008;138:459–463.
47. Shulman DH, Shipman B, Willis FB. Treating trismus with dynamic splinting: a cohort, case series. *Adv Ther.* 2008;25:9–15.

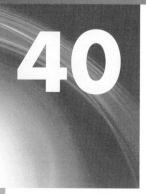

40

Exercise interventions in supportive oncology

Erin L. McGowan and Kerry S. Courneya

Advancements in the detection and treatment of cancer have resulted in an improvement in overall 5-year survival rate to about 66%.[1] However, cancer and its treatment can produce negative side effects that result in persisting physical and emotional challenges that may last well beyond cancer diagnosis and treatment.[2] In light of this, researchers are exploring the ability of behavioral strategies to manage symptoms arising from cancer and its treatment, in an attempt to improve the cancer survivor's quality of life (QoL) and disease outcome.[3] One such behavioral strategy that has received significant research attention is physical activity (PA) and exercise. PA is described as any movement created by the skeletal muscles that causes a substantial increase in energy expenditure.[4] Leisure-time PA represents any activity undertaken during free time based on a personal choice, but it does not include household and/or occupational activities. Exercise is a specific form of leisure-time PA that is performed on a repeated basis over an extended period of time, with the intention of improving fitness levels, performance, and/or health.[4] Another important concept is health-related fitness, which is composed of five related components: cardiorespiratory fitness, muscular strength, muscular endurance, flexibility, and body composition. These components represent important outcomes in cancer survivors that may mediate the influence of exercise on other supportive care and disease outcomes. For this chapter, cancer survivors will be defined as those diagnosed with cancer from the time of diagnosis and for the balance of their life.[5]

The purpose of this chapter is to provide an up-to-date overview of the role of PA and exercise in supportive care and disease endpoints in cancer survivors. Supportive care endpoints refer to indicators of the cancer survivor's generic and disease-specific QoL. In particular, QoL refers to overall well-being and happiness, and encompasses physical, functional, psychological, and social aspects.[6] Disease endpoints are indicators of the quantity of expected life, such as disease-free survival, cancer-specific mortality, and overall survival.[6] Because cancer includes many different diseases that may vary considerably based on the pathophysiology of the disease, prognosis, treatment received, side effects experienced, patient demographic profile (e.g., age, gender), medical profile (e.g., obesity, comorbidities), and behavioral profile (e.g., smoking history, alcohol consumption, past exercise behavior), the chapter will be organized by specific cancer groups. Additionally, the chapter will focus on PA and exercise motivation and behavior change in cancer survivors. When possible, systematic reviews are summarized first, before recent randomized controlled trials are reviewed.

EFFECTS OF PHYSICAL ACTIVITY ON SUPPORTIVE CARE OUTCOMES

Several systematic reviews have combined all cancer survivor groups when summarizing the effects of PA. Schmitz et al.[7] conducted a systematic qualitative and quantitative review of 32 controlled trials that examined the role of PA in cancer survivors (i.e., 72%, breast cancer) during and after treatment. In this review, small to moderate positive effects on PA behavior, cardiorespiratory fitness, physiologic outcomes, and symptoms/side effects during cancer treatment were found following PA interventions; moderate to large positive effects on cardiorespiratory fitness and vigor/vitality were noted following treatment. Additionally, quantitative null findings were found for the effect of PA on fatigue both during and following treatment.

Knols et al.[8] reviewed 34 randomized clinical and controlled clinical trials that examined the effects of exercise on physical functioning and psychological well-being in cancer survivors during and after treatment. Results during treatment in breast cancer survivors indicated statistically significant benefits for functional capacity, psychological well-being, and self-reported outcomes (e.g., nausea) favoring the exercise group. After treatment, significant differences in terms of aerobic capacity, cardiopulmonary changes, self-esteem, depression, and anxiety were noted for breast cancer survivors in the exercise groups. Finally, combined results during and after treatment indicated significant benefits favoring the exercise group for a variety of outcomes, including walking distance, QoL, fatigue, mood status, and strength. During bone marrow and peripheral stem cell transplantation, exercise was found to provide positive effects on body composition (e.g., fat-free mass), muscle strength, functional capacity, symptoms of medical treatment (e.g., pain, diarrhea), days in the hospital, and self-reported psychological well-being and mood status. With exercise during treatment in a mixed solid tumor population, benefits were reported for physical fitness, aerobic capacity, bone mineral density, shoulder range of motion, pain, fatigue, completion rate of the exercise program, and self-reported QoL and mood status. Finally, exercise after treatment in a mixed solid tumor population led to improved physical strength and aerobic capacity and decreased body fat, anxiety, sleeping problems, flexibility, and self-reported QoL. Overall, the pattern of results supports the benefits of exercise both during and following cancer treatment.

In a meta-analysis, Conn et al.[9] examined the effects of PA both during and following treatment. Most of the studies included in the meta-analysis contained exclusively ($k = 13$) or primarily ($k = 5$) breast cancer survivors. Other less commonly included cancer groups consisted of lymphoma ($k = 8$), lung ($k = 6$), hematologic ($k = 5$), gastrointestinal ($k = 4$), and prostate cancers ($k = 2$), and melanoma ($k = 1$). Medium standardized effects were found for physical functioning, and more modest effects were noted for body composition, mood, QoL, and fatigue. Overall results support the benefits of PA interventions, which were more favorable when delivered following cancer treatment. However, this was not the case for physical functioning, as it improved both during and following treatment.[9]

Knobf et al.[10] reviewed 25 studies that examined the effects of exercise interventions on physical, psychological, social, and spiritual QoL in a variety of cancer groups, including breast and endometrial cancer, non-Hodgkin's lymphoma, and prostate and colorectal cancer survivors. Results provided strong evidence supporting the positive effects of exercise on physical QoL (i.e., physical functioning, muscle strength, and weight management) and psychological QoL (i.e., emotional well-being, self-esteem, anxiety, depression, and fatigue). Additionally, the results suggested that exercise fosters improved social functioning. The authors recommend that more research is required to explore the relationship between exercise and spiritual well-being.

Schwartz[11] reviewed studies that examined the effects of exercise both during ($k = 35$) and after ($k = 38$) treatment on cancer survivors with any type or stage of cancer. During treatment, the studies explored a variety of exercise interventions, including home-based and supervised exercise programs and aerobic and resistance training; the duration of programs ranged from 2 to 52 weeks. Most studies that used exercise following treatment were supervised programs that included aerobic or resistance training, or a combination of these. The literature consistently found positive associations with QoL, cardiorespiratory fitness, muscle strength, flexibility, fatigue, anxiety, depression, anthropometric measures of body weight (e.g., body fat), and other health-related biomarkers followed during cancer treatment. Following cancer treatment, the benefits of exercise were not as great as during treatment; however, benefits were found in terms of cardiorespiratory fitness, muscle strength, fatigue, depression, anxiety, vigor and vitality, body image, body size, mental health, and QoL.

Cancer-related fatigue is a symptom that is frequently associated with cancer and its treatment. Cramp and Daniel[12] reviewed 28 randomized controlled trials that examined the effects of exercise on cancer-related fatigue both during and after treatment. Statistically significant improvements were noted after completion of an exercise program, regardless of when the exercise intervention was carried out during cancer treatment. Thus, exercise was found to improve cancer-related fatigue when performed both during and after treatment.

A recent systematic review conducted by Speck and colleagues[13] summarized 82 randomized and nonrandomized controlled trials of PA in cancer survivors. Most studies focused on or included breast cancer survivors (i.e., 83%); very few studies included other cancers (Fig. 40-1). The most common outcomes of these studies were aerobic fitness, overall QoL, functional QoL, fatigue, depression, and anxiety (Fig. 40-2). A large effect of PA was found on post–cancer treatment body strength (i.e., upper and lower); moderate effects were noted for fatigue and breast cancer–specific concerns. Small to moderate benefits were noted for aerobic fitness, PA level, muscular strength, functional QoL, anxiety, and self-esteem during cancer treatment. Effect size was generally greater for PA in survivors than when performed during the cancer treatment phase (Fig. 40-3). Exercise was well tolerated both during and after treatment.[13]

A large randomized trial recently conducted by Adamsen et al.[14] examined the benefits of a 6-week structured group exercise intervention on outcomes such as fatigue, QoL,

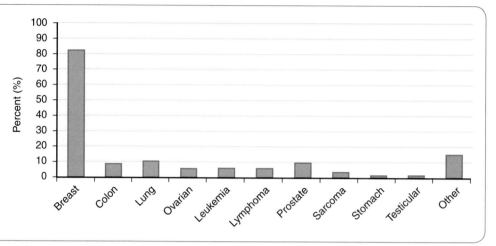

Fig. 40-1 The most common cancer diagnoses targeted in exercise trials. Percent (%) = the percentage of studies that include at least one participant with that particular cancer diagnosis. *(Data from Speck RM, Courneya KS, Masse LC, et al. An update of controlled physical activity trials in cancer survivors: a systematic review and meta-analysis. J Cancer Surv 2010. DOI 10.1007/ s11764-009-0110-5.)*

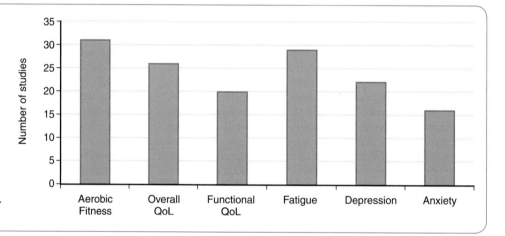

Fig. 40-2 The most common health outcomes targeted in exercise trials. *(Data from Speck RM, Courneya KS, Masse LC, et al. An update of controlled physical activity trials in cancer survivors: a systematic review and meta-analysis. J Cancer Surv 2010. DOI 10.1007/s11764-009-0110-5.)*

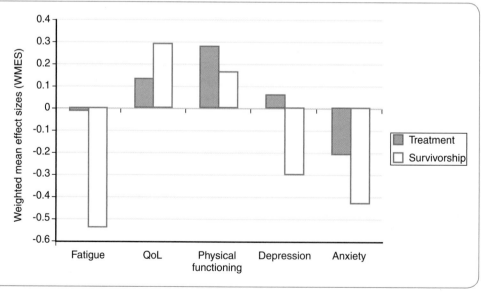

Fig. 40-3 Summary of weighted mean effect sizes by cancer phase (i.e., treatment or survivorship) for the most common patient-reported outcomes targeted in exercise trials. *(Data from Speck RM, Courneya KS, Masse LC, et al. An update of controlled physical activity trials in cancer survivors: a systematic review and meta-analysis. J Cancer Surv 2010. DOI 10.1007/s11764-009-0110-5.)*

general well-being, PA, and physical capacity. This was compared with conventional care provided for 269 cancer survivors from 21 different cancer groups. The exercise intervention consisted of high-intensity cardiovascular and resistance training, as well as low-intensity training (i.e., relaxation training, body awareness training, and restorative training), provided for a total of 9 hours per week. At 6 weeks, fatigue was reduced in the exercise intervention group. The intervention improved vitality, aerobic capacity, muscular strength, physical and functional activity, and emotional well-being in cancer survivors. However, no improvements in QoL were noted. The authors suggested that exercise consisting of high- and low-intensity components was both feasible and safe for cancer survivors while on treatment.

The previous reviews and trials did not separate studies by cancer group, despite the fact that significant differences between cancer groups have been observed. These mixed reviews have noted that most of the studies were conducted in early-stage breast cancer survivors. As such, the conclusions pertaining to the benefits of PA interventions are based largely on trials done in those with breast cancer and may not be generalizable to those with other cancer at other sites. Several recent reviews have focused on specific cancer groups, but the most common focus remains breast cancer.

BREAST CANCER

McNeely et al.[15] conducted a systematic review and meta-analysis of 14 randomized controlled trials to examine the effects of exercise intervention on 717 breast cancer survivors (i.e., stage 0–III). Exercise led to significant and meaningful improvements in QoL, physical functioning, cardiorespiratory fitness (i.e., peak oxygen consumption), and fatigue among breast cancer survivors. When body mass index (BMI) or body weight was assessed, no significant changes were found. However, when objective body composition was assessed using dual-energy X-ray absorptiometry (DEXA), changes in bone density and lean body mass were noted.

Markes et al.[16] reviewed nine controlled trials that assessed the effects of exercise interventions (i.e., aerobic and resistance) in 492 women who were stage I to III breast cancer survivors receiving adjuvant treatment. Exercise significantly improved cardiorespiratory fitness, which, in turn, led to improved ability to perform activities of daily living. Nonsignificant improvements were found for other outcomes, such as fatigue, anxiety, depression, strength, weight gain, and immune function. These mixed results could have been due to clinical heterogeneity in cancer treatment and exercise interventions.[16]

In a review of exercise during and after treatment of breast cancer, Kirshbaum[17] evaluated 29 articles, which reported that the benefits of aerobic exercise were consistently noted for breast cancer survivors during adjuvant therapy (i.e., chemotherapy or radiotherapy) rather than during the post-treatment period. Strong evidence supported the benefit of aerobic exercise in reducing cancer-related fatigue. Exercise had the potential to benefit other outcomes, such as QoL, self-esteem, health, strength, reduced weight gain, anxiety, depression, and tiredness. Kirshbaum[17] noted that additional studies of higher methodologic quality are warranted to validate results in survivor subgroups, such as advanced cancer survivors.

Finally, nine randomized controlled trials reviewed by Bicego et al.[18] examined the effects of exercise on QoL in women living with breast cancer. This review focused on structured exercise programs that lasted a minimum of 4 weeks and included women with all stages of breast cancer without regard for treatment status. Overall, exercise positively influenced QoL and mood by improving overall health through socialization, goal setting, participation, decreased body weight, and decreased fatigue.

In addition to the systematic reviews, several recent large randomized controlled trials warrant further discussion. Mutrie et al.[19] examined the benefits of a 12-week structured exercise program (i.e., aerobic and resistance) compared with usual care during treatment in 201 women with early-stage breast cancer (i.e., stage 0–III). Following a 12-week exercise program, the intervention group showed improvements in physical (e.g., aerobic fitness, shoulder mobility, breast cancer–specific symptoms) and psychological (i.e., depression and mood) functioning compared with the usual care group. Additionally, benefits noted at the end of the exercise program were largely maintained at the 6-month follow-up.

The Supervised Trial of Aerobic versus Resistance Training (START) trial is one of the largest multicenter studies conducted in breast cancer survivors undergoing adjuvant chemotherapy.[20] This trial was designed to compare the effects of aerobic and resistance exercise training versus usual care on physical functioning, body composition, psychosocial functioning, and QoL. Compared with usual care, aerobic exercise training led to improved self-esteem, aerobic fitness, and percent body fat; resistance exercise training led to improved self-esteem, muscular strength, lean body mass, and chemotherapy completion rate. Although not statistically significant, benefits for cancer-specific QoL, fatigue, depression, and anxiety were noted for the exercise groups.

Daley et al.[21] examined the effects of an 8-week aerobic exercise or flexibility exercise program versus usual care in 108 breast cancer survivors who had completed treatment within 12 to 36 months. Positive postintervention effects were found in terms of QoL, self-worth, fatigue, aerobic fitness, and depression. Additionally, beneficial effects on depression were maintained at the 6-month follow-up. The Weight Training for Breast Cancer Survivors (WTBS) study explored the effects of biweekly weight training on outcomes in 86 breast cancer survivors who completed treatment within 4 to 36 months. The results revealed no changes in depression; however, weight training had positive effects on physical and psychological QoL, lean body mass, and upper body strength.

COLORECTAL CANCER

No systematic reviews of exercise in colorectal cancer survivors are available because of the limited research in this group. In a prospective study, Courneya et al.[22] explored the impact of PA on QoL in colorectal cancer survivors. Fifty-three postsurgical colorectal cancer survivors participated and were assessed 2 months following surgery, and again 4 months later. Mildly intense exercise from before diagnosis to the time after surgery was associated with improvement in overall QoL.

In the only randomized controlled trial to date, Courneya et al.[23] examined the benefits for QoL of a home-based exercise intervention provided to recently resected colorectal cancer survivors. One hundred two participants were randomly assigned in a 2:1 ratio to an exercise or control group. Overall adherence to the exercise intervention was 75.8%, but significant contamination occurred in the control group. Intent-to-treat analysis found no significant difference between groups on any outcomes; however, ancillary analyses found that survivors who improved their cardiovascular fitness over the course of the study showed greater improvements in QoL, fatigue, depression, and anxiety than survivors whose fitness was reduced. The authors acknowledged problems with exercise adherence and contamination, and suggested the need for a better controlled trial.

Peddle et al.[24] conducted a study that examined QoL and fatigue in colorectal cancer survivors to see whether they were meeting public health exercise guidelines. Of 413 colorectal cancer survivors surveyed, only 25.9% met exercise guidelines. Those meeting exercise guidelines reported clinically and significantly superior QoL and fatigue compared with colorectal cancer survivors who did not meet guidelines.

In the largest prospective study to date, Lynch et al.[25] examined the relationship between PA and QoL for 2 years following a colorectal cancer diagnosis. Participants included 1966 colorectal cancer survivors who completed telephone interviews at 6, 12, and 24 months following diagnosis. A positive and clinically significant association between PA and QoL was found. Specifically, PA was consistently associated with QoL in that at any given time point, participants achieving at least 150 minutes of PA per week had an 18% higher QoL score when compared with those reporting less PA.

PROSTATE CANCER

Thorsen et al.[26] conducted a systematic review of PA in prostate cancer survivors. The review consisted of four randomized controlled trials, two single-arm trials, and three observational studies that examined PA outcomes. Most of the studies focused on prostate cancer survivors receiving androgen deprivation therapy. This review found that PA interventions, specifically, resistance training, may have a positive effect on health outcomes in prostate cancer survivors. Beneficial health outcomes included muscular fitness and improved physical functioning, fatigue, and health-related QoL. Since that time, several additional randomized controlled trials have focused on prostate cancer survivors (Table 40-1).

In a recent randomized controlled trial, Segal et al.[27] examined the effects of 24 weeks of resistance or aerobic training on fatigue, QoL, fitness, and body composition in prostate cancer survivors during radiation therapy with or without androgen deprivation therapy. One hundred twenty-one prostate cancer survivors were randomized to resistance exercise, aerobic exercise, or usual care. Adherence to the prescribed exercise program was 85.5%. Short-term resistance and aerobic exercise lessened fatigue in prostate cancer survivors. Resistance exercise produced longer-term improvements, as well as improved QoL and upper and lower body strength and reduced body fat.

In another recent randomized controlled trial, Galvao et al.[28] examined the impact of a combined resistance and aerobic exercise program on minimizing treatment side effects in prostate cancer survivors receiving androgen suppression therapy. Fifty-seven prostate cancer survivors undergoing androgen suppression therapy were randomized to a combined resistance and aerobic exercise program or to usual care for 12 weeks. Survivors in the exercise group had significantly improved total body and regional lean mass, muscular strength, functional performance, and balance, as well as improvement in several domains of QoL such as fatigue and general health compared with the usual care group.

LYMPHOMA CANCER

Lui et al.[29] conducted a systematic review of exercise interventions in hematologic cancer survivors. Ten studies were reviewed, including three randomized controlled trials, one nonrandomized controlled trial, and six single-group studies. A total of 194 survivors, including 159 adults and 35 children, participated. Encouraging results were reported for physical fitness (i.e., muscle strength and aerobic capacity), body composition (i.e., lean body weight) and fatigue, despite poor methodologic quality and study heterogeneity. Despite the limitations of the trials, findings suggested that it is safe and feasible to conduct exercise interventions in hematologic cancer survivors. The authors recommended better quality studies that would include larger samples, control groups, and validated outcome measures in this population.

Courneya et al.[30] published a randomized controlled trial examining exercise in lymphoma survivors, called the Healthy Exercise for Lymphoma Patients (HELP) trial. Following baseline testing, 122 survivors were stratified by major lymphoma category (i.e., Hodgkin's lymphoma, indolent non-Hodgkin's lymphoma, and aggressive non-Hodgkin's lymphoma) and treatment (i.e., chemotherapy or off treatment), and were randomly assigned to a 12-week aerobic exercise training or to usual care. The rate of adherence to the exercise program was 92%. Aerobic exercise training was superior to usual care for patient-rated physical functioning, overall QoL, fatigue, depression, general health, cardiovascular fitness, and lean body mass. At the 6-month follow-up, improvements in overall QoL, happiness, and depression favored the aerobic exercise training group. Major lymphoma category and treatment status did not influence the results, suggesting that exercise interventions are beneficial in all major subgroups of lymphoma survivors whether on or off treatment. Moreover, the intense exercise program did not interfere with the chemotherapy completion rate and did not adversely influence treatment response. In fact, although not statistically significant, the exercise group had a 46% complete response compared with only 30% for the control group (Fig. 40-4).

LUNG CANCER

Because of the limited number of studies, no systematic reviews have been published on exercise in lung cancer survivors. Jones et al.[31] conducted a prospective single-group study to investigate the benefits of preoperative structured exercise training for cardiorespiratory fitness in 25 lung cancer survivors undergoing thoracic surgery. The rate of adherence to the exercise program was 72%. Intent-to-treat analysis revealed that mean maximal oxygen uptake (VO_2 max) increased by 2.4 ml $\cdot$ kg^{-1} $\cdot$ min^{-1}, and 6-minute walking test distance increased by 40 m from baseline to presurgery assessment with exercise training. Individuals who attended ≥80% of the structured exercise sessions increased their peak VO_2 by 3.3 ml $\cdot$ kg^{-1} $\cdot$ min^{-1} and their 6-minute walking distance by 49 m. Of particular importance to note is that although presurgical fitness capacity decreased following surgery, it did not decrease beyond baseline values, suggesting that preoperative structured exercise training prevents reduced cardiorespiratory fitness in lung cancer survivors undergoing thoracic surgery.

Table 40-1 A review of randomized controlled trials of exercise interventions for prostate cancer survivors

Authors	Sample	Design	Exercise intervention	Outcomes and measures	Results
Segal et al.[82]	155 PC survivors Mean age = 67.9 years Receiving ADT	RCT	12-week supervised resistance training exercise program, 60%–70% 1 RM, 3/wk. Two sets of 8–12 reps of a variety of different resistance exercises	Fatigue, health-related QoL, muscular fitness (i.e., standard load test), body composition (i.e., body weight, BMI, waist circumference, and subcutaneous skin fold measurement)	Exercise group had significant improvements in terms of fatigue, health-related QoL, and muscular fitness compared with the control group. No group differences for body composition
Oliver[83]	9 PC survivors Mean age = 69.4 years Receiving ADT	RCT	12-week supervised progressive resistance training program, 80% 1 RM, 3/wk. Three sets of 8 reps were performed for 8 exercises for all major muscle groups	Body composition (i.e., lean mass, fat mass, and body water compartments using DEXA, physical function, habitual PA (senior fitness test and pedometer), fatigue (fatigue questionnaire), and health-related QoL	Exercise group had significant improvements in total lean mass, total body water, intracellular water, physical functioning, and upper body strength, as well as lower body flexibility, compared with the usual care group. Positive trends for fatigue and health-related QoL
Windsor et al.[84]	65 PC survivors Mean age = 68.8 years Receiving radiation therapy (RT)	RCT	4-week home-based unsupervised walking program for 30 min at least 3/wk at 60%–70% of HR maximum	Fatigue and physical functioning (modified shuttle test, resting HR, exercise HR)	Exercise group showed no significant change in fatigue during radiotherapy, while control group fatigue increased significantly. Exercise group had significant improvements in the modified shuttle test, and the control group distance decreased (trend effect). No differences in resting HR and exercise HR at baseline or at end of radiotherapy were observed.
Carmack-Taylor et al.[77]	134 PC survivors Mean age = 69.2 years Receiving continuous androgen ablation therapy	RCT	6-month group-based lifestyle intervention program that focused on cognitive-behavioral skills for increasing PA (i.e., self-monitoring, goal setting, problem solving, overcoming barriers, cognitive restructuring, and rewards)	Health-related QoL measures endurance, body composition, social support, PA, and theoretical mechanisms	No significant effects or changes were found for any of the health-related QoL measures, endurance, body composition, social support, or PA
Segal et al.[27]	121 PC survivors Mean age = 66.3 years Initiating RT with or without ADT	RCT	All exercise training interventions lasted 24 weeks. Resistance exercise training group: Performed 2 sets of 8–12 reps of 10 different exercises. 60%–70% of 1 RM, 3/wk. Aerobic exercise training group: Exercised 3/wk. Intensity started at 50%–60% of VO_2 peak for weeks 1–4 and progressed to 70%–75% for weeks 5–24. Duration began at 15 minutes and increased to 45 minutes	Fatigue, objectively measured outcomes (i.e., aerobic fitness, VO_2, strength 8 RM, body weight, body fat percentage, DEXA scan, serum lipids, PSA, testosterone, and hemoglobin)	Both resistance and aerobic exercise mitigated fatigue over the short term; resistance exercise also produced longer-term improvements in fatigue. Compared with the usual care group, resistance training improved QoL, aerobic fitness, upper and lower body strength and triglycerides, while preventing increases in body fat. Aerobic training was also found to improve fitness.
Galvao et al.[28]	57 PC survivors Mean age = 69.8 years Undergoing AST that commenced >2 months before	RCT	Combined progressive 12-week resistance and aerobic exercise program, 2/wk. The resistance program progressed from 12–6 RM for 2–4 sets. The aerobic component included 15–20 minutes of aerobic exercise at 65%–80% maximum HR	Body composition: DXA, muscular strength (i.e., 1 RM), muscle endurance (i.e., max reps at 70% of 1 RM), functional performance, balance, falling self-efficacy, fatigue, and general QoL. Blood samples examined testosterone, PSA, insulin, glucose, C-reactive protein, and lipid profile levels	Survivors in the exercise group had significant improvements in total body and regional lean mass, muscular strength, functional performance, balance, QoL, and fatigue, and decreased levels of C-reactive protein compared with the usual care group

ADT, Androgen deprivation therapy; *AST*, androgen suppression therapy; *BMI*, body mass index; *DEXA* or *DXA*, dual-energy X-ray absorptiometry; *HR*, heart rate; *PA*, physical activity; *PC*, prostate cancer; *PSA*, prostate-specific antigen; *QoL*, quality of life; *RCT*, randomized controlled trial; *Reps*, repetitions; *1 RM*, one-repetition maximum; *VO₂ peak*, peak O₂ consumption.

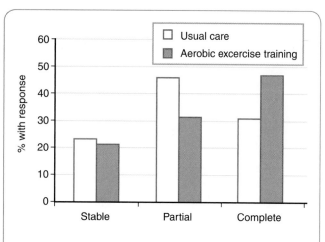

Fig. 40-4 Effects of aerobic exercise training on treatment response in the Healthy Exercise for Lymphoma Patients (HELP) trial. *(Data from Courneya KS, Sellar CM, Stevinson C, et al. Effects of aerobic exercise in physical functioning and quality of life in lymphoma patients. J Clin Oncol 2009b;27:1–9.)*

In a secondary analysis from the same study, Peddle et al.[32] explored the effects of a presurgical exercise training program on QoL and fatigue in survivors with suspected malignant lung lesions. The pilot study included nine individuals who provided complete data. Assessments of cardiovascular fitness and QoL were completed at baseline, presurgery, and post surgery. No statistically significant or clinically meaningful changes in QoL or fatigue were noted from baseline to presurgery; however, it is likely that the exercise program may have prevented the decline in QoL. To adequately answer this research question, the authors recommended randomized controlled trials.[32]

Most recently, Jones et al.[33] conducted a pilot study designed to examine the association between physical functioning (i.e., cardiorespiratory fitness), QoL, markers of systemic inflammation, and predictors of prognosis (i.e., performance status, weight loss, and lung function). Participants included 42 individuals with confirmed inoperable non–small cell lung cancer. Higher cardiorespiratory fitness levels were associated with a more favorable medical profile (e.g., lower BMI), lower systemic inflammation, and reduced fatigue.[33]

OTHER CANCERS

Preliminary evidence is mounting to support the benefits of PA for less common and more difficult cancers. Several observational studies using cross-sectional designs have examined the association between PA and QoL in certain cancer groups, such as multiple myeloma,[34] brain,[35] ovarian,[36,37] endometrial,[38] and bladder.[39] Jones et al.[34] examined the relationship between exercise and QoL in multiple myeloma cancer survivors both during and off treatment. A total of 88 individuals returned questionnaires by mail. Exercise both during active treatment and off treatment was associated with improved overall QoL and subdomains of QoL (i.e., social, functional, and emotional well-being, fatigue, depression, and anemia), except for physical well-being. However, a low percentage of multiple myeloma survivors were regularly exercising during

treatment (i.e., 6.8%) and off treatment (i.e., 20.4%). The results of this trial underscore the importance of exploring the effectiveness of PA habits in this population.

Jones et al.[35] conducted a study to examine the role of exercise in primary brain cancer survivors. One hundred six individuals returned mailed out questionnaires that assessed self-reported exercise at three time points (i.e., prediagnosis, during adjuvant therapy, and following adjuvant therapy). A relatively high percentage of brain tumor survivors were meeting exercise guidelines before diagnosis (i.e., 42%), during treatment (i.e., 38%), and following treatment completion (i.e., 41%). Younger male participants were at greater risk for decreased exercise levels following diagnosis. Future research is needed to explore the effects of exercise training on outcomes in brain cancer survivors.

Karvinen et al.[39] provided data exploring the association between exercise and QoL in bladder cancer survivors. Individuals with bladder cancer identified through a provincial cancer registry were mailed a survey. The response rate was 51%, with 525 bladder cancer survivors responding. Only 22.3% met exercise guidelines over the past month; 16.0% were insufficiently active, and 61.7% were completely sedentary. These results are unfortunate, as exercise was found to be positively associated with QoL, and those meeting the guidelines reported better QoL.

In a large population-based sample of ovarian cancer survivors, Stevinson et al.[36] explored PA prevalence and whether exercise has a dose-response relationship to QoL. Participants included 359 survivors who returned mailed questionnaires. Of those who returned questionnaires, 31.1% met exercise guidelines. Those meeting exercise guidelines reported significantly and meaningfully better QoL.

In a population-based sample of endometrial cancer survivors, Courneya et al.[38] examined the associations between exercise, body weight, and QoL. Three hundred eighty-six endometrial cancer survivors returned a mailed survey. Results revealed that 70% of the sample were not meeting exercise guidelines, and 72% were overweight or obese. Participants meeting exercise and body weight guidelines reported significantly and meaningfully better QoL. von Gruenigen et al.[40] explored the feasibility of lifestyle interventions to promote weight loss, healthy eating, and PA in obese endometrial cancer survivors. At 12 months, the intervention group lost 3.5 kg over the usual care group and showed significant improvement in PA. Weight loss was maintained for 6 months following completion of the intervention. Thus the results of the aforementioned studies demonstrate that a variety of cancer groups that met PA guidelines had improved supportive care outcomes.

DISEASE ENDPOINTS

Research on PA in cancer survivors has focused primarily on supportive care endpoints.[41] However, an emerging research interest involves whether PA reduces cancer recurrence and extends overall survival. Several large epidemiologic studies have investigated the association between postdiagnosis PA levels and disease endpoints in breast and colon cancer survivors, and have reported promising results.

From the Nurses Health Study, Holmes et al.[42] followed for a median of 8 years 2987 women diagnosed with stage I–III breast cancer between 1984 and 1998. Self-reported PA was assessed every 2 years, and analyses were adjusted for known prognostic factors, such as BMI. Women who reported accumulating more than nine metabolic equivalent task (MET) hours/wk of PA had a 25% to 50% reduced risk of recurrence, breast cancer–specific mortality, and all-cause mortality. Additionally, the benefits of PA were apparent for women with hormone-responsive tumors.

Postdiagnosis recreational PA and its association with survival were explored by Holick et al.[43] in a group of women with invasive breast cancer. This study followed 4482 breast cancer survivors between the ages of 20 and 79 years who were participating in the Women's Longevity study. Participants were followed for a maximum of 6 years. Women who participated in more PA had a lower risk of breast cancer mortality and all-cause death (by 40%–50%). These benefits remained significant even after adjustments were made for known prognostic factors, such as age, family history, disease stage, hormone therapy, types of treatments, energy intake, and BMI.

In the Life After Cancer Epidemiological study (LACE), Sternfeld et al.[44] prospectively studied the association between PA (i.e., recreational and nonrecreational), cancer recurrence, and all-cause mortality in women with early-stage breast cancer. Participants included 1970 women. Moderately intense PA increased the reduction in mortality; however, this was not the case for PA of vigorous intensity. Subgroup analyses found that the trend for risk reduction of all-cause mortality was significant only for postmenopausal women and estrogen/progesterone-positive status. Women with normal body weight experienced a risk reduction. Overall, the results suggest that regular PA for breast cancer survivors is beneficial, which reduces all-cause mortality, but it does not reduce breast cancer recurrence or breast cancer mortality.

Three prospective observational studies explored the relationship between PA and colon and colorectal cancer disease outcomes. Meyerhardt et al.[45] examined the influence of exercise on cancer survival in 573 women who were stage I–III colorectal cancer survivors from the Nurses Health Study. A significant negative correlation was found between postdiagnosis PA, cancer-specific risk, and overall mortality. In a similar study, Meyerhardt et al.[46] explored the impact of PA on cancer recurrence and survival in 832 stage III colon cancer survivors followed for a median of 3.8 years. A significant negative relationship was found between PA and recurrence-free survival, disease-free survival, and overall mortality. More recently, Meyerhardt et al.[47] examined cancer-specific and overall mortality in a cohort of 668 men with stage I–II colorectal cancer from the Health Professional Follow-up Study. Increased PA levels were significantly related to colorectal cancer specific–mortality and overall mortality (Fig. 40-5). PA benefits were reported regardless of age, disease stage, BMI, diagnosis year, tumor location, and prediagnosis PA. Taken together, these studies demonstrate that levels of exercise following colorectal and colon cancer diagnosis are associated with a risk reduction in cancer-specific mortality, recurrence, and overall mortality.

Observational studies suggest that PA is associated with a lower risk of disease recurrence and improved survival in breast and colon/colorectal cancer survivors. However, randomized controlled trials are needed to determine the causal benefits of PA on disease endpoints. The Colon Health and Life-Long Exercise Change (CHALLENGE) trial is a multicenter study

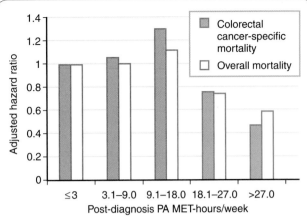

Fig. 40-5 Summary of hazard ratios for colorectal cancer–specific and overall mortality by postdiagnosis physical activity (PA). *(Data from Meyerhardt JA, Giovannucci EL, Ogino S, et al. Physical activity and male colorectal cancer survival. Arch Intern Med 2009;169:2102–2108.)*

designed to explore the benefits of a 3-year PA intervention for disease outcomes in a group of high-risk (i.e., stage II or III colon cancer) survivors who had completed adjuvant therapy within the previous 2 to 6 months.[48] Recruitment goals for the trial include 962 colon cancer survivors who will be randomized to a structured PA intervention or to health education materials. The goal of the PA intervention is to increase recreational PA from baseline by at least 10 MET hours/wk up to a maximum of 27 MET hours/wk using behavioral support sessions. The primary outcome is disease-free survival; secondary outcomes include patient-rated outcomes, physical functioning, biological correlative markers, and an economic analysis. If the results of this trial demonstrate that PA improves disease-free survival in colon cancer survivors, then similar research trials are warranted in other cancer survivor groups.[48]

SUMMARY/CLINICAL IMPLICATIONS

Based on the current research evidence, PA interventions are safe for many cancer survivors and result in beneficial improvement in several outcomes such as QoL and physical and psychological functioning when performed during and following treatment. Most studies have been conducted in breast cancer survivors, so the evidence of benefit of PA is most compelling for members of this population, who generally have a better prognosis and a higher level of functioning than those with other cancers. Positive benefits are also reported for colon/colorectal, prostate, lymphoma, lung, and other cancers. Additionally, for breast and colon cancer survivors, higher PA levels are associated with reduced risk of recurrence, cancer-specific mortality, and overall mortality.

The American Cancer Society recommends that cancer survivors engage in regular exercise.[49] The specific amount of PA depends on many factors, including where the cancer survivors are in the course of their disease (i.e., during or after treatment). Doing exercise during adjuvant therapy will be challenging; however, it is feasible and safe, as demonstrated in multiple studies. During treatment, it is generally recommended that low- to moderate-intensity exercise should be performed 3 to 5 days per week for 20 to 30 minutes.[3] However, this recommendation should be viewed only as a general guideline and may need to be modified or tailored on the basis of individual needs. Cancer survivors should be encouraged to reduce exercise intensity if they feel the need. Cancer treatment may lead to unfavorable changes in lean mass and body weight in some with breast and prostate cancer, such that resistance training will be beneficial to combat loss of lean body mass. Adjuvant therapy is associated with fatigue, such that progression or a prescribed routine likely will be unpredictable and will not follow a consistent pattern because of accumulated side effects that most experience with cancer therapies.[3]

After cancer treatment, cancer survivors should follow the exercise guidelines put forth by the U.S. Department of Health and Human Services.[50] Two different exercise guidelines have been proposed. The first, more traditional plan is to accumulate 75 minutes of vigorous-intensity exercise (i.e., ≥75% of maximal heart rate) over 3 days per week. The second is to accumulate 150 minutes of moderate-intensity exercise (i.e., 50%–75% of maximal heart rate) over at least 3 days per week in at least 10-minute increments. Exercise trials conducted in cancer survivors have generally involved the more traditional vigorous exercise guideline and have reported that QoL improvements may be incurred if strength and cardiovascular adaptations are realized.[3] Research is needed to explore whether one exercise guideline is superior to the other for a given cancer group at a given time point in the cancer trajectory for a given outcome. However, without confirmatory research evidence, it is reasonable to expect that both exercise routines will produce similar health benefits and outcomes. An important consideration is to develop exercise programs that are tolerable; thus the moderate-exercise routines may be more easily adopted by survivors.

PHYSICAL ACTIVITY MOTIVATION AND BEHAVIOR CHANGE IN CANCER SURVIVORS

It is important to understand the determinants of PA in the cancer population to develop interventions that promote PA after diagnosis. In this section, we review the research on PA prevalence, determinants, barriers and motives, and preferences, as well as behavior change interventions.

PA PREVALENCE

An important step in encouraging PA is to determine the extent to which cancer survivors are following the PA recommendations. Thus far, research exploring the prevalence of PA in cancer survivors has generally examined whether or not cancer survivors are meeting PA guidelines. Unfortunately, results based on studies from North America have demonstrated that up to 70% of cancer survivors are not sufficiently active.[51,52] Courneya et al.[53] found that in a population-based study in Canada, fewer than 22% of individuals were physically active. The lowest rates of PA were reported in females with colorectal cancer (i.e., 13.8%), breast cancer (i.e., 16.6%), melanoma (i.e., 19.1%), and male colorectal cancer (i.e., 20.1%). Similarly, Blanchard et al.[51] found that in a sample of individuals in America that surveyed six

cancer groups, it was found that a majority were not meeting the PA recommendations (i.e., 52.7% to 70.4%). Specifically, only 37.1% of breast, 43.2% of prostate, 35.0% of colorectal, 36.0% of bladder, 29.6% of uterine, and 47.3% of melanoma cancer survivors were meeting the PA recommendations. PA levels are below those determined from the general population, among whom 47.8% were meeting recommendations.[54] Finally, Coups et al.[55] reported that among a sample of lung cancer survivors, fewer than 30% met PA recommendations. Taken together, results from previously mentioned studies demonstrate that a substantial proportion of cancer survivors are not meeting PA guidelines, and thus are not sufficiently active to obtain health benefits.

These results are not all that surprising in that PA levels significantly decrease during treatment and do not return to prediagnosis levels following treatment.[56,57] This pattern has been consistent across various cancer groups.[58] Irwin et al.[59] examined PA levels in women with stage 0–IIIA breast cancer. Time spent being physically active decreased by about 2 hours/wk from prediagnosis to 3 years post diagnosis. Furthermore, being older and having a higher BMI were associated with greater levels of physical inactivity. Vallance and colleagues[58] also reported significant declines in exercise in non-Hodgkin's lymphoma survivors from prediagnosis to post diagnosis. Specifically, 33.8% of non-Hodgkin's lymphoma survivors were meeting PA guidelines; however, this decreased to 6.5% and 23.7% while survivors were on and off treatment, respectively. Finally, as in the general population, it is likely that cancer survivors overestimate their PA levels. Thus, PA prevalence rates for cancer survivors may actually be lower than reported.[58]

PA DETERMINANTS

Exercise adherence in cancer is complex. Exploring factors that influence PA and exercise behavior is essential for the successful development of effective behavior programs and interventions designed to increase PA and exercise behavior. Research has generally adopted theoretical models to guide the exploration into PA behavior in cancer survivors. Although we acknowledge the importance of theory-driven research, it is beyond the scope of this chapter to discuss all of the major social-cognitive theoretical models that have been used to study determinants of PA and exercise behavior in cancer survivors. Here, we provide a brief review of the theory of planned behavior (TPB),[60] one of the more common theories examined in PA and cancer survivorship research.[6]

The TPB is designed to explain volitional behavior and has been well studied and validated in exercise research.[61] TPB proposes that intention is a central determinant of actual behavior. This theory has three main constructs (i.e., attitude, subjective norm, and perceived behavioral control [PBC]) that influence an individual's intention to perform. Attitude represents the positive or negative evaluation of performing a behavior. Subjective norm reflects the perceived social pressure that individuals may feel to engage or not to engage in a behavior. Finally, PBC refers to an individual's perceptions of his or her ability (i.e., ease or difficulty) to perform a behavior. Within TPB, PBC is assumed to influence behavior directly or indirectly through intention. The constructs in the theory have been reconceptualized into a two-component model that divides attitudes into instrumental beliefs (i.e., benefits) and affective (i.e., enjoyment) components, norms into injunctive and descriptive components, and finally, PBC into perceived control and self-efficacy. This reconceptualization is supported by recent research.[62]

The TPB has been used to study PA and exercise behavior in several different cancer groups, such as colorectal,[62] breast,[63,64] lung,[32] and lymphoma cancer.[65] This section will review the research using TPB, as well as medical, demographic, and environmental determinants, to understand PA behavior in cancer survivors. PA determinant research is divided into two main categories: studies using observational designs (i.e., cross-sectional and prospective), which include cancer survivors not exercising and not necessarily trying to exercise; and studies testing interventions (i.e., randomized controlled trials or other intervention designs), which include exercise as part of an intervention study, usually with some behavioral support. The first group of studies can be thought of as "PA participation" studies, and the second group can be thought of as "PA adherence" studies.

DETERMINANTS OF PA PARTICIPATION

In a cross-sectional research study, Courneya et al.[66] used a TPB framework to explore the demographic, medical, and social cognitive correlates/determinants of PA intentions in 399 non-Hodgkin's lymphoma cancer survivors. TPB explained 55% of the response variance in lymphoma survivors' exercise intentions. Affect, PBC, and subjective norm accounted for most of the variance in exercise intentions.

Jones et al.[67] examined the determinants of exercise intention using TPB in 100 primary brain tumor survivors using a cross-sectional survey. The results of the study supported TPB, in that instrumental affective attitudes, subjective norms, and PBC in combination explained 32% of variance in exercise intention. The most important determinants of exercise intention in brain tumor survivors were found to be affective attitude and PBC. Past exercise behavior correlated with the TPB variables, and both medical and demographic variables were inconsistently related to TPB constructs. Male and overweight/obese survivors considered the health benefits of exercise to be more important. Finally, higher exercise behavior over the cancer trajectory was associated with more positive exercise beliefs.

In a population-based cross-sectional study, Stevinson et al.[36] explored the determinants of PA in a sample of ovarian cancer survivors. Participants included 359 ovarian cancer survivors who returned a mailed survey. Of those who returned the survey, 31.1% met PA guidelines. Younger age, higher education and income, being employed, lower BMI, absence of arthritis, longer time from diagnosis, earlier disease stage, and disease-free status were variables associated with meeting PA guidelines. TPB variables explained 36% of the variance in PA; however, intention was the only independent correlate.

Karvinen et al.[68] conducted a prospective study examining determinants of exercise behavior in a sample of 397 bladder cancer survivors. Intention, PBC, and planning explained 20.9% of the variance in exercise behavior over 3 months. PBC, affect and, descriptive norms explained 39.1% of the response variance in exercise intention. TPB variables mediate the relationship between adjuvant therapy, invasive disease, age, and exercise. Participants receiving adjuvant therapy and those with more invasive cancer reported less positive affect, which suggests that exercise is less pleasant for this group. Those with more invasive cancer reported lower instrumental attitude, suggesting that they perceived less benefit associated with exercise behavior. PBC was the strongest predictor of exercise behavior in older survivors (over the age of 65); for those who were younger, intention was the strongest predictor. Overall, TPB variables may be effective for promoting exercise behavior in bladder cancer survivors.[68]

DETERMINANTS OF PA ADHERENCE

In a single-arm prospective pilot study, Peddle et al.[69] examined demographic, medical, and social-cognitive determinants of adherence to a presurgical training intervention in 19 lung cancer survivors. The rate of adherence was 73%. PBC and subjective norms of the TPB correlated with exercise adherence. Survivors with greater than 80% adherence reported significantly higher PBC when compared with survivors with less than 80% adherence. Better adherence was seen in male than in female survivors. Coups et al.[55] reported that lung cancer survivors who reported a greater number of surgical complications engaged in less leisurely walking. Lung cancer survivors with lower reported QoL were found to have lower PA levels.

Courneya et al.[62] examined predictors of exercise adherence in 68 colorectal cancer survivors randomized to a home-based exercise intervention as part of the Colorectal Cancer and Home-Based Physical Exercise (CAN-HOPE) trial. The rate of adherence was 76%. The strongest predictors of adherence in the intervention group were exercise stage as determined by the Transtheoretical Model, employment status, treatment protocol, and PBC, which explained 39.6% of the response variance in exercise adherence. Cancer treatment had a significant negative impact on exercise adherence; participants in the exercise group on multimodal (i.e., chemotherapy or radiation) adjuvant therapy had lower adherence rates compared with those receiving a single treatment modality. As a consequence of this finding, Courneya et al.[62] advocate participant stratification based on treatment modality with randomization and additional support for colorectal cancer survivors receiving multimodal cancer treatment.

The START Trial[64] reported predictors of supervised exercise adherence in 160 breast cancer survivors randomized to resistance exercise or aerobic exercise during chemotherapy. Using objective adherence records, adherence was 70.2% and was predicted by location of the trial (i.e., differences across centers), higher cardiovascular fitness, lower body fat, more advanced disease stage, higher education, less depression, and nonsmoking status, but not by the TPB constructs.

Recently, Courneya et al.[65] reported predictors of supervised exercise adherence in 60 lymphoma survivors randomized to exercise as part of the HELP trial. Overall mean adherence to the HELP trial was 77.8% and was predicted by age, past exercise, previous treatment, BMI, and smoking history. Poorer adherence rates were found for those who were younger than 40 years old, insufficiently active at baseline, undergoing radiation therapy, and overweight or obese, and who were smokers; higher exercise adherence was observed in those who were older than 40, previous regular exercisers or completely sedentary, and disease-free stage IV, and who had a normal body weight and lower depression scores, were not receiving radiation therapy, and did not smoke. As in the START trial, TPB motivational variables did not predict exercise adherence. However, motivation tended to play a role in exercise adherence, although this was not statistically significant. Specifically, it was found that those who were extremely motivated had an 85% adherence rate, and those less motivated had a 66% adherence rate. Failure of the motivational variables to predict adherence was likely caused by the ceiling effect, which may be reflective of a motivational bias related to cancer survivors' willingness to participate in exercise studies.[6]

Results from the aforementioned studies demonstrate that demographic, medical, and TPB constructs are important determinants of PA participation and adherence. Developing interventions that focus on survivor demographics and medical and motivational variables that predict PA participation and adherence will be important.

PA AND EXERCISE BARRIERS AND MOTIVES

PA and exercise barriers and motivation research can be divided into two categories: (1) observational studies (i.e., cross-sectional and prospective), and (2) intervention studies (i.e., randomized controlled trials or other intervention designs). The first group of studies can be thought of as factors associated with barriers and motives to "PA participation"; the second group can be thought of as factors associated with barriers and motives to "PA adherence."

Barriers and motives to PA participation

To effectively promote PA and exercise behavior in cancer survivors, it is important to understand unique barriers that they encounter, as well as motives for exercise participation. Courneya and Friedenreich[70,71] reported that the main barriers to exercise participation for breast and colorectal cancer survivors were treatment side effects and symptoms (e.g., pain, nausea, fatigue). Additionally, these survivors reported that their motives for exercising were related to reasons other than fitness (i.e., taking their mind off of cancer and treatment, helping to cope with treatment).

Researchers are continuing to explore cancer survivor exercise barriers and motives with larger trials and in less-studied cancer groups. In a cross-sectional study of non-Hodgkin's lymphoma survivors, it was found that exercise motives were similar to those commonly reported in healthy populations (e.g., improved muscular strength and tone, increased energy, stress relief).[72] However, the most frequently reported exercise barriers were unique to cancer survivors (i.e., nausea, pain, weakness, and feeling ill).

Barriers and motives to PA adherence

In a randomized controlled trial, Courneya et al.[73] examined colorectal cancer survivors in the CAN-HOPE trial weekly to identify exercise barriers. Participants reported 37 different exercise barriers, with the three most common barriers being lack of time/too busy, treatment side effects, and fatigue, which accounted for 45% of the variance in missed exercise; the top 10 barriers included surgical complications, work responsibilities, progressing toward an exercise prescription, getting enough activity without formal exercise, diarrhea, flu,

and nausea, which accounted for almost 80% of all missed exercise weeks.

Courneya et al.[64] examined exercise barriers in breast cancer survivors receiving chemotherapy (i.e., START trial). Overall adherence to a structured exercise program was 70.2%. Breast cancer survivors identified 2090 reasons for missing an exercise session and 36 different exercise barriers, organized into three themes. These themes were (1) disease/treatment-related barriers (i.e., sickness, fatigue, and pain), (2) life-related barriers (e.g., weather, family illness), and (3) motivation (i.e., lack of time and lost interest), which represented 53%, 34%, and 13% of the listed barriers, respectively.

Taken together, cancer survivors share some PA and exercise barriers and motives with the general population; however, they also experience unique barriers and motives related to their cancer experience and treatment.[70,71]

BEHAVIOR CHANGE INTERVENTIONS

To explore the effectiveness of PA and exercise behavior change interventions in a variety of cancer survivor groups, research trials have employed a lifestyle interventional approach whereby diet and PA interventions are used to improve exercise and nutrition behavior in cancer survivors. Demark-Wahnefried et al.[74] explored whether a home-based diet and exercise program supported by telephone counseling and mailed materials would improve lifestyle behaviors and physical functioning among breast and prostate cancer survivors (Project LEAD). Participants were randomized to an interventional group involving exercise and diet information or to an attention control group that received general health information. Physical functioning, PA, and diet were assessed at baseline, 6 months, and 12 months (i.e., 6 months after the intervention). The intervention resulted in significant positive changes in diet at month 12; however, no change in PA was noted. The authors acknowledge that the outcome measure for PA (i.e., CHAMPS) and the low accrual rate, which underpowered the study, were limitations that may have played a role in the null findings for PA. Physical functioning was also in the expected direction and magnitude.

In another randomized controlled trial, Demark-Wahnefried et al.[75] explored the effects through diet and exercise in breast and prostate cancer survivors of information that was delivered exclusively via mailed print material. Outcomes were diet, PA behavior, and QoL. The trial, entitled FRESH START, randomized 306 breast and 237 prostate cancer survivors to a 10-month program of print material that promoted fruit and vegetable consumption, decreased total and saturated fat intake, and exercise, or to a 10-month program of nontargeted mailed materials on diet and exercise. The tailored intervention was matched to participant barriers, cancer coping style, change, and demographic characteristics, such as age, race, and gender. Telephone interviews assessed BMI, diet, PA, and psychosocial/ behavioral indices at baseline and 1 year later. Both groups significantly improved their lifestyle/behaviors. However, greater gains were seen in the FRESH START intervention group in terms of dietary behavior, total weekly PA minutes, fruit and vegetables servings per day, and BMI, but not in QoL.

von Gruenigen et al.[40] examined the feasibility of a lifestyle intervention designed to promote weight loss, improve eating behavior, and increase PA in obese endometrial cancer survivors. Forty-five early-stage endometrial cancer survivors were randomized to a 6-month lifestyle intervention or to usual care. The lifestyle intervention group received both group and individual counseling for 6 months that focused on nutrition and exercise. At 12 months, the lifestyle intervention group lost 3.5 kg, compared with the usual care group, which gained 1.4 kg and showed improvement in PA. The weight loss reported at 12 months was maintained 6 months after completion of the intervention.

Lifestyle interventions have not been examined and the effectiveness of PA and exercise behavior interventions has never been explored in a variety of cancer groups. In an early study, Jones et al.[76] examined the influence of an oncologist's recommendation to exercise on self-reported exercise behavior in newly diagnosed breast cancer survivors. Participants were randomized to one of three groups: (1) an oncologist's exercise recommendation only, (2) an oncologist's exercise recommendation and referral to an exercise specialist, and (3) usual care (i.e., no exercise recommendation). Participants in the groups that received the oncologist exercise recommendation reported significantly more exercise during a 6-month follow-up.

Carmack-Taylor et al.[77] conducted the first trial to evaluate the efficacy of a lifestyle PA intervention for prostate cancer survivors receiving continuous androgen ablation. This trial was designed to improve QoL (i.e., physical and emotional functioning). One hundred thirty-four prostate cancer survivors were randomized to one of three groups: (1) a lifestyle program focusing on self-efficacy and cognitive-behavioral skills needed to adopt and maintain PA, (2) educational support facilitating discussion and expert advice on prostate cancer treatment side effects, or (3) a standard care control group. The standard care group received a one-time mailing of educational materials and information on community services. No improvement in energy expenditure, days engaged in 30 minutes of moderate-intensity activity, social support, or QoL was observed for any condition. At 6 months, those in the lifestyle intervention group used significantly more cognitive and behavioral processes for change, which included more pros for PA, and a trend was noted for higher self-efficacy compared with the other groups. Similar results were found at 12 months; however, the additional pros for PA were no longer significant. Overall, results from the trial suggest that targeting cognitive-behavioral skills will not be sufficient for promoting routine PA behavior in prostate cancer survivors.

The Activity Promotion (ACTION) trial[78] randomized individuals with breast cancer to breast cancer–specific print materials and step pedometers and used PA and QoL as outcomes. Three hundred seventy-seven breast cancer survivors were randomized to one of four groups: (1) a standard public health recommendation for PA, (2) breast cancer–specific PA printed material, (3) a combination of breast cancer–specific print material plus step pedometers, and (4) step pedometers. Outcome assessments were conducted at baseline and post intervention (i.e., 12 weeks) and assessed self-reported moderate to vigorous PA minutes per week, QoL, fatigue, self-reported brisk walking, and objective step counts. Overall, breast cancer–specific print materials and step pedometers were found to increase PA and health-related QoL at 3 months post intervention. Specifically, moderate- to vigorous-intensity PA increased by 40 to 60 minutes/wk in the intervention group compared with control groups, and brisk walking improved by 60 to 90 minutes/wk in the intervention group. Finally, the group that had specific printed material and pedometers had better QoL and fatigue compared with the standard recommendation group.

Research personnel and healthcare providers usually advise behavior changes to improve PA in cancer survivors. Pinto et al.[79] conducted a pilot study to explore the feasibility of a telephone intervention by volunteers. The intervention was based on the Moving Forward Trial[80] and consisted of a 12-week theory-driven phone call intervention designed to encourage the adoption of moderate-intensity PA. Counseling focused on building rapport and motivational readiness, monitoring PA, identifying health concerns, and solving problems of barriers to PA. Participants were encouraged to gradually increase their intensity of PA over a 12-week period to 30+ minutes of PA on most days of the week. QoL, PA, mood, and fatigue outcomes were assessed at baseline and at 12 and 24 weeks. At 12 and 24 weeks, significant improvements in PA, fatigue, QoL, and vigor were found. The results show the feasibility and positive effects on PA and psychological outcomes of a volunteer-supported theory-driven PA intervention for breast cancer survivors.

Behavior change interventions for cancer survivors demonstrate that interventions involving lifestyle, PA, and exercise are effective in improving PA and nutrition behaviors.

FUTURE DIRECTIONS

Research has provided a greater understanding of the positive role of exercise in cancer survivors; however, numerous research questions remain unanswered. To date, most of the research has focused on exploring the effects of exercise on supportive care endpoints,[3] but several fruitful research avenues remain.

Future research should focus on exploring under-studied cancer groups (e.g., bladder, head and neck, liver), endpoints (e.g., sleep quality, pain), and time points (e.g., pretreatment, palliative settings). Research should focus on developing methodologically rigorous randomized controlled trials that include larger populations. Larger randomized controlled trials would allow researchers to explore subgroup analyses that may provide insight into which cancer survivors benefit the most from PA interventions. Most research has focused on aerobic exercise; the benefits of other types of exercise training (e.g., resistance, yoga) should also be explored. Randomized controlled trials designed to compare the benefits of different types of exercise training for cancer survivors, such as resistance versus aerobic versus yoga, and supervised exercise programs versus community-based programs are needed. PA preferences in cancer survivors should be explored more extensively, as it is likely that preferences will influence participant recruitment, adherence, and retention.

For breast and colon cancer survivors, greater prediagnosis and postdiagnosis PA levels are associated with risk reduction in recurrence, cancer-specific mortality, and overall mortality. Future research should examine the influence of prediagnosis and postdiagnosis PA levels on disease endpoints in under-studied cancer groups and should determine the specific exercise dose response (i.e., intensity, frequency, duration) and type of exercise (i.e., aerobic, resistance) required to reduce risk and potentially prevent cancer-specific mortality, recurrence, and mortality in a variety of cancer groups. Finally, randomized controlled trials, such as the CHALLENGE trial, are warranted to determine the causal effects of PA on disease endpoints in cancer survivors. It is also possible that greater PA is a reflection of better health and hence, better survival. In this case, PA could be an indicator of reduced recurrence and mortality, rather than a cause of reduced recurrence and mortality.

Research should explore the use of different models of intervention delivery to find the most cost-effective and beneficial means of improving PA. Traditionally, research staff and healthcare providers are involved in interventions provided through face-to-face interactions or mailings; interventions delivered over the Internet or by volunteers may be more feasible and cost-effective. Future research should explore the benefits of less time-consuming interventions (e.g., action and coping planning) for behavioral changes in cancer survivors, as these interventions have been found to be successful in cardiovascular patients.[81] Additionally, further exploration of factors (e.g., medical, demographic, behavioral variables, environment) that influence exercise behavior in a variety of cancer groups is needed to develop successful cancer-specific behavioral change interventions. Translation of research into ways of putting PA and exercise behavior interventions into practice to ensure that cancer survivors reap the benefits will be important.[3]

made possible by improvements in cancer survival, thereby creating an opportunity to explore the role of lifestyle factors such as PA in improving supportive care (i.e., QoL) and disease endpoints (i.e., overall survival, recurrence, cancer-specific mortality). Although, the most compelling evidence still remains to be discovered in breast cancer survivors, evidence for the benefits of PA is beginning to accumulate for other under-studied cancer groups, such as lymphoma, bladder, prostate, ovarian, and brain. Additionally, several recent large-scale prospective observational studies have been conducted to explore the impact of prediagnosis and postdiagnosis PA levels on disease recurrence, cancer-specific mortality, and overall survival in breast and colorectal cancer survivors. Promising results have been found that demonstrate an inverse relationship between PA and disease endpoints. Randomized controlled trials such as the CHALLENGE trial are warranted to explore the influence of PA programs following cancer diagnosis on recurrence, cancer-specific mortality, and overall survival. PA behavior interventions have been found to be effective for increasing PA and improving outcomes. The effectiveness of these programs will depend largely on cancer survivor motivation. Based on evidence from supportive care research, healthcare professionals should recommend PA to cancer survivors both during and after treatment to improve QoL outcomes and possibly disease endpoints.

SUMMARY

Although a great deal of research in the area of exercise and cancer remains to be conducted, great strides have been made in recent years to understand the beneficial role that PA plays in cancer survivors. These advancements have been

ACKNOWLEDGMENTS

Erin McGowan is supported by a postdoctoral fellowship from the Canadian Cancer Society Research Institute. Kerry Courneya is supported by the Canada Research Chairs Program.

REFERENCES

1. American Cancer Society. *Cancer facts and figures 2009*. Atlanta, GA: American Cancer Society; 2009.
2. Courneya KS, Freidenreich CM. Framework PEACE: an organizational model for examining physical exercise across the cancer experience. *Ann Behav Med*. 2001;23:263–272.
3. Courneya KS. Physical activity and exercise interventions in cancer survivors. In: Holland JC, et al., eds. *Psycho-Oncology*. 2nd ed.New York: Oxford Press; 1998.
4. Bouchard C, Shephard RJ. Physical activity, fitness and health: the model and key concepts. In: Bouchard C, Shephard RJ, Stephens T, eds. *Physical activity, fitness and health: international proceedings and consensus statement*. Champaign, IL: Human Kinetics; 1994:77–78.
5. National Coalition for Cancer Survivorship. *Glossary, vol 2009*. Silver Spring, MD: National Coalition for Cancer Survivorship; 2009.
6. Speed-Andrews AE, Courneya KS. Exercise psychology in cancer survivors. In: Acevedo EO, ed. *Oxford handbook of exercise psychology*. New York: Oxford University Press; in press.
7. Schmitz K, Holtzman J, Courneya K, et al. Controlled physical activity trials in cancer survivors: a systematic review and meta-analysis. *Cancer Epidemiol Biomarkers Prev*. 2005;14:1588–1595.
8. Knols R, Aaronson NK, Uebelhart D, et al. Physical exercise in cancer patients during and

after medical treatment: a systematic review of randomized and controlled clinical trials. *J Clin Oncol*. 2005;23:3830–3842.
9. Conn VS, Hafdahl AR, Porock DC, et al. A meta-analysis of exercise interventions among people treated for cancer. *Support Care Cancer*. 2006;14:699–712.
10. Knobf MT, Musanti R, Dorward J. Exercise and quality of life outcomes in patients with cancer. *Semin Oncol Nurs*. 2007;23:285–296.
11. Schwarz AL. Physical activity. *Semin Oncol Nurs*. 2008;24:164–170.
12. Cramp F, Daniel J. Exercise of the management of cancer-related fatigue in adults. Review. *Cochrane Database Syst Rev*. 2008;16:1–37.
13. Speck RM, Courneya KS, Masse LC, et al. An update of controlled physical activity trials in cancer survivors: a systematic review and meta-analysis. *J Cancer Surv*. 2010; doi: 10.1007/ s11764–009–0110–5.
14. Adamsen L, Quist M, Andersen C, et al. Effect of a multimodal high intensity intervention in cancer patients undergoing chemotherapy: randomised controlled trial. *Br Med J*. 2009;339:b3410.
15. McNeely ML, Campbell KL, Rowe BH, et al. Effects of exercise on breast cancer patients and survivors: a systematic review and meta-analysis. *Can Med Assoc J*. 2006;175:34–41.
16. Markes M, Brockow T, Resch KL. Exercise for women receiving adjuvant therapy for breast

cancer. *Cochrane Database Syst Rev*. 2006;(4): CD005001.
17. Kirshbaum M. A review of the benefits of whole body exercise during and after treatment for breast cancer. *J Clin Nurs*. 2007;6:104–121.
18. Bicego D, Brown K, Ruddick M, et al. Effects of exercise on quality of life in women living with breast cancer: a systematic review. *Breast J*. 2009;15:45–51.
19. Mutrie N, Campbell A, Whyte F, et al. Benefits of supervised group exercise programme for women being treated for early stage breast cancer: pragmatic randomized controlled trial. *Br Med J*. 2007;334:517–523.
20. Courneya KS, Segal RJ, Mackey JR, et al. Effects of aerobic and resistance exercise in breast cancer patients receiving adjuvant chemotherapy: a multicenter randomized controlled trial. *J Clin Oncol*. 2007;25:4396–4404.
21. Daley AJ, Crank H, Saxton JM, et al. Randomized trial of exercise therapy in women treated for breast cancer. *J Clin Oncol*. 2007;25:1713–1721.
22. Courneya K, Friedenreich CM, Arthur K, et al. Physical exercise and quality of life in postsurgical colorectal cancer patients. *Psychol Health Med*. 1999;4:181–187.
23. Courneya K, Friedenreich CM, Quinney HA, et al. A randomized trial of exercise and quality of life in colorectal cancer survivors. *Eur J Cancer Care*. 2003;12:347–357.

24. Peddle CJ, Au HJ, Courneya KS. Associations between exercise, quality of life, and fatigue in colorectal cancer survivors. *Dis Colon Rectum.* 2008;51:1242–1248.

25. Lynch BM, Cerin E, Owen N, et al. Prospective relationships of physical activity with quality of life among colorectal cancer survivors. *J Clin Oncol.* 2008;26:4480–4487.

26. Thorsen L, Courneya KS, Stevinson C, et al. A systematic review of physical activity in prostate cancer survivors: outcomes, prevalence, and determinants. *Support Care Cancer.* 2008;16:987–997.

27. Segal RJ, Reid RD, Courneya KS, et al. Randomized controlled trial of resistance and aerobic training in men receiving radiation therapy for prostate cancer. *J Clin Oncol.* 2009;27:344–351.

28. Galvao DA, Taaffe DR, Spry N, et al. Combined resistance and aerobic exercise program reverses muscle loss in prostate cancer without bone metastases: a randomized control trial. *J Clin Oncol.* 2010;28:340–347.

29. Lui RDKS, Chinapow MJM, Huijgens PC, et al. Physical exercise interventions in haematological cancer patients, feasible to conduct but effectiveness to be established: a systematic literature review. *Cancer Treat Rev.* 2009;35:185–192.

30. Courneya KS, Sellar CM, Stevinson C, et al. Effects of aerobic exercise in physical functioning and quality of life in lymphoma patients. *J Clin Oncol.* 2009;27:1–9.

31. Jones LW, Peddle CJ, Eves ND, et al. Effects of presurgical exercise training on cardiorespiratory fitness among patients undergoing thoracic surgery for lung lesions. *Cancer.* 2007;110:590–598.

32. Peddle CJ, Jones LW, Eves ND, et al. Effects of presurgical exercise training on quality of life in patients undergoing lung resection for suspected malignancy: a pilot study. *Cancer Nurs.* 2009;32:158–165.

33. Jones LW, Eves ND, Mackey JR, et al. Systematic inflammation, cardiorespiratory fitness, and quality of life in patients with advanced non-small cell lung cancer. *J Thorac Oncol.* 2008;3:194–195.

34. Jones LW, Courneya KS, Vallance JK, et al. Association between exercise and quality of life in multiple myeloma cancer survivors. *Support Care Cancer.* 2004;12:780–788.

35. Jones LW, Guill B, Keir ST, et al. Patterns of exercise across the cancer trajectory in brain cancer patients. *Cancer.* 2006;106:2224–2232.

36. Stevinson C, Faught W, Steed H, et al. Associations between physical activity and quality of life in ovarian cancer survivors. *Gynecol Oncol.* 2007;106:244–250.

37. Stevinson C, Tonkin K, Capstick V, et al. A population-based study of the determinants of physical activity in ovarian cancer survivors. *J Phys Activ Health.* 2009;6:339–346.

38. Courneya KS, Karvinen KH, Campbell KL, et al. Associations among exercise, body weight, and quality of life in a population based sample of endometrial cancer survivors. *Gynecol Oncol.* 2005;97:422–430.

39. Karvinen KH, Courneya KS, North S, et al. Associations between exercise and quality of life in bladder cancer survivors: a population based study. *Cancer Epidemiol Biomarkers Prev.* 2007;16:984–990.

40. von Gruenigen VE, Courneya KS, Gibbons HE, et al. Feasibility and effectiveness of a lifestyle intervention program in obese endometrial cancer patients: a randomized trial. *Gynecol Oncol.* 2008;109:19–26.

41. Courneya KS. Physical activity in cancer survivors: a field in motion. *Psychooncology.* 2009;18:337–342.

42. Holmes MD, Chen WY, Feskanich D, et al. Physical activity and survival after breast cancer diagnosis. *JAMA.* 2005;293:2479–2485.

43. Holick CN, Newcomb PA, Trentham-Dietz A. Physical activity and survival after diagnosis of invasive breast cancer. *Cancer Epidemiol Biomarkers Prev.* 2008;17:379–386.

44. Sternfeld B, Weltzien E, Quesenberry CP, et al. Physical activity and risk of recurrence and mortality in breast cancer survivors: findings from the LACE study. *Cancer Epidemiol Biomarkers Prev.* 2009;18:87–95.

45. Meyerhardt JA, Giovannucci EL, Holmes MD, et al. Physical activity and survival after colorectal cancer diagnosis. *J Clin Oncol.* 2006;24:3527–3534.

46. Meyerhardt JA, Heseltine D, Niedzwiecki D, et al. Impact of physical activity on cancer recurrence and survival in patients with stage III colon cancer: findings from CALGB 89803. *J Clin Oncol.* 2006;24:3535–3541.

47. Meyerhardt JA, Giovannucci EL, Ogino S, et al. Physical activity and male colorectal cancer survival. *Arch Intern Med.* 2009;169:2102–2108.

48. Courneya KS, Booth CM, Gill S, et al. The colon health and life-long exercise change trial: a randomized trial of the National Cancer Institute of Canada trials group. *Curr Oncol.* 2008;15:262–270.

49. Doyle C, Kushi L, Byers T, et al. Nutrition and physical activity during and after cancer treatment: an American Cancer Society guide to informed choices. *Cancer.* 2006;56:323–353.

50. U.S. Department of Health and Human Services. *Physical activity guidelines for Americans.* Washington, DC. Available at: www.health.gov/paguidelines; 2008.

51. Blanchard CM, Courneya KS, Stein K. Cancer survivors' adherence to lifestyle behavior recommendations and associations with health related quality of life: results from the American Cancer Society's SCS-II. *J Clin Oncol.* 2008;26:2198–2204.

52. Coups EJ, Ostroff JS. A population based estimate of the prevalence of behavioral risk factors among adult cancer survivors and noncancer controls. *Prev Med.* 2005;40:702–711.

53. Courneya KS, Katzmarzyk PT, Bacon E. Physical activity and obesity in Canadian cancer survivors: population-based estimates from the 2005 Canadian community health survey. *Cancer.* 2008;112:2475–2482.

54. Centers for Disease Control and Prevention. *Behavioral risk factor surveillance system survey data.* Atlanta, GA: U.S. Department of Health and Human Services, Centers for Disease Control and Prevention; 2005.

55. Coups EJ, Park BJ, Feinstein MB, et al. Correlates of physical activity among lung cancer survivors. *Psychooncology.* 2009;18:395–404.

56. Courneya KS, Friedenreich CM. Relationship between exercise pattern across the cancer experience and current quality of life in colorectal cancer survivors. *J Altern Complement Med.* 1997;3:215–226.

57. Courneya KS, Karvinen KH, Vallance JKH, eds. *Exercise motivation and behavior change.* New York: Springer; 2007.

58. Vallance JK, Courneya KS, Jones LW, et al. Differences in quality of life between non-Hodgkin's lymphoma survivors meeting and not meeting public health exercise guidelines. *Psychooncology.* 2005;14:979–991.

59. Irwin ML, McTiernan A, Bernstein L, et al. Physical activity levels among breast cancer survivors. *Med Sci Sports Exerc.* 2004;36:1484–1491.

60. Ajzen I. The theory of planned behavior. *Organ Behav Hum Decis Process.* 1991;50:179–211.

61. Ajzen I. Perceived behavioral control, self-efficacy, locus of control, and the theory of planned behavior. *J Appl Soc Psychol.* 2002;32:665–683.

62. Courneya K, Friedenreich C, Quinney H, et al. Predictors of adherence and contamination in a randomized trial of exercise in colorectal cancer survivors: an application of the theory of planned behavior and the five factor model of personality. *Ann Behav Med.* 2004;24:257–268.

63. Courneya KS, Reid RD, Friedenreich CM, et al. Understanding breast cancer patients' preferences for two types of exercise during chemotherapy in an unblinded randomized controlled trial. *Int J Nutr Phys Activ.* 2008;52:1–9.

64. Courneya KS, Segal RJ, Gelmon K, et al. Predictors of supervised exercise adherence during breast cancer chemotherapy. *Med Sci Sports Exerc.* 2008;40:1180–1187.

65. Courneya KS, Stevinson C, McNeely ML, et al. Predictors of adherence to supervised exercise in lymphoma patients participating in a randomized controlled trial. *Ann Behav Med.* 2010;40:30–39.

66. Courneya KS, Friedenreich CM, Quinney HA, et al. A longitudinal study of exercise barriers in colorectal cancer survivors participating in a randomized controlled trial. *Ann Behav Med.* 2005;29:147–153.

67. Jones LW, Guill B, Keir ST, et al. Using the theory of planned behavior to understand the determinants of exercise intention in patients diagnosed with primary brain cancer. *Psychooncology.* 2007;16:232–240.

68. Karvinen KH, Courneya KS, Plotnikoff RC, et al. A prospective study of the determinants of exercise in bladder cancer survivors using the theory of planned behavior. *Support Care Cancer.* 2009;17:171–179.

69. Peddle CJ, Jones LW, Eves ND, et al. Correlates of adherence to supervised exercise in patients awaiting surgical removal of malignant lung lesions: results of a pilot study. *Oncol Nurs Forum.* 2009;36:287–295.

70. Courneya KS, Friedenreich CM. Utility of the theory of planned behavior for understanding exercise during breast cancer treatment. *Psychooncology.* 1999;8:112–122.

71. Courneya KS, Friedenreich CM. Relationship between exercise during treatment and current quality of life among survivors of breast cancer. *J Psychosoc Oncol.* 1997;15:35–57.

72. Courneya K, Vallance JK, Jones L, et al. Correlates of exercise intentions in non-Hodgkin's lymphoma survivors: an application of the theory of planned behavior. *J Sport Exerc Psychol.* 2005;27:335–349.

73. Courneya KS, Friedenreich CM, Quinney HA, et al. A longitudinal study of exercise barriers in colorectal cancer survivors participating in a randomized controlled trial. *Ann Behav Med.* 2005;29:147–153.

74. Demark-Wahnefried W, Clipp EC, Morey MC, et al. Lifestyle intervention development study to improve physical function in older adults with cancer: outcomes from project lead. *J Clin Oncol.* 2006;24:3465–3473.

75. Demark-Wahnefried W, Clipp EC, Lipkus IM, et al. Main outcomes of the fresh start trial: a sequentially tailored, diet and exercise mailed print intervention among breast and prostate cancer survivors. *J Clin Oncol.* 2007;25:2709–2718.

76. Jones LW, Courneya KS, Fairey AS, et al. Effects of an oncologist's recommendation to exercise on self-reported exercise behavior in newly diagnosed breast cancer survivors: a single-blind, randomized controlled trial. *Ann Behav Med.* 2004;28:105–113.

77. Carmack-Taylor CL, Demoor C, Smith MA, et al. Active for life after cancer: a randomized trial examining a lifestyle physical activity program for prostate cancer survivors. *Psychooncology.* 2006;15:847–862.

78. Vallance JK, Courneya KS, Plotnikoff RC, et al. Randomized controlled trial of the effects of print materials and step pedometers on physical activity and quality of life in breast cancer survivors. *J Clin Oncol.* 2007;25:2352–2359.

79. Pinto BM, Rabin C, Abdow A, et al. A pilot study on disseminating physical activity promotion among cancer survivors: a brief report. *Psychooncology.* 2008;17:517–521.

80. Pinto BM, Frierson GM, Rabin C, et al. Home-based physical activity intervention for breast cancer patients. *J Clin Oncol.* 2005;23:3577–3587.

81. Sniehotta FF, Scholz U, Schwarzer R. Action plans and coping plans for physical exercise: a longitudinal intervention study in cardiac rehabilitation. *Br J Health Psychol.* 2006;11:23–37.

82. Segal RJ, Reid RD, Courneya KS, et al. Resistance exercise in men receiving androgen deprivation therapy for prostate cancer. *J Clin Oncol.* 2003;21:1653–1659.

83. Oliver SJ. *Physiological and psychological effects of progressive resistance training in elderly prostate cancer patients undergoing androgen deprivation therapy: a pilot study.* Bangor, United Kingdom: University of Wales; 2003 Thesis/dissertation.

84. Windsor PM, Nicol KF, Potter J. A randomized, controlled trial of aerobic exercise for treatment-related fatigue in men receiving radical external beam radiotherapy for localized prostate carcinoma. *Cancer.* 2004;101:550–557.

Late effects of chemotherapy and radiation

Wolfgang Dörr

41

Chemotherapy is administered as a systemic treatment in almost all instances, with a risk of early as well as late adverse events in a variety of organs and tissues. In contrast, radiotherapy is a local or regional approach, with organ injury occurring within the irradiated volume only; the latter, however, may have systemic consequences, such as hypertension after irradiation of the kidney. At the cellular level, chemotherapy and radiotherapy have largely similar effects, eventually resulting in proliferative sterilization of cells. At the tissue level, this can result in modulation of a variety of signaling cascades and modification of cellular function and interaction in various cell populations (see the section on pathogenesis of late complications of oncologic treatment). In contrast to the development of early complications, which are characterized by cell depletion as a lead mechanism, the pathogenetic pathways of chronic side effects are more complex. Here, the dominating processes occur in the parenchyma (i.e., the organ-specific compartments), but they also occur in the connective and vascular tissues.[1] Regularly, the immune system (macrophages, mast cells) also contributes to the tissue reaction. Besides the delayed clinical injury of tissues or organs, the induction of second primary tumors must be considered as a late consequence of both radiotherapy and chemotherapy,[2] as discussed in Chapter 44.

In comparison with radiation exposure, much less is known about chronic sequelae of specific classical chemotherapeutic agents—with the exception of a few organ systems, such as heart, kidney, bladder, central nervous system (CNS), and peripheral nerves—and their late toxicity in combination with radiotherapy.[3] To date, almost nothing is known about the late toxicity of novel, biologically targeted drugs such as specific antibodies or tyrosine kinase inhibitors, given alone or in combination with radiotherapy.[3]

In curative radiotherapy, despite optimum conformation of the treatment fields to the tumor and precise treatment planning and application, the target volume includes a substantial amount of normal tissue, for several reasons. First, malignant tumors usually infiltrate microscopically into normal structures, which hence must be included in the high-dose volume. Second, normal tissues within the tumor (e.g., soft tissue, blood vessels) are exposed to the full tumor dose. Third, normal structures in the entrance and exit channels of the radiation beam may be exposed to clinically relevant doses. Therefore, effective curative radiotherapy is unavoidably associated with an (accepted) risk for severe early and late adverse events to achieve adequate tumor cure rates. The optimum radiation dose in curative radiotherapy hence is defined as the dose that is associated with a certain low incidence of sequelae of defined severity in cured patients, in keeping with the concept of "complication-free tumor cure,"[4] as reviewed by Dörr et al.[3] The same statement holds for the optimum aggressiveness of radiochemotherapy or chemotherapy alone. The manifestation of side effects at a tolerated incidence hence is not a priori a consequence of incorrect treatment, but indicates optimum treatment and maximum tumor cure probability.[1]

Late (chronic) side effects of oncologic therapy usually become clinically manifest after symptom-free latent times of months to many years, but early (acute) side effects are observed during or shortly after treatment. The cutoff time between the onset of early and late sequelae has arbitrarily been defined as 90 days after the start of therapy.[1] This classification is based exclusively on the time course of the treatment response (i.e., the time since first diagnosis of specific pathologic changes). Late side effects can be observed in virtually all tissues and organs. With few exceptions they are, in contrast to early effects, irreversible and progressive in nature, with increasing severity over longer follow-up times.[1] Therefore, the longer the survival times and the higher the survival rates of patients (i.e., the better the oncologic therapy), the higher is the number of patients at risk for late reactions. A hazard for the manifestation of a chronic reaction remains throughout the life of the patient.[5] In consequence, lifelong follow-up of oncologic patients must be recommended.

Management of clinically manifest late effects of oncologic therapies (i.e., impairment or loss of organ function) at present is predominantly symptom oriented, independent of the initiating agent, and must follow general medical practice for the specific organ and symptom.

However, late adverse events represent the result of a multi-faceted response with various components and steps.[1,6] Hence, any element of these "damage processing" cascades, including particularly those that occur before the clinical manifestation of the complication, represents a potential target for a specific modification, aimed at postponement or amelioration of the tissue response. Currently, most of the studies into such strategies are purely experimental and have gathered very few clinical data. This chapter will summarize the principles that can be applied to modulate late treatment effects in normal tissues.

PATHOGENESIS OF LATE COMPLICATIONS OF ONCOLOGIC TREATMENT

Exposure to radiation or cytostatic/cytotoxic drugs injures parenchymal cells in any organ. The damage may occur only in the form of cell loss if the damaged cell attempts to divide; however, changes in cell function may occur. Both can result in parenchymal injury. It is also generally accepted that besides the parenchyma of the organs and the organ-specific cells, additional tissue structures and cell populations are involved in the pathogenesis, particularly of late effects, as described later.[1] These include predominantly vascular endothelial cells, mainly in small blood vessels and capillaries, and connective tissue fibroblasts. Moreover, macrophages, irradiated or recruited into the tissue after irradiation, are known to contribute to the pathophysiology of chronic radiation reactions (Fig. 41-1).

Reactive oxygen and nitrogen species and a perpetual cascade of cytokines,[7,8] chronically produced by various cell populations, in combination with chronic hypoxia, seem to play an essential role in the pathogenesis of chronic treatment sequelae.[1,6] The orchestrated response leads to progressive parenchymal damage and eventually to loss of tissue function—in cases of radiotherapy restricted to the irradiated volume. Clinical consequences depend on the proliferative and functional architecture of the organ and the relative or absolute volume of the organ involved.[9,10]

Irradiation causes changes in the function of endothelial cells.[1,11,12] Endothelial cell vacuolization and foci of endothelial detachment are accompanied by transudation of serum components into the vessel wall and subendothelial edema. Moreover, thrombus formation and occlusion of capillaries have been reported.[12] Leukocyte adhesion and infiltration into the vessel wall are regularly observed. Based on all these changes, treatment eventually results in progressive loss of capillaries, associated with a "sausage-like" appearance of the arterioles, blind-ending vessels, and arteriovenous shunts. In arterioles, progressive sclerosis of the tunica media is observed, presumably through direct radiation effects on the cells in the media layer, in combination with endothelial changes. All these changes indicate substantial impairment of local perfusion. An insufficient supply of oxygen (chronic hypoxia) and nutrients results in secondary atrophy of the downstream parenchyma. Telangiectasia, defined as the presence of pathologically dilated capillaries, is observed in all irradiated tissues and organs. The pathogenesis is unclear, but it is again assumed that endothelial cell damage is involved. Loss of smooth muscle cells surrounding larger capillaries and veins may also contribute to the development of telangiectasia. In the intestine, the urinary system, or the CNS,

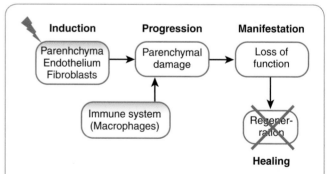

Fig. 41-1 Pathogenesis of late effects of oncologic treatment. Late effects of oncologic treatment are based on a complex interaction of several pathophysiologic processes. These involve changes in organ-specific parenchymal cells, vascular endothelial cells (loss of capillaries), and fibroblasts (differentiation, increased collagen deposition). All these cell populations, as well as macrophages, interact through a variety of signaling molecules. Their orchestrated response leads to progressive parenchymal damage and eventually to impairment or loss of tissue function for radiotherapy within the irradiated volume. Clinical consequences of the functional deficit depend on the architecture of the organ and the volume irradiated. Clinical symptoms, with few exceptions, are irreversible.

telangiectasia can be clinically relevant because of the tendency toward capillary hemorrhage. In the skin, telangiectasia can be a cosmetic problem.

Mammalian tissues display a balance between the number of mitotic fibroblasts and the number of postmitotic fibrocytes. Irradiation causes early differentiation of fibroblasts into fibrocytes, with the consequence of substantially increased collagen synthesis and deposition.[13,14] This also has an impact on organ function and is a major component of radiation-induced fibrosis. This process is substantially influenced by the synthesis and release of transforming growth factor-β (TGF-β) from various cell populations, which further triggers fibroblast differentiation.[14,15] Increased expression of TGF-β at the mRNA and protein level can be observed over long time intervals in various cell populations.[6]

For different organs, the relevance of the individual cell populations mentioned may vary. For example, in the liver, inactivation of parenchymal cells (hepatocytes) is less important than the vascular response to the clinical symptoms (i.e., veno-occlusive disease).[1] Similarly, the response of the kidney to oncologic treatment, at least at higher doses, is dominated by the vascular response. In the lung, type II pneumocytes (slowly turning-over tissue), endothelial cells, and fibroblasts seem to contribute equally to radiation-induced fibrosis.[7] In contrast, late fibrotic changes in the bladder occur secondary to functional impairment, which is based predominantly on urothelial (i.e., parenchymal) and endothelial changes, and does not represent a primary radiation effect.[1,16]

Each of the cell populations involved in a late effect responds specifically to cytotoxic treatment, with specific cell survival parameters. Only the interactive response, in combination with changes in cell function of surviving cells, defines the overall dose response, including tolerance, for the different clinical endpoints. Hence, it appears unlikely that the response can be predicted by cell survival measurements in only one cell population.

CONSEQUENTIAL LATE EFFECTS

Early and late normal tissue effects of oncologic therapies are primarily independent with regard to their pathogenesis and incidence, and in general, conclusions based on the severity of early reactions or on the risk of late effects should not be drawn. However, in particular situations, interactions between acute and chronic reactions can occur within a single organ, resulting in consequential late effects (CLEs).[1,17] This is the case when the early-responding tissue compartment (e.g., epithelium) serves a protective function against mechanical and/or chemical exposure of target structures for late complications (e.g., vasculo-connective tissue). This barrier function is impaired during the acute complication phase as the result of cell depletion and epithelial breakdown. In consequence, secondary trauma, mechanical and/or chemical, can have an impact on the target structures of late sequelae, in addition to direct effects of radiation on these tissue components, which can aggravate the late radiation response.[1,17] Consequential late effects have been demonstrated (Fig. 41-2) for intestine, urinary tract, oral mucosa, and particular skin locations with major mechanical (skin folds) or chemical (transpiration) stress, as well as for lung.[1,17,18] It must be emphasized that

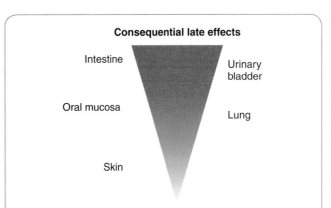

Fig. 41-2 Relevance of consequential late effects. Consequential late effects occur when the early (epithelial) reaction in the same organ is associated with loss of protective barrier function against mechanical and/or chemical stress. In intestine, oral cavity, and particularly exposed skin sites (e.g., folds), chemical and mechanical impacts are similarly important, but in the urinary bladder and the lung, chemical influences are relevant.

in the case of a relevant or even a dominating consequential component of a certain late effect, amelioration of the early response (e.g., by effective supportive care measures) will lead to reduced risk and/or reduced severity of late treatment sequelae in the same organ. This strategy may be followed already during treatment (e.g., at a time during which the patient is seen by the physician at regular, short intervals).

TIME COURSE AND DOCUMENTATION

The latent time for chronic radiation effects, as well as the rate at which the severity of clinical changes progresses, is dependent inversely on the aggressiveness of the treatment protocol, that is, the radiation dose.[1] This is based on several factors: Higher doses cause damage to a greater number of endothelial cells; hence the loss of capillaries eventually resulting in loss of tissue function occurs faster. Similarly, higher doses trigger more fibroblasts into differentiation, with a higher synthesis rate of collagen, and collagen accumulation levels associated with loss of tissue function will be noted earlier. Parenchymal radiation effects contribute to these dose-dependent changes in latent time in an organ-specific manner.

As a consequence of the inverse dose dependence of latent time and the progression rate, more and more treatment responses are seen at lower doses with increasing follow-up times. Hence, iso-effective doses for a defined clinical response decrease with increasing follow-up time. In consequence, the definition of tolerance doses for late effects always requires information about the follow-up time on which the estimate is based.[1]

Two aspects must be considered for the documentation and quantitation of normal tissue complications: the frequency of assessment, and the scoring system used. Because chronic radiation sequelae develop slowly and, more important, are usually irreversible, assessments should be repeated at intervals of several months after the end of radiotherapy to assess the dynamics of their development, and at later time points may be documented at annual intervals. The follow-up intervals may be adjusted to the organs at risk for a specific treatment protocol. It must be emphasized that for some chronic reactions, such as those occurring in the heart or the urinary bladder, the time to clinical manifestation of the reaction, particularly after low radiation doses, can be in the range of decades. Hence, lifelong follow-up of patients must be recommended.

Documentation of (late) normal tissue reactions must be suitable for comparison between investigators, institutions, and studies; hence, standardized classification systems have been established and should be applied. In general, complications are graded from 0 (no response) to 5 (lethality based on the complication). Supportive care must be adjusted to the severity of the changes. In general, grade 1 reactions (mild) do not require any specific therapeutic intervention. Grade 2 responses (moderate/clear) can be treated on an outpatient basis. In contrast, grade 3 effects (severe, pronounced) frequently require hospitalization and intense supportive care. Grade 4 reactions are life threatening and require immediate hospitalization and intense therapeutic interventions.

The most widely used classification systems include the following:

- RTOG/EORTC classification: Jointly developed by the Radiation Therapy and Oncology Group and the European Organisation for Research and Treatment of Cancer[19]
- CTCAE: Common Terminology Criteria for Adverse Events (in its current version, 4.0), developed by the National Cancer Institute (NCI) of the United States[20]
- WHO: World Health Organization classification[21]
- LENT/SOMA system: Late Effects in Normal Tissue/Subjective Objective Management Analytic, which was developed specifically for scoring late sequelae resulting from oncologic treatment[22]

For clinical reports on side effects, the scoring protocol used must be described in detail, particularly if modified versions of the original protocols are introduced. In principle, all these classification systems are comparable, and the scores from one system in many instances can be translated into the scores for another system, yet with exceptions. This translation is definitely precluded if sum scores are calculated, as was suggested initially for LENT/SOMA,[22] for which information on individual symptoms is lost; documentation of individual scores for each item rather than sum scores must be recommended.

LATE EFFECTS IN INDIVIDUAL ORGANS

In this section, the response and tolerance of some clinically important, dose-limiting late complications of radiotherapy will be reported briefly. A short description of radio(chemo)therapy effects in specific tissues and organs, on which this compilation is based, can be found in Dörr.[1] A more extensive characterization of the response of individual organ systems to radio-oncologic therapy is available in Scherer et al.[23] The detailed pathologic background is described in Fajardo et al.[12]

It must generally be assumed that additional chemotherapy aggravates some if not all of the late adverse events, at least those with a strong consequential component. At present, nothing is known about the impact of biologically targeted drugs on late treatment sequelae.

SKIN AND ADNEXAE

Chronic dermal fibrosis becomes clinically manifest as induration. This is based on an increase in collagen content and a reduction in fatty tissue. Usually, the reaction is associated with epithelial atrophy. The development of skin telangiectasia illustrates the progression of vascular injury in the dermis. With modern high-energy X-rays as produced by linear accelerators, in contrast to orthovoltage radiotherapy, the maximum dose is deposited below the surface, for physical reasons; therefore, late damage may occur even without preceding early reactions. In hair follicles, fractionated doses up to 40 Gy still allow hair regrowth within 1 year, which frequently is associated with discoloration. Complications of chemotherapy and/or radiotherapy have recently been summarized by Ulrich et al.[24]

ORAL CAVITY, ESOPHAGUS, AND GASTROINTESTINAL TRACT

Chronic effects of radiotherapy in the oral and esophageal mucosa include mucosal atrophy and ulceration and telangiectasia, with the consequence of greater vulnerability to secondary trauma. Any additional injury in the oral cavity, predominantly extraction of teeth, may secondarily result in infected osteo(radio)necrosis (IORN). In the esophagus, strictures may develop as a late consequence of oncologic treatment, with some consequential effects.

Salivary glands are sensitive to radiation: Even after the first week of therapy, with cumulative doses of 10 Gy, salivation decreases; after cumulative doses >40 Gy to both parotid glands, saliva production virtually ceases. No recovery is usually observed after doses >60 Gy. Volume effects are very pronounced, as the loss of function is restricted to the volume irradiated. Chronic xerostomia has a major impact on the quality of life of patients. It depends not only on reduced production of predominantly serous saliva in the parotid glands, but also on a decrease in mucin produced in the submandibular glands and reduced function of the small salivary glands. The latter usually is not considered in parotid gland sparing approaches to radiotherapy (e.g., by intensity-modulated radiotherapy [IMRT]).

Late effects of radiochemotherapy in the intestine include chronic epithelial atrophy and ulcers, based on an orchestrated response of all intestinal wall components, plus mechanical/chemical stress due to feces and to infection. Epithelial changes can result in chronic malabsorption. Fibrotic changes may result in stenosis and ileus. Frequently, telangiectasias are found; they are most obvious in the rectum and may cause bleeding. It has been demonstrated experimentally, through the inhibition of pancreatic function by somatostatin analogs, that pancreatic enzymes, acting as additional trauma, significantly contribute to manifestations of early effects. Hence, this treatment also reduces late fibrosis, emphasizing the strong consequential component of chronic treatment effects in the gut.

LIVER

Chronic hepatopathy obviously can develop only after partial organ irradiation; otherwise, lethal veno-occlusive disease occurs as an early adverse event. Latent time varies between 6 months and >1 year post irradiation, and progressive fibrotic changes are noted in both centrilobular and periportal areas. These alterations are accompanied by recanalization, or newly formed veins, and regenerative proliferation of hepatocytes and bile ducts.

NERVOUS SYSTEM

The nervous system is less sensitive to radiation injury than are some other late-responding tissues such as lung or kidney. However, damage to this organ (e.g., resulting in necrosis) has severe clinical consequences. The pathobiology is complex, with involvement of the vasculature and myelinated nerves, resulting (in an inversely dose-dependent manner) in white matter necrosis at 6 to 12 months, glial atrophy after >2 years, or late vasculopathy after 1 to 10 or more years.[1,25]

The most important radiation syndromes in the brain develop a few months to several years after therapy. Within the first 6 months, transient demyelination ("somnolence syndrome") or markedly more severe leukoencephalopathy can occur. Typical radiation necrosis can occur within 6 months until even several years after treatment. Histologically, changes within the first year are predominantly seen in the white matter. At later intervals, gray matter is involved, along with more pronounced vascular lesions (telangiectasia, focal hemorrhage). Radionecrosis of the brain with latent times of 1 to 2 years is associated with a mixture of histologic alterations. The brain of children is significantly more sensitive than that of adults. Functional deficits (i.e., cognitive impairment and reduced IQ) can be attributed at least in part to radiotherapy and/or chemotherapy.[10]

Radiation-induced changes in the spinal cord are similar to those in the brain with regard to latency, histopathology, and tolerance dose. Among the "early" effects, Lhermitte's syndrome is frequently observed as demyelination. It usually develops several months after completion of treatment and can last for a few months to longer than a year. It may occur after radiation doses as low as 35 Gy in 2-Gy fractions, when long segments of cord are irradiated. It is important to note that Lhermitte's syndrome is not predictive for the development of myelopathy. Similar to the brain, myelopathy includes two major effects: demyelination and necrosis of the white matter after ≈6 to 18 months, and vasculopathy after 1 to >4 years. With regard to tolerance radiation dose of the spinal cord (as in the brain), dose per fraction is the critical parameter. In contrast, variations in overall treatment time up to 10 to 12 weeks are largely irrelevant in conventional schedules using 1 fraction per day. With longer times or intervals, substantial recovery occurs, and this has important implications for retreatment.[26]

Radiation effects in peripheral nerves, significant for plexus and nerve roots, are probably more common than effects in the spinal cord but are less well documented. No clinical evidence indicates that peripheral nerves are more resistant to radiation than the spinal cord or the brain; in contrast, surrounding fibrosis may secondarily aggravate radiation effects in the nerves. As with all nervous tissues, a dose of 60 Gy in 2-Gy fractions is associated with less than 5% probability of injury, and the probability increases steeply with increasing radiation dose. The brachial plexus is often included in treatments of the axillary and supraclavicular nodes in breast cancer patients. Clinically, brachial plexopathy is characterized by mixed sensory and motor deficits, which develop after a latent period ranging from months to years. The pathobiology is based on vascular degeneration, fibrosis, and demyelination, with consequent loss of nerve fibers.

URINARY TRACT

The kidney is one of the most sensitive late-responding organs. However, late treatment-related injury may become clinically manifest only after several years. The most significant treatment parameters defining the clinical manifestations of radiation effects in the kidney are dose per fraction and exposed volume.

Clinical radiation nephropathy includes proteinuria, hypertension, and impairment in urine concentration. Associated anemia is based on both hemolysis and decreased production of erythropoietin. A mild form of nephropathy, presenting only as sustained proteinuria, may be observed over a period of many years. Parts of one or both kidneys can receive much higher doses without affecting excretory function. However, after partial kidney irradiation, hypertension may develop after a latent period of up to or beyond 10 years. The dose tolerated by the kidney in a scenario of retreatment does not increase with increasing time after oncologic treatment; it even declines because of continuous progression of damage after low doses that do not result in any functional changes. The pathogenesis of radiation nephropathy is complex. Most studies suggest glomerular endothelial injury as the initial event, resulting in glomerular sclerosis and subsequent tubulointerstitial fibrosis. Several experimental studies have shown the importance of the renin-angiotensin system in these processes via upregulation of plasminogen activator inhibitor-1 (PAI-1) and enhanced fibrin deposition.

Late changes in the urinary bladder are associated with a reduction in bladder storage capacity and, in consequence, an increase in micturition frequency. Latent times are inversely dependent on radiation dose and can last 10 years or longer after treatment. Initial late changes are based on progressive urothelial breakdown, ranging from superficial denudation to ulceration and even the formation of fistulas. These mucosal changes are frequently accompanied by urothelial areas of compensatory hyperproliferation, which may represent precancerous lesions with a risk of second cancer. Vascular changes in the bladder wall, with signs of local ischemia, have been reported. These processes progress into secondary fibrosis of the bladder wall. Telangiectasia can result in severe, treatment-refractory hemorrhage. A strong consequential component was demonstrated in experimental and clinical studies.

RESPIRATORY TRACT

The quality of the voice can be impaired after radiation doses >50 Gy, which must be considered in patients who depend on a functional ability to speak in their professional lives.

In the lung, although very early onset of subclinical changes has been described,[8] fibrosis develops slowly over several months to years, usually after a phase of pneumonitis within the irradiated volume. The lung displays a pronounced volume effect. Besides a reduction in irradiated volume, reduced doses per fraction are effective in avoiding severe (clinically manifest) lung reactions. The development of chronic fibrotic radiation pneumopathy follows the general principles described previously. The complexity of the underlying signaling cascades was reviewed by Dörr and Herrmann.[8] Local fibrotic responses must be expected in all patients with early pneumonitis, indicating a strong consequential component of the late reaction.[18]

HEART

At higher doses, morphologic changes can be observed in the heart.[27] The most common type of radiation-induced heart injury is pericarditis, which has a variable degree of pericardial effusion. This complication has a relatively early onset with latent times of 6 to 24 months. It is usually asymptomatic and resolves spontaneously. Cardiomyopathy presents as reduced ventricular ejection or as conduction block; it develops slowly over a 10 to 20 years. Current estimates of doses giving a 50% complication probability consist of approximately 50 Gy in 2-Gy fractions. However, with more recent long-term follow-up studies, an increased risk of cardiovascular disease after periods in clear excess of 10 years has been observed, as reviewed in Schultz-Hector and Trott.[28] The large variation in risk estimates reported in different studies suggests that volume effects are important, but that sensitive substructures are present: The heart auricles and the proximal parts of the coronary arteries seem to be particularly sensitive. Late damage to the myocardium is associated with diffuse interstitial and perivascular fibrosis, loss of cardiomyocytes, and vascular changes. However, the (molecular) pathophysiology of these effects at present remains unclear.

CARTILAGE AND BONE

Growing cartilage (i.e., the epiphyseal plate) is radiosensitive; single doses of 4 to 7 Gy are sufficient to reduce bone growth in children and adolescents; this is more pronounced at an earlier age. In contrast, adult cartilage (e.g., in joints, larynx, trachea), as well as adult bone, is relatively radiation resistant, presumably as the result of constitutive hypoxia. However, late sequelae in these structures, including osteoradionecrosis (ORN), must be considered as an interaction of parenchymal injury with vascular radiation effects. Most frequently, ORN is seen in the mandible and in the bones of the pelvic ring.

SENSE ORGANS

In the eye lens, cataract develops to varying degrees. Latent times are inversely related to dose and range from 6 months to several decades. Tolerance doses usually reported in textbooks are in the range of 4 to 5 Gy for fractionated irradiation, and around 1 to 2 Gy for single-dose exposure. However, recent epidemiologic analyses indicate a significantly lower tolerance.[29] The fractionation effect seems to be pronounced, but no long-term recovery can be expected. Management of cataracts with modern surgical techniques appears to be effective. Yet, secondary treatment-refractory posterior capsular opacification (PCO, secondary cataract) due to proliferation, migration, and myofibroblastic transformation of lens epithelial cells on the posterior capsule ranks as the number one complication following cataract surgery. The incidence of decreased visual acuity induced by PCO is 20% to 40% 2 to 5 years after surgery.[30]

Loss of function of the lacrimal glands and consequent changes in the cornea, depicted as "dry eye" syndrome, are often dose limiting. Even after moderate radiation doses, these can result in chronic corneal ulceration and loss of the eye.

In the ear, doses >30 Gy can result in direct effects on the inner ear, with the consequence of permanent hearing impairment.

Radiation effects on taste acuity involve a multifactorial process, including direct changes (cell loss) to taste buds, xerostomia with reduced cleansing of the taste buds, and changes in smelling ability. Taste impairment is usually observed after doses of around 30 Gy. Generally, changes in individual taste qualities resolve within the first year after treatment; however, a general increase in threshold concentration may be seen and must be considered in accordance with the taste function of patients in their professional lives.

AMELIORATION OF LATE EFFECTS AFTER ONCOLOGIC TREATMENT

Several general strategies may be followed to reduce the incidence and/or severity of late effects of oncologic treatment. With regard to the radiotherapy regimen, a reduction in dose per fraction is effective in most tissues and organs for decreasing the rate of late complications. Moreover, based on the architecture of the organ, changes in the spatial radiation dose distribution, exploiting the "volume effect,"[9] may reduce the risk for clinical manifestations of late complications. Eventually, a compromise in total dose may be considered, but it must be emphasized that recurrent tumors due to insufficient treatment will frequently result in markedly earlier symptoms and even death, compared with late adverse events. With regard to chemotherapy, if possible, drugs may be chosen that exert their major toxicity in tissues not included in the volume exposed to (high doses of) radiation. Moreover, a reduction in cumulative chemotherapy dose may be considered, particularly in patients already presenting with functional impairment in the organs at risk.

SYMPTOMATIC TREATMENT

Late changes to normal tissues (related to symptoms) after oncologic treatment in most cases are similar to impairment of organ function from other causes; hence, symptomatic management must follow general clinical rules. These involve pharmacologic treatment, dietary counseling and supplementation, nutritional support, physical therapies (lymphedema), psychosocial support, and others.[3] The symptomatic approach is not the focus of present considerations. Several management protocols are described in the chapters on individual organ toxicity.

BIOLOGY-BASED PROPHYLACTIC OR THERAPEUTIC APPROACHES

One promising field for the amelioration of adverse events from oncologic treatment involves interventions in "damage processing" events, as illustrated in Figure 41-3.[31,32] In all cell populations involved, the generation of radicals and aggressive reactive oxygen (ROS) and nitrogen species (NOS) by ionizing radiation or chemotherapeutic agents results, directly or indirectly, in DNA damage. In consequence, through multiple steps, activation of transcription factors (e.g., nuclear

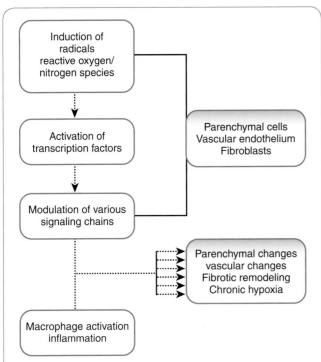

Fig. 41-3 "Damage processing" as a basis for biologically targeted modification of normal tissue complications. Radiation and some classical chemotherapeutic drugs induce free radicals, which then generate reactive oxygen and other reactive molecular species. Indirectly, this results in the activation of nuclear transcription factors, which consequently leads to modulation of various signaling chains. The orchestrated response of all tissue components, plus the contribution of macrophages and inflammatory changes, results in various changes at cellular and tissue levels.

factor [NF]-κB, activator protein 1 [AP-1]) occurs, leading to stimulation or modulation of a variety of signaling cascades (growth factors, interleukins, caspases, adhesion molecules, and others) within the tissue.[31] This can result in a perpetuating process that eventually may become clinically manifest as a late complication.

Here, only those strategies for biological response modification will be reviewed that have already been tested in preclinical investigations in experimental animals or in first clinical trials. It must be stressed that preclinical in vivo testing of these approaches should focus on clinically important endpoints for the individual organ or tissue, and should be performed with clinically relevant treatment protocols, including fractionated irradiation. A vast number of studies on normal tissue protection or mitigation of normal tissue complications performed in vitro in cell or tissue culture systems will not be included.

One major prerequisite for the reasonable application of normal tissue response modifiers is the association with therapeutic gain. This can be achieved by selectivity for normal tissues and hence exclusion of similar effects in tumors, or by a relatively higher effect on normal tissues compared with tumors. It must be emphasized that the tumor effects of any protective/mitigative approach should be thoroughly tested in adequate tumor systems (e.g., xenograft tumors in mice) with relevant fractionation protocols and analyses of appropriate endpoints (e.g., tumor control).

GROWTH FACTOR SIGNALING

Exogenous growth factors have been suggested to modify normal tissue effects of oncologic treatment. With regard to late complications in the lung, conflicting data have emerged from several studies using fibroblast growth factor-2.[33] For prevention or amelioration of late complications in the central nervous system and the kidney, insulin-like growth factor-1 (IGF-1) as an antiapoptotic factor for oligodendrocytes and their progenitor cells, as well as platelet-derived growth factor (PDGF) as a survival factor of progenitor cells, has been suggested.[33]

For late responding tissues, significant, long-lasting stimulation of transforming growth factor-β (TGF-β) has been reported (see earlier). These processes hence may be targeted to modify normal tissue radiation effects.[14] Although there are good indications for the relevance of TGF-β in the development of radiation-induced fibrosis, targeted approaches for inhibition of TGF-β signaling have been studied only recently. One strategy is to inhibit the activation of TGF-β from its latent form, which, at least in the lung, is regulated by a specific membrane receptor, the integrin $\alpha_v\beta_6$. Treatment of irradiated mice with a monoclonal antibody against this integrin prevented fibrosis.[34] Also, prevention of radiation-induced lung injury by an anti-TGF-β type 1 receptor inhibitor was recently demonstrated in a rat model of radiation pneumopathy.[35]

ANTIINFLAMMATORY STRATEGIES

Some preclinical studies addressed the potential for acetylsalicylic acid (ASA) to specifically target biological pathways of normal tissue complications. In an early study in mouse kidney, ASA was administered as an antithrombotic agent.[36] Treatment resulted in a significant delay in the clinical manifestations of renal failure.

Essential fatty acids (EFAs) are known to interact through arachidonic acid metabolism into synthesis of higher concentrations of antiinflammatory end products. In pig skin, oral administration of EFAs resulted in a clear reduction in the severity of early and late adverse events of irradiation.[37] Similarly, in mouse urinary bladder, EFA treatment yielded a reduction in the incidence of late radiation effects (Dörr et al., unpublished data).

ANTIOXIDATIVE APPROACHES

For late effects in normal tissues, long-lasting perpetuation of the production of reactive oxygen and nitrogen species appears to play an essential role. Therefore, antioxidative strategies have been developed to interrupt this chronic oxidative stress cascade, which has been tested for fibrotic changes in skin, using a combination of pentoxifylline (PTX) and tocopherol (vitamin E). Clear regression of clinically manifest fibrotic lesions was observed at 6 months after treatment with PTX and tocopherol in clinical trials.[38,39] These results, however, could not be confirmed in a larger, double-blind, placebo-controlled trial in breast cancer patients,[40] and inconclusive results were obtained in another trial in patients after pelvic radiotherapy.[41]

MODULATION OF ANGIOTENSIN

The renin-angiotensin system appears to be involved in the development of fibrosis, at least in lung and kidney, presumably through interactions with TGF-β signaling. Therefore, angiotensin-converting enzyme (ACE) inhibitors, such as captopril, and antagonists of the angiotensin II type 1 (AT1) and type 2 (AT2) receptor were tested for their potential to mitigate or treat late radiation effects, particularly in kidney and lung. In a rat model of radiation nephropathy after local or total body irradiation (followed by bone marrow transplantation), these drugs were shown to effectively prevent sequelae of irradiation in the kidney.[42] All drugs were also effective in the management of kidney damage. Obviously, different modes of action are relevant at different time periods (i.e., for mitigation and treatment). As a hypothesis,[42] mitigation may be based on suppression of the renin-angiotensin system, but treatment of established nephropathy is based on (additional) blood pressure control.

In two models of radiation injury of the lung (total body irradiation, hemithorax irradiation), inhibition of ACE or AT1 receptors was effective in the prevention of radiation pneumonitis and fibrosis.[43,44]

CONCLUSIONS

The "classical" view of the pathogenesis of normal tissue effects of oncologic therapies has been markedly refined over the last decade, with novel insights into "molecular" pathways at the tissue level involving a variety of cell populations, particularly for late complications. Their interactions, starting right from the time of exposure to cytotoxic agents, have been described to lead through a variety of pathophysiologic cascades during the clinically symptomless latent period—some general, some organ specific—to manifest adverse events after months to many years. These observations have opened innovative avenues for biologically targeted strategies for the prevention or amelioration of normal tissue adverse events. At present, such strategies in most instances are purely experimental, and a vast majority of studies are focusing on early effects; this may valuably assist in the reduction of consequential components of late treatment sequelae. However, some approaches have been developed, and others are emerging, for the specific modulation of late treatment sequelae. These include interventions in more general signaling pathways such as rho/rock-signaling[45] or the administration of adult mesenchymal or hematopoietic stem cells.[46] It is likely that some of these strategies will be transferred through clinical trials and will eventually be available for prevention, amelioration, or management of late effects of chemotherapy and/or radiotherapy.

REFERENCES

1. Dörr W. Pathogenesis of normal-tissue side-effects. In: Joiner M, Van der Kogel AJ, eds. *Basic clinical radiobiology.* 4th ed. London: Hodder Arnold; 2009: 169–190.

2. Trott KR. Second cancers after radiotherapy. In: Joiner M, Van der Kogel AJ, eds. *Basic clinical radiobiology.* 4th ed. London: Hodder Arnold; 2009:339–352.

3. Dörr W, Riesenbeck D, Nieder C. Early and late treatment-induced toxicity. In: Brown JM, Mehta MP, Nieder C, eds. *Multimodal concepts for integration of cytotoxic drugs.* Berlin: Springer; 2006:317–332.

4. Holthusen H. Erfahrungen über die Verträglichkeitsgrenze für Röntgenstrahlung und deren Nutzanwendung zur Verhütung von Schäden. *Strahlenther Onkol.* 1936;57:30–36.

5. Jung H, Beck-Bornholdt HP, Svoboda V, et al. Quantification of late complications after radiation therapy. *Radiother Oncol.* 2001;61:233–246.

6. Bentzen SM. Preventing or reducing late side effects of radiation therapy: radiobiology meets molecular pathology. *Nat Rev Cancer.* 2006;6:702–713.

7. Rubin P, Johnston CJ, Williams JP, et al. A perpetual cascade of cytokines postirradiation leads to pulmonary fibrosis. *Int J Radiat Oncol Biol Phys.* 1995;33:99–109.

8. Dörr W, Herrmann T. Pathogenetic mechanisms of lung fibrosis. In: Nieder C, Milas L, Ang KK, eds. *Biological modification of radiation response.* Berlin-Heidelberg-New York: Springer; 2003:29–36.

9. Dörr W, Van der Kogel AJ. The volume effect in radiotherapy. In: Joiner M, Van der Kogel AJ, eds. *Basic clinical radiobiology.* 4th ed. London: Hodder Arnold; 2009:191–206.

10. Marks LB, Ten Haken RK, Martel MK. Quantitative analysis of normal tissue effects in the clinic. *Int J Radiat Oncol Biol Phys.* 2010;76(3 suppl):S3–S9.

11. Schultz-Hector S. Radiation-induced heart disease: review of experimental data on dose response and pathogenesis. *Int J Radiat Oncol Biol Phys.* 1992;61:149–160.

12. Fajardo LF, Berthrong M, Anderson RE. *Radiation pathology.* New York: Oxford University Press; 2001.

13. Rodemann HP, Bamberg M. Cellular basis of radiation-induced fibrosis. *Radiother Oncol.* 1995;35:83–90.

14. Rodemann H-P. Role of radiation-induced signaling proteins in the response of vascular and connective tissues. In: Nieder C, Milas L, Ang KK, eds. *Modification of radiation response: cytokines, growth factors and other biological targets.* Berlin-Heidelberg-New York: Springer; 2003:29–36.

15. Hakenjos L, Bamberg M, Rodemann HP. TGF-beta1-mediated alterations of rat lung fibroblast differentiation resulting in the radiation-induced fibrotic phenotype. *Int J Radiat Oncol Biol Phys.* 2000;76:503–509.

16. Dörr W, Jaal J, Zips D. Prostate cancer: biological dose considerations and constraints in tele- and brachytherapy. *Strahlenther Onkol.* 2007;183(suppl 2): 14–15.

17. Dörr W, Hendry JH. Consequential late effects in normal tissues. *Radiother Oncol.* 2001;61:223–231.

18. Dörr W, Bertmann S, Herrmann T. Radiation induced lung reactions in breast cancer therapy: modulating factors and consequential effects. *Strahlenther Onkol.* 2005;181:567–573.

19. RTOG. *RTOG/EORTC late radiation morbidity scoring schema.* Available at: http://www.rtog.org/members/toxicity/late.html Accessed April 22, 2010.

20. National Cancer Institute. *Common terminology criteria for adverse events (CTCAE), version 4.0.* Washington, DC: 2009. Available at: http://ctep.cancer.gov/protocolDevelopment/electronic_applications/ctc.htm.

21. World Health Organization. *Handbook for reporting results of cancer treatment.* Geneva, Switzerland: World Health Organization; 1979 WHO Offset Publication 48.

22. Pavy JJ, Denekamp J, Letschert J, et al. EORTC Late Effects Working Group. Late effects toxicity scoring: the SOMA scale. *Radiother Oncol.* 1995;35:11–15.

23. Scherer E, Streffer C, Trott K.-R., eds. *Radiopathology of organs and tissues.* Berlin-Heidelberg-New York: Springer; 1991.

24. Ulrich J, Hartmann JT, Dörr W, et al. Skin toxicity of anti-cancer therapy. *J Dt Dermatol Gesellsch.* 2008;6:959–977.

25. Van der Kogel AJ. Central nervous system radiation injury in small animal models. In: Gutin PH, Leibel SA, Sheline GE, eds. *Radiation injury to the nervous system.* New York: Raven Press; 1991:91–111.

26. Dörr W, Stewart FA. Retreatment tolerance of normal tissues. In: Joiner M, Van der Kogel AJ, eds. *Basic clinical radiobiology.* 4th ed. London: Hodder Arnold; 2009:259–270.

27. Schultz-Hector S. Radiation-induced heart disease: review of experimental data on dose response and pathogenesis. *Int J Radiat Biol.* 1992;61:149–160.

28. Schultz-Hector S, Trott KR. Radiation-induced cardiovascular diseases: is the epidemiologic evidence compatible with the radiobiologic data? *Int J Radiat Oncol Biol Phys.* 2007;67:10–18.

29. Ainsbury EA, Bouffler SD, Dörr W, et al. Radiation cataractogenesis—a review of recent studies. *Radiat Res.* 2009;172:1–9.

30. Awasthi N, Guo S, Wagner BJ. Posterior capsular opacification: a problem reduced but not yet eradicated. *Arch Ophthalmol.* 2009;127:555–562.

31. Dörr W. Biological response modifiers: normal tissues. In: Joiner M, Van der Kogel AJ, eds. *Basic clinical radiobiology.* 4th ed. London: Hodder Arnold; 2009:301–315.

32. Nieder C, Milas L, Ang KK, eds. *Biological modification of radiation response*. Berlin-Heidelberg-New York: Springer; 2003.

33. Nieder C, Andratschke N, Ang KK. Mechanisms and modification of the radiation response of the central nervous system. In: Nieder C, Milas L, Ang KK, eds. *Modification of radiation response: cytokines, growth factors and other biological targets*. Berlin-Heidelberg-New York: Springer; 2003:73–88.

34. Puthawala K, Hadjiangelis N, Jacoby SC, et al. Inhibition of integrin alpha(v)beta6, an activator of latent transforming growth factor-beta, prevents radiation-induced lung fibrosis. *Am J Respir Crit Care Med*. 2008;177:82–90.

35. Anscher MS, Thrasher B, Zgonjanin L, et al. Small molecular inhibitor of transforming growth factor-beta protects against development of radiation-induced lung injury. *Int J Radiat Oncol Biol Phys*. 2008;71:829–837.

36. Verheij M, Stewart FA, Oussoren Y, et al. Amelioration of radiation nephropathy by acetylsalicylic acid. *Int J Radiat Biol*. 1995;67:587–596.

37. Hopewell JW, van den Aardweg GJ, Morris GM, et al. Amelioration of both early and late radiation-induced damage to pig skin by essential fatty acids. *Int J Radiat Oncol Biol Phys*. 1994;30:1119–1125.

38. Delanian S, Balla-Mekias S, Lefaix JL. Striking regression of chronic radiotherapy damage in a clinical trial of combined pentoxifylline and tocopherol. *J Clin Oncol*. 1999;17:3283–3290.

39. Delanian S, Porcher R, Balla-Mekias S, et al. Randomized, placebo-controlled trial of combined pentoxifylline and tocopherol for regression of superficial radiation-induced fibrosis. *J Clin Oncol*. 2003;21:2545–2550.

40. Gothard L, Cornes P, Earl J, et al. Double-blind placebo-controlled randomised trial of vitamin E and pentoxifylline in patients with chronic arm lymphoedema and fibrosis after surgery and radiotherapy for breast cancer. *Radiother Oncol*. 2004;73:133–139.

41. Gothard L, Cornes P, Brooker S, et al. Phase II study of vitamin E and pentoxifylline in patients with late side effects of pelvic radiotherapy. *Radiother Oncol*. 2005;75:334–341.

42. Moulder JE, Fish BL, Cohen EP. Treatment of radiation nephropathy with ACE inhibitors and AII type-1 and type-2 receptor antagonists. *Curr Pharm Des*. 2007;13:1317–1325.

43. Molteni A, Heffelfinger S, Moulder JE, et al. Potential deployment of angiotensin I converting enzyme inhibitors and of angiotensin II type 1 and type 2 receptor blockers in cancer chemotherapy. *Anticancer Agents Med Chem*. 2006;6:451–460.

44. Molteni A, Wolfe LF, Ward WF, et al. Effect of an angiotensin II receptor blocker and two angiotensin converting enzyme inhibitors on transforming growth factor-beta (TGF-beta) and alpha-actomyosin (alpha SMA), important mediators of radiation-induced pneumopathy and lung fibrosis. *Curr Pharm Des*. 2007;13:1307–1316.

45. Gervaz P, Morel P, Vozenin-Brotons MC. Molecular aspects of intestinal radiation-induced fibrosis. *Curr Mol Med*. 2009;9:273–280.

46. Coppes RP, van der Goot A, Lombaert IM. Stem cell therapy to reduce radiation-induced normal tissue damage. *Semin Radiat Oncol*. 2009;19:112–121.

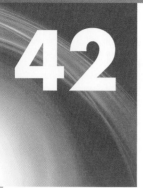

42 Bone health and prevention of treatment-induced osteoporosis in oncology

Ingo J. Diel

Osteooncology specializes in damage to the skeleton caused by tumors and their treatment. By definition, this does not refer to primary bone sarcoma, but rather to metabolic osteopathies such as tumor-induced and tumor treatment–induced osteoporosis and treatment of bone metastases and their impact. The concept of osteooncology should replace wordings such as "bone health in tumor patients" or "bone health and cancer care."[1]

Osteooncology is a typical interdisciplinary field. This means that representatives from different disciplines must share their knowledge to create guidelines, educate colleagues, and inform patients. Requirements for this include broad knowledge about the basic principles of bone metabolism and about the impact on the skeleton of tumor diseases and their treatment, as well as knowledge of diagnostics for osteoporosis and bone metastases and their prophylaxis and treatment.

BONE METABOLISM AND OSTEOPOROSIS

The function of the skeleton is obvious to both laypeople and physicians. It gives the body an inner supportive structure that is indispensable for upright walking and movement. Movement is facilitated by functioning of the muscles, which are attached to individual bones by tendons and exert their force via the joints. Furthermore, the bones protect the central nervous system, house the bone marrow, and serve as a mineral reservoir, in which 1 to 2 kg of calcium is stored (in addition to phosphate and magnesium).

Bone is a highly metabolically active organ. This means that bone is continually built up and broken down, and thus the possibility for change and adaptation is created. In the first two decades of life, the skeleton is built rapidly until a maximum weight is attained, the so-called peak bone mass. Starting in the third decade of life, the skeleton starts to lose mass, at first very slowly (about 1% annually); starting in middle age, loss of mass is more accelerated (Fig. 42-1).

Continuous reconstruction of bone (remodeling) is brought about by osteoclasts and osteoblasts, which are regulated in so-called bone multicellular units (BMUs) by higher-level systems and with millions constantly in action in the body. Osteoclasts and osteoblasts, whose molecular signal pathways have been explained only in recent years, are coupled in their functionality (coupling). Simply put, osteoblasts create substances that can activate and inhibit osteoclasts. For activation, receptor activator for nuclear factor κB ligand (RANKL) is produced and is tied receptor-like to RANKL on the surface of the clasts; this leads to new osteoclasts for recruiting and maturation. To curtail the activity of RANKL, the osteoblast can secrete osteoprotegerin (OPG), which blocks RANKL. But RANKL can also be created by other cells (fibroblasts and T cells, among others), and this makes things a lot more complicated (Fig. 42-2).[2,3]

Substances and hormones that have a stimulating effect on bones (testosterone and estradiol) lead to overproduction of osteoprotegerin and thus inhibit the activity of osteoclasts. On the other hand, this process is crucial for the development of postmenopausal osteoporosis.

In addition to genetic, traumatic, inflammatory, and neoplastic illnesses of the skeleton are numerous metabolic disturbances, of which osteoporosis is the most frequent. By definition, osteoporosis is a skeletal disorder that is characterized by decreased bone stability caused by low bone mass

438

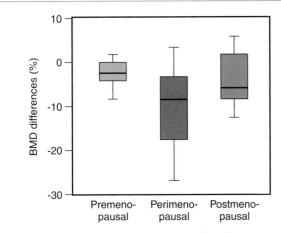

Fig. 42-1 Loss of bone mineral density. *(Data from Rosenbrock H, Seifert-Klauss V, Kaspar S, et al. Changes of biochemical bone markers during the menopausal transition. Clin Chem Lab Med 2002;40:143–151.)*

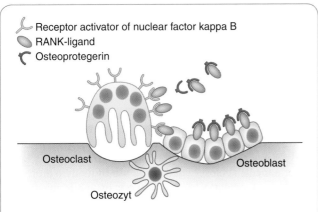

Fig. 42-2 Coupling of osteoblasts and osteoclasts. *(Courtesy Prof. Jakob, Würzburg, Germany.)*

Table 42-1   Risk factors for the development of osteoporosis

- Genetics
- Sex
- Familial tendency
- Nutrition
  - Calcium depletion
  - Phosphate enrichment
  - High alcohol consumption
  - Highly salted nutrition
  - High-level protein (animal)
- Lifestyle
  - Smoking
  - Reduced physical activity
  - Alcohol
- Endocrine factors
  - Estrogen decrease
  - Menstrual cycle disorders
  - Early ovariectomy
  - Body mass index (BMI)
- Medications
  - Corticosteroids
  - Chemotherapies
  - Endocrine therapies (gonadotropin-releasing hormone [GnRH], aromatase inhibitor [AI])
  - Heparin
  - Immunsuppressive therapy
  - Anticonvulsants
  - Thyroid medications

Table 42-2   Primary and secondary osteoporosis

Primary osteoporosis
- Senile osteoporosis
- Postmenopausal osteoporosis

Secondary osteoporosis
- Immobilization
- Medications (corticosteroids, chemotherapy, endocrine therapy)
- Malnutrition and malabsorption
- Infectious diseases, malignant diseases
- Hyperparathyroidism, etc.

and worsening of the microarchitecture with a subsequent related predisposition to fracture (World Health Organization [WHO] Definition, Consensus 2001). Many factors can play a role in the development of the disease (Table 42-1).

At the beginning, the osteoporosis is silent. With progressive development, especially in the vertebrae, fractures may lead to typical deformations, decreased height, immobility, and pain, all of which result in significant limitations in terms of quality of life. Also, the appearance of extravertebral fractures after minor trauma, especially in the hip, is typical and is associated with increased mortality. The risk of disability is present, as is the need for care.

Postmenopausal osteoporosis, similar to senile osteoporosis, which also affects men, is one of the primary osteoporoses. But many diseases and medications can cause an increase in the risk of osteoporosis and fracture (Table 42-2). The best known example is glucocorticoid-induced osteoporosis. This type of osteoporosis is known as secondary osteoporosis. In many older patients, secondary osteoporosis accompanies postmenopausal/senile osteoporosis and speeds up bone resorption.

TUMOR AND TUMOR TREATMENT–INDUCED OSTEOPOROSIS

Treatment certainly is by no means the only thing within the framework of a tumor disease that can lead to osteoporosis. It can be the underlying illness itself. Reduced physical activity, immobility, nausea, malnutrition, and direct effects of the tumor (Table 42-3) can lead to a reduction in bone mass.

Treatment with medication must be viewed as an independent risk factor. Numerous chemotherapeutics can damage the bone directly, even without shutting off gonadal activity.[4]

Table 42-3   Osteoporosis due to cancer and treatment

Cancer
- Reduced body activity, immobilization
- Inappetence, nausea, malnutrition, weight loss
- Cancer systemic effects

Cancer treatment
- Chemotherapy, glucocorticoids
- Secondary hypogonadism in men and women
- Negative effects of analgesia, sedation, hypnotics

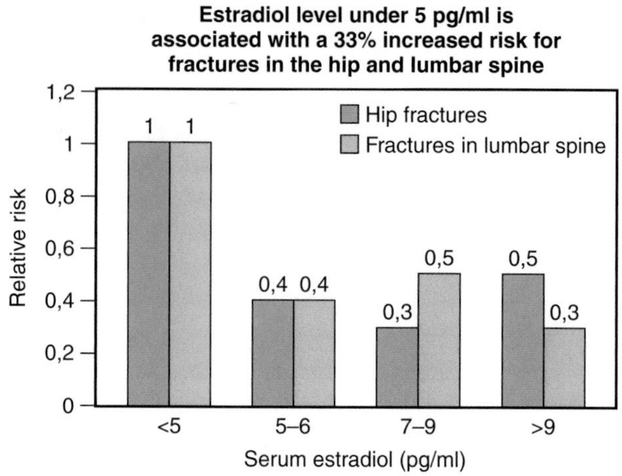

Estradiol level under 5 pg/ml is associated with a 33% increased risk for fractures in the hip and lumbar spine

Fig. 42-3   Low estrogen level increases the risk for osteoporotic fracture. (*Data from Cummings SR, Browner WS, Bauer D et al. Endogenous hormones and the risk of hip and vertebral fractures among older women. N Engl J Med 1998;339:733–738.*)

The best studied is the pathomechanism for methotrexate. In this way, the drug inhibits mineralization, disturbs coupling between bone cells, and reduces osteoblast recruitment. Similar mechanisms are described for doxorubicin, cyclophosphamide, ifosfamide, and docetaxel. Because chemotherapy is usually administered over a short time, direct damage is nevertheless limited.

Bone is much more sustainably damaged by hypogonadism, which is the desired and stated goal of treatment for patients with hormone-sensitive tumors. For breast cancer, three types of endocrine treatment are used: (1) blockade of hormone receptors, (2) elimination of the gonads through oophorectomy or gonadotropin-releasing hormone (GnRH) analogs, and (3) complete estrogen deprivation with aromatase inhibitors in the postmenopausal patient (i.e., a combination of castration and aromatase inhibitors given premenopausally) (Table 42-4).

Cummings et al.,[5] in their study of postmenopausal women, have shown impressively how much fracture risk depends on estrogen level (Fig. 42-3). An estradiol level below 5 pg/ml is associated with a 33% increased risk for hip and vertebral fracture, compared with higher levels.[5] Another study points to the direct dependence of falling bone density levels in the hip and calcaneus on falling estrogen levels in the blood.[6]

In 1999, Kanis et al.,[7] in an impressive study, described the fact that the risk that patients with breast cancer would suffer a fracture was significantly increased, whereby no distinction was made between the impact of treatment and the effects of illness. In nonmetastasized patients, a fivefold increased risk of vertebral fracture was calculated in comparison with the general population; for patients with advanced disease without bone metastases, the risk was increased 20-fold.[7] Many studies have confirmed the data from Kanis and thus emphasize

the influence of chemotherapy and endocrine treatment on rate of fracture in postmenopausal patients and bone density in premenopausal women.[8]

LOSS OF BONE MASS THROUGH TOTAL ESTROGEN DEPRIVATION

Total estrogen deprivation for adjuvant treatment of breast cancer patients is closely tied to the use of modern aromatase inhibitors. Aromatase inhibitors work by inhibiting the last step of conversion of estrone and estradiol from androgen precursors. Evidence of the aromatase gene (CYP19) has been found near the ovaries and in fat tissue, muscles, liver, skin, and other places. The distinction is made between reversible nonsteroidal aromatase inhibitors (anastrozole, letrozole) and irreversible steroidal aromatase inhibitors (exemestane). All three drugs lead to 96% inhibition of aromatase and suppression of the serum estradiol level to <5 pg/ml.[9-11] This enormous, complete estrogen blockade easily explains why osteoporosis and the resulting increase in frequency of fractures is one of the typical side effects of aromatase inhibitor treatment in patients with breast cancer (Fig. 42-4).

ANASTROZOLE

Already the first publication on the use of anastrozole versus tamoxifen in the treatment of postmenopausal women with primary breast cancer (ATAC Trial) has shown an increase in the ratio of women with osteoporosis and fracture (see Fig. 42-4).[12] Analysis of the bone substudy of anastrozole after only 2 years of treatment described a bone mass loss in all patients treated that ranged from negative 4.1% in the lumbar spine to negative 3.9% in the femoral neck, compared with bone growth of 2.2% and 1.2% in patients who received tamoxifen.[13]

After 5 years in a small portion of patients in the substudy (n = 308), it was shown that bone loss in women on anastrozole decreased even farther (≈-7%); however, for women on

Table 42-4   Tumor therapy–induced osteoporosis

Treatment-related hypogonadism

In women
- Bilateral oophorectomy
- Chemotherapy
- Gonadotropin-releasing hormone (GnRH) analogs
- Aromatase inhibitors

In men
- Castration
- Chemotherapy
- GnRH analogs
- Androgen deprivation

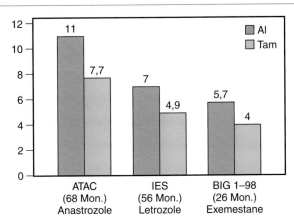

Fig. 42-4 Patients treated with aromatase inhibitors (AIs) are at risk for osteoporosis and fracture. *(Data from Howell A, Cuzick J, Baum M, et al. ATAC Trialists'Group: Results of the ATAC [Arimidex, Tamoxifen Alone or in Combination] trial after completion of 5 years' adjuvant treatment for breast cancer. Lancet 2005;365:60–62; Thuerlimann B, Keshaviah A, Coates AS, et al. A comparison of letrozole and tamoxifen in postmenopausal women with early breast cancer. N Engl J Med 2005;353:2747–2757; Coombes RC, Hall E, Gibson LJ, et al. A randomized trial of exemestane after two to three years of tamoxifen therapy in postmenopausal women with primary breast cancer. N Engl J Med 2004;350:1081–1092; Coombes RC, Kilburn LS, Snowdon CF, et al. Intergroup Exemestane Study. Survival and safety of exemestane versus tamoxifen after 2-3 years' tamoxifen treatment [IES]: a randomized controlled trial. Lancet 2007;369:559–570.)*

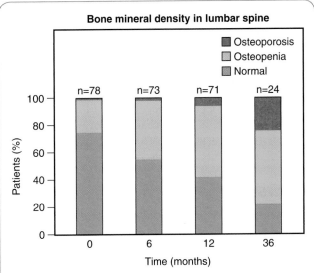

Fig. 42-5 Osteoporosis and osteopenia in premenopausal patients with total estrogen blockade. *(Data from Gnant MFX, Mlineritsch B, Luschin-Ebengreuth G, et al. Zoledronic acid prevents cancer treatment-induced bone loss in premenopausal women receiving adjuvant endocrine therapy for hormone-responsive breast cancer: a report from the Austrian Breast and Colorectal Cancer Study Group. J Clin Oncol 2007;25:820–828.)*

tamoxifen, it increased slightly (1%–2%).[14] However, the authors distinguished the results according to initial bone density values and point out that women with normal levels before treatment did not become osteoporotic. However after 5 years, 17% had osteopenic levels, and of the women with osteopenic starting levels, 5% had osteoporosis. It is interesting to note that the picture changed dramatically after treatment with anastrozole ended. In a reanalysis of patients after 100 months (5 years of treatment, 3–4 years of follow-up), the fracture rate fell below the risk before the start of treatment, even though women on average were 8 to 9 years older, and thus postmenopausally would have had physiologically higher osteoporosis and fracture risks.[15] This could be explained by the punctual use of bisphosphonates and the general change in attitude among patients with regard to maintenance of bone health using counteractive measures (e.g., activity, a calcium-rich diet).

But the havoc that a total estrogen block can wreak on the bones was shown in the work published in March 2007 by Gnant et al.,[16] who reported on premenopausal patients treated with anastrozole or tamoxifen simultaneously with goserelin. What was most impressive was the drop in bone density in the lumbar vertebrae of women in the anastrozole-treated group without bisphosphonate protection (Fig. 42-5). At the beginning of the study, 75% of patients showed normal bone density; however, after 3 years, bone density was only 20%. At the beginning of the study, 23% were osteopenic; after 3 years, 60% were osteopenic. At the end of follow-up, about 24% had osteoporotic values. At the beginning of the study, this number was 2%! T scores in the femoral neck were far

less dramatic; this can be easily explained by slower bone metabolism in the compact bones compared with trabecular metabolism in the lumbar spine.

Also in this study, the bone recovered after discontinuation of treatment after 2 to 3 years.[17] Initially, this does not seem unusual. Still, about 75% of women saw their period start again as a sign of ovarian recovery. To be sure, the authors point out that bone density values did not reach original levels, but this seems logical in that after the last measurement, recovery went up steeply, and the question may just be related to the short follow-up period. Nevertheless, the bone mineral density (BMD) values of women with continued zoledronate treatment significantly improved over baseline values obtained at the beginning of the study. The question remains open about the quality of the microarchitecture of bones that are strong again. Another question is this: What would happen to patient bone density if patients were treated longer with standard treatment? In the previous publication, only two fractures were reported in the group without bisphosphonates, and none were reported among the women on zoledronate.

LETROZOLE

Another study in which letrozole adjuvant was tested against tamoxifen came to the conclusion that the fracture risk in patients treated with letrozole was significantly increased when compared with women who took tamoxifen (see Fig. 42-4).[18]

Because a significant portion of distant recurrences of breast cancer occurred even 5 to 10 years after diagnosis, adjuvant endocrine treatment was suggested for this length of time. The design of the so-called MA17 Study corresponded to this expanded adjuvant design.[19] Patients who had already been treated for 5 years with tamoxifen were treated after randomization for another 5 years with letrozole or placebo. But here it was shown that patients who had a "protective factor" against bone mass loss with tamoxifen suffered bone damage with letrozole. To be sure, the fracture rate did not increase significantly, but clearly more patients were found to have osteoporotic bone density values. It is only a matter of time, especially if patients are treated for longer than 5 years, until more broken bones occur. The subanalysis on bone metabolism showed that in addition to increased bone remodeling in the letrozole-treated group, bone mass losses in the femoral neck of −3.6% and in the lumbar spine of −5.35%, in contrast to tamoxifen-treated patients, produced a slight increase in bone density (respectively, 0.7%).[20]

EXEMESTANE

Initially, it appeared that breast cancer patients who were treated with the third aromatase inhibitor exemestane had no increased risk for osteoporosis or fracture. In the so-called IES Study, all postmenopausal patients were initially pretreated with tamoxifen for 2 to 3 years.[21] This means that they received a relatively good osteoprotective effect from the medication and its known intrinsic estrogen residual activity. But after a longer follow-up period, even for the exemestane-treated patients the known bone disadvantages were evident (see Fig. 42-4). In a comprehensive study published in 2007 by Coleman et al.,[22] an immediate increase in bone remodeling markers was confirmed for all patients treated with the aromatase inhibitor exemestane. Also, bone density dropped, as is typical for patients with total estrogen deprivation, and the fracture risk was significantly increased for patients on exemestane (n = 162; 7%) compared with those on tamoxifen (n = 111; 5%; $P = .003$).

In the adjuvant study with exemestane without previous treatment with tamoxifen (TEAM), the bone-destroying effect after 12 months of treatment appeared to clearly slow down.[23–25] Patients treated with exemestane initially lost bone mass in the first year in a comparable way to those who took anastrozole or letrozole; afterward, the curve was significantly flatter, both for bone density and for resorption markers. The authors are assuming that exemestane because of its steroidal function has another, less damaging impact on bone density and structure. Only one study, which compared all three aromatase inhibitors (e.g., MA-27), can explain whether results will be different over the long term.

TREATMENT OPTIONS FOR TUMOR TREATMENT–INDUCED OSTEOPOROSIS

Briefly, the following is recommended (Table 42-5):

1. Regular physical activity: special training to increase muscle strength, balance, coordination, endurance, and performance
2. Avoiding immobility
3. Fall history and avoidance of fall risks
4. Adequate nutrition, avoidance of a body mass index <20
5. A calcium-rich diet with 1200 to 1500 mg/day as possible supplementation
6. Vitamin D supplementation (400–800 IE) with too little or too seldom sunlight exposure
7. No nicotine, and avoidance of excessive alcohol consumption

Table 42-5 Treatment and prevention of osteoporosis
Healthy lifestyle (sports, nutrition)
Physiotherapy
Avoidance of low body mass index (BMI)
Calcium and vitamin D
Hormones (estrogens, testosterone, calcitonin)
Antiresorptive agents (e.g., raloxifene, bisphosphonates)
Osteoanabolics (e.g., fluorides, anabolics, strontium)

PROPHYLAXIS AND TREATMENT WITH BISPHOSPHONATES

To be sure, many medication options are available for the treatment and prophylaxis of osteoporosis, but with no other drug class are the results as positive with tumor treatment–induced (TTI) osteoporosis as with the bisphosphonates.

The first studies were performed by the working group of Inkeri Eloma from Helsinki.[26,27] Breast cancer patients who were treated with endocrine treatment or with chemotherapy received 1600 mg clodronate orally daily, or placebo. In all examined bone sections, bone density was maintained or improved by clodronate. Powles et al.[28] had similarly positive results in their large prophylaxis study with clodronate that examined bone density. Even though the patient population in relation to tumor treatment was highly heterogeneous, in all measured bone sections, improvements were seen in T scores and clodronate (Fig. 42-6). Delmas et al. showed similarly positive results in patients on chemotherapy with the bisphosphonate risedronate. Risedronate, an aminobisphosphonate that in contrast to clodronate has been approved to treat osteoporosis, dramatically improved bone density when compared with placebo. When treatment ended after 2 years, bone density suddenly dropped (Fig. 42-7).[29]

The two most important studies on avoiding bone mass loss from aromatase inhibitors just came out in early 2007. The first, from Gnant et al.,[16] was already quoted in the previous chapter in a discussion of the dramatic drop in bone density seen in patients with total estrogen blockade. Nevertheless, the purpose of the four-arm study (n = 401) was to examine the protective function of the bisphosphonate zoledronate.

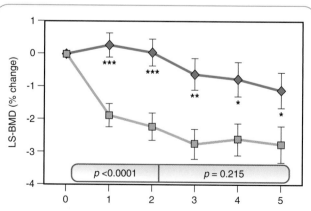

Fig. 42-6 Effects of adjuvant clodronate on cancer treatment–induced bone loss (CTIBL).

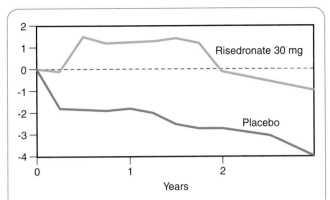

Fig. 42-7 Risedronate improves bone mineral density (BMD) in breast cancer patients. *(Data from Delmas PD, Balena R, Confravreux E, et al. Bisphosphonate risedronate prevents bone loss in women with artificial menopause due to chemotherapy of breast cancer: a double-blind, placebo controlled study. J Clin Oncol 1997;15:955–962.)*

Thus one patient population was respectively treated with anastrozole, and one with tamoxifen, respectively, along with 4 mg zoledronate IV every 6 months (all patients in addition received goserelin). In the figure on BMD results of the lumbar spine and the femoral neck (Fig. 42-8), bone density was completely maintained for longer than 36 months through the addition of a bisphosphonate. Because zoledronate, in contrast to high-dose treatment for bone metastases, was given only in low quantities, no cases of nephrotoxicity or osteonecrosis of the jaw were observed in this study.

Another study in postmenopausal patients treated with letrozole also examined the protective effects of zoledronic acid (4 mg IV every 6 months). In this approach, patients were treated from the start with zoledronate, or were treated only if T score fell below 2.0, or a fracture occurred.[30,31] After a 1-year follow-up, the bone density in those treated from the start was significantly better than in those with delayed treatment (Fig. 42-9). Also, no severe side effects were reported in this study.

Very good results were obtained in a study with oral ibandronate in patients with anastrozole-induced osteopenia.[32] Respectively, 25 women received 150 mg ibandronate orally once a month for 2 years. After this time, the bone density in the active control group increased by up to 3%, whereas in the placebo group over the same time period, a decrease of 3% to 4% was confirmed. At the same time, bone formation markers and bone resorption markers responded analogously.

This short but incomplete overview shows that bisphosphonate treatment, whether oral or IV, older or more recent, amino- or non–amino-BP, is effective, and destruction of bone through hormone deprivation is counteracted.[33-35] What's more, results on the osteoprotective effect in patients with prostate cancer and hormone ablation are comparable.

WHO SHOULD BE TREATED WITH MEDICATION?

The question of who should be treated is unclear. The American Society of Clinical Oncology (ASCO) recommends making prevention dependent on the progression of T scores: below negative 1, monitoring of progress with dual-energy X-ray absorptiometry (DEXA) measurements; below negative 2.5, treatment with medication; between negative 1 and 2.5, treatment based on individual risk factors.[36] When should bone density be measured? In women over 65, in women starting at 60 with familial risk of low body mass index (BMI) and prevalent fracture, and in women who were treated with aromatase inhibitors. Repeat at yearly intervals.

An expert opinion that was published in 2008 in the *Annals of Oncology* may be helpful.[37] According to this opinion, patients treated with aromatase inhibitors and those with a T score better than negative 2 should not be treated with bisphosphonates, but rather should be treated with calcium and vitamin D (in addition to being advised about greater movement

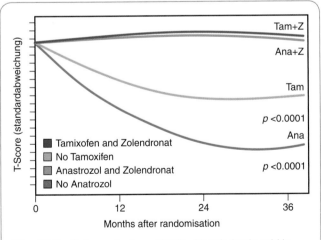

Fig. 42-8 Osteoprotection of BMD with zoledronic acid in patients with total estrogen blockade. *(Data from Gnant MFX, Mlineritsch B, Luschin-Ebengreuth G, et al. Zoledronic acid prevents cancer treatment-induced bone loss in premenopausal women receiving adjuvant endocrine therapy for hormone-responsive breast cancer: a report from the Austrian Breast and Colorectal Cancer Study Group. J Clin Oncol 2007;25:820–828.)*

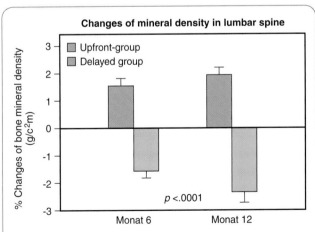

Fig. 42-9 Osteoprotection of postmenopausal breast cancer patients with zoledronic acid (lumbar spine). *(Data from Brufsky A, Harker WG, Beck JT, et al. Zoledronic acid inhibits adjuvant letrozole-induced bone loss in postmenopausal women with early breast cancer. J Clin Oncol 2007;25:829–836.)*

and activity). Patients with a bone density of negative 2 or worse should additionally receive a bisphosphonate that is approved for treatment of osteoporosis. Patients who, in addition to marginal bone density, have additional risk factors (treatment with corticosteroids, age over 65, low BMI, etc.) should also be treated with bisphosphonates (Fig. 42-10).

Also, the Gynecological Oncology Working Group (Arbeitsgemeinschaft für gynäkologische Onkologie [AGO-Breast Cancer]) has integrated treatment of TTI osteoporosis into its new guidelines (Fig. 42-11). In the guidelines, both bisphosphonates and the new RANKL antibodies are recommended for treatment and prophylaxis.

Ultimately, a lot depends on determination of bone density before and during treatment. Because in Germany this measurement is not paid for by statutory health insurance, many patients at risk for osteoporosis are not identified and suffer a fracture. It is important to heighten awareness of oncologists of these long-term complications and to closely monitor high-risk patients.

Given what we now know, we can hope to avoid metastasis through adjuvant use of bisphosphonates in a small but significant proportion of patients, and to avoid osteoporosis in even more women. A moderate risk profile of the drug class and falling treatment prices are good news for tumor patients.

DEVELOPMENT OF ANTIBODIES AGAINST RANKL

Very soon after the discovery of the RANK/RANKL/OPG-System in the mid-90s, the first recombinant proteins that inhibit the signaling pathways were developed. The first clinical trials with OPG showed a significant drop in bone resorption markers, and the remodeling markers were unaffected in postmenopausal women with osteoporosis.[38] This effect occurred quickly and enduringly after subcutaneous injection of OPG.

But first, the development of denosumab (AMG 162), which was shown to be more effective at decreasing the resorption marker at a lower dose, led to the first systematic trials in humans.[39] Denosumab is a fully human monoclonal antibody against RANKL and was generated by immunizing xenomice with human RANKL protein. The immunoglobulin (Ig)G_2 antibody (AMG 162) has an extremely high affinity for human RANKL and does not bind to tumor necrosis factor (TNF) or TNF-related apoptosis inducing ligand (TRAIL). The human antibody denosumab, a member of the TNF family, acts similarly to OPG. That means it interrupts signal transmission to RANK on osteoclasts and to the monocytic precursor cells. Thus fusion of osteoclasts is inhibited, as is the activity of mature multinucleated giant cells (Fig. 42-12). This mechanism of action interrupts both the vicious circle of metastasis-induced bone destruction and the increase in bone resorption in primary and secondary osteoporosis. Currently, more than 20,000 patients have already been treated with denosumab in clinical studies. Most patients have nonmalignant conditions (osteoporosis, rheumatoid arthritis, among others). In oncology, phase I and II trials for the treatment of metastatic bone disease have been completed and published as abstracts. The results of TTI osteoporosis have been published, as have full papers. Falling estrogen and androgen levels led to an increase in RANKL with a simultaneous drop in OPG. The use of RANKL antibodies, such as denosumab, thus seems useful for both tumor entities to avoid bone mass loss caused by treatment-induced hypogonadism.

TREATMENT OF TTI OSTEOPOROSIS WITH DENOSUMAB

Corresponding to the results of phase II and III studies for postmenopausal osteoporosis, the dose for TTI osteoporosis was set at 60 mg every 6 months. Ellis et al.[40] in 2008 published the first results of breast cancer patients with aromatase inhibitor–induced osteopenia. Women with a T score of −1.0 or −2.5 in the lumbar spine or in the femoral neck were treated

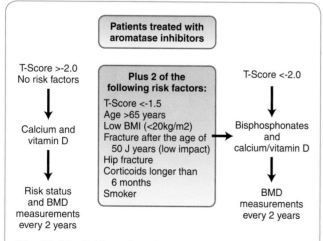

Fig. 42-10 Guidance from Expert Consensus 2008. *(Adapted from Hadji P, Body J-J, Aapro MS, et al. Practical guidance for the management of aromatase inhibitor-associated bone loss. Ann Oncol 2008;19:1407–1416.)*

Prevention and therapy of tumor therapy-induced bone loss	Oxford/AGO LoE/GR		
• Regular BMD-measurement recommended	2b	B	+
• Bisphosphonates	1b	B	+
• RANK-ligand antibody	2b	B	+
• HRT (independent from ER-status of BC)	5	D	−
Some data derived from steroid induced bone loss*:			
• Physical activity	4	C	++
• Calcium and vitamin D supplements	4	C	++
• Avoiding BMI <18	3b	C	++

Fig. 42-11 AGO Guidelines 2009, 2010 (www.ago-online.de). *(Data compiled from AGO guidelines [www.ago-online.de].)*

with denosumab (n = 127) or placebo injections (n = 125) for 2 years. Bone density measurements (DEXA) were performed at the beginning of the study and after 3, 6, 12, and 24 months. After a year, the difference was already 5.5%, to the benefit of women who took denosumab, whose gain after 24 months increased to 7.6% (Figs. 42-13 and 42-14). Almost all women who had received antibodies experienced an improvement in bone density. With the small number of patients in the study, no differences in the frequency of fractures were verifiable.

The study design for men with nonmetastatic prostate cancer was similar to that for women on aromatase inhibitors.[41] A total of 734 patients on androgen deprivation treatment received 60 mg denosumab every 6 months or received placebo injections (n = 734). Bone density in the lumbar spine and in the hip increased after 2 years by 5% to 7%, which is comparable to the breast cancer study findings (Fig. 42-15). Additionally, antibody treatment already after 12 months led to a significant reduction in the cumulative incidence of vertebral fractures (1.9% vs. 0.3%; $P = .004$), which was also true after 2 years (3.3% vs. 1.0%) and 3 years (3.9% vs. 1.5%) (Fig. 42-16). Surely, this good result is due to the large number of patients (6 times as many as in the breast cancer study).

The side effects in both studies with regard to treatment with denosumab were insignificant. Especially in comparison with trials of patients with bone metastases, no cases of osteonecrosis of the jaw occurred. These observations coincide with those from treatment with bisphosphonates. Also no osteonecrosis was observed with the osteoporosis dose that was only one sixth of the tumor dose (with denosumab one twelfth).

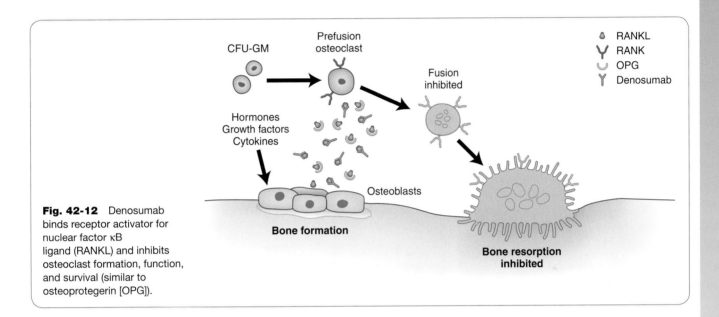

Fig. 42-12 Denosumab binds receptor activator for nuclear factor κB ligand (RANKL) and inhibits osteoclast formation, function, and survival (similar to osteoprotegerin [OPG]).

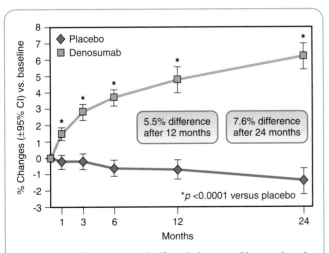

Fig. 42-13 Denosumab significantly increased bone mineral density (BMD) at 12 months in breast cancer. (*Data from Ellis G, Bone HG, Chlebowski R, et al. Randomized trial of denosumab in patients receiving adjuvant aromatase inhibitors for nonmetastatic breast cancer. J Clin Oncol 2008;26:4875–4882.*)

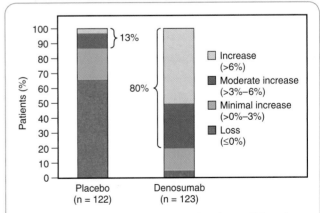

Fig. 42-14 Receptor activator for nuclear factor κB ligand (RANKL) inhibition in the treatment of aromatase inhibitor (AI)-induced bone loss in breast cancer patients; bone mineral density (BMD) in the lumbar spine after 24 months. (*Data from Ellis G, Bone HG, Chlebowski R, et al. Randomized trial of denosumab in patients receiving adjuvant aromatase inhibitors for nonmetastatic breast cancer. J Clin Oncol 2008;26:4875–4882.*)

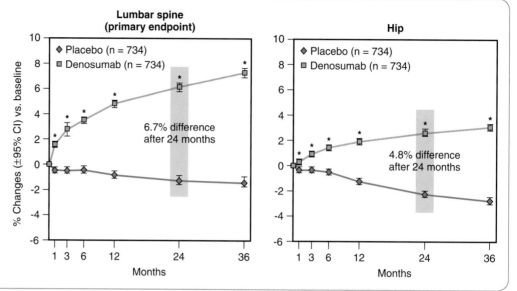

Fig. 42-15 Denosumab significantly increases bone mineral density in prostate cancer patients with androgen deprivation. *(Data from Smith MR, Egerdie B, Hernándes Toriz N, et al. Denosumab in men receiving androgen-deprivation therapy for prostate cancer. N Engl J Med 2009;361:745–755.)*

Denosumab is just as effective in combating TTI osteoporosis as in preventing subsequent fractures, as well as postmenopausal osteoporosis, and in treating both entities with bisphosphonates. This drug, because of its small number of side effects and its simple subcutaneous administration, has the potential to complement treatment with bisphosphonates or even to replace it when used in a pharmacoeconomically equivalent manner.

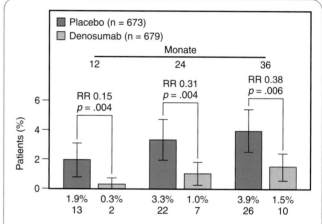

Fig. 42-16 Significantly decreased new vertebral fractures for prostate cancer patients with androgen deprivation. *(Data from Smith MR, Egerdie B, Hernándes Toriz N, et al. Denosumab in men receiving androgen-deprivation therapy for prostate cancer. N Engl J Med 2009;361:745–755.)*

REFERENCES

1. Theriault RL, Biermann S, Brown E, et al. NCCN Task Force report: Bone health and cancer care. *J Natl Compr Canc Netw.* 2006;4(suppl 2):S1–S24.
2. Boyle WJ, Simonet WS, Lacey DL. Osteoclast differentiation and activation. *Nature.* 2003;423:337–342.
3. Boyce BF, Xing L. Biology of RANK, RANKL and osteoprotegerin. *Arthritis Res Ther.* 2007;(suppl 1):1–7.
4. Pfeilschifter J, Diel IJ. Osteoporosis due to cancer treatment: pathophysiology and management. *J Clin Oncol.* 2000;18:1570–1593.
5. Cummings SR, Browner WS, Bauer D, et al. Endogenous hormones and the risk of hip and vertebral fractures among older women. *N Engl J Med.* 1998;339:733–738.
6. Stone K, Bauer DC, Black DM, et al. Hormonal predictors of bone loss in elderly women:

a prospective study. *J Bone Miner Res.* 1998;131:167–174.
7. Kanis J, McCloskey EV, Powles T, et al. A high incidence of vertebral fracture in women with breast cancer. *Br J Cancer.* 1999;79:1179–1181.
8. Chen Z, Maricic M, Bassford TL, et al. Fracture risk among breast cancer survivors: results from the Women's Health Initiative observational study. *Arch Intern Med.* 2005;165:552–558.
9. Shapiro CL, Manola J, Leboff M. Ovarian failure after adjuvant chemotherapy with rapid bone loss in women with early-stage breast cancer. *J Clin Oncol.* 2001;19:3306–3311.
10. Sverrisdottir A, Fornander T, Jacobsson H, et al. Bone mineral density among premenopausal woman with early breast cancer in a randomized trial of adjuvant endocrine therapy. *J Clin Oncol.* 2005;22:3694–3699.

11. Chien AJ, Goss PE. Aromatase inhibitors and bone health in women with breast cancer. *J Clin Oncol.* 2006;24:5305–5312.
12. The ATAC Trialists Group. Anastrozole alone or in combination with tamoxifen versus tamoxifen alone for adjuvant treatment of postmenopausal women with early breast cancer: first results of the ATAC randomised trial. *Lancet.* 2002;359:2131–2139.
13. Baum M, Buzdar A, Cuzick J, et al. Anastrozole alone or in combination with tamoxifen versus tamoxifen alone for adjuvant treatment of postmenopausal women with early-stage breast cancer: results of the ATAC trial efficacy and safety update analyses. *Cancer.* 2003;98:1802–1810.
14. Eastell R, Adams JE, Coleman RE, et al. Effect of anastrozole on bone mineral density: 5-year results from anastrozole, tamoxifen, alone or in combination trial 18233230. *J Clin Oncol.* 2008;26:1051–1058.

15. The Arimidex, Tamoxifen, Alone or in Combination (ATAC) Trialists Group. Effect of anastrozole and tamoxifen as adjuvant treatment for early-stage breast cancer: 100-month analysis of the ATAC trial. *Lancet Oncol.* 2008;9:45–53.

16. Gnant MFX, Mlineritsch B, Luschin-Ebengreuth G, et al. Zoledronic acid prevents cancer treatment-induced bone loss in premenopausal women receiving adjuvant endocrine therapy for hormone-responsive breast cancer: a report from the Austrian Breast and Colorectal Cancer Study Group. *J Clin Oncol.* 2007;25:820–828.

17. Gnant M, Mlineritsch B, Luschin-Ebengreuth G, et al. Adjuvant endocrine therapy plus zoledronic acid in premenopausal women with early breast cancer: 5-year follow-up of the ABCSG-12 bone-mineral density substudy. *Lancet Oncol.* 2008;9:840–849.

18. Thuerlimann B, Keshaviah A, Coates AS, et al. A comparison of letrozole and tamoxifen in postmenopausal women with early breast cancer. *N Engl J Med.* 2005;353:2747–2757.

19. Goss PE, Ingle JM, Martino S, et al. A randomized trial of letrozole in postmenopausal women after 5 years of tamoxifen therapy for early-stage breast cancer. *N Engl J Med.* 2003;349:1793–1802.

20. Goss PE, Ingle JM, Martino S, et al. Randomized trial of letrozole following tamoxifen as extended adjuvant therapy in receptor-positive breast cancer: updated findings from MCIC CTG MA.17. *J Natl Cancer Inst.* 2005;97:1262–1271.

21. Coombes RC, Hall E, Gibson LJ, et al. A randomized trial of exemestane after two to three years of tamoxifen therapy in postmenopausal women with primary breast cancer. *N Engl J Med.* 2004;350:1081–1092.

22. Coleman RE, Banks LM, Girgis SI, et al. Skeletal effects of exemestane on bone-mineral density, bone biomarkers and fracture incidence in postmenopausal women with early breast cancer participating in the Intergroup Exemestane Study (IES): a randomised controlled study. *Lancet Oncol.* 2007;8:119–127.

23. Jones S, Stokoe C, Sborov M, et al. The effect of tamoxifen or exemestane on bone mineral density during the first 2 years of adjuvant treatment of postmenopausal women with early breast cancer. *Clin Breast Cancer.* 2008;8:527–532.

24. Hadji P, Ziller M, Kieback DG, et al. The effect of exemestane or tamoxifen on markers of bone turnover: results of a German sub-study of the tamoxifen exemestane adjuvant multicentre (TEAM) trial. *The Breast.* 2009;18:159–164.

25. Hadji P, Ziller M, Kieback DG, et al. Effects of exemestane and tamoxifen on bone health within the tamoxifen exemestane adjuvant multicentre (TEAM) trial: results of a German, 12-month, prospective, randomised substudy. *Ann Oncol.* 2009;20:1203–1209.

26. Saarto T, Blomqvist C, Välimäki M, et al. Clodronate improves bone mineral density in postmenopausal breast cancer patients treated with adjuvant antioestrogens. *Br J Cancer.* 1997;75:602–605.

27. Saarto T, Blomqvist C, Välimäki M, et al. Chemical castration induced by adjuvant CMF chemotherapy causes rapid bone loss that is reduced by clodronate: a randomized study in premenopausal patients. *J Clin Oncol.* 1997;15:1341–1347.

28. Powles TJ, McCloskey E, Paterson AH, et al. Oral clodronate and reduction in loss of bone mineral density in women with operable breast cancer. *J Natl Cancer Inst.* 1998;90:704–708.

29. Delmas PD, Balena R, Confravreux E, et al. Bisphosphonate risedronate prevents bone loss in women with artificial menopause due to chemotherapy of breast cancer: a double-blind, placebo controlled study. *J Clin Oncol.* 1997;15:955–962.

30. Brufsky A, Harker WG, Beck JT, et al. Zoledronic acid inhibits adjuvant letrozole-induced bone loss in postmenopausal women with early breast cancer. *J Clin Oncol.* 2007;25:829–836.

31. Brufsky A, Bundred N, Coleman R, et al. Integrated analysis of zoledronic acid for prevention of aromatase inhibitor-associated bone loss in postmenopausal women with early breast cancer receiving adjuvant letrozole. *Oncologist.* 2008;13:503–514.

32. Lester JE, Dodwell DE, Purohit OP, et al. Prevention of anastrozole-induced bone loss with monthly oral ibandronate during adjuvant aromatase inhibitor therapy for breast cancer. *Clin Cancer Res.* 2008;14:6336–6342.

33. Bundred N. Aromatase inhibitors and bone health. *Curr Opin Obstet Gynecol.* 2009;21:60–67.

34. Pant S, Shapiro CL. Aromatase inhibitor-associated bone loss. *Drugs.* 2008;18:2591–2600.

35. Camacho PM, Dayal AS, Diaz JI, et al. Prevalence of secondary causes of bone loss among breast cancer patients with osteopenia and osteoporosis. *J Clin Oncol.* 2008;26:5380–5385.

36. Hillner BE, Ingle JN, Chlebowski RT, et al. American Society of Clinical Oncology 2003 update on the role of bisphosphonates and bone health issues in women with breast cancer. *J Clin Oncol.* 2003;21:4042–4057.

37. Hadji P, Body J-J, Aapro MS, et al. Practical guidance for the management of aromatase inhibitor-associated bone loss. *Ann Oncol.* 2008;19:1407–1416.

38. Bekker PJ, Holloway D, Nakanishi A, et al. The effect of a single dose of osteoprotegerin in postmenopausal women. *J Bone Miner Res.* 2001;16:348–360.

39. Bekker PJ, Holloway D, Rasmussen AS, et al. A single-dose placebo-controlled study of AMG 162, a fully human monoclonal antibody to RANKL in postmenopausal women. *J Bone Miner Res.* 2004;19:1059–1066.

40. Ellis G, Bone HG, Chlebowski R, et al. Randomized trial of denosumab in patients receiving adjuvant aromatase inhibitors for nonmetastatic breast cancer. *J Clin Oncol.* 2008;26:4875–4882.

41. Smith MR, Egerdie B, Hernándes Toriz N, et al. Denosumab in men receiving androgen-deprivation therapy for prostate cancer. *N Engl J Med.* 2009;361:745–755.

43 Cognitive function in cancer survivors

Janette Vardy and Haryana Dhillon

With patients enjoying improved survival rates from most common cancers, increasing attention has focused on longer-term side effects of cancer and/or cancer treatment. Cancer survivors have coined the terms "chemobrain" and "chemo-fog" to describe their experience of changes in memory and concentration during chemotherapy. Recent studies suggest that the cancer itself and/or cancer treatments may contribute to these cognitive changes. Fortunately, the cognitive symptoms are generally subtle and often improve after completion of treatment; however, for a subset of survivors, the impairment may be sustained, and even mild impairment may have an impact on quality of life and on a survivor's ability to function both at home and at work.[1,2]

This chapter will be limited to evaluating cognitive function in adult patients with solid tumors, with the exclusion of patients with primary brain tumors or central nervous system (CNS) involvement, and of adults who are survivors of childhood cancer.

INCIDENCE OF COGNITIVE IMPAIRMENT

The incidence of cognitive impairment in cancer survivors is unknown but likely varies with the criteria used to define cognitive impairment, the neuropsychological test battery administered, the method used for analysis, the timing of assessments after treatment, and the treatment regimen received.[3] Early cognitive studies were cross-sectional in design and reported that 15% to 75% of adjuvant breast cancer patients had impairment in neuropsychological performance on formal testing.[4-8] Many of these studies had various methodologic problems, including lack of appropriate control groups and heterogeneity of the patient population. No comparisons were made with pretreatment results; consequently, patients who were functioning at a high level before the time of diagnosis may have had a substantial decline in cognitive function but still scored within the normal range. Conversely, people may have had undiagnosed cognitive impairment before treatment that was then incorrectly attributed to their cancer treatment.

More recent studies that evaluated cognitive function after patients recovered from the acute effects of surgery, but before receipt of chemotherapy, have found that a third of patients have cognitive impairment before receiving chemotherapy.[9-12] The cause of this baseline impairment is not known, but hypotheses include that the cancer itself or surgery and anesthesia may contribute to the impairment, and/or that distress associated with the diagnosis may be involved. One study that briefly evaluated attention in patients before and after surgery did not find a significant decline post surgery.[13] Our own ongoing study in colorectal cancer patients found cognitive impairment in 36% of patients at baseline, with no difference between those assessed post surgery but before chemotherapy, and those assessed before receiving any neoadjuvant treatment (i.e., presurgery).[14] Researchers acknowledge that assessing patients early in their cancer journey is challenging as they are still coming to terms with the diagnosis of a potentially life-threatening illness.[11] Cognitive function might be confounded by a number of psychological variables. As discussed later, no association has been found between anxiety/depression and neuropsychological performance on formal cognitive testing, but there may be distress associated with a recent diagnosis that is not being identified.

Prospective, longitudinal studies have demonstrated that most cancer survivors' cognitive function remains stable or improves with time post chemotherapy, but a subgroup of survivors either experience cognitive decline or fail to demonstrate the expected practice effect (improvement due to patient familiarity with tests) on sequential testing.[15-18] After correcting for practice effect, one study found that 27% of patients had cognitive decline after chemotherapy.[12] A smaller study reported that 61% of adjuvant breast cancer patients had decline post chemotherapy.[15] Cross-sectional studies comparing cognitive function between chemotherapy- and nonchemotherapy-treated cancer populations have generally shown that chemotherapy patients have significantly greater cognitive impairment than those cancer survivors who did not receive chemotherapy.[4-6,19] Results from prospective, longitudinal studies are less consistent. One large study found no significant difference in cognitive function between groups of cancer patients that had received chemotherapy and those that had not; however, there was a trend for cancer patients to show greater decline on multiple measures compared with healthy controls.[18] One study reported decline in 25% of breast cancer patients receiving high-dose chemotherapy compared with 6.7% of healthy controls, but no significant difference was noted between cancer survivors receiving either standard-dose chemotherapy or no chemotherapy and healthy controls.[16] Another study found that breast cancer survivors who had received chemotherapy and those who had received radiotherapy alone had subtle impairment in verbal memory and fluency compared with healthy controls.[20]

The studies just discussed highlight the importance of having appropriate control groups who perform the same assessments as frequently as the group of interest. The ideal would be to have two control groups: a disease-specific group that does not receive chemotherapy (even though individuals are likely to have earlier-stage disease) and a healthy control group.[11] This allows comparison between groups that have and have not received chemotherapy, and between groups that do and do not have cancer, as well as assessment of individual changes in cognitive performance over time with adjustment for practice effect. Because cognitive impairment affects only a subgroup of survivors, it is important to also evaluate cognitive change in individuals over time.

DOSE RESPONSE TO CHEMOTHERAPY

It is likely that the chemotherapy regimen and the dose and duration of chemotherapy used influence the incidence and severity of cognitive impairment.[4,5] A Dutch group reported that patients receiving high-dose chemotherapy had worse cognitive impairment than those receiving standard doses 2 years after chemotherapy,[5] although another study found no statistical difference in cognitive impairment between high-dose and standard-dose chemotherapy 5 years after treatment.[17]

Breast cancer survivors assessed some time after completion of chemotherapy in earlier cognitive studies were likely to have received treatment with cyclophosphamide, methotrexate, and 5-fluorouracil (CMF).[4,6,7] It is possible that this chemotherapy regimen was more toxic than modern breast cancer chemotherapy regimens and may contribute to the lower incidence of cognitive impairment seen in contemporary studies.

DURATION OF COGNITIVE IMPAIRMENT

The duration of cognitive impairment after anticancer treatment appears to be variable. One study reported poorer cognitive function in breast cancer and lymphoma survivors who had received chemotherapy, compared with those who had not, up to 10 years after treatment.[4] Another found impairment in breast cancer survivors who had received chemotherapy at a median of 1.9 years after chemotherapy,[6] but no difference between the chemotherapy and nonchemotherapy survivors at 4 years post treatment.[21] A recent study reported that breast cancer patients who received chemotherapy were more likely to show cognitive decline a month after completing chemotherapy compared with women who received hormonal treatment only, but no difference was noted between the two groups in the percent of women showing cognitive decline 12 months later.[22] It is hoped that the results of ongoing longitudinal studies will help to determine the duration of cognitive impairment.

COGNITIVE DOMAINS AFFECTED

The cognitive domains that are consistently reported as being affected are those of working memory, executive function, information and processing speed, and memory retrieval.[11] The pattern of deficits generally seen in cancer survivors is a frontal subcortical pattern, as distinct from the cortical deficits seen in Alzheimer's dementia, in which orientation, memory storage, and language are the predominant features.[11]

SELF-REPORTED COGNITIVE FUNCTION

A 2007 online survey by the breast cancer advocacy group Hurricane Voices found that up to 96% of respondents (n = 471) reported changes in their thinking, memory, or attention during or after their cancer treatment, with more than 50% reporting that the symptoms were moderate to severe.[23] Although surveys of this type are subject to self-selection bias (i.e., people with the condition are more likely to complete the survey), the results highlight that survivors perceive cognitive impairment associated with cancer treatment as a major concern. A qualitative study involving in-depth interviews with cancer survivors found that many reported cognitive impairment to be the side effect that most affected their daily functioning and quality of life.[24] Survivors reported that the impairment they experienced was frustrating and frightening, and for some resulted in diminished independence.

In published studies, 30% to 70% of breast cancer survivors have self-reported cognitive impairment.[6,25] These studies have consistently failed to find an association between self-reported cognitive impairment and formally tested neuropsychological performance.[4-6,19,26] Self-reported cognitive function is strongly associated with symptoms of anxiety and depression and fatigue, and with poorer quality of life, but none of these variables has been found to be associated with neuropsychological performance.[5,6,18,19]

We studied 420 breast and colorectal cancer survivors who had completed 840 formal cognitive assessments, with concurrent questionnaires evaluating perceived cognitive function, quality of life, fatigue, and anxiety and depression. The relationship between self-reported cognitive impairment and neuropsychological test results was weak (r = 0.15; P = .001), as was the association between neuropsychological performance and each of anxiety and depression, quality of life, and fatigue. However, consistent with the published literature, the association between each of these factors and self-reported cognitive impairment was moderately strong (r = 0.43–0.51; P < .0001).[26]

This consistent apparent disconnect between neuropsychological performance and self-reported cognitive function suggests that tests are measuring different constructs, with fatigue and affective symptoms contributing to self-reported cognitive impairment but not to objective neuropsychological performance. Other possible explanations for the disparity are that the formal tests being used to assess cognitive function may not be sensitive to the types of cognitive impairment that survivors generally complain of, or that the conditions under which testing is performed (i.e., a quiet room with no external distractions) are not those most likely to reproduce their cognitive problems (i.e., the neuropsychological tests lack ecologic validity). Many breast cancer survivors complain of increased difficulty with multitasking, which becomes more noticeable once they try to resume their normal activities, in particular returning to work, especially for those in intellectually demanding occupations. Although these people may still score within the normal range on formal cognitive testing, any decline may be very noticeable to them if they were previously functioning at a higher level. Alternatively, they may have to work harder than before their cancer diagnosis to achieve the same level of neuropsychological performance and consequently report cognitive difficulties despite demonstrating performance within normal limits. It is also possible that people who have had a life-threatening illness attribute "normal" lapses or age-related decline in memory or concentration to the illness, particularly if they are aware that cognitive impairment is a potential side effect of treatment.

It is important for cancer survivors that their cognitive difficulties are acknowledged. Cancer survivors report frustration with the lack of recognition of their symptoms from treating doctors and allied health professionals.[24] Other survivors report that despite acknowledging the existence of symptoms, health professionals are rarely able to suggest strategies to help them cope with these changes.[24]

We recommend that all survivors who self-report cognitive impairment after cancer treatment should be evaluated for fatigue, anxiety, and depression. Appropriate management of these symptoms, if present, may improve the individual's perceived cognitive impairment and quality of life. Formal assessment of cognitive function is becoming more readily available and should be performed in those who continue to experience cognitive difficulties.

MECHANISMS OF COGNITIVE IMPAIRMENT

The cause of cognitive impairment in cancer survivors is unknown, but it is likely multifactorial. Possible mechanisms by which cancer or anticancer treatment might lead to cognitive dysfunction include direct neurotoxic effects (e.g., injury to neurons or surrounding cells, altered neurotransmitter levels)[27]; oxidative damage; indirect effects such as induced hormonal changes; immune dysregulation with release of cytokines; blood clotting in small vessels of the central nervous system (CNS); and anemia leading to reduced delivery of oxygen to the CNS.[11,28]

It can be difficult to establish causation, but chemotherapy may plausibly cause direct neurotoxic damage, with higher concentrations of anticancer drugs (including methotrexate, 5-fluorouracil [5-FU], and cisplatin) crossing the blood-brain barrier than had been recognized previously.[11] Support for a causal relationship between cognitive impairment and chemotherapy can be derived from animal models. With the exception of one study, investigators have consistently shown impairment in some cognitive domains following the administration of chemotherapy. Carmustine, cisplatin, cytosine arabinoside, and 5-FU all have been found to be toxic to the progenitor cells of the CNS and to nondividing progenitor cells, causing increased cell death and suppression of cell division in mice.[29] Han et al.[27] showed that 5-FU causes both acute CNS damage and a syndrome of delayed CNS damage, associated with slower impulse conduction in the auditory system. Other studies found that mice who received methotrexate and 5-FU performed worse on spatial memory, nonspatial memory, and conditional rule learning than mice randomized to receive normal saline,[30] and rats treated with methotrexate showed impairment of spatial memory and decreased performance of a novel object recognition task.[31,32] Our own group has shown that rats treated with single-agent 5-FU and/or oxaliplatin had impairment of spatial memory (measured on the Morris water maze) and worse performance on a novel object recognition task. These effects were seen acutely after chemotherapy and persisted as late effects of the treatment.[33]

Chemotherapy can damage blood vessels and interfere with blood perfusion. It may decrease blood flow to the small vessels of the CNS directly through the by-products of oxidative stress, or by increasing blood coagulation.[34]

Pro-inflammatory cytokines such as interleukin (IL)-1, IL-6, and tumor necrosis factor-alpha (TNF-α) cross the blood-brain barrier and have been associated with cognitive impairment and/or fatigue in other diseases. Support for this cytokine-immunologic prototype is seen in animal models in which "sickness behavior" is found after injection of infectious or inflammatory agents or some cytokines. It is also seen in patients treated with cytokine therapy (e.g., interferon, IL-2), in whom the rate-limiting toxicity often consists of severe fatigue, depressed mood, cognitive disturbance, and flu-like symptoms.[35,36]

Our ongoing studies show that serum levels of several cytokines are elevated in people with breast and colorectal cancer before chemotherapy and, compared with levels in healthy subjects, remain elevated at 2 years[35] (Fig. 43-1). Our preliminary results show a trend for an association between cytokine levels and cognitive function in breast cancer patients (Table 43-1),[8] but our more recent work in colorectal cancer patients before they receive chemotherapy does not support this association.

Women with breast cancer often experience early menopause secondary to chemotherapy. An early abrupt menopause induced by chemotherapy might contribute to cognitive impairment secondary to decreased estrogen, which is thought to be neuroprotective. Most cognitive studies in cancer survivors do not support this hypothesis. Tchen et al.[8] found no correlation between hormone levels or menopausal symptoms and cognitive function in breast cancer patients treated

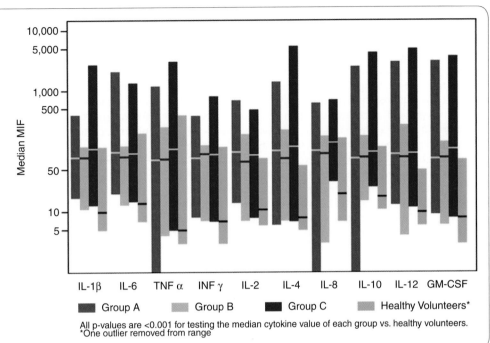

Fig. 43-1 Cytokines MIF (mean immunofluorescence) (in women with breast cancer compared with a noncancer control population.)

All p-values are <0.001 for testing the median cytokine value of each group vs. healthy volunteers.
*One outlier removed from range

Table 43-1 Association of cytokines with neuropsychological performance in breast cancer survivors

Cytokine	Spearman correlation	P value
IL-1b	0.27	.06
IL-2	0.32	.04
IL-4	0.44	.003
IL-6	0.27	.06
IL-8	0.25	.08
IL-10	0.45	.001
IL-12	0.39	.005
IFN-γ	0.34	.015
TNF-α	0.31	.03
GM-CSF	0.32	.25

GM-CSF, Granulocyte-macrophage colony stimulating factor; *IFN,* interferon; *IL,* interleukin; *TNF,* tumor necrosis factor.

with chemotherapy. Our ongoing study in men and women with colorectal cancer shows no association between cognitive function and sex hormone levels. One longitudinal study in breast cancer found a greater decline in multiple measures in women who underwent chemotherapy-induced menopause,[12] but another found no association between cognitive decline and chemotherapy-induced menopause.[1]

Anemia causing fatigue and decreased cerebral oxygenation may contribute to problems with cognitive function during chemotherapy but is unlikely to account for sustained cognitive impairment after completion of treatment when hemoglobin levels have normalized.

We do not know why only a subgroup of patients develop cognitive impairment, but it is possible that some patients have a genetic predisposition to cognitive impairment after cancer treatment. One study suggests greater cognitive impairment after chemotherapy in people with apolipoprotein (APO) ε4 genotypes, which is also associated with changes in magnetic resonance images of the brain.[28] Other genetic polymorphisms might increase the risk of cognitive impairment after cancer treatment in some individuals[28]: Possible mechanisms include decreased effectiveness of the blood-brain barrier due to less efficient efflux pumps or changes in transporters, decreased DNA or neuronal repair mechanisms, changes in levels or efficacy of neurotransmitters, shorter telomere length or less telomerase, and genetic polymorphisms affecting cytokine regulation.[35,37]

IMAGING AND ELECTROPHYSIOLOGIC STUDIES

Magnetic resonance imaging (MRI) and positron emission tomography (PET) are relatively new imaging techniques that allow brain activity to be investigated. Structural and functional brain imaging with MRI and PET supports a causal relationship for chemotherapy and cognitive impairment.[28] Changes seen in the brains of chemotherapy-treated cancer survivors compared with healthy controls include a reduction in the volume of brain structures and changes in white and gray matter.[35,37]

Functional MRI (fMRI) scans of the brain taken while the subject is performing a working memory task allow investigation of patterns of brain activation. On fMRI, chemotherapy-exposed cancer survivors have decreased activation in the mid frontal regions of the brain as the memory task increases in difficulty, compared with those who have not received che-motherapy.[37] Survivors who self-report cognitive function had increased activation in other regions of the frontal and parietal lobes, suggesting that they are able to perform the memory task but have to activate additional regions of the brain to do so (i.e., they are working harder, using more of their brain to complete the memory task).[38] A study that compared fMRI, neuropsychological performance, and self-report cognitive symptoms in a pair of monozygotic twins, one of whom had breast cancer and had received chemotherapy, and the other who did not have breast cancer, found that the twin with breast cancer self-reported more cognitive complaints, although only a minimal difference in neuropsychological performance between the two was noted. The twin with breast cancer had more white matter hyperintensities on MRI and greater areas of brain activation during the working memory task than her nonaffected twin[39] (Fig. 43-2). Silverman and colleagues were able to confirm abnormal activation in the inferior frontal cortex using PET imaging of chemotherapy-treated patients performing a working memory task[38] (Fig. 43-3). This group

also reported that patients who had received chemotherapy and tamoxifen had decreased metabolism in the basal ganglia compared with those who had received chemotherapy alone.

Neurophysiologic studies by Kreukels and colleagues show changes in electroencephalogram (EEG) and event-related potentials in survivors treated with chemotherapy, particu-larly high-dose chemotherapy, compared with those who did not receive chemotherapy.[39] However, it is difficult to inter-pret the clinical or functional significance of these changes, and more research in this area is required.

The findings just described imply that chemotherapy has an effect on cognitive function, in addition to any impact from cancer or from other anticancer treatments.

HORMONE THERAPY

Cognitive studies in breast cancer survivors have commonly included women treated with both chemotherapy and hormonal treatment; consequently, it is difficult to know the relative

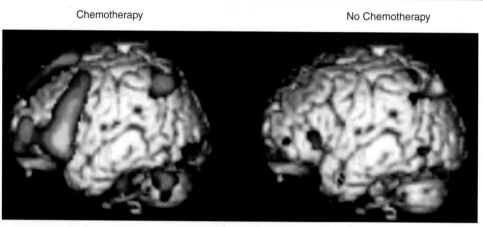

Fig. 43-2 Brain activation patterns in a chemotherapy-treated brain compared with one not exposed to chemotherapy. Abnormal activation can be seen in the inferior frontal cortex in the chemotherapy-treated survivor when performing a working memory task. *(Image used with permission of Dan Silverman, UCLA.)*

Chemotherapy   No Chemotherapy

Abnormal activation in inferior frontal cortex in CTh-treated survivors when performing working memory

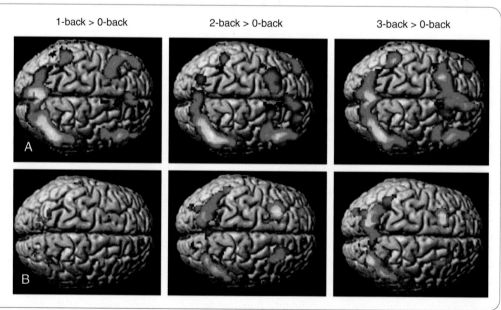

Fig. 43-3 Functional magnetic resonance images of 60-year-old identical twins during a working memory task with incrementally increasing levels of difficulty *(left to right)*. Colored regions denote increased brain activation during working memory relative to a simple vigilance task. **A,** Twin treated with chemotherapy. **B,** Twin who did not receive chemotherapy. Note the expanded spatial extent of cortical activation in the chemotherapy-treated twin. *(Image used with permission of Robert Ferguson, Andrew Saykin, and Tim Ahles, Memorial-Sloan Kettering, NY.)*

1-back > 0-back   2-back > 0-back   3-back > 0-back

contribution of each to objective or self-reported cognitive impairment after treatment. Three studies found no cognitive differences between patients who had received chemotherapy and tamoxifen compared with those who had received chemotherapy alone,[4,6,8] but one study found that patients who had received tamoxifen after chemotherapy had worse cognitive impairment.[40]

Two groups have investigated the impact of anticancer hormonal therapy on women with breast cancer who have not been treated with chemotherapy.[41] A British group reviewed cognitive performance in 94 breast cancer survivors in the Anastrozole, Tamoxifen, Alone or in Combination (ATAC) Trial, in which none of the participants in this substudy were treated with adjuvant chemotherapy, but more than two thirds had received radiotherapy. Women receiving these hormonal agents had specific impairments in verbal memory and information processing speed in comparison with a group of healthy postmenopausal controls.[41] A study by Collins et al.[42] reported that women receiving anticancer hormonal treatment (tamoxifen or anastrozole) were more likely to have experienced cognitive decline 5 to 6 months after starting hormonal treatment. As in Jenkins' study, Collins et al. found that the cognitive domains most affected were processing speed and verbal memory.

Two groups have performed large cognitive studies in postmenopausal women at increased risk of developing breast cancer. One evaluated cognitive performance in the Integrated Biomarker and Imaging Study (IBIS) 2 study, with women randomized to receive either prophylactic anastrozole or placebo. No statistically significant difference in cognitive function was found between the groups on formal neuropsychological testing,[43] but compliance was poor for longitudinal evaluation. Another study found no cognitive difference in women over 65 years who were randomized to receive tamoxifen or raloxifene, but no placebo control arm was included for comparison.[44]

INTERVENTIONS FOR COGNITIVE IMPAIRMENT AFTER CANCER TREATMENT

No interventions have been proven to prevent cognitive impairment due to cancer and/or its treatment, or to treat it once it has developed. Improved cognitive impairment in other disease states has been seen with methylphenidate,[42] the herb ginkgo biloba,[45] and anticholinesterase inhibitors such as donepezil.[46] Physical activity has also been shown to decrease cognitive decline in elderly people with mild cognitive impairment.[47] Randomized, placebo-controlled studies of methylphenidate,[48,49] erythropoietin, ginkgo biloba, and modafinil[50] in cancer survivors have failed to show a convincing improvement in cognitive function. However, several studies in cancer survivors have been underpowered and/or had methodologic limitations. Although evidence for use of these agents outside of a clinical trial is lacking, some warrant further investigation.

Candidate mechanisms for cognitive impairment associated with cancer and/or cancer treatment suggest that other pharmacologic agents that could be considered for future trials are antiinflammatory agents, cytokine inhibitors, antioxidants, and antiplatelet agents. Based on results in noncancer populations and our own work in animal cognitive models, physical activity may be a potential intervention for treating chemotherapy-induced cognitive impairment.

Rehabilitation interventions have been found to be effective in treating people with acquired cognitive impairment who do not have cancer; most programs focus on restoration of a specific cognitive function (e.g., attention) or compensatory training to help patients adapt to the presence of deficits.[51] Several groups, including our own, are investigating some of the following cognitive rehabilitation programs to determine whether they are able to improve perceived or measurable cognitive impairment and quality of life.

Stimulation of attentional systems is hypothesized to facilitate improvement in cognitive capacity.[52-55] Attention process training (APT) is an intervention that endeavors to restore damaged cognitive processes by using repetitive, hierarchical exercises designed to practice increasingly difficult attention tasks.[51,53] It has been used to rehabilitate people with traumatic brain injury and in those with cognitive problems associated with other disease states, such as stroke, psychiatric disorders, and human immunodeficiency virus (HIV).[51] Studies have documented that improvement in attention can also result in enhanced memory and executive function.[51] Patients with mild cognitive impairment, similar to the impairment found in cancer survivors, have derived a benefit from APT programs.[56-58] Studies in other populations have shown improvement in everyday functioning (e.g., driving, returning to work) after completion of APT programs.[59]

Compensatory strategies are designed to help patients adapt to living with impairment and function better through the systematic use of strategies (e.g., regulatory "self-talk," minimizing distractions) and the use of external aids (e.g., checklists, hand computers, diaries).[60] Most strategies target memory deficits, which generally are believed to be less amenable to restoration techniques.[61] Training to use these strategies is believed to require structured practice, adapted to situations in which patients may be experiencing problems.[61] Compensatory strategies have been found to be an effective form of cognitive rehabilitation in other patient groups, particularly for memory deficits.

Computer-based neurocognitive programs aimed at improving memory, attention, concentration, and visuospatial learning have been developed based on models of brain plasticity. These use adaptive exercises that target language or vocal or auditory systems and are designed to improve cognition by improving the speed and accuracy of information processing and by engaging neuromodulatory systems.[62] One such intervention has shown promise in a large, randomized, controlled trial in a healthy elderly population.[63] A small, single-arm, open-label study in breast cancer survivors who had received chemotherapy within the previous 5 years and self-reported cognitive deficits has been reported in abstract form only. Investigators found statistically significant improvement in participant-reported health-related quality of life, stress levels, and cognitive function.[63]

Finally, a cognitive-behavioral treatment program has been piloted that uses a memory and attention adaptation training (MAAT) intervention. This program includes education, self-awareness training, self-regulation and relaxation, and compensatory strategies. Improvement in self-reported cognitive function and neuropsychological performance was reported post intervention and was sustained at 6 months. Participants reported high satisfaction with the intervention.[61] Evaluation in a randomized controlled trial design is ongoing.

CONCLUSION

Cancer and cancer treatment can have cognitive sequelae for a subset of survivors that are detrimental to their ability to function in daily life and to their quality of life. The incidence, duration, and cause of cognitive impairment associated with cancer or cancer treatment are poorly defined, and no methods for treating it have been established. Several large, prospective longitudinal studies are currently being conducted in a range of tumor sites. It is hoped that these will provide some definitive evidence regarding the incidence of, risk factors for, and mechanisms of cognitive impairment in cancer survivors.

The International Cognition and Cancer Task Force (ICCTF) is a multidisciplinary group of researchers working to improve our understanding of the effects of cancer and cancer treatment on cognitive function in adults with non–central nervous system tumors.[64] Further information about this topic and the ICCTF can be found at their website (http://www.icctf.com).[64]

REFERENCES

1. Tannock IF, Ahles TA, Ganz PA, et al. Cognitive impairment associated with chemotherapy for cancer: report of a workshop. *J Clin Oncol*. 2004;22:2233–2239.
2. Ahles TA, Saykin A. Cognitive effects of standard-dose chemotherapy in patients with cancer. *Cancer Invest*. 2001;19:812–820.
3. Vardy J, Rourke S, Tannock IF. Evaluation of cognitive function associated with chemotherapy: a review of published studies and recommendations for future research. *J Clin Oncol*. 2007;25:2455–2463.
4. Ahles TA, Saykin AJ, Furstenberg CT, et al. Neuropsychologic impact of standard-dose systemic chemotherapy in long-term survivors of breast cancer and lymphoma. *J Clin Oncol*. 2002;20:485–493.
5. van Dam FS, Schagen SB, Muller MJ, et al. Impairment of cognitive function in women receiving adjuvant treatment for high-risk breast cancer: high-dose versus standard-dose chemotherapy. *J Natl Cancer Inst*. 1998;90:210–218.
6. Schagen SB, van Dam FS, Muller MJ, et al. Cognitive deficits after postoperative adjuvant chemotherapy for breast carcinoma. *Cancer*. 1999;85:640–650.
7. Brezden CB, Phillips KA, Abdolell M, et al. Cognitive function in breast cancer patients receiving adjuvant chemotherapy. *J Clin Oncol*. 2000;18:2695–2701.
8. Tchen N, Juffs HG, Downie FP, et al. Cognitive function, fatigue, and menopausal symptoms in women receiving adjuvant chemotherapy for breast cancer. *J Clin Oncol*. 2003;21:4175–4183.
9. Vardy JL, Rourke S, Pond GR, et al. Cognitive function and fatigue in cancer patients after chemotherapy: a longitudinal cohort study in patients with colorectal cancer (CRC). *ASCO Meeting Abstracts*. 2007;25:9099.
10. Wefel JS, Lenzi R, Theriault R, et al. 'Chemobrain' in breast carcinoma? A prologue. *Cancer*. 2004;101:466–475.
11. Vardy J, Wefel JS, Ahles T, et al. Cancer and cancer-therapy related cognitive dysfunction: an international perspective from the Venice cognitive workshop. *Ann Oncol*. 2008;19:623–629.
12. Hermelink K, Untch M, Lux MP, et al. Cognitive function during neoadjuvant chemotherapy for breast cancer: results of a prospective, multicenter, longitudinal study. *Cancer*. 2007;109:1905–1913.
13. Cimprich B, Ronis DL. Attention and symptom distress in women with and without breast cancer. *Nurs Res*. 2001;50:86–94.
14. Vardy JL, Dhillon H, Xu W, et al. Cognitive function and fatigue in colorectal cancer (CRC) patients: baseline assessments prior to chemotherapy. *ASCO Meeting Abstracts*. 2009;27:9557.

15. Wefel JS, Lenzi R, Theriault RL, et al. The cognitive sequelae of standard-dose adjuvant chemotherapy in women with breast carcinoma: results of a prospective, randomized, longitudinal trial. *Cancer*. 2004;100:2292–2299.
16. Schagen SB, Muller MJ, Boogerd W, et al. Change in cognitive function after chemotherapy: a prospective longitudinal study in breast cancer patients. *J Natl Cancer Inst*. 2006;98:1742–1745.
17. Scherwath A, Mehnert A, Schleimer B, et al. Neuropsychological function in high-risk breast cancer survivors after stem-cell supported high-dose therapy versus standard-dose chemotherapy: evaluation of long-term treatment effects. *Ann Oncol*. 2006;17:415–423.
18. Jenkins V, Shilling V, Deutsch G, et al. A 3-year prospective study of the effects of adjuvant treatments on cognition in women with early stage breast cancer. *Br J Cancer*. 2006;94:828–834.
19. Castellon SA, Ganz PA, Bower JE, et al. Neurocognitive performance in breast cancer survivors exposed to adjuvant chemotherapy and tamoxifen. *J Clin Exp Neuropsychol*. 2004;26:955–969.
20. Quesnel C, Savard J, Ivers H. Cognitive impairments associated with breast cancer treatments: results from a longitudinal study. *Breast Cancer Res Treat*. 2009;116:113–123.
21. Schagen SB, Muller MJ, Boogerd W, et al. Late effects of adjuvant chemotherapy on cognitive function: a follow-up study in breast cancer patients. *Ann Oncol*. 2002;13:1387–1397.
22. Collins B, Mackenzie J, Stewart A, et al. Cognitive effects of chemotherapy in post-menopausal breast cancer patients 1 year after treatment. *Psychooncology*. 2009;18:134–143.
23. Cognitive changes related to cancer treatment. *Hurricane Voices*. 2007;1–10.
24. Boykoff N, Moieni M, Subramanian SK. Confronting chemobrain: an in-depth look at survivors' reports of impact on work, social networks, and health care response. *J Cancer Surviv*. 2009;3:223–232.
25. Shilling V, Jenkins V. Self-reported cognitive problems in women receiving adjuvant therapy for breast cancer. *Eur J Oncol Nurs*. 2007;11:6–15.
26. Vardy JL, Xu W, Booth CM, et al. Relation between perceived cognitive function and neuropsychological performance in survivors of breast and colorectal cancer. *ASCO Meeting Abstracts*. 2008;26:9520.
27. Han R, Yang YM, Dietrich J, et al. Systemic 5-fluorouracil treatment causes a syndrome of delayed myelin destruction in the central nervous system. *J Biol*. 2008;7:12.
28. Ahles TA, Saykin AJ. Candidate mechanisms for chemotherapy-induced cognitive changes. *Nat Rev Cancer*. 2007;7:192–201.

29. Dietrich J, Han R, Yang Y, et al. CNS progenitor cells and oligodendrocytes are targets of chemotherapeutic agents in vitro and in vivo. *J Biol*. 2006;5:22.
30. Winocur G, Vardy J, Binns MA, et al. The effects of the anti-cancer drugs, methotrexate and 5-fluorouracil, on cognitive function in mice. *Pharmacol Biochem Behav*. 2006;85:66–75.
31. Seigers R, Schagen SB, Beerling W, et al. Long-lasting suppression of hippocampal cell proliferation and impaired cognitive performance by methotrexate in the rat. *Behav Brain Res*. 2008;186:168–175.
32. Vardy J, Tannock I. Cognitive function after chemotherapy in adults with solid tumours. *Crit Rev Oncol Hematol*. 2007;63:183–202.
33. Fardell J, Vardy J, Johnston I. *Oxaliplatin and 5-fluorouracil induced cognitive deficits in laboratory rodents*. Gold Coast: Clinical Oncological Society of Australia; 2009.
34. Seruga B, Zhang H, Bernstein LJ, et al. Cytokines and their relationship to the symptoms and outcome of cancer. *Nat Rev Cancer*. 2008;8:887–899.
35. Booth CM, Vardy J, Crawley A, et al. Cognitive impairment associated with chemotherapy for breast cancer: an exploratory case-control study. *J Clin Oncol (Meeting Abstracts)*. 2006;24:8501.
36. Vardy J, Booth C, Pond GR, et al. *Cytokine levels in patients with colorectal cancer and breast cancer and their relationship to fatigue and cognitive function*. Chicago, IL: American Society of Clinical Oncology; 2007.
37. Ferguson RJ, McDonald BC, Saykin AJ, et al. Brain structure and function differences in monozygotic twins: possible effects of breast cancer chemotherapy. *J Clin Oncol*. 2007;25:3866–3870.
38. Silverman DH, Dy CJ, Castellon SA, et al. Altered frontocortical, cerebellar, and basal ganglia activity in adjuvant-treated breast cancer survivors 5-10 years after chemotherapy. *Breast Cancer Res Treat*. 2007;103:303–311.
39. Kreukels BP, Schagen SB, Ridderinkhof KR, et al. Electrophysiological correlates of information processing in breast-cancer patients treated with adjuvant chemotherapy. *Breast Cancer Res Treat*. 2005;94:53–61.
40. Collins B, Mackenzie J, Stewart A, et al. Cognitive effects of hormonal therapy in early stage breast cancer patients: a prospective study. *Psychooncology*. 2009;18:811–821.
41. Jenkins VA, Ambroisine LM, Atkins L, et al. Effects of anastrozole on cognitive performance in postmenopausal women: a randomised, double-blind chemoprevention trial (IBIS II). *Lancet Oncol*. 2008;9:953–961.
42. Legault C, Maki PM, Resnick SM, et al. Effects of tamoxifen and raloxifene on memory and other cognitive abilities: cognition in the study

of tamoxifen and raloxifene. *J Clin Oncol.* 2009;27:5144–5152.

43. O'Shaughnessy JA, Vukelja SJ, Holmes FA, et al. Feasibility of quantifying the effects of epoetin alfa therapy on cognitive function in women with breast cancer undergoing adjuvant or neoadjuvant chemotherapy. *Clin Breast Cancer.* 2005;5:439–446.

44. Sohlberg M, Mateer CA. *Cognitive rehabilitation: an integrative neuropsychological approach.* New York: Guilford Press; 2001.

45. Birks J, Grimley EV, Van Dongen M. Ginkgo biloba for cognitive impairment and dementia. *Cochrane Database Syst Rev.* 2002;(4) CD003120.

46. Kwon JC, Kim EG, Kim JW, et al. Follow-up study for efficacy on cognitive function of donepezil in Binswanger-type subcortical vascular dementia. *Am J Alzheimers Dis Other Demen.* 2009;24:293–301.

47. Lautenschlager NT, Cox KL, Flicker L, et al. Effect of physical activity on cognitive function in older adults at risk for Alzheimer disease: a randomized trial. *JAMA.* 2008;300:1027–1037.

48. Mar Fan HG, Clemons M, Xu W, et al. A randomised, placebo-controlled, double-blind trial of the effects of d-methylphenidate on fatigue and cognitive dysfunction in women undergoing adjuvant chemotherapy for breast cancer. *Support Care Cancer.* 2008;16:577–583.

49. Lower EE, Fleishman S, Cooper A, et al. Efficacy of dexmethylphenidate for the treatment of fatigue after cancer chemotherapy: a randomized clinical trial. *J Pain Symptom Manage.* 2009;38:650–662.

50. Kohli S, Fisher SG, Tra Y, et al. The effect of modafinil on cognitive function in breast cancer survivors. *Cancer.* 2009;115:2605–2616.

51. Mateer CA, Kerns KA, Eso KL. Management of attention and memory disorders following traumatic brain injury. *J Learn Disabil.* 1996;29:618–632.

52. Sivak M, Hill CS, Olson PL. Computerized video tasks as training techniques for driving-related perceptual deficits of persons with brain damage: a pilot evaluation. *Int J Rehabil Res.* 1984;7:389–398.

53. Sohlberg MM, Mateer CA. *Cognitive rehabilitation: an integrative neuropsychological approach.* New York: Guilford Press; 2001.

54. Sohlberg MM, Mateer CA. Improving attention and managing attentional problems: adapting rehabilitation techniques to adults with ADD. *Ann N Y Acad Sci.* 2001;931:359–375.

55. Palmese CA, Raskin SA. The rehabilitation of attention in individuals with mild traumatic brain injury, using the APT-II programme. *Brain Inj.* 2000;14:535–548.

56. Cicerone KD, Dahlberg C, Kalmar K, et al. Evidence-based cognitive rehabilitation: recommendations for clinical practice. *Arch Phys Med Rehabil.* 2000;81:1596–1615.

57. Berg I, Konning-Haanstra M, Deelman M. Long term effects of memory rehabilitation: a controlled study. *Neuropsychol Rehabil.* 1991;1:97–111.

58. Consensus Conference. Rehabilitation of persons with traumatic brain injury: NIH Consensus Development Panel on Rehabilitation of Persons With Traumatic Brain Injury. *JAMA.* 1999;282:974–983.

59. Mahncke HW, Connor BB, Appelman J, et al. Memory enhancement in healthy older adults using a brain plasticity-based training program: a randomized, controlled study. *Proc Natl Acad Sci U S A.* 2006;103:12523–12528.

60. Kim S, Stasio C, Spina L. *Effects on health-related quality of life in individuals with "chemobrain" using a brain-plasticity-based training program.* Presented at: 36th Annual International Neuropsychological Society Meeting, Waikoloa, Hawaii. February 6-9; 2008.

61. Ferguson RJ, Ahles TA, Saykin AJ, et al. Cognitive-behavioral management of chemotherapy-related cognitive change. *Psychooncology.* 2007;16:772–777.

62. Buonomano DV, Merzenich MM. Cortical plasticity: from synapses to maps. *Annu Rev Neurosci.* 1998;21:149–186.

63. Smith GE, Housen P, Yaffe K, et al. A cognitive training program based on principles of brain plasticity: results from the improvement in memory with plasticity-based adaptive cognitive training (IMPACT) study. *J Am Geriatr Soc.* 2009;1–10.

64. Schagen SB. *International Cognition and Cancer Taskforce.* Amsterdam; 2010.

44

Secondary cancers in cancer survivors

Debra L. Friedman

In the United States, cancer survivors constitute 3.5% or 10 million of the population.[1] Because of advances in diagnosis and therapy, the 5-year rate of survival exceeds 60%[1]; however, this growing population can experience serious adverse physical and psychological effects from therapy. One of the most serious medical consequences of cancer therapy experienced by cancer survivors is a new or secondary cancer. Mariotto et al.[2] reported in 2006 that among those cancer survivors who were alive as of January 1, 2002, nearly 8% had experienced more than one form of cancer.[2] Secondary cancers are the leading cause of death among long-term survivors of many different types of cancers, including Hodgkin's lymphoma.[3-5] Secondary cancers can be sequelae of treatment with chemotherapy and radiation, but also can be a consequence of environmental exposures, lifestyle choices, and genetic predispositions. A recent review[6] examined secondary primary cancers and categorized them according to etiologic influences. These three etiologic categories were nonexclusive of one another: treatment-related events, genetic syndromes, and those due to shared factors. We will examine these categories in this chapter. Table 44-1 summarizes the major known groups of etiologic factors that contribute to increased risks of secondary malignancies among cancer survivors.

CUMULATIVE INCIDENCE OF SUBSEQUENT NEOPLASMS

INCIDENCE IN ADULT SURVIVORS

Second cancers account for approximately 1 in every 6 cancers reported to the National Cancer Institute's Surveillance, Epidemiology and End Results Program.[1] Fraumeni et al.[7] examined data from the National Cancer Institute's Surveillance, Epidemiology, and End Results (SEER) Program in 2006 and noted that among cancer survivors, there was a 14% higher risk of developing a new or secondary malignancy than would be expected in the general population. The SEER data revealed that an age effect was noted, with a sixfold relative risk of developing a secondary cancer for survivors of childhood cancer, a twofold to threefold increase for patients who were young adults (aged 18–39 years at initial diagnosis) treated for cancer, and a 1.5-fold increase for patients diagnosed between 40 and 59 years of age.[7] The SEER data also examined the time of development of a secondary cancer from initial diagnosis and noted that the risk of new cancer is highest in the first 5 years after diagnosis.[7]

Table 44-1 Factors associated with the risk of developing secondary malignancies

Factors	Examples
Therapy related	Radiotherapy
	Chemotherapy
Genetic syndromes	Fanconi's anemia
	Li-Fraumeni syndrome
	Bloom syndrome
	Hereditary nonpolyposis
	colorectal cancer
	BRCA1- or *BRCA2*-related
	cancers
	Xeroderma pigmentosa
Shared etiologic influences	
Lifestyle	Tobacco
	Alcohol
	Sun exposure
	Diet/nutrition
Host factors	Immune dysfunction
	Infection
	Immune suppression
	Genetics
	Hormones
Environment	Contaminants
	Occupation

Secondary malignancies were noted to have occurred in the same site or organ as the first primary cancer in 13.2% of the SEER patient population surviving 2 months or longer. Of these secondary malignancies, new tumors in the breast for females, colon cancers, lung cancers, and melanoma of the skin were the most common secondary cancers.[7]

Previous studies have shown that patients exposed to specific chemotherapeutic agents or radiation therapy and those with a known genetic predisposition are at a higher risk for secondary malignancies (SMNs). Testicular cancer and Hodgkin's lymphoma (HL) are both highly curable and typically affect younger individuals with a life expectancy that is close to that of the normal population. Of importance, secondary solid tumors are a leading cause of death among long-term survivors of HL, sarcoma, and bone tumor.[4,8,9] Radiotherapy-associated solid tumors typically develop after a long latency of 5 to 10 years from initial treatment of HL, and the risk persists for as long as 30 years post therapy.[10] The types of SMNs that affect survivors of testicular cancer include leukemia and solid tumors such as mesothelioma and cancers of the lung, thyroid, esophagus, stomach, pancreas, colon, rectum, kidney, bladder, and connective tissue.[11] The risk of developing an SMN is associated with a predisposing risk factor. This is observed in survivors of breast cancer who develop a contralateral breast cancer.[12-16] An article by Boice et al.[12] examined the risk factors for developing breast cancer and noted that the risk for contralateral breast cancer is twofold to fivefold greater among patients who have breast cancer. These can be to the result of a preexisting breast cancer risk factor, although radiation therapy may contribute some risk.

INCIDENCE IN CHILDHOOD SURVIVORS

Secondary malignancies (SMNs) that occur in childhood cancer survivors vary with diagnosis, use of chemotherapy and/or radiation, and time from initial treatment, as seen in Figure 44-1. The Childhood Cancer Survivor Study (CCSS) has involved the largest cohort of long-term survivors of childhood cancer and has examined the relationship between cancer treatment and development of SMN. In 2009, Meadows et al.[17] revealed that an excess of SMNs was observed in all primary childhood cancer diagnostic groups when compared with the general population. A 30-year cumulative incidence of SMN was 9.3%.[17] Among childhood survivor, a 16 times higher risk of developing breast cancer was noted, along with a 19 times higher risk of developing bone cancer and an 11 times higher risk of developing thyroid cancer.[17] Previous studies done by SEER revealed a greater than sixfold increase in incidence relative to the general population[18]; this was similar to the risks reported for three other large cohorts from North America,[19] Great Britain,[20] and the Nordic countries.[21]

The most common types of secondary cancers were of the female breast, brain, bone, thyroid gland, and soft tissue, as well as melanoma and acute nonlymphocytic leukemia.[17,18] The risk of developing a secondary breast cancer was highest among those childhood survivors who were treated with chest radiation for HL, non-Hodgkin's lymphoma (NHL), sarcoma, or Wilms' tumor.[22-24] Women with a family history of breast cancer had an almost threefold greater risk of breast cancer than the general population in the CCSS study.[17] The risk of sarcoma after an initial childhood cancer was ninefold greater than in the general population and was 24-fold greater in those with a primary diagnosis of soft tissue sarcoma. Subsequent central nervous system (CNS) gliomas were also predominant in the CCSS study, with those children diagnosed before the age of 5 at highest risk (standardized incidence ratio [SIR], 14.5). Risk factors for developing SMNs included younger age at time of diagnosis (specifically for thyroid and CNS SMN) and exposure to alkylating agents, anthracyclines, and epipodophyllotoxins.[17]

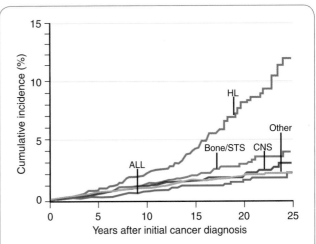

Fig. 44-1 The cumulative incidence of secondary cancers among children. (*Adapted from Inskip PA. New malignancies following childhood cancer. In Curtis RE, Ron E, Ries LAG, et al, editors. New malignancies among cancer survivors: SEER cancer registries, 1973-2000. Betheda, MD: National Cancer Institute; 2006.*)

ROLE OF CHEMOTHERAPY

Since chemotherapy agents were first introduced, reports of secondary malignancies have emerged. A review of the literature done in the early 1980s observed that alkylating agents such as melphalan, chlorambucil, and cyclophosphamide seemed to lead to the highest rate of secondary cancers, most of which were acute leukemias.[25]

ALKYLATING AGENTS

Alkylating agents that induce human leukemia include busulfan, carmustine, chlorambucil, cyclophosphamide, dihydroxybusulfan, lomustine, mechlorethamine, melphalan, prednimustine, and semustine. Following treatment with alkylating agents, the risk of leukemia begins to increase at 1 to 2 years, peaks at 5 to 10 years, and then decreases.[26] Many times, a preceding myelodysplastic syndrome is reported. Several chromosomal abnormalities are associated with the myelodysplastic syndrome, including unbalanced translocations or deletions involving portions of chromosome 5 and/or 7, consisting of loss of all or part of the long arm of the chromosome.[26,27] The risk of alkylating agent–related acute myeloid leukemia (AML) typically increases with the increasing cumulative dose or duration of therapy. During the early 1970s, several cooperative groups reported an excess risk of secondary AML in adults and children treated for HL with a combination of mechlorethamine, vincristine, procarbazine, and prednisone, or similar alkylating agents.[28–30] The Late Effects Study Group observed that survivors of HL who had been treated with alkylating agents before the age of 16 years had a relative risk of leukemia that was nearly 80 times that of population controls.[31] Leukemias that occur as the result of alkylating agent therapy usually are refractory to treatment and associated with poor survival.[32] A recent study by Ng et al.[33] examined the development of secondary leukemia among HL survivors and noted that the rate of survival was only 0.4 years, with a 5 year-survival rate of 4.9%. Patients with genetic syndromes such as Fanconi's anemia and neurofibromatosis I who develop a first cancer have an increased susceptibility to alkylating agent–induced leukemia.[26]

TOPOISOMERASE AGENTS

Topoisomerase II inhibitor–related AML develops after treatment with cytotoxic drugs that target DNA topoisomerase II, particularly the epipodophyllotoxins etoposide and tenoposide. Epipodophyllotoxin-induced leukemia was first described in the late 1980s.[34,35] Evidence suggests that anthracyclines such as doxorubicin may also be associated with this type of leukemia.[36] Leukemias induced by topoisomerase inhibitors tend to have a shorter induction period, with a median latency of only 2 to 3 years. Various risk factors have been documented that influence the risk of epipodophyllotoxin-related AML; these include frequency of administration,[26,37] prolonged administration of low dose,[38,39] use of cumulative dose,[40] concomitant administration of other chemotherapeutic regimens, and the genetic makeup of the individual. Morphology is usually monoblastic or myelomonocytic and frequently involves the MLL gene (11q23), t(9,11), t(11,19), and t(6,11) or 21q22.[36] Patients who develop these treatment-

related leukemias usually respond to therapy, in contrast to patients with de novo leukemia of the same type.[41]

Chemotherapy-induced leukemias also include acute lymphoblastic leukemia, which has been seen after topoisomerase II inhibitor therapy. This type of leukemia frequently shows a t(4;11)(q21;q23) chromosomal translocation.[36] Leukemia following chemotherapy for HL is perhaps the most studied treatment-associated malignancy. The cumulative risk of leukemia 15 years following therapy with MOPP (mechlorethamine, procarbazine, prednisone, and vincristine) is between 3% and 10%.[42,43]

ROLE OF RADIATION THERAPY

The role that radiotherapy plays in the development of second cancers has been the subject of many studies. We will summarize some of these findings. Radiation has been associated with many different types of cancers, including but not limited to breast, lung, and thyroid cancers and solid tumors. The risk of developing a secondary cancer from radiation exposure is highest when exposure occurs at a young age.[19,31] This risk increases with the cumulative dose of irradiation[44] and with increased follow-up time after radiation.[45]

DELAY BETWEEN RADIATION THERAPY AND EMERGENCE OF CANCER

The duration between radiation therapy and a secondary cancer is variable. When survivors of the A-bomb were studied, leukemia had developed between 5 and 15 years after the initial exposure; solid tumors were noted anywhere from 10 to 60 years after the initial exposure. Kirova et al.[46] noted the incidence of radiation-induced sarcoma after radiotherapy for breast cancer and found that the cumulative radiation-induced sarcoma incidence was 0.07% (±0.02) at 5 years, 0.27% (±0.05) at 10 years, and 0.48% (±0.11) at 15 years. Standardized incidence ratios were 10.2 (95% confidence interval [CI], 9.03%–11.59%) for irradiated patients and 1.3 (95% CI, 0.3%–3.6%) for nonirradiated patients. Perhaps the most compelling evidence comes from childhood HL survivors who received mantle radiation. Studies done by Bhatia et al.[31] have shown that girls who are between the ages of 10 and 16 years at the time of radiation therapy for HL are at greatest risk for developing breast cancer; the incidence of the estimated actuarial cumulative probability of breast cancer was 35% (95% CI, 17.4%–52.6%) at 40 years of age.[31]

INFLUENCE OF AGE AT IRRADIATION

Children and adolescents are at greater susceptibility to radiocarcinogenesis than adults. Cancers of the breast and thyroid are observed in children and adolescents treated with low doses of radiation (100 mGy), whereas adults do not develop cancers unless treated at higher doses.[19,45,47] The reason for these findings is unknown, although it is postulated that children and adolescents have higher numbers of stem cells in these tissues that are vulnerable to the effects of radiation.

INFLUENCE OF GENDER AT IRRADIATION

Various studies have shown that the incidence of secondary cancer is greater in women than in men following equal doses of radiation. It is unknown why this happens.

ORGANS RADIATED

The risk of secondary cancer in survivors of HL has been well established. Organs that are particularly sensitive to carcinogenic effects of radiation include breast and thyroid. In contrast to secondary leukemias, the latency period of therapy-associated solid tumors is usually much longer, greater than 10 years. Breast cancers have emerged as the most common solid tumor among survivors of HL.[4,31] This excess in breast cancer is largely due to the high-dose chest irradiation fields used to treat HL. The highest risks are observed among women treated for HL at <30 years of age.

Neglia et al.[44] investigated a cohort of 13,581 children in the Childhood Cancer Survivor Study who survived for longer than 5 years after treatment with a median follow-up time of 15 years.[44] The risk of leukemia peaked at between 5 and 8 years of follow-up, but the risk of solid tumors remained. The most common solid tumors were breast cancer, thyroid cancer, and CNS cancers. A study done in a cohort of 14,372 children to investigate sarcomas and brain tumors revealed that the risk of glioma was high in children irradiated at younger than 5 years of age, and secondary sarcomas occurred after a median delay of 11 years.[44] This was associated with high doses of radiation therapy (RT) but also with high doses of anthracyclines. The CCSS reported data from more than 13,000 childhood survivors and noted that secondary cancer risk varies according to the type of primary tumor.

RADIATION AND DOSE

Since the 1980s, several studies have shown that the risk of secondary cancers increases with the dose of radiation during therapy. In a study that included 100,000 survivors of cervical cancer, it was noted that secondary cancers are still occurring upward of 10 years after initial treatment.[48] Neglia et al.[44] revealed that the incidence of brain tumor in children treated with RT showed that no cancer was observed when the dose to the brain was <10 Gy, and that a maximal relative risk >10 was related to brain doses >30 Gy.[44] Dorr and Hermann[49] reported that a majority of second tumors are observed within the margin of the planned target volumes in regions receiving 6 Gy or more.[49] The relative risk per Gray of radiation received has been based on cancer risks observed among Japanese A-bomb survivors. In Japanese A-bomb survivors, it was estimated that at age 70, after exposure at age 30, solid cancer rates increased by about 35% per Gy.[50,51] Several studies have shown that the risk of secondary cancers increases with dose, at least until 80 Gy. However, the dose-response curve differs according to the tissue that is being irradiated, the histologic type of cancer, and the dose rate. Dose fractionation seems to be the main explanation for the much lower carcinogenic effect of medical irradiation. It is believed that this is due to a decrease in effectiveness in DNA repair during the time interval between sessions, as long as the delay is longer than 6 hours.[52] Despite DNA repair during the time interval between fractions, a cumulative effect of some residual damage seems to increase with the dose per fraction. Studies have shown that an excessive cancer risk is not detected below a cumulative dose of 0.6 Gy.[53] For doses between 0.6 Gy and 3.6 Gy, the risk of cancer is small but detectable.

GENETIC PREDISPOSITION

CANCER SYNDROMES

Hereditary susceptibility from genetic predisposition syndromes explains a small proportion of all secondary cancers. The most studied of these genetic predisposition syndromes are Li-Fraumeni syndrome, BRCA-related hereditary breast and/or ovarian cancer, and Fanconi's anemia. Common features of these syndromes are listed in Table 44-2.

The most common variant of Li-Fraumeni syndrome involves a germline mutation in the p53 tumor suppressor gene.[54,55] Gene mutation carriers are predisposed to a wide variety of tumors, including breast cancer, soft tissue sarcoma, brain tumor, and leukemia.[56,57] Most syndrome-associated cancers develop at younger than usual ages and affect family members throughout a lifetime. Members of families with Li-Fraumeni syndrome have reported an increased risk of subsequent cancer in survivors of childhood cancer.[58] The exact mechanism of how or why this syndrome inflicts a greater risk of cancer is still being studied, although theories have suggested that a germline mutation in the tumor suppressor gene may interact with therapeutic exposures, resulting in increased risk of second cancers.

Studies done by Metcalfe et al.[59] noted that the largest cumulative risk of secondary cancer for breast cancer survivors is a cancer in the contralateral breast associated with the BRCA mutation.

Table 44-2 Cancer syndromes and features

Syndrome	Mutation	Cancer predisposition
Li-Fraumeni syndrome	Germline mutation in p53 tumor suppressor gene	Breast cancer, osteosarcoma, soft tissue sarcoma, brain tumor, adrenocortical tumor, and leukemia
Hereditary breast cancer	BRCA1 or BRCA2 mutation	Breast cancer in contralateral breast, ovarian and uterine cancers, thyroid cancer, cancer of pancreas, gallbladder, stomach, and skin
Hereditary nonpolyposis colon cancer	Germline mutation in DNA, mismatch repair genes MLH1, MSH2, MSH6	Cancers of colon, endometrium, stomach, small intestine, hepatobiliary system, kidney, ureter, and ovary
Fanconi's anemia	Chromosomal instability, hypersensitivity to toxic effects of DNA cross-linking agents	Leukemia, cancers of head, neck, vulva, cervix, esophagus, liver, and brain
Retinoblastoma	RB-1 gene enhances risk of tumors arising in field of radiation	Osteosarcoma, soft tissue sarcoma, melanoma, cancers of brain, eye, orbit, and nasal cavity

The Breast Cancer Linkage Consortium also documented a three-fold to fivefold increased risk of subsequent cancers of prostate, pancreas, gallbladder, and stomach, and melanoma of the skin and uterus in carriers of the *BRCA2* mutation.[60]

Fanconi's anemia is a rare autosomal recessive syndrome characterized by chromosomal instability, cancer susceptibility, and hypersensitivity to the toxic effects of DNA cross-linking agents.[61] Patients with Fanconi's anemia are susceptible to leukemia and cancers of the head and neck, vulva, cervix, esophagus, liver, and brain.[62,63]

SECOND CANCERS CAUSED BY MULTIPLE FACTORS

As discussed previously, research has shown that both chemotherapy and radiotherapy have a role in the development of second cancers after treatment for pediatric and adult cancers. Late effects of treatment can be modified by moderate to low genetic traits or by gene-environment and gene-gene interactions. Various studies have reported 20% to 95% variability in the disposition and effects of cytotoxic drugs in different individuals.[64-66] Links have been found between polymorphisms in genes encoding selected drug-metabolizing enzymes such as glutathione S-transferase, cytochrome P450, and thiopurine methyltransferase, and the development of therapy-related cancers.[67-69] Perhaps the best studied example of this is the increased risk of acute myeloid leukemia after epipodophyllotoxin therapy.[70] Other treatment-related cancers are associated with variations in DNA repair after damage from radiotherapy and chemotherapy. Retinoblastoma serves as an example of how genetic mutations can influence the risk of radiotherapy-related cancers. Patients with hereditary retinoblastoma have a germline mutation in the *RB-1* gene that predisposes them to high risk of osteosarcomas, soft tissue sarcomas, melanomas, and cancers of the brain, nasal cavities, eye, and orbit. When the *RB* gene is mutated, it has an increased susceptibility to radiation damage; thus the risk of tumors arising in the radiation field is increased.[71]

TOBACCO AND ALCOHOL

Other factors that can lead to secondary cancers include tobacco and alcohol use. Tobacco and alcohol are major causes of cancer in the general population, but they also account for a large proportion of secondary malignancies among cancer survivors. Tobacco is a well-known cause of multiple primary cancers with well-established association with lung cancer, cancer of the upper digestive tract, and esophageal cancer.[72] Patients with lung cancer also have an increased risk of cancers of the lip and bladder and secondary primary lung cancers.[73] This risk is influenced by whether or not patients continue their tobacco habits after development of their first tobacco-related cancer. Alcohol is also associated with cancers of the upper digestive system and of the liver, breast, and colorectum.[74] Based on SEER data in 2006, upward of 35% of secondary cancers are related to tobacco and/or alcohol.[7]

NUTRITION AND HORMONES

Endocrine and dietary factors can influence the aggregation of cancers of the breast, uterus, ovary, and colon.[75] The Women's Healthy Eating and Living (WHEL) Study is a multisite randomized controlled trial that examined the effectiveness of a high-vegetable, low-fat diet aimed at markedly raising circulating carotenoid concentrations from food sources and reducing additional breast cancer events and early death in women with early-stage invasive breast cancer (within 4 years of diagnosis). This study randomly assigned 3088 such women to an intensive diet intervention or to a comparison group between 1995 and 2000 and followed them at different time intervals.[76] Recent examination of this cohort revealed that when assessed over time, a higher biological exposure to carotenoids was associated with a greater likelihood of breast cancer–free survival.[77] Other studies have observed an impact of obesity and endocrine issues from obesity on the risk of secondary malignancies. Calle et al.[78] examined prospectively the influence of body weight on death from cancer in 900,000 adults; they found that the heavier members of the cohort had 50% to 60% higher risk of death from all cancers than those of normal weight.[78] It seems likely that obesity and lifestyle factors may contribute to the development of secondary malignancies in cancer survivors.

INFECTION AND IMMUNE SUPPRESSION

Awareness that certain infectious agents such as human papillomavirus (HPV), Epstein-Barr virus (EBV), and human deficiency virus (HIV) may contribute to certain combinations of tumors[79] is growing. Studies have shown that cancers of the cervix and anogenital tract are more likely to occur in individuals who are infected with certain strains of HPV and have an underlying immunologic defect.[80] Studies done in bone marrow transplant survivors and immunosuppressed solid tumor survivors have shown an increase in cutaneous melanoma.[81]

IMPACT ON BURDEN OF DISEASE

CHRONIC HEALTH CONDITIONS

Several reports have described the burden of disease and chronic health problems that survivors of cancer experience and face.[82-84] These reports suggest that more than two thirds of survivors will experience at least one chronic medical condition, and one third will face a severe or life-threatening late effect. In a study conducted by Oeffinger et al.[82] that examined more than 10,000 adult survivors of childhood cancers, an upward of eightfold risk of a severe chronic health condition was reported when compared with age- and sex-matched siblings.[82] A study done by Meadows et al.[17] that examined secondary cancers in the CCSS cohort revealed that survivors had a 3.3-fold increased risk of a chronic health condition and an 8.2-fold increased risk of a life-threatening condition.[17]

SURVIVORSHIP CLINICS

The increased risk of subsequent malignancies among cancer survivors is well established. Continued long-term follow-up and careful documentation of treatment-related cancer risk as cancer therapies evolve will be critical for monitoring the patterns and temporal trends of excess subsequent cancers. Several key strategies are important in attempts to lessen the impact of secondary cancers on cancer survivors. Patient education and advocacy are important; patients need to be aware of their risks of secondary cancers and of long-term effects of their therapy. It is imperative that survivors be aware of healthy lifestyle practices that may affect their chances of secondary cancers, such as smoking cessation, sun safety awareness, and taking in alcohol in moderation. Screening for secondary cancers such as breast cancer via mammography and breast magnetic resonance imaging (MRI) is important. Primary care physicians and oncologists taking care of survivors need to be aware of screening guidelines (Table 44-3) that may differ as the result of chemotherapy and radiation exposure; for example, young women treated for HL who received radiation to their chest should be undergoing mammography and breast MRIs starting at age 30, or 10 years after their initial dose of radiation.[85] Providing appropriate health care for this heterogeneous population of cancer survivors is a challenge. The Institute of Medicine has recognized the need for systematic planning for lifelong surveillance that incorporates risks based on therapeutic exposures, genetic predispositions, health-related behaviors, and comorbid health conditions.[86] Optimal healthcare delivery to this heterogeneous population requires establishment of longitudinal care using a multidisciplinary team approach, with continuity provided by a single healthcare provider who coordinates needed services.

It is imperative that future research should address the development of interventions that mitigate excess cancer risks conferred by treatments in the past. These interventions need to focus on development of cancer screening and risk reduction strategies for high-risk cancer survivors based on treatment history and other risk factors. It is vital for cancer survivors and their caregivers to be educated about the risks of secondary cancer and the need to promote a healthier lifestyle and to adhere to screening guidelines. Consensus-based guidelines for specific patient populations and treatment exposures need to be developed, dispersed to primary care physicians and oncologists taking care of these survivors, and implemented.

Table 44-3 Screening recommendations from Children's Oncology Group for second cancer*

Therapeutic exposure	Potential late effect	Recommended screening
Etoposide	Acute myeloid leukemia	CBC, platelet, differential yearly for 10 years after exposure
Anthracyclines	Acute myeloid leukemia	CBC, platelet, differential yearly for 10 years after exposure
Alkylating agents	Acute myeloid leukemia/ myelodysplasia	CBC, platelet, differential yearly for 10 years after exposure
Radiation†	SMN in radiation field	Yearly history, physical examination with palpation of tissue in radiation field
Radiation of chest/breast	Breast cancer	Mammogram with adjunct MRI yearly, beginning 8 years after radiation or at age 25, whichever later
Radiation of abdomen/colon	Colorectal cancer	Colonoscopy every 5 years, beginning at 10 years after radiation or at age 35, whichever later

*Adapted from Children's Oncology Group Long Term Follow-up Guidelines. Available at: www.survivorshipguidelines.org.
†Specific recommendations for radiation fields are available and should be followed.
CBC, Complete blood count; MRI, magnetic resonance imaging; SMN, secondary malignancy.

REFERENCES

1. Ries LAG, Harkins D, Krapcho M, et al., eds. SEER cancer statistics review 1975-2003. Bethesda, MD: National Cancer Institute; 2006.
2. Mariotto AB, Rowland JH, Ries LA, et al. Multiple cancer prevalence: a growing challenge in long-term survivorship. *Cancer Epidemiol Biomarkers Prev.* 2007;16:566–571.
3. Aleman BM, van den Belt-Dusebout AW, Klokman WJ, et al. Long-term cause-specific mortality of patients treated for Hodgkin's disease. *J Clin Oncol.* 2003;21:3431–3439.
4. Dores GM, Metayer C, Curtis RE, et al. Second malignant neoplasms among long-term survivors of Hodgkin's disease: a population-based evaluation over 25 years. *J Clin Oncol.* 2002;20:3484–3494.
5. Travis LB, Hill D, Dores GM, et al. Cumulative absolute breast cancer risk for young women treated for Hodgkin lymphoma. *J Natl Cancer Inst.* 2005;97:1428–1437.
6. Travis LB, Rabkin CS, Brown LM, et al. Cancer survivorship—genetic susceptibility and second primary cancers: research strategies and recommendations. *J Natl Cancer Inst.* 2006;98:15–25.
7. Fraumeni JF, Edwards BK, Tucker MA, eds. *New malignancies among cancer survivors: SEER cancer registries, 1973-2000.* Bethesda, MD: National Cancer Institute; 2006 NIH Publ. No. 05-5302.
8. Ng AK, Travis LB. Second primary cancers: an overview. *Hematol Oncol Clin North Am.* 2008;22:271–289 vii.
9. Ng AK, Travis LB. Subsequent malignant neoplasms in cancer survivors. *Cancer J.* 2008;14:429–434.
10. Hodgson DC, Gilbert ES, Dores GM, et al. Long-term solid cancer risk among 5-year survivors of Hodgkin's lymphoma. *J Clin Oncol.* 2007;25:1489–1497.
11. Travis LB, Andersson M, Gospodarowicz M, et al. Treatment-associated leukemia following testicular cancer. *J Natl Cancer Inst.* 2000;92:1165–1171.
12. Boice Jr JD, Harvey EB, Blettner M, et al. Cancer in the contralateral breast after radiotherapy for breast cancer. *N Engl J Med.* 1992;326:781–785.
13. Gao X, Fisher SG, Emami B. Risk of second primary cancer in the contralateral breast in women treated for early-stage breast cancer: a population-based study. *Int J Radiat Oncol Biol Phys.* 2003;56:1038–1045.
14. Hemminki K, Ji J, Forsti A. Risks for familial and contralateral breast cancer interact multiplicatively and cause a high risk. *Cancer Res.* 2007;67:868–870.
15. Kirova YM, Gambotti L, DeRycke Y, et al. Risk of second malignancies after adjuvant radiotherapy for breast cancer: a large-scale, single-institution review. *Int J Radiat Oncol Biol Phys.* 2007;68:359–363.
16. Storm HH, Andersson M, Boice Jr JD, et al. Adjuvant radiotherapy and risk of contralateral breast cancer. *J Natl Cancer Inst.* 1992;84:1245–1250.
17. Meadows AT, Friedman DL, Neglia JP, et al. Second neoplasms in survivors of childhood cancer: findings from the Childhood Cancer Survivor Study cohort. *J Clin Oncol.* 2009;27:2356–2362.
18. Inskip PD, Cohen RJ, Curtis RE. New malignancies following childhood cancer. In: Curtis RE, Ron E, Ries LAG, et al., eds. *New malignancies among cancer survivors: SEER cancer registries, 1973-2000.* Bethesda, MD: National Cancer Institute; 2006:465–482.
19. Neglia JP, Friedman DL, Yasui Y, et al. Second malignant neoplasms in five-year survivors of childhood cancer: childhood cancer survivor study. *J Natl Cancer Inst.* 2001;93:618–629.
20. Jenkinson HC, Hawkins MM, Stiller CA, et al. Long-term population-based risks of second malignant neoplasms after childhood cancer in Britain. *Br J Cancer.* 2004;91:1905–1910.
21. Olsen JH, Garwicz S, Hertz H, et al. Second malignant neoplasms after cancer in childhood or adolescence. Nordic Society of Paediatric Haematology and Oncology Association of the Nordic Cancer Registries. *BMJ.* 1993;307:1030–1036.

22. Bhatia S, Yasui Y, Robison LL, et al. High risk of subsequent neoplasms continues with extended follow-up of childhood Hodgkin's disease: report from the Late Effects Study Group. *J Clin Oncol.* 2003;21:4386–4394.

23. Garwicz S, Anderson H, Olsen JH, et al. Second malignant neoplasms after cancer in childhood and adolescence: a population-based case-control study in the 5 Nordic countries. The Nordic Society for Pediatric Hematology and Oncology. The Association of the Nordic Cancer Registries. *Int J Cancer.* 2000;88:672–678.

24. Maule M, Scélo G, Pastore G, et al. Risk of second malignant neoplasms after childhood leukemia and lymphoma: an international study. *J Natl Cancer Inst.* 2007;99:790–800.

25. Rieche K. Carcinogenicity of antineoplastic agents in man. *Cancer Treat Rev.* 1984;11:39–67.

26. Davies SM. Therapy-related leukemia associated with alkylating agents. *Med Pediatr Oncol.* 2001;36:536–540.

27. Hijiya N, Ness KK, Ribeiro RC, et al. Acute leukemia as a secondary malignancy in children and adolescents: current findings and issues. *Cancer.* 2009;115:23–35.

28. Kushner BH, Zauber A, Tan CT. Second malignancies after childhood Hodgkin's disease. The Memorial Sloan-Kettering Cancer Center experience. *Cancer.* 1988;62:1364–1370.

29. Meadows AT, Baum E, Fossati Bellani F, et al. Second malignant neoplasms in children: an update from the Late Effects Study Group. *J Clin Oncol.* 1985;3:532–538.

30. Meadows AT, Obringer AC, Marrero O, et al. Second malignant neoplasms following childhood Hodgkin's disease: treatment and splenectomy as risk factors. *Med Pediatr Oncol.* 1989;17:477–484.

31. Bhatia S, Robison LL, Oberlin O, et al. Breast cancer and other second neoplasms after childhood Hodgkin's disease. *N Engl J Med.* 1996;334:745–751.

32. Michels SD, McKenna RW, Arthur DC, et al. Therapy-related acute myeloid leukemia and myelodysplastic syndrome: a clinical and morphologic study of 65 cases. *Blood.* 1985;65:1364–1372.

33. Ng AK, Bernardo MV, Weller E, et al. Second malignancy after Hodgkin disease treated with radiation therapy with or without chemotherapy: long-term risks and risk factors. *Blood.* 2002;100:1989–1996.

34. Pui CH, Behm FJ, Raimondi SC, et al. Secondary acute myeloid leukemia in children treated for acute lymphoid leukemia. *N Engl J Med.* 1989;321:136–142.

35. Winick N, Buchanan GR, Kamen BA. Secondary acute myeloid leukemia in Hispanic children. *J Clin Oncol.* 1993;11:1433.

36. Jaffe ES, Stein H, Vardiman JW. *World Health Organization classification of tumors: pathology and genetics of hematopoietic and lymphoid tissues.* Lyon: IARC Press; 2001.

37. Pui CH, Relling MV. Topoisomerase II. inhibitor-related acute myeloid leukaemia. *Br J Haematol.* 2000;109:13–23.

38. Chen CL, Fuscoe JC, Liu Q, et al. Relationship between cytotoxicity and site-specific DNA recombination after in vitro exposure of leukemia cells to etoposide. *J Natl Cancer Inst.* 1996;88:1840–1847.

39. Hijiya N, Gajjar A, Zhang Z, et al. Low-dose oral etoposide-based induction regimen for children with acute lymphoblastic leukemia in first bone marrow relapse. *Leukemia.* 2004;18:1581–1586.

40. Pui CH, Ribeiro RC, Hancock ML, et al. Acute myeloid leukemia in children treated with epipodophyllotoxins for acute lymphoblastic leukemia. *N Engl J Med.* 1991;325:1682–1687.

41. Pui CH, RElling MV, Rivera GK, et al. Epipodophyllotoxin-related acute myeloid leukemia: a study of 35 cases. *Leukemia.* 1995;9:1990–1996.

42. Devita Jr VT, Serpick AA, Carbone PP. Combination chemotherapy in the treatment of advanced Hodgkin's disease. *Ann Intern Med.* 1970;73:881–895.

43. Travis LB, Weeks J, Curtis RE, et al. Leukemia following low-dose total body irradiation and chemotherapy for non-Hodgkin's lymphoma. *J Clin Oncol.* 1996;14:565–571.

44. Neglia JP, Robison LL, Stovall M, et al. New primary neoplasms of the central nervous system in survivors of childhood cancer: a report from the Childhood Cancer Survivor Study. *J Natl Cancer Inst.* 2006;98:1528–1537.

45. de Vathaire F, Hawkins M, Campbell S, et al. Second malignant neoplasms after a first cancer in childhood: temporal pattern of risk according to type of treatment. *Br J Cancer.* 1999;79:1884–1893.

46. Kirova YM, Vilcoq JR, Asselain B, et al. Radiation-induced sarcomas after radiotherapy for breast carcinoma: a large-scale single-institution review. *Cancer.* 2005;104:856–863.

47. Cardis E, Kesminiene A, Ivanov V, et al. Risk of thyroid cancer after exposure to 131I in childhood. *J Natl Cancer Inst.* 2005;97:724–732.

48. Chaturvedi AK, Engels EA, Gilbert ES, et al. Second cancers among 104,760 survivors of cervical cancer: evaluation of long-term risk. *J Natl Cancer Inst.* 2007;99:1634–1643.

49. Dorr W, Herrmann T. Cancer induction by radiotherapy: dose dependence and spatial relationship to irradiated volume. *J Radiol Prot.* 2002;22:A117–A121.

50. Preston DL, Pierce DA, Shimizu Y, et al. Effect of recent changes in atomic bomb survivor dosimetry on cancer mortality risk estimates. *Radiat Res.* 2004;162:377–389.

51. Preston DL, Ron E, Tokuoka S, et al. Solid cancer incidence in atomic bomb survivors: 1958-1998. *Radiat Res.* 2007;168:1–64.

52. Hall EJ, Giaccia AJ. In: *Radiobiology for the radiologist.* 6th ed. Philadelphia: Lippincott Williams & Wilkins; 2006:ix.

53. Rubino C, de Vathaire F, Shamsaldin A, et al. Radiation dose, chemotherapy, hormonal treatment and risk of second cancer after breast cancer treatment. *Br J Cancer.* 2003;89:840–846.

54. Birch JM, Hartley AL, Tricker KJ, et al. Prevalence and diversity of constitutional mutations in the p53 gene among 21 Li-Fraumeni families. *Cancer Res.* 1994;54:1298–1304.

55. Frebourg T, Barbier N, Yan YX, et al. Germ-line p53 mutations in 15 families with Li-Fraumeni syndrome. *Am J Hum Genet.* 1995;56:608–615.

56. Li FP. Cancer families: human models of susceptibility to neoplasia—the Richard and Hinda Rosenthal Foundation Award lecture. *Cancer Res.* 1988;48:5381–5386.

57. Li FP, Fraumeni Jr JF, Mulvihill JJ, et al. A cancer family syndrome in twenty-four kindreds. *Cancer Res.* 1988;48:5358–5362.

58. Hisada M, Garber JE, Fung CY, et al. Multiple primary cancers in families with Li-Fraumeni syndrome. *J Natl Cancer Inst.* 1998;90:606–611.

59. Metcalfe K, Lynch HT, Ghadirian P, et al. Contralateral breast cancer in BRCA1 and BRCA2 mutation carriers. *J Clin Oncol.* 2004;22:2328–2335.

60. Thompson D, Easton DF. Cancer incidence in BRCA1 mutation carriers. *J Natl Cancer Inst.* 2002;94:1358–1365.

61. Garber JE, Offit K. Hereditary cancer predisposition syndromes. *J Clin Oncol.* 2005;23:276–292.

62. Alter BP, Greene MH, Velazquez I, et al. Cancer in Fanconi anemia. *Blood.* 2003;101:2072.

63. Rosenberg PS, Greene MH, Alter BP. Cancer incidence in persons with Fanconi anemia. *Blood.* 2003;101:822–826.

64. Dolan ME, Newbold KG, Nagasubramanian R, et al. Heritability and linkage analysis of sensitivity to cisplatin-induced cytotoxicity. *Cancer Res.* 2004;64:4353–4356.

65. Kalow W, Ozdemir V, Tang BK, et al. The science of pharmacological variability: an essay. *Clin Pharmacol Ther.* 1999;66:445–447.

66. Watters JW, Kraja A, Meucci MA, et al. Genome-wide discovery of loci influencing chemotherapy cytotoxicity. *Proc Natl Acad Sci U S A.* 2004;101:11809–11814.

67. Bhatia S, Sklar C. Second cancers in survivors of childhood cancer. *Nat Rev Cancer.* 2002;2:124–132.

68. Evans WE, Relling MV. Moving towards individualized medicine with pharmacogenomics. *Nature.* 2004;429:464–468.

69. Sparreboom A, Danesi R, Ando Y, et al. Pharmacogenomics of ABC transporters and its role in cancer chemotherapy. *Drug Resist Update.* 2003;6:71–84.

70. Relling MV, Yanishevski Y, Nemec J, et al. Etoposide and antimetabolite pharmacology in patients who develop secondary acute myeloid leukemia. *Leukemia.* 1998;12:346–352.

71. Marees T, Moll AC, Imhof SM, et al. Risk of second malignancies in survivors of retinoblastoma: more than 40 years of follow-up. *J Natl Cancer Inst.* 2008;100:1771–1779.

72. Begg CB, Zhang ZF, Sun M, et al. Methodology for evaluating the incidence of second primary cancers with application to smoking-related cancers from the Surveillance, Epidemiology, and End Results (SEER) program. *Am J Epidemiol.* 1995;142:653–665.

73. Do KA, Johnson MM, Lee JJ, et al. Longitudinal study of smoking patterns in relation to the development of smoking-related secondary primary tumors in patients with upper aerodigestive tract malignancies. *Cancer.* 2004;101:2837–2842.

74. Schottenfeld D. Alcohol as a co-factor in the etiology of cancer. *Cancer.* 1979;43(suppl 5):1962–1966.

75. Schottenfeld D, Fraumeni JF. In: *Cancer epidemiology and prevention.* 2nd ed. New York: Oxford University Press; 1996:xxi.

76. Pierce JP, Faerber S, Wright FA, et al. A randomized trial of the effect of a plant-based dietary pattern on additional breast cancer events and survival: the Women's Healthy Eating and Living (WHEL) Study. *Control Clin Trials.* 2002;23:728–756.

77. Rock CL, Natarajan L, Pu M, et al. Longitudinal biological exposure to carotenoids is associated with breast cancer-free survival in the Women's Healthy Eating and Living Study. *Cancer Epidemiol Biomarkers Prev.* 2009;18:486–494.

78. Calle EE, Rodriguez C, Walker-Thurmond K, et al. Overweight, obesity, and mortality from cancer in a prospectively studied cohort of U.S. adults. *N Engl J Med.* 2003;348:1625–1638.

79. Hisada M. Viral causes of cancer. In: Shields PG, ed. *Cancer risk assessment*. Taylor and Francis: Boca Raton; 2005:287–311.

80. de Araujo Souza PS, Sichero L, Maciag PC. HPV variants and HLA polymorphisms: the role of variability on the risk of cervical cancer. *Future Oncol*. 2009;5:359–370.

81. Schulz TF. Cancer and viral infections in immunocompromised individuals. *Int J Cancer*. 2009;125:1755–1763.

82. Oeffinger KC, Eshelman DA, Tomlinson GE, et al. Grading of late effects in young adult survivors of childhood cancer followed in an ambulatory adult setting. *Cancer*. 2000;88:1687–1695.

83. Sklar CA, Mertens AC, Mitby P, et al. Premature menopause in survivors of childhood cancer: a report from the childhood cancer survivor study. *J Natl Cancer Inst*. 2006;98:890–896.

84. Stevens MC, Mahler H, Parkes S. The health status of adult survivors of cancer in childhood. *Eur J Cancer*. 1998;34:694–698.

85. Children's Oncology Group. *Children's Oncology Group (COG)*. Bethesda, MD: Children's Oncology Group.

86. National Cancer Policy Board (U.S.), Weiner SL, Simone JV. In: *Childhood cancer survivorship: improving care and quality of life*. Washington, DC: National Academies Press; 2003:xvi.

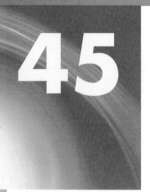

45

Complementary therapies in supportive oncology

Edzard K. Ernst

One possible definition of complementary therapies is treatments that are not normally used in conventional medicine. Because many centers now use complementary therapies routinely, this definition is problematic. Our own definition describes complementary medicine as "diagnosis, treatment, and/or prevention which complements mainstream medicine by contributing to a common whole, by satisfying a demand not met by orthodoxy, or by diversifying the conceptual frameworks of medicine."[1] Table 45-1 lists therapies that are among the most relevant in supportive oncology. Most of these treatments have not been associated with significant direct risks. However, a significant indirect risk would be associated with the use of any of them as an alternative to mainstream oncologic therapy. Fortunately, this is not a frequent occurrence in supportive oncology.

The aim of using these treatments in supportive oncology is to minimize the symptoms of the cancer or its treatment with a view toward enhancing well-being, reducing pain, and improving quality of life. Many cancer patients today use complementary therapies [2,3] but lack of information and misinformation are significant obstacles.[4] Cancer patients' reasons for trying complementary and alternative medicine (CAM) are complex, but rarely are they the expression of dissatisfaction with mainstream oncologic care.[2]

In the following sections, I will provide a brief description of the treatments listed in Table 45-1, as well as a summary of trial evidence related to these interventions. More detailed discussions can be found elsewhere.[5-7]

ACUPUNCTURE

DEFINITION

Acupuncture can be described as the insertion of a needle into the skin in special sites known as acupuncture points for therapeutic purposes.

BACKGROUND

The current flurry of interest in acupuncture started in the 1970s. Since then, its popularity has grown rapidly. A fundamental concept in acupuncture is "qi,"[8] often translated as "energy." Qi is thought to circulate through the body via 12 meridians, where 350 acupuncture points are located. Traditional acupuncturists view health as balance of the life forces yin and yang. It is believed that diseases are caused by an imbalance of these two opposites. Thus, every condition can be treated with acupuncture. No good evidence exists to confirm that qi or meridians are real.[9] Modern concepts explain the mode of action of acupuncture through neurophysiologic phenomena. For instance, acupuncture affects the

Table 45-1 Some of the treatments relevant in supportive oncology

Therapy	Percentage of hospices using this treatment*	Evidence	Significant direct risks (examples)
Acupuncture	32	Good only for chemotherapy-induced nausea and vomiting	Pneumothorax
Aromatherapy	45	Relaxation caused by gentle massage	None
Herbal medicine	n.i.	Mixed evidence, good for only a few herbs	Liver damage
Homeopathy	n.i.	No good evidence for highly diluted remedies	None
Hypnotherapy	16	Good evidence for reducing pain and anxiety	None
Imagery	45	May improve relaxation and reduce pain	None
Massage	87	Effective for a range of symptoms	None
Music therapy	74	Effective for pain reduction	None
Reflexology	19	A relaxing foot massage but nothing more	None
Relaxation therapy	n.i.	Conflicting results from clinical trials	None
Spiritual healing	65	No effect beyond placebo	None
Tai Chi	n.i.	Effects likely but may be due to flawed studies, not certain	None

*Data from ref Kozak LE, Kayes L, McCarty R, et al.[3]
n.i., No information

Table 45-2 Systematic reviews of acupuncture for supportive oncology

First author (year)[ref]	Subject	Number of primary studies	Conclusion (quote)
Lee (2009)[12]	Hot flashes in prostate cancer	6	The evidence is not convincing.
Lee (2009)[13]	Hot flashes in breast cancer	6	The evidence is not convincing.
Ezzo (2006)[14]	Chemotherapy-induced nausea and vomiting	11	[The evidence] suggests a biological effect on acupoint stimulation.
Lee (2005)[15]	Cancer pain	7	The notion that acupuncture is effective…is not supported by…rigorous clinical trials.
Jedel (2005)[16]	Xerostomia	3	…there is no evidence for the efficacy of acupuncture…

nervous and muscular systems[10] and releases neurotransmitters such as opioid peptides and serotonin.[10,11]

CLINICAL EVIDENCE

Table 45-2 is a summary of recent, high-quality systematic reviews of acupuncture trials pertaining to supportive oncology.[12-16]

These reviews reveal that, generally speaking, the evidence is weak and somewhat contradictory. Only for chemotherapy-induced nausea and vomiting do conclusively strong and positive data exist.[14] Because of numerous methodologic and other problems, current evidence allows ample room for interpretation. Clinical trials using sham devices (and thus controlling adequately for potential placebo effects) tend to show no or only small differences between real and sham acupuncture. These and other data[17] seem to suggest that the clinical effects of acupuncture are, to a large degree, the result of a placebo response.[18,19] Serious adverse effects of acupuncture (e.g., pneumothorax) are rare.

AROMATHERAPY

DEFINITION

Aromatherapy is defined as the controlled use of plant essences for therapeutic purposes.

BACKGROUND

Aromatherapists normally apply essential (the term is derived from *essence*) oils directly to the skin through gentle massage. This massage is claimed to be relaxing or stimulating, depending on the chemistry of the oil. The scent from the oil is believed to trigger the limbic system, which governs emotional responses. Essential oils are also absorbed through the skin and thus might have systemic pharmacologic effects. Yet the most important element in the relaxing action of aromatherapy seems to be the agreeably gentle manual massage.

CLINICAL EVIDENCE

A Cochrane review of 10 randomized controlled trials (RCTs) focused on aromatherapy and massage for symptom relief in patients with cancer. Reviewers found that "aromatherapy confers short-term benefits on psychological well-being, with the effect on anxiety supported by limited evidence."[20] Other RCTs fail to show benefit in terms of symptom control in cancer patients,[21] or pain control, anxiety, or quality of life in hospice patients.[22] One RCT tested whether the mere olfactory absorption of essential oils of lavender or rosemary affected pain sensitivity in healthy volunteers; the findings were negative.[23]

HERBAL MEDICINE

DEFINITION

Herbal medicine can be defined as the medical use of preparations that contain exclusively plant material.

BACKGROUND

Today, two very different types of herbal medicine are known. Modern herbalism (or phytomedicine) as practiced in many Western countries is integrated into conventional medicine. Other more traditional systems include Chinese herbal medicine, which is based on the concepts of yin and yang and qi energy (see earlier). In Japan, this system has evolved into kampo. Ayurveda, the traditional medical system of India, also frequently uses herbal mixtures. Characteristic of these traditional systems is a high degree of individualization of treatment (e.g., two patients with the same disease could receive two different herbal preparations). Contrary to modern phytomedicine, all traditional herbal medicine systems predominantly use complex mixtures of different herbs.

Herbal extracts contain pharmacologically active constituents. The active principle, which in many cases is unknown, may exert its effects at the molecular level. A single main constituent may be active, or, more often, a complex mixture of compounds produces a combined effect. Known active constituents or marker substances may be used to standardize herbal preparations.

CLINICAL EVIDENCE

The clinical evidence has to be evaluated according to each individual herbal preparation. In supportive oncology, preliminary evidence has been found for a range of herbal medicines.[6]

- Black cohosh *(Actaea racemosa)* has been shown to reduce hot flashes in breast cancer patients.
- *Calendula officinalis* cream alleviates radiation-induced dermatitis in breast cancer patients.
- Ginger reduces chemotherapy-induced nausea.[24]
- *Ginkgo biloba* reduces the symptoms of lymphedema after breast cancer therapy.
- Several Chinese herbal mixtures have improved the symptoms of cancer patients.

Contrary to this encouraging evidence for the rational use of herbal medicines, no good data are available to support the approach of individualized traditional herbalism (see earlier) for any condition.[25]

HOMEOPATHY

DEFINITION

Homeopathy is defined as a therapeutic method that usually uses highly diluted preparations of substances, whose effects, when administered to healthy subjects, correspond to manifestations of the disorder (symptoms, clinical signs, and pathologic states).

BACKGROUND

Homeopathy was developed by the German physician Samuel Hahnemann (1755–1843). Today, it is widely available again, not least because of a general trend toward alternative medicine. Homeopathy is based on two principles. The law of similars or "like cures like" principle states that a remedy that causes a certain symptom (e.g., a headache) in healthy volunteers can be used to treat a headache in a patient who suffers from it. According to the second principle, homeopathic remedies become more powerful when submitted to "potentization," that is, step-wise dilution of the remedy combined with vigorous shaking of the mixture. Thus, homeopaths believe that their remedies are clinically effective, even if they do not contain a single molecule of the original substance. Both principles fly in the face of science.

CLINICAL EVIDENCE

A Cochrane review investigated evidence for the notion that homeopathic medicines might reduce the adverse effects of cancer treatments.[26] Eight RCTs were reviewed, along with two studies that had a low risk of bias suggesting a clinical benefit: one of a calendula cream for the treatment of radiotherapy-induced dermatitis, and one of a proprietary mixed mouthwash for chemotherapy-induced stomatitis (Traumeels). Both of these preparations were not highly diluted, which is the hallmark of homeopathic remedies.

HYPNOTHERAPY

DEFINITION

Hypnotherapy is the induction of a trance-like state to facilitate relaxation and to treat psychological and medical conditions.

BACKGROUND

The Austrian physician Franz Anton Mesmer, in 1778, developed a treatment based on "magnetism." It was hugely successful until a Royal Commission investigated it and concluded that its effects were the result of the imagination. The goal of modern hypnotherapy is to gain self-control over behavior, emotions, or physiologic processes. This is achieved by inducing a hypnotic trance, whereby the patient's focus of attention is directed inward, thus allowing easier access to the noncritical unconscious mind.

CLINICAL EVIDENCE

Two meta-analyses[27,28] reported moderate to large analgesic effects of hypnotherapy. For pediatric oncology patients, a systematic review of eight clinical trials aimed to assess the effectiveness of hypnosis for procedure-related pain and distress.[29] This review concluded that hypnotherapy has considerable promise. A review of 15 clinical trials of hypnotherapy in children found promising but not compelling evidence for relief of pain, enuresis, and chemotherapy-related distress.[30] A further systematic review found no convincing evidence of effectiveness for terminally ill adult cancer patients.[31]

IMAGERY

DEFINITION

Imagery is a mind–body technique that uses the imagination and mental images of patients to generate relaxation.

BACKGROUND

Imagery is a visualization technique based on the idea that the mind can affect the functions of the body, and that stimulating the brain through visualization has direct effects on the endocrine and nervous systems.

CLINICAL EVIDENCE

A systematic review evaluating the evidence for imagery as a treatment for cancer patients concluded that it may be psychosupportive and may increase comfort.[32] Another systematic review reported that in patients near the end of life, relaxation/imagery can lessen pain from oral mucositis.[33] It has been suggested that the meaning of pain as a theme in patients' lives changes with the use of imagery.[34] Postoperatively, less pain and lower analgesic requirements attained through the use of imagery have been reported.[35,36]

MASSAGE

DEFINITION

Massage is a method of manipulating the soft tissue of body areas using pressure and traction.

BACKGROUND

The development of modern massage is attributed to the Swede Per Henrik Ling, who developed a system of massage and exercise termed Swedish massage. In the middle of the

19th century, it was introduced in the United States, and it was practiced predominantly by physicians until the early 20th century. Interest in massage therapy then gradually declined but increased again in the 1970s. Today, massage is considered a complementary therapy in most countries.

Various manual techniques are used to apply pressure and traction and to manipulate the soft tissues of the body. Mechanical pressure and friction on cutaneous and subcutaneous structures affect the circulation of blood and lymph and the nervous system, for instance, by reducing muscular tension.

CLINICAL EVIDENCE

A systematic review of 14 RCTs of massage therapy in supportive oncology showed a range of positive effects[37]: Massage effectively alleviated pain, nausea, anxiety, depression, anger, stress, and fatigue.

MUSIC THERAPY

DEFINITION

Music therapy can be defined as the use of music by an accredited professional to achieve individualized therapeutic goals.

BACKGROUND

Music therapy started to be recognized in North and South America in the 1940s. Music therapy is commonly based on psychoanalytic, humanistic, cognitive-behavioral, or developmental theory. Receptive music therapy includes listening to music played by the therapist for the patient or listening to recorded music selected by the therapist or the patient. In active music therapy, patients get involved in the music making. Sensations that accompany music therapy activate limbic or other areas of the brain related to the reward and motivation circuitry. Secondary physiologic changes and bodily reactions may follow.

CLINICAL EVIDENCE

A systematic review of the effectiveness of music as an intervention for hospital patients concluded that music may be an effective diversion.[38] Five RCTs found music therapy not to be superior to control interventions, and only one RCT reported less narcotic analgesia administered during the procedure via a patient-controlled device in the music group.

Several RCTs assessed the effect of music on patients undergoing surgery. Investigators found beneficial effects on pain after various types of operations[39-51] and procedures.[52-56]

REFLEXOLOGY

DEFINITION

Reflexology is a therapeutic method of applying manual pressure to specific areas of the feet that are believed to correspond to organs of the body.

BACKGROUND

In the early 20th century, William Fitzgerald discovered that the body was divided into 10 vertical zones, each represented by a part of the foot, including one toe. From this concept, the charts of bodily correspondences evolved. Reflexologists assume that the health of the body can be assessed by examining the feet to detect imbalances and obstructions to the flow of energy, which are expressed as tenderness or feelings of grittiness or crystal formation. Bodily functions are believed to be influenced by massaging these areas. No neurophysiologic basis for connections between organs or other body parts and specific areas of the feet is known. Reflexologists were no better than chance in identifying medical conditions in one blinded study.[57]

CLINICAL EVIDENCE

A recent systematic review included 18 RCTs of reflexology for any health problems and two RCTs for cancer palliation.[58,59] These results were contradictory, but the only placebo-controlled study failed to show positive effects. Thus the totality of the available data does not lend itself to a positive recommendation.

RELAXATION THERAPY

DEFINITION

Relaxation therapy uses techniques for eliciting the "relaxation response" of the autonomic nervous system.

BACKGROUND

Progressive muscle relaxation is one of the most commonly used relaxation techniques. It is based on the notion that it is impossible to be tense in any part of the body in which the muscles are completely relaxed. In addition, tension in involuntary muscles can be reduced if the associated skeletal muscles are relaxed. This technique is taught by tensing a muscle before relaxing it. Passive muscle relaxation involves the release of tension while focusing on muscle groups. Progressive muscle relaxation and other relaxation techniques generate a relaxation response, resulting in normalizing of the blood supply to the muscles, decreasing oxygen consumption, heart rate, respiration, and skeletal muscle activity and increasing skin resistance and alpha brain waves.

CLINICAL EVIDENCE

For patients with chronic cancer pain, an RCT reported positive effects of relaxation therapy.[60] However, an RCT testing imagery and progressive muscle relaxation for patients undergoing resections of colorectal cancer did not report differences related to analgesic consumption and pain intensity compared with a no-treatment control group.[61] A recent RCT of 150 breast cancer patients suffering from hot flashes suggested that relaxation training may effectively relieve this problem.[62]

SPIRITUAL HEALING

DEFINITION

Spiritual healing can be defined as the direct interaction between one individual (the healer) and a second (sick) individual with the intention of bringing about an improvement in the illness.[63]

BACKGROUND

Spiritual healing can be traced as far back as the Bible and has always had its adherents. In recent years, it has gained widespread popularity in the United States, the United Kingdom, and other countries. Spiritual healers believe that the therapeutic effect results from the channeling of healing "energy" from an assumed source via the healer to the patient. The central claim of healers is that they promote or facilitate self-healing in the patient. However, no scientific evidence is available to support the existence of this "energy," nor is there a scientific rationale for the concepts underlying spiritual healing.

CLINICAL EVIDENCE

A systematic review[64] of all types of healing included 23 placebo-controlled RCTs involving almost 3000 patients, many of them suffering from chronic pain. About half of these studies yielded a positive result. However, because of numerous methodologic limitations, no firm conclusions could be drawn. An update of this review included eight additional nonrandomized and nine randomized clinical trials.[65] These additional data collectively shifted the weight of evidence against the notion that healing involves more than a placebo. Cochrane reviews found no convincing evidence that intercessory prayer alleviates ill health of any type.[66] The largest RCT of intercessory prayer failed to show that healing is associated with specific therapeutic effects.[67] A recent RCT of 20 chronic pain patients showed that spiritual healing has no effect on pain over and above placebo.[68]

TAI CHI

DEFINITION

Tai Chi is a system of movements and postures rooted in ancient Chinese philosophy and martial arts aimed at enhancing mental and physical health.

BACKGROUND

Tai Chi has a long history in China, where it is widely practiced. Today, it is popular outside China as well. A number of different styles and forms comprising a series of postures are linked by gentle and graceful movements.

Tai Chi is based on the principles of yin and yang (see earlier). The slow movements of Tai Chi involve physical stimuli and have effects on the cardiovascular and muscular systems. These stimuli, much like other types of physical exercise, result in muscular adaptation. In addition to adaptation processes, these effects produce better cardiovascular function[69] and may enhance strength, balance, and coordination.[70]

CLINICAL EVIDENCE

A systematic review of health outcomes in patients with chronic conditions identified nine RCTs.[71] It concluded that Tai Chi generates physiologic and psychosocial benefits and is safe and effective in promoting balance control, flexibility, and cardiovascular fitness in older patients with chronic conditions. However, most of these studies were less than rigorous. Therefore, it is difficult to draw firm conclusions about the benefits reported. A systematic review of four clinical trials of Tai Chi in supportive oncology concluded that, because of the paucity and often low quality of primary data, the evidence is unconvincing.[72]

CONCLUSIONS

Cancer patients have many unmet supportive care needs.[73] Several treatments usually classified as complementary have shown considerable potential for meeting these needs. However, in most areas, the paucity and low quality of existing clinical trials prevent firm conclusions. In essence, this means that more research is required, particularly on those therapies that, so far, have generated the most encouraging results. To define the value of these treatments, we especially need studies that compare the effectiveness of conventional treatments to that of nonconventional therapies. Meanwhile, providers of supportive oncology need to be aware of existing evidence[74] and to use it wisely for the benefit of their patients.

REFERENCES

1. Ernst E, Resch KL, Mills S, et al. Complementary medicine—a definition. *Br J Gen Pract.* 1995;45:506.
2. Newsom-Davis T, Kenny L, Al-Shakarchi I, et al. Voodoo dolls and the cancer patient: patients do trust their doctors. *Q J Med.* 2009;(Jan):1–9.
3. Kozak LE, Kayes L, McCarty R, et al. Use of complementary and alternative medicine (CAM) by Washington state hospices. *Am J Hosp Palliat Care.* 2009;25:463–468.
4. Corner J, Yardley J, Maher EJ, et al. Patterns of complementary and alternative medicine use among patients undergoing cancer treatment. *Eur J Cancer Care.* 2009;18:271–279.
5. Ernst E, Pittler MH, Wider B, et al. *Complementary therapies for pain management.* St Louis: Mosby/Elsevier; 2007.
6. Ernst E, Pittler MH, Wider B, et al. *The desktop guide to complementary and alternative medicine.* 2nd ed. Edinburgh: Mosby/Elsevier; 2006.

7. Ernst E, Pittler M, Wider B, et al. *The Oxford handbook of complementary medicine.* Oxford: Oxford University Press; 2008.
8. Kaptchuck TJ. Acupuncture: theory efficacy and practice. *Ann Intern Med.* 2002;136:374–383.
9. Ramey DW. Acupuncture points and meridians do not exist. *Sci Rev Alt Med.* 2001;5:140–145.
10. Han J, Terenius L. Neurochemical basis of acupuncture analgesia. *Ann Rev Pharmacol Toxicol.* 1982;22:193–220.
11. Andersson S, Lundeberg T. Acupuncture—from empiricism to science: functional background to acupuncture effects in pain and disease. *Med Hypotheses.* 1995;45:271–281.
12. Lee MS, Kim K-H, Shin B-C, et al. Acupuncture for treating hot flushes in men with prostate cancer: a systematic review. *Support Care Cancer.* 2009;17:763–770.
13. Lee MS, Shin B-C, Ernst E. Acupuncture for treating menopausal hot flushes: a systematic review. *Climacteric.* 2009;12:16–25.

14. Ezzo JM, Richardson MA, Vickers A. et al. Acupuncture-point stimulation for chemotherapy-induced nausea or vomiting. *Cochrane Database Syst Rev.* 2006;19:CD002285.
15. Lee H, Schmidt K, Ernst E. Acupuncture for the relief of cancer-related pain—a systematic review. *Eur J Pain.* 2005;9:437–444.
16. Jedel E. Acupuncture in xerostomia—a systematic review. *J Oral Rehabil.* 2005;32:392–396.
17. Kaptchuk TJ, Stason WB, Davis RB, et al. Sham device and inert pill: randomised controlled trial of two placebo treatments. *BMJ.* 2006;332:391–397.
18. Ernst E. Acupuncture—a critical analysis. *J Intern Med.* 2006;259:125–137.
19. Moffet HH. Sham acupuncture may be as efficacious as true acupuncture: a systematic review of clinical trials. *J Altern Complement Med.* 2009;15:213–216.
20. Fellowes D, Barnes K, Wilkinson S. Aromatherapy and massage for symptom relief in patients with cancer. *Cochrane Database Syst Rev.* 2004; CD002287.

21. Wilcock A, Manderson C, Weller R, et al. Does aromatherapy massage benefit patients with cancer attending a specialist palliative care day centre? *Palliat Med.* 2004;18:287–290.

22. Soden K, Vincent K, Craske S, et al. A randomized controlled trial of aromatherapy massage in a hospice setting. *Palliat Med.* 2004;18:87–92.

23. Gedney JJ, Glover TL, Fillingim RB. Sensory and affective pain discrimination after inhalation of essential oils. *Psychosom Med.* 2004;66:599–606.

24. Levine ME, Gillis MG, Koch SY, et al. Protein and ginger for the treatment of chemotherapy-induced delayed nausea. *J Altern Complement Med.* 2008;14:545–551.

25. Guo R, Canter PH, Ernst E. A systematic review of randomised clinical trials of individualised herbal medicine in any indication. *Postgrad Med.* 2007;83:633–637.

26. Kassab S, Cummings M, Berkovitz S, et al. Homeopathic medicines for adverse effects of cancer treatments. *Cochrane Database Syst Rev.* 2009;(2) CD004845.

27. Montgomery GH, DuHamel KN, Redd WH. A meta-analysis of hypnotically induced analgesia: how effective is hypnosis? *Int J Clin Exp Hypn.* 2000;48:138–153.

28. Montgomery GH, David D, Winkel G, et al. The effectiveness of adjunctive hypnosis with surgical patients: a meta-analysis. *Anesth Analg.* 2002;94:1639–1645.

29. Richardson J, Smith JE, McCall G, et al. Hypnosis for procedure-related pain and distress in pediatric cancer patients: a systematic review of effectiveness and methodology related to hypnosis interventions. *J Pain Symptom Manage.* 2006;31:70–84.

30. Milling LS, Costantino CA. Clinical hypnosis with children: first steps toward empirical support. *Int J Clin Exp Hypn.* 2000;48:113–137.

31. Rajasekaran M, Edmonds PM, Higginson IL. Systematic review of hypnotherapy for treating symptoms in terminally ill adult cancer patients. *Palliat Med.* 2005;19:418–426.

32. Roffe L, Schmidt K, Ernst E. A systematic review of guided imagery as an adjuvant cancer therapy. *Psychooncology.* 2005;14:607–617.

33. Pan CX, Morrison RS, Ness J, et al. Complementary and alternative medicine in the management of pain, dyspnea, and nausea and vomiting near end of life: a systematic review. *J Pain Symptom Manage.* 2000;20:374–387.

34. Lewandowski W, Good M, Draucker CB. Changes in the meaning of pain with the use of guided imagery. *Pain Manag Nurs.* 2005;6:58–97.

35. Tusek DL, Church JM, Strong SA, et al. Guided imagery: a significant advance in the care of patients undergoing elective colorectal surgery. *Dis Colon Rectum.* 1997;40:172–178.

36. Laurion S, Fetzer SJ. The effect of two nursing interventions on the postoperative outcomes of gynaecologic laparoscopic patients. *J Perinesth Nurs.* 2003;18:254–291.

37. Ernst E. Massage therapy for cancer palliation and supportive care: a systematic review of randomised clinical trials. *Support Care Cancer.* 2009;17:333–337.

38. Evans D. The effectiveness of music as an intervention for hospital patients: a systematic review. *J Adv Nurs.* 2002;37:8–18.

39. Good M, Anderson GC, Stanton-Hicks M, et al. Relaxation and music reduce pain after gynecologic surgery. *Pain Manag Nurs.* 2002;3:61–70.

40. Good M, Anderson GC, Ahn S, et al. Relaxation and music reduce pain following intestinal surgery. *Res Nurs Health.* 2005;28:240–251.

41. Good M, Stanton-Hicks M, Grass JA, et al. Relaxation and music to reduced postsurgical pain. *J Adv Nurs.* 2001;33:215.

42. Good M, Stanton-Hicks M, Grass JA, et al. Relief of postoperative pain with jaw relaxation, music and their combination. *Pain.* 1999;81:163–172.

43. Kshettry VR, Carole LF, Henly SJ, et al. Complementary alternative medical therapies for heart surgery patients: feasibility, safety, and impact. *Ann Thorac Surg.* 2006;81:201–205.

44. Nilsson U, Rawal N, Unosson M. A comparison of intra-operative or postoperative exposure to music—a controlled trial of the effects on postoperative pain. *Anaesthesia.* 2003;58:699–703.

45. Nilsson U, Rawal N, Enqvist B, et al. Analgesia following music and therapeutic suggestions in the PACU in ambulatory surgery: a randomized controlled trial. *Acta Anaesthesiol Scand.* 2003;47:278–283.

46. Nilsson U, Unosson M, Rawal N. Stress reduction and analgesia in patients exposed to calming music postoperatively: a randomized controlled trial. *Eur J Anaesthesiol.* 2005;22:96–102.

47. Menegazzi JJ, Paris PM, Kersteen CH, et al. A randomized, controlled trial of the use of music during laceration repair. *Ann Emerg Med.* 1991;20:348–350.

48. Nilsson U, Rawal N, Unestahl LE, et al. Improved recovery after music and therapeutic suggestions during general anaesthesia: a double-blind randomised controlled trial. *Acta Anaesthesiol Scand.* 2001;45:812–817.

49. Voss JA, Good M, Yates B, et al. Sedative music reduces anxiety and pain during chair rest after open-heart surgery. *Pain.* 2004;112:197–203.

50. Heitz L, Symreng T, Samman FL. Effect of music therapy in the postanesthesia care unit: a nursing intervention. *J Post Anesth Nurs.* 1992;7:22–31.

51. Cepeda MS, Diaz JE, Hernandez V, et al. Music does not reduce alfentanil requirement during patient-controlled analgesia (PCA) use in extracorporeal shock wave lithotripsy for renal stones. *J Pain Symptom Manage.* 1998;16:382–387.

52. Chan YM, Lee PW, Ng TY, et al. The use of music to reduce anxiety for patients undergoing colposcopy: a randomized trial. *Gynecol Oncol.* 2003;91:213–217.

53. Lee DW, Chan KW, Poon CM, et al. Relaxation music decreases the dose of patient-controlled sedation during colonoscopy: a prospective randomized controlled trial. *Gastrointest Endosc.* 2002;55:33–36.

54. Uedo N, Ishikawa H, Morimoto K, et al. Reduction in salivary cortisol level by music therapy during colonoscopic examination. *Hepatogastroenterology.* 2004;51:451–453.

55. Kwekkeboom KL. Music versus distraction for procedural pain and anxiety in patients with cancer. *Oncol Nurs Forum.* 2003;30:433–440.

56. Jacobson AF. Intradermal normal saline solution, self-selected music, and insertion difficulty effects on intravenous insertion pain. *Heart Lung.* 1999;28:114–122.

57. White AR, Williamson J, Hart A, et al. A blinded investigation into the accuracy of reflexology. *Complement Ther Med.* 2000;8:166–172.

58. Ernst E. Is reflexology an effective intervention? A systematic review of randomised controlled trials. *Med J Aust.* 2009;191:263–266.

59. Hodgson H. Does reflexology impact on cancer patients' quality of life? *Nurs Stand.* 2000;14:33–38.

60. Reinhardt U. Investigations into synchronisation of heart rate and musical rhythm in a relaxation therapy in patients with cancer pain. [In German]. *Forsch Komplementarmed.* 1999;6:135–141.

61. Haase O, Schwenk W, Hermann C, et al. Guided imagery and relaxation in conventional colorectal resections: a randomized, controlled, partially blinded trial. *Dis Colon Rectum.* 2005; online. doi:10.1007/s10350-005-0114-9.

62. Fenlon DR, Corner JL, Haviland JS. A randomized controlled trial of relaxation training to reduce hot flashes in women with primary breast cancer. *J Pain Symptom Manage.* 2009;35:397–405.

63. Hodges RD, Scofield AM. Is spiritual healing a valid and effective therapy? *J Roy Soc Med.* 1995;88:203–207.

64. Astin J, Harkness E, Ernst E. The efficacy of spiritual healing: a systematic review of randomised trials. *Ann Intern Med.* 2000;132:903–910.

65. Ernst E. Distant healing—an "update" of a systematic review. *Wien Klin Wochenschr.* 2003;115:241–245.

66. Roberts L, Ahmed I, Hall S. Intercessory prayer for the alleviation of ill health. *Cochrane Database Syst Rev.* 2000;(2) CD000368.

67. Krucoff MW, Crater SW, Gallup D, et al. Music, imagery, touch, and prayer as adjuncts to interventional cardiac care: the Monitoring and Actualisation of Noetic Trainings (MANTRA) II randomised study. *Lancet.* 2005;366:211–217.

68. Lyvers M, Barling N, Harding-Clark J. Effect of belief in "psychic healing" on self-reported pain in chronic pain sufferers. *J Psychosom Res.* 2006;60:59–91.

69. Taylor-Piliae RE, Froelicher ES. Effectiveness of Tai Chi exercise in improving aerobic capacity: a meta-analysis. *J Cardiovasc Nurs.* 2004;19:48–57.

70. Wolfson L, Whipple R, Derby C, et al. Balance and strength training in older adults: intervention gains and Tai Chi maintenance. *J Am Geriatr Soc.* 1996;44:498–506.

71. Wang C, Collet JP, Lau J. The effect of Tai Chi on health outcomes in patients with chronic conditions: a systematic review. *Arch Intern Med.* 2004;164:493–501.

72. Lee MS, Pittler M, Ernst E. Is tai chi an effective adjunct in cancer care? A systematic review of controlled clinical trials. *Support Care Cancer.* 2007;15:597–601.

73. Harrison JD, Young KJM, Price MA, et al. What are the unmet supportive care needs of people with cancer? A systematic review. *Support Care Cancer.* 2009;17:1117–1128.

74. Broom A, Adams J. Oncology clinicians' accounts of discussing complementary and alternative medicine with their patients. *Health.* 2009;13:317–336.

COMMUNICATION AND DECISION MAKING

SECTION OUTLINE

46 Prognostic assessment of the cancer patient

Sheldon Kwok, Nadia Salvo, Jocelyn Pang, and Edward Chow

"Doctor, how long do I have to live?" This question, commonly asked by patients with advanced cancer, is feared by many healthcare practitioners.[1,2] Predicting how much time a patient has to live is arguably one of the most difficult tasks a practitioner will face. Knowing how much time one has left is of great importance to patients and their family members for making important medical and end-of-life decisions.[3,4]

Prognostication encompasses more than predicting a range of the time one has remaining. It is a term used in epidemiology for estimating the relative probabilities of several natural courses a disease may take; thus, prognoses can be made in a variety of situations.[2] Prognosis, diagnosis, and treatment are traditional clinical skills that are essential for high-quality medical practice.[1,5] Among these skills, the least amount of research has been conducted on prognostication.[2,6] The literature often ignores issues related to prognosis, and medical schools do not offer formal education on the topic.[6]

Prognostication is defined as the act of predicting an event, such as death, and is usually undertaken by a physician, but it can be done by other healthcare professionals as well.[6] A major difference between diagnostication and prognostication is that the former is static, but the latter is dynamic in nature. A diagnosis usually remains the same over time, whereas a prognosis may change many times over the course of a patient's disease.[2]

PROGNOSTICATION DEFINED

Prognostication is important in patients with advanced cancer because it allows healthcare professionals, patients, and family members to make important clinical decisions, plan for palliative care and supportive services, and prepare for the dying process.[1,3,4,7] Arriving at a prognosis for a patient with advanced cancer differs from making a prediction in earlier stages of the disease. Prognosis is no longer based on tumor site and stage in advanced phases; rather, it relies upon patient-related factors such as symptoms and measures of performance status.[8,9]

Knowledge of one's prognosis is important because a prognosis provides an estimate of when one should seek additional home care and possible placement in palliative or hospice care settings. Appropriate use of healthcare programs will decrease economic burden and provide optimal end-of-life care.[1] Patients are able to make informed decisions regarding treatment while weighing the benefits of prolonging life along with the risks of unwanted symptoms associated with life-extending therapies. Furthermore, practitioners may guide patients toward supportive treatments or services that would improve quality of life when increasing quantity of life is unlikely.[8,10] When patients are misinformed of their prognosis, they may have unrealistic treatment expectations.[4] Additionally, accurate prognoses would aid clinical decision making with regard to clinical trials or the design of new trials for terminal cancer patients.

CHALLENGES WITH PROGNOSTICATION

A clinician can never be exact in his or her estimation of life expectancy. Prognoses must be presented as probabilities rather than as individual estimates. A problem with presenting probabilities is that they can never be taken literally and are often based on studies with a small sample size that comprises patients who may not represent the general population.[2] It is important for clinicians to understand inherent biases within the literature. When formulating a prognosis, clinicians must consider that many individuals who meet study criteria are those with better prognoses who are quite different from the group of patients who were not eligible for participation in the studies.[2] This indicates that prognoses found in study populations may not apply to the general advanced cancer population.

Providing hope when delivering prognoses is a challenge for many clinicians.[2] It is important to maintain hope for patients with limited life expectancy,[11,12] while offering a realistic picture of the situation and not creating unlikely expectations.[13,14] Research has shown that clinicians are overly optimistic and often overestimate their prognoses.[3,7,15,16] This may lead to late referrals to palliative care and hospice, as well as delayed end-of-life care.[7]

Sensitivity to cultural differences is important when providing prognostic information. In some cultures, it is normal to provide information regarding diagnosis and prognosis to family members only, who may or may not choose to share the information with the patient. Mindfulness of such differences and avoidance of cultural stereotypes may be challenging to clinicians already burdened with the difficult task of prognostication.[2] The act of telling someone how long he or she has to live is challenging in itself. Although it is a challenge for the clinician to formulate (foresee) a prognosis, it is more difficult for many clinicians to discuss (foretell) this information with a patient.[2]

PATIENT UNDERSTANDING OF PROGNOSIS

Literature suggests that patients commonly misinterpret the prognostic information provided to them.[17,18] A number of studies in breast cancer have demonstrated patients' limited understanding of their prognosis.[19-23] Patients tend to remain overly optimistic regarding their prognoses even after discussing them with their physician.[24]

A study by Weeks et al.[25] evaluated the correlation between patients' understanding of their prognosis and their preference for comfort measures versus life-extending therapy. Investigators found that most patients believed there was a 90% chance or greater that they would be alive in 6 months, and thus were more likely to favor life-extending therapy over comfort measures. Weeks also found that patients who opted for life-extending therapy were 1.6 times more likely than those who chose comfort measures to have a hospital admission, attempted resuscitation, or death on a ventilator. Their 6-month survival was not statistically different from those who chose comfort measures only.

This chapter is written for clinicians, including physicians, nurses, counselors, and other professionals who work with advanced cancer patients. Our goal is to outline important factors that are shown to be associated with life expectancy in patients at advanced stages of cancer. We hope to provide useful prognostic models that have been validated in a hospice or a palliative outpatient setting, which you may consult when forming prognoses in the future.

The chapter is organized into the following headings:

- Clinical Predictions of Survival
- Prediction Factors
- Prognostic Tools and Models
- Communicating Prognosis
- Ethical Issues
- Conclusion

CLINICAL PREDICTIONS OF SURVIVAL

Clinical predictions of survival (CPS) influence medical decisions and help in planning of supportive care and allocation of resources.[26] They are crucial for patients and their families, allowing them to make the most of what time they have left. Clinicians are required to predict survival for patients to be considered for phase I clinical trials, as well as for hospice referrals.[27] Despite the consensus that end-of-life care should be supportive and aimed at managing symptoms,[28,29] few patients die at home, the preferred place of death[30]; less than 20% receive hospice care,[31] and the majority die in acute care hospitals.[30,32] One possible explanation for these findings is the inaccuracy of CPS.[3,7,15,16]

ACCURACY OF CPS

In 2001, Chow et al.[3] conducted a systematic review to examine the accuracy of CPS in terminally ill cancer patients. They identified 12 studies conducted between 1980 and 1999, 9 of which revealed that survival estimates tended to be inaccurate in an optimistic direction; however, the methods of obtaining CPS and the definition of errors in CPS varied from study to study. Nevertheless, Chow et al. expressed concern over the use of CPS alone for survival prediction, in that inaccurate survival predictions often result in inadequate delivery and choice of palliative care.

A study by Weeks et al.[25] in 1998 suggested that patients with overly optimistic prognostic estimates were much more likely to request highly aggressive, yet futile, life-extending therapy over palliative care that focuses on relief of pain and discomfort. The results of these studies demonstrate the need for an accurate predictive model in palliative settings that not only relies on CPS but takes into account other clinical symptoms such as performance status and weight loss.[33]

An updated systematic review was conducted by Glare et al.[1] in 2003 to examine the accuracy of CPS in terminally ill cancer patients. This review identified eight evaluable studies between 1972 and 2000 that provided 1563 individual prediction-survival dyads. The median CPS among these studies was found to be 42 days, and the median actual survival (AS) was 29 days, demonstrating the overly optimistic nature of CPS. Glare and associates also determined that the longer the CPS, the greater the variability in actual survival, with any CPS exceeding 6 months having no predictive value for actual survival. The authors, however, found that the log transformation of CPS was significantly correlated with the log transformation of AS in the eight studies, suggesting that despite its limitations, CPS was still one of the best predictors of survival, and that clinicians are still able to sense when things begin to go wrong. A similar conclusion was made in a previous systemic review by Vigano et al. in 2000.[34]

One theory that has been documented in relation to survival prediction is the "horizon effect," an analogy to meteorology, in which short-term forecasts are usually more accurate than long-term forecasts.[3,34,35] The horizon effect observed in prognostication suggests that CPS is more accurate when short-term predictions are made, such as toward the end of a patient's life, than long-term survival predictions of several months or longer. The systematic review by Glare et al.[1] supports the concept of the horizon effect for CPS, but other studies have arrived at conflicting conclusions.[36-39] Other trends that have been observed include improved prediction with repeated estimates, as well as with physician experience[3,8]; also, decreased accuracy is noted with stronger doctor-patient relationships.[40]

Research has shown that CPS and Karnofsky performance status* (KPS) were closely related (r = 0.61), suggesting that clinicians take into account patient performance status when making survival predictions.[8,41] This demonstrates the need for more research on this topic to better understand the rationale behind CPS.

FORESEEING AND FORETELLING

In addition to the difficulty of forming an accurate CPS, prognostication requires clinicians to perform an additional, perhaps even more challenging, task: communicating the prognosis to their patients. Lamont and Christakis[27] divided prognostication into two separate categories: foreseeing and foretelling. Foreseeing is the survival estimate that practitioners determine; foretelling involves communicating that prognosis to the patient. Their study suggests that physicians not only make overly optimistic errors in foreseeing patient's prognoses, but they make equally large optimistic errors in foretelling their predictions to patients. A potential reason for this error in foretelling is clinicians' desire to provide hope.[42] The need for hope and optimism is an ideal supported by both doctors and patients. However, there is a fine line between fostering realistic hope and creating unrealistic expectations and perhaps encouraging futile treatments.[13]

Past studies have focused on investigating patient preferences for prognosticating cancer survival in the advanced setting. Most patients desired detailed information about their disease, but preferred to negotiate the format, extent, and timing of the information they receive from their caregivers.[43-45] Patients with higher depression scores were found to be more likely to want to know the shortest time to live without treatment, but patients with lower depression scores preferred to never discuss expected survival.[43] Patients who were expected to live longer were more likely to discuss prognosis at their first consultation, but patients with children preferred to discuss prognosis later or never.[43]

Despite patients' desire to know how long they have to live, studies have shown infrequent communication of prognostic information between doctors and patients.[47,48] Concern is noted in the literature over whether patients fully understand the information that is given to them.[18,49] It is evident that communicating prognostic information is difficult for both patients and clinicians, and it becomes increasingly difficult as the news gets worse.[42]

A study by Butow et al.[13] in 2002 identified seven themes related to disclosure of prognostic information to patients with metastatic disease:

1. Communication within a caring, trusting, long-term relationship
2. Open and repeated negotiations regarding patient preferences for information
3. Clear, straightforward presentation of prognosis where desired
4. Strategies to ensure patient understanding
5. Encouragement of hope and a sense of control
6. Consistency of communication within the multidisciplinary team
7. Communication with and care of other members of the family, whose needs may differ from those of the patient

Communicating a prognosis to an advanced cancer patient is a challenging task, and clinicians must remember that each patient is unique and has specific needs and preferences that may change during the course of their disease.[50]

NEED FOR MODELS

As a result of difficulties faced and overall inaccuracies that result for clinicians in both foreseeing and foretelling patient prognosis, increasing focus has been placed on identifying predictors of survival that could aid clinicians in their prognostic estimates for similar patients.[51] The main advantages of CPS as a prognostic tool are its flexibility and availability,[8] but additional research in clinical psychology has shown that statistical methods are generally superior to CPS in predicting survival and other human behaviors.[52] In their systematic review, Maltoni et al.[9] recommended that CPS should be used in combination with other prognostic factors or scores to improve survival predictions.

PREDICTION FACTORS

Multiple causes of death have been identified in patients with terminal cancer. Predictors of these causes are often unapparent.[34] Prognostic factors are important to recognize in the advanced cancer population because they differ from those seen in early-stage disease.[8,9] Although diagnostic, pathologic, and treatment-related factors are important in early-stage cancers,

---

*A standard measure of performance. Ranges from 0 to 100, with the highest score being the best performance and 0 being death.[46]

they do not contribute to prognostication accuracy for terminal patients.[8] Identifying predictive factors for life expectancy is important to ensure that ethical and clinical decisions are made appropriately and resources are used most efficiently. Knowledge of these factors will also improve communication between physician and patient when discussing prognosis.[53]

Clinician predictions of survival (CPS), when used alone, are often imprecise.[53] Research has suggested that CPS is 3 to 5 times greater than actual survival, and clinicians underestimate only 20% of the time.[53] To improve clinicians' predictions, many research groups have studied specific prognostic factors to determine which correlate with actual survival.[54]

Two systematic reviews summarize the prognostic factors that have been identified as good predictors of life expectancy in advanced cancer patients.[9,34] Vigano et al.[34] examined 22 studies in which a total of 136 factors were investigated for correlation with survival. Qualitative review of these studies yielded factors that were described as "possibly" or "definitely" associated with decreased life expectancy. Factors that were possibly correlated include gender, primary tumor location, pain, serum albumin, and tachycardia. Those that were considered definitely linked are low performance status, CPS, cognitive impairment, anorexia, dyspnea, xerostomia, weight loss, and dysphagia. In a similar, more recent review by the Steering Committee of the European Association for Palliative Care,[9] physical, psychological, and biological factors were identified that were associated with limited survival. Items listed as having a definite correlation with prognosis included CPS, performance status, signs and symptoms of cancer anorexia-cachexia syndrome (including weight loss, dysphagia, and xerostomia), delirium, dyspnea, leukocytosis, lymphocytopenia, C-reactive protein levels, and prognostic scores. The authors also listed a variety of factors for which a correlation has been indicated but not yet confirmed.*

Based on the research, the following predictive factors are identified as highly correlated with prognosis and therefore will be discussed in greater detail: performance status, anorexia-cachexia syndrome, dyspnea, delirium, and biological factors.

PERFORMANCE STATUS

Performance status is the most extensively studied factor in prognostication and has been shown to consistently correlate with survival prediction.[8] A review by Maltoni et al.[9] found 20 studies that identified performance status as prognostically significant. Tools commonly used to evaluate patient performance status include KPS and the Palliative Performance Scale (PPS).[53] Among these tools, KPS is the most commonly used for quantifying performance status in the cancer population.[3] A KPS score of less than 50 is associated with decreased life expectancy[8]; however, initially high performance status does not indicate increased survival.[9] Although performance status is regarded as one of the most important prognostic factors, it accounts for only a small percentage of the variability in actual survival.[8]

PPS was developed as a modification of KPS by Anderson et al.[55] Similar to KPS, PPS rates patients from 0 (death) to 100

(normal functioning), adding categories for oral intake and level of consciousness.[55] PPS scores correlate strongly with KPS and also function as a good prognostic indicator. Some argue whether PPS scores represent distinct survival deciles or rather represent three prognostic groups: 1 week, 1 month, and 3 months (PPS 10–20, 30–50, and 60–70, respectively).[8] Similar to CPS, performance status as a prognostic indicator increases in accuracy with assessment of other predictive factors.[53]

ANOREXIA-CACHEXIA SYNDROME

The anorexia-cachexia syndrome, which includes weight loss, dysphagia, and xerostomia, is a commonly observed symptom; the prevalence of cachexia is greater than 80% in advanced cancer patients.[53] A patient who presents with anorexia, dysphagia, and weight loss may be described by some as having the "terminal cancer syndrome."[56] Weight loss has been associated with short- and long-term survival differences and has been reported to worsen side effects of cancer treatment and decrease functional status.[57] One study reported weight loss of greater than 5% in the preceding 6 months to be prognostically significant and to carry a prognostic value independent of other factors.[58] Weight loss in the cancer population is unlike that of a normal population; weight loss in cancer patients leads to wasting of lean muscle mass, rather than to a decrease in adipose tissue. Because lean muscle is responsible for a variety of bodily functions essential to life, those who lose an excessive amount of lean tissue (>40%) have a decreased survival period.[57] Weight loss is of great concern to patients because it is a visible sign that symbolizes proximity to death and loss of control.[59] Furthermore, pharmacologic interventions have little effect on weight loss in advanced cancer patients in terms of limiting or arresting the symptom.

DYSPNEA

Dyspnea, also referred to as breathlessness, is common in patients with advanced cancer.[60] It has been described as awareness of one's breathing and is an unpleasant feeling for those who experience it.[53] Approximately 21% to 71% of cancer patients will experience dyspnea; it most often occurs with greater severity near the end of life.[53,60] Dyspnea has been proven to be highly correlated with muscle wasting and weakness in terminal cancer patients.[56] Compared with other predictive factors, dyspnea is most associated with a short prognosis.[56] A study conducted by Hardy et al.[61] on patients admitted to a palliative care unit in a cancer hospital showed breathlessness to be one of two factors with the highest relative risk of death in multivariate analysis. The pathophysiology of dyspnea is not well understood; thus it remains a symptom that is poorly treated. To improve the use of dyspnea as a prognostic symptom, it is important to develop a more effective method of revealing its presence because it is difficult to identify.[56]

DELIRIUM

In the cancer population, delirium is defined as "an acutely disordered state of mind involving disturbances of consciousness and either perception or cognition, including confusion, disorientation, and changes in attention, memory, psychomotor behavior, emotion and the sleep-wake cycle."[62] Delirium is a very informative predictor of imminent death, as it is commonly

---

*Factors for which a correlation is indicated but not confirmed include pain, nausea, tachycardia, fever, neoplastic pattern (primary and secondary sites), comorbidity, anemia, hypoalbuminemia, prehypoalbuminemia, proteinuria, serum calcium level, serum sodium level, lactate dehydrogenase and other enzymes, and demographic characteristics.[34]

seen as the neuropsychiatric manifestation of the dying process. Delirium has frequently been proven to be an independent prognostic indicator for survival.[53,62] Causes of delirium in palliative patients are multifactorial in two thirds of cases and include opioids, metabolic disorders, infection, recent anesthetic or surgery, dehydration, organ failure, and corticosteroid therapy, among others. It is important to recognize reversible delirium by capturing appropriate patient histories to treat the symptom and gather crucial prognostic information.[62]

BIOLOGICAL FACTORS

The three most commonly reported biological factors with prognostic significance are leukocytosis, lymphocytopenia, and elevated C-reactive protein levels.[9,53,63] These biological parameters have also been proven to be prognostically significant in patients at less advanced stages of disease.[9] It is often difficult to study biological factors in the terminally ill cancer population as this requires more invasive blood testing, which may be undesirable to the patient if unnecessary.[9] Additional studies are needed to assess the role of biological prognostic factors; however, studies that have looked at these to date commonly reveal the three aforementioned parameters as prognostically valid.[34]

Many factors have been studied as predictive factors for prognosis. Consensus in the literature indicates that prognostic factors for those with advanced cancer are different from predictive factors of prognosis in early-stage disease.[53] Because terminally ill cancer patients represent such a heterogeneous group, it is difficult to recognize and study predictive factors that retain high external validity across settings.[4] Because of this, models that have been established and validated use certain predictive factors identified through statistical means as highly correlated with prognosis in specific populations.

PROGNOSTIC TOOLS AND MODELS

Prognostic tools have been developed over the years to enhance the accuracy of survival predictions. With clinicians reported to be consistently overestimating survival,[3,15,16,32] predictive models are needed not only to improve the decision making of healthcare providers, but to benefit patients and families who wish to maximize remaining time.[31] Traditionally, prognosis for cancer patients is determined by tumor-related factors, including clinical, imaging, laboratory, pathologic, and molecular features. Unfortunately, these models would require tests not suitable for a palliative population and would be less precise in predicting the short-term outcomes of patients with advanced cancer.[64] As a result, newer models for patients with terminal cancer have been developed that incorporate patient-related prognostic factors that have been shown to correlate with survival. However, because of the inconsistency of prognostic variables between cancer patients and the inaccuracy of CPS, no single prognostic tool has been universally successful and useful in predicting patient outcomes in the advanced cancer setting.[65] Several validated prognostic models will be discussed, including the Palliative Prognostic (PaP) Score, the Palliative Performance Index (PPI), and a predictive model for survival of outpatients in a palliative radiotherapy clinic. The PaP score and the PPI were the two prognostic scores or indices recommended for use by the European Association for Palliative Care in a systematic review of prognostic factors.[9]

PALLIATIVE PROGNOSTIC (PaP) SCORE

The Palliative Prognostic (PaP) Score was developed in 1999 in an effort to identify both clinical and biological prognostic factors that predict survival in terminally ill cancer patients.[65,66] Pirovano et al.[66] enrolled 540 eligible patients from 22 Italian hospice centers from October 1992 to November 1993 and identified statistically significant factors from individual multivariate analyses based on various clinical and biological parameters. The PaP score was then developed by integrating resulting factors into a separate exponential regression model. These factors, each of which was observed to have independent prognostic value, included anorexia, CPS, dyspnea, KPS, lymphocyte percentage, and total white blood count. Each factor is allocated a certain partial score, and these subscores are summed to obtain the final PaP score (Table 46-1). PaP scores from 0 to 5.5 were classified as Group A (survival at 30 days >70%), from 5.6 to 11.0 as Group B (survival at 30 days 30%–70%) and >11.0 as Group C (survival at 30 days <30%). Figure 46-1 demonstrates the very different survival experiences that each risk group had, which led investigators to believe that the PaP Score model could help clinicians classify patients in prognostically homogeneous classes. This could facilitate treatment decisions and patient consultation.

The same team of Italian researchers validated the PaP score by testing it on a similar but independent population of 451 evaluable patients in 14 Italian hospice centers from January to August 1996.[63] By applying the same previously used scoring system, patients were classified into three groups that had survival probability at 30 days of 86.6%, 51.6%, and 16.9%, respectively. These results matched the expected results outlined by the model and were remarkably similar to those of the original set (82.0%, 52.7%, and 9.6%). The authors noted that the CPS used to calculate the PaP score in both case series were made by physicians who had sufficient knowledge and experience. An additional question is whether the CPS given by a referring physician or a physician untrained in palliative care would be as accurate. However, an advantage of the PaP score is that it does not rely on CPS alone, potentially "correcting" any inaccuracies of CPS with other prognostic variables, all of which again have independent prognostic value.[63]

In an effort to determine the effectiveness of the PaP score in a different setting from which it was originally developed, Glare and Virik validated the PaP score within a heterogeneous population of 100 terminally ill patients at a university teaching hospital in Australia.[67] They determined the percentage survival at 30 days for the three groups to be 66%, 54%, and 5%, respectively; these rates were relatively similar to the previous case series done by the team of Italian doctors. The authors concluded that the PaP score appeared to be a reasonably robust model for prognostication in advanced cancer independent of the setting. A later study by Glare et al.[68] also showed the PaP score to be accurate in predicting survival in patients with less advanced disease still under the care of an oncologist. Glare concluded that the PaP score was a simple yet valid tool that can be used by busy clinicians to formulate a prognosis.[68] Nevertheless, concerns over use of the PaP score include its heavy dependence on CPS,[67,69] the fact that it requires blood tests that may not be appropriate for a palliative population,[3,67] the omission of delirium as a symptom,[52] and the fact that its clinical usefulness is limited by its ability to predict survival probability of only 1 month.[68]

Table 46-1 Computing the PaP score

Factor	Partial score
Dyspnea	
No	0
Yes	1
Anorexia	
No	0
Yes	1.5
KPS	
≥30%	0
10–20	2.5
CPS	
>12	0
11–12	2
7–10	2.5
5–6	4.5
3–4	6
1–2	8.5
Total WBC	
Normal (4800–8500 cells/mm³)	0
High (8501–11,000 cells/mm³)	0.5
Very high (>11,000 cells/mm³)	2.5
Lymphocyte percentage	
Normal (20.0%–40.0%)	0
Low (12.0%–19.9%)	1
Very low (0–11.9%)	2.5
Risk groups	**Total score**
A (30 day survival probability > 70%)	0–5.5
B (30 day survival probability 30-70%)	5.6–11
C (30 day survival probability <30%)	11.5–17.5

Source: Adapted from Table 3 of Maltoni M, Nanni O, Pirovano M, et al. Successful validation of the palliative prognostic score in terminally ill cancer patients. Italian Multicenter Study Group on Palliative Care. J Pain Symptom Manage 1999;17:240-7.
CPS, Clinical prediction of survival; KPS, Karnofsky performance status; PaP, Palliative Prognostic Score; WBC, white blood cell count.

PALLIATIVE PROGNOSTIC INDEX (PPI)

The Palliative Prognostic Index (PPI) was developed by Japanese researchers in 1999 in response to the need for an accurate method of predicting survival to effectively plan palliative care.[70,71] Morita et al. determined from experience that whether a patient dies within a few weeks or lives for longer than a month is clinically significant. The goal of the PPI was to act as a simple judgment tool to predict 3- and 6-week survival.

Similar to the development of the PaP score, researchers first performed a prospective study on 150 hospice inpatients and established five factors as independent predictors of survival: PPS (Palliative Performance Scale), appetite loss, edema, dyspnea at rest, and delirium.[70] In their initial study, Morita et al. created a classification system based solely on the presence or absence of clinical symptoms (Table 46-2). This classification system successfully predicted 3- and 6-week survival with a sensitivity and specificity of greater than 70%.[70]

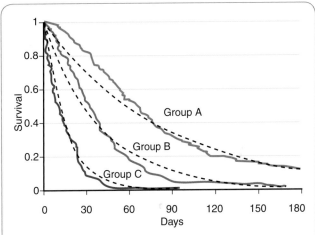

Fig. 46-1 Survival experience of the three groups of patients identified by the Palliative Prognostic (PaP) score. Survival probabilities were estimated by the exponential model (dotted lines) and by the Kaplan-Meier method (continuous lines). Log rank = 294.8 (2 df), P < .001. Risk groups' total score: A (178 patients), 30-day survival probability >70%, 0 to 5.5; B (205 patients), 30-day survival probability 30% to 70%, 5.6 to 11.0; and C (136 patients), 30-day survival probability <30%, 11.1 to 17.5. (Redrawn from Maltoni M, Nanni O, Pirovano M, et al. Successful validation of the palliative prognostic score in terminally ill cancer patients. Italian Multicenter Study Group on Palliative Care. J Pain Symptom Manage 1999;17:240-247.)

Table 46-2 Classification for survival prediction: statistically significant prognostic factors

<3 weeks survival	<6 weeks survival
PPS = 10–20	PPS = 10–20
Dyspnea at rest	Dyspnea at rest
Delirium	Delirium
	Edema

Sources: Stone CA, Tiernan E, Dooley BA. Prospective validation of the palliative prognostic index in patients with cancer. J Pain Symptom Manage 2008;35:617-22; Alloway L, Minton O. The accuracy of the clinical prediction of survival: a comparison of doctors' and nurses' estimations and the failure to validate the Palliative Prognostic Score. (PaP). Palliat Med 2004;18:155.
PPS, Palliative Performance Status.

With the development of the PaP score, Morita et al.[71] decided to develop and validate a similar scoring system with the same prognostic factors that were previously determined.[71] The authors noted that Maltoni et al., in their development of the PaP score, had not confirmed nor optimized cutoff points for actual survival prediction and as a result developed the Palliative Prognostic Index (PPI) with an appropriate cutoff point. Patients from a palliative care unit were initially enrolled in a training set to determine and construct the prognostic scoring system. Subsequent patients were enrolled into a second independent set to test the prognostic indicator (Table 46-3). Figure 46-2 illustrates the survival curves in the training set with different PPI scores. Researchers suggested using

Table 46-3 Calculating the Palliative Performance Index

Factor	Partial score
PPS 10%–20%	4
PPS 30%–50%	2.5
PPS >50%	0
Oral intake, mouthfuls or less	2.5
Oral intake, moderately reduced	1
Oral intake, normal	0
Edema	1
Dyspnea at rest	3.5
Delirium	4

Source: Adapted from Table 3 in Stone CA, Tiernan E, Dooley BA. Prospective validation of the palliative prognostic index in patients with cancer. *J Pain Symptom Manage.* 2008;35:617–622.

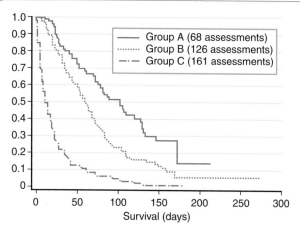

Fig. 46-2 Survival curves of groups with different scores on the Palliative Prognostic Index (PPI): Group A, PPI ≤2.0; Group B, 2.0<PPI≤4.0; and Group C, PPI >4.0. *(Redrawn from Stone CA, Tiernan E, Dooley BA. Prospective validation of the palliative prognostic index in patients with cancer. J Pain Symptom Manage 2008;35:617-22. Source: Chow E, Abdolell M, Panzarella T, et al. Predictive model for survival in patients with advanced cancer. J Clin Oncol 2008;26:5863–5869.)*

a PPI of greater than 4 as a cutoff point for 6-week survival (positive predictive value [PPV] of 0.76, negative predictive value [NPV] of 0.85), and a PPI of 6 or more as a cutoff point for 3 week survival (PPV of 0.83, NPV of 0.71). The high positive and negative predictive values led the authors to conclude that their scoring system was suitable for predicting short-term survival of patients with advanced cancer.[65,71]

A later study by the same research team compared the accuracy of the CPS recorded by a physician who had a reference to the patient's PPI score versus a CPS recorded by a physician who did not know the patient's PPI score.[72] The study suggested that PPI does contribute to improvement in physicians' ability to predict survival in terminally ill cancer patients, after significant reductions in differences between actual survival and CPS were observed. The most recent validation of PPI was done in Ireland by Stone et al. in 2008.[69] One hundred ninety-four patients from a hospital, a hospice home care service, and hospice inpatient units were enrolled in the study, and PPI scores were recorded. Predictions of survival of less than 3 and 6 weeks were found to be highly specific but only moderately sensitive, suggesting that although the PPI is fairly accurate in patients with a short prognosis, it does not identify all patients with a short prognosis. However, it was evident that PPI remained valid even in a different population and over a variety of care settings.[69]

Potential issues of the PPI model include that the patients used to construct the indicator (from Japan) may not be representative of a general population of patients with advanced cancer,[69,72] and that survival prediction of patients whose PPI was near cutoff points may not be practical.[72] Overall, a major advantage of PPI is that it does not require any invasive tests, such as blood sampling, making it a potentially easy, objective, and accurate scoring system to help clinicians plan medical treatment or collect homogeneous patients for an intervention trial.[69,71-73] In fact, Stone et al. proposed that the PPI has numerous advantages over the PaP score, including ease of use, reliability, and breadth of validity.[73] Currently, no studies have been conducted to compare the efficacy of different scores.[9,69]

PREDICTIVE MODEL FOR OUTPATIENT SURVIVAL IN A PALLIATIVE RADIOTHERAPY CLINIC

Optimal dose fractionation for radiotherapy is often based on the radiation oncologist's estimate of patients' survival. A prognostic model using six prognostic factors (primary cancer site, site of metastases, KPS, and three symptoms from the Edmonton Symptom Assessment Scale* [ESAS]: fatigue, appetite, and shortness of breath) was designed to predict the survival of English-speaking outpatients in a palliative radiotherapy clinic in Canada.[4] Unfortunately, gathering information on these six factors may be difficult because of language barriers or inability to complete the ESAS due to illness or lack of assistance. Thus, a simpler model using three readily available parameters (primary cancer site, sites of metastases, and KPS) was developed by the same group with the same method

*The Edmonton Symptom Assessment Scale (ESAS) is a tool for self-reporting of symptom intensity, designed for advanced cancer patients. It consists of numerical rating scales for nine common symptoms from 0 to 10.[74]

Table 46-4   Three-variable model for outpatients at palliative radiotherapy clinic

Survival prediction score (SPS) method		Number of risk factors (NRF) method
Sum of partial scores		*Risk factors*
Primary cancer site		1. Nonbreast cancer
Breast	0	2. Sites of metastases other than bone only
Prostate	2	3. Karnofsky performance status (SPS) ≤60
Lung	3	
Others	3	
Sites of metastases		
Bone metastases only	0	
Others	2	
KPS		
>60	0	
≤60	3	

Survival probabilities			
Group A (SPS ≤4)		**Group 1 (NRF ≤1)**	
3 month survival	83%–96%	3 month survival	80%–87%
6 month survival	64%–72%	6 month survival	63%–73%
12 month survival	51%–53%	12 month survival	53%–54%
Group B (SPS = 5)		**Group 2 (NRF = 2)**	
3 month survival	69%–78%	3 month survival	68%–76%
6 month survival	48%–53%	6 month survival	45%–52%
12 month survival	23%–25%	12 month survival	23%–26%
Group C (SPS ≥6)		**Group 3 (NRF = 3)**	
3 month survival	40%–46%	3 month survival	34%–44%
6 month survival	17%–28%	6 month survival	14%–27%
12 month survival	7%–13%	12 month survival	3%–11%

Source: Chow E, Abdolell M, Panzarella T, et al. Predictive model for survival in patients with advanced cancer. J Clin Oncol 2008;26:58.

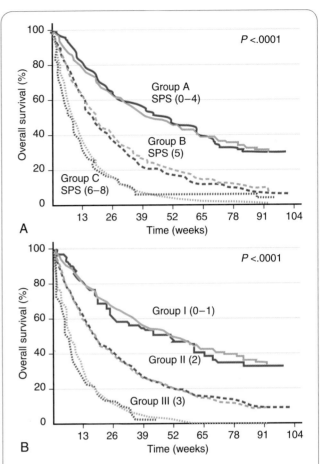

Fig. 46-3   Three- factor model: **A,** Survival prediction score (SPS) model developed from 1999 data. **B,** Number of risk factors (NRF) model developed from 1999 data. Estimated survival probabilities from Cox's model *(dotted lines)* and actual outcomes estimated by the Kaplan-Meier method *(solid lines)* are shown.

to determine median survival times and probability of survival at 3, 6, and 12 months for patients with advanced cancer.[75]

Using data from 395 patients from 1999, two risk group stratification methods were developed (Table 46-4): survival prediction score (SPS) and number of risk factors (NRF). The SPS ranged from 0 to 8 and was used to form three risk groups: Group A (SPS ≤4), Group B (SPS = 5), and Group C

(SPS ≥6). This led to fair separation of survival curves, as can be seen in Figure 46-3, *A*.

Three factors were identified for the NRF model: nonbreast cancer, sites of metastases other than bone, and KPS ≤60. Group 1 consisted of patients with 0 or 1 risk factor; Group 2 patients had 2 risk factors; Group 3 patients had all 3 risk factors. This, similar to the SPS model, led to fair separation of survival curves, as can be seen in Figure 46-3, *B*.

The three-variable model was validated by applying the SPS and NRF stratifications to two different datasets of similar patient characteristics. Similar survival probability at 3 months was observed in temporal, external, and training datasets. For the SPS method, survival probability at 3 months ranged from 80% to 96% in Group A, from 69% to 78% in Group B, and from 40% to 46% in Group C. For the NRF method, 3-month survival probability ranged from 80% to 87% in Group 1, from 68% to 76% in Group 2, and from 34% to 44% in Group 3 (see Table 46-4). The performance of this three-variable model was measured using a simple index of separation (PSEP) between prognostic groups. The PSEP (Table 46-5) is the difference between Pworst (the predicted probability of dying for a patient in the group with the

Table 46-5 Three-variable model for outpatients at palliative radiotherapy clinic: summary of median survival, survival probability and PSEP of the training, temporal, and external validation sets

Predictive model	Training set 1999 (n = 395)	Temporal validation set 2000 (n = 445)	External validation set 2002 (n = 467)
Partial score method			
Median survival (95% CI), weeks			
Group A (SPS ≤4)	60 (41%–70%)	53 (36%–75%)	64 (28%–undefined)[6]
Group B (SPS 5)	26 (19%–31%)	21 (18%–32%)	29 (23%–34%)
Group C (SPS ≥6)	10 (8%–13%)	11 (9%–13%)	10 (8%–15%)
Survival probability at 3,6, and 12 months, respectively, %			
Group A (SPS ≤4)	82, 70, and 52	96, 72, and 51	83, 64, and 53
Group B (SPS 5)	71, 51, and 24	69, 48, and 25	78, 53, and 23
Group C (SPS 6–8)	40, 17, and 7	42, 21, and 8	46, 28, and 13
PSEP, %			
At 3 months	42	44	37
At 6 months	53	51	36
At 12 months	45	43	40
Number of risk factors method			
Median survival (95% % CI), weeks			
Group 1 (NRF ≤1)	60 (37%–70%)	55 (37%–91%)	64 (28%–undefined)*
Group 2 (NRF = 2)	26 (20%–31%)	19 (17%–28%)	28 (22%–34%)
Group 3 (NRF = 3)	9 (6%–11%)	9 (7%–11%)	10 (8%–13%)
Survival probability at 3,6, and 12 months, respectively, %			
Group 1 (NRF ≤1)	80, 68, and 53	87, 73, and 54	83, 63, and 53
Group 2 (NRF = 2)	73, 51, and 26	68, 45, and 23	76, 52, and 25
Group 3 (NRF = 3)	35, 14, and 3	34, 17, and 4	44, 27, and 11
PSEP, %			
At 3 months	45	53	39
At 6 months	54	56	36
At 12 months	50	50	42

Source: Chow E, Abdolell M, Panzarella T, et al. Predictive model for survival in patients with advanced cancer. *J Clin Oncol.* 2008;26:5863–5869.
*The upper range of the median survival groups A and 1 in the external validation set was undefined because of the small effective sample size, as individuals assigned to those groups have longer survival times.
CI, Confidence interval; *NRF*, number of risk factors method; *PSEP*, simple index of separation; *SPS*, survival prediction score.

worst prognosis) and Pbest (the predicted probability of dying for a patient in the group with the best prognosis). The PSEP was maintained throughout the three sets, suggesting that the model is not overly optimistic.

Generalized R squared* values were 0.23, 0.24, and 0.15 for the training, temporal, and external validation sets, respec-tively, for the three-variable model. This was low in com-parison with the original six-factor model, with R^2 values ranging from 0.27 to 0.31. This relatively small reduction in correlation revealed lower predictive powers; however,

*The multiple correlation coefficient ranges from 0 (no correlation) to 1 (perfect fit).

the three-variable model is clinically simpler and more user friendly, outweighing the disadvantage shown by the decrease in R^2. Also, in terms of usability, Chow et al. recommended the NRF model over the SPS stratification as it avoids the need to remember the partial score for each prognostic variable.[75] It is also important to note that the small R^2 calculations do not invalidate the three factors identified as predictors in this model; rather, they are a reminder that it is unrealistic to predict survival for an individual patient with a high degree of accuracy.[76]

Successful validation of the proposed model in two different settings with sufficient sample sizes supports its use in different clinical situations. In fact, Bruera and Hui[64] commented on the model's generalizability, suggesting that the choice to study patients referred for palliative radiation represents a relatively homogeneous time point along cancer patients' disease trajectory, thus increasing the potential for the model to be applied in other settings and countries. However, the model was developed using only mentally capable, English-speaking patients from two palliative radiation clinics in Canada; therefore, it may not be applicable to the general population of patients with metastatic disease. Also, the model does not account for factors that have indicated significance in survival predictors by other studies, including weight loss, delirium, and patient-reported quality of life.[4,77] Nevertheless, the model proposed by Chow et al.[75] has many practical implications for oncologists. The validated predictive model is able to provide a high degree of discrimination between the three groups, while giving the median survival and survival probabilities for each prognostic group. Furthermore, the model could help radiation oncologists make appropriate treatment decisions.

OTHER MODELS

A variety of other prognostic indicators have been developed, but many of these models are not widely established or validated and require further research with larger sample sizes or within different populations and ethnicities.[53] The poor prognostic indicator described by Bruera et al. in 1992 includes prognostic factors of activity, pain, nausea, depression, weight loss, and cognitive status.[73] The Terminal Cancer Prognostic (TCP) score of Yun et al., developed in 2001, included factors of severe anorexia, severe diarrhea, and mild confusion.[78] The prognostic score used by Chuang et al., created in 2004, consisted of liver and lung metastases, functional performance status, weight loss, edema, cognitive impairment, tiredness, and ascites.[79] The most recently developed prognostic scale, first explored in 2007 as a simple prognostic indicator and amended into a new prognostic index in 2008, utilizes the vitamin B_{12}/C-reactive index (BCI), a product of serum vitamin B_{12} and serum C-reactive protein level (a higher index indicates a poorer prognosis), along with primary lung cancer, secondary liver cancer, and poor performance status.[80,81]

It is clear that creating an easy to use and accurate prognostic model for use in various populations and clinical settings is a challenging and complex task. A recent systematic review of prognostic tools cited the need for further validation, even for more established models such as PPI and PaP, and consistent reporting of prognosis, so tools can be compared.[82] The authors also raised the question of whether the predictive accuracy of models can be improved through repeated measures.

Currently, survival prediction begins with an initial group of factors when the clinician first sees the patient. Would predicting survival be more accurate if patients are assessed multiple times, and are any changes that are seen significant in prognostication? Future prognostic tools will include survival prediction risk calculators that can already be found and assessed online,[8] including a new interactive multimedia prognostic tool called "The Prognostigram," which generates individualized survival curves based on previous data and taking into account comorbid health information.[65]

LIMITATIONS OF MODELS

Most prognostic models are best for predicting at the group level, rather than the individual level.[76] This is demonstrated by the fact that R squared values remain low, even if the model is successfully validated.[75] It is crucial for the clinician to emphasize such a distinction to patients and their families when they are informed of a prognosis made by a particular model.[83] There will always be uncertainty in survival prediction, with many characteristics and potential complications affecting when the patient could die.[82,83]

Clinicians should also consider the limitations and consequences of using a prognostic model. Five key questions identified by Braitman and Davidoff[84,85] for clinicians to consider before using a prognostic model for prognosis for a particular patient are as follows:

1. Would your patient have been eligible for the study that led to the model?
2. Does the outcome variable in the prognostic model reflect the clinical outcome you want to predict?
3. Are values for all prognostic factors available for your patients where and when you need to use the model?
4. Will the predicted probability help in prognosis, choice of treatment, or other aspects of patient care?
5. Is the uncertainty in the predicted probability small enough for that estimate to aid in making a specific prognosis?

Future research in prognostication will continue to focus not only on developing models that provide accurate survival predictions while remaining simple enough for busy clinicians to use, but also on how prognostic information is best communicated to patients.[64]

COMMUNICATING PROGNOSIS

As previously mentioned, communication plays a critical role in foretelling a prognosis, potentially contributing to the inaccuracy of CPS. It is important to consider the communication of prognosis from a patient perspective, as the content and style of the information presented will affect how patients live the rest of their lives.[8] A study by Aabom et al.[86] found that an "explicit terminal diagnosis" reduced patients' admission rates to hospital and increased the likelihood of dying at home. Additionally, a study by Field et al.[87] documented psychological consequences, including increased mistrust and feelings of abandonment due to inadequate communication of prognosis. Other studies have shown that almost all patients want at least some prognostic information, often because they wish to optimize the time they have remaining. This evidence emphasizes the need for patients to have awareness of their disease prognosis.[88]

Unfortunately, past research has shown major inadequacies in doctor-patient communication regarding prognosis for patients with advanced cancer.[89] Two recent systematic reviews have investigated advanced cancer patients' preferences for prognostic information.[50,88] Both reviews emphasize the importance of individualized assessment and warn against making assumptions of patient preference based on demographic characteristics or cultural background. Clinicians must have a good understanding of the goals and needs of their patients and must tailor prognostic information accordingly, while recognizing that patient needs may change over the course of their disease. Clinicians must decide how much information to give to patients and the best way to deliver it, as unwanted information has been shown to diminish hope. The communication of a prognosis must occur in a conversation between practitioner and patient and is a process that must constantly be negotiated and repeated to meet patient and practitioner needs.

In terms of the style of communication preferred, Innes and Payne[88] recognized two potential paradoxes that clinicians commonly face: hope versus realism and honesty versus ambiguity. These seemingly contradictory patient preferences may be best mitigated if considerable planning occurs before the discussion takes place. This may include negotiating the extent of the information given and the appropriate setting for the discussion to take place.[50] In general, patients prefer a clinician to provide information in small portions, while offering empathy, compassion, and honesty. Honesty is desired by almost all patients, but only when balanced with sensitivity and hope, such as providing assurance that the patient will not suffer.[90,91] Most patients also favor words and numbers to diagrams and pie charts. Older patients were more likely to choose 100-person diagrams, and those with higher education levels desired pie charts.[8] It is important to ensure that patients understand what has been said by inviting questions and even writing information down for them to take home.[42]

Discussing prognosis with patients may be even harder than predicting their survival. Prognosis should be communicated only after patients first understand the nature of what they are to hear and subsequently indicate their desire to receive the information.[42]

ETHICAL ISSUES

Traditional medical practice favored a paternalistic culture, in which practitioners were reluctant to disclose unfavorable information, especially regarding limited life expectancy.

Modern practice has witnessed a movement away from paternalism toward patient autonomy, where practitioners are more honest regarding prognosis and treatment options.[88] Today, the law demands that patient information is provided; this is considered a basic human right in countries such as Germany, the United States, and England. Lenience is granted when physicians feel that disclosure may cause additional harm to the patient. In Canada and some American states, communication of prognosis should occur only when the needs of the "reasonable patient" are considered. This can create an ethical dilemma because abiding by this rule may fail to protect patients who may have concerns, apprehensions, religious or cultural beliefs, or personal values that differ from mainstream society.[42] Although it is important to recognize that patients have the right to be informed of their prognosis, it is essential to realize that they also have the right to refuse information regarding their prognosis or any aspect of their diagnosis or treatment.[92]

CONCLUSION

Prognostication remains a difficult topic for clinicians and for patients and their families. The advanced cancer population represents a heterogeneous group of people; thus it has been a challenging task for researchers to develop common prognostic factors for such diverse people. Research has been conducted over the last two decades to identify ways of improving the accuracy of clinical predictions of survival and to develop prognostic tools to aid in the foreseeing and foretelling of predictions. Many of these prognostic tools are beneficial for a specific population, and currently we are unable to recommend one specific tool to function as a universal method of prognostication. Common factors have been identified in systematic reviews as good indicators of prognosis; however, the subjectivity of many of the factors leads to limitations in their applicability. When communicating a prognosis, clinicians must consider cultural and personal differences, as well as patients' wishes regarding the method of delivery and the amount of information they wish to receive. More research is needed to demonstrate the use of both validated prediction models with clinical predictions of survival, as well as other prognostic indicators, in various advanced cancer populations.

REFERENCES

1. Glare P, Virik K, Jones M, et al. A systematic review of physicians' survival predictions in terminally ill cancer patients. *BMJ.* 2003;327:195–198.
2. Glare P, Christakis N. Overview: advancing the clinical science of prognostication. In: Glare P, ed. *Prognosis in advanced cancer.* 1st ed. New York: Oxford University Press; 2008:79–87.
3. Chow E, Harth T, Hruby G, et al. How accurate are physicians' clinical predictions of survival and the available prognostic tools in estimating survival times in terminally ill cancer patients? A systematic review. *Clin Oncol (R Coll Radiol).* 2001;13:209–218.
4. Chow E, Fung K, Panzarella T, et al. A predictive model for survival in metastatic cancer patients attending an outpatient palliative radiation clinic. *Int J Radiat Oncol Biol Phys.* 2002;53:1291–1302.
5. Christakis NA. Prognostication and bioethics. *Daedalus.* 1999;128:197–214.
6. Christakis NA, Sachs GA. The role of prognosis in clinical decision making. *J Gen Intern Med.* 1996;11:422–425.
7. Chow E, Davis L, Panzarella T, et al. Accuracy of survival prediction by palliative radiation oncologists. *Int J Radiat Oncol Biol Phys.* 2005;61:870–873.
8. Glare P, Sinclair C, Downing M, et al. Predicting survival in patients with advanced disease. *Eur J Cancer.* 2008;44:1146–1156.
9. Maltoni M, Caraceni A, Brunelli C, et al. Prognostic factors in advanced cancer patients: evidence-based clinical recommendations—a study by the Steering Committee of the European Association for Palliative Care. *J Clin Oncol.* 2005;23:6240–6248.
10. Chow E, Abdolell M, Panzarella T, et al. Validation of a predictive model for survival in metastatic cancer patients attending an outpatient radiotherapy clinic. *Int J Radiat Oncol Biol Phys.* 2009;73:280–287.

11. Girgis A, Sanson-Fisher RW, Schofield MJ. Is there consensus between breast cancer patients and providers on guidelines for breaking bad news? *Behav Med.* 1999;25:69–77.

12. Koopmeiners L, Post-White J, Gutknecht S, et al. How healthcare professionals contribute to hope in patients with cancer. *Oncol Nurs Forum.* 1997;24:1507–1513.

13. Butow PN, Dowsett S, Hagerty R, et al. Communicating prognosis to patients with metastatic disease: what do they really want to know? *Support Care Cancer.* 2002;10:161–168.

14. Kutner JS, Steiner JF, Corbett KK, et al. Information needs in terminal illness. *Soc Sci Med.* 1999;48:1341–1352.

15. Parkes CM. Accuracy of predictions of survival in later stages of cancer. *Br Med J.* 1972;2:29–31.

16. Tanneberger KS, Pannuti F, Malavasi I, et al. New challenges and old problems: end of life care and the dilemma of prognostic accuracy. *Adv Gerontol.* 2002;10:131–135.

17. Eidenger RN, Schapira DV. Cancer patients' insight into their treatment, prognosis and unconventional therapies. *Cancer.* 1984;53:2736–2740.

18. Lobb EA, Butow PN, Kenny DT. Communicating prognosis in early breast cancer: do women understand the language used? *Med J Aust.* 1999;171:290–294.

19. Siminoff LA, Fetting JH, Abeloff MD. Doctor-patient communication about breast cancer adjuvant therapy. *J Clin Oncol.* 1989;7:1192–1200.

20. Bernheim JL, Ledure G, Souris M, et al. Differences in perception of disease and treatment between cancer patients and their physicians. *Monogr Ser Eur Organ Res Treatment Cancer.* 1987;17:285–295.

21. Pronzato P, Bertelli G, Losardo P, et al. What do advanced cancer patients know of their disease? A report from Italy. *Support Care Cancer.* 1994;2:242–244.

22. Eidinger RN, Schapira DV. Cancer patients' insight into their treatment, prognosis and unconventional therapies. *Cancer.* 1984;53:2736–2740.

23. Yellen SB, Cella DF. Ignorance is bliss? Beliefs about illness and perception of well being. In: *Program and abstracts of the Fourth International Society of Behavioural Medicine.* Washington, DC: March 13–16, 1996. Abstract 45B.

24. Seale C. Communication and awareness about death: a study of a random sample of dying people. *Soc Sci Med.* 1992;32:943–952.

25. Weeks JC, Cook EF, O'Day SJ, et al. Relationship between cancer patients' predictions of prognosis and their treatment preferences. *JAMA.* 1998;279:1709–1714.

26. Maher EJ. How long have I got doctor? *Eur J Cancer.* 1994;30A:283–284.

27. Lamont EB, Christakis NA. Some elements of prognosis in terminal cancer. *Oncology (Williston Park).* 1999;13:1165–1170; discussion 1172–4, 1179–80.

28. Steinhauser KE, Christakis NA, Clipp EC, et al. Factors considered important at the end of life by patients, family, physicians, and other care providers. *JAMA.* 2000;284:2476–2482.

29. Steinhauser KE, Clipp EC, McNeilly M, et al. In search of a good death: observations of patients, families, and providers. *Ann Intern Med.* 2000;132:825–832.

30. Gott M, Seymour J, Bellamy G, et al. Older people's views about home as a place of care at the end of life. *Palliat Med.* 2004;18:460–467.

31. McCarthy EP, Burns RB, Ngo-Metzger Q, et al. Hospice use among Medicare managed care and fee-for-service patients dying with cancer. *JAMA.* 2003;289:2238–2245.

32. Higginson IJ, Astin P, Dolan S. Where do cancer patients die? Ten-year trends in the place of death of cancer patients in England. *Palliat Med.* 1998;12:353–363.

33. den Daas N. Estimating length of survival in end-stage cancer: a review of the literature. *J Pain Symptom Manage.* 1995;10:548–555.

34. Viganò A, Dorgan M, Buckingham J, et al. Survival prediction in terminal cancer patients: a systematic review of the medical literature. *Palliat Med.* 2000;14:363–374.

35. Stanski HR, Wilson LJ, Burrows WR. *Survey of common verification methods in meteorology.* MSRB; Environment Canada Atmospheric Environment Service Research Report. 1989:89–95.

36. Viganò A, Dorgan M, Bruera E, et al. The relative accuracy of the clinical estimation of the duration of life for patients with end of life cancer. *Cancer.* 1999;86:170–176.

37. Zahuranec DB, Brown DL, Lisabeth LD, et al. Early care limitations independently predict mortality after intracerebral hemorrhage. *Neurology.* 2007;68:1651–1657.

38. Gripp S, Moeller S, Bölke E, et al. Survival prediction in terminally ill cancer patients by clinical estimates, laboratory tests, and self-rated anxiety and depression. *J Clin Oncol.* 2007;25:3313–3320.

39. Wildman MJ, Sanderson C, Groves J, et al. Implications of prognostic pessimism in patients with chronic obstructive pulmonary disease (COPD) or asthma admitted to intensive care in the UK within the COPD and asthma outcome study (CAOS): multicentre observational cohort study. *BMJ.* 2007;335:1132.

40. Christakis NA, Lamont EB. Extent and determinants of error in doctors' prognoses in terminally ill patients: prospective cohort study. *BMJ.* 2000;320:469–472.

41. Maltoni M, Nanni O, Derni S, et al. Clinical prediction of survival is more accurate than the Karnofsky performance status in estimating life span of terminally ill cancer patients. *Eur J Cancer.* 1994;30A:764–766.

42. Butow P, Hagerty R, et al. Foretelling. In: Glare P, ed. *Prognosis in advanced cancer.* 1st ed. New York: Oxford University Press; 2008:33–53.

43. Hagerty RG, Butow PN, Ellis PA, et al. Cancer patient preferences for communication of prognosis in the metastatic setting. *J Clin Oncol.* 2004;22:1721–1730.

44. Butow P, Tattersall MHN. Talking prognosis with cancer patients. *Aust Doctor.* 2002;(17 May):1–8.

45. Kaplowitz SA, Campo S, Chui WT. Cancer patients' desire for communication of prognosis information. *Health Commun.* 2002;14:221–241.

46. Crooks V, Waller S, Smith T, Hahn TJ. The use of the Karnofsky Performance Scale in determining outcomes and risk in geriatric outpatients. *J Gerontol.* 1991;46:M139–M144.

47. The AM, Hak T, Koëter G, et al. Collusion in doctor-patient communication about imminent death: an ethnographic study. *West J Med.* 2001;174:247–253.

48. Bradley EH, Hallemeier AG, Fried TR, et al. Documentation of discussions about prognosis with terminally ill patients. *Am J Med.* 2001;111:218–223.

49. Gattellari M, Butow PN, Tattersall MH, et al. Misunderstanding in cancer patients: why shoot the messenger? *Ann Oncol.* 1999;10:39–46.

50. Parker SM, Clayton JM, Hancock K, et al. A systematic review of prognostic/end-of-life communication with adults in the advanced stages of a life-limiting illness: patient/caregiver

51. Lamont E. Foreseeing. In: Glare P, ed. *Prognosis in advanced cancer.* 1st ed. New York: Oxford University Press; 2008:25–32.

52. Steyerberg E, Harrell F. Statistical models for prognostication. In: Max M, Lynn J, eds. *Symptom research: methods and opportunities.* 2002. Available at: http://symptomresearch.nih.gov.

53. Ripamonti CI, Farina G, Garassino MC. Predictive models in palliative care. *Cancer.* 2009;115(suppl 13):3128–3134.

54. Stone PC, Lund S. Predicting prognosis in patients with advanced cancer. *Ann Oncol.* 2007;18:971–976.

55. Anderson F, Downing GM, Hill J, et al. Palliative performance status (PPS): a new tool. *J Palliat Care.* 1996;12:5–11.

56. Vigano A, Donaldson N, Higginson IJ, et al. Quality of life and survival prediction in terminal cancer patients. *Cancer.* 2004;101:1090–1098.

57. Jatoi A, Nguyen P. Weight Loss. In: Glare P, ed. *Prognosis in advanced cancer.* 1st ed. New York: Oxford University Press; 2008:395–399.

58. Dewys WD, Begg C, Lavin PT, et al. Prognostic effect of weight loss prior to chemotherapy in cancer patients. Eastern Cooperative Oncology Group. *Am J Med.* 1980;69:491–497.

59. Hopkinson J, Wright D, Corner J. Exploring the experience of weight loss in people with advanced cancer. *J Adv Nurs.* 2006;54:304–312.

60. Alloway L, Keeley V, Higginson I. Breathlessness. In: Glare P, ed. *Prognosis in advanced cancer.* 1st ed. New York: Oxford University Press; 2008:371–379.

61. Hardy JR, Turner R, Saunders M, et al. Prediction of survival in a hospital-based continuing care unit. *Eur J Cancer.* 1994;30A:284–288.

62. Friedlander M, Kissane D. Delirium. In: Glare P, ed. *Prognosis in advanced cancer.* 1st ed. New York: Oxford University Press; 2008:380–394.

63. Maltoni M, Nanni O, Pirovano M, et al. Successful validation of the palliative prognostic score in terminally ill cancer patients. Italian Multicenter Study Group on Palliative Care. *J Pain Symptom Manage.* 1999;17:240–247.

64. Bruera E, Hui D. Practical model for prognostication in advanced cancer patients: is less more? *J Clin Oncol.* 2008;26:5843–5844.

65. Piccirillo J, Vlahiotis A. Tools for formulating prognosis. In: Glare P, ed. *Prognosis in advanced cancer.* 1st ed. New York: Oxford University Press; 2008:79–87.

66. Pirovano M, Maltoni M, Nanni O, et al. A new palliative prognostic score: a first step for the staging of terminally ill cancer patients. Italian Multicenter and Study Group on Palliative Care. *J Pain Symptom Manage.* 1999;17:231–239.

67. Glare P, Virik K. Independent prospective validation of the PaP score in terminally ill patients referred to a hospital-based palliative medicine consultation service. *J Pain Symptom Manage.* 2001;22:891–898.

68. Glare PA, Eychmueller S, McMahon P. Diagnostic accuracy of the palliative prognostic score in hospitalized patients with advanced cancer. *J Clin Oncol.* 2004;22:4823–4828.

69. Stone CA, Tiernan E, Dooley BA. Prospective validation of the palliative prognostic index in patients with cancer. *J Pain Symptom Manage.* 2008;35:617–622.

70. Morita T, Tsunoda J, Inoue S, et al. Survival prediction of terminally ill cancer patients by

clinical symptoms: development of a simple indicator. *Jpn J Clin Oncol.* 1999;29:156–159.

71. Morita T, Tsunoda J, Inoue S, et al. The Palliative Prognostic Index: a scoring system for survival prediction of terminally ill cancer patients. *Support Care Cancer.* 1999;7:128–133.

72. Alloway L, Minton O. The accuracy of the clinical prediction of survival: a comparison of doctors' and nurses' estimations and the failure to validate the Palliative Prognostic Score (PaP). *Palliat Med.* 2004;18:155.

73. Bruera E, Miller MJ, Kuehn N, et al. Estimate of survival of patients admitted to a palliative care unit: a prospective study. *J Pain Symptom Manage.* 1992;7:82–86.

74. Watanabe S, Nekolaichuk C, Beaumont C, et al. The Edmonton symptom assessment system— what do patients think? *Support Care Cancer.* 2009;17:675–683.

75. Chow E, Abdolell M, Panzarella T, et al. Predictive model for survival in patients with advanced cancer. *J Clin Oncol.* 2008;26:5863–5869.

76. Toscani F, Brunelli C. Predicting survival in terminal cancer patients: clinical observation or quality-of-life evaluation? *Palliat Med.* 2005;19:220–227.

77. Christakis NA, Escarce JJ. Survival of Medicare patients after enrollment in hospice programs. *N Engl J Med.* 1996;335:172–178.

78. Yun YH, Heo DS, Heo BY. Development of terminal cancer prognostic score as an index in terminally ill cancer patients. *Oncol Rep.* 2001;8:795–800.

79. Chuang RB, Hu WY, Chiu TY, et al. Prediction of survival in terminal cancer patients in Taiwan: constructing a prognostic scale. *J Pain Symptom Manage.* 2004;28:115–122.

80. Kelly L, White S, Stone PC. The B12/CRP index as a simple prognostic indicator in patients with advanced cancer: a confirmatory study. *Ann Oncol.* 2007;18:1395–1399.

81. Stone P, Kelly L, Head R, et al. Development and validation of a prognostic scale for use in patients with advanced cancer. *Palliat Med.* 2008;22:711–717.

82. Lau F, Cloutier-Fisher D, Kuziemsky C, et al. A systematic review of prognostic tools for estimating survival time in palliative care. *J Palliat Care.* 2007;23:93–112.

83. Campos S, Hird A, Flynn C, et al. The not-so-crystal ball: the ongoing challenge of physician prognostication. *J Psychosom Res.* 2008;65:67–69.

84. Gimotty P. Statistical concepts and issues related to prognostic models. In: Glare P, ed. *Prognosis in advanced cancer.* 1st ed. New York: Oxford University Press; 2008:55–62.

85. Braitman LE, Davidoff F. Predicting clinical states in individual patients. *Ann Intern Med.* 1996;125:406–412.

86. Aabom B, Kragstrup J, Vondeling H, et al. Defining cancer patients as being in the terminal phase: who receives a formal diagnosis, and what are the effects? *J Clin Oncol.* 2005;23:7411–7416.

87. Field D. Awareness and modern dying. *Mortality.* 1996;1:255–265.

88. Innes S, Payne S. Advanced cancer patients' prognostic information preferences: a review. *Palliat Med.* 2009;23:29–39.

89. Gysels M, Richardson A, Higginson I. Communication training for health professional who care for patients with cancer: a systematic review of effectiveness. *Support Care Cancer.* 2004;12:692–700.

90. Rose KE. A qualitative analysis of the information needs of informal cancer of terminally ill cancer patients. *J Clin Nurs.* 1999;8:81–88.

91. Kirk P, Kirk I, Kristjanson LJ. What do patients receiving palliative care for cancer and their families want to be told? A Canadian and Australian qualitative study. *BMJ.* 2004;328:1343–1347.

92. Broeckaert B, Glare P. Ethical perspectives. In: Glare P, ed. *Prognosis in advanced cancer.* 1st ed. New York: Oxford University Press; 2008:89–94.

Communicating difficult news supportively: a practical approach

Robert Buckman

NEED FOR STRATEGIES, NOT SCRIPTS

The simple fact about breaking bad news is that, unfortunately, there is no such thing as a universal formula of words and sentences that we can use in every situation. There is no infallible script that possesses magical "one size fits all" capabilities.

No matter how extensive our clinical experience is, or how many times we have held discussions about difficult news, the process of breaking bad news in oncology is never easy.[1] Part of what makes it so difficult is that the reactions of our patients (and/or their friends and family) often seem both unpredictable and highly charged with emotion, so that we frequently feel unprepared to deal with the situation or to help the patient to cope.

However, as we shall see here, there are strategies and techniques that can help us to be supportive for patient and family, even when we are the bearers of bad news, and are therefore in danger of being identified with it, or blamed for it.

This chapter will first define bad news and will summarize the major factors that make it so difficult; it will then describe the six-point strategy, known by the acronym SPIKES, which is an aide-memoire that offers a practical and easily memorized logical approach to these difficult discussions.

WHAT IS BAD NEWS AND WHAT MAKES IT SO BAD?

Bad news can be defined in pragmatic terms as any information that seriously and adversely changes a person's view of his future. In other words, bad news is any new information that markedly lowers a person's expectations.[2]

Hence, the gap between a person's expectations of the situation and the actual medical realities can be thought of as a measure of the "badness" of the bad news to the patient, and is a likely indication of whether the impact of the news will be overwhelming or not. This conceptual framework of difficult news also offers a practical way of approaching breaking bad news, because we cannot have even the most approximate estimate of the impact of the news until we know what the individual patient is expecting. Therefore, the above definition of bad news suggests the approach of *"Before you tell, ask,"* a strategy that is incorporated into the SPIKES strategy.

Sharing bad news is always difficult, and, from our point of view as healthcare professionals, several components contribute to this. It is worthwhile considering these factors in some detail, as this may inform and reinforce the objectives of the strategy and the techniques necessary to counteract them.

The components that contribute to the difficulties involved in breaking bad news are best considered under the following seven headings.

BLAMING THE MESSENGER

Bad news, as implied in the above definition, is almost always accompanied by a feeling of disappointment. Much of this, of course, has its origins in the news itself and the implications of it.

485

Yet, despite the fact that the news itself is the precipitant of much of the emotion, it seems to be a normal and human reaction to "blame the messenger for the message." That is not necessarily the fault of the messenger's manner of transmitting the message; it is simply a human mechanism for coping with abstract bad news.

The process is often called "personification." It is a human trait as old as our history, and it seems to be one way in which most of us deal with the abstract idea of bad news.

We all react in this way to minor reversals of fortune almost daily, often without fully realizing that we are doing it. For example, most of us react to seeing an officer write out a parking ticket for our parking infraction by expressing blame and anger at the officer who is writing the ticket. This reaction is facilitated by the fact that the officer is wearing the uniform of the Parking Department, so we can feel that we are blaming "Officer Smith of City Hall," and not the person, John Smith.

Hence, when we are in the role of giving medical bad news—which is, of course, of considerably greater significance than a parking ticket—we may expect a similar response from our patients. Furthermore, the symbols and badges of our role (whether or not we are actually wearing a white coat or other uniform) make it easier for the patient or family to vent their feelings about the news itself on us, as we share the facts.

Anticipation of being blamed is therefore a factor that contributes to the difficulty we perceive in discussing the news.

STRONG EMOTIONS

Perhaps the most important factor in these discussions, however, is the emotional state that is created by the news. Most of us in nonpsychiatric specialties have not had a great deal of training in emotion handling, and we find the prospect of dealing with this emotional turbulence difficult. The more accomplished we are in our own field, the more difficult it is to accept that we have not been shown how to do an apparently simple task such as dealing with a patient who is crying or shouting, or who remains completely silent. In general, physicians, similar to most other people, do not relish having to do something that they feel relatively unskilled at, so this is another factor that causes us to flinch mentally as we come to impart bad news.

OUR FEELINGS IN SYMPATHY

Another factor that makes breaking bad news difficult is the onset of similar feelings that we ourselves may experience when our patient experiences the disappointment or pain of the news. The feelings that we experience as echoes or resonances of the other person's feelings are called "feelings in sympathy," and of course the extent to which we, as professionals, have these feelings varies widely. Some of us experience these feelings frequently, some experience them rarely, and some not at all. In itself, that variability is not important. The physician who experiences greater feelings in sympathy is not necessarily a better (or worse) physician because of them. However, it is important to be aware of these feelings simply because if they are uncomfortable, this will be another factor that contributes to making these discussions difficult.[3]

FEELINGS OF PROFESSIONAL FAILURE

Healthcare professionals want to solve their patients' problems, and they enjoy doing so. Hence, if the bad news that we impart includes problems that are incurable or unfixable, we are likely to feel a sense of professional failure, which may spill over into a sense of personal inadequacy.

Even if we know that we have used the best available treatment for this patient's condition, there still may lurk a vague and unspoken fear that somewhere, some other physician may have a miraculous remedy for precisely this problem.

This sense of professional unease is another factor that makes discussions of all conditions for which no major medical remedy is available even more uncomfortable.

MEDICO-LEGAL FACTORS AND THE WORD "SORRY"

Until recently, the threat of medico-legal (and financial) implications loomed large in discussions about bad news and made it extremely difficult to discuss freely, for example, a poor prognosis. It seemed almost as if, for any adverse medical event, even a totally natural one, there must be <u>someone</u> to blame: someone who had made errors of commission or of omission.

The situation has improved over the past decade or so, nevertheless there is still a fear of medico-legal consequences hanging over any discussion of bad news, along with a fear of being held responsible for the medical condition itself.

Furthermore, the ambiguity of the word "sorry" has added to the difficulty. The word "sorry" has two distinct meanings. When used as in "*I am sorry for you,*" it is an expression of a feeling that is commonly termed sympathy. But when the same word is used in "*I am sorry that I did this,*" it implies regret and responsibility (or, in medico-legal terms, culpability or "exposure"). Hence, even when we begin to express human sympathy for the feelings of the other person, we may inadvertently be perceived as taking responsibility if we say "*I am sorry,*" instead of the clearer but clumsier "*I am sorry for the way you're feeling.*"

Another advantage of the empathic response—as we shall see—is that it makes explicit the emotion that is being expressed, as well as the immediate cause of that emotion. Then by stating overtly the connection between the two, a sentence such as "*This is clearly awful for you*" avoids the ambiguities entailed in the simple single word "sorry."

DEALING WITH HOPE

Then there is the problem of dealing with hope. It is often stated as a maxim of medical practice that we should "never take away all hope." This principle has often been used as a reason (or, more likely, an excuse), by professionals who find these conversations difficult, for not telling the truth to patients and/or family. The implication is that by telling the patient nothing, you are thereby protecting the patient from losing all hope in the aftermath of the news.

Now this difficulty—the fear of destroying hope—is at its greatest if we erroneously equate truth telling with the destruction of all hope. If you happen to think that disclosure of a diagnosis that includes the word "cancer," for example, is tantamount to abolishing all hope, then you will avoid using the word (as 90% of physicians did in the 1960s[4]).

In practice, discussing the facts by no means inevitably implies the abolition of all hope. As you will see, the central purpose of the SPIKES protocol is to enable us, as professionals, to discuss the medical facts openly and honestly, and at the same time to acknowledge the impact that those facts produce. This process could be termed "sensitive truth telling."

By contrast, one could characterize the ways of dealing with bad news several decades ago, perhaps until even the late 1970s, as being of two types: concealing the information (perhaps best described as "sensitive concealment" or as "protective patronizing") or else a form of simply blurting out the bad news, which perhaps could be termed "insensitive truth telling," meaning that the facts are stated without regard to their impact on the patient.

We can legitimately claim to have made considerable progress in clinical communication since that time.[5] Even so, dealing with hope is never easy. It is a most important point to realize that hope is not a single monolithic entity. Many components make up any individual's hope in a situation, some of which may be unattainable (e.g., cure); other hopes are realistic and are directed at reachable goals (e.g., control of many physical symptoms, fixing the fear of being abandoned, resolving family conflicts).

The problem of dealing with hope is not a trivial one, and we need to be aware of the fear of abolishing all hope as another deterrent to our breaking bad news.

CHALLENGES TO OUR PERSONAL SENSE OF INVULNERABILITY

It has been suggested that many physicians first decided on a career in health care in part to diminish their own personal anxieties about disease and death (in other words, we may be partially driven by counter-phobic motives).

Of course, the importance of these particular motives in any individual's psychological makeup will vary from being a major factor in some people to being negligible or even absent in others. So, for some of us, dealing with our own fear of disease or death (even if it is subconscious) may be a significant factor. Whether this motive plays a big or a small role, a discussion about disease progression or terminal illness will challenge any denial that we may have about death. Further, the more that we seem to have in common with the patient, the greater this challenge will be. If a particular patient happens to remind us in some way of ourselves, a discussion about bad news may become even more difficult, as the awareness of "there, but for fortune. . . " develops.

For this reason, identifying with the plight of the patient—an activity that in itself has many potential benefits for both parties—may create a hazard by challenging our own view of our future. Simply being aware of this complication is helpful and may reduce its effect as an obstacle in breaking bad news.

ETHICS AND MEDICAL POLITICS OF TRUTH TELLING

In addition to all of these factors that affect the doctor-patient relationship is the issue of whether the physician is obliged to tell the truth to the patient. After many centuries of debate and controversy, clear and explicit legal regulations about this question have been defined.[6]

In most countries nowadays, the mentally competent patient has the legal right to any information concerning his medical condition if he wants to know it.[7] Hence, the current clinical question is not *whether* to tell a mentally competent patient the medical facts, but *how* to do it supportively—if a patient asks, we are obliged to tell and need to do it well. A practical strategy for approaching this task—as will be set out in the next part of this chapter—is important.

However, we are not obliged to give details, including the diagnosis, if the patient specifically does *not* want the information given to him. Even then, most ethicists would agree that if a mentally competent patient does not want the diagnosis named, we are obliged to describe, at the least, the seriousness of the condition, the nature of the treatment we propose, and the consequences of not getting that treatment, as well as the consequences (including side effects) of receiving that treatment.

Most authorities agree that those are our obligations. Of course, other circumstances may have an influence: For example, most clinical trials specify in the entry criteria that the patient must know the diagnosis (particularly true in oncology). If the patient does not want the diagnosis named or discussed, entry to that clinical trial is not possible, although, of course, treatment for that condition is possible with regimens outside the clinical trial.

Furthermore, most authorities would also agree that if a patient insists on not knowing the diagnosis—a rare event nowadays, but it still happens occasionally—we are obligated to ask whether there is someone else (a daughter or son or close friend perhaps) with whom the patient would like us to discuss the diagnosis or treatment. In many cases, but not in all, we will be asked to talk to another person. In my own hospital practice, I have encountered a few patients who specified that they did not want the diagnosis named, and were comfortable making decisions about their treatment and other aspects of care without involvement of any third party.

In addition to all these issues that affect doctor-patient communication, sometimes problems are created by what might be termed "local medical politics," meaning discussions with, and care plans for, the patient by other professionals that may conflict with your view of the situation and plan.[8]

For example, a patient may tell you of views expressed, or of implicit promises made, by other physicians involved in clinical management (*"But the surgeon said he'd got it all"*). This type of situation requires a tactful and careful strategic approach. In brief, it is important to achieve three objectives: First, you have to acknowledge the emotions that the patient experienced when hearing the news and/or is experiencing now (see the E of SPIKES below); second, you have to encourage the patient to describe what the other person said, and what the patient understood from it, and what it implies to the patient; and finally, you can describe your own assessment of the patient's clinical situation, emphasizing your view of the way the tumor is likely to behave, and what steps are most likely to be helpful. This all may sound difficult, but it isn't—as you can see in the filmed and unscripted scenario of this situation.[9]

More frequently, however, turbulence arises not from other healthcare professionals but from the patient's family members.[10] An example is when a son states, *"My mother is not to be told."* This can be a situation fraught with high emotion and conflict. Although the basic principle of the patient having primacy (and therefore access to the facts if that is what she desires) is clear, a tactical and productive approach to this situation does require some care and sensitivity. The main objective here is to acknowledge the relative's feelings and also their importance as part of the patient's support system, but at the same time to make sure the relative understands that the patient's choice does indeed have primacy over anyone else's. In other words, you are trying to persuade the relative to change his or her viewpoint and agree that the patient can be asked whether or not she wants to know the details of the diagnosis. You will find that this strategy is illustrated in an unscripted and unrehearsed videotaped scenario.[11]

As will be seen in the next section, the SPIKES six-step protocol provides a systematic approach that includes an invitation to share the information, so that if the patient specifically does not want the information at that particular moment, a discussion can be opened at a later date, when and if the patient so wishes.

SPIKES STRATEGY FOR BREAKING BAD NEWS: "BEFORE YOU TELL, ASK"

As suggested by the above definition, the impact of the bad news is correlated with the size of the gap between the expectations of the patient and the medical reality. In practical terms, this means that as clinicians, we have to deal with two components of the discussion at the same time: (1) the facts of the clinical situation and the care plan, and (2) the patient's (and/or friends') emotional responses to those facts. These and other aspects of communication skills have been shown to be teachable and learnable.[12]

As will be seen in what follows, the six-step protocol[13] known by the acronym SPIKES has two important features.[14]

First, this approach provides a methodical way of assessing the patient's perception of the situation before going on to give information (*"Before you tell, ask"*—the second step or the "P" of SPIKES). Second, it stresses the central importance of acknowledging the patient's (or friends') emotional reactions to the news as it emerges (the "E" of SPIKES).

The six steps of the SPIKES strategy are summarized in Table 47-1 and are discussed in the following sections.

S—SETTING
The physical components of the discussion—the setting of the interview, including body language, eye contact, interpersonal distance, touch, and others—have a material effect on the results of, and on the patient's satisfaction with, the dialogue.

In practical terms, the act of optimizing the physical setting of the discussion helps both parties to the conversation. It helps us, as professionals, because by doing this we feel in greater control of the situation and more confident. In turn, this increased confidence is perceived by the patient and/or friends as an indication of greater competence.

The details of the physical setting of the dialogue may initially seem perhaps trivial or fussy, nevertheless, a few seconds spent on the following aspects (also summarized in Table 47-2) makes a great deal of difference.[15]

The main points that deserve attention are these:

Privacy: It is worth spending a few seconds in trying to establish a degree of privacy (e.g., in the hospital setting, draw the curtains around the bed).

Table 47-1 The SPIKES protocol for breaking bad news

		Topics covered in this chapter
S	**S**ETTING AND STARTING	Sit down, body language, eye contact, touch. Open questions, silence and repetition.
P	**P**ERCEPTION	Assess what patient knows or suspects, listen to vocabulary and comprehension.
I	**I**NVITATION	Obtain permission to share knowledge or set agenda.
K	**K**NOWLEDGE	Align with patient's understanding; plain language, small chunks.
E	**E**MOTIONS	Acknowledge major emotions as they arise.
S	**S**TRATEGY AND SUMMARY	Set out plan of medical management. Close with précis, any questions, and contract for next contact.

Distance: It is worthwhile to ensure that the physical distance between you and the patient is less than 4 feet. The interpersonal distance for personal conversation varies with culture and country, but generally it is thought that between 3 and 4 feet is satisfactory in most cases.[16,17]

Eye Contact: The most important feature of the physical setting is to maintain good eye contact; this is made easier if your eyes are on the same level as the patient. Almost always this means that you have to sit down. In some cultures, direct eye contact is not regarded as demonstrating attention, but is interpreted as invasive or impolite.[18]

Neutral Body Posture: In general, it is worth adopting the so-called neutral body posture (feet flat on the ground, knees together, hands on lap or else on desk) because this does not transmit any signals of anxiety or stress.[19]

Facial Expression: Perhaps the most useful practical tip is this: Be prepared to smile. Often this simple act, although it is a matter of personal style and choice, is perceived as being friendly and courteous.

Touch: Touching the forearm of the patient (a nonthreatening are of the body) is valuable if you are comfortable doing this. If the patient withdraws the arm or in some way shows aversion, then do not repeat it.[20]

Listening Skills (Facilitation Techniques): The many techniques that facilitate a discussion represent an entire topic in themselves.[21] Of all the techniques described, two are best incorporated into every clinical interview: **silence** (not interrupting the patient while he is talking)[22] and **repetition** (using a key word from the patient's last sentence in your first sentence). Silence has also been shown to facilitate empathic communication.[23]

P—PERCEPTION
Perhaps the most important practical point in beginning discussions about difficult news is to determine where to start: to find the optimal level of information at which to begin the discussion.

Table 47-2 Optimizing the setting (physical components) of the interview

Technique	Central feature	Notes
Greeting	Make sure you use the person's name,	A simple way of establishing "person" as well as "problem."
Introduce yourself	Very briefly, say who you are and what you do.	Merely courteous.
Shake hands	Actual contact.	Do not do this during flu season, or if you or the patient has a cold!
Sit down	Bring your eyes to the same level as the other person's.	Essential.
Don't be too far away	Have less than 4 feet of space between you.	The exact optimal distance varies with gender and culture, but 3 feet is rarely wrong.
Neutral body posture	Look relaxed or at least not too anxious or irritated.	Even if you do not feel relaxed (and most of us don't at these times), try to adopt a neutral body posture and look relaxed.
Lean forward	Do not sit back all the way against the chair.	Studies show that patients recognize this as a sign of being interested in them.
Be ready to smile	Smiling may not be your usual "thing," but it helps if you can manage it.	If you do smile, try to "smile with your whole face."
Switch on your listening skills	Silence and repetition.	Consciously maintain silence as the patient starts to talk, then in your first sentence of response, use a word or phrase from the patient's last sentence.

In practical terms, this means finding out what the patient already knows or suspects about the condition, so that you can continue from that starting point (*"Before you tell, ask"*). The words that you use in assessing the patient's perception are not crucial. There is no "magic formula of words" that suits every person or that works every time when other phrases do not.

A few examples are set out in Table 47-3. The idea behind all of them is the same, and you can use these or any phrasings that feel comfortable.

As the patient replies and describes what he knows or has been told, it is important to focus on two things:

1. The Vocabulary and The Comprehension

Try to assess at what level the patient understands the situation.[24] Well-informed patients might say something such as, "The surgeon said it was breast cancer, less than 2 centimeters, and it hadn't spread to the lymph nodes, and it did have those hormone receptors on it." It is valuable to hear this from

Table 47-3 Some suggested phrases for assessing patient's perception

So what do you make of the situation?	Tell me what you think is going on.
What did Dr. X tell you when he/she sent you here?	What have you been told about the medical situation?
When you first had that chest pain/found that breast lump, did you think it was something serious?	Tell me what you've been thinking about the medical situation.
Why don't you tell me what you understand about the situation, and I'll go on from there.	

the patient because so much of the explaining has already been done, hence it would be appropriate to respond with words to the effect of, "That's right. Now if it's less than 2 centimeters, we'd regard that as quite small, which is good, and when it hasn't spread to the lymph nodes, that's also good."

On the other hand, occasionally a patient with, say, lung cancer will say something such as *"My GP said they saw a shadow on the chest X-ray, but it didn't sound serious or anything."* In this case, the gap between perception and reality is wide, and the task of breaking the difficult news is likely to be harder (see later for one approach to this).

As the patient describes the level of comprehension, it is valuable to make note of his vocabulary, the words that he uses, so that you can later line up and align your description of the situation when you come to it (in the K for Knowledge) with the patient's perception.

This process of aligning[25] your language and vocabulary is a useful way of responding to the patient, and is helpful in reinforcing your relationship.

2. The Presence of Denial

It may happen that the referring physician has said in the referral letter that he or she did tell the patient what was going on, yet despite that, the patient says to you that he has not been told anything.

Clearly, the patient is exhibiting denial. When this happens (even though you might be holding the referring letter stating that the diagnosis has been discussed), you simply need to note the denial at this point, just as you would note any other symptom such as pain. You need not (and should not) confront the denial directly at this early stage of the discussions.[26]

So if the patient says, *"They didn't tell me anything at that other clinic,"* it would be counterproductive to reply, *"Actually they did."* It would be more helpful to acknowledge the patient's perception of what he was told (i.e., that he believes he was told nothing) and then go on to ask him (the I of SPIKES) what he would like to know (if anything) about his condition now.

I—INVITATION

At the moment at which you ask the patient whether he wants you to go on to describe the medical facts, you are of course simultaneously offering him a chance <u>not</u> to hear the exact details of the diagnosis if that is what he wishes.[27,28]

Even if the invitation is as brief as *"I'd like to tell you the results of the test. Is that OK?"* you are still involving the patient in taking the next step. You are engaging in shared decision making.[29]

The exact words you use are not critical; a few examples are provided in Table 47-4. The significance of your question is that you are asking for the patient's collaboration. It may sound like a simple matter and just courtesy or common sense, but it will not be forgotten.

K—KNOWLEDGE

Having obtained a clear invitation to share the information—or at least having obtained agreement to the agenda that you have proposed—you can now start giving the medical facts.[30]

As you do so, these guidelines may be helpful (Table 47-5):

Table 47-4 Some suggested phrases for obtaining an invitation to share news

How would you like me to deal with this? Shall I tell you what we know so far?	Are you the kind of person who'd like to know the details as far as we know them?
Is it OK if I go ahead and tell you what we know about your situation so far?	I'll go ahead and talk about the results of the biopsy/scan/blood test. Is that OK?
Would you like me to go ahead and tell you the results of the biopsy/scan/ blood test?	How would you like me to handle the information? Shall I go ahead and tell you what we know?

Table 47-5 Some guidelines for giving medical facts (K – Knowledge)

Align your language with the patient's vocabulary.	Use similar (or the same) words at the same level as you heard the patient use them.
Give the facts in small chunks.	Don't give a long monologue; the patient may drift off or be totally at sea.
Check the patient's understanding.	You can use phrases such as "Does that make sense?" "Do you follow me?" or "Is that clear so far?"
Use plain language, not technical jargon.	It is an effort to deliberately translate technical Medspeak into everyday language, but it is worthwhile.
Respond to the patient's intense emotions as they are expressed.	See next section, E – Emotions.

■ Align your vocabulary with the patient's, and use plain language.

As you begin to describe the bad news, try to use the same level of vocabulary that you hear the patient use when describing his perception of the situation. If, for example, the patient says that he was told that the X-ray shows "a shadow," you can start with the word "shadow" and say something such as *"Yes, and I don't know if it was mentioned, but shadows can be caused by several different things, some serious, some not."*

■ Next, as you go on to describe the difficult news, make sure that you express the facts in plain language, not in esoteric technical jargon.

The basic problem is that our medical technical jargon is very useful for rapid transmission of information, but it is usually unintelligible to the patient. For example, in a medical emergency, our technical jargon ("Medspeak") is a brilliant and efficient way of transferring a large amount of information in a very few words. Consider the wealth of information that is carried in *"Chemotherapy 10 days ago. WBC 0.2. Temp 39.8, systolic is 80 and falling."* In a few seconds, an accurate picture emerges of probable septic shock.

Justifiably, we are proud of our ability to speak and understand Medspeak: It is unambiguous, precise, hard to learn (at first), and immensely valuable. The problem is that our patients do not speak it or understand it, so that we must make a conscious effort to translate what we want to say into plain language.

Some patients will want to advance the vocabulary to a more technical level. For this reason, you may, if you wish, use the technical word first and then go on to translate it into plain language. For example, you might say, *"The bone scan is reported as negative—in other words, it doesn't show anything wrong."* This shows that you clearly know the technical words, but you are also making an effort to ensure that the patient understands their meaning.

This is why it is so valuable to check that your patient understands what you are saying. If you check with the patient and the patient is comfortable with the technical words, it is relatively simple to move from plain language to technical language thereafter.

On the other hand, if you do not check with the patient, it is then difficult to move down from technical jargon to plain language because you will not know that the patient does not understand the facts—hence the importance of the guideline.

■ Give the information in small chunks, and check that it is being understood.

It is most important when giving information that the information is given in small (digestible) chunks. Try to avoid a long monologue (even though you might well be justifiably proud of the amount you know about the condition). Make a conscious effort to pause every few sentences, and check that patient is still with you and "on the same page."[31]

If you do not do this, the patient may well drift away and start thinking about the worst possible consequences of your opening statement. Thus, while you are trying to present the rather reassuring facts about, for example, ductal cancer in situ of the breast, the patient may be imagining the worst consequences associated with the word "cancer." Hence it is useful to prevent yourself from giving a long monologue by checking the patient's comprehension.

The words that you use for this are entirely a matter of personal style. Examples include the following: "Is this all making sense so far?" "Do you see what I mean?" "Are you with me so far?" and "Any questions so far?"

These details may appear to be minor or even trivial, but they make a great difference to the patient's perception of how the interview is being tailored and made specific to his understanding of the news.

E—EMOTIONS

Responding to the emotional content of the interaction is the most important component of a supportive doctor-patient relationship[32]; the three-step technique known as the empathic response is the best and easiest way of achieving this.[33]

Failure to acknowledge a strong emotion when it is expressed or demonstrated will have adverse effects on the interview. The patient will likely regard the physician as cold or insensitive. This applies to every stage of the interview, from the beginning onward, particularly if, as happens frequently, the patient asks an anxious question as you enter the room.

The most important advantage of the empathic response is that frequently the act of acknowledging the patient's emotion is all that is required.[34] The easiest and most straightforward way of doing this is the empathic response, which consists of the following three steps.

Step 1: Identify One of the Emotions.

Most emotions occur in groups. In fact, almost all emotions are "mixed emotions." For example, when a patient hears bad news, he may react with anger and also feel shock, disbelief (implying inability to take the news in), or denial (implying a desire not to take the news in), as well as fear, bewilderment, guilt, and other feelings. All of those emotions might coexist behind a shocked "Oh no!"

So when the patient shows an emotional response (such as "Oh no!"), you simply need to decide on <u>one</u> of the emotions being expressed. Furthermore, the fact that you can see the emotional expression shows that it is a "big" experience (i.e., something that the patient feels intensely and deeply).

Having decided on one of the more prominent emotions in the mixture, then name that emotion in your own mind. In other words, say to yourself, *"This patient is clearly shocked,"* or *"He's really angry now,"* or *"She's having difficulty believing what I just said."* It is useful to use plain-language words with wide all-inclusive meanings such as "shock" or "distress" or "upset" in your own mental description, because that will help you in Step 3.

Then, after you have mentally identified one of the emotions, proceed to Step 2.

Step 2: Identify the Cause of That Emotion.

The second step is to focus on the event that precipitated or triggered the emotion. Usually, the immediate cause of the emotion is the piece of news that you have just given or the topic that one of you has just raised.

You may not need to be more precise than that. You are not required to perform a miracle of psychoanalysis (*"This man is upset because he now sees his career and relationships as total failures and is doubtful that he can recreate his lost youth"*) to make an effective empathic response. All you need do in Step 2 is to pinpoint the immediate cause of the emotional reaction; very often it will be the news that you have just given.

Step 3: Respond in a Way That Shows You Have Made the Connection Between Steps 1 and 2.

In other words, tell the patient that you have observed his feelings, and that you are aware of what started that emotion off. Empathic responses (and there are hundreds) usually take the form of, *"Clearly that's a major shock,"* or *"You are obviously very upset by this,"* or *"I do realize that this is awful for you,"* or *"This is difficult to take in, isn't it?"*

When you respond to a patient's feelings with an empathic response, you achieve three objectives simultaneously:

1. **You legitimize that person's feelings:** You are telling the patient that the emotion he is experiencing is an understandable response to the situation. In doing this, you show that you are not making a judgment about the emotion.
2. **You are also telling the patient that it is permissible to discuss those feelings:** In other words, you are demonstrating that feelings are legitimate items on the agenda between the two of you, in the words of the cliché, *"We can talk about this."*
3. **You change the subject:** For this moment, you are not talking about the infarct or the hypertension or the bowel cancer; you are talking about how the patient feels now in response to the information.

In other words, you are showing the patient that you have noted his feelings—however briefly—and are including them as part of your approach to care.

Furthermore, it is worth emphasizing that the empathic response—simply identifying the emotion that is there—is nonjudgmental. You may (appropriately) be forming a judgment of the situation in your own mind and might be thinking, *"This patient is making a very big fuss over a small problem"*), but your response does not express that judgment. When you make an empathic response, you are not stating judgment on the emotion, and you not stating whether the emotion is appropriate (in your view) or in proportion (in your view) to the import of the news. You are simply stating that you have seen that the patient is experiencing it. That is one of the main features of the empathic response—you are acknowledging the existence of the patient's emotion and are not stating your own assessment of the appropriateness of that emotion. The empathic response is discussed in greater detail and is illustrated with examples of ways of phrasing it, both in diagram form and in videotaped scenarios on DVD.[35]

S—STRATEGY AND SUMMARY

The next step of the discussion—arriving at a strategy for clinical management and summarizing the whole discussion—is of course the "meat" of the discussion in terms of the treatment. This is the part of the discussion for which we have received the most training—determining the extent of the disease, the precise causes of the symptoms, the treatment, and all the other clinical features of the situation. Almost always, emotions will arise as these points are discussed; those reactions require acknowledgement as they arise.

The closing of the interview—the summary—should contain three components:

1. A Précis.

It is important to summarize in a few sentences the major points that have been covered.

2. "Any further points?"

Before closing the discussion, it is worthwhile to ask *"Are there any other major points that we need to discuss right now?"* If you have run out of time (as we all do!), then you can at least set the agenda for the next meeting.

3. Next contact.

Finally, close the interview with a clear "contract for the next contact" (*"So, we'll start the treatment next Tuesday, and I'll see you in 3 weeks. Goodbye for now."*)

CONCLUSION: THE PRACTICALITIES OF BREAKING BAD NEWS

Discussions of difficult news are an important part of the relationship between clinician and patient.[36,37] Each discussion is unique and individual, just as patients are unique and individual. Nevertheless, strategies and procedures can be used to optimize these discussions, just as strategies and procedures may be used to examine the cranial nerves or to assess the musculoskeletal system in the legs. Standardization of the approach is what allows accurate assessment and appropriate response in these physical examples, and the same is true of discussing difficult news. The strategy outlined above does not mean that you will use the same words every time, but it does mean that you will be able to assess the patient's comprehension of the situation and—more important—will respond to the way that each individual patient reacts to the news.[38] Furthermore, this strategy is teachable and helpful to students.[39]

The way in which we discuss difficult news with our patients has a major effect on the way they perceive us and our care from that moment on.[40] As is often said about communication, *"If we do it badly, they may never forgive us; if we do it well, they may never forget us."*[41]

REFERENCES

1. Wallace JA, Hlubocky FJ, Daugherty CK. Emotional responses of oncologists when disclosing prognostic information to patients with terminal disease: results of qualitative data from a mailed survey to ASCO members. *J Clin Oncol.* 2006;24:18S.
2. Buckman R. Breaking bad news: why is it still so difficult? *BMJ.* 1984;288:1597–1599.
3. Gorlin R, Zucker HD. Physicians' reactions to patients. *N Engl J Med.* 1983;308:1059–1063.
4. Oken D. What to tell cancer patients: a study of medical attitudes. *JAMA.* 1961;175:86–94.
5. Novack DH, Plumer R, Smith RL, et al. Changes in physicians' attitudes toward telling the cancer patient. *JAMA.* 1979;241:897–900.
6. Goldie U. The ethics of telling the patient. *J Med Ethics.* 1982;8:128–133.
7. Lichter I. Rights of the individual patient. In: Stoll BA, ed. *Ethical dilemmas in cancer care.* London: Macmillan; 1989:7–16.
8. Rockwell LE. Truthtelling. *J Clin Oncol.* 2007;25:454–455.
9. Buckman R. *"But the surgeon said he'd got it all."* Scenario #5, DVD, Practical plans for difficult conversations in medicine. Baltimore, MD: Johns Hopkins University Press; 2010.
10. Northouse PG, Northouse LU. Communication and care: issues confronting patients, health professionals and family members. *J Psychosoc Oncol.* 1987;5:17–45.
11. Buckman R. *"My mother's not to be told."* Scenario #6, DVD, Practical plans for difficult conversations in medicine. Baltimore, MD: Johns Hopkins University Press; 2010.
12. Maguire P, Faulkner A. How to do it: communicate with cancer patients. Handling bad news and difficult questions. *BMJ.* 1988;297:907–909.
13. Buckman R, Kason Y. *How to break bad news: a guide for health care professionals.* Baltimore, MD: Johns Hopkins University Press; 1992.
14. Baile WF, Buckman R, Lenzi R, et al. SPIKES—A six-step protocol for delivering bad news:
application to the patient with cancer. *Oncologist.* 2000;5:302–311.
15. DiMatteo MR, Taranta A, Friedman HS, et al. Predicting patient satisfaction from physicians' non-verbal communication skills. *Med Care.* 1980;18:376–387.
16. Knapp ML, Hall JA. *Nonverbal communication in human interactions.* 5th ed. Wadsworth, UK: Thomas Learning; 2007.
17. Hall ET. *The silent language.* New York: Doubleday; 1959 Reprinted Anchor, 1981.
18. Galanti G-A. *Caring for patients from different cultures.* 4th ed. Philadelphia: University of Pennsylvania Press; 2008.
19. Kleinsmith A, Bianchi-Berthouze N. Recognizing affective dimensions in body language. In: *Lecture Notes in Computer Science.* Berlin, Heidelberg: Springer; 2007.
20. Older J. Teaching touch at medical school. *JAMA.* 1984;252:931–933.
21. Maguire P. Communication skills. In: *Patient care health care and human behaviour.* London: Academic Press; 1984:153–173.
22. Frankel RM, Beckman HB. The pause that refreshes. *Hosp Pract.* 1988;(Sept 30):64–67.
23. Back AL, Bauer-Wu SM, Rushton CH, et al. Compassionate silence in the patient-clinician encounter: a contemplative approach. *J Palliat Med.* 2009;12:1113–1117.
24. Billings A. Sharing bad news. In: Billings A, ed. *Out-patient management of advanced malignancy.* Philadelphia: Lippincott; 1985:236–259.
25. Maynard DW. On clinicians co-implicating recipients perspective in the delivery of bad news. In: Drew P, Heritage J, eds. *Talk at work: social interaction in institutional settings.* Cambridge, UK: Cambridge University Press; 1992:331–358.
26. Maguire P, Faulkner A. How to do it: communicate with cancer patients. Handling uncertainty, collusion and denial. *BMJ.* 1988;297:972–974.
27. McIntosh J. Patients' awareness and desire for information about diagnosed but undisclosed malignant disease. *Lancet.* 1976;ii:300–303.
28. Jones JS. Telling the right patient. *BMJ.* 1981;283:291–292.
29. Saunders JM, McCorkle R. Models of care for persons with progressive cancer. *Nurs Clin North Am.* 1985;20:365–377.
30. Premi JN. Communicating bad news to patients. *Can Fam Physician.* 1981;27:837–841.
31. Reynolds PM, Sanson-Fisher RW, Poole AD, et al. Cancer and communication: information giving in an oncology clinic. *BMJ.* 1981;282:1449–1451.
32. Hockley JM, Dunlop R, Davies RJ. Survey of distressing symptoms in dying patients and their families in hospital and the response to symptom control team. *BMJ.* 1988;296:1715–1717.
33. Buckman R, Baile WB. Truth telling: yes, but how? *J Clin Oncol.* 2007;11:6814.
34. Maguire P, Pitceathly C. Key communication skills and how to acquire them. *BMJ.* 2002;325:697–700.
35. Buckman RDVD. *Practical plans for difficult conversations in medicine.* Baltimore, MD: Johns Hopkins University Press; 2010.
36. Kaplan SH, Greenfield S, Ware JE. Impact of the doctor-patient relationship on the outcomes of chronic disease. In: Stewart M, Roter D, eds. *Communicating with medical patients.* Newbury Park, CA: Sage Publications; 1989:228–245.
37. DiMatteo MR, Prince LM, Taranta AJ. Patients' preceptions of physicians' behaviour: determinants of patient commitment to the therapeutic relationship. *Commun Health.* 1979;4:280–290.
38. Maynard D. Breaking bad news in clinical settings. In: Dervin B, ed. *Progress in communication sciences.* Norwood, NJ: Ablex Publishing Co; 1989:161–163.
39. Garg A, Buckman R, Kason Y. Teaching medical students how to break bad news. *CMAJ.* 1997;6:1159–1164.
40. Radovsky SS. Bearing the news. *N Engl J Med.* 1985;513:586–588.
41. Buckman R. Communications and emotions: skills and effort are key. *BMJ.* 2002;325:672.

Assessing decision-making capacity

48

Martin L. Smith

Medical-surgical discoveries, advancements, and innovations have become commonplace during the past 50 years. Parallel to these significant medical-surgical developments has been an increased emphasis on patient participation and partnership in healthcare decision making. The bioethical terms emerging during these recent decades and reflecting this parallel development include "patient autonomy," "patient self-determination," "informed consent," "informed refusal," and "patient rights."[1]

But before these developments and for the first half of the 20th century, healthcare decision making was characterized (some might say, stereotyped) as "paternalistic,"[2] meaning that physicians viewed themselves akin to "fathers" (*pater* in Latin) or parents, and patients viewed themselves (or at least were viewed by their "fatherly" physicians) as unquestioning, child-like followers of medical directives. In this model of decision making, physicians had almost all of the authority, power, and control over medical decisions and provided directives that patients were expected to follow obediently. A minimum of selected information and explanation had to be provided by physicians to patients because patients were not viewed as capable of understanding much of the complex clinical information associated with their diagnoses and treatments. Patients were expected to comply with recommended interventions and medical regimens that physicians judged to be best. Ultimately, medical decisions were made almost unilaterally by physicians whose duty it was to promote and uphold their patients' best interests (i.e., maximize patient benefits; duty of beneficence) while minimizing patient harm (duty of nonmaleficence), with limited patient participation.[3]

But in the second half of the 20th century, this paternalism paradigm gave way to a partnership model for decision making in health care. In this newer model of decision making, the expertise of physicians (encompassing their knowledge and skills) remains essential. However, the expertise of patients has come to be recognized as significant as well.[4] Patients, after all, are experts regarding their own values, lifestyles, activities of daily living, relationships, the meaning that illness has for them, and their own meaning-generating interests and activities. In such a partnership model, the voice of physicians regarding medical assessments, options, and recommendations must be heard in conjunction with the voice of patients regarding their own goals, preferences, and wishes. Quill and Brody, envisioning a similar model for healthcare decision making, have described an "enhanced autonomy" model that encourages patients and physicians to actively exchange ideas, explicitly negotiate differences, and share power and influence to serve the patient's best interests.[5]

A partnership or enhanced autonomy model for medical decision making places significant emphasis on the doctrine, practice, and process of informed consent, and therefore on the possibility of informed refusal.[6] Patients need basic and understandable information about recommended treatments, specifically, the nature, purpose, risks, benefits, and alternatives of proposed interventions. More important, patients need to understand, in a transparent way, the thinking of their physicians[7] (i.e., how their physicians arrived at the treatment options and recommendations being presented). Only with this type of disclosed information and explanation (in language understandable to patients), coupled with patients' own goals and values, can patients make good and appropriate healthcare decisions that are in concert with and promote their own best interests.

In the context of a partnership or enhanced autonomy model for healthcare decision making, a moral maxim or "rule of thumb" has emerged:

Informed patients with decision-making capacity (DMC) and freedom of choice have the right to consent to and refuse recommended treatments, even when treatments are life-saving or life-sustaining.

Of course, exceptions exist for this assertion (e.g., the need for urgent, life-saving interventions when patient preferences or wishes are unknown), but in general, the moral maxim holds for most clinical situations and circumstances.

This paradigm shift from paternalism to partnership has profoundly changed the practice of medicine. Clinical "standards of care" now include patients' active participation in their own healthcare decisions.

A foundational element for operationalizing this partnership model, in concrete circumstances for a specific patient, is whether the patient has appropriate cognitive skills to participate actively in his or her own healthcare decisions. A core question, then, is this: In this specific clinical situation and for this specific clinical decision, does the patient have sufficient DMC to participate in this decision? Related and intertwined questions include these: If doubts or concerns exist about a patient's DMC, how should an assessment of DMC be performed? What cognitive skills does a patient need to demonstrate to be judged as having DMC? Who should perform such assessments and make such judgments about a patient's DMC? Who has ultimate responsibility for these assessments and determinations? If a patient is judged to lack DMC, how are decisions to be made if the decisions are to be consistent with a partnership or enhanced autonomy model as described previously? This chapter aims to answer these questions.

DECISION-MAKING CAPACITY DESCRIBED AND DISTINGUISHED

Decision-making capacity (DMC) refers to a set of cognitive skills that a patient possesses and demonstrates, and that are sufficient for the patient to make a specific healthcare decision. Admittedly, the phrase "decision-making capacity" is somewhat clumsy and awkward. A more frequently used short-hand term is "competence," which is used to describe whether a patient is viewed as capable of making his or her own healthcare decisions. But this use of "competence" to describe "decision-making capacity" is inaccurate and can be misleading.

Technically, "competence" and "incompetence" are legal determinations usually based on jurisdictional legislation or resulting from judicial proceedings.[8] In most governmental jurisdictions, persons are viewed as competent once they reach a specified chronological age of majority (usually 18 years). Before the specified age, under the law, a person is a minor and is incompetent, unless declared otherwise by a judge or by circumstances described in applicable law. Additionally, a court or a judge can conclude and declare an adult person as incompetent and therefore in need of a court-appointed guardian for decision making and protection. Expert opinions from physicians and psychiatrists are often used by judges during such competency hearings and determinations. But in clinical settings, unless a judicial intervention has resulted in a declaration of competence or incompetence, the more

appropriate term for describing a patient's ability to make a specific clinical decision is "decision-making capacity."

Four cognitive abilities and skills have been identified and associated with DMC: (1) the ability to express a choice, (2) the ability to understand relevant information, (3) the ability to appreciate the situation and its consequences, and (4) the ability to reason with relevant information.[9] Each skill is important and can be distinguished from the others, as will become clearer later when the assessment of each skill is discussed. Also, in a very real sense, all four skills are "relational" in that they can be assessed only in relation to a specific clinical intervention or decision with its own specific nature, purpose, risks, benefits, potential outcomes, and alternatives. For this reason, assessment of DMC should always be related and specific to a particular healthcare decision and the relevant information and consequences of that decision. Assessments of DMC, then, are narrow, specific, and limited to the decision at hand, in contrast to "competency" determinations, which are usually more generic judgments that apply to wide-ranging spheres of persons' lives.

TRIGGERS FOR ASSESSING DECISION-MAKING CAPACITY

Multiple forces and factors can have an impact on or compromise a patient's DMC. Such factors include powerful medications for cancer pain (e.g., opioids), dementia, delirium, intractable or untreated mental illness, debilitating depression, traumatic brain injury and stroke, mental retardation and developmental delay, prolonged stay in an intensive care unit ("ICU psychosis"), extreme fatigue, and emotional immaturity. Many of these factors can be temporary and reversible, but many can also be permanent.

Simply because a patient refuses recommended treatment does not mean that the patient lacks DMC. Treatment refusals by patients can be made for a variety of reasons, including deeply personal values, religious beliefs, misinformation, the influence of others, or idiosyncratic reasoning. Many patients who refuse treatment may have diminished decision-making abilities, but nevertheless, a refusal of treatment in and of itself is not sufficient grounds for concluding that a patient lacks DMC. The reasons for the refusal need to be explored before such a conclusion can be reached.

The reverse is also true: Because a patient is agreeable to and cooperative with recommended treatment does not mean that the patient possesses adequate DMC for the decision at hand. Patients can easily nod their heads as if in agreement with what they do not understand, or can provide affirmative answers to leading-type questions despite an absence of appreciation of risks and alternatives (*"You really do want us to remove that tumor before it gets any bigger, don't you?"*).

A patient who carries a diagnosis of a psychiatric illness (e.g., schizophrenia) does not necessarily lack DMC. The psychiatric illness could be under control as the result of effective medications, or the psychiatric illness could impede a patient from being able to make highly risky medical decisions but not impede the same patient from making low-risk, high-benefit decisions (see later for a discussion of a "sliding scale" model of DMC). Similarly, patients who are involuntarily committed to a psychiatric inpatient unit (often because they are a danger to themselves or others, or because they are unable to care for themselves) do not necessarily lack DMC for all healthcare decisions.

At least four triggers should prompt assessment of a patient's DMC.[10] The presence of these triggers does not mean that the patient does in fact lack DMC, but their presence can raise questions and concerns about cognitive abilities and therefore can prompt a more careful evaluation of the patient's DMC. These four triggers are (1) abrupt changes in a patient's mental status, (2) a patient's refusal of recommended treatment, (3) a patient's consent to treatment that will be especially invasive or risky, and (4) the presence of any of the risk factors noted in the first paragraph of this section.

ASSESSING DECISION-MAKING CAPACITY

Grisso and Appelbaum assert that an appropriate assessment of DMC can be performed only after a process of information disclosure regarding a specific procedure, treatment, or decision.[11] Their assertion is consistent with an understanding that DMC is not a global or generic determination regarding decision making, but a determination of cognitive abilities related to a particular decision to be made by a patient.

In an oncology setting, then, one can easily imagine a patient whose DMC may be uncertain being educated by members of a healthcare team about treatment options related to breast cancer or prostate cancer. The patient's medical condition and diagnosis are reviewed with the patient in understandable language. Chemotherapeutic, radiologic, and surgical options are presented and described, and their purposes are explained (e.g., curative vs. palliative). Short-term, longer-term, and permanent risks as well as benefits of each option are noted. The patient's questions are solicited and answered. A particular treatment option may be recommended by the physician, whose reasons for the recommendation are explained and made transparent to the patient. Only after satisfactory completion of this process of education and information disclosure is a DMC assessment performed.

Toward that end, Grisso and Appelbaum recommend a set of questions aimed at assessing each of the four cognitive skills noted above.[12] For example, for *the ability to express a choice*, the patient could be asked: Have you decided whether to go along with your doctor's suggestions for treatment? Can you tell me what your decision is? For the *ability to understand relevant information*, the patient could be instructed as follows: Tell me in your own words what your doctor told you about the nature of your condition, the recommended treatment (or diagnostic test, or research protocol), the possible benefits of the treatment (or test or research), the possible risks or discomforts of the treatment (or test or research), the possible risks and benefits of alternative treatments, and the possible risks and benefits of no treatment at all. Further, the patient could be asked this question: Your doctor told you of a percentage chance that [named risk] might occur with treatment. In your own words, how likely do you think the occurrence of [named risk] might be? Why is your doctor giving you all this information? What will happen if you decide not to go along with your doctor's recommendation?

Pertaining to the ability to appreciate the situation and its consequences, the patient could be instructed and then asked as follows: Tell me what you really believe is wrong with your health now. Do you believe that you need some kind of treatment? What is the treatment likely to do for you? Why do you think it will have that effect? What do you think will happen if you are not treated? Why do you think your doctor has recommended [specific treatment] for you? And finally, for the patient to demonstrate the *ability to reason with relevant information*, the patient could be requested in this way: Tell me how you reached the decision to accept [or reject] the recommended treatment. What were the factors that were important to you in reaching the decision? How did you balance those factors?

One additional and significant note regarding assessments of DMC is that an assessment should not depend on the patient's ability to vocalize or orally communicate. Patients can participate in DMC assessments via alternate means of communication such as sign language, hand signals, writing, "lip reading," computer keyboard use, eye blinking, or head nodding and shaking. Clearly, communication and assessments using these alternate means can be challenging, but not impossible.

RESPONSIBILITY FOR ASSESSING DECISION-MAKING CAPACITY

Ultimately, the patient's primary or treating physician is responsible for determining and judging whether a patient has DMC. Through training programs or continuing education, physicians should develop a basic competency for doing such assessments. Ideally and practically, a patient's primary or treating physician is the best professional to assess DMC because this physician (1) should already know the patient's medical circumstances and the decision(s) to be made; (2) may be most familiar with the patient's and family's personal, cultural, and religious values and views; (3) knows the patient's history and can place the assessment in the context of previous interactions; and (4) can reevaluate DMC in the future as needed because of an going physician-patient relationship.[13]

But primary or treating physicians need not shoulder the burden of decision-making assessments totally on their own. Many mental health professionals (including psychiatrists, neuropsychologists, and social workers), as a result of their training and expertise, can provide consultative opinions and insight into a patient's mental and emotional state and cognitive abilities. Further, nurses, clergy, and even family members who are familiar with the patient's baseline cognition and thought processes can provide "impressions" about the patient's cognitive functioning. Because a patient's DMC can fluctuate ("wax and wane") from moment to moment, thus making assessment even more challenging, input from professionals who have routine interactions with a patient (e.g., bedside nurses) can be especially valuable.

In many clinical settings, a routine practice has emerged for requesting formal assessments of DMC by consultative liaison psychiatrists. In many cases, a psychiatric consultation can have dual purposes: (1) to assess DMC, and (2) to assess diagnostically and make treatment recommendations for any underlying depression, delirium, or mental illness that may be affecting the patient's DMC. Primary or treating physicians requesting psychiatric consultations for their patients should be clear for which of these two purposes (or both) the consultation is being requested. Also, primary or treating physicians should be mindful that a broad request to assess "whether the patient has DMC" is insufficient; the question to the consultant should be whether the patient has DMC for deciding about a specific treatment or procedure (e.g., palliative radiation to a specific part of the body), with a specific set of known risks and alternatives. Only with this type of specificity can the consultant assess the patient's choice, understanding, appreciation, and reasoning related to the particular decision.

A SLIDING SCALE FOR ASSESSING DECISION-MAKING CAPACITY

Drane has proposed a sliding scale for assessing DMC.[14] An underpinning for this proposal is that an assessment of DMC is not a generic or global judgment about cognitive function but (as noted above) is focused on and related to a specific clinical decision in which the patient is asked to participate. A second underpinning of a sliding-scale approach is that DMC is not an "all or nothing" phenomenon.

Clinical decisions can vary significantly with regard to their benefits and risks. For example, a decision by a patient to authorize a blood test to check for neutropenia has a vastly different benefit-to-burden ratio than a decision about enrolling in a phase I research protocol studying a new combination of chemotherapeutic agents being tried in human subjects for the first time. Because of such wide-ranging variances related to possible benefits, burdens, and likely outcomes, clinical decisions can be located along a continuum determined by the likely effectiveness or ineffectiveness and benefits and burdens of a proposed treatment or intervention, and whether a patient consents to or refuses the treatment or intervention.

Drane suggests that the continuum of decisions can be gradated according to minimal, median, and maximum requirements for cognitive skills that a patient must demonstrate and be judged as having for a specific decision. For example, minimal requirements of awareness of one's medical condition coupled with a simple agreement to proceed with a treatment or diagnostic procedure are all that would be required if the treatment is highly likely to be effective for an acute illness, or if the treatment has few alternatives, or if the procedure has high diagnostic certainty with low risk. Similarly, only a minimal standard of DMC would be required for a patient's refusal of a likely ineffective treatment. On the other end of the continuum, maximum requirements of appreciation and understanding of the illness and treatment and rational decisions accompanied by clear justifications based on beliefs and values would be required for patient consent for likely ineffective treatment, or for refusal of an effective treatment for an acute illness, or for refusal of a treatment with high benefits and insignificant risks. Other decisions with a more balanced benefit-risk ratio (i.e., likely effective but more burdensome) or treatments with high risk but the only hope of benefit would fall into the median range of the continuum. For this middle range of decisions, the patient would be expected to demonstrate a basic understanding of the medical situation and proposed treatment, and to make a choice based on known medical outcomes.

For this sliding-scale model for assessing DMC, the four core cognitive skills previously discussed would continue to provide the framework for the DMC assessment. However, the rigor by which each skill would be assessed and the benchmarks that a patient would be expected to meet for each skill would vary, depending on the decision to be made and whether it fell within minimal, median, or maximum requirements.

STANDARDIZED TOOLS FOR ASSESSING COGNITIVE FUNCTION

Despite the significance that DMC holds for an effective and interactive physician-patient partnership and for actualizing an enhanced autonomy model of decision making, "there are currently no formal guidelines from professional societies for the assessment of a patient's capacity to consent to treatment."[15] As previously discussed, this chapter has endorsed as a clinically useful framework the Grisso-Appelbaum model of assessment for four delineated cognitive skills. However, a variety of standardized tests for assessing DMC have gained recognition in practice and in the published literature.[16]

One such tool is the Mini Mental State Examination (MMSE). It is an 11-question screening instrument that measures multiple areas of cognitive function: Orientation, Registration, Attention and Calculation, Recall, and Language. Each correct answer given by the patient is awarded 1 point, with an achievable maximum score of 30. For Orientation, the patient is asked the year, date, day of the week, and month, as well as the state, country, city, hospital, and floor. For Registration, the examiner names three objects (e.g., pencil, chair, bed), and the patient is asked to repeat the names until he or she gets them correct; attempts by the patient to learn three objects are counted and recorded. For Attention and Calculation, the patient is asked to count in multiples of 7 through five answers, or is asked to spell the word "world" backward. For Recall, the patient is asked to repeat the three objects learned during the Registration component. For Language, a series of six questions and directives are presented to the patient, including "Read and obey the following: CLOSE YOUR EYES," "Name a pencil and watch," and "Write a sentence." Significant for any assessment of DMC is that the MMSE may be useful as a generic screening tool to distinguish patients with and without cognitive impairments. MMSE scores lower than 19 are highly associated with the absence of DMC.[17,18] However, the MMSE is not a substitute for a formal assessment of DMC for a specific clinical decision. No components of the MMSE are flexible enough to allow an assessment of patients' understandings of particular clinical circumstances and the specific decisions to be made. Further, as can be concluded from the description of the various components of the MMSE, it relies significantly on verbal responses, reading, and writing. For patients with hearing or visual impairment, with marginal English language skills, or who are intubated, MMSE scores may indicate that patients have significant cognitive impairment, whereas in reality they may have adequate cognitive skills to make specific decisions. The usefulness of the MMSE, then, is as an initial screening tool that may lead to a more formal assessment of DMC for specific decisions in which the patient is asked to participate.

A second screening instrument that is structured in accord with the Grisso-Appelbaum four cognitive skills framework is the MacArthur Competence Assessment Tool for Treatment (MacCAT-T).[19] This instrument uses a structured interview incorporating specific information related to the particular decision a patient is asked to make. Quantitative scores are generated for each of the four cognitive skills being evaluated

(Choice, Understanding, Appreciation, and Reasoning). For an experienced evaluator, the MacCAT-T takes about 20 minutes to administer and score. Unlike the MMSE, the MacCAT-T can be an effective tool for assessing DMC.

ASSESSING ADOLESCENTS FOR DECISION-MAKING CAPACITY

If legally adult patients (i.e., those who have chronologically reached the age of majority) can be judged to lack DMC for specific decisions, can the opposite also be true? Can legally "minor" patients (usually below the age of 18) be judged to have the requisite cognitive skills to be viewed as having DMC for specific decisions? With some nuances, the answer is yes.

Cases not being addressed here are those in which persons younger than the age of majority have become emancipated minors, that is, they are already viewed by a court or society as having authority over their own persons and affairs. Depending on the legal jurisdiction, a chronologically minor-aged person can become emancipated by marrying, joining the military, being self-supporting, or being declared emancipated by a court. Such an adolescent would be viewed legally as competent, although he or she too could lack DMC, depending on the person's clinical condition and the specific healthcare decision to be made. For example, an emancipated minor's cognitive abilities could be compromised or diminished by the presence of a brain tumor, and the patient may be asked to consent to surgical resection with significant risks.

Regarding the presence or absence of DMC in adolescents, the more problematic and controversial cases involve adolescent patients who legally are still minors. These patients are the focus of this section of the chapter.

For pediatric decision making, the American Academy of Pediatrics (AAP) distinguishes parental permission, pediatric patient assent, and informed consent.[20] Most pediatric healthcare decisions, in a shared responsibility or partnership model of decision making, involve and include parental involvement and permission (i.e., authorization by the patient's parents to proceed with recommended treatments or diagnostic procedures), based on what is judged (by professionals and parents together) to be in the patient's best interests. Generally, informed parental permission should be sought in cases involving healthcare decisions for infants and young children. Of course, seeking parental authorization also implies the possibility of parental refusal of recommended interventions.

For older children and adolescents, the AAP recommends that, to the greatest extent feasible, decision making should include the assent of the patient, as well as the participation of parents and professionals. At a minimum, this means "helping the patient achieve a developmentally appropriate awareness of the nature of his or her condition," and "soliciting an expression of the patient's willingness to accept the proposed care."[21] Similar to the permission-refusal possibility for parents, pediatric patient assent or agreement to accept recommended treatment implies the possibility of patient dissent or refusal to assent. Here, the AAP accords significant weight to the patient's dissent under some clinical circumstances:

There are clinical situations in which a persistent refusal to assent (i.e., dissent) may be ethically binding. This seems most obvious in the context of research (particularly that which has no potential to directly benefit the patient). A patient's reluctance or refusal to assent should also carry considerable weight when the proposed intervention is not essential to his or her welfare and/or can be deferred without substantial risk... Coercion in diagnosis or treatment is a last resort.[22]

In the context of promoting pediatric inclusion, participation, and assent-dissent related to healthcare decisions, the AAP affirms the possibility that adolescents, for some specific clinical decisions, may be able to provide an authentic informed consent. This affirmation implies that some adolescents for some decisions under some circumstances can be judged to have DMC. Limited relevant empirical studies conclude that some adolescents, approximately age 14 and older, may have sufficiently developed cognitive skills to make informed healthcare decisions,[23] especially if the patient has had long-standing experiences in dealing with a chronic illness or disability for which decisions need to be made.[24] The AAP encourages continued parental involvement even in such cases, yet states "no additional requirement to obtain parental permission exists."

An assessment of DMC for specific decisions to be made by adolescents should follow the same format, framework, and guidelines as discussed previously. After a process of education and information disclosure, the adolescent patient should be assessed for abilities to express a choice, understand relevant information, appreciate the clinical situation and its circumstances, and reason with relevant information. A "sliding scale" of decision making, based on a benefit-risk analysis and ratio, would also apply to adolescent decision making and assessments of DMC.

DECISION MAKING FOR PATIENTS LACKING DECISION-MAKING CAPACITY

The "gold standard" for professional-patient decision making includes active participation of informed patients who have DMC for specific decisions and who have expertise regarding their own values, preferences, and wishes. But if a patient is judged to lack DMC for a specific clinical decision, an alternate decision-making process and standard need to be used, especially if a partnership model of decision making is to be upheld.

The "silver standard" (second best) for decision making includes involving surrogate or proxy decision makers (often family members or friends) who can provide a reasonable approximation of what patients would have wanted if they had DMC and could speak for themselves at the time. A surrogate decision maker should be asked to provide a substituted judgment on behalf of a patient, that is, the surrogate should substitute himself or herself in the place of the patient and make decisions based on the formerly capacitated patient's inferred values and wishes. An appropriate question to a surrogate could be this: "Knowing what we know about this person's behavior, values, and prior decisions, what do you think she would want in these circumstances?"[25] The goal, then, of surrogate decision makers is to make judgments and decisions in accord with what they think patients would have decided under the current clinical conditions and circumstances.

In emergency, life-threatening situations, the standard for decision making is usually for healthcare professionals to act to protect, promote, and preserve physiologic life, unless a clear directive to the contrary (e.g., a Do-Not-Resuscitate

[DNR] order) is provided. The prevailing standard under these circumstances is the "best interests"[26] of the patient. This same standard of best interests would also apply if a surrogate decision maker is available but the surrogate is unable to identify patient wishes or preferences (e.g., "We never talked about this clinical situation"). Finally, the best interest standard would also apply if the patient lacks DMC and a surrogate cannot be found. Under such circumstances, even in non–life-threatening situations but when informed consent (by patient or surrogate) would ordinarily be obtained before proceeding, clinical management of the patient should still proceed and not be significantly delayed. Healthcare professionals and multi-disciplinary teams should continue rigorous efforts to learn a patient's social and medical history, to identify a surrogate, and possibly to seek a court-appointed guardian.[27] But in the interim, based on patient best interests, there is ethical support for continuing "professional only" patient management decisions with appropriate safeguards in place. These safeguards could include a second medical opinion (documented in the patient's medical record) concurring with the management plan and recommendations of the primary or treating physician, and review by an ethics consultation team,[28] especially if decisions to be made could result in the patient's death (e.g., writing of a DNR order, withdrawal of a ventilator).

CONCLUSION

Multiple myths exist and prevail with regard to assessing DMC.[29] Eight of those myths are as follows: (1) DMC and legal competence are the same, (2) absence of DMC can be presumed when patients refuse recommended treatments or procedures, (3) patients who agree to and cooperate with

medical recommendations have DMC, (4) DMC is an "all or nothing" phenomenon, (5) patients lack DMC if they have a mental illness or a psychiatric disorder, or have been involuntarily committed, (6) absence of DMC is permanent and irreversible, (7) adolescents lack DMC simply because they are not legally adults, and (8) only mental health professionals can assess DMC. This chapter has provided information and explanations that should have dispelled all of these myths.

This chapter has consistently asserted that DMC is a relational reality, such that an assessment of DMC can only be properly done in relationship to a specific clinical decision in which a patient is asked to participate. Because of the relational nature of DMC assessments, DMC is not an "all or nothing" phenomenon, but rather is appropriately viewed on a continuum or "sliding scale," conditioned primarily by the likely benefit-risk ratio of the decision presented to the patient. Depending on the benefit-risk ratio, patients should be expected to demonstrate variable degrees of four cognitive abilities associated with DMC: (1) express a choice, (2) understand relevant information, (3) appreciate the situation and its consequences, and (4) reason with relevant information.

Finally, this chapter acknowledges the special expertise that psychiatrists and other mental health professionals may have for assessing DMC. The impressions and insights of clergy, social workers, nurses, and family members regarding a patient's cognitive functioning can also be helpful. Nevertheless, the ultimate responsibility for assessing DMC lies with a patient's primary or treating physician, who should, as a core clinical competency, be able to perform DMC assessments. Although there is no "gold standard" as to how such assessments should be done, this chapter has provided recommendations and resources for physicians to obtain or enhance this clinical competency.

REFERENCES

1. Smith ML, Eves M. Patient rights. In: Kattan M, ed. *Encyclopedia of medical decision making*. Thousand Oaks, CA: SAGE Publications, Inc; 2009:862–866.
2. Beauchamp TL, Childress JF. *Principles of biomedical ethics*. 5th ed. New York: Oxford University Press; 2001:176–187.
3. Emanuel EJ, Emanuel LL. Four models of the physician-patient relationship. *JAMA*. 1992;267:2221–2226.
4. Lidz CW, Appelbaum PS, Meisel A. Two models of implementing informed consent. *Arch Intern Med*. 1988;148:1385–1389.
5. Quill TE, Brody H. Physician recommendations and patient autonomy: finding a balance between physician power and patient choice. *Ann Intern Med*. 1996;125:763–769.
6. Connelly JE. Informed consent, an improved perspective. *Arch Intern Med*. 1988;148:1266–1268.
7. Brody H. Transparency: informed consent in primary care. *Hastings Cent Rep*. 1989;19:5–9.
8. Boyle RJ. Determining patients' capacity to share in decision making. In: Fletcher JC, Hite CA, Lombardo PA, et al., eds. *Introduction to clinical ethics*. Frederick, MD: University Publishing Group, Inc; 1995:65–79.
9. Appelbaum PS, Grisso T. Assessing patients' capacities to consent to treatment. *N Engl J Med*. 1988;319:1635–1638.

10. Tunzi M. Can the patient decide? Evaluating patient capacity in practice. *Am Fam Physician*. 2001;64:299–306.
11. Grisso T, Appelbaum PS. *Assessing competence to consent to treatment, a guide for physicians and other health professionals*. New York: Oxford University Press; 1998:83–84.
12. Grisso T, Appelbaum PS. In: *Assessing competence to consent to treatment, a guide for physicians and other health professionals*. New York: Oxford University Press; 1998:86–90.
13. Tunzi M. Can the patient decide? Evaluating patient capacity in practice. *Am Fam Physician*. 2001;64:299–306.
14. Drane JF. The many faces of competency. *Hastings Cent Rep*. 1985;15:17–21.
15. Appelbaum PS. Assessment of patients' competence to consent to treatment. *N Engl J Med*. 2007;357:1838.
16. Dunn LB, Nowrangi MA, Palmer BW, et al. Assessing decisional capacity for clinical research or treatment: a review of instruments. *Am J Psychiatry*. 2006;163:1323–1334.
17. Kim SYH, Caine ED. Utility and limits of the Mini Mental State Examination in evaluating consent capacity in Alzheimer's disease. *Psychiatr Serv*. 2002;53:1322–1324.
18. Karlawish JHT, Casarett DJ, James BD, et al. The ability of persons with Alzheimer's disease (AD)

to make a decision about taking an AD treatment. *Neurology*. 2005;64:1514–1519.
19. Grisso T, Appelbaum PS. *Assessing competence to consent to treatment, a guide for physicians and other health professionals*. New York: Oxford University Press; 1998:101–126, 173–200.
20. Committee on Bioethics of the American Academy of Pediatrics. Informed consent, parental permission, and assent in pediatric practice. *Pediatrics*. 1995;95:314–317.
21. Committee on Bioethics of the American Academy of Pediatrics. Informed consent, parental permission, and assent in pediatric practice. *Pediatrics*. 1995;95:315.
22. Committee on Bioethics of the American Academy of Pediatrics. Informed consent, parental permission, and assent in pediatric practice. *Pediatrics*. 1995;95:316.
23. Weithorn LA, Campbell SB. The competency of children and adolescents to make informed treatment decisions. *Child Dev*. 1982;53:1589–1598.
24. Alderson P, Sutcliffe K, Curtis K. Children's competence to consent to medical treatment. *Hastings Cent Rep*. 2006;36:25–34.
25. Post LF, Blustein J, Dubler NN. *Handbook for health care ethics committees*. Baltimore, MD: The Johns Hopkins University Press; 2007:31.

26. Beauchamp TL, Childress JF. *Principles of biomedical ethics*. 5th ed. New York: Oxford University Press; 2001:102–103.

27. Sadovnikoff N, Jurchak M. Substituted judgments in the absence of surrogates. Letter to the Editor. *Crit Care Med*. 2007;35:2467.

28. Lo B. Ethics committees and ethics consultations. *Resolving ethical dilemmas: a guide for clinicians*. 3rd ed. Philadelphia: Lippincott Williams & Wilkins; 2005:111–116.

29. National Ethics Committee of the Veterans Health Administration. Ten myths about decision-making capacity. 2002. Available at: http://www.ethics.va.gov/docs/necrpts/NEC_Report_20020201_Ten_Myths_about_DMC.pdf Accessed 03.01.10.

49

Discussion of treatment options in supportive oncology

Heather L. Shepherd and Martin H. N. Tattersall

Patients with cancer and their families face many instances when decisions are made about treatments. The outpatient cancer consultation is generally the arena in which these decisions are discussed, made, and reviewed. As the management of cancer has evolved, the range of available treatment options has increased. Additionally, the move toward a multidisciplinary team approach, involving collaboration with other health professionals to plan care, has increased the opportunity and the relevance of shared decision making.[1] The rise of evidence-based medicine and an increased focus on patient-centered care have increased the importance of information exchange between cancer doctors and their patients.

Treatment decision-making models in health care are generally described in terms of the roles taken by participants—the doctor and the patient—in the interaction and the resulting treatment decision.[2,3]

Several key pieces of information and interventions are required to reach a decision about treatment. The notion of involving patients in this process is one of the core themes behind the concept of patient-centered care. Patient-centered care supports the notion of sharing information, with clinicians having the ability to empower patients and to share power within their relationship with patients. This entails a change to the traditional view of a doctor-patient relationship.[4]

WHAT CONSTITUTES A TREATMENT OPTION?

In circumstances for which a clearly superior treatment is available, clinicians believe that patient preferences can contribute little to clinical decision making.[5] In other situations, particularly where the benefit-cost ratio of a treatment option is small, where options produce similar survival but different quality-of-life outcomes, or where no clear data on outcomes are available, preference about treatments will vary substantially. In these cases—called preference sensitive decisions—the preferences that drive decision making must be those of the patient, because patient and clinician preferences may be in disagreement. Examples include decisions about whether to have a mastectomy versus a lumpectomy plus radiotherapy for early-stage breast cancer. It has been reported that those patients offered choices show better psychological adjustment, and those who feel they have little control over their disease and treatment have a poorer psychosocial outcome.[6,7]

A survey of 100 patients and 156 clinical specialists regarding preferences for different surgical options for managing large-bowel cancer found that preferences differed significantly between them.[8] Thus it is important to identify preference sensitive decisions (in the opinion of both patients and clinicians) and to target interventions to elicit these preferences effectively. Preference sensitive decisions include not only decisions in which all options provide active treatment. Other clinical scenarios may pose decisions between an "active" cancer treatment and no treatment either as "watchful waiting" or as an option not to undergo anticancer therapy now. Examples of these clinical scenarios are treatment decisions in early prostate cancer, treatment decisions in advanced cancer with no cancer-related symptoms, and treatment decisions with older patients with cancer with comorbid illness.

Another context in which discussion of treatment options is particularly important is the transition from curative to palliative care. Discussing when to stop curative treatment is a difficult and emotionally charged task. Surveys of cancer doctors have found that emotionally charged situations and communicating bad news are reported as being significantly challenging.[9,10] Knowing when to broach this topic and how to introduce the palliative treatment option is important. Schofield and colleagues offer guidance on this discussion (Box 49-1).[11]

Not having this discussion can lead to futile therapy. Earle and colleagues reported increasing use of futile therapies in oncology, with an estimated 10% of patients receiving chemotherapy in their last 2 weeks of life, nearly one third visiting the emergency department, and approximately 10% being admitted to intensive care units at the end of life.[12] Improved

---

BOX 49-1 Guidance on Discussing the Transition From Curative to Palliative Care

Elicit the person's understanding of his/her situation and preferences before discussing clinical decisions.
Provide information.
Respond to the person's emotional reaction.
Negotiate new goals of care.
Ensure continuity of care.
Address family concerns.
Acknowledge cultural and linguistic diversity.

---

understanding of the goals and outcomes of therapy may minimize aggressive treatment at the end of life, where it rarely if ever improves outcome.

STEPS TO REACHING A TREATMENT DECISION IN CANCER CARE

Reaching a treatment decision requires a number of steps that have been highlighted in models of decision making. These models all incorporate the fundamental aspect of information exchange. Cancer doctors need to provide information concerning the clinical status of the patient and should explain what each or any treatment option would mean for the patient.[2] They need to guide the patient through the cognitive processes that result in a treatment decision.[13] In the context of treatment decision making, the most important information is often referred to as risk communication, which allows decisions by both parties to be based on knowledge of benefits, harms, and the probabilities of the choices and possible outcomes of those choices.[14,15]

After treatment options and their relative merits have been identified, a second step in selecting a treatment is the need to discuss values and preferences.

The literature usually focuses on two key areas: (1) treatment decision making, and (2) communication. These concepts in the context of cancer care bring attention to patient preferences, in terms of preferences for information and preferences for involvement. It is this terminology that has been used most frequently in the literature to determine current practice and behavior in cancer consultations. One of the most important messages research in this area consistently reports is that making decisions for patients without consideration of patient preferences is no longer acceptable in the current climate of patient-centered care.

In addition to providing information, cancer clinicians should explore patients' preferences for involvement in choosing a treatment.[15,16] Preferences may relate to the amount of information presented and involvement in making a decision, as well as to the particular treatment options being considered. Preferences for a specific treatment option in particular will be influenced by patient values. In cancer care, this may mean discussing prognosis, disease recurrence, and the harms and benefits of each treatment option, both physically and psychologically, as these will differ between individuals.

CANCER DOCTORS' ACKNOWLEDGMENT OF TREATMENT OPTIONS

A survey of doctors treating different cancer types in Australia regarding their usual approach to treatment decision making and their comfort with decision-making styles showed that doctor specialization in breast or urologic cancer compared with other cancer types, high case load, and female gender were all independently associated with the likelihood of using a shared approach to reaching a treatment decision.[17] More positive attitudes toward sharing treatment decisions with patients were expected in breast surgeons because for many patients, a clear choice of surgical treatment for early breast cancer exists, as had been reported by Charles et al.[18] The observation that urologists were more comfortable with sharing treatment decisions with their patients is similarly not unexpected. However, it is notable that medical oncologists treating breast cancer were less supportive of sharing treatment decisions than were breast surgeons, possibly because of the statistically significant improved outcome from adjuvant systemic therapy, even though many patients have prolonged survival without treatment. These findings add weight to the view that shared decision making is possible only when real options of clinical equipoise or clinical uncertainty exist, and the doctor is happy to allow the patient to be involved in the process.[5]

MAKING A TREATMENT RECOMMENDATION: THE DOCTOR'S PERSPECTIVE

The range of factors that can affect a doctor's treatment recommendation for a particular patient is wide. They can be considered under several categories (Box 49-2).

Research evidence informs the efficacy and side effects of treatment in the treated population, and depending on trial design, these outcomes may be compared with those of a control population. The extent to which the particular patient under consideration is close to the typical patient in the trial

---

BOX 49-2   Factors Influencing a Doctor's Treatment Recommendation

Research evidence
- Applicability to the particular patient

Disease factors
- History of illness
- Presence of measurable disease
- Presence or absence of symptoms due to cancer
- Previous outcomes of treatments

Patient factors
- Family history
- Past medical history and comorbidities
- Experience with previous treatments and their side effects

Expectations for longevity, and remaining life goals
- Attitude toward uncertainty, personality, attitudes of caregivers/relatives
- Geographic considerations

System factors
- Relevant skills locally

Waiting lists
- Costs

---

must be considered because the balance of benefits and side effects may be changed.

Disease factors that may have an impact on the treatment recommendation include the "pace" of disease and the length of history compared with the typical patient, the presence of measurable disease or "insurance policy" treatment, the tolerance and outcome of previous treatments, the presence or absence of disease-related symptoms, and the likelihood of symptom improvement with "effective" treatment. Consideration should also be given to whether treatment directed at symptom control rather than at the cancer may be as effective in palliating symptoms.

Patient factors include medical and family history, the presence of comorbidities that may influence life expectancy and tolerance of treatment, previous treatment and tumor response and tolerance, and patient expectations for longevity based on premorbid factors such as family longevity, social situations, and life goals. Patient attitudes toward uncertainty and side effects of treatments influence recommendations for toxic treatment, and available support from caregivers and geographic factors that can affect the ease of treatment delivery may influence the feasibility of frequent outpatient visits.

System factors include availability of skills to effect results similar to available evidence, the time scale of treatment availability, and the costs of treatment, including those that must be borne by the patient.

PATIENT AWARENESS OF TREATMENT CHOICE

Elit et al.[19] interviewed women with advanced ovarian cancer to identify the extent to which they perceived they had treatment options, understood treatment-related risks and benefits, and preferred to participate in treatment decision making. Most women felt that they made their treatment decision, but most believed they did not have a treatment choice. Women reported trust and hope in describing the patient-doctor interaction, but did not describe doctor exploration of patient preferences or values. Investigators observed that women with advanced epithelial ovarian cancer did not describe treatment decision making as shared, but rather as an interaction that was directed largely by the doctor. They concluded that the onus is on the doctor to provide an environment for shared decision making in the event that the patient is interested in such an interaction.

A survey of oncologists involved in breast cancer care in Ontario, Canada,[18] reported that patient involvement in decision making was less than the oncologist would like. This finding suggests that patients need to be prepared for their potential role in decision making. Studies suggest that doctors need to play a major role in this preparation.

SHARED DECISION MAKING

Shared decision making (SDM) is perceived by many as the preferred way for health professionals and patients to approach treatment decisions. This approach to decision making with patients reflects the move toward patient-centered care. The public expectation to be fully informed about health care and available options has increased over recent years, and acceptance of paternalism, highlighted in references to patients as consumers in the medical ethics and healthcare literature, is decreasing.[20]

One central idea is that of equal contribution, whereby doctor and patient are equal partners in the decision process.[21] This notion of partnership and of power being interchangeable in the doctor-patient relationship is also used to describe SDM.[22] SDM lies between paternalism and informed decision making and can be considered an important component of patient-centered care.[23] SDM involves two steps: presentation of facts about treatment options and discussion of preferences, with the doctor's and the patient's values together determining the final decision.[24]

One of the earliest descriptions of SDM was seen in a deliberative model.[2] Today, the most commonly cited model of SDM in the context of patients with life-threatening disease and different treatment options is that of Charles et al.[25] This model has four essential characteristics:

1. At least two people are involved in the decision-making process.
2. Both patient and doctor take part in treatment decision making.
3. Two-way flow of information occurs between the clinician and the patient.
4. A treatment decision is made when the clinician and the patient agree on the most appropriate treatment.

These four characteristics demonstrate collaboration between doctor and patient through exchange of information, personal values, and preferences related to potential treatment options. However, in many situations, more than two parties are involved. Examples of these include a newly diagnosed breast cancer patient who consults a medical oncologist, a radiation oncologist, and a surgeon, in addition to her family physician or general practitioner. Likewise, in situations of serious illness, significant others of the patient are often involved in making treatment decisions every step of the way.

Information sharing is fundamental to SDM, and the model requires that patients contribute information, including details of their illness or information they may have obtained from other sources such as Internet sites, friends, or disease-related pamphlets and consumer groups. This information sharing assists in communication of individual values and preferences, thereby developing mutual trust and respect. The final component described by Charles et al. is that of agreement by both (or more) parties to the decision reached. This consensus is a defining feature of SDM. This model accepts that the treatment decided upon may not necessarily be the option that either participant considers to be optimal, but it is the one that both support.

Following further research with breast cancer patients and doctors, Charles and colleagues[26] added to their model. The resulting new framework illustrated three stages of the decision-making process: information exchange, deliberation, and the decision of which treatment to implement. This updated model was reported to be more user friendly as a teaching tool for doctors and in assisting them in identifying their own and their patients' preferences for involvement in the process. Further, the authors acknowledged the dynamism of decision making and the likelihood that the preferences of either party change along the process, either within a consultation or at subsequent meetings. In 2003, the model was refined again, emphasizing the importance of doctor facilitation of SDM by encouraging patients to take sufficient time to make decisions, by tailoring information to patients' needs, and by

reinforcing the importance of patients' values in determining the optimal treatment.[27]

Other models of SDM have been presented.[16,28-30]

Current debate around the concept

Since the introduction of the term SDM and the models that describe this approach to decision making and communication with patients, discussion has included interpretation of SDM and what elements identify a decision as shared. Authors have discussed whether SDM is appropriate in all circumstances, whether SDM describes the decision about a treatment or test being made equally by the healthcare provider and the patient, and whether SDM is the process that leads to a treatment or test decision.[28,31-33]

According to Whitney, SDM is feasible only in medical decisions of low certainty, with high or low risk, where two or more alternatives are available. Thus the appropriateness of SDM may vary according to the diagnosis, the type of decision being made, and the context (e.g., general practice vs. specialist care). Patients may prefer to be the decision makers for treatment decisions in chronic but not life-threatening disease situations, but in instances that are considered urgent or life threatening, or with diseases for which the outcome of choice will be more significant, such as cancer, patients may prefer the clinician to take the lead.[23] Edwards asserts that an SDM approach is more likely in contexts where decisions may affect the risk of diseases such as hypertension or ischemic heart disease at a later stage, or when decisions are made about screening in which the risks and benefits of the intervention need to be considered by the doctor and the patient.[23]

The benefits of sharing treatment decisions

One benefit of patient participation is increased patient satisfaction.[21,34,35] Gattellari reported that patients with cancer who jointly decided on treatment with their oncologist experienced better outcomes. A match between preferred and perceived roles in decision making was found for just over one third of patients, with 29% more active than preferred, and 37% participating to a lesser degree than preferred. Patients whose level of participation was less than desired were significantly less satisfied. Irrespective of preference, patients who reported a shared role in decision making were more satisfied with their consultation, with their oncologist, and with information about treatment and emotional support.[21] Other studies have shown greater patient satisfaction when doctors actively encourage patients to participate, regardless of the patients' participation preferences,[36] when patients take an active role in decision making,[37] and when doctors display an enhanced participatory style.[38] These studies suggest that given appropriate support, patients may find value in an SDM approach, even if they initially feel unable to be actively involved in their treatment decisions.

Improved patient physical health outcomes have been reported in studies where patients played an active role in decisions about their treatment.[7,39] Greater adherence to the treatment plan was demonstrated in patients who were more involved in decisions about their treatment.[38] Similarly, Jahng et al.[34] reported agreement on involvement preferences between doctor and patient correlated with adherence and health perception.

Some studies suggest that SDM leads to enhanced psychological outcomes. For women with early breast cancer, being offered a treatment choice or seeing a surgeon who acknowledged treatment options correlated with better patient psychological outcomes, including lower levels of depression.[6,7,39,40] However, this significant difference did not persist 3 years postoperatively.[6] Anxiety levels were found to be lower in more educated patients who believed they had participated in decision making, and in those patients who reported a passive coping style but had received information or had been involved in decision making.[41] However, a study of initial consultations of 96 cancer patients in the Netherlands showed no significant relationship between clinicians' communication behavior and patients' quality of life.[42]

Can SDM improve discussion about treatment options?

Shared decision making is a process that in many respects represents a response to, and an acknowledgment of, the right of patients to be informed of potential healthcare interventions and to choose between them. The philosophy of patient-centered care embraces the notion that the patient has a role to play in this process; however, the expertise that clinicians bring to the process, above and beyond information giving, should not be ignored. From the clinician's perspective, SDM is a useful way of presenting to patients the reality that outcomes in medicine are not certain. SDM is particularly appropriate in instances in which more than one clinically reasonable treatment option is available, or when uncertainty about the outcome of a particular intervention exists.[43,44]

Shared decision making draws attention to the importance of communication and information sharing. The challenges for the clinician are to minimize patients' misunderstanding and misinterpretation of risks or benefits of treatment and to avoid imposing his or her own treatment preferences onto the patient. It is these skills that are required for discussion of treatment options and subsequent decisions, and that enable SDM.

Skills and competences required to practice shared decision making

One of the major challenges in implementing SDM is ensuring that both parties participate in the process. Shared decision making is extremely difficult for the patient to instigate and requires health professionals and particularly the doctor to be supportive of this approach.[25] Health professionals need to create a consultation environment in which patients sense that their input is valued, and that their views and concerns about potential treatment options and outcomes are welcome. Health professionals need skills to elicit preferences from the patient, as well as skills to communicate complex information concerning risks and benefits and probabilities of treatment success or failure.

The skills and competences generally agreed to be necessary are outlined in Boxes 49-3, 49-4, and 49-5.[45,46]

HOW INVOLVED DO CANCER PATIENTS WANT TO BE IN DISCUSSING AND MAKING TREATMENT DECISIONS WITH THEIR CANCER CARE TEAM?

Information preferences

Most studies reveal that patients have a strong desire for maximum information. In an Australian study of 65 female cancer patients, more than 80% wanted to receive as many details

---

BOX 49-3 Competencies of Physicians for Informed Shared Decision Making[45]

1. Develop a partnership with the patient.
2. Establish or review the patient's preferences for information (such as amount or format).
3. Establish or review the patient's preferences for a role in decision making (such as risk taking and degree of involvement of self and others) and the existence and nature of any uncertainty about the course of action to take.
4. Ascertain and respond to patient's ideas, concerns, and expectations (such as about disease management options).
5. Identify choices (including ideas and information that the patient may have), and evaluate the research evidence in relation to the individual patient.
6. Present (or direct patient to) evidence, taking into account competencies 2 and 3 and framing effects (how presentation of the information may influence decision making, etc.). Help patient to reflect on and assess the impact of alternative decisions with regard to his or her values or lifestyle.
7. Make or negotiate a decision in partnership with the patient, and resolve conflict.
8. Agree on an action plan and complete arrangements for follow-up.
   a. Informed shared decision making may also
      i. Involve a team of health p rofessionals
      ii. Involve others (partners, family)
      iii. Differ across cultural, social, and age groups

BOX 49-4 Competencies of Patients for Informed Shared Decision Making*[45]

1. Define (for oneself) the preferred doctor-patient relationship.
2. Find a physician, and establish, develop, and adapt a partnership.
3. Articulate (for oneself) health problems, feelings, beliefs, and expectations in an objective and systematic manner.
4. Communicate with the physician to understand and share relevant information (such as from competency 3) clearly and at the appropriate time in the medical interview.
5. Access information.
6. Evaluate information.
7. Negotiate decisions, give feedback, resolve conflict, and agree on an action plan.

*Preliminary list.

---

as possible, and more than 85% wanted as much information as possible, before and after initial consultations with their oncologists.[47] A study of 2231 patients in the United Kingdom found that 87% preferred to have as much information as possible, good or bad.[48] More than 90% of subjects stated that they "absolutely needed" or "would like to have" information concerning all possible treatments, all possible side effects, and how the treatments work.

Involvement preferences

Patients vary in the extent to which they wish to participate in decisions and in the decisions in which they wish to participate. Patients in the developed world are increasingly health consumers. A European survey of 8119 adults reported that more than 50% of the sample preferred to share decisions with their healthcare provider,[49] with highest rates (74%) found in the younger age group (<35 years). In contrast, few patients report achieving the level of involvement in clinical decision making that they would like.[21]

Involvement preferences of patients with cancer have varied, perhaps because of different disease types and stages among the samples involved. However, in most studies, a majority of patients prefer SDM to passivity or complete autonomy. An Australian study reported that decisional preferences were lower than preferences for information, with 52% wishing to share the decision equally with their doctor, 16% wishing to make the decision themselves after strongly considering the doctor's opinion, and 27% wishing the doctor to make the decision but with consideration of their needs and priorities.[47] Studies of breast cancer patients report that from 48%[50] to 66%[51] to 89%[52] want to play an active or a shared role in decision making. A study in lung cancer patients revealed that 57% wished to play an active or collaborative role in decision making about treatment.[53] Gwede et al.[54] reported that 63% of prostate cancer patients preferred an active role in decision making, 29% preferred a collaborative role, and just 9% preferred a passive role. Beaver et al.[55] reported differences in involvement preferences of patients with different cancer types: 78% of colorectal cancer patients preferred a passive role compared with 52% of breast cancer patients. Pieterse et al.[56] interviewed rectal cancer patients and cancer doctors, finding that 11% of patients preferred "to leave the decision about my treatment to my doctor," and the remainder (89%) of respondents preferred the patient and clinician to share the decision. Studies of heterogeneous samples of cancer patients have reported that 41%,[57] 69%,[58] and 88%[35] preferred a collaborative or active role. In another study, participation in decision making was broken down into knowledge, options, and decision, with 52% preferring to leave final decisions to the doctor.[59]

Patients tend to leave doctors who fail to involve them in decisions.[38] Responding to the growing expectations of patients to participate in medical care decisions creates significant difficulties for healthcare providers in many countries.[60,61]

Cancer patients' expectations for information and involvement in decision making have changed rapidly; only 50 years ago, most patients in the United States were not told their cancer diagnosis, and the doctor's role was to participate in a conspiracy of silence or euphemism, and to decide treatment in the best interests of the patient. Now, most cancer patients are told the diagnosis and expect to be informed about their disease and its management.

FACTORS AFFECTING PATIENT INVOLVEMENT (PARTICIPATION)

Factors that may influence patient involvement in decision making include the context of the treatment decision, the disease type or stage, system issues, and patient and clinician characteristics, such as age, gender, experience, and cultural background.

Context

For clinicians, the idea of involving patients in the decision-making process appears to depend on the existence of options that are clinically equivalent, or on professional uncertainty about the best course of action.

Disease

Studies have reported that the more serious the illness, the less patients prefer to participate in decision making.[62] In one study, only 25% of participants with "serious" illness wanted full information about their illness but did not want to be involved in treatment decisions.[58] These patients were generally male, older, and sicker. Participants with "benign" disease showed more enthusiasm for participation in treatment decisions, with 69% preferring an active or shared role.[50,57] Similarly, in a prospective study, as patients' cancer status worsened, their involvement preference trended toward greater passivity.[63] In contrast, a more recent study found that the desire to participate in decision making increased along the disease trajectory, with 76% of end-stage renal patients preferring to have an active or shared role in decisions.[64]

System factors

Lack of time in the cancer consultation was one of the more frequently experienced barriers to treatment decision making reported by Australian cancer physicians. Physicians with less experience reported system issues as difficult more often. The authors concluded that this might be because physicians with greater experience are more patient-centered in their approach to consultations or have become skilled at overcoming system issues.[65] Numerous studies have reported that collaborative decision making does not increase consultation time and may save time in the long run, in that thorough initial discussion enables subsequent consultations to be more succinct.[66-68]

Patient factors

Studies have identified some predictors of involvement preference, with educational achievement most commonly associated with a desire to play a more active role in the process.[56,69]

Age and education level have been found to correlate with desire for patient participation.[57,62,64,70-72] Younger people, those with more education, and women show a greater inclination toward a collaborative or active role in decision making than older people, those with less education, and men.[57,59,72]

Additional predictors of greater patient involvement include psychological factors such as anxiety, self-efficacy, and locus of control. Data reporting the link between these factors and patients' preferences for involvement in decision making are limited, although these factors are alluded to in studies identifying improved psychological outcomes as a result of greater involvement.

Australian cancer doctors reported that patient anxiety and misconception of their disease or treatment were two of the most frequent barriers to sharing decision making.[65] In Gravel et al.'s review of barriers to implementing SDM, lack of applicability of the process due to patient characteristics, such as anxiety, featured strongly.[73]

Clinician factors

As patient involvement and the consumer role in health care grow,[74] the importance of physicians gaining their patients' trust may increase. Previous studies suggest that trust develops through excellent communication and by response to patient preferences for information and involvement.[75-77] Shepherd et al.[65] investigated cancer doctors' perceptions of factors that may facilitate patient involvement in decision making. Providing written information about treatment options (choices), making another appointment to reach a treatment decision, encouraging the patient to speak with his or her family doctor, and the presence of a third person during the consultation were believed to encourage patient involvement and reflection on treatment choice.

Cultural factors

Cultural norms also play a role in influencing patients' or health professionals' willingness or resistance to involvement in treatment discussions. Eliciting preferences is even more difficult when communication is limited because patients and their cancer care team do not share a common language. Much of the research investigating patient attitudes toward involvement excluded those without sufficient ability in English, although interest in this topic is increasing, and work in these previously neglected populations is under way.

MEASURING SHARED DECISION MAKING: IS IT OUT THERE?

A number of measures have been developed to evaluate the decision-making process. Dy[78] found 11 instruments that focussed on preferences for roles and information. Observational instruments include those reviewed by Elwyn et al.[79] and additional ones listed by Dy.[78,80,81]

Other instruments, which measure other aspects of decision making, have also been developed. These include measures of decision self-efficacy, emotional control, decision regret, decisional conflict, and decisional attitude.

- Decision Emotional Control Scale—Bunn and O'Connor (1996)
- Decision Regret Scale—Brehaut et al. (2003)

- Decision Self-Efficacy Scale—Bunn and O'Connor (1996)
- Decisional Conflict Scale (O'Connor)—O'Connor (1995)
- Decision Attitude Scale—Sainfort and Booske (2000)
- Satisfaction With Decision Scale—Holmes-Rovner et al. (1996)
- Health Care Professionals' Provider Decision Process Assessment Instrument—Dolan (1999)

Alternative ways of evaluating the decision-making process include interaction analysis techniques such as coding systems for use with audio- or video-recorded consultations. Transcripts of the audio or video recordings are analyzed to determine which of the derived elements are present or absent in each consultation.

Does evidence reveal that cancer doctors use an SDM approach when discussing treatment options?

Analysis of 59 consultations between cancer patients and 10 Australian oncologists showed that SDM was introduced in only 24% of oncology consultations and was rated as poor in 75%; preferences for involvement were checked in 10%, and information preferences were checked in 40%.[82] The choice between standard treatment and no treatment was explicitly offered in only 19% of consultations, and an explicit choice between standard treatment and clinical trial participation was presented in 32%. Decisional delay was offered in 78% of consultations. Understanding was verified on one occasion in 46% of consultations, and more than once in 15% of consultations. Questions were invited in 60% of consultations. Thus some but not all elements of SDM models were present in most of these consultations, but a high level of skill was rarely displayed.

Analysis of 118 audio-taped consultations with advanced cancer patients discussing treatment options found that just 14% were given information about life expectancy with and without treatment, 57% were not given any prognostic information, and acknowledgment of trade-offs, one of the characteristics of informed treatment decision making, was presented in 60% of consultations.[83] Patient understanding was checked in 10% of consultations, and even though patients' views were expressed in 75% of cases, in only a third did the doctor invite these opinions.

Tools to monitor patient involvement

The OPTION tool, developed for use in general practice or family medicine[80] to measure evidence of SDM, uses a five-point Likert scale (strongly agree to strongly disagree) for 12 items identified as required components of an SDM consultation (Box 49-3). This tool has been translated into a number of European languages. Other tools developed to measure SDM include the Decision Analysis System for Oncology (DAS-O)[82] and the Decision Support Analysis Tool (DSAT).[84] These three tools have recently been compared by coding transcriptions of audio-recorded consultations of 55 women with early-stage breast cancer. All three coding systems revealed a low score for SDM behaviors[85] (Table 49-1).

Much literature has documented the decision-making style evidenced by patients through their reports post consultation, most commonly using the five-point involvement preferences scale developed by Degner and Sloan[57,86] (Fig. 49-1). This scale, although originally designed to elicit involvement preferences, is commonly used as a descriptive tool to report

Table 49-1 Shared decision making (SDM) scores from the three coding systems

	DAS-O	DSAT	Option
Mean (SD)	34.42 (9.1)	5.35 (1.9)	11.25 (4.4)
Observed range of scores	11–63	0.1–10	5–21
Full scale range	0–78	0–12	0–48
Percentage of score range (mean/highest possible score × 100)	44	46	23

DAS-O, Decision Analysis System for Oncology; DSAT, Decision Support Analysis Tool.

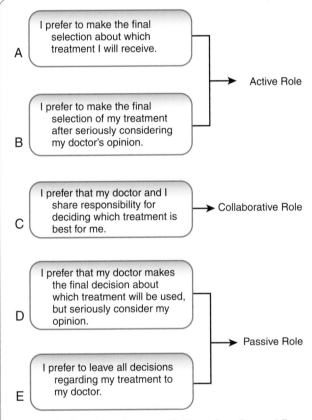

Fig. 49-1 Control preferences. *(Redrawn from Degner LF, Sloan JA. Decision making during serious illness: what role do patients really want to play? J Clin Epidemiol 1992;45:941–950.)*

what actually happened. Often these two results have been compared to determine whether patient preferences have been met. Many of these studies show that many patients do not achieve their desired level of involvement.[21,52,87]

Studies of cancer patients' recall of their role in decision making

A study of patients with lung cancer who were asked to recall their actual involvement found that 33% perceived the doctor

had made the decision, 43% believed the doctor had made the decision but considered their opinion, 9% recalled a shared decision, and 14% recalled making the decision after considering the doctor's views.[53] Most breast cancer patients (40%) recalled that they had made the decision once all options were presented, a third (33%) reported a collaborative experience, and 27% recalled a doctor-led experience that was presented with a recommendation to accept or reject, or in which the surgeon outlined treatment, and then treatment proceeded.[35]

Measuring outcomes or measuring process?

Some currently available measures seek to measure the process, but others measure the outcome (i.e., how the decision is reached or who made the decision). An ongoing question is whether SDM requires the decision itself to be shared, as in "The doctor and the patient made the decision together," or whether an SDM process can occur as long as information, preferences, and negotiation are involved. A further challenge to researchers and health professionals is determining whether process or outcome is more important. This issue is particularly relevant when interventions designed to support SDM are evaluated and their consequences are demonstrated in clinical practice.

DO CANCER DOCTORS SUPPORT AN SDM APPROACH WHEN DISCUSSING TREATMENT OPTIONS?

Three studies investigating clinicians' views of patient involvement in treatment decision making have targeted health professionals who specialize in breast cancer care. One of the earliest studies in the United States[88] invited oncologists, nurses, and patients to complete the 15-item Locus of Decisional Authority in Decision Making survey. For each item, three responses were possible: 0 = doctor should make the decision, 1 = doctor and patient should make the decision, 2 = patient should make the decision. A score of 15 indicated that respondents believed that all decisions should be shared. Total scores for the three groups were below 15, indicating that doctors should have overall decisional authority, with the doctors' group mean score being the lowest—10.23 compared with 12.49 for the patient group and 13.74 for the nurses. Attitudes of the different clinical disciplines represented in the sample were also reported; surgical oncologists were more supportive of patient involvement than were medical and radiation oncologists. No significant differences were found in attitude toward patient involvement in terms of patient age or physician gender; however, older clinicians (both nurses and doctors) were less supportive of patient involvement.

A cross-sectional survey completed in Canada and Australia explored the views and understanding of cancer doctors toward SDM.[17,18,89] In Canada and Australia, 56% and 62% of oncologists and 69% and 72% of surgeons stated that their usual approach to a decision-making consultation was most similar to SDM. Breast cancer doctors in Australia and Canada strongly endorsed SDM,[18] suggesting a similar culture surrounding treatment decision making in the two countries. The Australian survey found that doctors who treated patients with breast cancer or urologic cancer were more likely to report using SDM than their colleagues who cared

Table 49-2 Discrepancy between high comfort level and reported use of shared decision making (SDM)

	Usual approach, N (%)	High level of comfort, N (%)	Mismatch
Tumor type			
Breast	202 (67.1)	266 (86.9)	19.8
Colorectal	36 (46.2)	51 (67.1)	20.9
Leukemia/ lymphoma	39 (47.0)	18 (81.8)	34.8
Gynecologic	11 (40.7)	24 (88.9)	48.2
Urologic	84 (81.6)	94 (89.5)	7.9
Doctor type			
Medical oncologists	91 (65.0)	105 (89.0)	24.0
Radiation oncologists	26 (50.0)	39 (78.0)	28.0
Hematologists	29 (47.5)	4 (66.7)	19.2
Pediatric oncologists	4 (28.6)	9 (81.8)	53.2
Surgeons	231 (69.2)	296 (84.3)	15.1

From Shepherd HL, Tattersall MHN, Butow PN.[17]

for patients with colorectal, gynecologic, and hematologic cancers (Table 49-2). These findings suggest that cancer doctors may feel more inclined to share decision making when a treatment decision involves a real choice between two options with similar survival outcomes.[43] Examples include mastectomy versus breast conservation and radical prostatectomy versus hormone therapy and brachytherapy for prostate cancer. It seems that colorectal and gynecologic oncologists and hematologists may feel that their patients need more direction because of the lack of treatment options available with similar outcomes.

Charles' survey[18] was completed by breast cancer doctors in France, Canada, and Australia (Table 49-3). Differences reported between the French sample and the Australian and Canadian samples are perhaps reflective of the cultural norms of the relevant populations, as well as the usual clinical practice of cancer surgeons in the different countries. (Data reported at EACH 2008 Symposium: Shared decision-making in general and hospital practice: physicians' and patients' points of views in Canada, France, Australia, Germany, and Switzerland.[90])

STRATEGIES TO ENHANCE DISCUSSION OF TREATMENT OPTIONS

As the interest around SDM and patient participation has grown, methods to improve the discussion of treatment options have been developed and evaluated. These methods generally focus on the patient and family or on the health professional, and they may target different time points (before, during, or after the consultation).

Strategies include tools to prepare patients for their consultation and communication training for health professionals that will assist them in discussing important issues when presenting treatment options. The following section will outline some of the interventions that have been developed and evaluated.

PREPARING PATIENTS FOR THEIR CANCER CONSULTATION
Question prompt lists

Question prompt lists (QPLs) are simple tools designed to assist the patient in obtaining information by listing questions pertinent to the consultation and allowing the patient to raise these during the consultation.[91-95] Patients who received QPLs asked significantly more questions, particularly about difficult and emotional subjects such as prognosis. Endorsement of the QPL by the doctor was found in another study to increase the number of questions asked and to improve patient recall of information; another positive outcome in terms of implementation was that the intervention decreased the consultation length.[92] Similarly, Bruera et al.'s study comparing a question prompt sheet versus a general information sheet found no increase in consultation duration.[96]

A recent review of QPLs as a method to empower cancer patients to ask relevant questions found that QPLs

Table 49-3 Breast cancer doctors' self-reported use of decision-making approaches

	France*	Australia*†		Canada†‡	
	Breast surgeons, n (%)	Breast surgeons, n (%)	Oncologists, n (%)	Breast surgeons, n (%)	Oncologists, n (%)
Some sharing	39 (56)	20 (12)	26 (18)	39 (17)	27 (27)
Shared	16 (23)	115 (72)	87 (62)	158 (69)	56 (56)
Paternalistic	14 (20)	0 (0)	5 (3)	5 (2)	1 (1)
Informed	0 (0)	17 (11)	13 (9)	17 (7)	8 (8)

*French and Australian data presented at EACH 2008.[90]
†Percentages do not add up to 100%, as data do not include the doctors who responded in the "none/other" category.
‡Canadian data published.[18]

BOX 49-6

BOX 49-6 Recommendations for Implementation of QPLs in Australia

1. Provide education, training sessions, and reminders for health providers and administrative staff to improve understanding of the scientific evidence supporting the utility of the QPL, and to help foster a culture where health providers support patients in using the QPL and in asking questions.
   - Interactive training sessions allow staff to ask questions, exchange views, and develop an interest in the intervention. This will help foster a culture among health providers to support question asking by patients. Reminders for doctors to ask patients if they have any questions from the list should be incorporated via signs placed in doctors' consulting rooms. Information packages appear to have limited utility in educating staff about QPLs, as they are not often read.

2. Allow staff at each site to develop the implementation process and procedures to suit their individual needs.
   - Involving all staff in this process, rather than using a top-down approach, was more beneficial, as it increased a sense of ownership in the implementation at a number of staff levels.

3. Enlist the support of active clinical champions from within each discipline to encourage clinic-wide acceptance at all levels.
   - Champions should be sought from among department heads, influential clinical staff specialists, and allied health and administrative staff.

4. Provision of QPLs should be targeted toward patients when they first visit the clinic through an information pack mailed out to them before the consultation.
   - A QPL mailed to new patients in an information pack before the first consultation allows them time to properly consider the questions listed. However, this should be supplemented with distribution of the QPL by administrative and allied health staff.

5. Educate patients about the QPL, and encourage them to ask for, take, and use the QPL.
   - A project assistant and cancer care coordinators would facilitate the process of encouraging and educating patients about the utility of the QPL at the cancer center. Working with champions from consumer lobby groups and promoting awareness of the QPL via the media will encourage patients to ask for the QPL.

QPL, Question prompt list.

increased asking of questions about prognosis.[97] Cancer doctors and their patients reportedly avoid this topic in consultations.[98-100] Subsequent to work in this field performed in Australia, implementation in different cancer clinics was evaluated. This work produced five recommendations[101] (Box 49-6).

Decision support tools (DSTs)

One tool that can enhance patient understanding and involvement and the quality of decision making is the use of decision aids. Decision support tools (DSTs) or decision aids (DAs) are designed to help people make choices by providing relevant information on potential options and health outcomes. DAs are standardized, evidence-based tools that aid achievement of an informed, value-based choice among treatment options, one of which could be watching and waiting.[102] A Cochrane systematic review identified 34 randomized trials of DAs and reported positive outcomes compared with standard care in terms of knowledge, patient comprehension of probable outcomes, agreement between personal values and choices made, decisional conflict, and the number of patients who could not make a decision.[103] Anxiety was not increased in those patients who participated in decision making.

A randomized trial of a DA for cancer patients considering adjuvant chemotherapy reported significantly improved knowledge of disease and treatment options and improved satisfaction with the decision making itself.[104]

A recent systematic review of the effectiveness of cancer-related DAs reported that despite the small number of trials available in the context of prevention and treatment decision making, the DAs improved knowledge, without increasing anxiety, and with a trend toward improved decisional conflict.[105] Decision aids for use in advanced cancer have been developed and piloted in breast and lung cancer.[106,107] A randomized trial of DA in advanced colorectal cancer found that patients receiving the DA demonstrated a greater increase in understanding of prognosis, options, and benefits and higher overall understanding ($P < .0001$). Decisional conflict and treatment decisions made were similar between the groups. Anxiety was similar and decreased over time.[108]

Increasing evidence-based online information summarizing outcomes of different treatments for patients with common cancers has been incorporated into oncologist discussions with individual patients (e.g., http://www.adjuvantonline.com). Commonly, a printout is given to the patient to take away, so that he or she can reflect on personal values and attitudes toward treatments with differing side effects and often small differences in disease-free or overall survival. Often, these printouts inform uncertainty about the future and enable patients to understand that a treatment choice is available in which they may choose to play a major role.

Consultation planning/coaching

A program incorporating consultation planning, recording, and summarizing (CPRS) by trained facilitators has been implemented at a breast cancer clinic in the United States. This program provides patients with a consultation planning sheet based on concerns and questions that the patient and his or her companion voice to the facilitator before consultation with the cancer doctor. The consultation is then audio recorded, and the facilitator provides a summary of the consultation and the responses to questions raised at the outset by the patient. Despite scheduling difficulties and concerns about disruption of clinic flow, evaluation of this program as part of a clinical service reported that the clinic staff, physicians, and patients support continuation of the CPRS program.[109]

Despite the development of different effective interventions in different contexts of cancer care, a challenge remains to increase their adoption in routine clinical practice. In Australia, cancer doctors were not very supportive of some of the interventions outlined here (Table 49-4).

Table 49-4 Interventions that physicians would support to encourage patient involvement and reflection[65]

N = 415*	Yes N (%)
Offering the patient written information about available treatment options	321 (81.1)
Having a third person in the room	273 (68.9)
Input from Cancer Nurse Coordinator (CNC) before consultation	196 (49.5)
Booklet explaining clinical decision making	135 (34.1)
Preparing patient for a greater role in decision making by offering question prompt lists before the consultation	124 (31.3)
Booklet about patient roles explaining shared decision making (SDM)	111 (28.0)
Access for medical practitioners to training to enhance skills in meeting patients' preferences for SDM	99 (25.0)
Explicitly negotiating SDM	89 (22.5)
Input from CNC post consultation	50 (12.6)
Follow-up appointment to make a decision	381 (96.2)
Giving written information highlighting treatment options	356 (89.9)
Encouraging patient to talk to treatment team and general practitioner	288 (72.7)
Worksheets for the patient to help him/her articulate what is important for him/her	77 (19.4)
Audio taping of consultation	64 (16.2)
Telephone follow-up to discuss treatment decision	54 (13.6)

*Breast and urologic cancer physicians only.

SUMMARY

Facilitating involvement is inextricably linked to the clinician's motivation to involve patients.[110] The difficulties we report emphasize system and patient attributes that prove challenging for physicians. Changing established practice and successfully implementing evaluated communication interventions remains difficult. Perhaps greater success will be realized by aiming strategies at patients or at the system.[111]

REFERENCES

1. Stevenson FA, Barry CA, Britten N, et al. Doctor-patient communication about drugs: the evidence for shared decision making. *Soc Sci Med.* 2000;50:829–840.
2. Emanuel EJ, Emanuel LL. Four models of the physician-patient relationship. *JAMA.* 1992;267:2221–2226.
3. Wirtz V, Cribb A, Barber N. Patient-doctor decision-making about treatment within the consultation—a critical analysis of models. *Soc Sci Med.* 2006;62:116–124.
4. Stewart M, Brown JB, Weston WW, et al. *Patient-centered medicine: transforming the clinical method.* 2nd ed. Patient-Centered Care Series. Abingdon: Radcliffe Medical Press; 2003.
5. Whitney SN, McGuire AL, McCullough LB. A typology of shared decision making, informed consent, and simple consent. *Ann Intern Med.* 2004;140:54–59.
6. Fallowfield LJ, Hall A, Maguire P, et al. Psychological effects of being offered choice of surgery for breast cancer. *BMJ.* 1994;309:448.

7. Morris J, Royle GT. Offering patients a choice of surgery for early breast cancer: a reduction in anxiety and depression in patients and their husbands. *Soc Sci Med.* 1988;26:583–585.
8. Solomon MJ, Pager CK, Keshava A, et al. What do patients want? Patient preferences and surrogate decision making in the treatment of colorectal cancer. *Dis Colon Rectum.* 2003;46:1351–1357.
9. Dimoska A, Girgis A, Hansen V, et al. Perceived difficulties in consulting with patients and families: a survey of Australian cancer specialists. *Med J Aust.* 2008;189:612–615.
10. Baile WF, Lenzi R, Parker PA, et al. Oncologists' attitudes toward and practices in giving bad news: an exploratory study. *J Clin Oncol.* 2002;20:2189–2196.
11. Schofield P, Carey M, Love A, et al. Would you like to talk about your future treatment options?' Discussing the transition from curative cancer treatment to palliative care. *Palliat Med.* 2006;20:397–406.

12. Earle CC, Neville BA, Landrum MB, et al. Trends in the aggressiveness of cancer care near the end of life. *J Clin Oncol.* 2004;22:315–321.
13. Feldman-Stewart D, Brundage MD, McConnell BA, et al. Practical issues in assisting shared decision-making. *Health Expect.* 2000;3:46–54.
14. Elwyn G, Edwards A, Kinnersley P. Shared decision-making in primary care: the neglected second half of the consultation. *Br J Gen Pract.* 1999;477–482.
15. Coulter A. Patient information and shared decision-making in cancer care. *Br J Cancer.* 2003;89(suppl 1): S15–S16.
16. Coulter A. Partnerships with patients: the pros and cons of shared clinical decision-making. *J Health Serv Res Pol.* 1997;2:112–121.
17. Shepherd HL, Tattersall MHN, Butow PN. The context influences doctors' support of shared decision making in cancer care. *Br J Cancer.* 2007;97:6–13.
18. Charles C, Gafni A, Whelan T. Self-reported use of shared decision-making among breast cancer specialists and perceived barriers and facilitators

to implementing this approach. *Health Expect.* 2004;7:338–348.

19. Elit L, Charles C, Gold I, et al. Women's perceptions about treatment decision making for ovarian cancer. *Gynecol Oncol.* 2003;88:89–95.

20. Shotton L. *Health care law and ethics.* Katoomba NSW: Social Science Press; 1997.

21. Gattellari M, Butow PN, Tattersall MHN. Sharing decisions in cancer care. *Soc Sci Med.* 2001;52:1865–1878.

22. Trevena L, Barratt A. Integrated decision making: definitions for a new discipline. *Pt Educ Couns.* 2003;50:265–268.

23. Edwards A, Evans R, Elwyn G. Manufactured but not imported: new directions for research in shared decision making support and skills. *Pt Educ Couns.* 2003;50:33–38.

24. Eddy DM. Clinical decision making: from theory to practice. Anatomy of a decision. *JAMA.* 1990;263:441–443.

25. Charles C, Gafni A, Whelan T. Shared decision-making in the medical encounter: what does it mean? (or it takes at least two to tango). *Soc Sci Med.* 1997;44:681–692.

26. Charles C, Gafni A, Whelan T. Decision-making in the physician-patient encounter: revisiting the shared treatment decision-making model. *Soc Sci Med.* 1999;49:651–661.

27. Charles CA, Whelan T, Gafni A, et al. Shared treatment decision making: what does it mean to physicians? *J Clin Oncol.* 2003;21:932–936.

28. Makoul G, Clayman ML. An integrative model of shared decision making in medical encounters. *Pt Educ Couns.* 2006;60:301–312.

29. Elwyn G, Edwards A, Gwyn R, et al. Towards a feasible model for shared decision making: focus group study with general practice registrars. *BMJ.* 1999;319:753–756.

30. Siminoff LA, Step MM. A communication model of shared decision making: accounting for cancer treatment decisions. *Health Psychol.* 2005;24:S99–S105.

31. Whitney SN. A new model of medical decisions: exploring the limits of shared decision making. *Med Decis Making.* 2003;23:275–280.

32. Elwyn G, Edwards A, Kinnersley P, et al. Shared decision making and the concept of equipoise: the competencies of involving patients in healthcare choices. *Br J Gen Pract.* 2000;50:892–897.

33. McNutt RA. Shared medical decision making: problems, process, progress. *JAMA.* 2004;292:2516–2518.

34. Jahng KH, Martin LR, Golin CE, et al. Preferences for medical collaboration: patient-physician congruence and patient outcomes. *Pt Educ Couns.* 2005;57:308–314.

35. Keating NL, Guadagnoli E, Landrum MB, et al. Treatment decision making in early-stage breast cancer: should surgeons match patients' desired level of involvement? *J Clin Oncol.* 2002;20:1473–1479.

36. Golin C, DiMatteo MR, Duan N, et al. Impoverished diabetic patients whose doctors facilitate their participation in medical decision making are more satisfied with their care. *J Gen Intern Med.* 2002;17:866–875.

37. Lam W, Fielding R, Chan M, et al. Participation and satisfaction with surgical treatment decision-making in breast cancer among Chinese women. *Breast Cancer Res Treat.* 2003;80:171–180.

38. Kaplan SH, Greenfield S, Gandek B, et al. Characteristics of physicians with participatory decision-making styles. *Ann Intern Med.* 1996;124:497–504.

39. Morris J, Ingham R. Choice of surgery for early breast cancer: psychosocial considerations. *Soc Sci Med.* 1988;27:1257–1262.

40. Fallowfield LJ, Hall A, Maguire GP, et al. Psychological outcomes of different treatment policies in women with early breast cancer outside a clinical trial. *BMJ.* 1990;301:575–580.

41. Margalith I, Shapiro A. Anxiety and patient participation in clinical decision-making: the case of patients with ureteral calculi. *Soc Sci Med.* 1997;45:419–427.

42. Ong LML, Visser MRM, Lammes FB, et al. Doctor-patient communication and cancer patients; quality of life and satisfaction. *Pt Educ Couns.* 2000;41:145–156.

43. Whitney SN, McGuire AL, McCullough LB. A typology of shared decision making, informed consent, and simple consent. *Ann Intern Med.* 2003;140:54–59.

44. Kaplan RM. Shared medical decision making: a new tool for preventive medicine. *Am J Prev Med.* 2004;26:81–83.

45. Towle A, Godolphin W. Framework for teaching and learning informed shared decision making. *BMJ.* 1999;319:766–771.

46. Elwyn G, Edwards A, Kinnersley P, et al. Shared decision making and the concept of equipoise: the competences of involving patients in healthcare choices. *Br J Gen Pract.* 2000;50:892–897.

47. Brown RF, Butow PN, Sharrock MA, et al. Education and role modelling for clinical decisions with female cancer patients. *Health Expect.* 2004;7:303–316.

48. Jenkins V, Fallowfield L, Saul J. Information needs of patients with cancer: results from a large study in UK cancer centres. *Br J Cancer.* 2001;84:48–51.

49. Coulter A, Jenkinson C. European patients' views on the responsiveness of health systems and healthcare providers. *Eur J Public Health.* 2005;15:355–360.

50. Beaver K, Luker KA, Owens RG, et al. Treatment decision making in women newly diagnosed with breast cancer. *Cancer Nurs.* 1996;19:8–19.

51. Degner LF, Kristjanson LJ, Bowman D, et al. Information needs and decisional preferences in women with breast cancer. *JAMA.* 1997;277:1485–1492.

52. Bruera E, Willey JS, Palmer JL, et al. Treatment decisions for breast carcinoma: patient preferences and physician perceptions. *Cancer.* 2002;94:2076–2080.

53. Davidson JR, Brundage MD, Feldman-Stewart D. Lung cancer treatment decisions: patients' desires for participation and information. *Psychooncology.* 1999;8:511–520.

54. Gwede CK, Pow-Sang JJ, Seigne P, et al. Treatment decision-making strategies and influences in patients with localized prostate carcinoma. *Cancer.* 2005;104:1381–1390.

55. Beaver K, Bogg J, Luker KA. Decision-making role preferences and information needs: a comparison of colorectal and breast cancer. *Health Expect.* 1999;2:266–276.

56. Pieterse A, Baas-Thijssen M, Marijnen C, et al. Clinician and cancer patient views on patient participation in treatment decision-making: a quantitative and qualitative exploration. *Br J Cancer.* 2008;99:875–882.

57. Degner LF, Sloan JA. Decision making during serious illness: what role do patients really want to play? *J Clin Epidemiol.* 1992;45:941–950.

58. Blanchard CG, Labrecque MS, Ruckdeschel JC, et al. Information and decision-making preferences

of hospitalized adult cancer patients. *Soc Sci Med.* 1988;27:1139–1145.

59. Levinson W, Kao A, Kuby A, et al. Not all patients want to participate in decision making: a national study of public preferences. *J Gen Intern Med.* 2005;20:531–535.

60. Braddock III CH, Edwards KA, Hasenberg NM, et al. Informed decision making in outpatient practice: time to get back to basics. *JAMA.* 1999;282:2313–2320.

61. Barry M. Involving patients in medical decisions: how can physicians do better? *JAMA.* 1999;282:2356–2357.

62. Ende J, Kazis L, Ash A, et al. Measuring patients' desire for autonomy: decision making and information-seeking preferences among medical patients. *J Gen Intern Med.* 1989;4:23–30.

63. Butow PN, Maclean M, Dunn SM, et al. The dynamics of change: cancer patients' preferences for information, involvement and support. *Ann Oncol.* 1997;8:857–863.

64. Orsino A, Cameron JI, Seidl M, et al. Medical decision-making and information needs in end-stage renal disease patients. *Gen Hosp Psychiatry.* 2003;25:324–331.

65. Shepherd HL, Tattersall MHN, Butow PN. Physician-identified factors affecting patient participation in reaching treatment decisions. *J Clin Oncol.* 2008;26:1724–1731.

66. Edwards A, Elwyn G, Mulley A. Explaining risks: turning numerical data into meaningful pictures. *BMJ.* 2002;324:827–830.

67. Say RE, Thomson R. The importance of patient preferences in treatment decisions—challenges for doctors. *BMJ.* 2003;327:542–545.

68. Greenfield S, Kaplan S, Ware Jr JE. Expanding patient involvement in care: effects on patient outcomes. *Ann Intern Med.* 1985;102:520–528.

69. Degner LF, Kristjanson LJ, Bowman D, et al. Information needs and decisional preferences in women with breast cancer. *JAMA.* 1997;277:1485–1492.

70. Thompson SC, Pitts JS, Schwankovsky L. Preferences for involvement in medical decision-making: situational and demographic influences. *Pt Educ Couns.* 1993;22:133–140.

71. Cassileth BR, Zupkis RV, Sutton-Smith K, et al. Information and participation preferences among cancer patients. *Ann Intern Med.* 1980;92:832–836.

72. Arora NK, McHorney CA. Patient preferences for medical decision making: who really wants to participate? *Med Care.* 2000;38:335–341.

73. Gravel K, Legare F, Graham I. Barriers and facilitators to implementing shared decision-making in clinical practice: a systematic review of health professionals' perceptions. *Implement Sci.* 2006;1:16.

74. Coulter A. Paternalism or partnership? *BMJ.* 1999;319:719–720.

75. Keating NL, Green DC, Kao AC, et al. How are patients' specific ambulatory care experiences related to trust, satisfaction, and considering changing physicians? *J Gen Intern Med.* 2002;17:29–39.

76. Thom DH, Physicians STS. Physician behaviors that predict patient trust. *J Fam Pract.* 2001;50:323–328.

77. Trachtenberg F, Dugan E, Hall MA. How patients' trust relates to their involvement in medical care: trust in the medical profession is associated with greater willingness to seek care and follow recommendations. *J Fam Pract.* 2005;54:344–353.

78. Dy SM. Instruments for evaluating shared medical decision making: a structured literature review. *Med Care Res Rev.* 2007;64:623–649.

79. Elwyn G, Edwards A, Mowle S, et al. Measuring the involvement of patients in shared decision-making: a systematic review of instruments. *Pt Educ Couns*. 2001;43:5–22.

80. Elwyn G, Edwards A, Wensing M, et al. Shared decision making: developing the OPTION scale for measuring patient involvement. *Qual Saf Health Care*. 2003;12:93–99.

81. Elwyn G, Hutchings H, Edwards A, et al. The OPTION scale: measuring the extent that clinicians involve patients in decision-making tasks. *Health Expect*. 2005;8:34–42.

82. Brown RF, Butow PN, Ellis P, et al. Seeking informed consent to cancer clinical trials: describing current practice. *Soc Sci Med*. 2004;58:2445–2457.

83. Gattellari M, Voigt KJ, Butow PN, et al. When the treatment goal is not cure: are cancer patients equipped to make informed decisions? *J Clin Oncol*. 2002;20:503–513.

84. Guimond P, Bunn H, O'Connor AM, et al. Validation of a tool to assess health practitioners' decision support and communication skills. *Pt Educ Couns*. 2003;50:235–245.

85. Butow P, Juraskova I, Chang S, et al. Shared decision making coding systems: how do they compare in the oncology context? *Pt Educ Couns*. 2010;78:261–268.

86. Degner LF, Russell CA. Preferences for treatment control among adults with cancer. *Res Nurs Health*. 1988;11:367–374.

87. Davison BJ, Gleave ME, Goldenberg SL, et al. Assessing information and decision preferences of men with prostate cancer and their partners. *Cancer Nurs*. 2002;25:42–49.

88. Beisecker AE, Helmig L, Graham D, et al. Attitudes of oncologists, oncology nurses, and patients from a women's clinic regarding medical decision making for older and younger breast cancer patients. *Gerontologist*. 1994;34:505–512.

89. Shepherd HL, Tattersall MHN, Butow PN. *Australian oncologists' views and use of shared decision-making (SDM): means of reducing some of the perceived barriers to SDM*. Basel, Switzerland: European Association of Communication in Healthcare; 2006.

90. Charles C, Charvet A, Gafni A, et al. *Shared decision-making in general and hospital practice: physicians' and patients' points of views in Canada, France, Australia, Germany and Switzerland*. Oslo, Norway: International Conference on Communication in Healthcare; 2008.

91. Clayton J, Butow PN, Tattersall MH, et al. Asking questions can help: development and preliminary evaluation of a question prompt list for palliative care patients. *Br J Cancer*. 2003;89:2069–2077.

92. Brown RF, Butow PN, Dunn SM, et al. Promoting patient participation and shortening cancer consultations: a randomised trial. *Br J Cancer*. 2001;85:1273–1279.

93. Brown R, Butow PN, Boyer MJ, et al. Promoting patient participation in the cancer consultation: evaluation of a prompt sheet and coaching in question-asking. *Br J Cancer*. 1999;80:242–248.

94. McJannett M, Butow P, Tattersall MH, et al. Asking questions can help: development of a question prompt list for cancer patients seeing a surgeon. *Eur J Cancer Prev*. 2003;12:397–405.

95. Butow PN, Dunn SM, Tattersall MHN, et al. Patient participation in the cancer consultation: evaluation of a question prompt sheet. *Ann Oncol*. 1994;5:199–204.

96. Bruera E, Sweeney C, Willey J, et al. Breast cancer patient perception of the helpfulness of a prompt sheet versus a general information sheet during outpatient consultation: a randomized, controlled trial. *J Pain Symptom Manage*. 2003;25:412–419.

97. Dimoska A, Tattersall MHN, Butow PN, et al. Can a "prompt list" empower cancer patients to ask relevant questions? *Cancer*. 2008;113:225–237.

98. The A, Hak T, Koeter G, et al. Collusion in doctor-patient communication about imminent death: an ethnographic study. *Western J Med*. 2001;174:247–253.

99. Koedoot C, de Haan RJ, Stiggelbout A, et al. Palliative chemotherapy or best supportive care? A prospective study explaining patients treatment preference or choice. *Br Med J*. 2003;89:2219–2226.

100. Butow PN, Kazemi JN, Beeney L, et al. When the diagnosis is cancer: patient communication experiences and preferences. *Cancer*. 1996;77:2630–2637.

101. Dimoska A, Tattersall MH. *Implementing question prompt lists into routine cancer care in NSW*. Sydney: Medical Psychology Research Unit, University of Sydney; Cancer Institute NSW; 2008:78.

102. O'Connor AM, Graham ID, Visser A. Implementing shared decision making in diverse health care systems: the role of patient decision aids. *Pt Educ Couns*. 2005;57:247–249.

103. O'Connor AM, Stacey D, Entwistle V, et al. Decision aids for people facing health treatment or screening decisions. *Cochrane Database Syst Rev*. 2003;(2):CD001431.

104. Whelan T, Sawka C, Levine M, et al. Helping patients make informed choices: a randomized trial of a decision aid for adjuvant chemotherapy in lymph node-negative breast cancer. *J Natl Cancer Inst*. 2003;95:581.

105. O'Brien M, Whelan T, Villasis-Keever M. Are cancer-related decision aids effective? A systematic review and meta-analysis. *J Clin Oncol*. 2009;27:974–985.

106. Leighl N, Shepherd FA, Zawiska D, et al. Enhancing treatment decision-making: pilot study of a treatment decision aid in stage IV non-small cell lung cancer. *Br J Cancer*. 2008;98:1769–1773.

107. Chiew KS, Shepherd H, Vardy J, et al. Development and evaluation of a decision aid for patients considering first-line chemotherapy for metastatic breast cancer. *Health Expect*. 2008;11:35–45.

108. Leighl N, Shepherd H, Butow P, et al. *When the goal of treatment is not cure: a randomized trial of a patient decision aid in advanced colorectal cancer*. Presented at: ASCO, June 1-5, Chicago, IL: 2007.

109. Belkora JK, Lotha MK, Volza S, et al. Implementing decision and communication aids to facilitate patient-centered care in breast cancer: a case study. *Pt Educ Couns*. 2009;77:360–368.

110. Entwistle VA, Watt IS. Patient involvement in treatment decision-making: the case for a broader conceptual framework. *Pt Educ Couns*. 2006;63:268–278.

111. Holmes-Rovner M, Valade D, Orlowski C, et al. Implementing shared decision-making in routine practice: barriers and opportunities. *Health Expect*. 2000;3:182–191.

Communication about palliative care and end-of-life planning

50

Camilla Zimmermann, Amanda Caissie, and Orit Freedman

Despite advances in the diagnosis and cure of cancer, close to half of patients diagnosed with cancer ultimately will not be cured.[1,2] Discussions about end-of-life planning and palliative care therefore should be a routine component of the practice of oncology. However, these conversations are emotionally taxing for oncology professionals, patients, and their families. The discomfort that many feel when discussing these topics often results in procrastination and delay until late in the disease course, when palliative care becomes an urgent necessity rather than a planned process. Other chapters in this section have discussed strategies for the supportive communication of difficult news, discussing treatment options, and communicating prognosis. Here we discuss the communication of information regarding palliative care and end-of-life planning.

DISCUSSING END-OF-LIFE PLANNING

The focus of end-of-life planning discussions is often on an endpoint of a formal written document such as an advance directive or a code status order. However, more important than the actual written directive or order are the discussions that lead up its completion. End-of-life decision making involves the discussion of many preferences, including the extent of investigations, the aggressiveness of treatment, hospice enrollment, the preferred place of death, organ donation, and religious rites before or after death. For these discussions to be meaningful, the patient needs to gain an appreciation for the extent of his or her underlying illness, and the potential benefit or lack thereof of a given intervention. Similarly, the physician needs to understand the cultural and individual preferences of the patient, and family members need to be brought into the discussion, so that they are familiar with the patient's wishes. Thus end-of-life discussions are conversations that involve input from patient, family, and health care providers and take place over a period of time rather than during a single patient encounter.

ADVANCE DIRECTIVES

The completion of advance directives allows patients to state their preferences while they have the ability to do so, so that care proceeds according to their wishes in the event that they no longer have decision-making capacity. In the United States, the Patient Self-Determination Act became effective in 1991; it requires that Medicare and Medicaid providers (e.g., hospitals, nursing homes, home health agencies) provide information to patients at the time of enrollment on their rights regarding advance directives.[3] These include the right to participate in their health care decisions; the right to accept or refuse treatment; the right to prepare an advance directive; and the right to information on providers' policies regarding these rights. Unlike other legally binding documents, advance directives can be completed without an attorney, which facilitates their implementation. Advance directives typically consist of a living will and the assignment of a substitute decision maker, or durable power of attorney, who will make decisions for a patient in the case of incompetence.

513

LIVING WILL

The living will states the patient's preferences for care and serves not only to maintain patient autonomy, but also to minimize the burden of decision making on families faced with the emotionally charged situation of having a loved one who is near death. Typically, the directive includes instructions regarding whether or not life-sustaining treatment should be given, and it may have specific directions regarding the use of cardiopulmonary resuscitation, mechanical ventilation, tube feeding, and antibiotics. For these directives to be meaningful, it is important to explain to patients what these various life-sustaining procedures are, and how they would or would not contribute to quality and/or quantity of life in the patient's situation.

In a study of 728 patients in Oregon that assessed understanding of legal options at the end of life,[4] 69% understood options regarding refusal of treatment, but only 46% understood options for withdrawal of treatment, 23% for assisted suicide, and 32% for active euthanasia. Better understanding was associated with white race, higher education, and having been a proxy for health care decisions. It is interesting to note that personal experience with illness, death or illness of a loved one, and authoring an advance directive were not associated with advanced knowledge of these end-of-life options. Thus it is important to educate patients and their family members, so that the directive is completed with sufficient knowledge of the content and meaning of the document being completed.

DURABLE POWER OF ATTORNEY

Regardless of whether or not a living will is completed, it is important for patients to assign a durable power of attorney. If patients have not made such an assignment, then the law in some countries (e.g., Canada, certain areas of the United States) outlines a hierarchy of substitute decision makers for patients who are incapacitated. Typically, this starts with the spouse and proceeds to an adult child, parent, sibling, and, finally, a more distant relative.[5] If several family members have the same priority, then decisions may be made by consensus, by majority, or by choosing one member who is responsible for making decisions on behalf of the group. Although this procedure is intended to reflect the typical order of priority that would be assigned by a patient, the first person on a legally assigned hierarchy list may not necessarily be the one the patient would have chosen, and may or may not share similar viewpoints or values. It is also possible in the situation of having no assigned power of attorney for a critically ill patient who lacks decision-making capacity, that the attending physician makes the decision of whether or not to limit life support.[6]

Whether or not they have been assigned by the patient as substitute decision makers, family members often inaccurately predict the patient's wishes[7,8]; the same is true for patients' physicians.[8] In a recent study, Hauser and colleagues interviewed 893 patients and their caregivers, 50% of whom had cancer, and assessed concordance for preferences of care. The proportion of concordant responses ranged from 53% to 66%; patients were more likely to express concern about domains that might impose on caregivers, and caregivers were more likely to express concern about patients' physical suffering.[9] Thus it is important to emphasize to patients that they need to explicitly discuss their treatment preferences with their family members, as well as with their physicians. Once a power of attorney has been chosen, it is useful for the patient and power of attorney to meet with the patient's oncologist to discuss the patient's wishes for care.

OVERCOMING BARRIERS TO THE COMPLETION OF ADVANCE DIRECTIVES

Although the number of patients with completed advance directives in the United States has increased substantially since the passage of the Patient Self-Determination Act, approximately half of all severely or terminally ill patients still lack advance directives.[10] In a recent survey of 75 consecutive patients admitted to a cancer inpatient service, 40% had an advance directive and 7% had discussed advance directives with their oncologist. However, 95% thought that discussing advance directive issues was very or somewhat important, and almost 90% thought it was acceptable to discuss advance directives with the admitting physician, with whom they had no prior relationship.[11] Although only 23% stated that they would like to discuss advance directives with their oncologist, when asked specifically with which physician they would *choose* to have this discussion, 48% preferred to discuss advance directives with their oncologist, and 35% preferred to have this discussion with their family physician. A survey performed a decade ago in a different population admitted to an inpatient oncology ward similarly found that 33% had completed an advance directive, 9% had discussed preferences with their clinical oncologist, and 23% wished to do so. However, 58% would support a policy under which medical house staff would offer to discuss advance directives as part of the admission history.[12]

The findings from these surveys are consistent with those from previous studies, which showed that patients are unlikely to initiate discussions about advance care directives but are willing to complete them if their physicians initiate the discussion.[13] Reliance on patients to bring up discussions about advance directives will result in only a small percentage of patients completing these documents because of lack of familiarity with these documents and the process for their completion,[14] or a perceived lack of relevance to their situation.[15] Patients who complete advance directives tend to be white, educated, and of higher socioeconomic status[16]; minority groups are less likely to be familiar with these documents. Still other patients may complete advance directives and not inform their physicians that they have done so.[17]

Although there may be a fear on the part of patients that completion of an advance directive will hasten their death, the opposite has been found: In a study of patients undergoing hematopoietic stem cell transplantation, patients without advance directives had twice the risk of death compared with those who had an advance directive in place.[18] Although the authors emphasize that this association is not causal, it does demonstrate that discussing advance directives is not associated with increased mortality. It is appropriate for physicians to proactively bring up the topic of advance directives for all patients with cancer. If the patient already has an advance directive, physicians should still discuss the directive and clarify any misconceptions. The patient's wishes can then be documented in the living will, as well as in the patient's chart, to avoid misunderstandings and ensure that future care proceeds as the patient desires.

WHEN SHOULD THE DISCUSSION OF ADVANCE DIRECTIVES OCCUR?

There is a dearth of evidence for implementation of advance care planning at specific times in the cancer trajectory; however, it is generally agreed that this process should occur early, and be updated regularly. Oncology practice guidelines recommend that advance care planning should be discussed at the diagnosis of advanced cancer and at sentinel events during the cancer course.[19] These events include the initiation of invasive procedures, the first diagnosis of central nervous system disease, the initiation of a new chemotherapy regimen, an admission to hospital or to an intensive care unit, the initiation of mechanical ventilation, and the decision to undergo major surgery (Table 50-1). It is also recommended to discuss advance directives before an expected death from cancer, although this is likely to result in leaving the discussion for too late, in that prognostication by physicians is notoriously optimistic.[20]

FRAMEWORK FOR ADVANCE DIRECTIVES DISCUSSIONS

Discussion of advance directives is best initiated by the physician in a routine manner incorporated into the cancer treatment plan. Routinely discussing advance directives and preferences for care at the time of diagnosis of cancer normalizes this process for both patients and physicians. The discussion itself need not take place in a single appointment time; it is useful to broach the subject during one visit and encourage the patient to reflect on his or her own views and discuss them with family members. During the next patient encounter, the document can be reviewed and placed in the medical record. The directive will need to be rediscussed and updated from time to time, even if the patient's status is stable. For a patient who has a prognosis measured in years, this can occur every 1 to 2 years.[21] For patients who are more ill, the discussion should occur during sentinel events, as suggested above. Lastly, it is important to ensure the availability and use of these documents when they are needed.[22]

Table 50-1 Recommendations for care planning in patients with advanced cancer

Timing	Recommendation	Evidence*
Within 1 month of new diagnosis of advanced cancer	Discuss prognosis and advance care planning	II
Within 48 hours of any hospital admission	Document patient's goals or preferences for care	III
Within 48 hours of admission to an intensive care unit and before mechanical ventilation	Document patient's goals or preferences for care	III
New diagnosis of CNS metastases or beginning a new chemotherapy regimen	Discuss prognosis and advance care planning	II
Patient beginning high-dose opioids	Discuss advance care planning	II
Patient undergoing new hemodialysis, pacemaker, or implantable cardioverter-defibrillator placement; major surgery; or gastric tube placement	Discuss goals of care and preferences for interventions	II
When death is expected	Document advance directive or SDM	II

Adapted from Walling A, Lorenz KA, Dy SM, et al. Evidence-based recommendations for information and care planning in cancer care. *J Clin Oncol.* 2008;26:3896–3902.
*Level I: randomized clinical trials; level II: nonrandomized controlled trials; level III: descriptive studies, opinions, and textbooks.
CNS, Central nervous system; *SDM,* substitute decision maker.

CODE STATUS

Cardiopulmonary resuscitation (CPR) was initially introduced in the 1960s, and in 1974, the American Medical Association issued a recommendation that code status be documented in the medical record.[23] Success rates of CPR are low, with a chance of survival to discharge from hospital of approximately 17%.[24,25] In patients with cancer, this percentage is reduced to approximately 10%,[26] and metastatic disease, renal failure, sepsis, and reduced performance status reduce the prognosis considerably.[27,28] In a study of 243 inpatients who experienced cardiac arrest at a comprehensive cancer center, 16 of 73 patients (22%) who had unanticipated cardiac arrests survived to be discharged, and none of the 171 patients who experienced an anticipated arrest survived.[29] Thus it is important to assess code status in all patients with cancer, particularly those with advanced disease or an anticipated decline in status.

Despite recommendations that discussions regarding preferences for care should occur within 48 hours of admission,[19] most do-not-resuscitate (DNR) orders are written after the patient loses decision-making capacity, meaning that the patient had no input into this decision.[30] In some cases, DNR decisions are made on an institutional basis without input from the patient.[31] Although only about a third of patients with advanced cancer have discussed their CPR preferences with their physicians, most have thought about their CPR preferences and are willing to discuss them.[32] However, patients have a very poor understanding of CPR and its outcomes,[32,33] even after discussion with their physicians,[33] and physicians' confidence in their ability to conduct these discussions compared with other medical discussions is low.[34] In some cases, there are differences in the perceived outcome of a CPR discussion between patients and physicians.[35] This may be avoided by conducting code status discussions in the context of an overall plan of care, and explaining procedures and their outcomes thoroughly. If available, a specialized palliative care team can help with these discussions.[36] Nurses are more likely than physicians to consider DNR discussions rewarding experiences,[37] and the role of nurses in the DNR communication process is worthy of further exploration.

The approach to discussing code status is important and may dictate the outcome. A framework for code status discussions is provided in Box 50-1. Ideally, code status preferences are already indicated in a living will, and it is important to ask on admission to hospital whether or not an advance directive exists. If so, then the advance directive should be reviewed and the patient's preferences documented. If there is no advance directive, then a discussion needs to take place with the patient and/or power of attorney to review the patient's underlying condition and overall prognosis, explain what is involved in CPR, and outline what the outcomes typically are for patients in their situation.

Increasingly, hospitals and other health care institutions have protocols regarding code status, including which exact order should be written. However, one should not assume that because a DNR order exists, the patient does not desire any other therapeutic interventions.[36] Specific treatments should be discussed in detail with the patient or substitute decision maker, so that a complete understanding of what is desired can be reached. This also serves to allay fears of patients that their care will be inferior if a DNR order exists. Finally, it is important to emphasize that the patient will not be abandoned, and that care will continue for pain and symptom management, as will support for the patient and family.

BOX 50-1   A Framework for Discussions of Code Status[23,30]

- Determine whether the patient has an advance directive or assigned power of attorney.
- Ask if the patient would like particular family members or friends to be present.
- Ask about patients' understanding of their illness, their cultural preferences, and their goals of care.
- Clarify any misunderstandings in patients' perceptions of their medical condition and prognosis.
- Explain that the discussion of code status is routine (e.g., "I routinely discuss CPR with all my patients who are admitted to hospital. Do you know what CPR is?")[30]
- Explain procedures involved in CPR and its likely outcomes.
- Check for comprehension of information, and assess preferences.
- Summarize what will or will not be done, and answer any questions.
- Provide assurance that the patient's comfort and dignity will be respected, and that appropriate management of symptoms will continue.
- Inform patients of how to contact you if they have further questions.
- Document the discussion and outcome in the patient's medical record.
- Continue to review and revise the plan as needed.

CPR, Cardiopulmonary resuscitation.

DISCUSSING HOSPICE AND PALLIATIVE CARE

Similar to discussions of advance care planning, discussions of palliative care and hospice are often delayed until a crisis arises. Although international and national guidelines recommend involvement of palliative care early in the cancer trajectory, this is not what currently occurs in practice. In the next section, we discuss possible reasons for this divide and ways in which it can be overcome.

DEFINITIONS OF PALLIATIVE CARE AND HOSPICE

Most patients and their families, and many health care professionals, associate palliative care with care for the patient who is imminently dying. This association stems from the origins of the hospice and palliative care movements, which were developed initially in the 1960s and 1970s with a focus on care at the end of life. However, palliative care has since evolved to encompass treatment along the continuum of incurable disease. The World Health Organization (WHO) currently defines palliative care as "an approach that improves the quality of life of patients and their families facing the problems associated with life-threatening illness, through the prevention and relief of suffering by means of early identification and impeccable assessment and treatment of pain and other problems: physical, psychosocial, and spiritual."[38] The WHO definition also states explicitly that palliative care "is applicable early in the course of illness, in conjunction with other therapies that are intended to prolong life, such as chemotherapy or radiation therapy, and includes those investigations needed to better understand and manage distressing clinical complications."[38]

Hospice is an equally confusing term because it too is evolving and refers to different services in different countries. For example, in the United Kingdom and in Canada, hospice generally refers to a service consisting of a freestanding unit, often with home nurses providing outreach (in the United Kingdom, day care is also available), which is funded both by the government and by charities.[39] In the United States, hospice refers to a program of care that is covered by the Medicare Hospice Benefit, which was established in 1983. Unlike in the United Kingdom and Canada, where hospice is available to all patients with a life-limiting illness, patients enrolled in the U.S. hospice program must have a prognosis of 6 months or less, and must sign a statement choosing hospice care instead of standard Medicare benefits for the terminal illness.[40,41]

Both palliative care and hospice use an interdisciplinary approach with expertise from fields such as medicine, nursing, social work, physiotherapy, occupational therapy, and spiritual care. Care is provided by multidisciplinary teams, which provide support to the patient and family in an inpatient facility or in the home setting.

TREATMENT TRANSITIONS AND GOALS OF CARE

The "transition from curative to palliative care" is in many ways an artificial one, considering that many cancers are not curable at diagnosis, and the transition referred to is usually one of stopping palliative chemotherapy—which is by definition not of curative intent—and simultaneously referring to specialized palliative care or hospice.[42,43] In reality, treatment of the patient with advanced cancer involves a series of transitions.[44] These include transitions from one line of chemotherapy to the next, to perhaps starting on a clinical trial, to finally stopping therapy altogether; the transition of having disease progression or new sites of metastases; the transition from being able to conduct self-care to being dependent on others; the transition of awareness that the cancer is incurable; and the transition of referral to palliative care and/or hospice. Some of these transitions may occur simultaneously, and it is important at each point to take the time to assess understanding, clearly communicate the news, and appropriately support the patient and family.

Miscommunication around the goals of treatment is common; one study showed that although more than 90% of physicians believed that they had accurately conveyed the extent of disease and the intent of treatment, almost one third of patients with metastatic disease thought that their disease was localized, and almost one third of patients receiving palliative treatment thought that the intent was curative.[45] In a Canadian study, 30% of patients receiving palliative radiation therapy thought that their disease was curable,[46] and a recent Australian study similarly found that 30% of patients receiving palliative treatment believed that the goal was cure.[47] Furthermore, understanding of treatment goals differed between patients and their caregivers: In 39% of cases, only one member of the couple understood that the treatment was not intended to cure the disease; in 15%, both patient and caregiver believed the goal was to cure.[48]

Such misunderstanding about treatment goals can obstruct the process of obtaining proper informed consent, and may influence treatment decisions. Weeks and colleagues found that patients overestimated their prognosis, whereas physicians' estimates were more accurate; these overestimates by patients influenced treatment decisions, with optimistic patients being more likely to undergo aggressive care despite a lack of difference in survival.[49] Illness may also change one's perceptions and treatment preferences. Patients with advanced cancer are more willing to undergo treatments with only slight potential benefit and substantial potential side effects, in contrast to what oncologists or healthy counterparts might imagine accepting in the patient's situation.[50,51]

Miscommunication about treatment goals can result from failure to accurately present information, misunderstanding of the information that is being presented, or an inability to process the information that is being provided. If the goals of care are clarified each time a new treatment is offered, then the eventual transition to entirely stopping anticancer treatment will not be as traumatic. Schofield and colleagues have published evidence-based recommendations for communication during the "transition from curative treatment to palliative care."[43] As mentioned previously, this is not actually a transition that occurs at one particular time; it generally occurs in multiple steps over a number of months, or in some cases years (e.g., in metastatic prostate or breast cancer, in patients with myeloma in whom the disease is treatable for years but is not actually curable). In Box 50-2, we have adapted these recommendations, which are applicable during any discussion along this transition process.

BOX 50-2 Communication During Transitions in Palliative Anticancer Treatment

Prior to discussion
  Review all relevant information from records and test results.
  Ensure that the discussion takes place in a private place with adequate uninterrupted time.
  Invite the person to bring family to the consultation.
Elicit the patient's understanding.
  Ask open-ended questions to determine understanding of the disease.
  Ask about feelings, concerns, and goals.
  Assess preferences for information.
Provide information.
  Use simple honest communication, avoiding lay terms and euphemisms.
  Content may include disease progression, treatment efficacy, and symptom management.
Respond to the emotional reaction.
  Allow and encourage expression of feelings.
  Express empathy and listen actively.
  Wait until emotions subside before continuing.
Negotiate new goals of care.
  Ask whether the patient would like to discuss future treatment options now or later.
  Provide relevant information about the role of palliative care services, if these have not been provided.
  Provide realistic hopes for the future (e.g., effective symptom management).
Continuity of care
  Explicitly state to the patient and family that they will not be abandoned.
  Refer to the palliative care professionals as part of the multidisciplinary team.
Address family concerns and acknowledge cultural diversity.
  Ask about concerns for the family and for children, and clarify assistance required.
  Acknowledge cultural diversity.
Concluding the discussion
  Summarize main points and check understanding.
  Provide a written summary or other information tailored to patient preferences.
  Ask about the need for referrals to other services such as home care, social work, spiritual care, or child psychology.
  Ask whether there are further questions.

Adapted from Schofield P, Carey M, Love A, et al. "Would you like to talk about your future treatment options?" Discussing the transition from curative cancer treatment to palliative care. Palliat Med 2006;20:397-406.

Similar to the SPIKES (setting, perception, invitation, knowledge, emotions, strategy and summary) general strategy for breaking bad news,[52] the steps suggested by Schofield et al. involve ensuring a private setting and appropriate support; assessing the patient's knowledge of the situation; providing information simply and honestly; responding to emotional content of the interaction; and negotiating new goals of care. It is important to communicate information about disease progression and goals of care in a manner that is sensitive but clear. Overly optimistic information protects the patient and family from bad news in the short term, but denies them the opportunity to reorganize and adapt their lives toward the attainment of achievable goals.[42] On the other hand, providing exact survival periods and stating that nothing further can be done is very distressing for patients and families.[53] Patients vary in their understanding of medical information, and some patients may need to maintain ambiguity for the future; this need can be respected while still providing prognostic information that is important in the context of each patient's individual aspirations.[54]

The need for information is as important for the family as for the patient. Family members will have increasing involvement as caregivers and need to be provided with assistance and support to achieve this. Caregiver burden is common and is often overlooked.[55] If the patient has young or adolescent children, then planning for the future is especially important, and appropriate resources should be recommended. A wide range of cultural attitudes toward death and customs surround prognostic disclosure, and although this should be kept in mind, it should also be remembered that the differences between individuals may be as marked as those between cultures.[56] It is appropriate to ask at the beginning of the clinical encounter whether there are any cultural or religious preferences that one should be aware of as health care provider.[57]

REFERRAL TO SPECIALIZED PALLIATIVE CARE AND HOSPICE

National and international organizations such as the American Society of Clinical Oncology, the European Society for Medical Oncology, the National Comprehensive Cancer Network (NCCN), and the World Health Organization all support introducing palliative care concurrently with cancer-directed care.[38,58,59] A recent evidence-based review recommended that patients should have a comprehensive palliative care assessment as a routine part of their cancer care.[19] NCCN oncology practice guidelines recommend integration of palliative care into general oncology care and consultation, and informing patients and families that palliative care is an integral part of their comprehensive cancer care.[58] According to NCCN guidelines, patients should have access to palliative care services from the initial visit, and should be screened for palliative care needs throughout the course of their illness.

Contrary to the integrated process suggested earlier, the process of referral to palliative care most often occurs late in the course of illness, with time from referral to death of less than 2 months.[60-62] A recent survey of American physicians caring for cancer patients revealed that most physicians would not discuss end-of-life options with terminally ill patients who are feeling well; instead they would wait for symptoms or until no further treatment could be offered.[63] In the United States, hospice referrals typically occur very late, and only approximately one third of Americans die while under hospice care.[64,65]

Patients vary in their preferences for timing of communication about palliative care, depending on how the information is presented. In one survey of patients with metastatic cancer,[66] 33% wanted to discuss "dying and palliative care services" when first told that the cancer had spread, 19% in the next few consultations, 33% later upon their request, 11% never, and 10% were unsure. However, the pairing of "dying" with "palliative care services" undoubtedly influenced these responses, and more than 80% said they wished to discuss "treatment goals and options" and "symptoms of the cancer and side effects of treatment" when first diagnosed with metastatic disease. Given these responses, the concept of palliative care is best introduced early in the course of the illness, so that patients are aware of their options and of the availability of services. Referral can then be made at a time negotiated between physician and patient.

Patients may benefit from early referral to palliative care services, before stopping cancer-directed treatment, for several reasons. Palliative care clinics can improve symptom control,[67] and early referral has been shown to be feasible in studies of simultaneous care for patients enrolled in clinical trials[68] and for patients newly diagnosed with advanced lung cancer.[69] In a study focusing on American veterans who had died from cancer, bereaved family members reported higher satisfaction with end-of-life care when the patient had a palliative care consultation or hospice referral.[70] Early referral to palliative care also avoids the need to go through two simultaneous transitions of stopping chemotherapy and introducing a new team, and joint care by the oncology and palliative care teams may prevent patient fears of abandonment. Indeed, if the palliative care team is involved early, it can help support the patient and family through the difficult stage of stopping antineoplastic treatment. In the United States, the involvement of palliative care services before the discussion of hospice takes place may help with this transition and improve the timeliness of hospice referrals.[40]

When discussing a possible referral to specialized palliative care, it should be kept in mind that the term "palliative care" may be confusing and at times frightening to patients[71]; therefore, clarifying the goals of palliative care with an emphasis on active symptom management and quality of life is appropriate. One approach is to ask the patient open-ended questions about how the patient is feeling, focusing on current symptoms. Patients can then be asked whether they would like to hear more about supportive care options. Emphasizing what can be done to address and improve physical symptoms and exploring realistic goals for the future have been shown to enhance coping among patients with advanced cancer.[72] Just as each patient has likely had many physicians already playing a role in their treatment (surgeon, radiation oncologist, medical oncologist), palliative care can be introduced as another specialty to help support patients during the course of their illness.

SUPPORTING HOPE

Clinicians may be concerned that by discussing referral to a palliative care service, patients may lose hope.[73] However, not discussing palliative care and end-of-life issues can deprive the patient and family of the opportunity to plan ahead,[74] and palliative care provides an additional source of support at a time when this is particularly important. In a qualitative study conducted in Australia, focus groups and individual interviews were conducted with patients with advanced cancer, their caregivers, and palliative care professionals regarding ways to foster coping and allow hope when discussing prognosis and end-of-life issues.[72] Themes identified were an emphasis on what can be done (i.e., control of symptoms, emotional support, and practical support); exploring realistic goals; and discussing day-to-day living. The spectrum of hope included hope for a miracle cure, hope of living longer than expected, hope in finding meaning in life, hope in relationships with family/friends, hope in finding spiritual meaning, and hope for a peaceful death. Early palliative care planning can occur simultaneously with maintaining hope by emphasizing what can be done and by being sensitive to the readiness of individual patients to receive information.[44]

Some patients and families may understand the palliative nature of the medical treatment, but hope for a miracle or cure. It is important for clinicians to realize that such seemingly contradictory thinking is common and is a manner of coping with the illness. Often patients or families will ask several clinicians the same questions about prognosis; it is therefore important that all members of a clinical team are communicating the same information in a consistent fashion. An approach that is helpful for patients and families struggling with accepting that the cancer is not curable is "hope for the best, prepare for the worst,"[75] which acknowledges that hope can be sustained while planning for the occurrence of clinical situations that may evolve quickly. Wish statements can also help to express empathy, while also tacitly conveying that the wish unfortunately is not a reality.[76] Box 50-3 shows examples of these approaches.

CONCLUSION

Patients with advanced cancer are involved in multiple transitions in terms of their treatment, their physical status, and their treatment goals and expectations. Introduction of palliative care can help patients cope with physical symptoms and

---

BOX 50-3   Statements Acknowledging Hope[75,76]

Patient statement:
   "I can't give up hope that I'm going to be cured. I refuse to believe there is no treatment out there that can cure my cancer."
Physician responses:
   Wish statement: *"I wish there were treatments that could cure your cancer."*
   Hope for the best, plan for the worst: *"I agree that hope is so important and nobody can take that away from you. It's important for us also to discuss what we will do if the cancer does continue to progress, so that plans are in place for you and your family."*

---

psychosocial distress; advance care planning ensures that an appropriate plan is in place in the event of a rapid decline in function. Both can be introduced proactively as options that help to support the patient with advanced disease. Although patients vary in their desire for information and in their capacity for internalizing it, they generally will not ask for information about palliative care and advance care planning, and instead rely on their clinical team to offer it. As well, they may not understand its relevance if the current goals of care are not clear to them, or if they associate palliative care only with the very end of life. It is therefore up to us as oncology clinicians to routinely check for patient understanding of the goals of care, clarify any discrepancies, explain the scope of palliative care, and engage patients and their families in proactive planning discussions.

REFERENCES

1. Jemal A, Thomas A, Murray T, et al. Cancer statistics, 2002. *CA Cancer J Clin.* 2002;52:23–47.
2. Canadian Cancer Society's Steering Committee. Canadian cancer statistics 2009. Toronto: Canadian Cancer Society; 2009. Available at: www.cancer.ca/statistics Accessed February 24, 2010.
3. Omnibus Reconciliation Act. Congressional Record. *October.* 1990;26:12638.
4. Silveira MJ, DiPiero A, Gerrity MS, et al. Patients' knowledge of options at the end of life: ignorance in the face of death. *JAMA.* 2000;284:2483–2488.
5. Government of Ontario. *A guide to advance care planning.* Ontario, Quebec, Canada: Queen's Printer for Ontario; last updated July 30, 2007. Available at: http://www.culture.gov.on.ca/seniors/english/programs/advancedcare/dontappoint.shtml Accessed February 24, 2010.
6. White DB, Curtis JR, Lo B, et al. Decisions to limit life-sustaining treatment for critically ill patients who lack both decision-making capacity and surrogate decision-makers. *Crit Care Med.* 2006;34:2053–2059.
7. Emanuel EJ, Emanuel LL. Proxy decision making for incompetent patients: an ethical and empirical analysis. *JAMA.* 1992;267:2067–2071.
8. Seckler AB, Meier DE, Mulvihill M, et al. Substituted judgment: how accurate are proxy predictions? *Ann Intern Med.* 1991;115:92–98.
9. Hauser JM, Chang CH, Alpert H, et al. Who's caring for whom? Differing perspectives between

seriously ill patients and their family caregivers. *Am J Hosp Palliat Care.* 2006;23:105–112.
10. Saraiya B, Bodnar-Deren S, Leventhal E, et al. End-of-life planning and its relevance for patients' and oncologists' decisions in choosing cancer therapy. *Cancer.* 2008;113:3540–3547.
11. Dow LA, Matsuyama RK, Ramakrishnan V, et al. Paradoxes in advance care planning: the complex relationship of oncology patients, their physicians, and advance medical directives. *J Clin Oncol.* 2010;28:299–304.
12. Lamont EB, Siegler M. Paradoxes in cancer patients' advance care planning. *J Palliat Med.* 2000;3:27–35.
13. Johnston SC, Pfeifer MP, McNutt R. The discussion about advance directives: patient and physician opinions regarding when and how it should be conducted. End of Life Study Group. *Arch Intern Med.* 1995;155:1025–1030.
14. Pollack KM, Morhaim D, Williams MA. The public's perspectives on advance directives: implications for state legislative and regulatory policy. *Health Policy.* 2010;96:57–63.
15. Kierner KA, Hladschik-Kermer B, Gartner V, et al. Attitudes of patients with malignancies towards completion of advance directives. *Support Care Cancer.* 2009;18:367–372.
16. Hanson LC, Rodgman E. The use of living wills at the end of life: a national study. *Arch Intern Med.* 1996;156:1018–1022.

17. Ozanne EM, Partridge A, Moy B, et al. Doctor-patient communication about advance directives in metastatic breast cancer. *J Palliat Med.* 2009;12:547–553.
18. Ganti AK, Lee SJ, Vose JM, et al. Outcomes after hematopoietic stem-cell transplantation for hematologic malignancies in patients with or without advance care planning. *J Clin Oncol.* 2007;25:5643–5648.
19. Walling A, Lorenz KA, Dy SM, et al. Evidence-based recommendations for information and care planning in cancer care. *J Clin Oncol.* 2008;26:3896–3902.
20. Glare P, Virik K, Jones M, et al. A systematic review of physicians' survival predictions in terminally ill cancer patients. *BMJ.* 2003;327:195.
21. Emanuel LL, Emanuel EJ, Stoeckle JD, et al. Advance directives: stability of patients' treatment choices. *Arch Intern Med.* 1994;154:209–217.
22. Emanuel LL. Advance directives. *Annu Rev Med.* 2008;59:187–198.
23. Loertscher L, Reed DA, Bannon MP, et al. Cardiopulmonary resuscitation and do-not-resuscitate orders: a guide for clinicians. *Am J Med.* 2010;123:4–9.
24. Ehlenbach WJ, Barnato AE, Curtis JR, et al. Epidemiologic study of in-hospital cardiopulmonary resuscitation in the elderly. *N Engl J Med.* 2009;361:22–31.
25. Peberdy MA, Kaye W, Ornato JP, et al. Cardiopulmonary resuscitation of adults in

the hospital: a report of 14720 cardiac arrests from the National Registry of Cardiopulmonary Resuscitation. *Resuscitation*. 2003;58:297–308.

26. Vitelli CE, Cooper K, Rogatko A, et al. Cardiopulmonary resuscitation and the patient with cancer. *J Clin Oncol*. 1991;9:111–115.

27. Levy PD, Ye H, Compton S, et al. Factors associated with neurologically intact survival for patients with acute heart failure and in-hospital cardiac arrest. *Circ Heart Fail*. 2009;2:572–581.

28. Ebell MH. Prearrest predictors of survival following in-hospital cardiopulmonary resuscitation: a meta-analysis. *J Fam Pract*. 1992;34:551–558.

29. Ewer MS, Kish SK, Martin CG, et al. Characteristics of cardiac arrest in cancer patients as a predictor of survival after cardiopulmonary resuscitation. *Cancer*. 2001;92:1905–1912.

30. Ebell MH. Practical guidelines for do-not-resuscitate orders. *Am Fam Physician*. 1994;50:1293–1294.

31. van Delden JJ, Lofmark R, Deliens L, et al. Do-not-resuscitate decisions in six European countries. *Crit Care Med*. 2006;34:1686–1690.

32. Heyland DK, Frank C, Groll D, et al. Understanding cardiopulmonary resuscitation decision making: perspectives of seriously ill hospitalized patients and family members. *Chest*. 2006;130:419–428.

33. Fischer GS, Tulsky JA, Rose MR, et al. Patient knowledge and physician predictions of treatment preferences after discussion of advance directives. *J Gen Intern Med*. 1998;13:447–454.

34. Sulmasy DP, Sood JR, Ury WA. Physicians' confidence in discussing do not resuscitate orders with patients and surrogates. *J Med Ethics*. 2008;34:96–101.

35. Deep KS, Griffith CH, Wilson JF. Discussing preferences for cardiopulmonary resuscitation: what do resident physicians and their hospitalized patients think was decided? *Patient Educ Couns*. 2008;72:20–25.

36. Smith CB, Bunch OL. Do not resuscitate does not mean do not treat: how palliative care and other modalities can help facilitate communication about goals of care in advanced illness. *Mt Sinai J Med*. 2008;75:460–465.

37. Sulmasy DP, He MK, McAuley R, et al. Beliefs and attitudes of nurses and physicians about do not resuscitate orders and who should speak to patients and families about them. *Crit Care Med*. 2008;36:1817–1822.

38. World Health Organization. WHO definition of palliative care. 2002. Available at: www.who.int/cancer/palliative/definition/en. Accessed February 24, 2010.

39. Higginson IJ. End-of-life care: lessons from other nations. *J Palliat Med*. 2005;8(suppl 1):S161–S173.

40. Finlay E, Casarett D. Making difficult discussions easier: using prognosis to facilitate transitions to hospice. *CA Cancer J Clin*. 2009;59:250–263.

41. Hospice Net. *Medicare hospice benefits*. Available at:http://www.hospicenet.org/html/medicare.html Accessed February 24, 2010.

42. Fallowfield LJ, Jenkins VA, Beveridge HA. Truth may hurt but deceit hurts more: communication in palliative care. *Palliat Med*. 2002;16:297–303.

43. Schofield P, Carey M, Love A, et al. "Would you like to talk about your future treatment options?" Discussing the transition from curative cancer treatment to palliative care. *Palliat Med*. 2006;20:397–406.

44. Evans WG, Tulsky JA, Back AL, et al. Communication at times of transitions: how to help patients cope with loss and re-define hope. *Cancer J*. 2006;12:417–424.

45. Mackillop WJ, Stewart WE, Ginsburg AD, et al. Cancer patients' perceptions of their disease and its treatment. *Br J Cancer*. 1988;58:355–358.

46. Chow E, Andersson L, Wong R, et al. Patients with advanced cancer: a survey of the understanding of their illness and expectations from palliative radiotherapy for symptomatic metastases. *Clin Oncol (R Coll Radiol)*. 2001;13:204–208.

47. Craft PS, Burns CM, Smith WT, et al. Knowledge of treatment intent among patients with advanced cancer: a longitudinal study. *Eur J Cancer Care (Engl)*. 2005;14:417–425.

48. Burns CM, Broom DH, Smith WT, et al. Fluctuating awareness of treatment goals among patients and their caregivers: a longitudinal study of a dynamic process. *Support Care Cancer*. 2007;15:187–196.

49. Weeks JC, Cook EF, O'Day SJ, et al. Relationship between cancer patients' predictions of prognosis and their treatment preferences. *JAMA*. 1998;279:1709–1714.

50. Balmer CE, Thomas P, Osborne RJ. Who wants second-line, palliative chemotherapy? *Psychooncology*. 2001;10:410–418.

51. Matsuyama R, Reddy S, Smith TJ. Why do patients choose chemotherapy near the end of life? A review of the perspective of those facing death from cancer. *J Clin Oncol*. 2006;24:3490–3496.

52. Baile WF, Buckman R, Lenzi R, et al. SPIKES—a six-step protocol for delivering bad news: application to the patient with cancer. *Oncologist*. 2000;5:302–311.

53. Morita T, Akechi T, Ikenaga M, et al. Communication about the ending of anticancer treatment and transition to palliative care. *Ann Oncol*. 2004;15:1551–1557.

54. Innes S, Payne S. Advanced cancer patients' prognostic information preferences: a review. *Palliat Med*. 2009;23:29–39.

55. Braun M, Mikulincer M, Rydall A, et al. Hidden morbidity in cancer: spouse caregivers. *J Clin Oncol*. 2007;25:4829–4834.

56. Bosma H, Apland L, Kazanjian A. Cultural conceptualizations of hospice palliative care: more similarities than differences. *Palliat Med*. 2010;24:510–522.

57. Mitchell BL, Mitchell LC. Review of the literature on cultural competence and end-of-life treatment decisions: the role of the hospitalist. *J Natl Med Assoc*. 2009;101:920–926.

58. National Comprehensive Cancer Network. *Practice guidelines in oncology, version 1*. 2009. Available at: http://www.nccn.org/professionals/physician_gls/f_guidelines.asp Accessed February 24, 2010.

59. Cherny NI, Catane R, Kosmidis PA, ESMO Palliative Care Working Group. *ESMO policy on supportive and palliative care*. European Society for Medical Oncology; 2010. Available at: http://www.esmo.org/fileadmin/media/pdf/policies/PolicySupportivePalliativeCare.pdf. Accessed February 24, 2010.

60. Cheng WW, Willey J, Palmer JL, et al. Interval between palliative care referral and death among patients treated at a comprehensive cancer center. *J Palliat Med*. 2005;8:1025–1032.

61. Good PD, Cavenagh J, Ravenscroft PJ. Survival after enrollment in an Australian palliative care program. *J Pain Symptom Manage*. 2004;27:310–315.

62. Morita T, Akechi T, Ikenaga M, et al. Late referrals to specialized palliative care service in Japan. *J Clin Oncol*. 2005;23:2637–2644.

63. Keating NL, Landrum MB, Rogers Jr SO, et al. Physician factors associated with discussions about end-of-life care. *Cancer*. 2010;116:998–1006.

64. Younis T, Milch R, Abul-Khoudoud N, et al. Length of survival of patients with cancer in hospice: a retrospective analysis of patients treated at a major cancer center versus other practice settings. *J Palliat Med*. 2007;10:381–389.

65. Christakis NA, Escarce JJ. Survival of Medicare patients after enrollment in hospice programs. *N Engl J Med*. 1996;335:172–178.

66. Hagerty RG, Butow PN, Ellis PA, et al. Cancer patient preferences for communication of prognosis in the metastatic setting. *J Clin Oncol*. 2004;22:1721–1730.

67. Follwell M, Burman D, Le LW, et al. Phase II study of an outpatient palliative care intervention in patients with metastatic cancer. *J Clin Oncol*. 2009;27:206–213.

68. Meyers FJ, Linder J, Beckett L, et al. Simultaneous care: a model approach to the perceived conflict between investigational therapy and palliative care. *J Pain Symptom Manage*. 2004;28:548–556.

69. Temel JS, Jackson VA, Billings JA, et al. Phase II study: integrated palliative care in newly diagnosed advanced non-small-cell lung cancer patients. *J Clin Oncol*. 2007;25:2377–2382.

70. Finlay E, Shreve S, Casarett D. Nationwide veterans affairs quality measure for cancer: the family assessment of treatment at end of life. *J Clin Oncol*. 2008;26:3838–3844.

71. van Kleffens T, Van Baarsen B, Hoekman K, et al. Clarifying the term "palliative" in clinical oncology. *Eur J Cancer Care (Engl)*. 2004;13:263–271.

72. Clayton JM, Butow PN, Arnold RM, et al. Fostering coping and nurturing hope when discussing the future with terminally ill cancer patients and their caregivers. *Cancer*. 2005;103:1965–1975.

73. Fadul N, Elsayem A, Palmer JL, et al. Supportive versus palliative care: what's in a name? A survey of medical oncologists and midlevel providers at a comprehensive cancer center. *Cancer*. 2009;115:2013–2021.

74. Apatira L, Boyd EA, Malvar G, et al. Hope, truth, and preparing for death: perspectives of surrogate decision makers. *Ann Intern Med*. 2008;149:861–868.

75. Back AL, Arnold RM, Quill TE. Hope for the best, and prepare for the worst. *Ann Intern Med*. 2003;138:439–443.

76. Quill TE, Arnold RM, Platt F. "I wish things were different": expressing wishes in response to loss, futility, and unrealistic hopes. *Ann Intern Med*. 2001;135:551–555.

Spirituality in supportive oncology

51

Susan E. McClement and Harvey M. Chochinov

The consequences of cancer and its treatment are substantial.[1] In addition to the burden caused by a multitude of physical symptoms, individuals living with cancer also experience psychosocial and spiritual concerns.[2–4] If left unaddressed, these can create distress and can greatly impair patients' quality of life and that of their families.[4]

The importance of spirituality and religion to health has been extensively explored in the literature.[5,6] Cancer patients with an enhanced sense of spiritual well-being are described as being able to cope more effectively with the process of living with cancer and have a better quality of life.[7]

A recent consensus conference aimed at improving the quality of spiritual care as a dimension of palliative care recommended that spirituality be considered a patient vital sign that is screened routinely, and that spiritual distress or religious struggle be treated with the same urgency as pain or any other medical problem.[8] Not all patients will have spiritual needs that require attention all of the time, nor will they look to health care providers to help meet these needs.[9] However, some patients will be desirous of having their spiritual needs addressed during clinical encounters.[10] Moreover, literature documents patients' desire to have their spiritual needs openly discussed by their health care providers, particularly when facing a potentially incurable disease.[11] It is thus imperative that supportive oncology care address the physical, psychological, and *spiritual issues* that arise within this patient population.

Evidence in the literature suggests that a variety of disciplines endorse, at least in principle, the importance of spiritual care provision as part of their professional work.[12,13] However, there has been minimal corresponding dialogue regarding how such care might be operationalized in supportive oncology practice. Germane to such discussions are conceptual understandings of spirituality, the types of spiritual needs that patients have, and approaches for detecting, exploring, and responding to these needs. Therefore, the purposes of this chapter are (1) to consider definitions of, and the discourse about, spirituality as discussed in the health care literature; (2) to examine the ways in which spirituality and spiritual needs might be assessed in clinical practice; and (3) to describe some empirically based interventions aimed at enhancing the spiritual care of those living with life-threatening illness. The chapter concludes with a brief discussion of the implications that the mandate to provide spiritual care will have for individual clinicians, the wider multidisciplinary team, and health care institutions.

SPIRITUALITY: DEFINITION AND DISCOURSE

Attending to patients' spiritual needs presupposes that clinicians have a clear working definition of what spirituality is. However, evidence in the general health and palliative care literature demonstrates that the term *spirituality* is plagued by conceptual ambiguity.[14] Some scholars have concluded that the intangible and highly individualized ways in which people experience spirituality render it resistant to language.[15] Such a response is of little help to health care providers in trying to communicate with patients about spiritual needs, and in developing interventions to address those needs.

Far from being resistant to language, definitions of spirituality found in diverse professional health literature and in research conducted with dying patients speak to issues of meaning, purpose, connectedness, and transcendence, and thereby suggest what a definition of spirituality (albeit broad) might include. A consensus conference was convened in February 2009 to identify points of agreement about spirituality in health care and to make recommendations to advance the delivery of quality spiritual care in the context of palliative care.[8] Building on previous literature and informed by the philosophical, religious, spiritual, and existential issues that arise in clinical practice, an expert advisory group defined spirituality as "the aspect of humanity that refers to the way individuals seek and express meaning and purpose, and the way they experience their connectedness to the moment, to self, to others, to nature, and to the significant or sacred"[8] (p. 886). Although this definition may not be satisfactory to all, it does represent the outcome of a systematic, deliberative, interdisciplinary approach aimed at identifying points of agreement about spiritual care within a palliative care context, and it provides a basis from which ongoing dialogue about spiritual care issues can occur.

Discussions of spirituality often include its relationship to the concept of religion, which is characterized as having foundations in established traditions arising from a group of people with common beliefs and practices concerning the sacred.[16,17] Spirituality and spiritual care have historically been firmly rooted in religion[16–18]; however, spirituality is now described in the health care literature as a concept that is related to, but distinct from, religion.[19]

What might account for this shift in conceptualization? Two influences merit comment. First, the ascendancy of reason and science in the Enlightenment period eroded the social and political authority that religion held in most of Western society. Because it could not be proven by reason, or verified through scientific methods, religion was relegated to the sphere of private and personal belief.[20,21] Second, reaction to the Enlightenment and its claims of scientific rationalization spawned the philosophical romanticism movement, in which strong emphasis came to be placed on individual expression of emotion, imagination, and feeling. Within this context, spirituality came to be understood in terms of positive emotional esthetic experiences of the individual.[22,23]

It may be argued that because of significant congregational decline in mainline Catholic and Protestant churches, and census data reporting markedly fewer numbers of individuals laying claim to a particular faith tradition, the adoption of a more secularized approach to spirituality poses minimal challenges for health professionals involved in the provision of spiritual care. However, Reimer-Kirkham[47] and others[16,20] challenge assertions that society is becoming more secularized and note that increased church attendance among evangelical denominations and increasing migration trends among those adhering to non-Christian religions should challenge us to think about the seeming irrelevance of religion to public life. If some segments of society have become secularized, but religious resurgence has occurred in others, discussions of spirituality in the health care literature characterizing it as largely devoid of religion will need to be rethought.[10]

Given the historical and social context of conceptualizations of spirituality and religion as previously discussed, critical reflection regarding the discourse about spirituality and religion in the health care literature is warranted. More than just a verbal exchange of ideas, discourse shapes and creates meaning. Ideas that gain the status of "truth" dominate how people define themselves and their social world.[21,22] Although discourse can foster the production of new knowledge and can help illuminate differences, it can also result in the marginalization and silencing of other ways of experiencing the world.

Although attempts among scholars to distinguish the concepts of spirituality and religion are important in the service of obtaining conceptual clarity, we believe that they have had significant consequences. Reviewing the discourse about spirituality and religion in health care reveals that religion has been depicted as a narrow, prescriptive, restrictive, codified set of communal beliefs and practices that tend to suppress personal spiritual exploration through concern with maintaining the boundaries of a particular institution.[16,20,24] In contrast, spirituality is characterized as being dissociated from religion and religious community; it is free from prescriptive boundaries, self-directed, and concerned about discovery of meaning in the context of the person. Cast in these terms, religion is negatively portrayed as reductive, old fashioned, and communal, whereas spirituality has been characterized as contemporary and more highly evolved.[10,16,25]

Rather than advancing our understanding of the important interrelatedness of religion and spirituality, an unwitting consequence of this type of discourse has been to dichotomize and polarize these two concepts. Dichotomy has been described as the "usual pathway to vulgarization"[26] (p. 7), in which a complex set of arguments are divided into two polarized positions—them against us. We portray "them" as a foolish caricature of extremes to put "us" in a better light. Intentional or not, is this what has happened to the concept of religion vis à vis the larger discussion of spirituality and spiritual care?

Some authors posit that the expansion of spirituality in health care beyond its traditional religious roots represents an attempt to be more inclusive in pluralistic health care settings and to find common ground for diverse beliefs.[18] In so doing, however, references to things explicitly religious have been largely muted, ostensibly out of concern that emphasizing religious understandings of spirituality in the clinical encounter might disadvantage or offend patients for whom a nonreligious orientation is relevant. Paradoxically, however, spiritual care that preferentially places nonreligious notions of spirituality above traditional religious understandings is equally alienating and disenfranchising to patients for whom the religious remains a relevant concern. It can be argued that to move away from discussions that are characterized as "religious," simply because they are religious, obviates health care professional claims of providing holistic care.

A final, ironic consequence of dichotomizing religion and spirituality needs to be considered. The nebulous nature of spirituality that has defied strict definition in any traditional sense would, it seem, be part of its attraction to those who eschew notions of orthodoxy and orthopraxy. Yet a burgeoning wave of scholarly activity is aimed at better understanding and ordering spirituality into an organized typology of antecedents, attributes, and empirical referents[12,24]—the very things that have rendered religion unfashionable in Western society. Pesut observes that secularization has paradoxically contributed to the sacralization of the public domain.[27] One might rightly ask whether spirituality, as it is defined in contemporary terms, will experience a similar conceptual fate and become the "new" religion.

SPIRITUAL ASSESSMENT

Cancer patients can experience a plethora of spiritual concerns, including, but not limited to, existential concerns, feelings of abandonment by God or others, conflicted or challenged belief systems, and feelings of hopelessness, despair, and shame.[3,8] From the previous discussion, it is evident that although some patients see themselves as both religious and spiritual, others may self-identify as being highly spiritual, yet not religious. This creates an interesting tension for clinicians who care for both patients whose spirituality is primarily expressed through religious practice and those whose spirituality is understood in individualistic, secular terms. There may be patients who conflate notions of spirituality and religiosity such that the language of spirituality—even for those patients who view it in a very secular fashion—is heard as "religious" and thus alienating. To avoid inadvertently closing the door on further dialogue, clinicians must themselves be clear regarding a given patient's personal integration of religiosity and spirituality. Asking a simple, time-efficient questions such as "Is religion or spirituality important in your life?" or "What are the things that continue to have meaning and purpose in your life?" may be helpful in this regard.[10] A follow-up query as to how well religious and/or spiritual resources are working for the patient can provide insights regarding the need for more in-depth assessment within the context of a spiritual history.

Conducting a formal spiritual history with patients is a recommendation endorsed by the consensus conference report on ways to improve the quality of spiritual care within palliative care. Set within the context of a comprehensive examination, the spiritual history invites patients to share their own definitions of spirituality, and to identify beliefs and practices that are important in clinical decision making and care planning.[10]

A variety of approaches have been developed that can facilitate the collection of a patient's spiritual history. Familiarity with some of these approaches will enable clinicians to critically appraise their appropriateness for use in a given clinical context with a given patient. The approach of Taylor and colleagues[27] to spiritual history taking examines (1) areas of connection with other persons, other communities, and a power greater than self; (2) assessment; (3) experiences of meaning and joy; (4) sources of strength and comfort; and (5) hopes and concerns.

The mnemonic SPIRIT offered by Maugans[28] offers six components of a spiritual assessment that clinicians should address. These include (1) spiritual belief systems, which refer to issues of theology and a person's religious affiliation; (2) personal spirituality, which concerns the spiritual views that are individual to the patient that need not necessarily be associated with religion; (3) integration and involvement of the individual with a spiritual community that may serve as a source of spiritual support; (4) ritualized practices and lifestyle activities that may influence the person's health; (5) the influence of spiritual beliefs and practices on patients' desire to participate in health care; and (6) terminal events planning related to end-of-life concerns that the patient may have.

The mnemonic "FICA" developed by Puchalski and Romer[29] considers the following dimensions:

F, representing faith and belief, explores the extent to which patients consider themselves spiritual or religious, and asks what gives the person's life meaning
I, importance, asks the importance of faith or belief in the person's life
C, community, elicits whether or not the person is part of a spiritual or religious community
A, standing for Address/Action in care, prompts clinicians regarding what needs to be done with the information collected.

Information gleaned from the history will help clinicians understand patients' sources of spiritual support and distress. Those patients in need of a more comprehensive spiritual assessment can then be referred to a member of the health care team who has specific training and expertise in the identification and exploration of spiritual care issues.[10] The need for such expertise among the health care team is an important consideration in the provision of spiritual care, and is related to the issue of who exactly should be involved in the planning and provision of such care.

Some authors argue that spiritual care should be the ambit of any member of the health care team[29]; others caution that the delivery of such care can be experienced as burdensome and daunting for those who feel ill equipped to do so.[30] Several factors identified in the literature may contribute to the reticence of health care providers to engage in the provision of spiritual care. A qualitative study conducted by Chibnall and associates[30] with physicians at a university-based hospital revealed that psychosocial and spiritual care was devalued in their medical training, and that physicians lacked both a safe environment and sufficient time in which to discuss spiritual matters. In a descriptive phenomenologic study that examined how family practice physicians, nurse practitioners, and physician assistants incorporate spiritual care in practice, barriers identified included lack of formal training in spiritual issues and concern that raising such issues would be perceived by patients as "pushing religion."[32]

Although each member of the health care team should be able to listen respectfully to patients' individual expressions of their spirituality, it does not logically follow that each member of the team is equipped to conduct a formal spiritual assessment. Special clinical training and preparation are needed to skillfully and sensitively appraise and explore spiritual needs and concerns.[10] Thus a more rational and balanced approach to the organization of spiritual care provision would see the responsibility of spiritual care shared among specially prepared spiritual care providers and the collective members of the team, in response to the needs of the patient.

Sinclair and colleagues[32] offers a cautionary note regarding potential issues of overlap when spiritual care is provided by oncology members within an interdisciplinary setting. When multiple members of the health care team have a potential role in providing spiritual care, confusion over, and concerns about, professional turf may arise. Research examining the ecology of team science[34] indicates that communication among team members enhances team cohesion and performance and encourages feelings of trust and psychological safety. Therefore, any turf issues need to be superseded by open, respectful communication among the team, in which the roles of each team member can be articulated and the insights and proficiencies that each brings can be clarified and used for the benefit of the patient.

SPIRITUAL CARE INTERVENTIONS

Information gleaned from spiritual assessments provides the foundation from which specifically tailored interventions can be implemented and evaluated. Rousseau[34] has advanced a framework that offers practical guidance for the treatment of spiritual suffering among dying patients. This involves a blend of religious expression and psychotherapeutic approaches and consists of the following: (1) control of physical symptoms; (2) providing a supportive presence; (3) encouraging life review to assist in recognizing purpose, value, and meaning; (4) exploring guilt, remorse, forgiveness, and reconciliation; (5) facilitating religious expression; (6) reframing goals; and (7) encouraging meditative practices that focus on healing rather than on cure. Such approaches are consistent with the broad range of spiritual health interventions identified and recommended in the consensus report to improve the quality of spiritual care in palliative care.[8]

Short-term psychotherapeutic interventions aimed at addressing issues such as purpose and meaning in advanced cancer patients have been empirically examined.

Research evaluating meaning-centered therapy[36] and dignity therapy[37–40] represents particularly exciting, viable approaches to reducing common elements of existential distress in advanced cancer patients. Drawing on Frankl's concepts of meaning-based psychotherapy, Breitbart and colleagues[35] used meaning-centered group psychotherapy with a group of ambulatory advanced cancer patients. The intervention consisted of eight weekly manualized sessions conducted by experienced psychiatrists or psychologists, who used a combination of instruction, discussion, and experiential exercises, each organized around a specific meaning-centered theme. Patients with advanced solid tumor cancers (n = 90) were randomly assigned to meaning-centered group psychotherapy or supportive group psychotherapy. Outcome measures of spiritual well-being as captured by the FACIT (Functional Assessment of Chronic Illness Therapy) Spiritual Well-Being Scale—meaning, hopelessness, desire for death, optimism/pessimism, anxiety, depression, and overall quality of life—were assessed at baseline, at the end of 8 weeks, and 2 months after the intervention. Although attrition and potential sample bias affect the generalizability of the findings, compared with those receiving supportive group therapy, patients in the treatment group demonstrated greater improvement in the sense of meaning and spiritual well-being that persisted over 2 months post evaluation. The treatment group also demonstrated significant improvement in anxiety and a decreased desire for death that strengthened over time.

The programmatic research conducted by Chochinov and associates[36–41] to examine issues of dignity in end-of-life care from the perspective of dying patients produced an empirically derived model that provides clinicians with a framework from which to understand and explore a broad range of physical, psychological, social, and spiritual issues that may affect patients' perceptions of this construct. From this foundational work, dignity therapy, a unique, individualized, brief psychotherapy, was developed for the purpose of relieving distress and bolstering quality of life among patients nearing death. Dignity therapy provides patients an opportunity to reflect on things that matter most to them, or that they would most want remembered. Questions informing the content of the therapeutic process are flexible so as to accommodate patients' particular needs and choices regarding what they specifically wish to address, and have been published elsewhere.[38] Conversations arising out of dignity therapy are audio-recorded and transcribed, and an edited version of the transcript is returned to patients to share or bequeath to individuals of their choice.

In a phase I trial of dignity therapy[38] that included a sample of 100 terminally ill patients, 91% reported being satisfied with the therapy; 76% reported a heightened sense of dignity; 68% an increased sense of purpose; 67% a heightened sense of meaning; and 47% an increased will to live; 81% indicated that it had been or would be of help to their family. Modest significant improvements were also seen in postintervention measures of suffering and depressive symptoms. Family members of patients also found dignity therapy helpful: 78% stated that it enhanced patient dignity, 72% reported that it heightened the meaning of life for the patient, 78% said that the document produced from the therapy session was a comfort to them in their time of grief, and 95% stated that they would recommend dignity therapy to other patients and families.[41] Evaluation of the efficacy of dignity therapy in alleviating existential concerns of advanced cancer patients in the context of an international, multicenter, randomized, controlled trial is currently under way.

Rigorously evaluated psychotherapeutic interventions demonstrated to bolster a sense of meaning, purpose, and spiritual well-being among advanced cancer patients represent important therapeutic options that can be used to mitigate spiritual distress and constitute significant contributions to the evidence base informing supportive care.[42]

PROVIDING SPIRITUAL CARE: INDIVIDUAL, TEAM, AND INSTITUTIONAL IMPLICATIONS

Tending to the spiritual needs of cancer patients has implications for individual clinicians, the health care team, and the institution. Participation in spiritual care will require that clinicians have some comfort with and acumen in connecting with others and engaging in the processes of active listening, valuing, and empathizing. The extent to which these abilities reside within the individual will influence the extent to which he or she is able to provide a compassionate presence, and underscores the importance of clinicians' engaging in careful self-reflection to identify their strengths and learning needs in providing spiritual care.[43]

Healthcare teams will need to embrace the challenging but necessary work of discussing the diverse and potentially contradictory perspectives that each discipline brings to the provision of spiritual care. Rather than looking for synthesis and common ground among disciplines, Swinton[44] advocates the need for dialogue and dialectic. Such an approach may prevent domination of the loudest or most powerful discipline within the team, while preventing neglect or disregard of potentially important ideas, thus resulting in the co-creation of a spiritual care plan that "supports the dignity of each patient by honouring the inherent value of that person, their beliefs and values that support them and their practices that enable them to find meaning and hope in the midst of suffering."[45]

The wider institutions within which health care and thus spiritual care are provided must endorse an ethos of respect for personhood and attention to whole person care. This endorsement must transcend words within an institutional mission and values statement and must include what Sinclair and colleagues have described as the "brick, mortar, and governance of spiritual care programs."[46] Administrators will need to grapple with providing more open and inclusive spiritual care programs while still respecting religious traditions; will make decisions about how spiritual care programs will be funded; will decide how staff will be educated to provide spiritual care; will determine what the reporting structure for such programs will be within the organizational chart; and will consider the role and placement of sacred spaces within public venues such as hospitals or clinics.[46]

CONCLUSION

Individuals living with cancer experience a multitude of issues and concerns, including those of a spiritual nature. Provision of holistic care requires that these concerns be identified, explored, and addressed. Important headway has been made regarding approaches to spiritual assessment, and empirically sound approaches for addressing spiritual issues have been identified. Ongoing work will be needed as health care providers strive to deliver skilled, sensitive, and culturally relevant spiritual care within a context of global migration and increasing ethnic, linguistic and religious diversity.[47]

REFERENCES

1. Holland J, Weiss T. The new standard of quality cancer care: integrating the psychosocial aspects in routine cancer from diagnosis through survivorship. *Cancer J.* 2008;14:425–428.
2. Bradley N, Davis L, Chow E. Symptom distress in patients attending an outpatient palliative radiotherapy clinic. *J Pain Symptom Manage.* 2005;30:123–131.
3. Chochinov HM, Cann BJ. Interventions to enhance the spiritual aspects of dying. *J Palliat Med.* 2005;8:S103–S115.
4. Moadel A, Morgan C, Fatone A, et al. Seeking meaning and hope: self-reported spiritual and existential needs among an ethnically-diverse cancer patient population. *Psychooncology.* 1999;8:378–385.
5. Chida Y, Steptoe A, Powell LH. Religiosity/ spirituality and mortality: a systematic quantitative review. *Psychother Psychosom.* 2009;78:81–90.
6. Townsend M, Kladder V, Ayele H. Systematic review of clinical trials examining the effects of religion on health. *South Med J.* 2002;95:1429–1434.
7. Cohen SR, Leis A. What determines the quality of life of terminally ill cancer patients from their own perspective? *J Palliat Care.* 2002;18:48–58.
8. Puchalski C, Ferrell B, Virani R, et al. Improving the quality of spiritual care as a dimension of palliative care: the report of the Consensus Conference. *J Palliat Med.* 2009;12:885–904.
9. McSherry W, Ross L. Dilemmas of spiritual assessment: considerations for nursing practice. *J Adv Nurs.* 2002;38:479–488.
10. Sinclair S, Pereira J, Raffin S. A thematic review of the spirituality literature within palliative care. *J Palliat Med.* 2006;9:464–479.
11. Balboni TA, Vanderwerker LC, Block SD, et al. Religiousness and spiritual support among advanced cancer patients and associations with end-of-life treatment preferences and quality of life. *J Clin Oncol.* 2007;25:555–560.
12. Ledger SD. The duty of nurses to meet patients' spiritual and/or religious needs. *Br J Nurs.* 2005;14:220–225.
13. D'Souza R. The importance of spirituality in medicine and its application to clinical practice. *Med J Aust.* 2007;186(suppl 10):S57–S59.
14. Vachon M, Fillion L, Achille M. A conceptual analysis of spirituality at the end of life. *J Palliat Med.* 2009;12:53–59.
15. Koenig HG. Research on religion, spirituality, and mental health: a review. *Can J Psychiatry.* 2009;54:283–291.

16. McBrien B. A concept analysis of spirituality. *Br J Nurs.* 2006;15:42–45.
17. Patterson S, Balducci L, Meyer R. The book of Job: a 2,500-year-old current guide to the practice of oncology: the nexus of medicine and spirituality. *J Cancer Educ.* 2002;17:237–240.
18. Emblen J. Religion and spirituality define according to current use in nursing literature. *J Prof Nurs.* 1992;8:41–47.
19. Pesut B, Fowler M, Taylor EJ, et al. Conceptualising spirituality and religion for healthcare. *J Clin Nurs.* 2008;17:2803–2810.
20. Bell C. Paradigms behind (and before) the modern concept of religion. *History and Theory.* 2006;45:27–46.
21. Aléx L, Hammarström A. Shift in power during an interview situation: methodological reflections inspired by Foucault and Bourdieu. *Nurs Inq.* 2008;15:169–176.
22. Meraviglia MG. Critical analysis of spirituality and its empirical indicators. *J Holist Nurs.* 1999;17:18–33.
23. Tanyi RA. Towards clarification of the meaning of spirituality. *J Adv Nurs.* 2002;39:500–509.
24. Clarke J. Religion and spirituality: a discussion paper about negativity, reductionism and differentiation in nursing texts. *Int J Nurs Stud.* 2006;43:775–785.
25. Kristjanson LJ. Conceptual issues related to measurement in family research. *Can J Nurs Res.* 1992;24:37–52.
26. Pesut B. Ontologies of nursing in an age of spiritual pluralism: closed or open worldview? *Nurs Philos.* 2010;11:15–23.
27. Taylor P. Issues of suffering at the end of life. In: Poor B, Porrier GP, eds. *End of life nursing care.* Boston: Jones and Bartlett; 2001:175–187.
28. Maugans TA. The SPIRITual history. *Arch Fam Med.* 1996;5:11–16.
29. Puchalski C, Romer AL. Taking a spiritual history allows clinicians to understand patients more fully. *Palliat Med.* 2000;3:129–137.
30. Chibnall JT, Bennett ML, Videen SD, et al. Identifying barriers to psychosocial spiritual care at the end of life: a physician group study. *Am J Hosp Palliat Care.* 2004;21:419–426.
31. Tanyi RA, McKenzie M, Chapek C. How family practice physicians, nurse practitioners, and physician assistants incorporate spiritual care in practice. *J Am Acad Nurse Pract.* 2009;21:690–697.
32. Sinclair S, Raffin S, Pereira J, et al. Collective soul: the spirituality of an interdisciplinary palliative care team. *Palliat Support Care.* 2006;4:13–24.

33. Stokols D, Misra S, Moser RP, et al. The ecology of team science: understanding contextual influences on transdisciplinary collaboration. *Am J Prev Med.* 2008;35(suppl 2):S96–S115.
34. Rousseau P. Spirituality and the dying patients. *J Clin Oncol.* 2003;1:21(9 suppl):54s–56s.
35. Breitbart W, Rosenfeld B, Gibson C, et al. Meaning-centered group psychotherapy for patients with advanced cancer: a pilot randomized controlled trial. *Psychooncology.* 2010;19:21–28.
36. Chochinov HM, Hassard T, McClement S, et al. The landscape of distress in the terminally ill. *J Pain Symptom Manage.* 2009;38:641–649.
37. Chochinov HM, Hassard T, McClement S, et al. The patient dignity inventory: a novel way of measuring dignity-related distress in palliative care. *J Pain Symptom Manage.* 2008;36:559–571.
38. Chochinov HM, Hack T, Hassard T, et al. Dignity therapy: a novel psychotherapeutic intervention for patients near the end of life. *J Clin Oncol.* 2005;23:5520–5525.
39. Chochinov HM, Hack T, Hassard T, et al. Dignity in the terminally ill: a cross-sectional, cohort study. *Lancet.* 2002;360:2026–2030.
40. Chochinov HM, Hack T, McClement S, et al. Dignity in the terminally ill: a developing empirical model. *Soc Sci Med.* 2002;54:433–443.
41. McClement S, Chochinov HM, Hack T, et al. Dignity therapy: family member perspectives. *J Palliat Med.* 2007;10:1076–1082.
42. McClement SE. Acquiring an evidence-base in palliative care: challenges and future directions. *Expert Rev Pharmacoecon Outcomes Res.* 2006;6:37–40.
43. Gordon A. Competency model for the assessment and delivery of spiritual care. *Palliat Med.* 2004;18:646–651.
44. Swinton J. Identity and resistance: why spiritual care needs "enemies". *J Clin Nurs.* 2006;15:918–928.
45. Puchalski CM, Lunsford B, Harris MH, et al. Interdisciplinary spiritual care for seriously ill and dying patients: a collaborative model. *Cancer J.* 2006;12:398–416.
46. Sinclair S, Mysak M, Hagen NA. What are the core elements of oncology spiritual care programs? *Palliat Support Care.* 2009;7:415–422.
47. Reimer-Kirkham S. Lived religion: implications for nursing ethics. *Nurs Ethics.* 2009;16:406–417.

PSYCHOSOCIAL ONCOLOGY

SECTION OUTLINE

52 Depression and anxiety in supportive oncology

Madeline Li, Virginia Boquiren, Christopher Lo, and Gary Rodin

Emotional distress is a universal response to the trauma of cancer. The prolonged and cumulative exposure to multiple stressors associated with this disease contributes to elevated risk for psychological distress, specifically, symptoms of anxiety and depression, and for the development of clinically significant anxiety and depressive disorders.[1-3] Distress of this type deserves attention not only because of its impact on quality of life,[4] but also because of its potential adverse effects on medical treatment compliance,[5] health care utilization,[6] the risk of suicide and the desire for hastened death,[7-9] and the risk of death from all causes.[10,11] This chapter is focused on anxiety and depression in the context of cancer, addressing their clinical features, detection, prevalence, pathogenesis, and treatment. It focuses attention on the role of routine screening for these symptoms and early clinic-based intervention.

The severity and persistence of psychological distress associated with cancer are related to the physical, psychological, and social stressors associated with the disease and to the other risk and protective factors in these domains.[12] The physical burden of cancer and its treatment typically interfere with the ability to engage in activities of daily living and in occupational and recreational activities, and with role functioning in the family, in intimate relationships, and in the community. A variety of fears and concerns are common, including uncertainty about the future, loss of the sense of autonomy and control, alterations in anticipated life trajectory, existential concerns related to perceived foreshortening of life, and fear of dying.[3,13] These concerns typically evoke at least transient feelings of anxiety, grief, and sadness, which can be regarded as normative and nonpathologic.[13] However, in a substantial minority of individuals with cancer, clinically significant symptoms of anxiety or depression may develop.

CONTINUUM OF DISTRESS: FROM "NORMAL" TO DISORDER

The *Diagnostic and Statistical Manual of Mental Disorders, Fourth Edition, Text Revision (DSM-IV-TR)*[14] outlines the core criteria that must be present to diagnose a psychiatric disorder. However, although clear DSM criteria have been put forth for full syndrome disorders, such as major depression, the diagnostic threshold that demarcates "normality" from a subthreshold or so-called "minor disorder" is not well established.[15-17] This is especially problematic in the evaluation of distress in medical populations, in whom psychological symptoms most often fall into a mid range of severity. For this reason, a categorical approach to the diagnosis of psychological disturbances in this mid range of severity may have less validity and utility than one that considers such disturbances on a continuum. Disturbances may range from symptoms of nonpathologic sadness, grief, or anxiety, to symptoms that meet criteria for an adjustment disorder or a subthreshold disorder, to those that clearly meet diagnostic criteria for a formal depressive or anxiety disorder as specified in the DSM. These categories are described in the following sections.

ADJUSTMENT DISORDER

Adjustment disorder refers to a state of persistent distress that occurs within 3 months of onset of a stressor, such as cancer, and that is associated with significant impairment in social, psychological, or occupational functioning.[14] This condition, which can be categorized with specifiers of anxious and/or depressed mood, lies on the continuum of distress between nonpathologic distress and a major psychiatric disorder. However, there is a lack of precision in its diagnostic criteria and boundaries, and its validity is unclear in the context of a medical illness, such as cancer, in which distress is normative.[15] Although the evidence base for this disorder is not well established,[18,19] the heuristic appeal and nonstigmatizing nature of this diagnostic category have lent it great popularity to capture prodromal or transient states of distress that are amenable to preventive or early intervention. For these reasons, and because psychological disturbances are so common in the mid range of severity in this population, adjustment disorder is the most commonly reported psychiatric diagnosis in patients with cancer.[20,21]

DEPRESSIVE DISORDERS

The five major categories of depressive disorders as specified in the DSM-IV-TR include (1) major depressive disorder (MDD), (2) dysthymic disorder (DD), (3) mood disorder due to a (specified) general medical condition (GMC), (4) substance-induced mood disorder, and (5) depressive disorder not otherwise specified (NOS), which specifies research criteria for minor depression.[14] The diagnostic and clinical features of MDD and of the subthreshold mood disorders, DD and minor depression, are briefly described.

Major depressive disorder and subthreshold mood disorders

A categorical diagnosis of MDD, based on DSM-IV-TR criteria,[14] requires the presence of five or more symptoms, which must include depressed mood or anhedonia for at least 2 weeks, representing a significant change from previous functioning. Neurovegetative symptoms specified in the diagnostic criteria include impairment in sleep or appetite, loss of energy, and psychomotor retardation or agitation. Psychological criteria include feelings of worthlessness, hopelessness or excessive guilt, cognitive impairment, and recurrent suicidal ideation. The rubric of subthreshold depressive disorders, which includes minor depression, refers to the presence of two to four depressive symptoms present

for longer than 2 weeks. DD is characterized by symptoms of depression that are less severe than those of MDD, but that have been continuously present for at least 2 years. A chronic depressive disorder, such as DD, may be likely to occur in association with cancer because of the persistence, repetitiveness, and progression of the stressors associated with it. Subthreshold disorders that do not meet full criteria for MDD can nevertheless substantially impair quality of life and the capacity to comply with medical treatment.

DIAGNOSTIC COMPLEXITY OF MDD IN CANCER

Oncologists and oncology mental health professionals are faced with multiple diagnostic challenges in the assessment of mood disturbances in cancer patients. One of these stems from the overlap between symptoms of depression and those of cancer. For example, fatigue, anorexia, weight loss, insomnia, psychomotor retardation, and cognitive impairment may arise secondary to MDD, to the cancer, and/or to its treatment. This symptom overlap may lead to overdiagnosis of depression, with the false attribution of cancer symptoms to a mood disturbance, or to underdiagnosis, with symptoms of depression mistaken for symptoms of the disease or its treatment. Although the distinction between cancer-related symptoms and depression may be difficult, somatic symptoms that are disproportionate to the medical condition may be a clue to the presence of depression. The clinician must also be alert to atypical presentations of depressive symptoms in cancer, such as those seen in treatment noncompliance or refusal. Depression, which denotes a primary disturbance in mood, must also be distinguished from states of demoralization characterized by feelings of incompetence, hopelessness, and existential despair.[22]

ANXIETY

Research on anxiety disorders in cancer has been much less developed than that on depression. The DSM lists eight major categories of anxiety disorders relevant to cancer[13]: (1) panic disorder with/without agoraphobia, (2) specific phobia, (3) generalized anxiety disorder (GAD), (4) acute stress disorder (ASD), (5) posttraumatic stress disorder (PTSD), (6) anxiety disorder due to a GMC, (7) substance-induced anxiety disorder, and (8) anxiety disorder NOS. Subthreshold anxiety disorders fall under anxiety disorder NOS, comparable with the classification of depressive disorders, but their clinical features and diagnostic thresholds have not been well described. In consideration of anxiety in this chapter, we have focused on panic disorder and specific phobias, GAD, and ASD/PTSD.

PANIC DISORDER AND SPECIFIC PHOBIAS

Panic disorder frequently occurs in association with depressive disorders, or with other anxiety disorders. Panic attacks are characterized by discrete episodes of intense anxiety or a sense of impending doom, associated with physical symptoms such as shortness of breath, heart palpitations, chest pain, sweating, shaking, nausea, and light-headedness. Distinct from the persistent anxiety seen in GAD, panic symptoms peak acutely and then resolve over several minutes. Panic disorder is diagnosed when panic attacks are recurrent and unexpected, and are associated with concern about having additional attacks, worry about the consequences of an attack, or significant resultant behavioral change such as agoraphobia. In cancer patients, isolated panic attacks may be precipitated by specific cancer-related worries or may be associated with blood or needle phobias or claustrophobia related to radiation therapy or medical imaging machines, or may occur as part of the phenomena of anticipatory or conditioned nausea and vomiting associated with chemotherapy.[23] Panic disorder may manifest in cancer patients as avoidance of coming to hospital for treatment, or sudden treatment refusal and an urgent desire to leave hospital against medical advice.

GENERALIZED ANXIETY DISORDER (GAD)

GAD associated with cancer may be diagnosed when symptoms persist for longer than 6 months and are free-floating, without a particular trigger or pattern. Anxiety in cancer may be most closely related to GAD, whose features may be detected with the State-Trait Anxiety Inventory.[24] Patients with GAD typically experience exaggerated anxiety and worry about everyday life events. In cancer patients, this may be manifest in unrealistic fears of being left without emotional, financial, or practical support. However, the diagnosis of GAD may be more difficult to ascertain when repetitive stressors are related to pain or other symptoms, recurrence, treatment side effects, or multiple medical complications. In addition, physical symptoms of GAD, such as restlessness, muscle tension, shortness of breath, heart palpitations, sweating, dizziness, and fatigue,[14] may both exacerbate and mimic cancer-related physical symptoms.

ACUTE STRESS DISORDER (ASD) AND POSTTRAUMATIC STRESS DISORDER (PTSD)

It has only recently been recognized in the DSM that cancer may represent a traumatic stressor that can precipitate ASD or PTSD. Its belated inclusion in the DSM may be explained by the unique characteristics of cancer as a trauma that distinguishes it from traumatic events that are more discrete, acute, and external. By contrast, the nature of the threat in cancer is often uncertain, intangible, and anticipatory in nature because the disease trajectory of cancer is often unpredictable, with long periods of remission interrupted by periods of illness and active disease, and with threats of recurrence, progressive deterioration, and death that may never be eliminated.

ASD refers to a constellation of symptoms that occur following exposure to a traumatic event that involves threatened death or serious injury, both of which are common in patients with cancer. Diagnostic symptoms for ASD[14] include (1) dissociative symptoms, such as a subjective sense of numbing, detachment, or experiences of unreality; (2) persistent reexperiencing of a traumatic event through recurrent images, thoughts, dreams, or flashback episodes; (3) marked avoidance of stimuli associated with the trauma; and (4) marked symptoms of anxiety or hyperarousal, which may manifest in hypervigilance, sleep disturbance, and irritability. The diagnosis of ASD can be made when these symptoms are associated with significant distress and impairment in social, occupational, or other important areas of functioning, and when they occur within 4 weeks of the trauma and last from 2 days to 4

weeks. A diagnosis of PTSD can be made if the symptoms persist for longer than 1 month. Subcategorizations of PTSD are based on whether the symptoms are acute (i.e., less than 3 months) or chronic (i.e., longer than 4 months) in duration.[14]

MIXED ANXIETY AND DEPRESSIVE SYMPTOMS

Mixed states of anxiety and depression have recently been identified as a common manifestation of distress in cancer patients.[25] These mixed states may occur both because of the comorbid association of anxiety and depressive disorders and because these symptoms may arise within a single clinical presentation. Mixed anxiety and depressive states can be diagnosed within the category of adjustment disorder, subthreshold disorder that does not meet Axis I criteria for any disorder (NOS categorization), or MDD with a comorbid anxiety disorder, listed as two primary Axis I disorders. However, the high rate of comorbidity and shared temperamental and risk factors for anxiety and depression have prompted a proposal for a new mixed anxiety/depression diagnostic category in the DSM-V, to be released in 2013.[26] In a large cross-sectional study (n = 8265), Brintzenhofe-Szoc et al.[25] found mixed symptoms of anxiety and depression in 12.4% of patients, depressive symptoms in 18.3%, and anxiety symptoms in 24.0%. Rates of mixed anxiety/depression symptoms were found to be higher in stomach, pancreatic, head and neck, and lung cancers, and lower in breast cancer. Such mixed states have been associated with less improvement after treatment,[25,27,28] poorer treatment compliance,[25] slower rates of recovery,[25,29] and worse quality of life[25] than are found in cancer patients without such comorbid symptoms.

CAUSES

A biopsychosocial perspective, with attention to subsystems of variables that are relevant in this context, is helpful to understand the development of anxiety and depressive disorders in cancer patients.[3,12,30] As illustrated in Figure 52-1, the emergence of significant mood and anxiety disorders in cancer patients may be understood as a final common pathway resulting from the interaction of multiple risk and protective factors. The nature, intensity, and duration of the distress response elicited by cancer are jointly determined by individual characteristics, in biological and psychosocial domains, that may amplify or buffer the stress response. Anxiety is a response to perceived immediate threat, whereas depression may be a more delayed response to the meaning of illness and to its cumulative burden.

TRAJECTORY OF DISTRESS RESPONSE

The diagnosis of a potentially fatal disease such as cancer is inevitably threatening to an individual's sense of safety and security. Fears of disability, dependency, suffering, disfigurement, and death may evoke profound feelings of anxiety. Discrete psychological stressors, such as diagnostic investigation, intensive treatments, communication of worrisome test results, or evidence regarding disease recurrence and progression, frequently trigger anxiety related to the perceived threat. In this regard, symptoms of anxiety have been observed to peak early after diagnosis and to subside over the course of the

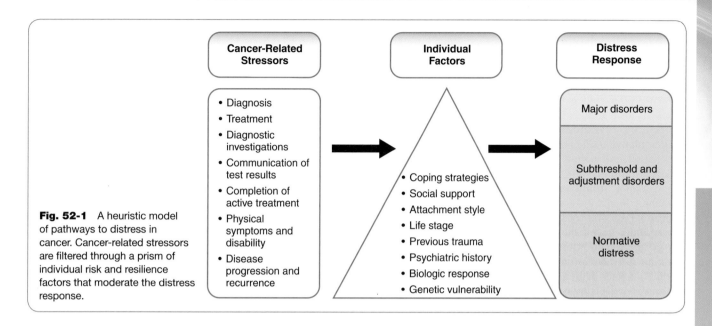

Fig. 52-1 A heuristic model of pathways to distress in cancer. Cancer-related stressors are filtered through a prism of individual risk and resilience factors that moderate the distress response.

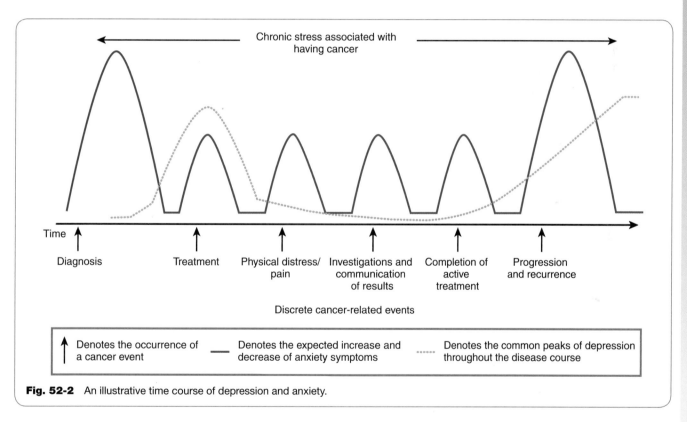

Fig. 52-2 An illustrative time course of depression and anxiety.

disease (Fig. 52-2).[31–33] Full or subthreshold ASD and PTSD are more likely to occur early in the cancer course, in response to the confrontation with numerous acute cancer-related stressors. Prospective studies have shown that PTSD symptoms substantially decrease 3 months after diagnosis and after treatment completion,[34–37] although avoidance and intrusive symptoms may fluctuate over the cancer course.[34]

Whereas discrete and acute stressors tend to trigger anxiety or fear related to the perception of immediate and inescapable threat, depression may be a more delayed response related to the personal meaning of the illness and to the multiple losses associated with it. Nondiscrete and chronic stressors, including

disability and loss of role functions, fears of death and dying, and the burden of living with unending uncertainty about the future, all may heighten the risk of depression. Depressive symptoms and disorders tend to occur later, in response to greater reflective awareness of the losses associated with the illness, the recognition that it may not be reversible, and the inability to find support or meaning when all of the domains that sustain identity and well-being are in jeopardy. Indeed, the inability to find meaning, reflected in the construct of spiritual well-being, has been shown to predict depression in cancer patients with advanced disease.[38] Persistent and severe depression reflects a relative inability to modulate and process feelings of grief, sadness, and loss, also referred to as failure to neutralize the stress or "dysallostatic load" of chronic illness.[39,40]

Depressive symptoms tend to peak initially during adjuvant treatment with chemotherapy or radiation, approximately 4 to 5 months after diagnosis, with a second peak occurring 6 to 7 months later at the completion of all active treatments (see Fig. 52-2).[31–33] Posttreatment depression may be a response to the cumulative burden of the disease and its treatment, and to the challenge of adjusting to a new phase of the cancer trajectory. Additional stressors at this time may include diminishing support from family and friends, after the acute phase of treatment, and growing awareness of the impact of the illness on all domains of life. In some cases, self-reflection has been avoided during the initial phase after diagnosis, when all energy and attention are directed toward the treatment, and does not fully begin until later. Further, as the frequency of medical contact decreases, during the surveillance phase of treatment, patients may also begin to worry more about recurrence. It is not surprising that rates of depression increase with disease recurrence, advancement of cancer, and increasing proximity to death.[38]

RISK AND RESILIENCE FACTORS

Demographic variables, such as age, gender, and socioeconomic status, influence the risk of mood and anxiety disorders, because of their association with biological and biopsychosocial factors. A consistent finding in recent studies has been the inverse relationship between age and the severity of mood disturbance.[41,42] Hypotheses that have been advanced to explain this finding include the greater disruption in occupational activities and in the anticipated life trajectory caused by cancer in younger individuals and unique concerns in such individuals regarding financial security, the welfare of their children, sexual functioning, and child-bearing ability.[41] Older cancer patients may report less distress because of a greater perceived stigma associated with emotional distress in this age cohort and a biologically determined reduction in affective intensity in older populations. We have observed[41] that the greater attachment security and spiritual well-being of older individuals may provide greater protection from emotional distress.

A well-established finding in the general population is an increased prevalence of mood and anxiety disorders in women. Biological factors and the disproportionate existence of lower education and socioeconomic status, as well as a greater number of adverse life events, have been proposed as explanations for this gender effect in women. However, many studies in cancer have not found a gender difference in the prevalence of anxiety or depression.[43–47] We have postulated[44] that the disproportionate exposure to social adversity may account for the gender effect in other populations, and that the overriding and common stressors related to cancer obliterate differences due to gender.

Social supports, both instrumental and emotional, have been shown to "buffer" the stresses associated with chronic illness[48] and may moderate the impact of other social risk factors such as prior experience of trauma, difficulties in social and work relationships, financial strain, and poor communication with medical caregivers. Positive social support has been consistently associated with decreased levels of anxiety and depression in cancer patients across the disease course in numerous cross-sectional and prospective studies.[49,50] More recent evidence suggests that expectations of support and the capacity for flexible use of social support, captured in the construct of attachment security, may serve a protective function in the development of anxiety and depressive symptoms in cancer.[43] Furthermore, these individuals with less attachment security may be in double jeopardy because they may also have less ability to attract and to experience social support.[43] These psychological and social risk factors contribute to individual vulnerability by contributing to feelings of isolation and meaninglessness, by limiting instrumental support that is available, and by diminishing the capacity to buffer emotional reactivity.

A variety of biological factors related to cancer, the treatment of cancer, or to comorbid medical conditions may also contribute to the onset or persistence of depression and anxiety in this population. Many medications have been associated with symptoms of anxiety and depression, although clear causal relationships have been identified for only a few. Symptoms of anxiety are associated with bronchodilators and psychostimulants, and antiemetics such as prochlorperazine can induce akathisia, which may be perceived as anxiety. Anxiety is also common in the context of the use of substances such as alcohol, barbiturates, and nicotine, or with opioid withdrawal, a condition that is often unrecognized in cancer patients. Some evidence suggests that corticosteroids, gonadotropin-releasing hormone agonists, mefloquine, interferon-alpha and interleukin-2 may contribute to both depression and anxiety.[51] Significantly, interferons and interleukins are cytokine immunomodulatory agents that may result in so-called "sickness behaviors" that affect or mimic disturbances in mood. These sickness behaviors include symptoms such as anhedonia, fatigue, cognitive disturbance, anxiety, irritability, psychomotor slowing, anorexia, and sleep alterations.[52] In this regard, a few studies have demonstrated increases in the proinflammatory cytokine interleukin-6 in cancer patients with depression.[53] Our cross-sectional and longitudinal research with patients with metastatic gastrointestinal and lung cancer has found that greater disease burden is associated with higher levels of depression.[12,38] Depression and anxiety in patients with more advanced disease may be related not only to the attendant psychological distress, but also to the tumor cell burden and tissue destruction that contribute to the release of proinflammatory cytokines.

Genetic vulnerability may contribute to the risk of anxiety and depression through the heritable predisposition to a neurobiological sensitivity and to temperamental traits that increase the risk of mood and anxiety disorders, in interaction with environmental and other factors. Temperament shapes emotional experience by determining emotional reactivity—the tendency for an individual to experience a greater than normal level of distress in response to a stressful event. This tendency is associated with distinctive cognitive-processing styles such as catastrophizing and looming,[54] with trait anxiety[55] and anxiety sensitivity,[56] and with lack of effective coping and emotion regulation skills. Other psychological vulnerabilities include factors such as self-esteem and spirituality[43] and the capacity to express affect.[57] Positive emotional expressivity is commonly observed in resilient individuals, who tend to pay greater attention to their affective states and to make more successful attempts at repairing and/or maintaining their positive mood when encountering distressing situations.[49] The literature has also linked specific coping strategies to depression,[58] although it has been difficult in some studies to distinguish what is a cause from what is an effect of depression. These mechanisms may additively elevate the response to cancer-related stressors above the critical threshold for the emergence of a mood or anxiety disorder.

EPIDEMIOLOGY
Depressive disorders

The reported prevalence of clinically significant depression in cancer patients has ranged from 8% to 57%, depending on the cancer type, the demographics of the population studied, hospitalization status, diagnostic criteria and strategy applied, timing and method of assessment (self-report vs. structured interview), measurement tools used, diagnostic thresholds, and stage and severity of cancer.[59,60] The timing of the assessment of depression in cancer is relevant because the presence and severity of depressive symptoms may mirror the fluctuating disease status, the functional level of the patient, and the patient's current psychosocial environment. Moreover, no validated cutoff points demarcate the threshold between normative and pathologic symptoms of depression in association with cancer.

We found clinically significant depressive symptoms, based on a self-report measure, to be present in almost one quarter of outpatients with metastatic gastrointestinal or lung cancer.[7] These results are similar to the recent findings of Ell et al.,[61] who found that 23% of 2330 cancer patients receiving acute medical treatment or follow-up care met the criteria for MDD. We also observed that depressive symptoms became 3 times more common toward the end of life,[38] and a recent review by Clarke and Currie[62] showed a higher prevalence rate of depression in cancers with poorer prognoses, such as pancreatic, oropharyngeal, and breast cancer.[63] These overall rates of depression in cancer are approximately 2 to 4 times that found in the adult U.S. population.[64] Although longitudinal studies indicate that most cases of minor depression do not progress to MDD, family psychiatric history and chronic illness have been shown to be risk factors for conversion. The prevalence of subthreshold depressive disorders, estimated at up to 58%, is much greater than that observed in MDD, although the psychopathologic significance and treatment of subthreshold states are not clear.[59,65]

Anxiety disorders

Significant symptoms of anxiety have been reported in up to 25% of cancer patients.[20,65] However, as with depressive disorders, subthreshold anxiety syndromes are much more common than the more severe anxiety disorders, ranging in frequency from 20% in early-stage cancer patients[66] to over 40% in patients with recent recurrence of disease.[45,67] GAD has been found in from 6% to 10% of early breast cancer patients.[68,69] One study reported a 28% prevalence rate of ASD in newly diagnosed cancer.[70] The prevalence rates of PTSD in cancer are lower than those of ASD, but have been found to be higher than those in the general population.[71] Full-syndrome PTSD has been identified in 3% to 4% of newly diagnosed, early-stage cancers[66] and in 35% of patients after treatment.[35] The variability in reported prevalence rates of anxiety is most likely due to a variety of factors, such as type of cancer studied, stage of disease, use of different scales to measure anxiety, and diagnostic criteria used.

ASSESSMENT

Various strategies have been proposed for diagnosing a psychological disorder in the general context of medical illness, none of which has demonstrated consistent validity.[72] The inclusive approach includes all symptoms in the diagnosis, regardless of whether they are attributed to the mental disorder or to the physical illness, minimizing the likelihood of missing cases. The DSM-IV utilizes the etiologic approach, in which symptoms are counted only if they are clearly not due to the cancer. However, this distinction relies heavily on inference by an experienced clinician to determine the relevant attributions. The exclusive approach considers only symptoms that are more frequent in patients with the psychological disorder than in those without. This approach, which identifies only the most severe cases of the psychological disorder, may be preferred in specific research applications in which there is a wish to minimize false-positive diagnoses. Finally, a substitutive approach, which replaces confounding physical symptoms with symptoms that are more affective and cognitive in nature (e.g., indecisiveness, irritability, social withdrawal) has also been advocated. However, no standards or criteria have been established for which symptoms should be selected as substitutes. Experienced clinicians combine these approaches, typically excluding symptoms such as anorexia, weight loss, and fatigue from the diagnosis of depression unless they are significantly disproportionate to the stage or extent of disease. Further, attention is paid to the duration, severity, and persistence of depressive symptoms, which help to distinguish depressive disorders from normative distress.

Self-report rating measures can also be helpful in assessing symptoms of anxiety and depression in both clinical and research settings. Several such measures have been widely used and validated in cancer populations; some of these are detailed in Table 52-1.[73–88] The cutoff scores utilized with depression and anxiety measures determine their sensitivity and specificity, and therefore, the proportion of false-negative and false-positive cases. Higher cutoffs are more likely to yield true prevalence rates of anxiety/depression in cancer and may be preferable for research studies and for the determination of resource allocation; lower thresholds may be preferable in treatment settings in which there is a high priority on not missing cases and identifying subthreshold disorders. The use of anxiety or depression rating scales ensures that relevant symptoms are assessed comprehensively and in a standardized fashion and provides consistency of assessment across time and across examiners. Such tools can be used for multiple clinical purposes, including measuring symptom severity or change over time, or they can be used as diagnostic aids or as screening tools to identify patients in need of further assessment. Most tools demonstrate good reliability and validity for measuring and monitoring symptom severity in populations with diagnosed mood disorders. However, they cannot be used independently to establish a diagnosis of anxiety or depression. Because clinical interviews are considered the gold standard for the diagnosis of depression and anxiety in cancer patients, a two-stage approach is required. A first-stage screen can be used to identify individuals likely to have anxiety or depressive disorders; this is followed by a second-stage clinical diagnostic interview.

Table 52-1 Commonly used assessment measures for depression and anxiety in cancer

Measure	Brief description	Practical issues	No. of items	Range of scores	Cutoff
Depression					
CES-D: Center for Epidemiologic Studies Depression Scale[73]	• Developed to measure depressive symptoms in community populations • Does not include items that assess changes in appetite or sleep, guilt, psychomotor changes, suicidal thoughts	Time: 5 min Self-report	20	0–60	17[74]
BDI-II: Beck Depression Inventory-II[75]	• Newer version of the BDI • Developed to better reflect DSM-IV criteria • 13 of the 21 items assess somatic symptoms	Time: 10-15 min Self-report	21	0–63	22[74]
PHQ-9: Patient Health Questionnaire-9[76]	• The depression module of the Patient Health Questionnaire, a self-report version of the PRIME-MD • Scores each of the nine DSM-IV diagnostic criteria for a major depressive episode	Time: 5 min Self-report	9	0–27	10[77]
HADS: Hospital Anxiety and Depression Scale[78]	• Designed for use in primary care or hospital settings • Two 7-item subscales for anxiety and depression	Time: 2-5 min Self-report	14	0–21 (for each subscale)	15[79]
Anxiety					
STAI: Spielberger State-Trait Anxiety Inventory[80]	• Composed of two 20-item scales that measure (1) transient, state-dependent anxiety, (2) stable trait anxiety	Time: 10-20 min Self-report	40	20–80	State: 30 Trait: 39[24]
GAD-7: Generalized Anxiety Disorder-7[81]	• Primarily designed to screen and assess severity of GAD symptoms • Also shown to have moderately good operating characteristics for panic disorder, social anxiety disorder, and PTSD	Time: 5 min Self-report	7	0–21	10[82]
BAI: Beck Anxiety Inventory[83]	• Measures the frequency of anxiety symptoms experienced in the past week • Evidence suggests it is best at assessing panic symptoms[84]	Time: 10-15 min Self-report	21	0–63	10[74]
IES-R: Impact of Events Scale-Revised[85]	• Revised version of the original IES[86] • Developed to parallel DSM-IV criteria for PTSD • Assesses subjective distress for any specific life event • 3 subscales: intrusions, avoidance, hyperarousal	Time: 10-15 min Self-report	22	Total: 0–88 intrusion: 0–32 avoidance: 0–32 hyperarousal: 0–24	+
SASRQ: Stanford Acute Stress Reaction Questionnaire[87]	• Evaluates anxiety and dissociation symptoms associated with a trauma • Follows DSM-IV criteria for acute stress disorder (ASD) • Items concern dissociative, intrusive, avoidant, and hyperarousal symptoms	Time: 5-15 min Self-report	30	0–150	18*[88]

+,No clinical cutoffs for cancer population were available.
*Based on the DSM-IV, individuals were identified as having clinical ASD if they endorsed (1) at least three highly rated (score of 3–5) dissociative symptoms; (2) at least one highly rated intrusive symptom; (3) at least one highly rated avoidant symptom; and (4) at least one highly rated hyperarousal symptom.
DSM-IV, Diagnostic and Statistical Manual of Mental Disorders, Fourth Edition, Text Revision; *GAD,* generalized anxiety disorder; *PRIME-MD,* The Primary Care Evaluation of Mental Disorders; *PTSD,* posttraumatic stress disorder.

Distress screening

Missed diagnoses of anxiety or depression in cancer represent lost opportunities to treat these conditions and thereby to improve quality of life, treatment compliance, length of hospital stays, and suicide risk. However, the time constraints in oncology clinic visits may limit the opportunity for patients to disclose or elaborate psychological symptoms. Some patients may minimize distress or be reluctant to disclose psychological symptoms for fear of being judged as weak or inadequate, or because of their own lack of knowledge about the importance and availability of treatment for anxiety or depression. In addition, some clinicians avoid inquiry because of their discomfort or lack of experience with responding to emotional reactions in patients. These factors may result in variability and failure to detect emotional distress in cancer patients. In a recent study of referral patterns to specialized psychosocial oncology care at a comprehensive Canadian cancer treatment center before the initiation of routine distress screening,[89] we found that only about 40% of depressed patients with metastatic gastrointestinal or lung cancer were referred. Most striking, we found a fivefold difference in the rate of referral between depressed elderly and younger patients. Routine screening for psychological symptoms, which we have since initiated, can address such disparities and improve the detection and treatment of unrecognized distress. A screening program that uses measures that are accurate, brief, acceptable to patients, and easy to administer and score can also facilitate both psychosocial resource planning and referral of patients for psychosocial and psychiatric treatment.

A large number of emotional distress screening instruments have been validated in cancer populations, and have been described in a recent systematic review.[90] More comprehensive cancer-specific distress screening tools, which include physical symptoms and social needs, such as the "How Can We Help You and Your Family?" instrument,[91] have recently been developed, but require further validation and refinement to establish their clinical utility. Screening for psychological disturbances, such as anxiety and depression, in cancer is now recognized as an essential part of comprehensive patient care. In this regard, emotional distress has been officially endorsed as a sixth vital sign,[92] and most national cancer organizations now recommend routine distress screening in cancer as part of standard care.[93–96] Guidelines for distress screening advocate comprehensive distress assessment, including patients' emotional, physical, and social or practical needs—all elements that may interfere with the ability to cope effectively with cancer and to participate in treatment.[97] However, screening will have a positive effect on patient outcomes only if screening programs are paired with a strong institutional commitment to providing adequate treatment resources and longitudinal follow-up.[98,99]

INTERVENTIONS

Consistent with their shared origins, depressive and anxiety disorders respond to common treatment approaches. However, the evaluation of their effectiveness in cancer patients has been limited by a variety of methodologic problems, including variability in methods used to measure distress and uncertainty about symptom attribution and diagnostic criteria. Evidence regarding the treatment of anxiety and depression in cancer patients, based on studies in cancer and in other medical populations, is discussed later. Unrelieved pain and other physical distress are the most common causes of anxiety and depression in cancer patients, particularly in those with advanced disease. Treatment of these symptoms and their underlying causes may be a matter of highest priority in cancer patients who are distressed.

Psychological interventions

A variety of general and specific psychotherapeutic interventions have been used in the treatment of depressive and anxiety symptoms in cancer patients. Most important is that relationships with healthcare providers and with disease-specific support groups may protect patients from depression and anxiety by maintaining morale, diminishing stigmata, and promoting self-efficacy and a sense of mastery. Further, limited evidence indicates that psychological interventions may reduce or prevent the emergence of depressive symptoms in patients with cancer.[100] Patients with more severe and persistent distress may benefit from referral to a mental health practitioner, optimally one specialized in psychosocial oncology. Psychological therapies for anxiety and depression have several advantages over pharmacologic therapies in medical illness, in that they are free of physical side effects and drug-drug interactions. Also, they can be used to treat depressive and anxiety symptoms and to modify health behaviors that may adversely affect disease outcomes. However, their use may be limited in patients with significant pain, fatigue, cognitive impairment, or more severe illness, or when there is a lack of interest or motivation on the part of the patient to participate in psychological treatment.

A recent review[101] suggests that there are no large differences in efficacy between the major psychotherapies for mild to moderate depression. However, the optimal type and target of specific psychotherapy will most likely be influenced by the severity of anxiety or depressive symptoms, the stage of disease, functional status, and the patient's motivation to participate in psychological treatment. For example, patients who are at the beginning of their cancer experience may benefit from psychoeducation, from assistance in managing anxiety symptoms associated with cancer-related events, and from adapting to the new demands and circumstances imposed by the disease. Patients who have more advanced disease may benefit from psychotherapy that focuses on processing fears associated with dying, death anxiety, spiritual crises, and other existential concerns.[1] Some of the psychotherapeutic interventions used to treat depression in patients with cancer, not all of which have been empirically validated in this population, are described in the following sections.

Cognitive-behavioral therapy (CBT) is based on the assumption that anxiety and depressive symptoms arise from maladaptive or irrational beliefs or thoughts. CBT can help cancer patients examine their anticipatory fears of pain, helplessness, dependency on others, recurrence, and death, and to recognize maladaptive tendencies to overgeneralize and catastrophize.[1] Relaxation techniques, such as active and passive muscle relaxation and visualization, and relatively newer techniques, such as mindfulness-based stress reduction, may also helping to reduce mood disturbances.[1,60,102] CBT and relaxation techniques can be particularly helpful for patients with anticipatory nausea and vomiting and with specific phobias or panic disorder related to treatment. Problem-solving therapy, based on the assumption that more efficient problem solving can relieve psychological distress, has been shown to be effective in the treatment of depression in cancer patients.[77,103] Psychoeducation has been shown to relieve distress, especially in early-stage cancer.[104] Interpersonal therapy (IPT) has been used to relieve depression by resolving interpersonal conflicts, grief, and life-stage transitions.[105] Behavioral activation, an approach that encourages social engagement and activity, has also been shown to relieve depressive symptoms.[105]

A recent Cochrane review of the effect of psychotherapy on depression among incurable cancer patients concluded that psychotherapy is effective in decreasing depressive symptoms in this population, although none of the studies in that review focused on psychotherapy for the syndrome of MDD in advanced cancer.[106] We have developed a manualized individual intervention referred to as CALM (Managing **C**ancer **A**nd **L**iving **M**eaningfully) to treat depression by addressing the problems that affect patients with advanced cancer. These include symptom control and negotiations with health care providers, sense of self and relationships with others, spiritual well-being, and mortality-related concerns.[105,106a] Preliminary results indicate a high degree of patient satisfaction with this intervention.

Considerable debate is ongoing over the effectiveness and acceptability of psychosocial interventions for reducing emotional distress and improving quality of life of adult cancer patients. Some researchers[107] argue that the evidence is not compelling enough to warrant investment in psychosocial interventions, whereas others[108] argue instead that the preponderance of evidence supports the benefit of psychosocial interventions. As Schneider et al.[109] aptly point out, there is a dire need for investigation and systematic review of the need-benefit relationship in psychosocial interventions for cancer patients. Most psychological intervention studies in cancer have been conducted in patients who do not meet diagnostic criteria for a mood or anxiety disorder. Studies without such inclusion criteria are unlikely to show treatment efficacy in relieving distress.[109] Many psychological intervention studies in cancer have been based on the hypothesis that psychotherapeutic treatment can prolong survival. The psychotherapy and cancer survival question has been the subject of extensive debate,[110,111] but the preponderance of evidence does not support an effect on survival in advanced cancer.[112] More recent, larger studies and meta-analyses have not demonstrated a survival benefit from maintaining or promoting optimism or a "fighting spirit."[113] Further, considering the proposed immunologic mechanisms and the potential effect size of psychological factors on them, it does not seem biologically plausible that psychological therapies could have a significant impact on disease progression in patients with advanced cancer. Cancer patients should be relieved of the "tyranny of optimism"[114] that may result from the belief that positive thinking or psychological growth can affect survival. Instead, psychological interventions in cancer should be recommended based on their potential to reduce anxiety and depressive symptoms, and to improve quality of life.

Pharmacologic interventions
DEPRESSION

The effectiveness of antidepressant treatment has been demonstrated for many medical disorders,[115] although several recent systematic reviews of the treatment of depression in cancer suggest that the evidence for antidepressant treatment effect is positive but limited.[116] This weak evidence base calls for more robust research in the treatment of depression in illness to inform the development of effective practice guidelines. Further, some forms of cancer-related depression may be pathophysiologically distinct from depression in nonmedical

populations, and it is possible that tailored pharmacologic and psychological interventions may be most effective.

Several pharmacologic classes of antidepressants are currently available, not one of which has been shown to be most effective for treating depression in illness,[117] and all of which have differing risks and benefits in specific medical disorders. Classes with particular relevance in cancer patients are described later.

Tricyclic/Heterocyclic Antidepressants (TCAs) and Monoamine Oxidase Inhibitors (MAOIs)

These older classes of antidepressants have demonstrated effectiveness for the treatment of depression in multiple medical conditions, as well as for neuropathic pain syndromes and for the treatment of insomnia, which frequently accompanies medical conditions. However, they are discontinued before treatment completion in one third of medical patients, as a result of adverse effects related to the central and peripheral anticholinergic and antihistaminic effects of these drugs, as well as their strong antagonist effect on alpha-adrenergic receptors. Of even greater concern is that both TCAs and MAOIs can be lethal in overdose. For these reasons, in the treatment of depression in illness, they have largely been replaced by newer classes of antidepressants, which have wider therapeutic windows and are better tolerated and easier to administer.

Selective Serotonin Reuptake Inhibitors (SSRIs)

The SSRIs are generally regarded as first-line treatment for MDD in cancer[60] because of their relative safety and tolerability. SSRIs may have additional benefits beyond treating depression in cancer. Paroxetine and sertraline effectively reduce hot flashes in women with breast cancer related to tamoxifen use, and in men requiring hormone therapy for prostate cancer. Despite their benefits, caution must be exercised with SSRIs in cancer, particularly in the presence of hepatic disease, because of their significant potential for drug interactions and altered pharmacokinetics. For example, paroxetine can decrease plasma concentrations of endoxifen (an active tamoxifen metabolite associated with the CYP2D6 genotype) by a genetic polymorphism and is a strong inhibitor of the cytochrome P450-2D6 enzyme. Inhibition of this enzyme would affect the catalysis of tamoxifen and thus decrease levels of its active metabolite.[60] Sertraline and citalopram appear to present the lowest risk of drug interaction. Short-term adverse effects of SSRIs include nausea and gastrointestinal disturbance, anxiety, headache, sedation, and tremor. Long-term potential side effects include sexual dysfunction, weight gain, the syndrome of inappropriate antidiuretic hormone secretion, and platelet dysfunction leading to bleeding.

Novel Antidepressants

Other pharmacologic classes of antidepressants commonly used in cancer include the serotonin-norepinephrine reuptake inhibitors (SNRIs; e.g., venlafaxine, duloxetine), norepinephrine and dopamine modulators (NDMs; e.g., bupropion), and noradrenergic and specific serotonergic antidepressants (NaSSAs; e.g., mirtazapine). These agents are increasingly used as alternatives to SSRIs in medical populations, although empirical evidence for their safety and efficacy in these patients remains limited.

Dual-action agents such as the SNRIs may be more effective than SSRIs for remission of depression. Similar to the SSRIs, venlafaxine is effective for hot flashes in breast cancer,[118] and both venlafaxine and duloxetine are effective for the treatment of neuropathic pain.[119–121] The main adverse effects of these medications are hypertension with high doses of venlafaxine, and possible elevation of serum transaminases and bilirubin with duloxetine, which limits its use in patients with hepatic insufficiency or significant renal impairment.

Buproprion has a favorable side effect profile in cancer, in that it is nonsedating and may alleviate the prominent fatigue and neurovegetative symptoms of cytokine-induced depression. At higher doses, buproprion is associated with seizure risk and therefore is best avoided in patients with brain tumors or a history of seizures. Mirtazapine is highly sedating, increases appetite, and has antiemetic effects, making it an optimal choice for the treatment of depression in cancer patients with significant insomnia, cachexia, and nausea. Unlike the SSRIs, buproprion and mirtazapine do not cause gastrointestinal disturbance or anxiety or sexual dysfunction, and they are associated with minimal drug interactions.

Augmenting Agents

Psychostimulants such as methylphenidate or modafinil are often used to treat depressive symptoms in advanced illness and in palliative care settings because of their rapid onset of action and their limited side effects. They can be used as single agents or in combination with other antidepressant medications. Methylphenidate has been observed to elevate mood rapidly, increase appetite, diminish fatigue, improve attention and concentration, and decrease sedation from opiates, although its efficacy in the treatment of depression in patients with advanced disease has not yet been established with randomized controlled trials. In addition, atypical antipsychotics such as olanzapine and Seroquel can be used to augment antidepressant action, with the added benefits of their off-label use in advanced cancer to stimulate appetite, promote sleep, reduce anxiety, and relieve chemotherapy-related nausea.[122,123]

New directions in the treatment of depression in patients with cancer may target more specific illness-related pathophysiology, such as cytokine antagonists or neuropeptide systems.[124–126] The question of whether pharmacologic agents are effective for subthreshold symptoms also requires further study. In this regard, Navari et al.[127] recently published a placebo-controlled study demonstrating the efficacy of 6 months of fluoxetine in reducing subthreshold depressive symptoms in 357 early-stage breast cancer patients. Fluoxetine-treated patients demonstrated significant improvement in quality of life and in completion of treatment with hormonal therapy and/or chemotherapy. In addition, new approaches to neurostimulation techniques such as deep brain stimulation, transcranial magnetic stimulation, and electroconvulsive therapy have been developed for severe or treatment-resistant depression.[128] These modalities may have applicability in cancer patients in whom intolerable side effects or medical comorbidity (e.g., severe renal, cardiac, or hepatic disease) contraindicates the use of antidepressant medication. Depression in medical illness may be more treatment resistant when comorbid with anxiety.[129] Optimal and possibly more effective treatment approaches in cancer patients would combine judicious use of pharmacologic interventions with psychological approaches.

ANXIETY

Relatively few randomized, controlled trials (RCTs) have investigated the use of antidepressants in patients with MDD and cancer,[116] and there has been a virtual absence of such treatment studies for anxiety in cancer.[130] The pharmacologic treatment of anxiety in cancer patients has been evaluated in some trials that simultaneously assessed treatment effects on depression. In general, antidepressants such as TCAs, SSRIs, and SNRIs have been shown to have some anxiolytic effects. In fact, some studies have demonstrated the amelioration of anxiety symptoms in patients diagnosed with primary depression, which may argue for their use in cancer patients with comorbid anxiety and depression.[130] Jacobsen et al.[100] systematically reviewed the literature from 1980 to 2003 and found eight RCTs that examined the effects of anxiolytics (e.g., lorazepam, alprazolam) and antidepressants (e.g., fluoxetine, paroxetine) in reducing anxiety. These trials produced a total of 16 anxiety outcomes, of which 7 yielded a significant treatment effect. These results are very similar to the positive but limited evidence of efficacy for antidepressant medications.

Panic Attacks and Treatment-Related Anxiety

Many cancer patients experience situational anxiety related to treatment. This includes anxiety related to blood and needle phobias and claustrophobia associated with medical machinery that requires immobilization of the patient. Benzodiazepines are considered first-line anxiolytics to be used in short-term treatment of situational anxiety.[130] They may be used on an acute basis to interrupt panic attacks, or as a single dose simply carried with the patient at all times to be used to prevent the onset of a panic attack. Having the knowledge that a panic attack can be aborted with medication, if breathing and cognitive strategies fail, may in itself prevent panic attacks and diminish the risk of associated agoraphobia. Benzodiazepines should be used cautiously to treat anxiety in palliative patients, or in those with compromised hepatic or pulmonary function, because these agents may affect mental status, amplifying confusion and impaired memory and concentration, and may suppress central respiratory mechanisms. If panic attacks are severe and frequent enough to interfere with daily functioning, SSRIs and/or CBT is the treatment of choice.

Generalized Anxiety Disorder

Although benzodiazepines have been the mainstay of treatment for GAD, their potential for tolerance and addiction, as well as predisposition to delirium in elderly patients and those with advanced disease, precludes their regular use in cancer patients. Buspirone, a nonbenzodiazepine anxiolytic without sedative or cognitive side effects, can also be used in the treatment of GAD, although its effectiveness is reduced in patients previously treated with benzodiazepines. In addition to psychological interventions, SSRIs are used as the main treatment for GAD in cancer, although specific evidence of their effectiveness in this patient population is lacking. Evidence from placebo-controlled RCTs supports the effectiveness of antidepressants, including imipramine, venlafaxine, and paroxetine, for GAD in primary psychiatric populations.[131]

POSTTRAUMATIC STRESS DISORDER

Evidence from placebo-controlled RCTs suggests the effectiveness of SSRIs in improving the three symptom clusters of PTSD, with an additional beneficial impact on sleep disturbances and impulsivity.[2,132] The U.S. Food and Drug Administration has approved the SSRIs, sertraline and paroxetine, for the treatment of PTSD. In addition, venlafaxine is considered a recommended psychopharmacotherapy for PTSD treatment,[133] and atypical neuroleptics (risperidone and olanzapine) are considered as adjunctive agents for reexperiencing symptoms.[134] However, specific evidence for the effectiveness of these agents in PTSD associated with cancer is missing.

SUMMARY AND CONCLUSIONS

Anxiety and depression are common psychological responses to cancer that may reach clinically significant thresholds of severity in the context of multiple risk factors. These include physical distress, social isolation, attachment anxiety, impaired spiritual well-being, and poor relationships and communication with health care providers. Anxiety is typically a response to an immediate threat in the course of the disease, whereas depression is more often a response to the cumulative burden and stress of the disease, and to its reflected meaning for that individual. Specific biological factors related to cancer and its treatment may contribute to symptoms of anxiety or depression. A holistic approach to psychological distress is important in cancer because pain and other physical symptoms are some of the most common precipitants of depression and anxiety, and these symptoms may be mutually reinforcing. Meticulous attention to pain and symptom control may be one of the most important primary interventions in anxious or depressed cancer patients. The relationship of the patient to the healthcare team may also provide important protection from unmanageable distress in the course of the disease.

Evidence regarding the treatment of distress in cancer patients has been limited by a variety of methodologic issues. However, current evidence suggests that a variety of psychological and pharmacologic treatments for depression and anxiety are effective. Psychotherapeutic approaches include psychoeducation, relaxation therapies, and other active approaches early in the course of the disease, as well as meaning-centered approaches later in the course of the disease. SSRI medication is the mainstay of pharmacologic treatment for both anxiety and depression in cancer patients, although a variety of other medications have been used. These include benzodiazepines for anxiety and psychostimulants for the treatment of depression in advanced disease. Identification of specific biological markers for depression in cancer also holds the potential for the development of novel agents. The introduction of routine distress screening methods has the potential to increase awareness of psychological disturbances such as anxiety and depression in cancer patients. However, their effectiveness will be entirely dependent on education and other resources applied to ensure that appropriate treatment follows from the identification of distress. Distress in cancer patients should be considered as a final common pathway resulting from multiple interacting factors. A comprehensive approach to the detection, assessment, and treatment of distress holds the greatest possibility for successful outcomes that protect and maintain quality of life.

REFERENCES

1. Roth AJ, Massie MJ. Anxiety and its management in advanced cancer. *Curr Opin Support Palliat Care*. 2007;1:50–56.
2. Desaive P, Ronson A. Stress spectrum disorders in oncology. *Curr Opin Oncol*. 2008;20:378–385.
3. Lo C, Li M, Rodin G. The assessment and treatment of distress in cancer patients: overview and future directions. *Minerva Psichiatr*. 2008;49:129–143.
4. Grassi L, Indelli M, Marzola M, et al. Depressive symptoms and quality of life in home-care assisted cancer patients. *J Pain Symptom Manage*. 1996;12:300–307.
5. Colleoni M, Mandala M, Peruzzotto G, et al. Depression and degree of acceptance of adjuvant cytotoxic drugs. *Lancet*. 2000;356:1326–1327.
6. Prieto JM, Blanch J, Atala J, et al. Psychiatric morbidity and impact on hospital length of stay among hematologic cancer patients receiving stem-cell transplantation. *J Clin Oncol*. 2002;20:1907–1917.
7. Rodin G, Zimmermann C, Rydall A, et al. The desire for hastened death in patients with metastatic cancer. *J Pain Symptom Manage*. 2007;33:661–665.
8. Chochinov HM, Wilson KG, Enns M, et al. Desire for death in the terminally ill. *Am J Psychiatry*. 1995;152:1185–1191.
9. Chochinov HM, Tataryn D, Clinch JJ, et al. Will to live in the terminally ill. *Lancet*. 1999;354:816–819.
10. Stommel M, Given BA, Given CW. Depression and functional status as predictors of death among cancer patients. *Cancer*. 2002;94:2719–2727.
11. Faller H, Bulzebruck H, Drings P, et al. Coping, distress, and survival among patients with lung cancer. *Arch Gen Psychiatry*. 1999;56:756–762.
12. Rodin G, Lo C, Mikulincer M, et al. Pathways to distress: the multiple determinants of depression, hopelessness and the desire for hastened death in metastatic cancer patients. *Soc Sci Med*. 2009;68:562–569.
13. Li M, Rodin G. Depression and illness. In: Suls JM, Davidson KW, Kaplan RW, eds. *Handbook of health psychology and behavioral medicine*. New York: Guilford Press; 2010.
14. American Psychiatric Association. *Diagnostic and statistical manual of mental disorders*. 4th ed. Text revision (DSM-IV-TR). Washington, DC: American Psychiatric Association Press; 2000.
15. Li M, Hales S. Adjustment disorders. In: Holland J, Breitbert W, Jacobsen P. et al., ed. *Psycho-oncology*. 2nd ed. New York, NY: Oxford University Press; 2010:303–310.
16. Kleinman A. The normal, the pathological, and the existential. *Compr Psychiatry*. 2008;49:111–112.
17. Horwitz AV, Wakefield JC. *The loss of sadness: how psychiatry transformed normal sorrow into depressive disorder*. New York, NY: Oxford University Press; 2007.
18. Casey P, Dowrick C, Wilkinson G. Adjustment disorders: fault line in the psychiatric glossary. *Br J Psychiatry*. 2001;179:479–481.
19. Strain JJ, Diefenbacher A. The adjustment disorders: the conundrums of the diagnoses. *Compr Psychiatry*. 2008;49:121–130.
20. Derogatis L, Morrow GR, Fetting J, et al. The prevalence of psychiatric disorders among cancer patients. *JAMA*. 1983;249:751–757.
21. Strain JJ, Smith GC, Hammer JS, et al. Adjustment disorder: a multisite study of its utilization and interventions in the consultation-liaison psychiatry setting. *Gen Hosp Psychiatry*. 1998;20:139–149.
22. Kissane DW, Clarke DM, Street AF. Demoralization syndrome—a relevant psychiatric diagnosis for palliative care. *J Palliat Care*. 2001;17:12–21.
23. Aapro MS, Molassiotis A, Olver I. Anticipatory nausea and vomiting. *Support Care Cancer*. 2005;13:117–121.
24. Stark D, Kiely M, Smith A, et al. anxiety disorders in cancer patients: their nature, associations, and relation to quality of life. *J Clin Oncol*. 2002;20:3137–3148.
25. Brintzenhofe-Szoc KM, Levin TT, Li Y, et al. Mixed anxiety/depression symptoms in a large cancer cohort: prevalence by cancer type. *Psychosomatics*. 2009;50:383–391.
26. American Psychiatric Association. *DSM-5 development. DSM-5: The future of psychiatric diagnosis*. Available at: www.DSM5.org; accessed April 20, 2010.
27. Coryell W, Endicott J, Andreasen NC, et al. Depression and panic attacks: the significance of

overlap as reflected in follow-up and family study data. *Am J Psychiatry*. 1998;145:293–300.

28. Fava M, Uebelacker LA, Alpert JE, et al. Major depressive subtypes and treatment response. *Biol Psychiatry*. 1997;43:568–576.

29. Brown C, Schulberg HC, Madonia MJ, et al. Treatment outcomes for primary-care patients with major depression and lifetime anxiety disorders. *Am J Psychiatry*. 1996;153:1293–1300.

30. Kendler KS. Explanatory models for psychiatric illness. *Am J Psychiatry*. 2008;165:695–702.

31. Annunziata MA, Muzzatti B, Bidoli E. Psychological distress and needs of cancer patients: a prospective comparison between the diagnostic and therapeutic phase. *Support Care Cancer*. 2010 Feb 5 [Epub ahead of print].

32. Hinnen C, Ranchor AV, Sanderman R, et al. Course of distress in breast cancer patients, their partners, and matched control couples. *Ann Behav Med*. 2008;36:141–148.

33. Stanton AL, Ganz PA, Rowland JH, et al. Promoting adjustment after treatment for cancer. *Cancer*. 2005;104(suppl 11):2608–2613.

34. Kangas M, Henry JL, Bryant RA. Posttraumatic stress disorder following cancer: a conceptual and empirical review. *Clin Psychol Rev*. 2002;22:499–524.

35. Mundy EA, Blanchard EB, Cirenza E, et al. Posttraumatic stress disorder in breast cancer patients following autologous bone marrow transplantation or conventional cancer treatments. *Behav Res Ther*. 2000;38:1015–1027.

36. Tjemsland L, Soreide JA, Malt UF. Traumatic distress symptoms in early breast cancer. I: Acute response to diagnosis. *Psychooncology*. 1996a;5:1–8.

37. Tjemsland L, Soreide JA, Malt UF. Traumatic distress symptoms in early breast cancer. II: Outcome six weeks postsurgery. *Psychooncology*. 1996b;5:295–303.

38. Lo C, Zimmermann C, Rydall A, et al. Longitudinal study of depressive symptoms in patients with metastatic gastrointestinal and lung cancer. *J Clin Oncol*. 2010;28:3084–3089.

39. Breslau N, Davis GC, Peterson EL, et al. A second look at comorbidity in victims of trauma: the posttraumatic stress disorder-major depression connection. *Biol Psychiatry*. 2000;48:902–909.

40. Ronson A. Psychiatric disorders in oncology: recent therapeutic advances and new conceptual frameworks. *Curr Opin Oncol*. 2004;16:318–323.

41. Lo C, Lin J, Gagliese L, et al. Age and depression in patients with metastatic cancer: the protective effects of attachment security and spiritual well-being. *Ageing Society*. 2010;30:325–336.

42. Hopwood P, Haviland J, Mills J, et al. START Trial Management Group. The impact of age and clinical factors on quality of life in early breast cancer: an analysis of 2208 women recruited to the UK START Trial (Standardisation of Breast Radiotherapy Trial). [Erratum appears in *Breast* 2008;17:115. Note: START Trial Management Group added]. *Breast*. 2007;16:241–251.

43. Rodin G, Walsh A, Zimmermann C, et al. The contribution of attachment security and social support to depressive symptoms in patients with metastatic cancer. *Psychooncology*. 2007;16:1080–1091.

44. Miller S, Lo C, Gagliese L, et al. Patterns of depression in cancer patients: an indirect test of gender-specific vulnerabilities to depression. *Soc Psychiatry Psychiatr Epidemiol*. 2010 Jun 25 [Epub ahead of print].

45. Gurevich M, Devins GM, Rodin G. Stress response syndromes and cancer: conceptual and assessment issues. *Psychosomatics*. 2002;43:259–281.

46. Carlson LE, Angen M, Cullum J, et al. High levels of untreated distress and fatigue in cancer patients. *Br J Cancer*. 2004;90:2297–2304.

47. Cheung WY, Le LW, Gagliese L, et al. Age and gender differences in symptom intensity and symptom clusters among patients with metastatic cancer. *Support Care Cancer*. 2010 Mar 24 [Epub ahead of print].

48. Parker PA, Baile WF, De Moor C, et al. Psychosocial and demographic predictors of quality of life in a large sample of cancer patients. *Psychooncology*. 2003;12:183–193.

49. Manne S, Rini C, Rubin S, et al. Long-term trajectories of psychological adaptation among women diagnosed with gynaecological cancers. *Psychosom Med*. 2008;70:677–687.

50. Helgeson VS, Snyder P, Seltman H. Psychological and physical adjustment to breast cancer over 4 years: identifying distinct trajectories of change. *Health Psychol*. 2004;23:3–15.

51. Patten SB, Barbui C. Drug-induced depression: a systematic review to inform clinical practice. *Psychother Psychosom*. 2004;73:207–215.

52. Dantzer R, O'Connor JC, Freund GG. From inflammation to sickness and depression: when the immune system subjugates the brain. *Nat Rev Neurosci*. 2008;9:46–56.

53. Miller AH, Ancoli-Israel S, Bower JE, et al. Neuroendocrine-immune mechanisms of behavioral comorbidities in patients with cancer. *J Clin Oncol*. 2008;26:971–982.

54. Levin TT, Riskind JH, Li Y. Looming threat-processing style in a cancer cohort. *Gen Hosp Psychiatry*. 2007;29:32–38.

55. De Vries J, Van der Steeg AF, Roukema JA. Trait anxiety determines depressive symptoms and fatigue in women with an abnormality in the breast. *Br J Health Psychol*. 2009;14:143–157.

56. Asmundson GJG, Dristi DW, Hadjistavropoulos HD. Anxiety sensitivity and disabling chronic health conditions: state of the art and future directions. *Scand J Behav Ther*. 2000;29:100–117.

57. Classen CC, Kraemer HC, Blasey C, et al. Supportive-expressive group therapy for primary breast cancer patients: a randomized prospective multicenter trial. *Psychooncology*. 2008;17:438–447.

58. Roesch SC, Adams L, Hines A, et al. Coping with prostate cancer: a meta-analytic review. *J Behav Med*. 2005;28:281–293.

59. Massie MJ. Prevalence of depression in patients with cancer. *J Natl Cancer Inst Monogr*. 2004;32:57–71.

60. Reich M. Depression and cancer: recent data on clinical issues, research challenges and treatment approaches. *Curr Opin Oncol*. 2008;20:353–359.

61. Ell K, Quon B, Quinn DI, et al. Improving treatment of depression among low-income patients with cancer: the design of the ADAPt-C study. *Gen Hosp Psychiatry*. 2007;29:223–231.

62. Clarke DM, Currie KC. Depression, anxiety and their relationship with chronic diseases: a review of the epidemiology, risk and treatment evidence. *Med J Aust*. 2009;7:S54–S60.

63. Evans DL, Charney DS, Lewis L, et al. Mood disorders in the medically ill: scientific review and recommendations. *Biol Psychiatry*. 2005;58:175–189.

64. Kessler RC, Chiu WT, Demler O, et al. Prevalence, severity, and comorbidity of twelve-month DSM-IV disorders in the National Comorbidity Survey Replication (NCS-R). *Arch Gen Psychiatry*. 2005;62:617–627.

65. Miovic M, Block S. Psychiatric disorders in advanced cancer. *Cancer*. 2007;110:1665–1676.

66. Green BL, Rowland JH, Krupnick JL, et al. Prevalence of posttraumatic stress disorder in women with breast cancer. *Psychosomatics*. 1998;9:102–111.

67. Okamura H, Watanabe T, Narabayashi M, et al. Psychological distress following first recurrence of disease in patients with breast cancer: prevalence and risk factors. *Breast Cancer Res Treat*. 2000;61:131–137.

68. Mehnert A, Koch U. Prevalence of acute and post-traumatic stress disorder and comorbid mental disorders in breast cancer patients during primary cancer care: a prospective study. *Psychooncology*. 2007;16:181–188.

69. Gandubert C, Carriere I, Escot C, et al. Onset and relapse of psychiatric disorders following early breast cancer: a case-control study. *Psychooncology*. 2009;18:1029–1037.

70. Kangas M, Henry J, Bryant R. Correlates of acute stress disorder in cancer patients. *J Trauma Stress*. 2007;20:325–334.

71. Gudmundsdottir H, Gudmundsdottir A, Gudmundsdottir D. PTSD and psychological distress in Icelandic parents of chronically ill children: does social support have an effect on parental distress? *Scand J Psychol*. 2006;47:303–312.

72. Trask PC. Assessment of depression in cancer patients. *J Natl Cancer Inst Monogr*. 2004;32:80–92.

73. Radloff L. The CES-D scale: a self-report depression scale for research in the general population. *Appl Psychol Meas*. 1977;1:385–401.

74. Hopko DR, Bell JL, Armento ME, et al. The phenomenology and screening of clinical depression in cancer patients. *J Psychosoc Oncol*. 2008;26:31–51.

75. Beck AT, Steer RA, Brown GK. *Manual for Beck Depression Inventory-II*. San Antonio, TX: Psychological Corporation, Harcourt Brace and Company; 1996.

76. Spitzer RL, Kroenke K, Williams JB. Validation and utility of a self-report version of PRIME-MD: the PHQ primary care study. Primary Care Evaluation of Mental Disorders. Patient Health Questionnaire. *JAMA*. 1999;282:1737–1744.

77. Ell K, Xie B, Quon B, et al. Randomized controlled trial of collaborative care management of depression among low-income patients with cancer. *J Clin Oncol*. 2008;26:4488–4496.

78. Zigmond AS, Snaith RP. The hospital anxiety and depression scale. *Acta Psychiatr Scand*. 1983;67:361–370.

79. Walker J, Postma K, McHugh GS, et al. Performance of the Hospital Anxiety and Depression Scale as a screening tool for major depressive disorder in cancer patients. *J Psychosom Res*. 2007;63:83–91.

80. Spielberger CD. *Manual for the State-Trait Anxiety Inventory*. Palo Alto, CA: Consulting Psychologists Press; 1983.

81. Spitzer RL, Kroenke K, Williams JB, et al. A brief measure for assessing generalized anxiety disorder: the GAD-7. *Arch Intern Med*. 2006;166:1092–1097.

82. Kroenke K, Spitzer RL, Williams JBW, et al. Anxiety disorders in primary care: prevalence, impairment, comorbidity, and detection. *Ann Intern Med*. 2007;146:317–325.

83. Beck AT, Steer RA. *Beck Anxiety Inventory: Manual*. San Antonio, TX: The Psychological Corporation, Harcourt Brace and Company; 1993.

84. Leyfer OT, Ruberg JL, Woodruff-Borden J. Examination of the utility of the Beck Anxiety Inventory and its factors as a screener for anxiety disorders. *J Anxiety Disord*. 2006;20:444–458.

85. Weiss DS, Marmar CR. The Impact of Event Scale-Revised. In: Wilson JP, Keane TM, ed. *Assessing psychological trauma and PTSD.* New York, NY: The Guilford Press; 1997:399–412.

86. Horowitz M, Wilner N, Alvarez W. Impact of Event Scale: a measure of subjective stress. *Psychosom Med.* 1979;41:209–218.

87. Cardena E, Koopman C, Classen C, et al. Psychometric properties of the Stanford Acute Stress Reaction Questionnaire (SASRQ): a valid and reliable measure of acute stress. *J Trauma Stress.* 2000;13:719–734.

88. Pedersen AF, Zachariae R. Cancer, acute stress disorder, and repressive coping. *Scand J Psychol.* 2010;51:84–91.

89. Ellis J, Lin J, Walsh A, et al. Predictors of referral for specialized psychosocial oncology care in patients with metastatic cancer: the contributions of age, distress, and marital status. *J Clin Oncol.* 2009;27:699–705.

90. Vodermaier A, Linden W, Siu C. Screening for emotional distress in cancer patients: a systematic review of assessment instruments. *J Natl Cancer Inst.* 2009;101:1–25.

91. Loscalzo MJ, Clark KL. Problem-related distress in cancer patients drives requests for help: a prospective study. *Oncology.* 2007;21:1133–1138.

92. Holland JC, Bultz BD. The NCCN guideline for distress management: a case for making distress the sixth vital sign. *J Natl Compr Canc Netw.* 2007;5:3–7.

93. Institute of Medicine. *Cancer care for the whole patient: meeting psychosocial health needs: Institute of Medicine report.* Washington, DC: The National Academies Press; 2007.

94. National Comprehensive Cancer Network (NCCN) Clinical Practice Guidelines in Oncology. NCCN Guidelines for Supportive Care: Distress Management. Version 1.2011. Available at: http://www.nccn.org; accessed November 24, 2010.

95. National Institute for Clinical Excellence (NICE). *Guidance on cancer services.* London, UK: NICE; 2004.

96. Canadian Association of Psychosocial Oncology (CAPO). National Psychosocial Oncology Standards of Canada; 1999. Principle 7: Assessment of need. Available at: http://www.capo.ca; accessed November 24, 2010.

97. Canadian Partnership Against Cancer. *Guide to implementing screening for distress: the 6th vital sign moving towards person-centered care.* Toronto, Ontario, Canada: Cancer Journey Action Group, Canadian Partnership Against Cancer; 2009.

98. Palmer SC, Coyne JC. Screening for depression in medical care: pitfalls, alternatives, and revised priorities. *J Psychosom Res.* 2003;54:279–287.

99. Schade CP, Jones Jr ER, Wittlin BJ. A ten-year review of the validity and clinical utility of depression screening. *Psychiatr Serv.* 1998;49:55–61.

100. Jacobsen PB, Donovan KA, Swaine ZN, et al. Management of anxiety and depression in adult cancer patients: toward an evidence-based approach. In: Change AE, Hayes DF, Pass HI, et al., eds. *Oncology: an evidence-based approach.* Philadelphia, PA: Springer; 2006:1552–1579.

101. Cuijpers P, van Straten A, Andersson G, et al. Psychotherapy for depression in adults: a meta-analysis of comparative outcome studies. *J Consult Clin Psychol.* 2008;76:909–922.

102. Garland SN, Carlson LE, Cook S, et al. A nonrandomized comparison of mindfulness-based stress reduction and healing arts programs for facilitating posttraumatic growth and spirituality in cancer outpatients. *Support Care Cancer.* 2007;15:949–961.

103. Strong V, Waters R, Hibberd C, et al. Management of depression for people with cancer (SMaRT oncology 1): a randomised trial. *Lancet.* 2008;372:40–48.

104. Dolbeaut S, Cayrou S, Brédart A, et al. The effectiveness of a psycho-educational group after early-stage breast cancer treatment: results of a randomized French study. *Psychooncology.* 2009;18:647–656.

105. Kissane DW, Levin T, Hales S, et al. Psychotherapy for depression in cancer and palliative care. In: Kissane DW, Maj M, Sartorius N, eds. *Depression and cancer.* Chêne-Bourg, Switzerland: World Psychiatric Association; 2011; p. 177–206.

106. Akechi T, Okuyama T, Onishi J, et al. Psychotherapy for depression among incurable cancer patients. *Cochrane Database Syst Rev.* 2008;(2) CD005537.

106a. Hales S, Lo C, Rodin G. *Managing Cancer and Living Meaningfully (CALM) treatment manual: an individual psychotherapy for patients with advanced cancer.* Toronto, Canada: Psychosocial Oncology and Palliative Care, Princess Margaret Hospital, University Health Network; 2010.

107. Coyne JC, Lepore SJ, Palmer SC. Efficacy of psychosocial interventions in cancer care: evidence is weaker than it first looks. *Ann Behav Med.* 2006;32:104–110.

108. Andrykowski MA, Manne SL. Are psychological interventions effective and accepted by cancer patients? I. Standards and levels of evidence. *Ann Behav Med.* 2006;32:93–97.

109. Schneider S, Moyer A, Knapp-Oliver S, et al. Pre-intervention distress moderates the efficacy of psychosocial treatment for cancer patients: a meta-analysis. *J Behav Med.* 2010;33:1–14.

110. Coyne JC, Stefanek M, Thombs BD, et al. Time to let go of the illusion that psychotherapy extends the survival of cancer patients: reply to Kraemer, Kuchler, and Spiegel. *Psychol Bull.* 2009;135:179–182.

111. Kraemer HC, Kuchler T, Spiegel D. Use and misuse of the consolidated standards of reporting trials (CONSORT) guidelines to assess research findings: comment on Coyne, Stefanek, and Palmer. *Psychol Bull.* 2009;135:173–178.

112. Kissane D. Beyond the psychotherapy and survival debate: the challenge of social disparity, depression and treatment adherence in psychosocial cancer care. *Psychooncology.* 2009;18:1–5.

113. Coyne JC, Tennen H. Positive psychology in cancer care: bad science, exaggerated claims, and unproven medicine. *Ann Behav Med.* 2010;39:16–26

114. Aspinwall LG, Tedeschi RG. The value of positive psychology for health psychology: progress and pitfalls in examining the relation of positive phenomena to health. *Ann Behav Med.* 2010;39:4–15.

115. Krishnan KR. Treatment of depression in the medically ill. *J Clin Psychopharmacol.* 2005;25 (4 suppl 1):S14–S18.

116. Rodin G, Lloyd N, Katz M, et al. The treatment of depression in cancer patients: a systematic review. *Support Care Cancer.* 2007;15:123–136.

117. Rayner L, Price A, Evans A, et al. Antidepressants for depression in physically ill people. *Cochrane Database Syst Rev.* 2010;(3) CD007503.

118. Loprinzi CL, Kugler JW, Sloan JA, et al. Venlafaxine in management of hot flashes in survivors of breast cancer: a randomised controlled trial. *Lancet.* 2000;356:2059–2063.

119. Davis JL, Smith RL. Painful peripheral diabetic neuropathy treated with venlafaxine HCl extended release capsules. *Diabetes Care.* 1999;22:1909–1910.

120. Jann MW, Slade JH. Antidepressant agents for the treatment of chronic pain and depression. *Pharmacotherapy.* 2007;27:1571–1587.

121. Muller N, Schennach R, Riedel M, et al. Duloxetine in the treatment of major psychiatric and neuropathic disorders. *Expert Rev Neurother.* 2008;8:527–536.

122. Von Roenn J, ed. Observation: olanzapine and mirtazapine for multiple palliation. *J Support Oncol.* 2003;1:64.

123. Tan L, Liu J, Liu X, et al. Clinical research of Olanzapine for prevention of chemotherapy-induced nausea and vomiting. *J Exp Clin Cancer Res.* 2009;28:131.

124. Holmes A, Heilig M, Rupniak NM, et al. Neuropeptide systems as novel therapeutic targets for depression and anxiety disorders. *Trends Pharmacol Sci.* 2003;24:580–588.

125. Kramer MS, Winokur A, Kelsey J, et al. Demonstration of the efficacy and safety of a novel substance P (NK1) receptor antagonist in major depression. *Neuropsychopharmacology.* 2004;29:385–392.

126. Nemeroff CB. New directions in the development of antidepressants: the interface of neurobiology and psychiatry. *Hum Psychopharmacol.* 2002;17(Suppl1):S13–S16.

127. Navari RM, Brenner MC, Wilson MN. Treatment of depressive symptoms in patients with early stage breast cancer undergoing adjuvant therapy. *Breast Cancer Res Treat.* 2008;112:197–201.

128. Fitzgerald PB, Daskalakis ZJ. The use of repetitive transcranial magnetic stimulation and vagal nerve stimulation in the treatment of depression. *Curr Opin Psychiatry.* 2008;21:25–29.

129. Iosifescu DV. Treating depression in the medically ill. *Psychiatr Clin North Am.* 2007;30:77–90.

130. Roy-Byrne PP, Davidson KW, Kessler RC, et al. Anxiety disorders and comorbid medical illness. *Gen Hosp Psychiatry.* 2008;30:208–225.

131. Kapczinski FK, Silva de Lima M, dos Santos Souza JS, et al. Antidepressants for generalized anxiety disorder. *Cochrane Database Syst Rev.* 2003;(2) CD003592.

132. Stein DJ, Ipser JC, Seedat S. Pharmacotherapy for post traumatic stress disorder (PTSD). *Cochrane Database Syst Rev.* 2006;(1) CD002795.

133. American Psychiatric Association. *Treatment of patients with acute stress disorder and posttraumatic stress disorder.* Available at:http://www.psychiatryonline.com/pracGuide/pracGuideTopic_11.aspx; accessed April 22, 2010.

134. Canadian Psychiatric Association. *Clinical practice guidelines: management of anxiety disorders—posttraumatic stress disorder.* Available at:http://publications.cpa-apc.org/media.php?mid=446; accessed April 23, 2010.

Delirium 53

William Breitbart and Yesne Alici

Delirium is a common and often serious neuropsychiatric complication in the management of cancer patients that should be prevented, identified, and treated vigorously. Delirium is often underrecognized or misdiagnosed and inappropriately treated or untreated in the medical setting. It is characterized by abrupt onset of a disturbance of consciousness, with reduced ability to focus, sustain, or shift attention, and with changes in cognition or perceptual disturbances that occur over a short period of time and tend to fluctuate over the course of the day. Delirium is considered a medical emergency and indicates a significant physiologic disturbance that usually involves multiple medical causes, including infection, organ failure, and medication adverse effects.[1-10] Delirium can interfere with the recognition and control of other physical and psychological symptoms, such as pain, fatigue, and depression.[10-13] It is associated with increased morbidity and mortality, causing distress in patients, caregivers, and clinicians.[7,10,14-18] Delirium has been shown to increase length of hospital stay, risk for falls, and fall-related injuries.[19,20] It is a prognostic indicator for approaching death in terminally ill cancer patients.[21] Thus it is important for clinicians who are treating cancer patients to recognize and diagnose delirium accurately, undertake appropriate assessment of causes, and be familiar with the pharmacologic and nonpharmacologic interventions currently available for managing delirium. This chapter presents an overview of delirium in cancer patients, including its prevalence, pathophysiology, clinical features, diagnostic criteria, assessment methods, causes, and differential diagnosis, as well as a concise review of nonpharmacologic and pharmacologic treatment of delirium.

PREVALENCE

Delirium is one of the most prevalent neuropsychiatric disorders in oncology inpatient settings. The reported prevalence of delirium varies widely in the medical literature because of the diverse and complex nature of delirium, the assessment scales used, and the heterogeneity of populations studied.[7]

The prevalence of delirium at hospital admission ranges from 14% to 24%, and the incidence of delirium during hospitalization ranges from 6% to 56% among general hospital populations.[7,9,10] Old age is a well-known risk factor for delirium because of increased medical comorbidities, physical frailty, and increased risk of dementia.[22] Community data from the Eastern Baltimore Mental Health survey showed a lower prevalence of delirium in younger populations compared with older patients, with a significant increase in prevalence with advancing age. The prevalence was 0.4% in patients over the age of 18, 1.1% in patients over the age of 55, and 13.6% in patients over the age of 85.[23] Studies of hospitalized elderly patients estimate that 30% to 50% of patients age 70 years or older develop delirium at some point during hospitalization.[24] Postoperative patients and cancer and AIDS patients are also at greater risk for delirium. Delirium occurs in up to 51% of postoperative patients.[25] Approximately 30% to 40% of hospitalized AIDS patients develop delirium.[7] Delirium is present in 26% to 44% of cancer patients at the time of admission to an acute care hospital or palliative care unit.[26–28] The highest prevalence and incidence of delirium are reported in terminally ill cancer patients; it occurs in up to 88% of patients in the last weeks of life.[10,26,29,30] Prospective studies conducted in inpatient palliative care units have found an occurrence rate of delirium ranging from 20% to 42% on admission,[2,5,29,31] and an additional 32% to 45% of patients developing delirium during the week before death.[2,22,31] Advanced or severe illness involving multiorgan systems increases the risk of developing delirium. Therefore, it is not surprising that the highest rates of delirium are reported in hospices among terminally ill patients.[10]

PATHOPHYSIOLOGY

Delirium is a syndrome of generalized brain dysfunction, affecting multiple regions of the brain, that translates into a complex phenomenology characterized by disturbances in level of consciousness, attention, thinking, perception, cognition, psychomotor behavior, mood, and the sleep-wake cycle. Fluctuations of these symptoms, as well as abrupt onset of such disturbances, are critical features of delirium.[8,9] Despite many different possible causes of delirium, it has been postulated through brain imaging and lesion studies that dysfunction of a final common neuroanatomic and neurochemical pathway could be responsible for the core features of delirium, including disturbances in higher cortical functioning (e.g., language, thought process), attention, and the sleep-wake cycle, in addition to disturbances in level of consciousness.[32,33] The final common pathway has been postulated to involve the prefrontal cortex, posterior parietal cortex, temporo-occipital cortex, anteromedial thalamus, and right basal ganglia, with an imbalance in the neurotransmitters acetylcholine and dopamine.[32,34–36] Insufficient cholinergic transmission is implicated in many causes of delirium, including delirium due to metabolic disturbances such as thiamine deficiency, hypoxia, and hypoglycemia; in delirium due to medications with anticholinergic activity[37,38,71] and in delirium due to structural lesions as evidenced by lesion studies.[32] The cholinergic hypothesis is not separable from dopamine (DA), as these two neurotransmitters interact closely and usually reciprocally in the brain. Dopamine excess can precipitate delirium as seen with dopamine agonists, cocaine, and possibly electroconvulsive therapy (ECT).[39–41] The acetylcholine-dopamine hypothesis may explain the efficacy of dopamine antagonists in the treatment of delirium by regulating the imbalance between cholinergic and dopaminergic activity, while the underlying cause is being treated.[32]

Many other neurotransmitter systems, including the serotonergic, noradrenergic, opiatergic, glutamatergic, GABAergic, and histaminergic systems, may contribute to delirium as a syndrome.[32,42] Cytokines, including interleukin-1 (IL-1), IL-6, IL-8, interferon, and tumor necrosis factor, chronic hypercortisolism, and high-dose interleukin therapy have all been suggested to play a role in the pathophysiology of delirium.[43–45] Cytokines may act as neurotoxins or alter glial function by disrupting the blood-brain barrier and cholinergic transmission.[44] Current literature on the pathophysiology of delirium remains limited at best. The study of the pathophysiology of delirium is vital to our understanding of the phenomenology, prognosis, treatment, and prevention of delirium.

CLINICAL FEATURES

The clinical features of delirium are numerous and include a variety of neuropsychiatric symptoms that are common to other psychiatric disorders, such as depression, cognitive disturbances, and psychotic symptoms[9,10] (Table 53-1). Main features of delirium include prodromal symptoms (e.g., restlessness, anxiety, sleep disturbances, irritability); a rapidly fluctuating course; abrupt onset of symptoms; attention disturbances (e.g., distractibility); altered level of consciousness; increased or decreased psychomotor activity; disturbances in sleep-wake cycle; affective symptoms (e.g., emotional lability, depressed mood, irritability, euphoria); perceptual disturbances (e.g., misperceptions, illusions, hallucinations); delusions; disorganized thinking; incoherent speech; and cognitive impairment.[10,16] Cognitive impairment can take the form of language disturbances (such as dysnomia, dysgraphia, dysphasia), apraxia, disorientation, agnosia, memory problems, and/or executive dysfunction. A variety of nonspecific neurologic abnormalities can be seen during an episode of delirium, including tremor, asterixis, myoclonus, frontal release signs, muscle tone, and reflex changes.[10]

Cognitive impairment was found to be the most common symptom in phenomenology studies, with disorientation occurring in 78% to 100% of patients with delirium, attention deficit

---

Table 53-1 Common clinical features of delirium

Disturbance in level of alertness (consciousness)

Attention disturbance

Rapidly fluctuating course and abrupt onset of symptoms

Increased or decreased psychomotor activity

Disturbance in sleep-wake cycle

Mood symptoms

Perceptual disturbances

Disorganized thinking

Incoherent speech

Disorientation and memory impairment

Other cognitive impairments (e.g., aphasia, agnosia, executive dysfunction, dysgraphia, constructional apraxia, dysnomia)

Asterixis, myoclonus, tremor, frontal release signs, changes in muscle tone

in 62% to 100%, memory deficit in 62% to 90%, and diffuse cognitive deficit in 77%.[46] Disturbance of consciousness was recorded in 65% to 100% of patients with delirium. In addition, disorganized thinking was found in 95%, language abnormalities in 47% to 93%, and sleep-wake cycle disturbances in 49% to 96%. Less common symptoms included affective lability (43%), delusions (18%–62%), and hallucinations (4%–77%).[46] A recent phenomenology study by Meagher and colleagues[33] has shown that sleep-wake cycle abnormalities (97%) and inattention (97%) were the symptoms experienced most frequently by patients with delirium; disorientation was the least common symptom.

The clinical presentation of delirium may vary according to the age of the patient. A phenomenology study of different age groups has shown that childhood delirium is more likely to present with severe perceptual disturbances, visual hallucinations, severe delusions, severe lability of mood, and agitation when compared with delirium in adult and geriatric patient populations.[47] More severe cognitive symptoms have been observed in geriatric patients with delirium.[47]

DIAGNOSTIC CRITERIA

The *Diagnostic and Statistical Manual of Mental Disorders*[8] outlines the diagnostic criteria for delirium as follows:

1. Disturbance in consciousness with reduced ability to focus, sustain, or shift attention.
2. Change in cognition that is not better accounted for by a preexisting, established, or evolving dementia or development of a perceptual disturbance.
3. Development of the disturbance over a short period of time, usually hours to days, and fluctuation of symptoms during the course of the day.
4. Evidence from the history, physical examination, or laboratory tests that the delirium is a direct physiologic consequence of a general medical condition, substance intoxication or withdrawal, use of a medication, or toxin exposure, or a combination of these factors.

The disturbance in consciousness is manifested by reduced clarity of awareness of the environment. Because of the disturbance in consciousness and impaired attention, questions must be repeated, because the individual's attention wanders, or the individual may perseverate with an answer to a previous question rather than appropriately shifting attention. Patients with delirium may be easily distracted by outside stimuli or may become over-absorbed in a task, such as picking at the bed sheet, which makes it difficult to engage the person in conversation.[10] Clinicians may ask patients to describe their surroundings with their eyes closed or may directly ask patients if they are feeling 100% awake to test for level of alertness.[10] Forward and backward digit span testing is a useful bedside examination tool for assessment of attention.[10]

An accompanying change in cognition (which may include memory impairment, disorientation, or language disturbances) or development of a perceptual disturbance may occur. Memory impairment in recent memory is most commonly evident and can be tested by asking the person to remember several unrelated objects or a brief sentence, and then to repeat them after a few minutes of distraction. Disorientation is usually manifested by the individual's disorientation to time or to place. In mild delirium, disorientation to time may be the first symptom to appear. Clinicians should test the limits of orientation (e.g., year, month, date, day, time). It is often misleading to assume full orientation when patients answer the year and the month correctly.[10] Disorientation to self is less common. Language disturbance may be evident as dysnomia (i.e., the impaired ability to name objects) or dysgraphia (i.e., the impaired ability to write). In some cases, speech is rambling and irrelevant; in others, pressured and incoherent. It may be difficult for the clinician to assess changes in cognitive function because the individual may be inattentive and incoherent. Under these circumstances, it is helpful to review carefully the individual's history and to obtain information from family members or other caregivers.[10] Perceptual disturbances may include misinterpretations, illusions, or hallucinations. Although sensory misperceptions are most commonly visual, they may occur in other sensory modalities as well. Misperceptions range from simple and uniform to highly complex. Abrupt onset and fluctuation of symptoms are integral parts of the diagnostic criteria. The disturbance develops over a short period of time and tends to fluctuate during the course of the day. For example, the person may be coherent and cooperative during the morning hospital rounds, but at night might be pulling out intravenous lines and insisting on going home. Although the *Diagnostic and Statistical Manual of Mental Disorders,* Fourth Edition (DSM-IV) places less diagnostic emphasis on incoherent speech, disorganized thinking, disturbance in the sleep-wake cycle, and disturbances in psychomotor activity, it is important for clinicians to assess these symptoms for prompt recognition of delirium in the medically ill.[16] Clinicians should also carefully assess for a subsyndromal delirium (i.e., delirium that does not meet the full DSM-IV criteria for a diagnosis of delirium) or prodromal signs of delirium in palliative care settings.[48]

SUBTYPES OF DELIRIUM

Based on psychomotor behavior and level of alertness, two clinical subtypes of delirium have been described: the hyperactive subtype and the hypoactive subtype.[33,49] A third subtype, namely, the mixed subtype, has been proposed, with alternating features of the hyperactive and hypoactive subtypes. The hypoactive (hypoalert) subtype is characterized by psychomotor retardation, lethargy, sedation, and reduced awareness of surroundings.[5,33,50,51] Hypoactive delirium is often mistaken for depression and is difficult to differentiate from sedation due to opioids, or obtundation in the last days of life.[52] The hyperactive (hyperalert) subtype is commonly characterized by restlessness, agitation, hypervigilance, hallucinations, and delusions.[50,51] The hyperactive delirium is more easily recognized by clinicians. Mittal et al. studied delirium subtypes in patients referred to a psychiatric consultation service in a veterans' hospital, and found that patients with hyperactive delirium were more likely than patients with other subtypes of delirium to be referred to psychiatry.[53]

Most episodes of delirium are of the hypoactive or mixed subtype.[5] Despite the frequency of hypoactive delirium, Fang et al. reported that hypoactive delirium was significantly underdetected when compared with the detection rates of hyperactive and mixed subtypes of delirium in palliative care settings.[54] In a prospective study by Lawlor et al., 48 of 71 patients (68%) were found to have a mixed subtype of delirium.[2] A meta-analysis of delirium subtypes has shown a mean prevalence of hypoactive delirium to be 48% (range, 15%–71%),[50] while the prevalence of hyperactive delirium ranged from 13% to 46%.[50] A systematic review of delirium subtypes by de Rooij et al. has identified 10 studies[55] conducted in different settings, predominantly among older, medically ill patients. The authors concluded that because of the lack of a standardized classification method, and because different results were obtained, it was difficult to draw any firm conclusions regarding the frequency of the three motoric subtypes of delirium and their association with specific prognoses, etiologic factors, and therapeutic consequences. Peterson et al. studied delirium subtypes in patients admitted to a medical intensive care unit and found that those aged 65 and older were almost twice as likely to have hypoactive delirium as younger patients.[56] In the palliative care setting, hypoactive delirium is most common. Spiller and Keen found a delirium prevalence of 29% in 100 acute admissions to a hospice center; 86% of these had the hypoactive subtype. The authors emphasized the need for comprehensive assessment of patients in palliative care settings to minimize misdiagnosis of hypoactive delirium as depression or profound fatigue.[5]

Evidence suggests that different subtypes of delirium may be related to different causes and may have different treatment responses. The hyperactive and mixed subtypes are highly associated with medication side effects, alcohol and drug withdrawal, and drug intoxication, whereas hypoactive delirium is most often associated with hypoxia, dehydration, metabolic disturbances, and hepatic encephalopathy.[4,50,52,57] Regardless of the treatment response, patients with hyperactive delirium are more likely to receive psychotropic medications in clinical settings.[58] A randomized controlled trial of haloperidol and chlorpromazine found that these medications were equally effective in hypoactive and hyperactive subtypes of delirium.[59] However, in an open-label trial, the hypoactive subtype was associated with poorer treatment response to olanzapine.[60] The hypoactive subtype of delirium is associated with higher mortality risk compared with hyperactive delirium.[9,10,54,59,61] Kiely and colleagues[57] studied 1-year mortality among 457 patients with hypoactive, hyperactive, and mixed subtypes of delirium and found that all three psychomotor disturbance subtypes were associated with an elevated risk of mortality during 1-year follow-up. The hypoactive group had the highest mortality and was the only group with a significantly increased risk of mortality compared to the group with normal psychomotor activity.

It is important to note that despite differences in origin, phenomenology, treatment response, and prognosis between different subtypes of delirium, both hypoactive and hyperactive subtypes of delirium have been shown to cause distress in patients, family members, and clinicians.[14]

EXPERIENCE OF DELIRIUM FOR PATIENTS, FAMILY MEMBERS, CLINICIANS, AND STAFF

Delirium is associated with increased morbidity, which causes distress in patients, family members, clinicians, and staff.[14,15,17,62] In a study of 99 patients with advanced cancer, 74% were able to recall their delirium episode after recovery from delirium. Recall was not significantly different according to the delirium subtype. Eighty-one percent of patients with delirium recall reported that the experience was distressing versus 42% of patients with no recall. Patients who recalled their delirium episodes had significantly higher levels of distress.[17] In a study of 101 terminally ill cancer patients, Breitbart et al.[14] found that 54% of patients recalled their delirium experience after recovering from the episode. The more severe the episode, the less likely the patient was to recall it. The presence of hallucinations and delusions made delirium more likely to be recalled (and to be reported as distressing). Distress related to the episode was rated by patients on a 0 to 4 numeric rating scale (with 4 being most severe). Patients who recalled the delirium episode rated their distress on average at 3.2. Patients with hypoactive delirium were just as distressed as patients with hyperactive delirium, highlighting the importance of treating the causes and controlling the symptoms of delirium in both hypoactive and hyperactive subtypes. DiMartini and colleagues reported the development of posttraumatic stress disorder in patients who experienced hallucinations and delusions during delirium.[62]

Recent studies suggest that the experience of family members caring for a delirious patient is perhaps even more distressing than the experience of the patient with delirium.[14,63] In a study of delirium-related caregiver distress, Breitbart et al.[14] found that spouses and family caregivers rated their distress (on a 0 to 4 scale) at 3.75, and nurses at 3.1—just below the average patient rating of 3.2. Predictors of nurse distress included delirium severity, the presence of perceptual disturbances, paranoid delusions, and sleep-wake cycle disturbance. For the nursing staff, an agitated, severely delirious patient with hallucinations, delusions, and disrupted sleep is a significant nursing care challenge and in fact can consume many hours of nursing time, which is often associated with great anxiety, frustration, helplessness, and even fear. Breitbart et al.[14] have shown that predictors of spouse distress included the patient's Karnofsky performance status (the lower the Karnofsky, the worse the spouse distress) and the presence of hyperactive delirium, as well as delirium related to brain metastases.[14] Bruera et al.,[17] in their study of caregiver distress due to delirium, found that family caregivers recalled more delirium-related symptoms than patients, nurses, or physicians; this suggests that family caregivers provide the most accurate information regarding the frequency of delirium-related symptoms. Among individuals caring for a patient with delirium, family caregivers experienced higher levels of distress than did nurses or physicians.[17] Morita and colleagues, in their survey of 300 bereaved Japanese families, found that two thirds of families reported delirium in their loved ones as highly distressing. Symptoms that caused the most distress included agitation and cognitive impairment.[15] In a recent study, caregivers of terminally ill patients with delirium were found to have a 12 times increased risk of developing an anxiety disorder compared with caregivers of patients without delirium.[63]

Often, family members are uneducated about the high prevalence of delirium, the medical nature of delirium, and the potential course of delirium in the palliative care setting. It is important for the clinician to explain the medical nature of delirium and the potential for treatment and control of symptoms. Several inpatient hospice centers and palliative care units have taken the step of developing delirium education pamphlets for family members, so that families are prepared and informed and have the ability to discuss delirium treatment options while the patient still has the capacity to participate in these discussions.

ASSESSMENT OF DELIRIUM

The diagnostic gold standard for delirium is the clinician's assessment utilizing the DSM-IV criteria as outlined above.[8,9] Several delirium screening and evaluation tools have been developed to maximize diagnostic precision for clinical and research purposes, and to assess delirium severity.[10,64–72] A detailed review of these assessment tools is available elsewhere.[64] Mini-Mental State Examination (MMSE),[73] despite its common use in clinical settings, is helpful merely in assessment of cognitive functioning without addressing other aspects of delirium. Several examples of delirium assessment tools currently used in cancer patients and in palliative care settings include the Memorial Delirium Assessment Scale (MDAS),[67,68] the Delirium Rating Scale-Revised 98 (DRS-R-98),[66] and the Confusion Assessment Method (CAM).[70]

The Memorial Delirium Assessment Scale (MDAS) is designed to be administered repeatedly within the same day, to allow objective measurement of changes in delirium severity in response to medical changes or clinical interventions. The MDAS is a 10-item, 4-point clinician-rated scale (possible range, 0–30) designed to quantify the severity of delirium; it has been validated among hospitalized patients with advanced cancer and AIDS.[67] Items included in the MDAS reflect the diagnostic criteria for delirium in the DSM-IV, as well as symptoms of delirium from earlier or alternative classification systems (e.g., DSM-III, DSM-III-R, International Classification of Diseases [ICD]-9). The MDAS is both a good delirium diagnostic screening tool and a reliable tool for assessing delirium severity among patients with advanced disease. Scale items assess disturbances in level of consciousness, as well as in several areas of cognitive functioning (memory, attention, orientation, disturbances in thinking) and psychomotor activity.[67] A cutoff score of 13 is diagnostic of delirium. The MDAS has advantages over other delirium tools in that it is both a diagnostic and a severity measure that is ideal for repeated assessments and for use in treatment intervention trials. The MDAS has been re-validated among advanced cancer patients in inpatient palliative care settings with a sensitivity of 98% and a specificity of 96% at a cutoff score of 7.[68]

The Delirium Rating Scale (DRS)[65] is based on the DSM-III-R diagnostic criteria for delirium. It is a 10-item scale, with items scored from 0 to 3 or 0 to 4 in the following domains: (1) temporal onset, (2) perceptual disturbance, (3) hallucinations, (4) delusions, (5) psychomotor behavior, (6) cognitive status, (7) physical disorder, (8) sleep-wake cycle disturbance, (9) lability of mood, and (10) fluctuation of symptoms.[65] A score of 12 or greater is diagnostic of delirium. DRS-R-98 is the revised version of the DRS.[66] It includes more items than the DRS and was designed for phenomenologic and treatment research, although it may be used clinically. The summation of the first 13 item scores provides a total severity score (range, 0–39); the last three (temporal onset and fluctuation of symptoms and the presence of a physical disorder) can be exclusively used for diagnostic purposes. The DRS-R-98 is a valid, sensitive, and reliable instrument for rating delirium severity.[66]

The Confusion Assessment Method (CAM) is used mainly for delirium screening. It is a nine-item delirium diagnostic scale based on the DSM-III-R criteria for delirium.[70] A unique and helpful feature of the CAM is that it has been simplified into a diagnostic algorithm that includes only four items of the CAM designed for rapid identification of delirium by nonpsychiatrists. The four-item algorithm requires the presence of (1) acute onset and fluctuating course, (2) inattention, and either (3) disorganized thinking or (4) altered level of consciousness. The Confusion Assessment Method has recently been validated in the palliative care setting with a sensitivity of 0.88 (range, 0.62–0.98) and a specificity of 1.0 (range, 0.88–1.0) when used by clinicians trained in its administration.[72]

DIFFERENTIAL DIAGNOSIS

Many of the clinical features of delirium can also be associated with other psychiatric disorders, such as depression, mania, psychosis, and dementia. It is important to recognize that not all patients with agitation have delirium. The diagnosis is reserved for those who meet the diagnostic criteria and present with the clinical syndrome described above. Patients may become agitated for a variety of reasons such as fecal impaction, urinary retention, uncontrolled pain, or clinical syndromes such as akathisia, panic attacks, and mania.[10] On the other hand, patients with fecal impaction, urinary retention, and uncontrolled pain may also develop delirium when these conditions are left untreated.[10]

When delirium presents with mood symptoms such as depression, apathy, euphoria, or irritability, these symptoms are not uncommonly attributed to depression or mania, especially in patients with a past psychiatric or family history of these conditions.[9] The hypoactive subtype of delirium is commonly misdiagnosed as depression.[10,55,74] Symptoms of major depression, including decreased psychomotor activity, insomnia, reduced ability to concentrate, depressed mood, and even suicidal ideation, can overlap with symptoms of delirium. In distinguishing delirium from depression, particularly in the context of advanced cancer, an evaluation of the onset and the temporal sequencing of depressive and cognitive symptoms is particularly helpful. It is important to note that the degree of cognitive impairment is much more pronounced in delirium than in depression, with a more abrupt onset. Also, in delirium the characteristic disturbance in level of consciousness is present, but it is usually not a feature of depression. Leonard et al. assessed 100 consecutive palliative care admissions for symptoms of depression and delirium. Most patients with delirium also met criteria for major depressive illness, and 50% of those with depression had delirium or subsyndromal delirium. The authors concluded that delirium should be considered in patients with altered mood states, and screening for depression should initially rule out delirium.[75]

A manic episode may share some features of delirium, particularly a hyperactive or mixed subtype of delirium. Again, the temporal onset and course of symptoms, the presence of a disturbance in level of consciousness as well as cognition, and the identification of a presumed medical cause for delirium are helpful in differentiating these disorders. Symptoms such as severe anxiety and autonomic hyperactivity can lead the clinician to an erroneous diagnosis of panic disorder, or medication-induced akathisia.[10] Delirium that is characterized by vivid hallucinations and delusions must be distinguished from a variety of psychotic disorders such as schizophrenia. Delusions in delirium tend to be poorly organized and of abrupt onset, and hallucinations are predominantly visual or tactile, rather than auditory, as is typical of schizophrenia. Acute onset, fluctuating course, and disturbances in cognition and consciousness, in the presence of one or more medical causes, are characteristic in the diagnosis of delirium.[9,10]

The most challenging differential diagnostic issue is whether the patient has delirium, dementia, or a delirium superimposed on a preexisting dementia. Both delirium and dementia are disorders of cognition and share common clinical features, such as disorientation, memory impairment, aphasia, apraxia, agnosia, and executive dysfunction.[9,10] Impairments in judgment and abstract thinking, as well as disturbances in thought process, are seen in both disorders. Delusions and hallucinations can be central features of certain types of dementia. It is the abrupt onset, fluctuating course, and disturbances of consciousness that differentiate delirium from dementia.[9] Dementia with Lewy bodies, a form of dementia characterized by visual hallucinations, parkinsonism, and a fluctuating course, is particularly difficult to differentiate from an episode of delirium. The temporal onset of symptoms in dementia is more subacute and chronically progressive. In delirium superimposed on an underlying dementia, such as in the case of an elderly patient, an AIDS patient, or a patient with a paraneoplastic syndrome, differential diagnosis becomes even more challenging. Delirium, unlike dementia, is by definition reversible, although in terminally ill patients or in patients with preexisting cognitive impairment, delirium may be irreversible.[9] A phenomenology study of 100 patients with delirium has shown that patients with comorbid dementia had significantly greater levels of disturbance in consciousness and impairment in all cognitive domains when compared with patients without preexisting dementia. No significant differences were found between the two groups in terms of the presence or the severity of hallucinations, delusions, psychomotor behavior, and sleep-wake cycle disturbances.[76]

INTERFERENCE OF DELIRIUM WITH ASSESSMENT AND MANAGEMENT OF PAIN

It is well recognized that success in the treatment of cancer pain is highly dependent on proper assessment. However, assessment of pain intensity becomes very difficult in patients with delirium. Delirium can interfere dramatically with the recognition and control of pain, along with other physical and psychological symptoms in advanced cancer patients, particularly in the terminally ill.[10–12] It has been shown that because of reversal of the sleep-wake cycle, patients with delirium use a significantly greater number of "breakthrough" doses of opioids at nights compared with patients without delirium.[13] On the other hand, agitation may be misinterpreted as uncontrolled pain, resulting in inappropriate escalation of opioids, potentially exacerbating delirium.[12,18] Accurate pain reporting depends on the ability to perceive pain normally and to communicate the experience appropriately. Delirium may impair the ability to both perceive and report pain accurately. It has been shown that the ability to communicate pain is frequently impaired among terminally ill hospice patients, with the degree of impairment related to both delirium and opioid dosage.[18,77] Efforts have been made to improve assessment of pain in nonverbal palliative care patients.[78]

CAUSES AND REVERSIBILITY OF DELIRIUM

Delirium can have multiple potential causes. In patients with cancer, delirium can result from the direct effects of cancer on the central nervous system (CNS), or from indirect CNS effects of the disease or its treatments (e.g., medications, electrolyte imbalance, dehydration, major organ failure, infection, vascular complications, paraneoplastic syndromes)[1,2,4–6,10,55,79] (Table 53-2).

The diagnostic workup of delirium should include an assessment of potentially reversible causes of delirium. The clinician should obtain a detailed history from family and staff of the patient's baseline mental status and should verify the current fluctuating mental status. It is important to inquire about alcohol and other substance use disorders in hospitalized cancer patients to be able to recognize and treat alcohol or other substance-induced withdrawal delirium appropriately.[9] A full physical examination should assess for evidence of sepsis, dehydration, or major organic failure (renal, hepatic, and pulmonary).[9]

Medications that could contribute to delirium should be reviewed. Opioid analgesics, benzodiazepines, and anticholinergic drugs are common causes of delirium, particularly in the elderly and the terminally ill.[6,9,79,80] In palliative care settings, medications used for symptom control (e.g., antihistamines, opioids, tricyclic antidepressants, corticosteroids) have been shown to significantly increase the overall burden of anticholinergic adverse effects, thus increasing the risk of delirium.[81] Delirium, sedation, myoclonus, hyperalgesia, allodynia, and even seizures caused by opioid analgesic use have been described.[16,82] The term *opioid-induced neurotoxicity* has been used to describe a syndrome of neuropsychiatric side effects seen with opioid therapy.[18] Reducing the dose of opioids or switching to another opioid has been demonstrated to reverse delirium due to opioids.[18] However, assessing the role of opioid therapy in an episode of delirium is often compounded by the presence of many other potential contributors to cognitive impairment, such as infection, metabolic

Table 53-2   Causes of delirium in cancer patients
Direct effects of cancer on the central nervous system (CNS)
Primary CNS tumors
Metastatic brain tumors
Leptomeningeal carcinomatosis
Indirect effects of cancer or treatments on the CNS
Major organ failure (e.g., pulmonary, renal, hepatic)
Electrolyte imbalances
Medications (including chemotherapeutic agents)
Infections
Hematologic abnormalities
Paraneoplastic syndromes

disturbance, dehydration, or other medication effects. Chemotherapeutic agents known to cause delirium include methotrexate, fluorouracil, vincristine, vinblastine, bleomycin, carmustine (BCNU), cis-platinum, ifosfamide, asparaginase, procarbazine, and glucocorticosteroids.[16] A screen of laboratory parameters will allow assessment of the possible role of metabolic abnormalities, such as hypercalcemia, and other problems, such as hypoxia or disseminated intravascular coagulation. In some instances, an electroencephalogram (EEG) (to rule out seizures), brain imaging studies (to rule out brain metastases, intracranial bleeding, or ischemia), or lumbar puncture (to rule out leptomeningeal carcinomatosis or meningitis) may be appropriate.[9,10]

When assessing causes of delirium, an important challenge is the clinical differentiation of delirium as a reversible complication of cancer or as an integral element of the dying process in terminally ill patients. The potential utility of a thorough diagnostic assessment has been demonstrated in patients with advanced cancer. When diagnostic information points to a likely cause, specific therapy may be able to reverse delirium. Debate is ongoing as to the appropriate extent of diagnostic evaluation that should be pursued in a terminally ill patient with delirium.[10] A survey of 270 physicians from four disciplines (palliative care, medical oncology, geriatrics, and geriatric psychiatry) found that about 85% of specialists would order basic blood tests when confronted with delirium in advanced cancer; on the other hand, more than 40% of specialists reported that they would not do any investigation in patients with terminal delirium.[83] When confronted with delirium in the terminally ill patient, the clinician must take a more individualized and judicious approach, consistent with the goals of care. Most clinicians would undertake diagnostic studies only when a clinically suspected cause can be identified easily, with minimal use of invasive procedures, and treated effectively with simple interventions that carry minimal burden or risk of causing further distress.[10] Diagnostic workup in pursuit of an origin for terminal delirium may be limited by practical constraints such as the setting (home, hospice) or by the focus on patient comfort, so that invasive diagnostics may be avoided.[16] Most often, however, the cause of terminal delirium is multifactorial or may not be determined.

Bruera et al. reported that a cause was discovered in 43% of terminally ill patients with delirium, and one third of the patients with delirium improved following treatment of the specific causes.[84] One study found that 68% of delirious cancer patients had a reversible medical cause underlying delirium, despite a 30-day mortality of 31%.[85] Lawlor and colleagues explored the etiologic precipitants and the potential reversibility of delirium in advanced cancer patients admitted to a palliative care unit for symptom control, and found an overall reversibility rate of 49%.[2] No difference was found in reversibility rates for delirium present on admission and that which developed subsequently. However, a significant difference was observed in the reversibility of initial (56%) compared to repeated episodes (6%). The median duration of reversible delirium was 3.5 days, as opposed to a median duration of 6 days with irreversible delirium. The median number of precipitating factors for both reversible and irreversible delirium was 3 (range, 1–6). The application of standardized criteria resulted in a classification of causative factors in 78% of episodes of reversible delirium

and in 59% of irreversible cases. Reversibility of delirium was significantly associated with opioids, other psychoactive medications, and dehydration. In contrast, the irreversibility of delirium was significantly associated with hypoxic encephalopathy and metabolic factors related to major organ failure, including hepatic and renal insufficiency, as well as refractory hypercalcemia.[2] Gaudreau et al. prospectively studied the association of medication use with the development of delirium in 43 patients with cancer, and found that daily doses of benzodiazepines (oral lorazepam equivalent) above 2 mg, corticosteroids (oral dexamethasone equivalent) above 15 mg, and opioids (subcutaneous morphine equivalent) above 90 mg were associated with increased risk of delirium. The authors emphasized that most of these precipitants were amenable to correction.[1]

Ljubisavljevic and Kelly prospectively assessed the development of delirium in oncology patients, and found a delirium occurrence rate of 18% (26 out of 145 patients) and a reversal rate of 84.6% (22 out of 26 patients).[3] Morita examined factors associated with the reversibility of delirium in a population of advanced cancer patients admitted to hospice.[4] This study's overall delirium reversibility rate was 20%—lower than that reported in prior studies. Patients with delirium had a 30-day mortality rate of 83% and a 50-day mortality rate of 91%. Although reversibility of delirium was significantly associated with medications (37%) or hypercalcemia (38%), irreversibility was associated with infection (12%), hepatic failure, hypoxia, disseminated intravascular coagulation, and dehydration (<10%).

Leonard and colleagues[61] found a 27% recovery rate from delirium among patients in palliative care. Patients with irreversible delirium experienced greater disturbances in sleep and cognition. Mean time until death was 39.7 days (SD, 69.8 days) in patients with reversible delirium (n = 33) versus 16.8 days (SD, 10.0 days) in patients with irreversible delirium (n = 88).[61]

Older hospitalized patients are specifically identified as a high-risk population for persistent, chronic, or irreversible delirium.[86] Patients with underlying cognitive impairment are less likely to recover from an episode of delirium.[7]

A recent review of 1322 patients with delirium from 18 studies found that the combined proportions of patients with persistent delirium at discharge and at 1, 3, and 6 months were 44.7% (95% confidence interval [CI], 26.8%–63.7%), 32.8% (95% CI, 18.4%–47.2%), 25.6% (95% CI, 7.9%–43.4%) and 21% (95% CI, 1.4%–40.6%), respectively. The outcomes (mortality, nursing home placement, function, cognition) of patients with persistent delirium were consistently worse than the outcomes of patients who had recovered from delirium.[82]

In light of several studies on the reversibility of delirium, the prognosis of patients who develop delirium is dependent on several factors, including the patient's baseline physiologic susceptibility to delirium (e.g., predisposing factors), the precipitating causes, and any response to treatment of the underlying causes. If a patient's susceptibility or resilience is modifiable, then targeted interventions may reduce the risk of delirium upon exposure to a precipitant and enhance the capacity to respond to treatment of the precipitating causes.[16] Conversely, if a patient's vulnerability is high and resistant to modification, then exposure to precipitants enhances the risk of developing delirium and decreases the likelihood of complete restoration of cognitive function.[16]

MANAGEMENT OF DELIRIUM IN ADVANCED CANCER PATIENTS

The standard approach to managing delirium includes a search for underlying causes, correction of those factors, and management of the symptoms of delirium.[9] Treatment of the symptoms of delirium should be initiated, together with a diagnostic assessment of the causes, to minimize distress to patients, staff, and caregivers.[9] In palliative care settings, the desired and often achievable outcome is a patient who is awake, alert, calm, comfortable, not in pain, cognitively intact, not psychotic, and communicating coherently with family and staff. In the terminally ill patient who develops delirium in the last days of life, the management of delirium is unique, presenting a number of dilemmas, and the desired clinical outcome may be significantly altered by the dying process.[10] The goal of care in the terminally ill may shift to providing comfort through the judicious use of sedatives, even at the expense of alertness.[10]

NONPHARMACOLOGIC INTERVENTIONS

Nonpharmacologic and supportive therapies play an essential role in the treatment of cancer patients with delirium, especially in patients with terminal delirium.[30] Nonpharmacologic interventions have been shown to result in faster improvement of delirium symptoms and slower deterioration in cognition.[30,87-90] However, these interventions have not been found to have any beneficial effects on mortality or health-related quality of life when compared with usual care.[87-90]

Nonpharmacologic interventions include oxygen delivery, fluid and electrolyte administration, ensuring bowel and bladder function, nutrition, mobilization, pain treatment, frequent orientation, use of visual and hearing aids, and environmental modifications (e.g., quiet, well-lit room with familiar objects, a visible clock or calendar) to enhance a sense of familiarity.[10] One-to-one nursing may be necessary for observation of agitated patients with delirium. Physical restraints should be avoided, when possible. The use of physical restraints has been identified as an independent risk factor for persistence of delirium at the time of hospital discharge.[88] Physical restraints should be used only when a patient represents a clear, imminent risk of harm to self and a less restrictive alternative is not available. Restraint orders should be time-limited, and the patient's condition should be monitored closely.

Education and psychosocial support for the family, caregivers, nurses, and patients play an essential role in alleviating the distress due to delirium; thus they should be an integral part of nonpharmacologic management of delirium in palliative care settings.

PHARMACOLOGIC INTERVENTIONS

Nonpharmacologic interventions and supportive measures alone are often not effective in controlling the symptoms of delirium. Symptomatic treatment with psychotropic medications is often essential to control the symptoms of delirium, although no medications have been approved by the U.S. Food and Drug Administration (FDA) for the treatment of delirium.

Antipsychotic medications

Antipsychotics are considered to be first-line agents in the pharmacologic management of delirium. The American Psychiatric Association (APA) practice guidelines provide directions for the use of antipsychotics in the treatment of delirium, and growing evidence supports their use[10,59,91-93] (Table 53-3).

Haloperidol, a "typical" antipsychotic, is often the gold standard medication for the treatment of delirium among cancer patients, because of its efficacy and safety (e.g., few anticholinergic effects, lack of active metabolites, availability in different routes of administration).[10] Haloperidol in low doses, 1 to 3 mg per day, is usually effective in targeting agitation and psychotic symptoms. In general, doses of haloperidol do not exceed 20 mg in a 24-hour period; however, some clinicians advocate higher doses in selected cases.[94] In severe agitation related to delirium, clinicians may add lorazepam to haloperidol. This combination may be more effective in rapidly sedating patients and may help minimize any extrapyramidal adverse effects of haloperidol.[10] The FDA has issued a warning about the risk of QT interval prolongation and torsades de pointes with intravenous haloperidol; thus monitoring QT intervals daily among medically ill patients receiving intravenous haloperidol has become standard clinical practice.[95]

Oral or intravenous (IV) chlorpromazine, at doses of 12.5 to 50 mg every 4 to 12 hours, is considered to be an effective alternative to haloperidol (with or without lorazepam) when increased sedation is required, especially in the intensive care unit (ICU) setting, where close blood pressure monitoring is feasible, and for severe agitation in terminally ill patients to decrease distress for the patient, family, and staff. It is important to monitor the anticholinergic and hypotensive side effects of chlorpromazine, particularly in elderly patients.[10]

In a double-blind, randomized comparison trial (n = 30) of haloperidol, chlorpromazine, and lorazepam, Breitbart and colleagues[59] demonstrated that lorazepam alone, in doses up to 8 mg in a 12-hour period, was ineffective in the treatment of delirium, and in fact sometimes worsened it. Both haloperidol and chlorpromazine, in low doses (approximately 2 mg of haloperidol equivalent per 24 hours), were effective in controlling the symptoms of delirium and in improving cognitive function in the first 24 hours of treatment.[59] Both hyperactive and hypoactive subtypes of delirium were equally responsive to treatment with haloperidol or chlorpromazine. A systematic review of pharmacologic therapies for delirium in the terminally ill concluded that haloperidol was the most suitable medication for the treatment of patients with delirium near the end of life, with chlorpromazine being an acceptable alternative.[93]

Atypical antipsychotic agents (i.e., risperidone, olanzapine, quetiapine, ziprasidone, and aripiprazole) are increasingly used in the treatment of delirium in cancer patients because of a lower risk of extrapyramidal adverse effects.[58] Several researchers have published their favorable experiences in case reports, case series, and open-label studies on the treatment of delirium and agitation with atypical antipsychotics, including olanzapine,[60,96-99] risperidone,[99-102] quetiapine,[103,104] ziprasidone,[105,106] and aripiprazole.[107] In a double-blind comparative delirium intervention study assessing the efficacy of haloperidol versus risperidone, Han and Kim demonstrated, in a small sample of 24 oncology patients, that there was no

Table 53-3 Antipsychotic medications in the treatment of delirium

Medication	Dose range	Routes of administration	Side effects	Comments
Typical antipsychotics				
Haloperidol	0.5–2 mg every 2–12 hours	PO, IV, IM, SC	Extrapyramidal adverse effects can occur at higher doses. Monitor QT interval on ECG	Gold standard treatment for delirium
Chlorpromazine	12.5–50 mg every 4–6 hours	PO, IV, IM, SC, PR	More sedating and anticholinergic compared with haloperidol	May be preferred in agitated patients because of its sedative effect
Atypical antipsychotics				
Olanzapine	2.5–5 mg every 12–24 hours	PO,* IM	Sedation is the main dose-limiting side effect in short-term use	Older age, preexisting dementia, and hypoactive subtype of delirium have been associated with poor response
Risperidone	0.25–1 mg every 12–24 hours	PO*	Extrapyramidal adverse effects can occur with doses >6 mg/day. Orthostatic hypotension	Clinical experience suggests better results in patients with hypoactive delirium
Quetiapine	12.5–100 mg every 12–24 hours	PO	Sedation, orthostatic hypotension.	Sedating effects may be helpful in patients with sleep-wake cycle disturbance
Ziprasidone	10–40 mg every 12–24 hours	PO, IM	Monitor QT interval on ECG	Evidence is limited to case reports
Aripiprazole	5–30 mg every 24 hours	PO,* IM	Monitor for akathisia	Evidence is limited to case reports and case series

*Risperidone, olanzapine, and aripiprazole are available in orally disintegrating tablets.
ECG, Electrocardiography.

significant difference in clinical efficacy or response rate. The mean risperidone dose was 1.02 mg, and the mean haloperidol dose was 1.71 mg. MDAS scores improved significantly in both groups. No significant difference in adverse effects was observed. However, despite the double-blind design of this study, authors acknowledged that they were not able to obtain identical looking tablets of haloperidol and risperidone.[108]

A randomized controlled trial[109] comparing olanzapine (n = 75), haloperidol (n = 72), and placebo (n = 29) in the treatment of delirium among hospitalized patients (mean olanzapine dose of 4.5 mg/day, and a haloperidol dose of 7 mg/day) has demonstrated an improvement in DRS scores with olanzapine and haloperidol—significantly higher in the olanzapine (72%) and haloperidol (70%) groups compared with placebo (29.7%) (P < .01). Increased rates of extrapyramidal symptoms were observed in the haloperidol group. However, haloperidol was administered intramuscularly, which makes it difficult to reliably interpret the study results.

A randomized, placebo-controlled study of quetiapine versus placebo as add-on treatment to "as-needed" haloperidol for treatment of delirium among 36 intensive care unit patients has shown faster delirium resolution (1 vs. 4.5 days; P = .001), reduced duration of delirium (36 vs. 120 hours; P = .006), less agitation, and a greater rate of transfer to home or rehabilitation.[110] However, concurrent use of haloperidol limits

the interpretation of results in this study. A double-blind, randomized, placebo-controlled trial with haloperidol and ziprasidone to demonstrate the feasibility of a placebo-controlled trial of antipsychotics for delirium in the intensive care unit has not been able to show any difference between haloperidol, ziprasidone, and placebo groups in the number of days alive without delirium, hospital length of stay, or mortality.[111] The study results are confounded by the use of open-label haloperidol in the placebo and ziprasidone groups.

A Cochrane review comparing efficacy and the incidence of adverse effects between haloperidol and atypical antipsychotics concluded that, similar to haloperidol, selected newer atypical antipsychotics (risperidone, olanzapine) were effective in managing delirium.[91] Haloperidol doses greater than 4.5 mg/day were more likely to result in increased rates of extrapyramidal symptoms compared with atypical antipsychotics, but low-dose haloperidol (i.e., less than 3.5 mg/day) did not result in a greater frequency of extrapyramidal adverse effects.[91] The APA guidelines for the treatment of delirium recommend use of low-dose haloperidol (i.e., 1–2 mg PO every 4 hours as needed, or 0.25–0.5 mg PO every 4 hours for the elderly) as the treatment of choice in cases where medications are necessary.[9]

Based on the existing literature, risperidone may be used in the treatment of delirium, starting at doses ranging from

0.25 to 1 mg and titrated up as necessary, with particular attention to the risks of extrapyramidal symptoms (EPS), orthostatic hypotension, and sedation at higher doses. Olanzapine can be started at between 2.5 and 5 mg nightly and titrated up with sedation being the major limiting factor, which may be favorable in the treatment of hyperactive delirium. The current literature on the use of quetiapine suggests a starting dose of 25 to 50 mg and a titration up to 100 to 200 mg a day (usually at twice-daily divided doses). Sedation and orthostatic hypotension are the main dose-limiting factors. Case reports suggest a starting dose of 10 to 15 mg daily for aripiprazole, with a maximum dose of 30 mg daily.[10,58,92] Olanzapine, aripiprazole, and ziprasidone are available in intramuscular form. However, no published trials have assessed the efficacy and safety of intramuscular forms of any of those medications in the treatment of delirium.

Important considerations in starting treatment with any antipsychotic for delirium may include EPS risk, sedation, anticholinergic side effects, cardiac arrhythmias, and possible drug-drug interactions. The FDA has issued a "black box" warning of increased risk of death associated with the use of typical and atypical antipsychotics in elderly patients with dementia-related psychoses.[112,113] The initial warning for atypical antipsychotics was based on a meta-analysis by Schneider et al.[114] of 17 placebo-controlled trials involving patients with dementia. The risk of death in patients treated with atypical antipsychotic agents was 1.6 to 1.7 times greater than in those who received placebo. Most deaths were associated with cardiovascular disease or infection. A second, retrospective study of nearly 23,000 older patients found higher mortality rates associated with typical than with atypical antipsychotics—whether or not patients had dementia.[115] This finding has led to an extension of the FDA warning to typical antipsychotics. A retrospective study comparing the mortality risk among elderly patients with delirium who were treated with antipsychotics versus those who did not receive antipsychotics did not find an increased risk of mortality with the use of antipsychotics in this patient population.[116]

Psychostimulants

Some clinicians have suggested that the hypoactive subtype of delirium may respond to psychostimulants such as methylphenidate, or combinations of antipsychotics and psychostimulants or antipsychotics and wakefulness agents such as modafinil.[117,118] Studies with psychostimulants in treating delirium are limited to case reports and one open-label study.[117,118] No randomized controlled trials have supported the use of psychostimulants in the treatment of delirium. The risks of precipitating agitation and exacerbating psychotic symptoms should be carefully evaluated when psychostimulants are considered in the treatment of delirium in cancer patients.

Cholinesterase inhibitors

Impaired cholinergic function has been implicated as one of the final common pathways in the neuropathogenesis of delirium, which led researchers to consider cholinesterase inhibitors as a treatment option for delirium.[32] Despite case reports of beneficial effects of donepezil and rivastigmine in the treatment of delirium, a Cochrane review concluded that currently no evidence from controlled trials supports the use of cholinesterase inhibitors in the treatment of delirium.[119–121]

Dexmedetomidine

Dexmedetomidine, a selective alpha-2 agonist with sedative and analgesic properties, has been shown to decrease the prevalence and duration of delirium in mechanically ventilated patients in open-label trials.[122] In an open-label study among 20 patients in the ICU with hyperactive delirium, dexmedetomidine was found to shorten the time to extubation and to decrease the length of stay in the ICU when compared with haloperidol.[123] A double-blind, randomized controlled trial comparing the efficacy and safety of sedation with dexmedetomidine versus midazolam for mechanically ventilated patients assessed the prevalence and duration of delirium as secondary outcome measures of the study. The prevalence of delirium was 54% (n = 244) in the dexmedetomidine-treated group compared with 76.6% (n = 122) in the midazolam-treated group (difference 22.6% [95% CI, 14%–33%]; $P < .001$). Patients treated with dexmedetomidine had more delirium-free days than those treated with midazolam (2.5 days vs. 1.7 days; $P = .002$).[124] The use of dexmedetomidine in the treatment of delirium among mechanically ventilated ICU patients was associated with an increased number of delirium-free days compared with lorazepam-treated patients in a randomized controlled trial.[125] It is important to note that dexmedetomidine has been studied primarily for use in sedation of critically ill patients in ICU settings; the feasibility of its use in the treatment of delirium in palliative care settings or in palliative sedation remains to be explored.

Benzodiazepines

Benzodiazepines are commonly used in the treatment and prevention of alcohol withdrawal delirium. A controlled trial comparing the effectiveness of lorazepam, haloperidol, and chlorpromazine in the treatment of delirium among hospitalized AIDS patients has shown increased confusion associated with the use of lorazepam.[59] A systematic review of the use of benzodiazepines in the treatment of delirium that is not related to alcohol or benzodiazepine withdrawal concluded that no controlled trials support the use of benzodiazepines.[126]

CONTRIBUTION OF DELIRIUM TO PROGNOSIS

Delirium is an independent predictor of mortality in patients with advanced cancer, as well as among hospitalized patients.[5,21,127] Advanced age, greater cognitive impairment, and organ failure have been significantly associated with shorter survival among hospitalized palliative care patients with delirium.[61] Delirium in terminally ill cancer patients is also a reliable predictor of approaching death in the coming days to weeks.[30,128]

The death rates among hospitalized elderly patients with delirium over the 3-month postdischarge period range from 22% to 76%.[9] In the palliative care setting, several studies provide support that delirium reliably predicts impending death in patients with advanced cancer. Bruera and colleagues[84] demonstrated a significant association between delirium and increased risk of mortality within 4 weeks. Morita and colleagues[129] found that delirium predicted poor short-term prognosis in patients admitted to a hospice in Japan. Caraceni and colleagues[21] evaluated the impact of delirium on patients for whom chemotherapy was no longer considered effective and who had been referred to palliative care programs. Length of survival of patients with delirium differed significantly from those without delirium. Compared with an overall median survival of 39 days in their study, delirious patients died, on average, within 21 days.

Recognizing an episode of delirium, in the late phases of palliative care, is critically important in treatment planning and in advising family members on what to expect. If advanced care planning has not taken place before an episode of delirium in a terminally ill patient, it is often too late to do so. However, some patients with mild delirium can still participate in limited decisions such as naming a health care proxy. Additionally, given the fact that delirium is so common in the terminally ill, and is so often a harbinger of impending death, it is critical for the clinician to make every effort to ask the patient, while he or she has the capacity to make treatment decisions, about preferences for the management of delirium.[10]

CONTROVERSIES IN THE MANAGEMENT OF TERMINAL DELIRIUM

The use of antipsychotics and other pharmacologic agents in the management of delirium in the dying patient remain controversial.[16] Some controversy remains among different specialties regarding the pharmacologic management of terminal delirium. According to a survey of 270 physicians from different disciplines, medical oncologists were found to be more likely to manage terminal delirium with benzodiazepines or benzodiazepine and antipsychotic combinations. On the other hand, palliative care physicians were more likely to use antipsychotics to manage delirium symptoms, including the hypoactive subtype of delirium.[83] Researchers have argued that pharmacologic interventions are inappropriate in the dying patient. Delirium is viewed by some as a natural part of the dying process that should not be altered. In particular, some clinicians who care for the dying view hallucinations and delusions as an important element in the transition from life to death. Clearly, many patients experience hallucinations and delusions during delirium that are pleasant and in fact comforting, and many clinicians question the appropriateness of intervening pharmacologically in such instances. Another concern is that these patients are so close to death that aggressive treatment is unnecessary, and antipsychotics or sedatives may be mistakenly avoided because of exaggerated fears that they might hasten death through hypotension or respiratory depression.[16]

Clinical experience in managing delirium in dying patients suggests that the use of antipsychotics in the management of agitation, paranoia, hallucinations, and altered sensorium is safe, effective, and often quite appropriate. Management of delirium on a case-by-case basis seems wise. The agitated, delirious dying patient should probably be given antipsychotics to help restore calm. A "wait-and-see" approach may be appropriate with some patients who have a lethargic or somnolent presentation of delirium, or who are having frankly pleasant or comforting hallucinations. However, this wait-and-see approach must be tempered by the knowledge that a lethargic or hypoactive delirium may very quickly and unexpectedly become an agitated or hyperactive delirium that can threaten the serenity and safety of the patient, family, and staff. It is important to remember that, by their nature, the symptoms of delirium are unstable and fluctuate over time.[16]

Perhaps the most challenging clinical problem is the management of the dying patient with a terminal delirium that is unresponsive to standard pharmacologic interventions. Approximately 30% of dying patients with delirium do not have their symptoms adequately controlled by antipsychotic medications.[130–132] In such cases, a reasonable choice is the use of sedative agents such as benzodiazepines (e.g., midazolam, lorazepam), propofol, or opioids.[130–132] In studies on the use of palliative sedation for symptom control, delirium was identified as the target symptom in up to 82% of cases.[130,131,133] Clinicians are sometimes concerned that the use of sedating medications may hasten death via respiratory depression, hypotension, or even starvation. However, studies have found that the use of opioids and psychotropic agents in hospice and palliative care settings is associated with longer rather than shorter survival.[131–137] Ethical concerns related to palliative sedation have been reviewed by Lo and Rubenfeld.[138]

Before undertaking interventions such as midazolam or propofol infusions, where the best achievable goal is a calm, comfortable, but sedated and unresponsive patient, the clinician must first take several steps. The clinician must have a discussion with the family (and the patient if there are lucid moments when the patient appears to have capacity), eliciting their concerns and wishes for the type of care that can best honor their desire to provide comfort and symptom control during the dying process. The clinician should describe the optimal achievable goals of therapy as they currently exist. Family members should be informed that the goal of sedation is to provide comfort and symptom control and not to hasten death. The distress and confusion that family members can experience during such a period can be ameliorated by including the family in the decision making and by emphasizing shared goals of care. Sedation in such patients is not always complete or irreversible; some patients have periods of wakefulness despite sedation, and many clinicians periodically lighten sedation to reassess the patient's condition.[10]

Ultimately, the clinician must always keep in mind the goals of care and communicate these goals to staff, patients, and family members. The clinician must weigh each of the issues outlined here in making decisions on how to best manage the dying patient who presents with delirium in a way that preserves and respects the dignity and values of that individual and family.[10]

PREVENTION OF DELIRIUM

Several researchers have studied both pharmacologic and nonpharmacologic interventions in the prevention of delirium among older patient populations, particularly in surgical settings.[139–144] The applicability of these interventions to the prevention of delirium in cancer patients or in palliative care settings has not been studied.

Antipsychotic medications (i.e., haloperidol) and cholinesterase inhibitors (donepezil and rivastigmine) have been studied in randomized controlled trials for their effectiveness in the prevention of postoperative delirium. Both groups of medications have failed to reduce the incidence of delirium in patients undergoing elective cardiac or joint replacement surgery.[139,140,144] Geriatric consultations and a multicomponent intervention program have reported reduced numbers and duration of episodes of delirium among hospitalized older patients. However, a systematic review of all existing delirium prevention studies concluded that current evidence on the effectiveness of interventions to prevent delirium was limited.[142] In a randomized, placebo-controlled, double-blind clinical trial in elderly hip surgery patients, low-dose haloperidol (1.5 mg/day) prophylaxis was not found effective for the prevention of postoperative delirium; however, it markedly reduced the severity and duration of delirium, and no drug-related side effects were noted.[144]Two randomized placebo-controlled prevention trials with donepezil among surgical patients undergoing total joint replacement surgery failed to show a difference in the incidence of delirium and the duration of hospitalization.[139,140] In another randomized controlled trial, proactive geriatric consultations (mainly nonpharmacologic interventions) were found to be effective in reducing the incidence and severity of delirium in a population of patients undergoing surgery for hip fracture.[143] Inouye and colleagues[141] reported on a successful multicomponent intervention program to prevent delirium

in hospitalized older patients. This program focused on a set of risk factors that were highly predictive of delirium in the elderly, including preexisting cognitive impairment, visual impairment, hearing impairment, sleep deprivation, immobility, dehydration, and severe illness. Interventions directed at constant orientation, correction of hearing and visual impairment, reversal of dehydration, and early mobilization appeared to significantly reduce the number and duration of episodes of delirium in hospitalized older patients.

CONCLUSION

Clinicians commonly encounter delirium as a major complication of cancer and its treatments, particularly in palliative care settings. Proper assessment, timely diagnosis, and management of delirium are essential in improving quality of life and minimizing morbidity in cancer patients, as well as in reducing distress among families and caregivers.

REFERENCES

1. Gaudreau JD, Gagnon P, Harel F, et al. Psychoactive medications and risk of delirium in hospitalized cancer patients. *J Clin Oncol.* 2005;23:6712–6718.
2. Lawlor PG, Gagnon B, Mancini IL, et al. Occurrence, causes, and outcome of delirium in patients with advanced cancer: a prospective study. *Arch Intern Med.* 2000;160:786–794.
3. Ljubisavljevic V, Kelly B. Risk factors for development of delirium among oncology patients. *Gen Hosp Psychiatry.* 2003;25:345–352.
4. Morita T, Tei Y, Tsunoda J, et al. Underlying pathologies and their associations with clinical features in terminal delirium of cancer patients. *J Pain Symptom Manage.* 2001;22:997–1006.
5. Spiller JA, Keen JC. Hypoactive delirium: assessing the extent of the problem for inpatient specialist palliative care. *Palliat Med.* 2006;20:17–23.
6. Stiefel FC, Breitbart WS, Holland JC. Corticosteroids in cancer: neuropsychiatric complications. *Cancer Invest.* 1989;7:479–491.
7. Inouye SK. Delirium in older persons. *N Engl J Med.* 2006;354:1157–1165.
8. American Psychiatric Association. *Diagnostic and statistical manual of mental disorders.* 4th ed. text revision. Washington, DC: American Psychiatric Association Press; 2000.
9. American Psychiatric Association. Practice guidelines for the treatment of patients with delirium. *Am J Psychiatry.* 1999;156:S1–S20.
10. Breitbart W, Alici Y. Agitation and delirium at the end of life: "we couldn't manage him." *JAMA.* 2008;300:2898–2910.
11. Bruera E, Fainsinger RL, Miller MJ, et al. The assessment of pain intensity in patients with cognitive failure: a preliminary report. *J Pain Symptom Manage.* 1992;7:267–270.
12. Coyle N, Breitbart W, Weaver S, et al. Delirium as a contributing factor to "crescendo" pain: three case reports. *J Pain Symptom Manage.* 1994;9:44–47.
13. Gagnon B, Lawlor PG, Mancini IL, et al. The impact of delirium on the circadian distribution of breakthrough analgesia in advanced cancer patients. *J Pain Symptom Manage.* 2001;22:826–833.
14. Breitbart W, Gibson C, Tremblay A. The delirium experience: delirium recall and delirium-related

distress in hospitalized patients with cancer, their spouses/caregivers, and their nurses. *Psychosomatics.* 2002;43:183–194.
15. Morita T, Hirai K, Sakaguchi Y, et al. Family-perceived distress from delirium-related symptoms of terminally ill cancer patients. *Psychosomatics.* 2004;45:107–113.
16. Breitbart W, Friedlander M. Confusion/delirium. In: Bruera E, Higginson I, Ripamonti C, et al., eds. *Palliative medicine.* London, UK: London Hodder Press; 2006:688–700.
17. Bruera E, Bush SH, Willey J, et al. Impact of delirium and recall on the level of distress in patients with advanced cancer and their family caregivers. *Cancer.* 2009;115:2004–2012.
18. Bush SH, Bruera E. The assessment and management of delirium in cancer patients. *Oncologist.* 2009;14:1039–1049 Epub 2009 Oct 6.
19. Siddiqi N, House AO, Holmes JD. Occurrence and outcome of delirium in medical in-patients: a systematic literature review. *Age Ageing.* 2006;35:350–364 Epub 2006 Apr 28.
20. Pautex S, Herrmann FR, Zulian GB. Factors associated with falls in patients with cancer hospitalized for palliative care. *J Palliat Med.* 2008;11:878–884.
21. Caraceni A, Nanni O, Maltoni M, et al. Impact of delirium on the short term prognosis of advanced cancer patients. Italian Multicenter Study Group on Palliative Care. *Cancer.* 2000;89:1145–1149.
22. Caraceni A, Simonetti F. Palliating delirium in patients with cancer. *Lancet Oncol.* 2009;10:164–172.
23. Folstein MF, Bassett SS, Romanoski AJ, et al. The epidemiology of delirium in the community: the Eastern Baltimore Mental Health Survey. *Int Psychogeriatr.* 1991;3:169–176.
24. Warshaw GA, Moore JT, Friedman SW, et al. Functional disability in the hospitalized elderly. *JAMA.* 1982;248:847–850.
25. Tune LE. Postoperative delirium. *Int Psychogeriatr.* 1991;3:325–332.
26. Massie MJ, Holland J, Glass E. Delirium in terminally ill cancer patients. *Am J Psychiatry.* 1983;140:1048–1050.
27. Pereira J, Hanson J, Bruera E. The frequency and clinical course of cognitive impairment in patients with terminal cancer. *Cancer.* 1997;79:835–842.

28. Centeno C, Sanz A, Bruera E. Delirium in advanced cancer patients. *Palliat Med.* 2004;18:184–194.
29. Minagawa H, Uchitomi Y, Yamawaki S, et al. Psychiatric morbidity in terminally ill cancer patients: a prospective study. *Cancer.* 1996;78:1131–1137.
30. Casarett DJ, Inouye SK. American College of Physicians-American Society of Internal Medicine End-of-Life Care Consensus Panel. Diagnosis and management of delirium near the end of life. *Ann Intern Med.* 2001;135:32–40.
31. Gagnon P, Allard P, Mâsse B, et al. Delirium in terminal cancer: a prospective study using daily screening, early diagnosis, and continuous monitoring. *J Pain Symptom Manage.* 2000;19:412–426.
32. Trzepacz PT. Is there a final common neural pathway in delirium? Focus on acetylcholine and dopamine. *Semin Clin Neuropsychiatry.* 2000;5:132–148.
33. Meagher DJ, Moran M, Raju B, et al. Phenomenology of delirium: assessment of 100 adult cases using standardised measures. *Br J Psychiatry.* 2007;190:135–141.
34. Trzepacz PT. Update on the neuropathogenesis of delirium. *Dement Geriatr Cogn Disord.* 1999;10:330–334.
35. Gaudreau JD, Gagnon P. Psychotogenic drugs and delirium pathogenesis: the central role of the thalamus. *Med Hypotheses.* 2005;64:471–475.
36. Trzepacz PT. The neuropathogenesis of delirium: a need to focus our research. *Psychosomatics.* 1994;35:374–391.
37. Karlsson I. Drugs that induce delirium. *Dement Geriatr Cogn Disord.* 1999;10:412–415.
38. Tune LE, Egeli S. Acetylcholine and delirium. *Dement Geriatr Cogn Disord.* 1999;10:342–344.
39. Rudorfer MV, Manji HK, Potter WZ. Bupropion, ECT, and dopaminergic overdrive. *Am J Psychiatry.* 1991;148:1101–1102.
40. Wetli CV, Mash D, Karch SB. Cocaine-associated agitated delirium and the neuroleptic malignant syndrome. *Am J Emerg Med.* 1996;14:425–428.
41. Ishihara K, Sasa M. Mechanism underlying the therapeutic effects of electroconvulsive therapy (ECT) on depression. *Jpn J Pharmacol.* 1999;80:185–189.

42. Inouye SK, Ferrucci L. Elucidating the pathophysiology of delirium and the interrelationship of delirium and dementia. *J Gerontol A Biol Sci Med Sci*. 2006;61:1277–1280.

43. Trzepacz P, van der Mast R. The neuropathophysiology of delirium. In: Lindesay J Rockwood K, Macdonald A, eds. *Delirium in old age*. Oxford, UK: Oxford University Press; 2002:51–90.

44. Adamis D, Treloar A, Martin FC, et al. APOE and cytokines as biological markers for recovery of prevalent delirium in elderly medical inpatients. *Int J Geriatr Psychiatry*. 2007;22:688–694.

45. de Rooij SE, van Munster BC, Korevaar JC, et al. Cytokines and acute phase response in delirium. *J Psychosom Res*. 2007;62:521–525.

46. Meagher DJ, Trzepacz PT. Delirium phenomenology illuminates pathophysiology, management, and course. *J Geriatr Psychiatry Neurol*. 1998;11:150–156.

47. Leentjens AF, Schieveld JN, Leonard M, et al. A comparison of the phenomenology of pediatric, adult, and geriatric delirium. *J Psychosom Res*. 2008;64:219–223.

48. Gagnon PR. Treatment of delirium in supportive and palliative care. *Curr Opin Support Palliat Care*. 2008;2:60–66.

49. Lipowski ZJ. *Delirium: acute confusional states*. New York: Oxford University Press; 1990.

50. Ross CA, Peyser CE, Shapiro I, et al. Delirium: phenomenologic and etiologic subtypes. *Int Psychogeriatr*. 1991;3:135–147.

51. Meagher DJ, O'Hanlon D, O'Mahony E, et al. Relationship between symptoms and motoric subtype of delirium. *J Neuropsychiatry Clin Neurosci*. 2000;12:51–56.

52. Stagno D, Gibson C, Breitbart W. The delirium subtypes: a review of prevalence, phenomenology, pathophysiology, and treatment response. *Palliat Support Care*. 2004;2:171–179.

53. Mittal D, Majithia D, Kennedy R, et al. Differences in characteristics and outcome of delirium as based on referral patterns. *Psychosomatics*. 2006;47:367–375.

54. Fang CK, Chen HW, Liu SI, et al. Prevalence, detection and treatment of delirium in terminal cancer inpatients: a prospective survey. *Jpn J Clin Oncol*. 2008;38:56–63.

55. de Rooij SE, Schuurmans MJ, van der Mast RC, et al. Clinical subtypes of delirium and their relevance for daily clinical practice: a systematic review. *Int J Geriatr Psychiatry*. 2005;20:609–615.

56. Peterson JF, Pun BT, Dittus RS, et al. Delirium and its motoric subtypes: a study of 614 critically ill patients. *J Am Geriatr Soc*. 2006;54:479–484.

57. Kiely DK, Jones RN, Bergmann MA, et al. Association between psychomotor activity delirium subtypes and mortality among newly admitted postacute facility patients. *J Gerontol A Biol Sci Med Sci*. 2007;62:174–179.

58. Seitz DP, Gill SS, van Zyl LT. Antipsychotics in the treatment of delirium: a systematic review. *J Clin Psychiatry*. 2007;68:11–21.

59. Breitbart W, Marotta R, Platt M, et al. A double-blind trial of haloperidol, chlorpromazine, and lorazepam in the treatment of delirium in hospitalized AIDS patients. *Am J Psychiatry*. 1996;153:231–237.

60. Breitbart W, Tremblay A, Gibson C. An open trial of olanzapine for the treatment of delirium in hospitalized cancer patients. *Psychosomatics*. 2002;43:175–182.

61. Leonard M, Raju B, Conroy M, et al. Reversibility of delirium in terminally ill patients and predictors of mortality. *Palliat Med*. 2008;22:848–854.

62. DiMartini A, Dew MA, Kormos R, et al. Posttraumatic stress disorder caused by hallucinations and delusions experienced in delirium. *Psychosomatics*. 2007;48:436–439.

63. Buss MK, Vanderwerker LC, Inouye SK, et al. Associations between caregiver-perceived delirium in patients with cancer and generalized anxiety in their caregivers. *J Palliat Med*. 2007;10:1083–1092.

64. Smith M, Breitbart W, Platt M. A critique of instruments and methods to detect, diagnose, and rate delirium. *J Pain Symptom Manage*. 1994;10:35–77.

65. Trzepacz P, Baker R, Greenhouse J. A symptom rating scale of delirium. *Psychiatry Res*. 1988;23:89–97.

66. Trzepacz PT, Mittal D, Torres R, et al. Validation of the Delirium Rating Scale-revised-98: comparison with the delirium rating scale and the cognitive test for delirium. *J Neuropsychiatry Clin Neurosci*. 2001;13:229–242.

67. Breitbart W, Rosenfeld B, Roth A. The Memorial Delirium Assessment Scale. *J Pain Symptom Manage*. 1997;13:128–137.

68. Lawlor P, Nekolaichuck C, Gagnon B, et al. Clinical utility, factor analysis and further validation of the Memorial Delirium Assessment Scale (MDAS). *Cancer*. 2000;88:2859–2867.

69. Albert M, Levkoff S, Reilley C. The delirium symptom interview: an interview for the detection of delirium symptoms in hospitalized patients. *J Geriatr Psychiatry Neurol*. 1991;5:14–21.

70. Inouye B, Vandyck C, Alessi C. Clarifying confusion: the confusion assessment method, a new method for the detection of delirium. *Ann Intern Med*. 1990;113:941–948.

71. Hart R, Levenson J, Sessler C, et al. Validation of a cognitive test for delirium in medical ICU patients. *Psychosomatics*. 1996;37:533–546.

72. Ryan K, Leonard M, Guerin S, et al. Validation of the confusion assessment method in the palliative care setting. *Palliat Med*. 2009;23:40–45.

73. Folstein M, Folstein S, McHugh P. "Mini-Mental Status": a practical method for grading the cognitive state of patients for clinicians. *J Psychiatr Res*. 1975;12:189–198.

74. Nicholas LM, Lindsey BA. Delirium presenting with symptoms of depression. *Psychosomatics*. 1995;36:471–479.

75. Leonard M, Spiller J, Keen J, et al. Symptoms of depression and delirium assessed serially in palliative-care inpatients. *Psychosomatics*. 2009;50:506–514.

76. Boettger S, Passik S, Breitbart W. Delirium superimposed on dementia versus delirium in the absence of dementia: phenomenological differences. *Palliat Support Care*. 2009;7:495–500.

77. Morita T, Tei Y, Inoue S. Impaired communication capacity and agitated delirium in the final week of terminally ill cancer patients: prevalence and identification of research focus. *J Pain Symptom Manage*. 2003;26:827–834.

78. Morrison RS, Meier DE, Fischberg D, et al. Improving the management of pain in hospitalized adults. *Arch Intern Med*. 2006;166:1033–1039.

79. Bruera E, Macmillan K, Hanson J, et al. The cognitive effects of the administration of narcotic analgesics in patients with cancer pain. *Pain*. 1989;39:13–16.

80. Jackson N, Doherty J, Coulter S. Neuropsychiatric complications of commonly used palliative care drugs. *Postgrad Med J*. 2008;84:121–126 quiz 125.

81. Agar M, Currow D, Plummer J, et al. Changes in anticholinergic load from regular prescribed medications in palliative care as death approaches. *Palliat Med*. 2009;23:257–265.

82. Lawlor PG, Bruera ED. Delirium in patients with advanced cancer. *Hematol Oncol Clin North Am*. 2002;16:701–714.

83. Agar M, Currow D, Plummer J, et al. Differing management of people with advanced cancer and delirium by four sub-specialties. *Palliat Med*. 2008;22:633–640.

84. Bruera E, Miller L, McCallion J, et al. Cognitive failure in patients with terminal cancer: a prospective study. *J Pain Symptom Manage*. 1992;7:192–195.

85. Tuma R, DeAngelis L. Acute encephalopathy in patients with systemic cancer. *Ann Neurol*. 1992;39:13–16.

86. Cole MG, Ciampi A, Belzile E, et al. Persistent delirium in older hospital patients: systematic review of frequency and prognosis. *Age Ageing*. 2009;38:19–26.

87. Cole MG, McCusker J, Bellavance F, et al. Systematic detection and multidisciplinary care of delirium in older medical inpatients: a randomized trial. *CMAJ*. 2002;167:753–759.

88. Inouye SK, Zhang Y, Jones RN, et al. Risk factors for delirium at discharge: development and validation of a predictive model. *Arch Intern Med*. 2007;167:1406–1413.

89. Pitkälä KH, Laurila JV, Strandberg TE, et al. Multicomponent geriatric intervention for elderly inpatients with delirium: a randomized, controlled trial. *J Gerontol A Biol Sci Med Sci*. 2006;61:176–181.

90. Pitkala KH, Laurila JV, Strandberg TE, et al. Multicomponent geriatric intervention for elderly inpatients with delirium: effects on costs and health-related quality of life. *J Gerontol A Biol Sci Med Sci*. 2008;63:56–61.

91. Lonergan E, Britton AM, Luxenberg J, et al. Antipsychotics for delirium. *Cochrane Database Syst Rev*. 2007;(2) CD005594.

92. Boettger S, Breitbart W. Atypical antipsychotics in the management of delirium: a review of the empirical literature. *Palliat Support Care*. 2005;3:227–237.

93. Jackson KC, Lipman AG. Drug therapy for delirium in terminally ill patients. *Cochrane Database Syst Rev*. 2004;(2) CD004770.

94. Fernandez F, Holmes V, Adams F, et al. Treatment of severe refractory agitation with a haloperidol drip. *J Clin Psychiatry*. 1988;49:239–241.

95. Information for healthcare professionals: haloperidol (marketed as Haldol, Haldol Decanoate and Haldol Lactate). U.S. Food & Drug Administration Web page. Available at: http://www.fda.gov/CDER/DRUG/InfoSheets/HCP/haloperidol.htm.

96. Sipahimalani A, Massand P. Olanzapine in the treatment of delirium. *Psychosomatics*. 1998;39:422–430.

97. Kim KS, Pae CU, Chae JH, et al. An open pilot trial of olanzapine for delirium in the Korean population. *Psychiatry Clin Neurosci*. 2001;55:515–519.

98. Skrobik YK, Bergeron N, Dumont M, et al. Olanzapine vs haloperidol: treating delirium in a critical care setting. *Intensive Care Med*. 2004;30:444–449.

99. Liu CY, Juang Y, Liang H, et al. Efficacy of risperidone in treating the hyperactive symptoms of delirium. *Int Clin Psychopharmacol*. 2004;19:165–168.

100. Horikawa N, Yamazaki T, Miyamoto K, et al. Treatment for delirium with risperidone: results of a prospective open trial with 10 patients. *Gen Hosp Psychiatry*. 2003;25:289–292.

101. Mittal D, Jimerson N, Neely E, et al. Risperidone in the treatment of delirium: results from a prospective open-label trial. *J Clin Psychiatry*. 2004;65:662–667.

102. Parellada E, Baeza I, de Pablo J, et al. Risperidone in the treatment of patients with delirium. *J Clin Psychiatry*. 2004;65:348–353.

103. Schwartz TL, Masand PS. Treatment of delirium with quetiapine. *Prim Care Companion J Clin Psychiatry*. 2000;2:10–12.

104. Kim KY, Bader G, Kotlyar V, et al. Treatment of delirium in older adults with quetiapine. *J Geriatr Psychiatry Neurol*. 2003;16:29–31.

105. Leso L, Schwartz T. Ziprasidone treatment of delirium. *Psychosomatics*. 2002;43:61–62.

106. Young CC, Lujan E. Intravenous ziprasidone for the treatment of delirium in the intensive care unit. *Anesthesiology*. 2004;101:794–795.

107. Straker DA, Shapiro PA, Muskin PR. Aripiprazole in the treatment of delirium. *Psychosomatics*. 2006;47:385–391.

108. Han CS, Kim Y. A double-blind trial of risperidone and haloperidol for the treatment of delirium. *Psychosomatics*. 2004;45:297–301.

109. Hu H, Deng W, Yang H. A prospective random control study comparison of olanzapine and haloperidol in senile delirium. *Chongging Med J*. 2004;8:1234–1237.

110. Devlin JW, Roberts RJ, Fong JJ, et al. Efficacy and safety of quetiapine in critically ill patients with delirium: a prospective, multicenter, randomized, double-blind, placebo-controlled pilot study. *Crit Care Med*. 2010;38:419–427.

111. Girard TD, Pandharipande PP, Carson SS, et al. Feasibility, efficacy, and safety of antipsychotics for intensive care unit delirium: the MIND randomized, placebo-controlled trial. *Crit Care Med*. 2010;38:428–437.

112. U.S. Food and Drug Administration. *Deaths with antipsychotics in elderly patients with behavioral disturbances*. Silver Spring, MD: U.S. Food and Drug Administration; 2005. Available at: http://www.fda.gov/Drugs/DrugSafety/PublicHealthAdvisories/ucm053171.htm Accessed 13.02.10.

113. U.S. Food and Drug Administration. *Conventional antipsychotics—healthcare professional sheet text version*. Silver Spring, MD: U.S. Food and Drug Administration; 2008. Available at: http://www.fda.gov/Drugs/ResourcesForYou/HealthProfessionals/ucm124830.htm Accessed 13.02.10.

114. Schneider LS, Dagerman KS, Insel P. Risk of death with atypical antipsychotic drug treatment for dementia: meta-analysis of randomized placebo-controlled trials. *JAMA*. 2005;294:1934–1943.

115. Wang PS, Schneeweiss S, Avorn J, et al. Risk of death in elderly users of conventional vs atypical antipsychotic medications. *N Engl J Med*. 2005;353:2335–2341.

116. Elie M, Boss K, Cole MG, et al. A retrospective, exploratory, secondary analysis of the association between antipsychotic use and mortality in elderly patients with delirium. *Int Psychogeriatr*. 2009;21:588–592.

117. Keen JC, Brown D. Psychostimulants and delirium in patients receiving palliative care. *Palliat Support Care*. 2004;2:199–202.

118. Morita T, Otani H, Tsunoda J, et al. Successful palliation of hypoactive delirium due to multi-organ failure by oral methylphenidate. *Support Care Cancer*. 2000;8:134–137.

119. Mukadam N, Ritchie CW, Sampson EL. Cholinesterase inhibitors for delirium: what is the evidence? *Int Psychogeriatr*. 2008;20:209–218.

120. Overshott R, Karim S, Burns A. Cholinesterase inhibitors for delirium. *Cochrane Database Syst Rev*. 2008;(1) CD005317.

121. Kalisvaart CJ, Boelaarts L, de Jonghe JF, et al. Successful treatment of three elderly patients suffering from prolonged delirium using the cholinesterase inhibitor rivastigmine. *Ned Tijdschr Geneeskd*. 2004;148:1501–1504.

122. Maldonado JR, Wysong A, van der Starre PJ, et al. Dexmedetomidine and the reduction of postoperative delirium after cardiac surgery. *Psychosomatics*. 2009;50:206–217.

123. Reade MC, O'Sullivan K, Bates S, et al. Dexmedetomidine vs. haloperidol in delirious, agitated, intubated patients: a randomised open-label trial. *Crit Care*. 2009;13:R75.

124. Riker RR, Shehabi Y, Bokesch PM, et al. SEDCOM (Safety and Efficacy of Dexmedetomidine Compared With Midazolam) Study Group. Dexmedetomidine vs midazolam for sedation of critically ill patients: a randomized trial. *JAMA*. 2009;301:489–499.

125. Pandharipande PP, Pun BT, Herr DL, et al. Effect of sedation with dexmedetomidine vs lorazepam on acute brain dysfunction in mechanically ventilated patients: the MENDS randomized controlled trial. *JAMA*. 2007;298:2644–2653.

126. Lonergan E, Luxenberg J, Areosa Sastre A. Benzodiazepines for delirium. *Cochrane Database Syst Rev*. 2009;(4) CD006379.

127. Maltoni M, Caraceni A, Brunelli C, et al. Steering Committee of the European Association for Palliative Care. Prognostic factors in advanced cancer patients: evidence-based clinical recommendations—a study by the Steering Committee of the European Association for Palliative Care. *J Clin Oncol*. 2005;23:6240–6248.

128. Dhillon N, Kopetz S, Pei BL, et al. Clinical findings of a palliative care consultation team at a comprehensive cancer center. *J Palliat Med*. 2008;11:191–197.

129. Morita T, Tsunoda J, Inoue S, et al. Validity of the palliative performance scale from a survival perspective. *J Pain Symptom Manage*. 1999;18:2–3.

130. Fainsinger RL, Waller A, Bercovici M, et al. A multicentre international study of sedation for uncontrolled symptoms in terminally ill patients. *Palliat Med*. 2000;14:257–265.

131. Rietjens JA, van Zuylen L, van Veluw H, et al. Palliative sedation in a specialized unit for acute palliative care in a cancer hospital: comparing patients dying with and without palliative sedation. *J Pain Symptom Manage*. 2008;36:228–234.

132. Connor SR, Pyenson B, Fitch K, et al. Comparing hospice and nonhospice patient survival among patients who die within a three-year window. *J Pain Symptom Manage*. 2007;33:238–246.

133. Elsayem A, Curry Iii E, Boohene J, et al. Use of palliative sedation for intractable symptoms in the palliative care unit of a comprehensive cancer center. *Support Care Cancer*. 2009;17:53–59.

134. Sykes N, Thorns A. Sedative use in the last week of life and the implications for end-of-life decision making. *Arch Intern Med*. 2003;163:341–344.

135. Morita T, Chinone Y, Ikenaga M, et al. Efficacy and safety of palliative sedation therapy: a multicenter, prospective, observational study conducted on specialized palliative care units in Japan. *J Pain Symptom Manage*. 2005;30:320–328.

136. Bercovitch M, Adunsky A. Patterns of high-dose morphine use in a home-care hospice service: should we be afraid of it? *Cancer*. 2004;101:1473–1477.

137. Vitetta L, Kenner D, Sali A. Sedation and analgesia-prescribing patterns in terminally ill patients at the end of life. *Am J Hosp Palliat Care*. 2005;22:465–473.

138. Lo B, Rubenfeld G. Palliative sedation in dying patients: "We turn to it when everything else hasn't worked." *JAMA*. 2005;294:1810–1816.

139. Liptzin B, Laki A, Garb JL, et al. Donepezil in the prevention and treatment of post-surgical delirium. *Am J Geriatr Psychiatry*. 2005;13:1100–1106.

140. Sampson EL, Raven PR, Ndhlovu PN, et al. A randomized, double-blind, placebo-controlled trial of donepezil hydrochloride (Aricept) for reducing the incidence of postoperative delirium after elective total hip replacement. *Int J Geriatr Psychiatry*. 2007;22:343–349.

141. Inouye SK, Bogardus Jr ST, Charpentier PA, et al. A multicomponent intervention to prevent delirium in hospitalized older patients. *N Engl J Med*. 1999;340:669–766.

142. Siddiqi N, Stockdale R, Britton AM, et al. Interventions for preventing delirium in hospitalised patients. *Cochrane Database Syst Rev*. 2007;(2) CD005563.

143. Marcantonio ER, Flacker JM, Wright RJ, et al. Reducing delirium after hip fracture: a randomized trial. *J Am Geriatr Soc*. 2001;49:516–522.

144. Kalisvaart KJ, de Jonghe JF, Bogaards MJ, et al. Haloperidol prophylaxis for elderly hip-surgery patients at risk for delirium: a randomized placebo-controlled study. *J Am Geriatr Soc*. 2005;53:1658–1666.

54

Clinical counseling and applied psychotherapy in supportive oncology

David W. Kissane and Matthew Doolittle

High rates of distress are found in cancer care, with the need for all members of the treatment team to help ameliorate the suffering being experienced.[1] Existential distress with the fear of recurrence and dying, related uncertainty about what the future holds, and grief at loss and change are universally present at some level for all.[2] Specifically, between 15% and 40% of cancer patients will develop significant anxiety or depressive disorders, although rates of true major depression

are lower.[3] Caregivers and family members share in the distress of illness, are second-order patients in their own right, and are deserving of care from the whole team.[4] Person-centered, family-centered, and culturally sensitive philosophies of care must prevail.

The approach to counseling will vary depending on needs, the skills of the providers, and the service model in use at any treatment center. Comprehensive programs present broad psychoeducational and supportive approaches across disease teams, with all physicians, surgeons, nurses, and related psychosocial staff being skilled at patient and family support. More specialized psychological and psychiatric care is targeted to higher-risk individuals, couples, and families when distress is intense or psychiatric disorder emerges. Models of counseling can be applied individually or to couples, groups, and families, depending on clinical need and staffing availability.

In this chapter, we review common issues and concerns that suggest an indication for counseling, models of intervention that can be applied, techniques and process issues for clinicians who deliver counseling, and evidence of effective outcomes.

PATIENT ISSUES, CONCERNS, DIAGNOSES

Patients will often have a worry or concern, sometimes will complain of specific symptoms, and, more rarely, will present with a specific disorder. Whether their issue is buried among questions, presents as a perplexed look, or is directly raised as their current concern, the clinician needs to recognize the cues and respond to each request for help. Understanding each person and his or her gamut of life experiences, successes and failures, accomplishments and omissions, shame and secrets, and health and illness is central to being able to truly respond to this person as a unique individual within the family, culture, and social world.[5]

Clinicians will be helped by some organizational schema that helps them plan interventions in response to patient concerns. Themes are generally extracted as the clinician listens to the patient's narrative and are arranged into groups. Common themes relevant to supportive counseling include

(1) loss and change, (2) emotional response, (3) associated meaning, and (4) coping efforts. Grief at loss and change is universal and occurs on many levels at which the illness is experienced—loss of health, fitness, capacity, and functionality, through to loss of dreams, relationships, work, and multiple sources of fulfillment in life. Where the illness occurs within the life cycle also has major relevance to acceptance and coping. Clinicians do well to always ask how each patient is coping emotionally, and what attributions of meaning he or she is assigning to the illness. Offering a name for the coping style that is evident and validating its appropriateness are helpful ways to support the confidence of the patient in dealing with the disease.

The biopsychosocial model is an integrating framework for organizing the common issues that present for counseling. In oncology, the addition of an existential or spiritual dimension ensures the comprehensiveness of this approach. Table 54-1 illustrates the typical issues and concerns that arise.

In response to these challenges, counseling serves as an important part of treatment for five key groups in the oncology setting.

- *Help with coping:* The stress of the illness and its associated threats create the first group of patients who need assistance with coping. Emotions commonly experienced include worry, fear, limited understanding of the illness and its treatment, desire to make sense of the biology, impact of work and family, and feeling overwhelmed with it all. Patients can experience a new traumatic reaction from the illness or treatments, or the retriggering of existing trauma might occur. For instance, the exposure required for staging studies in breast cancer may trigger symptoms in a patient who has been sexually abused. Often, distress may not be burdensome during the active stage of treatment for serious illness, because multiple appointments and procedures prove containing and hope sustaining. However, during transition to survivorship, when treatments are reduced, symptoms may begin to appear or to worsen, and patients may perceive abandonment.

- *Preexisting psychiatric illness:* Patients who have been diagnosed with prior psychiatric illness are an important subset. Patients with mood or anxiety disorders will be vulnerable to recurrence, at risk for drug interactions, and in need of special expertise. In many cases, patients with established psychiatrists or therapists will continue to work with them; others will seek expert psycho-oncologic care. Patients with schizophrenic spectrum illnesses constitute a small but vulnerable subset. The common use of steroids in oncology creates a hazard for patients with bipolar disorder.

- *New psychiatric disorder:* Common diagnoses that arise in cancer care include adjustment disorders (e.g., intense grief, social withdrawal, demoralization), anxiety disorders (e.g., panic attacks), mood disorders (e.g., major depression, bipolar disorder), psychotic disorders (e.g., paranoid states), organic psychiatric disorders (e.g., delirium, frontal lobe syndrome), relational disorders (e.g., sexual dysfunction), and existential distress (e.g., obsessional control).

- *Couple or family needs:* The fourth group that may be referred for psychosocial intervention consists of those who have spousal or family issues. Relationships may be strained. Relatives may be distressed at impending loss, may have difficulty coping with caregiving, may feel angry or resentful about change, or may be concerned about exacerbation of existing relationship issues. Family members may also experience new psychiatric illness or increased difficulty in controlling a prior one. In addition, families may seek treatment, as interactions and resources are strained through care provision. Families with young children may seek help about what to tell their children about the illness. Teenage children can be challenged as they try to integrate the developmental tasks of adolescence with parental needs.

- *Professional caregivers and team support:* The challenges of death and dying are not limited to patients and families, as professionals in cancer care may be at risk for burnout.

Assessment and diagnosis should occur before specific counseling is undertaken, because planning for treatment

Table 54-1 The biopsychosocial and existential approach to patients and families

Biological	Psychological	Social	Existential
The cancer: stage, prognosis, genetics	*The person:* age, gender, self-esteem, confidence	*Role and occupation:* job, education level, lifestyle issues	*Life cycle:* meaning of illness, aging, youth
Symptoms: pain, dyspnea, fatigue, insomnia	*Distress:* grief, fear, depression, anxiety	*Culture:* health beliefs, attitudes, access to care	*Angst:* death anxiety, uncertainty, aloneness, global meaning
Functioning: frailty, disfigurement, disabilities, impairments	*Coping:* pessimist, fatalist, denier, stoic, courage, acceptance	*Family and friends:* level of support, marital/sexual relationships	*Spirituality:* use of religion, philosophy, freedom of choice, and mastery
Treatments: surgery, chemotherapy, hormone, radiation therapy	*Decision making:* level of understanding, goals of care, treatment adherence	*Instrumental care:* nursing, pharmacy, aids, appliances, respite needs	*Rituals:* prayer, church or temple, chaplain, community involvement
Outcomes: sepsis, anemia, DVT, cure or control	*Quality of life:* stigma, shame, traumatic	*Survivorship:* financial impact, burden, outcomes	*Dignity:* sense of respect and accomplishment

DVT, Deep vein thrombosis

flows naturally from the process of diagnosis. In a patient with a medical illness who is fatigued and has deficits in concentration, for instance, active listening and a thorough interview will allow the clinician to distinguish between medical symptoms and depression. In a patient who is frightened, delineating between an anxiety disorder and reasonable fear will clarify treatment choices. In a patient who is concerned about being a burden to family members, a detailed understanding of circumstances will allow a guilt-ridden depression to be distinguished from deep-seated deficits in self-esteem. The process of diagnosis and biopsychosocial formulation requires appreciation of the "four P's," that is, the factors predisposing to, precipitating, perpetuating, or protecting from distress or psychiatric illness. Appreciating how these elements interact through the discipline of professional diagnosis will allow careful selection of the most helpful aspects of psychosocial intervention.

Research has repeatedly highlighted how often psychiatric disorders are missed in cancer care.[6] Screening for distress as the sixth vital sign becomes an important mechanism to recognize and triage psychosocial care.[7] A randomized controlled trial of computer-assisted screening and referral for intervention has demonstrated an ability to reduce depressive symptoms in oncology outpatients.[8] Patients with mild levels of distress are often triaged to social workers; those with more severe levels of distress are assigned to psychology and psychiatry.

MODELS OF PSYCHOTHERAPY

Counselors choose strategies from a variety of schools of psychotherapy, applying their techniques eclectically to meet the predicaments, coping styles, and needs of any patient, couple, or family. Moreover, combinations of approach (e.g., individual and family therapy) may be needed, depending on circumstances. Let us consider each approach in turn.

PSYCHOEDUCATIONAL INTERVENTIONS

Psychoeducation, an organized process of imparting information about illness to sufferers, their families, and sometimes to staff members, is an element of virtually all types of therapy, and in some cases, it can be a modality in itself.[9] Studies of psychoeducation using successful acquisition of new knowledge as endpoints show good effect size in meta-analytic work.[10] Lack of information, particularly shortly after a grave or serious diagnosis, is a major unmet need and offers one of the clearest opportunities for intervention.[11] Quality of life for both patients and caregivers can be much improved by informing them about predictable symptoms or likely stages of illness. In particular, they can be reassured by learning about the likelihood of pain or other symptoms, and for those close to death, clear information about the physiologic changes that may attend death can relieve anxiety in the immediate term, and help the family better recognize the process of dying. In patients who are not hospitalized, advice about possible changes in condition or symptoms that should result in a return to inpatient care is both appropriate and tends to relieve anxiety. In general, psychoeducation seeks both to elicit and to predict questions and fears that patients may have, and seeks to identify and anticipate the needs of caregivers, identifying appropriate services and resources. Engaging patients and their families in this way in a discussion of pragmatic aspects of illness can lead to improved adherence to treatments that may be complicated and onerous.

SUPPORTIVE COUNSELING

Similar to psychoeducational approaches, the set of techniques that fall under the rubric "supportive" is utilized in nearly every therapeutic interaction. Supportive work focuses on active listening, clarification, and reflection with the purpose of emphasizing any evidence of strong coping and adaptive interactions to encourage and reinforce them, and thus increase the patient's sense of self-efficacy.[12] Such support can become meaningful only if it is plausible, that is, the reactions and suggestions of the therapist should occur in a setting of trust, established and maintained by the therapist's compassionate and reliable regard for suffering. The physical and psychological environment should invite the articulation of emotions and descriptions of behaviors and relationships. After a therapeutic alliance is established, the patient can be encouraged to realize and to mobilize supports through articulation of appropriate goals and improved coping with illness. In cases of grave illness, another role of supportive treatment is to "detoxify" death, that is, to help the patient observe the process of death as part of life—a part that can be managed admirably by the patient as it has been managed admirably by others.

Supportive-expressive group therapy

One notable form of structured supportive therapy, supportive-expressive group therapy (SEGT), has been used in the field of oncology to aid management of medical symptoms through a group process that creates a "medicalized" culture. Based on Yalom's work[13] in existential therapy and elaborated by David Spiegel and colleagues,[14] SEGT was devised with the goal of improving quality of life by establishing unique social supports to sustain advanced cancer patients through illness and death. Groups are larger than usual at 10 to 12 members to allow for absence due to illness, with new members joining 2 or 3 at a time to replace deceased members. As a way of emphasizing social support and group cohesion, therapists allow and even encourage contact among members outside of the group, with the understanding that members will discuss these out-of-session interactions and bring up relevant concerns during group time. Sessions generally take place weekly at a clinical location, but when a member becomes gravely ill, groups may meet at the hospital or at the home of the dying member to sustain their connectedness. Therapists and group members also routinely attend funerals. The effective group helps members move from a mindset of ambivalence about illness to one better focused on creative living, evidenced by humor, celebration, assertiveness, altruism, worthwhile pursuits, and eventually courageous acceptance of dying.[15] Co-therapy is essential for groups, allowing one therapist to have greater expertise about cancer and the other about psychotherapy, if this balance works. The primary task of the therapists is to ensure that feelings are shared alongside medical information, and that attitudes to treatment emerge in group discussions, allowing an appreciation of the diversity of views in the group and the modeling of alternative behavior and coping approaches. Although the long-term nature of the group allows members to observe a range of experiences and to recognize demoralization or "burnout," one danger of the long-term nature of the treatment is that group members will become complacent.

Rather than let the group function as just a social gathering, therapists are responsible for keeping the focus on cancer and on connectedness, both within and between members of the group and their families. Mature groups may be able to achieve these goals through genuine humor (not an expression of an awkward defensiveness), celebration of life's milestones, rehearsal of assertive and effective medical interactions, development of creativity in group members, altruism representing kindness to others to whom the members feel connected, and finally acceptance of dying with courage when that time finally comes.

Clinicians face the possibility of negative transference reactions that may be masked in the criticism of other doctors, as well as the risk of an idealized transference in which the therapist is given too much authority, with the possibility that the work of the group as well as the treatment of cancer may be impeded. These challenges can be further magnified by the relatively loose boundaries of the group work and the emotional intensity of death. Regular supervision and frequent coordination between co-therapists are therefore critical to this work. Early findings that similar forms of therapy were associated with increased survival have long been disconfirmed,[16,17] but the medicalizing approach in SEGT may promote treatment adherence.[18] Multiple studies have shown that SEGT improves quality of life in cancer patients and may reduce anxiety and depression.[19,20] Indeed, the Melbourne-based SEGT study prevented new onset of depression compared with patients in the control arm.[18]

COGNITIVE-BEHAVIORAL THERAPY

The goal of the therapist in cognitive-behavioral therapy (CBT) is to act as a tutor or coach, helping the patient identify and document patterns connecting thoughts, feelings or sensations, and actions. Through a collaborative approach and Socratic questioning, "negative automatic thoughts" are identified, along with a connection to the patient's behaviors and feelings.[21] By recording thoughts, feelings, and actions as they occur on a daily basis, the patient is guided in identifying maladaptive patterns and, during sessions and homework exercises, alternative thoughts and outcomes are imagined and rehearsed, leading the patient to a sense of mastery. Here is an illustrative example:

Mrs. T is a 49-year-old divorced, female patient, treated for stage III breast cancer, who also had a history of well-documented childhood sexual abuse. Post initial treatment, she began to experience pain in her neck, shortness of breath, and nightmares about her childhood trauma. She also began to avoid neighborhoods that were associated with the attack and eventually was unable to leave her house or to sleep for longer than 3 hours at a time. The physical symptoms correlated well with choking and other injuries sustained during the attacks, and the patient was diagnosed with posttraumatic stress disorder. She entered into structured CBT. She reported, "I shouldn't be feeling this way. I should be grateful that the cancer is under control," and "I just have to do this, I just have to feel differently." The identification of these cognitive distortions associated with her repeated use of the terms "should" and "have to" made up an important part of the treatment. By tracking the occurrence of these thoughts, she was able to identify an underlying fear that her teenage son would not love her if she were not a "perfect mother." Having cancer meant that "there's something wrong with me, my body isn't right. I'm not good enough. I'm not perfect." Through a graded series of exercises, she was able to leave the house for medical follow-ups and ultimately return to work.

General cognitive strategies for the treatment of anxiety and depression are readily adapted for use in supportive cancer care.[22] The focus is on identifying emotions and distress associated with illness, and using tracking, reframing, and grounding, relaxation, or breathing exercises and exposure to reduce symptoms. One traditional focus of CBT has been on identifying catastrophic thinking, mind reading, overgeneralization, and other maladaptive patterns, and using gentle but persistent questioning to encourage reality-based thinking.[23] Rather than assessing a thought for its logic or rationality, the standard of "Is this realistic?" is appropriate for cancer care. See examples in Table 54-2. In the medically ill, this exploration can be a sensitive process because the reality may not be comforting, but focusing on patterns that exacerbate anxiety, as well as on guilt, a sense of responsibility for being ill, fear of rejection by others, and fear of the process of death, may give the patient needed skills to develop active coping and face significant illness. Cognitively oriented group therapy has been applied to women with early-stage breast cancer.[24]

In addition, cancer or another grave diagnosis may be a schema-discrepant crisis, leaving patients with the deep belief that the entire world is a bad place, or that they are deeply flawed, with resulting anxiety and fear or pervasive guilt preventing them from engaging fully with the remainder of their lives. CBT has been shown to improve anxiety and depression in patients with cancer,[25,26] and more recent work has developed its role in the setting of palliative care.[27,28] For instance, one 16-week cluster randomized trial involving 80 patients in an inpatient hospice setting utilized simplified CBT delivered by clinical nurse specialists, and showed a reduction in anxiety but not in depression.[29] In the SMaRT (Symptom Management Research Trial) oncology trial,[30,31] 16% of participants had advanced cancer, and in the trial by Ell and colleagues,[32] 28% had metastatic disease. These collaborative care models, with strong contributions from nursing and a range of health professionals, use CBT principles as they seek to redress inadequate depression care. CBT interventions have much to offer, as they shift cognitive distortions and guide patients toward a more realistic appreciation of what is happening.

INTERPERSONAL PSYCHOTHERAPY

Interpersonal psychotherapy (IPT) focuses on improving patients' relationships, supporting their grief, and helping them to cope better through examination of life and its role transitions, any disrupted or contentious relationships, and any tendency to be overly sensitive.[33] In general, these latter vulnerabilities are addressed through a confident alliance with the therapist, and by coming to a detailed understanding of the role of trusting relationships and disrupted trust in the patient's biography. An interpersonal exploration of expectations and patterns of communication in both satisfactory and

Table 54-2 Examples from cognitively oriented therapy of realistic reframes used to counter the negative automatic thoughts found commonly in cancer care

Type of negative automatic thought (NAT)	Examples of NATs from patients	Examples of realistic cognitive reframes
1. *Catastrophization*—the worst case scenario is considered	"This cancer will gallop through me. My situation is hopeless. I'm sure to die soon."	"My cancer is indolent and well controlled by chemotherapy. I'll have a long life ahead."
2. *Magnification*—blowing out of perspective	"This backache will be the cancer back again. Here come the secondaries!"	"I've been straining my back doing the vacuuming. It will be gone tomorrow. I'll see my doctor if it persists next week."
3. *Pessimism*—predicting the future negatively	"My hair will fall out with chemotherapy, and then my husband will leave me."	"*Look good, feel better* teaches me confidence in wearing a wig. I'll maintain my femininity."
4. *Selective attention*—focused negativity	"The side effects of chemotherapy are certain to make me miserable."	"Chemotherapy is strong insurance. I'll put up with any side effects to gain this benefit."
5. *All-or-nothing thinking*—a black or white world	"If I can't be cured, there is no point in living anymore."	"Although incurable, my cancer can be managed as a chronic illness for several years."
6. *Habitual negative labeling*—repeatedly putting oneself down	"I'm useless. I'm such a coward. I can't cope with this pain."	"Inflammation from the radiation causes pain that can be controlled with painkillers."
7. *Expectations* declared through use of verbs "should" and "ought"—may be unreasonable	"I should be able to do all that I did before cancer. I'm so frustrated by this."	"The fatigue comes from a mild anemia due to the chemotherapy. Gentle exercise will protect against muscle wasting."
8. *Personalization*—taking responsibility when not appropriate	"All the stress in my life has caused this cancer. It's all my fault … I'm to blame."	"Random DNA changes cause cancer. It is an old myth that stress causes cancer."
9. *Emotional reasoning*—negative feelings serving as a causal basis for events	"Because I feel terrible, I must be performing so poorly at work. This cancer will cost me my job."	"My supervisor is very supportive. My self-esteem is separate from my job. I'll manage OK at work."
10. *Illogical thinking*—making flawed attributions	"If I can't feel better soon, I'll never get over this cancer."	"I need patience for the treatments to help. In time, I will feel stronger again."

unsatisfactory relationships may be helpful as patients strive to mend relationships. Role playing may be helpful both in bringing patterns to light and in modeling alternative behaviors, often in anticipation of joint sessions, when the patient is able to engage in interpersonal work directly.

The focus on role transitions involves identifying and reframing negative attitudes toward the anticipated role, and supporting self-esteem and mastery, with an emphasis on moving away from one thing and moving toward another. In the setting of palliative care, role transitions often involve loss of cherished aspects of identity and health, and the goal is to assist the patient in accepting some of the limitations of illness while not exaggerating the negative aspects of the new role or feeling helpless in the transition. This focused exploration using IPT is manageable in the setting of acute medical illness. IPT proved better than placebo in 8 of 13 studies.[34]

PSYCHODYNAMIC PSYCHOTHERAPY

Similar to supportive techniques, psychodynamic principles are used in almost every type of therapy, as the patterns of early parent-child relationships repeat themselves in later life.[35] In the setting of supportive care, dynamic approaches are most often used to identify and evaluate defenses that may be helping or harming the patient, and to work with transference and countertransference reactions.[36] In some cases, it may be possible to examine long-term conflicts with the hope of building understanding and resolution before the patient's death.

In existential work, the concept of self-awareness gives rise to a celebration of freedom and choices, but also an awareness of death.[13] The therapist helps the patient come to terms with losses, loneliness, demoralization, or spiritual despair by deploying confrontation and reaction formation, and inviting choice about those aspects of life that should be most valued. In other palliative care work informed by psychodynamic ideas, defenses may be adaptive or maladaptive, and the clinician's role is to respond to these defenses in a way that alleviates the patient's distress. In a gravely ill or dying patient, for instance, denial may be used intermittently in a manner that alleviates symptoms of depression, anxiety, or other distress, but also allows participation in care during those periods when denial is not so evident. Similarly, regression may be an adaptive response to the isolation and privations of illness. If, on the other hand, the patient's defenses prevent participation in care or necessary preparation for death, the defenses may become more of a focus of therapy, and education of treating clinicians about the role of the patient's defenses may be helpful.

Transference and countertransference are examined in the same way as would happen in the general setting, and often examination of these issues can guide even a brief treatment.

Anger, helplessness, and other negative emotions experienced by therapists treating critically ill patients may reflect the patient's own feelings and can thus increase understanding and focus treatment when time is short.

NARRATIVE THERAPIES

Narrative therapy seeks to help patients arrive at a methodical understanding of their life philosophies, values and accomplishments. The therapist listens to, evaluates, and then summarizes the patient's life story, affirming successful developments and cherished roles and relationships, and identifying patterns in accounts of past and present adversities that may finally allow a purpose to be discerned.[37] The process involves the therapist in much questioning, which helps the patient order his or her story, and reaches consensus about the sources of fulfillment and life's meaning.[38] This collaborative approach makes the therapist an editor and, in some cases, a scribe in the authorship of the patient's life story to achieve the central goal, which is to develop a narrative authentic to an individual patient.[39] Here is an illustrative case example:

> Mr. D. was a 54-year-old married male patient, who was diagnosed with pancreatic cancer. After many aggressive treatments, he was referred because of ongoing fatigue that spoiled life for him. Initially, treatment involved psychostimulants and antidepressants, but little gain was seen in his energy level. In reviewing his life as an accountant, he commented on adolescent dreams of becoming a photographer. The idea of creating a photo album to leave to his children held instant appeal. He asked his relatives to provide photographs for a book. As his interest grew, he retrieved his old camera and began photographing varied aspects of everyday life. Over several weeks, he engaged in the production of his album and eventually added a narrative, with his interest and energy invested in this blossoming. The patient's wife and children all worked with him to complete the project and expressed gratitude for this opportunity to reminisce together. Ten days after completing and sharing this legacy, he died.

Therapy that is informed in keeping with this philosophy of authenticity through the process of lending a voice to the patient has been studied increasingly, exemplified by the dignity-conserving and meaning-centered forms of psychotherapy discussed in the following section.

The incorporation of hope into narrative therapy has also been further developed. Some researchers have attempted to use formal measures to identify hope, for instance, finding that patients receiving palliative care did not score significantly differently from patients being treated curatively in their degree of hopefulness for cure, other positive health outcomes, emotional well-being, return to previous function, or interpersonal goals.[40] The theme of hope has then been incorporated into a treatment program, which includes watching an inspirational video and then engaging in hope-focused activities such as writing a letter, collecting objects associated with one's hope, and incorporating these into one's life story. More than 60% of patients undergoing the hope-generating exercises reported higher levels of hope.[41]

DIGNITY THERAPY

Building on work about the concept of the "good death" and on efforts to define and preserve quality of life, dignity-conserving treatment is designed to recognize that one's life has been and continues to be worthwhile, even though this may seem to be challenged by terminal illness.[42] Starting with the idea that sustaining self-worth and respect is critical to the goal of helping patients to die with dignity, and that this goal is the basic tenet of palliative care, researchers first developed a framework for evaluating and advancing dignity in terminal patients. An in-depth, qualitative study of 50 patients identified three major domains contributing to dignity: (1) *illness-related concerns,* including physical symptoms, cognitive and functional capacity, coping or psychological distress, and degree of uncertainty about medical elements or anxiety about death itself; (2) *dignity-conserving repertoire,* which includes a subjective sense of autonomy, resilience, acceptance of condition, and pride in past accomplishments, and the sense of continuity between those accomplishments and the present situation, that is, the ability to maintain a routine, to participate in spiritual life, and to live in the moment; and (3) *social dignity inventory,* primarily consisting of such environmental factors as social support and ability to maintain privacy, but also including subjective assessments of the current social condition of the patient, including the degree to which the patient feels a burden and the patient's concerns for the aftermath of death.[43] As a validation of this conceptualization of dignity, a further study involving 211 palliative care patients validated a quantitative measure, the Patient Dignity Inventory.[44]

Dignity therapy is a structured intervention designed to enhance the patient's sense of generativity by providing orderly assistance in the production of a legacy document to leave to those being left behind. Using a protocol consisting of 12 questions about their lives (Table 54-3), the therapist interviews patients believed to be near the end of life.[45] Patients are asked about when they felt most alive, their important roles and accomplishments, and the things that they may still wish to say to loved ones before they die. The videotape then is transcribed and read back to the patient, who joins with the therapist in a process of editing the narrative. At the end of this process, the final document is given to the patient, who may use it as a legacy for survivors. Whether in hospice or hospital, dignity therapy and related approaches to narrative psychotherapy offer important ways of reducing distress and providing tangible resources to assist not only patients but their survivors.

MEANING-CENTERED THERAPY

Meaning-centered psychotherapy is designed to renew a sense of purpose and moral connectedness with the world through a set of exercises emphasizing the articulation of experiences and the ability of such articulation to identify unique worth to which the patient may not previously have been paying attention. Breitbart and colleagues developed a psychoeducational model of meaning-centered group therapy from Victor Frankl's logotherapy, which emphasized the holistic nature of the person as a physical, psychological, and spiritual being.[46] Similar to logotherapy, meaning-centered

Table 54-3   Questions asked in dignity therapy

1. Can you tell me a little about your life history, particularly those parts that you remember most or think are the most important?

2. When did you feel most alive?

3. Are there specific things that you would want your family to know about you, and are there things you would want them to remember?

4. What are the most important roles (e.g., family, vocational, community service) that you have played in life?

5. Why are they so important to you, and what do you think you accomplished in those roles?

6. What are your most important accomplishments, and what do you feel most proud of?

7. Are there particular things that you feel still need to be said to your loved ones, or things that you would want to take the time to say once again?

8. What are your hopes and dreams for your loved ones?

9. What have you learned about life that you would want to pass along to others?

10. What advice or words of guidance would you wish to pass along to your____ (son, daughter, husband, wife, parents, other[s])?

11. Are there words or perhaps even instructions that you would like to offer your family, to provide them with comfort or solace?

12. Are there other things that you would like to include?

Reprinted from Chochinov HM, Hack T, Hazard T, et al.[42]

Table 54-4   Themes in Meaning-Centered Group Psychotherapy (MCGP) covered in weekly psychoeducational sessions

1. Concepts of meaning and sources of meaning

2. Cancer and meaning, meaning and the historical context of life

3. Storytelling and life project

4. Limitations and the finiteness of life

5. Responsibility, creativity, and deeds

6. Experience of nature, art, and humor

7. Goodbyes and hopes for the future

psychotherapy (MCGP) program are presented in Table 54-4. Acceptance of the reality of grave illness and working within that limitation to recognize unique and valuable aspects of experiences empower an active and creative response to each person's life. MCGP does not seek to be explicitly religious, but among patients who are religious, disruption of the human will to meaning may be experienced as a spiritual crisis or a crisis of faith. In people who are not religious, the same destruction may be experienced as purposelessness and hopelessness. The principles of MCGP have been applied not only to the treatment of the dying patient, but to the treatment of caregivers in palliative care as a strategy for preventing burnout. Initial studies, for instance, showed that a modified version of MCGP administered to palliative care nurses by licensed psychologists over four 2-hour sessions improved the nurses' tendency to perceive benefits of working in palliative care at 3-month follow-up, and all measures of quality of life were unaffected.[47] As a brief, structured intervention, MCGP might be well adapted to the palliative care setting logistically; further effectiveness studies are ongoing, and this is a promising area for future work.

psychotherapy proposes that the central aspect of human consciousness is the ability to find meaning, that all human beings seek to find this meaning—a "will to meaning"—and that all human beings have an inherent knowledge that life has meaning.[47,48] Logotherapy holds that human beings are not merely driven by events, but are naturally motivated to move toward something called *meaning,* the fulfillment of which can take place only with the exercise of one's basic will to make decisions and to take action. Within this framework, the word *meaning* not only refers to a set of cherished beliefs associated with positive emotions, but also includes a sense of motivation and striving toward valued goals. Meaning is thus expressed through creativity, or what material contribution people make to the world; through experience of the world (observing a sunset) that becomes consciously valued through attention (appreciating the beauty of the sunset as a joyful gift of life); and in the ability to accept the limitations of human life.[49]

Meaning-centered psychotherapy is delivered as a series of six to eight weekly, 90-minute sessions that include teaching on the philosophy of meaning, discussion of such topics as "the good death," engagement in experiential exercises intended to enhance participants' ability to attend to psychological and material observations, and home exercises that reinforce similar themes.[50] Key topics covered in the meaning-centered group

COUPLES THERAPY

The needs of patients and their partners are highly correlated and reciprocally interdependent.[51] The key targets of couples therapy in supportive oncologic care are relationship enhancement and protection against relational distress. Thus, the relationship serves as the main source of mutual support, and fostering open communication promotes mastery and improved coping. In the breast cancer setting, a randomized controlled trial of an active coping intervention for couples relative to usual care showed a reduction in women's depressive symptoms up to 6 months post treatment.[52] Couples therapy in prostate cancer is illustrated by the FOCUS intervention, which targets Family involvement, Optimistic attitude, Coping effectiveness, Uncertainty reduction, and Symptom management.[53] Spouses improved their quality of life and reduced hopelessness, likely gaining some protection against depressive outcomes.

Couples therapy promotes adaptation when changes in body image occur (e.g., mastectomy, colostomy, ileal conduit, limb amputation), sexuality is affected (e.g., erectile dysfunction after prostate cancer, dyspareunia after gynecologic cancers), infertility results (e.g., chemotherapy, castration surgery), or shame, guilt, despair, or depression arise, and the partner is a prime source of support. In the setting of advanced cancer, couples therapy shifts its emphasis to caregiving, anticipated loss, and existential concerns.[54] Despite the separation anxiety associated with the potential loss of a key attachment figure, emotion-focused couples therapy that seeks to address threats to emotional engagement by recognizing distancing interactions and promoting closeness was effective in reducing depression.[55]

Effective mutual support results when individuals in couples are securely attached to each other. In contrast, for the distressed couple, separation protest develops as a pattern of demand-withdraw, leading to disengagement and diminished safety, which increases risk. Couples therapy that identifies existential fears and supports intimacy in the face of death can do much to harness resilience and protect against demoralization and depression.

FAMILY THERAPY

Therapists may also choose to involve patients and caregivers directly in family treatments when end-of-life care warrants consideration, when children or adolescents are involved in the family, or when genetic issues have salience for those with familial disease. Work with the patient's nuclear family, siblings, parents, or entire family of origin may assist in the adjustment to changing goals and expectations, as well as in supporting grief in families of the critically ill.[56] In general, any family work would take into consideration that family members take on an important role in caring for patients, evaluating symptoms, and, in some cases, directly providing treatments.

Family systems theory recognizes the concept of homeostasis, or the pull to create a balance between change and stability. Attention to alliances and subsystems within the overall family hierarchy and awareness of the boundaries between these subsystems are critical for the therapist to remain neutral and to understand the family-as-a-whole. Transgenerational patterns of relating within families become evident across generations, as do the ways in which the illness of one family member may reinforce or change such patterns.[57]

Most families will function adequately when a member becomes ill, and will be able to manage grief effectively. However, vulnerable families may not be able to maintain connectedness or homeostasis during illness and bereavement, and significant suffering and morbidity may result. One model that provides a methodical way to identify vulnerable families and to train therapists and administer effective time-limited treatment is family-focused grief therapy (FFGT), which commences during palliative care and continues into bereavement.[58,59] By using the Family Relationships Index (FRI), a validated, 12-item, self-report measure, individual members of families are assessed, and their perspective of family functioning is scored on cohesion, communication, and conflict.[60] Therapists who undergo training in the manualized model meet with families 6 to 10 times over 6 to 18 months for 90-minute sessions. The assessment phase takes place over two weekly sessions and allows identification of family patterns and concerns, leading to the development of the treatment plan collaboratively with the family. The intervention phase consists of 4 to 6 monthly sessions during which the treatment plan is put into action, with particular focus on improving communication, enhancing cohesiveness, fostering conflict resolution, and promoting shared grief. One or two termination sessions occur as more widely spaced booster sessions over the next 4 to 6 months to allow review and articulation of progress and desired change.

In a randomized controlled trial of FFGT targeting "at risk" families preventively, family therapy that aimed to optimize family functioning through promotion of effective communication, enhanced cohesion, and adaptive resolution of conflict was shown to reduce depression and support mourning arising from family loss due to cancer.[61] The more pronounced the relational dysfunction, the greater the number of family sessions that are needed across the bereavement phase. In general, mild family dysfunction can be aided by 4 to 6 sessions, whereas 10 to 12 sessions are likely needed for those with pronounced dysfunction. Openness to discussion of death and dying and early containment of conflict prove beneficial, until improved communication and closeness help family members to tolerate any differences of opinion.[62] Therapists make use of circular questions to reveal family dynamics and offer regular summaries as a means to help families integrate understanding of their patterns of relating and coping with loss and change.[63] Commencing therapy with the cancer patient still alive and present to voice his or her opinion establishes a model of family care that is preventive and cost-effective and enables continuity of support to be carried into bereavement.

A schema for running a family meeting is presented in Table 54-5. The facilitator moves from direct linear questions that seek information from an individual, to sequentially constructed circular questions that ask family members to express opinions about one another. Inviting this reflection about how members are coping generally fosters a dynamic of mutual support as the family-as-a-whole begins to consider its overall functioning, teamwork, and problem-directed activities. Therapists avoid giving the family advice, remain neutral in not taking the side of any member, and through asking questions, encourage family members to seek solutions and reflect more deeply as to how they could respond as a group to the predicament under review. As the family becomes more generative in the direction of its problem solving, the therapist affirms that movement as creative and likely beneficial.

When families have very high levels of conflict and hostility that have resulted in considerable alienation and separation, the goals of any family work need to be modest. In practice, progress will often occur only with an available subgroup of the family. Clinicians do well to avoid unrealistic rescue fantasies. Moreover, distance between family members may be an effective solution for families unable to tolerate differences. On the other hand, families with less openly expressed anger but with poor communication and reduced cohesion may benefit significantly from an intervention such as FFGT.

COLLABORATIVE TEAM CARE MODELS OF SUPPORT

Recently, supportive care approaches have been enriched by a series of projects (e.g., SMaRT oncology) demonstrating the effectiveness of collaborative care.[64-65] Elements of collaborative care incorporated into problem-solving therapy (PST) include the use of clinic distress screening to identify depressed patients,[54] communication with primary care doctors and oncologists about the patient's depressive symptoms,[54] use of trained health professionals from social work, nursing, and psychiatry in the delivery of manualized

Table 54-5   Guidelines for running family meetings in supportive care

Strategy of therapist	Example of questions or comments
1. Establish meeting goals and shared agenda with the family.	• In meeting together, we want to reach consensus about our goals of care for [patient's name]. • Do any of you have questions or concerns that you'd like us to talk about?
2. Clarify seriousness of illness and current goals of care.	• [Name of offspring or partner], tell me what you understand about the seriousness of X's cancer. Ask family members sequentially. • [Patient's name], how well has your family grasped what is happening with your illness? • Can any of you tell me what the goal of our current treatment is?
3. Check for issues/symptoms of concern.	• Are there key symptoms that are a concern to any of you? • What is most challenging in caring for [patient's name]?
4. Clarify family's view of future.	• Has it been possible to talk about [patient's name] wishes toward the end of life? • Appoint a health care proxy? • Have you made an advance directive that tells the family about your wishes in the event of complications, or if you are dying? • What are your thoughts about dying at home versus dying in hospital?
5. Review coping/emotions.	• [Patient's name], how is your partner coping? How will he/she manage in the future? • [Partner's name], how is X coping? • How does the family know when to be strong and when to talk about your fears? • Is there the potential to grow closer, or do different styles need to be respected? • How do you resolve differences of opinion?
6. Create mutually agreed upon plans.	• We are actively treating the pain and helping X set the right pace to manage the fatigue. You've built a roster to better coordinate your support. I want to congratulate you on the teamwork I see emerging and how openly you've talked about the challenges and fears.
7. Check understanding and summarize.	• Before we close, let's review our understanding of the goals of care and treatment plans. [Name of partner], can you summarize what you understand our goals of care to be? • We are working as a team here to support [name of patient] with this illness and to optimize his/her quality of life so that life can be lived out fully and well. Our control of [key symptoms] is a prime target here. We'll review how our medication adjustments work out in the days ahead. I'm there for you all and want you not to hesitate to contact me if new concerns emerge.

psychosocial and pharmacologic treatment,[54,67] patient monitoring after treatment end,[54,57] and assistance in navigating and accessing community services.[57] The use of social workers and nurses in the delivery of PST also increases the feasibility of interventions in institutions with limited resources and staffing for psychosocial care. Another collaborative care model developed in Toronto is Managing **C**ancer **A**nd **L**iving **M**eaningfully (CALM) therapy, which seeks to promote active coping strategies.

CALM THERAPY

CALM is an individual model of focused psychotherapy developed in Toronto, which was designed to address the specific problems and risk factors that contribute to distress and depressive symptoms[66] in patients with advanced disease, but with a life expectancy greater than 6 months. The model is based on several broad theoretical traditions, including attachment theory and existential psychotherapy.[67,68] It is important to note that it attends to symptom management and navigation of the health care system, while prioritizing attention to the emotional, existential, and meaning-based aspects of coping. Individual sessions can be complemented by couple or family work.

CALM is embedded within a collaborative care context and consists of 3 to 6 individual sessions delivered over 3 months, with 2 booster sessions offered in the subsequent 3 months. It comprises four empirically derived domains of concern (Table 54-6), which serve as a framework to address the common and interrelated stressors that patients with advanced cancer face.[69-70] The time devoted to each domain varies, based on the needs and concerns of the individual patient, who prioritizes the issues. Research has consistently highlighted that symptom management and effective relationships with health care providers, including clear communication, contribute to decision making and individualized care and are major concerns for patients facing advanced disease and the end of life.[72] Key attention to optimal symptom management is therefore imperative for other aspects of psychotherapeutic work to proceed.

Increased dependency and role and identity changes are common experiences of the advanced cancer patient. An individual's expectations of social support and his or her capacity to make use of this support, reflected in attachment style, have been shown to modulate the expression of distress. Practical issues such as division of household labor, financial responsibilities, and parenting roles intersect with a variety of relational themes connected to attachment security, intimacy, and

Table 54-6 Domains of focus in CALM therapy (Cancer And Living Meaningfully)

Domain of attention	Goals of therapy	Therapist activity	Desired outcomes
1. Optimal symptom management and effective communication with health care providers	To explore the experience of symptoms and to support active engagement in all treatment modalities, fostering a sense of partnership with the treatment team	• Therapist works to maintain a balanced patient perspective • Acts as an advocate between the patient and other caregivers	• Improved adherence to symptom management regimens • Improved teamwork; better coordination of care • Clearer agreement about the goals of care
2. Adaptation to any changes in self and relations with close others resulting from the illness	To explore altered body image and self-esteem, and alterations in social and intimate relationships resulting from the disease or its treatment	• Promote expressions of grief, and encourage coping strategies • Provide couples or family sessions to explore relational dynamics • Promote realistic acceptance of the challenges and tasks that lie ahead	• Better understanding and consensus about the goals of care • Improved relational communication, cohesion, and mutual support
3. Support for spirituality and awareness of sense of meaning and purpose	To explore the patient's spiritual beliefs and/or sense of meaning and purpose in life in the face of suffering and advanced disease	• Facilitate and support meaning making as an adaptive strategy • Foster sense of fulfillment • Promote mastery over what one can control and acceptance of what one cannot	• Validation and/or reevaluation of priorities and goals • An active approach to the end-of-life experience • Sense of courage, peace, and contentment
4. Thinking of the future, hope, and mortality	To explore anticipatory fears and provide a forum for discussion of life closure and death preparation activities	• Normalize anxieties regarding dying and death • Normalize sadness and grief • Support open communication about the future and planning	• Acceptance of agreed goals of care • A balance between tasks of living and dying

emotional communication. The timing and nature of disclosure to children and other family members about the prognosis and ways to support them through the illness process are also commonly addressed.

Issues of spirituality, meaning, and purpose are often of increased importance near the end of life, and, in the medically ill, meaning, purpose in life, and faith have been found to be inversely correlated with depression.[71] For some, the crisis of illness and dying may strengthen long held religious or philosophical views. For others, unanswerable questions such as "Why me?" "What comes next?" or "Why must my family suffer?" trigger distress and challenge existing beliefs. Working through these issues with the patient leads to reevaluation of priorities and focus for the future. CALM therapy helps patients to focus not only on the closure of their life, which is approaching, but on the life that can be lived.[72]

COMPLEMENTARY APPROACHES TO CONVENTIONAL THERAPY

Many complementary interventions helpfully supplement conventional psychotherapies and will be chosen by many patients; these include relaxation, meditation and hypnosis, massage and aromatherapies, art and music therapies, exercise and behavioral activation, and yoga and a wide range of Eastern approaches. One meta-analysis on the effectiveness of relaxation therapy showed a moderate amelioration of depression.[73] Paced abdominal breathing, progressive muscle relaxation with guided imagery, and coping self-statements were combined in a single stress management intervention that reduced anxiety and depressive symptoms for patients receiving chemotherapy.[74] Behavioral activation, although usually a key component of

CBT, has been tested independently with a focus on scheduling, self-monitoring by rating the level of pleasure achieved in daily activities, and role playing to optimize the strategies used to engage in social activities.[75] Behavioral activation has proven effective in ameliorating the severity of depression.[76]

Aerobic exercise has been shown to improve cardiopulmonary function and decrease body fat in women receiving treatment for breast cancer.[77] Exercise is an important adjunct to psychological therapies for patients troubled by fatigue, although its use alone has yielded nonsignificant effect sizes.[78] On meta-analysis, exercise interventions show clear benefit in terms of physical functioning and a small gain in symptom control for symptoms other than fatigue.[79] Exercise also assists the sense of well-being in cancer survivors.[80]

Music therapy has long been appreciated as a helpful intervention in palliative care.[81-82] Art therapy has been similarly used to help with expression of feelings.[83,84] One study using the Edmonton Symptom Assessment Scale saw a reduction in symptom intensity following art therapy in palliative care.[85] Aromatherapy and massage therapy feature prominently in most palliative care programs.[86]

EFFECTIVENESS OF COUNSELING AND APPLIED PSYCHOTHERAPIES IN SUPPORTIVE CARE

Meta-analyses have established strong evidence for the effectiveness of psychological therapies in assuaging distress, reducing anxiety, and relieving depression.[10,87,88] Couples therapy has also been shown to effectively reduce distress.[89] Group therapy is at least as effective and often more powerful than individual therapy.[91] What emerges is the importance of the length of psychotherapy, with longer therapies increasing effect size over brief interventions.[91] For instance, in reducing anxiety, more than 8 hours of therapy generates an effect size of 1.01, compared with 0.41 when between 4 and 7 hours is given ($P = .002$).

The skill of the therapist also stands out as a determinative finding in meta-analytic reviews. More experienced therapists increase the effect size in treating anxiety (experienced, d = 0.57 vs. inexperienced, d = 0.10; $P = .054$) and depression (d = 0.43 vs. d = -0.18; $P = .038$) when compared with less experienced or trainee therapists.[10] Oncology and supportive care programs are challenged to hire properly trained and experienced therapists to care for these patients and their families.

As with all treatments in medicine, counseling and applied psychotherapy have the potential to do harm. Research over several decades has suggested that 10% of psychotherapy interventions cause unwanted effects such as worsening anxiety, depression, or marital and family conflict.[90] Psychotherapy interventions for cancer patients have much to offer in helping ameliorate suffering, albeit with well-trained and experienced therapists.[91]

CONCLUSION

The art of psychotherapy in supportive care is the strategic and yet eclectic selection of components from several models that are targeted to the needs and coping styles of individual patients and their family members. Integrated care that makes appropriate use of concomitant pharmacology and thoughtfully plans the psychotherapeutic approach must also remain cognizant of the cancer, any progression, poorly controlled physical symptoms, unaddressed systemic issues, or confounding spiritual or social issues—whole-person–centered and family-centered care is provided by psycho-oncologists in an experienced treatment team. There is much to do to foster the living until that final moment, when each life stops.

REFERENCES

1. Zabora J, Brintzenhofezock S, Curbow B, et al. The prevalence of psychological distress by cancer site. *Psychooncology.* 2001;10:19–28.
2. Morita T, Kawa M, Honke Y, et al. Existential concerns of terminally ill cancer patients receiving specialized palliative care in Japan. *Support Cancer Care.* 2004;12:137–140.
3. Miller K, Massie MJ. Depression and anxiety. *Cancer J.* 2006;12:388–397.
4. Kissane DW, Bloch S, Burns WI, et al. Psychological morbidity in the families of patients with cancer. *Psychooncology.* 1994;3:47–56.
5. Cassell EJ. *The nature of suffering and the goals of medicine.* New York: Oxford University Press; 1991.
6. Carlson LE, Angen M, Cullum J, et al. High levels of untreated distress and fatigue in cancer patients. *Br J Cancer.* 2004;90:2297–2304.
7. Jacobsen PB, Donovan KA, Trask PC, et al. Screening for psychologic distress in ambulatory cancer patients. *Cancer.* 2005;103:1494–1502.
8. McLachlan SA, Allenby A, Matthews J, et al. Randomized trial of coordinated psychosocial interventions based on patient self-assessments versus standard care to improve the psychosocial functioning of patients with cancer. *J Clin Oncol.* 2001;19:4117–4125.
9. Burton M, Watson M. *Counselling people with cancer.* Chichester: Wiley; 1998.
10. Devine EC, Westlake SK. The effects of psychoeducational care provided to adults with cancer: meta-analysis of 116 studies. *Oncol Nurs Forum.* 1995;22:1369–1381.
11. Newell S, Sanson-Fisher RW, Girgis A, et al. The physical and psychosocial experiences of patients attending an outpatient medical oncology department: a cross-sectional study. *Eur J Cancer.* 1999;8:73–82.
12. Bloch S, ed. *An introduction to the psychotherapies.* 3rd ed. Melbourne: Oxford Medical Publications; 1996.
13. Yalom ID. *Existential psychotherapy.* New York: Basic Books; 1980.
14. Spiegel D, Classen C. *Group therapy for cancer patients.* New York: Basic Books; 2000.
15. Kissane DW, Grabsch B, Clarke DM, et al. Supportive-expressive group therapy: the transformation of existential ambivalence into creative living while enhancing adherence to anti-cancer therapies. *Psychooncology.* 2004;11:755–768.
16. Kissane DW. Letting go of the hope that psychotherapy prolongs cancer survival. *J Clin Oncol.* 2007;25:5689–5690.
17. Goodwin PJ, Leszcz M, Ennis M, et al. The effect of group psychosocial support on survival in metastatic breast cancer. *N Engl J Med.* 2001;345:1719–1726.
18. Kissane DW, Grabsch B, Clarke DM, et al. Supportive-expressive group therapy for women with metastatic breast cancer: survival and psychosocial outcome from a randomized controlled trial. *Psychooncology.* 2007;16:227–286.
19. Classen C, Butler LD, Koopman C, et al. Supportive-expressive group therapy and distress in patients with metastatic breast cancer: a randomized clinical intervention trial. *Arch Gen Psychiatry.* 2001;58:494–501.
20. Andersen BL, Farrar WB, Golden-Kreutz D, et al. Distress reduction from a psychological intervention contributes to improved health for cancer patients. *Brain Behav Immun.* 2007;21:953–961.
21. Beck J. *Cognitive therapy: basics and beyond.* New York: Guilford Press; 1995.
22. Moorey S, Greer S. *Cognitive behavior therapy for people with cancer.* 2nd ed. Oxford: Oxford University Press; 2002.
23. White CA. *Cognitive behavior therapy for chronic medical problems: a guide to assessment and treatment in practice.* Chichester: Wiley; 2001.
24. Kissane DW, Bloch S, Miach P, et al. Cognitive-existential group therapy for patients with primary breast cancer—techniques and themes. *Psychooncology.* 1997;6:25–33.
25. Clum GA, Suris R. A meta-analysis of treatments for panic disorder. *J Consult Clin Psychol.* 1993;61:317–326.
26. Gloaquenu K, Cotraux J, Cucherat M, et al. A meta-analysis of the effects of cognitive therapy with depressed patients. *J Affect Disord.* 1998;49:59–72.
27. Savard J, Simard S, Giguere I, et al. Randomized clinical trial of cognitive therapy for depression in women with metastatic breast cancer: psychological and immunological effects. *Palliat Support Care.* 2006;4:219–237.
28. Edelman S, Bell DR, Kidman AD. A group cognitive behavior therapy programme with metastatic breast cancer patients. *Psychooncology.* 1999;8:295–305.
29. Moorey S, Cort E, Kapari M, et al. A cluster randomized controlled trial of cognitive behavior therapy for common mental disorders in patients with advanced cancer. *Psychol Med.* 2009;39:713–723.
30. Strong V, Waters R, Hibberd C, et al. Management of depression for people with cancer (SMaRT oncology 1): a randomized trial. *Lancet.* 2008;372:40–48.
31. Walker J, Sharpe M. Depression for people with cancer: a collaborative care intervention. *Gen Hosp Psychiatry.* 2009;31:436–441.
32. Ell K, Xie B, Quon B, et al. Randomized controlled trial of collaborative care management of depression among low-income patients with cancer. *J Clin Oncol.* 2008;26:4488–4496.
33. Weissman MM, Markowitz JC, Klerman GL. *Comprehensive guide to interpersonal psychotherapy.* New York: Basic Books; 2000.
34. De Mello M, de Jesus MJ, Bacaltchuk J, et al. A systematic review of research findings on the efficacy of interpersonal therapy for depressive disorder. *Eur Arch Psychiatr Clin Neurosci.* 2005;255:75–82.
35. Straker N. Psychodynamic psychotherapy for cancer patients. *J Psychother Pract Res.* 1989;7:1–9.
36. McDougall J. *Theatres of the body: a psychoanalytic approach to psychosomatic medicine.* London: Free Association Press; 1989.
37. White M. *Narrative means to therapeutic ends.* New York: Norton; 1990.
38. Viederman M. Psychodynamic life narrative in a psychotherapeutic intervention useful in crisis situations. *Psychiatry.* 1983;46:236–246.
39. White M. *Narratives of therapists' lives.* Dulwich: Adelaide; 1997.
40. Sanatani M, Schreier G, Stitt L. Level and direction of hope in cancer patients: an exploratory longitudinal study. *Support Care Cancer.* 2008;16:493–499.

41. Duggleby WD, Degner L, Williams A, et al. Living with hope: initial evaluation of a psychosocial hope intervention for older palliative home care patients. *J Pain Symptom Manage*. 2007;33:247–257.

42. Chochinov HM, Hack T, Hazard T, et al. Dignity therapy: a novel psychotherapeutic intervention for patients near the end of life. *J Clin Oncol*. 2005;23:5520–5525.

43. Chochinov HM, Hack T, McClement S, et al. Dignity in the terminally ill: a developing empirical model. *Soc Sci Med*. 2002;54:433–443.

44. Chochinov HM, Kristjanson LJ, Hack TF, et al. Dignity in the terminally ill: revisited. *J Palliat Med*. 2006;9:666–672.

45. Chochinov HM, Hack T, Hassard T, et al. Dignity therapy: a novel psychotherapeutic intervention for patients near the end of life. *J Clin Oncol*. 2005;23:5520–5525.

46. Breitbart W, Heller KS. Reframing hope: meaning-centered care for patients near the end of life. *J Palliat Med*. 2003;6:979–988.

47. Fillion L, Dupuis R, Tremblay I, et al. Enhancing meaning in palliative care: a meaning-centered intervention to promote job satisfaction. *Palliat Support Care*. 2006;4:333–344.

48. Frankl VF. *Man's search for meaning*. 4th ed. Boston: Beacon Press; 1992.

49. Breitbart W, Gibson C, Poppito S, et al. Psychotherapeutic interventions at the end of life: a focus on meaning and spirituality. *Can J Psychiatry*. 2004;49:366–372.

50. Breitbart W. Spirituality and meaning in supportive care: spirituality- and meaning-centered group psychotherapy interventions in advanced cancer. *Support Cancer Care*. 2002;10:272–280.

51. Hagedoorn M, Sanderman R, Bolks HN, et al. Distress in couples coping with cancer: a meta-analysis and critical review of role and gender effects. *Psychol Bull*. 2008;134:1–30.

52. Manne SL, Ostroff JS, Winkel G, et al. Couple-focused group intervention for women with early stage breast cancer. *J Consult Clin Psychol*. 2005;73:634–646.

53. Northouse LL, Mood DW, Schafenacker A, et al. Randomized clinical trial of a family intervention for prostate cancer patients and their spouses. *Cancer*. 2007;110:2809–2818.

54. McLean LM, Jones JM. A review of distress and its management in couples facing end-of-life cancer. *Psychooncology*. 2007;16:603–616.

55. McLean LM, Nissim R. Marital therapy for couples facing advanced cancer: case review. *Palliat Support Care*. 2007;5:303–313.

56. Kissane DW, Lichtenthal WG, Zaider T. Family care before and after bereavement. *Omega*. 2007–2008;56:21–32.

57. Chan EK, O'Neill I, McKenzie M, et al. What works for therapists conducting family meetings: treatment integrity in family focused grief therapy during palliative care and bereavement. *J Pain Symptom Manage*. 2004;27:502–512.

58. Kissane DW, Bloch S, Burns WI, et al. Perceptions of family functioning and cancer. *Psychooncology*. 1994;3:259–269.

59. Kissane DW, Bloch S, Dowe DL, et al. The Melbourne family grief study, I: perceptions of family functioning in bereavement. *Am J Psychiatry*. 1996;153:650–658.

60. Kissane DW, Bloch S. *Family focused grief therapy: a model of family-centered care during palliative care and bereavement*. Buckingham: Open University Press; 2002.

61. Kissane DW, McKenzie M, Bloch S, et al. Family focused grief therapy: a randomized, controlled trial in palliative care and bereavement. *Am J Psychiatry*. 2006;163:1208–1218.

62. Zaider T, Kissane DW. Resilient families. In: Monroe B, Oliviere D, eds. *Resilience in palliative care*. Oxford: Oxford University Press; 2007.

63. Dumont I, Kissane DW. Techniques for framing questions in conducting family meetings in palliative care. *Palliat Support Care*. 2009;7:163–170.

64. Sharpe M, Strong V, Allen K, et al. Major depression in outpatients attending a regional cancer centre: screening and unmet treatment needs. *Br J Cancer*. 2004;90:314–320.

65. Walker J, Sharpe M. Depression care for people with cancer: a collaborative care intervention. *Gen Hosp Psychiatry*. 2009;31:436–441.

66. Rodin G, Lo C, Mikulincer M, et al. Pathways to distress: multiple determinants of depression, hopelessness and the desire for hastened death in metastatic cancer patients. *Soc Sci Med*. 2009;68:562–569.

67. Rodin G, Walsh A, Zimmermann C, et al. The contribution of attachment security and social support to depressive symptoms in patients with metastatic cancer. *Psychooncology*. 2007;16:1080–1091.

68. Lo C, Walsh A, Mikulincer M, et al. Measuring attachment security in patients with advanced cancer: psychometric properties of modified and brief experiences in close relationships scale. *Psychooncology*. 2009;18:490–499.

69. Hales S, Zimmermann C, Rodin G. The quality of dying and death. *Arch Intern Med*. 2008;168:912–918.

70. Lo C, Li M, Rodin G. The assessment and treatment of distress in cancer patients: overview and future directions. *Minerva Psychiatr*. 2008;49:129–143.

71. McClain CS, Rosenfeld B, Breitbart W. Effect of spiritual well-being on end-of-life despair in terminally-ill cancer patients. *Lancet*. 2003;362:1603–1607.

72. Rodin G, Zimmermann C. Psychoanalytic reflections on mortality: a reconsideration. *J Am Acad Psychoanal Dynamic Psychiatry*. 2008;36:181–196.

73. Luebbert K, Dahme B, Hasenbring M. The effectiveness of relaxation training in reducing treatment-related symptoms and improving emotional adjustment in acute non-surgical cancer treatment: a meta-analytical review. *Psychooncology*. 2001;10:490–502.

74. Jacobsen PB, Meade CD, Stein KD, et al. Efficacy and costs of two forms of stress management training for cancer patients undergoing chemotherapy. *J Clin Oncol*. 2002;20:2851–2862.

75. Dimidjian S, Hollon SD, Dobson KS, et al. Randomized trial of behavioral activation, cognitive therapy, and antidepressant medication in the acute treatment of adults with major depression. *J Consult Clin Psychol*. 2006;74:658–670.

76. Dobson KS, Hollon SD, Dimidjian S, et al. Randomized trial of behavioral activation, cognitive therapy, and antidepressant medication in the prevention of relapse and recurrence in major depression. *J Consult Clin Psychol*. 2008;76:468–477.

77. Kim CJ, Kang DH, Park JW. A meta-analysis of aerobic exercise interventions for women with breast cancer. *Western J Nurs Res*. 2009;31:437–461.

78. Jacobsen PB, Donovan KA, Vadaparampil ST, et al. Systematic review and meta-analysis of psychological and activity-based interventions for cancer-related fatigue. *Health Psychol*. 2007;26:660–667.

79. Conn VS, Hafdahl AR, Porock DC, et al. A meta-analysis of exercise interventions among people treated for cancer. *Support Care Cancer*. 2006;14:699–712.

80. Speck RM, Courneya KS, Mâsse LC, et al. An update of controlled physical activity trials in cancer survivors: a systematic review and meta-analysis. *J Cancer Surv*. 2010;4:87–100.

81. O'Callaghan C. Clinical issues: music therapy in an adult cancer inpatient treatment setting. *J Soc Integr Oncol*. 2006;4:57–61.

82. O'Callaghan C, O'Brien E, Magill L, et al. Resounding attachment: cancer inpatients' song lyrics for their children in music therapy. *Support Care Cancer*. 2009;17:1149–1157.

83. Heywood K. Introducing art therapy into the Christie Hospital, Manchester, UK, 2001–2002. *Complement Ther Nurs Midwifery*. 2003;9:125–132.

84. Jones G. An art therapy group in palliative cancer care. *Nurs Times*. 2000;96:42–43.

85. Nainis N, Paice JA, Ratner J, et al. Relieving symptoms in cancer: innovative use of art therapy. *J Pain Symptom Manage*. 2006;31:162–169.

86. Buckley J. Massage and aromatherapy massage: nursing art and science: Review. *Int J Palliat Nurs*. 2002;8:276–280.

87. Sheard T, Maguire P. The effect of psychological interventions on anxiety and depression in cancer patients: results of two meta-analyses. *Br J Cancer*. 1999;80:1770–1780.

88. Osborn R, Demoncada A, Feuerstein M. Psychosocial interventions for depression, anxiety, and quality of life in cancer survivors: meta-analyses. *Int J Psychol Med*. 2006;36:13–34.

89. Hagedoorn M, Sanderman R, Bolks HN, et al. Distress in couples coping with cancer: a meta-analysis and critical review of role and gender effects. *Psychol Bull*. 2008;134:1–30.

90. Miller K, Kissane DW. Counseling in palliative care (Chapter 74). In: Bruera E, et al., eds. *Textbook of palliative medicine*. London: Hodder Arnold; 2006:705–717.

91. Daniels J, Kissane DW. Psychosocial interventions for cancer patients. *Curr Opin Oncol*. 2008;20:367–371.

Substance abuse in supportive oncology

Amy E. Lowery, Kenneth L. Kirsh, and Steven D. Passik

Cancer pain management utilizes opioid medications as its foundation. These medications are being prescribed far more commonly for noncancer pain than ever before. The co-occurring growth of prescription drug abuse now contextualizes all opioid prescribing. For clinicians working with cancer patients who are in pain, concern about drug abuse and addiction to medications is a serious and complicated matter. Although a vast majority of patients do not experience any problems in this arena, others may develop or exacerbate an existing drug abuse or misuse problem. Although this percentage of patients is small, the problem is becoming increasingly common. Younger cancer patients are particularly more challenging in this regard, as they are exposed to these medications before their genetic predisposition and other risk factors have been fully expressed.

Individualizing care for these patients is essential. Specialized programs can aid in managing this small but labor-intensive subset of higher addiction risk patients in cancer centers. However, further work is needed to integrate pain management and addiction medicine, as well as train medical professionals in these areas. In this chapter, we will examine the prevalence of prescription drug abuse in general and cancer populations; explore common misconceptions of terms and labels related to substance abuse; describe confounding clinical issues, such as comorbid psychological disorders, aberrant drug-related behaviors, and primary and secondary abuse; list the various subgroups of pain patients and nonmedical users; illustrate assessment strategies and tools; and discuss effective psychotherapeutic and pharmacologic interventions.

PREVALENCE

Nonmedical use of prescription pain killers is a national epidemic with important implications for pain management. The incidence has quadrupled over the past decade from 573,000 in 1990 to 2.5 million in 2002,[1] and 2.4 million new cases of prescription drug abuse were reported in 2004, exceeding illicit drugs, including marijuana (2.1 million) and cocaine (1 million).[2] The high prevalence of prescription drug abuse is a source of much concern in the medical setting, where not only adults but even children with cancer pain may be at risk for developing an addiction. The therapeutic use of such potentially abusable drugs and the abuse of these drugs are complex processes that must be understood if optimal patient care is to be provided.[3] When working with patients with progressive life-threatening disease who have a remote or current history of drug abuse, physical and psychosocial concerns that could potentially affect pain management and treatment must be addressed.

The prevalence of substance abuse in the cancer population is relatively low. In 1990, only 3% of inpatient and outpatient consultations performed by the Psychiatry Service at

Memorial Sloan-Kettering Cancer Center (MSKCC) included a request for management of issues related to substance abuse. This number is significantly lower than the overall prevalence of substance use disorders found in society, general medical populations, and emergency medical departments.[4–8] The Psychiatric Collaborative Oncology Group study assessed psychiatric diagnoses in ambulatory cancer patients from several tertiary care hospitals and reported a similarly low prevalence rate.[6] In an early study using structured clinical interviews for assessment, less than 5% of 215 cancer patients met the *Diagnostic and Statistical Manual for Mental Disorders* (DSM) Third Edition criteria for a substance use disorder.[9] Although a more current replication of this study has not been conducted, it is likely that the prevalence data do not accurately capture substance use disorder in today's cancer population, particularly among those who are community based. In a survey of patients admitted to a palliative care unit, 25% had a current or remote history of alcohol abuse.[10]

The relatively low prevalence of substance abuse among cancer patients treated in tertiary care hospitals where opioid prescriptions are abundant may not seem conceptually intuitive, but may be the result of a variety of factors. First, there may be institutional biases or a tendency toward patient underreporting in these settings. It has been shown that a high percentage of drug abusers fall into the lower socioeconomic bracket, feel alienated from the health care system, and may not seek care in tertiary centers. Therefore, they may show hesitation to report a history of drug abuse because of the potential for stigmatization. A study by Bruera and colleagues[10] of 100 terminally ill alcoholic cancer patients found that despite multiple hospital admissions and screenings, only one third had documentation of alcoholism in their medical records. The fact that cancer patients are generally older (50 years and older) may also explain the low addiction rate, as most addictions are manifested by age 35.[12] If a patient has never had a problem with drugs or alcohol use before cancer in mid or late life, it is highly unlikely that a new problem will develop. Additional studies are needed to clarify the epidemiology of substance abuse and addiction in cancer patients and other populations with progressive medical diseases.

TOLERANCE, DEPENDENCE, AND ADDICTION

A major obstacle of managing substance abuse within the cancer pain population is the inconsistent and overlapping terminology.[13] Although epidemiologic studies and clinical management depend on an accepted, valid nomenclature for substance abuse and addiction, the current terminology is highly problematic. Because many clinicians are not trained in and do not specialize in treating co-occurring substance abuse, they may confuse common behaviors associated with tolerance and dependence with those of abuse and addiction.[13] Defining abuse and addiction in medically ill populations, specifically oncology, poses additional challenges because these terms were originally developed to assess the general population of addicts without the addition of a painful coexisting medical illness. Clarifying these terms and applying them appropriately will improve the diagnosis and management

of substance abuse and will promote pain management and overall patient care.

TOLERANCE

Tolerance is a pharmacologic phenomenon characterized by the need to increase doses to maintain the effects of the medication.[14,15] It is a frequent concern of both clinicians and patients that a tolerance to analgesics will develop, compromising the therapeutic benefits and requiring progressively higher, and ultimately unsustainable, doses. However, although it is frequently associated with increasing pain or disease progression, tolerance is not automatically a sign of abuse or addiction.[16–24] This resulting need to increase doses may be an important element in the pathogenesis of addiction.[25]

In spite of these concerns, extensive clinical experience with opioid drugs in the medical context suggests that tolerance rarely leads to substantial problems, including addiction.[17,20] Tolerance to a variety of opioid effects can be reliably observed in animal models,[26] and tolerance to nonanalgesic effects, such as respiratory depression and cognitive impairment,[27] occurs regularly in the clinical setting. Analgesic tolerance does not appear to routinely interfere with the clinical efficacy of opioid drugs. Research has shown that most patients can manage stable doses of opioids and maintain a balance between analgesia and side effects for prolonged periods. Unlike tolerance to the side effects of opioids, clinically meaningful analgesic tolerance seems to be a rare phenomenon and is infrequently the cause for dose escalation.[16,18,19,21–24]

Clinical observation does not support the assumption that analgesic tolerance is a significant contributor to the development of addiction. Generally, addicts who present without a co-occurring medical condition may or may not have any of the manifestations of analgesic tolerance. Occasionally, opioid-treated patients present manifestations consistent with analgesic tolerance. However, they typically do so without evidence of abuse or addiction.[3,26]

PHYSICAL DEPENDENCE

Physical dependence is characterized by the occurrence of a withdrawal syndrome that follows a rapid decrease in dosage or administration of an antagonist.[14,15,28] Many clinicians find the differential properties of physical dependence and addiction unclear. Although physical dependence is an element of addiction,[29,30] it is theorized that the behavioral contingencies of the avoidance of withdrawal reinforce drug-seeking behavior.[25] Physical dependence does not necessarily impede the discontinuation of opioids in patients with nonmalignant pain,[31] and cessation of opioid therapy commonly occurs without difficulty in cancer patients whose pain is diminished after completion of antineoplastic therapy. Circuitous evidence for a primary distinction between physical dependence and addiction has been provided by animal models of opioid self-administration, which have demonstrated that chronic drug taking behavior can be maintained in the absence of physical dependence.[32]

ERRORS IN LABELING

Misuse of definitions, such as tolerance and physical dependence, highlights the difficulty in accurately classifying and thereby treating substance-related problems. Particularly problematic are the terms "addiction" and "addict," which have an inaccurate tendency to be applied to describe both aberrant drug use (such as those behaviors that characterize active abusers of illicit drugs) and phenomena related to tolerance or physical dependence. Clinicians and patients may use the word "addicted" to describe compulsive drug taking in one patient and nothing more than the "potential for withdrawal" in another. This lack of universal understanding of these terms fosters concern among patients, families, and staff about the outcomes of opioid treatment.[33]

Patients who are perceived to have the capacity for an abstinence syndrome should never be labeled as "addicts" or as having an "addiction." Rather, these patients should be identified as "physically dependent." The term "habituation" should not be used, so as to reduce any further confusion.[3] Additionally, applying the label "dependent" alone is discouraged because it creates confusion between physical dependence and psychological dependence (a component of addiction).

CLINICAL ISSUES

Many patient characteristic variables may have an impact on the management of pain in cancer patients with a history of addiction.

COMORBID PSYCHIATRIC DISORDERS

Individuals with alcoholism are at higher risk for other comorbid psychiatric disorders.[34] Anxiety disorder (19.4%), antisocial personality disorder (14.3%), affective disorder (13.4%), and schizophrenia (3.8%) are among the most common of these.[35] This co-occurrence may result in poor treatment compliance and lack of success caused by cognitive limitations and premorbid (in relation to the diagnosis of cancer) pain and neurologic deficits. The same is true of opioid abuse; 85% of addicts have a comorbid, non–drug-related psychological disorder.[36] This highlights the importance of assessing and treating any preexisting addiction or alcoholism in cancer patients.

ABERRANT DRUG-RELATED BEHAVIORS

Hesitancy to treat pain with potentially abusable medications, specifically opioids, may stem from concerns regarding aberrant drug-related behavior, addiction, and abuse. Problematic behaviors that are indicative of abuse are ambiguous to many clinicians. This fact is complicated by the lack of empirical information that helps to distinguish such behaviors. Aberrant behavior can be described as any questionable drug-related behavior exhibited by a patient that is suggestive of abuse.[33] Such behaviors vary significantly in severity or frequency and should be viewed along a continuum that ranges from mild or limited (e.g., use of a prescribed dose to self-medicate a problem not intended by the clinician, such as insomnia) to more severe or overwhelming behaviors (e.g., injection of an oral formulation) and have the potential to predict addiction[37]

Table 55-1 The spectrum of aberrant drug-related behaviors

Aberrant drug-related behaviors more suggestive of addiction	Aberrant drug-related behaviors less suggestive of addiction
Selling prescription drugs	Aggressive complaining about need for higher doses
Prescription forgery	Drug hoarding during periods of reduced symptoms
Stealing or borrowing another patient's drugs	Requesting specific drugs
Injecting oral formulation	Acquisition of similar drugs from other medical sources
Obtaining prescription drugs from nonmedical sources	Unsanctioned dose escalation, 1–2 times
Concurrent abuse of related illicit drugs	Unapproved use of the drug to treat another symptom
Multiple unsanctioned dose escalations	Reporting psychic effects not intended by the clinician
Recurrent prescription losses	

(Table 55-1). The issue of noncompliance must be stressed early on and at length between patients and clinicians.

An assessment is used to determine the underlying nature of a problem, which will foster development of an appropriate therapeutic intervention.[38,39] Accurate identification of aberrant behaviors will lead the clinician to formulate a differential diagnosis and distinguish between a "true" addiction (a substance use disorder) and a "pseudoaddiction" (desperate behaviors motivated by unrelieved pain). Escalating drug-seeking behaviors may be exhibited in patients with addiction disorders as a result of untreated pain, reflecting both addiction and pseudoaddiction. This distinction is among the most confounding differential diagnoses.[40] Impulsive or inappropriate drug use may also be rooted in an underlying psychiatric disorder. For example, a patient with borderline personality disorder may engage in aberrant drug use to relieve boredom or to convey fear or anger. Likewise, a patient suffering from depression, anxiety, or insomnia may self-medicate with prescription drugs to obtain relief from the discomfort of symptoms.[37] Other possible causes of aberrant drug use include criminal intent (drug diversion) and familial dysfunction (family members taking the patient's medication for their own use).[38,41]

Aberrant drug-related behaviors in medically ill populations

A variety of personal and psychological characteristics have been found to be related to substance abuse in medically ill populations with the presence of pain.

A study by Passik and colleagues[42] looked at the prevalence and correlates of aberrant drug-taking behaviors in two populations: patients with HIV-related pain and a history of substance abuse (n = 73), and patients with cancer pain and no history of substance abuse (n = 100). This study used a

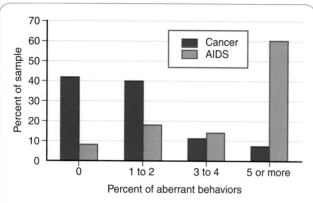

Fig. 55-1 Aberrant behaviors in cancer and AIDS. *(From Passik SD, Kirsh KL, Donaghy KB, et al.[42])*

Primary or secondary abuse

The relationship between drug or alcohol abuse and coexisting psychiatric conditions is complex. Although some patients' abuse is primary, which results in mood and anxiety syndromes, other patients experience secondary abuse, reflecting out-of-control self-medication for preexisting mood and anxiety disorders.[43–45] Whether alcohol or substance use is primary or secondary or whether it can be targeted for appropriate treatment is difficult to determine unless the patient's drug or alcohol use can be controlled. For example, a patient with insomnia may experience it as a primary symptom or as a result of withdrawal or intoxication (secondary). The distinction between primary and secondary symptoms can be made only once control over the patient's abusive behaviors can be attained.[46]

battery of questionnaires to assess substance abuse history and levels of pain, depression, distress, and other related variables. Results from both groups showed that (1) expressing anxiety or depression over recurrent symptoms, and (2) hoarding medications were the two most frequent aberrant behaviors. More specifically, the AIDS subgroup showed significantly greater use of potentially aberrant behaviors than was seen in the cancer group (Fig. 55-1), as well as a lower percentage of pain relief from current analgesic therapy, increased opioid doses without doctors' orders, use of more opioids than recommended, use of opioids to treat other nonrelated symptoms, and admitting to family members that they use other street drugs to relieve pain. In the cancer group, drinking alcohol to relieve pain was the only aberrant behavior significantly related to a low percentage of pain relief from current analgesic therapy. Additionally, AIDS patients showed higher levels of psychological distress, depression, and interference related to residual pain when compared with cancer patients. Overall, the results of this study suggest that aberrant behaviors may be more influenced by substance abuse history and psychosocial distress than by pain and analgesic variables.

Another study by Passik and colleagues[33] examined self-reported attitudes toward aberrant drug-taking behaviors in a sample of cancer (n = 52) and AIDS (n = 111) patients and found that patients in both groups reported past drug use and abuse more frequently than present drug use and abuse. However, in the context of unrelieved pain, patients would consider engaging in aberrant drug use, or conceivably would excuse others from engaging in these behaviors for the same reason. The authors also found that aberrant behaviors and attitudes were endorsed more frequently by women in the AIDS group than by patients in the cancer group. Moreover, patients significantly overestimated addiction risk in pain treatment.

These studies suggest that "red flag" behaviors may vary by specific diagnoses in different populations. Much too frequently, clinicians' perspectives on these behaviors are shaped by anecdotal accounts. Some behaviors have been almost universally regarded as problematic despite the support of systematic data (e.g., a patient's request for a specific dose). These behaviors may appear to be aberrant based on their face value, but have limited predictive validity for true addiction, and may, in fact, be more indicative of patients who are knowledgeable about what works for them.

CANCER PAIN PATIENTS VERSUS NONMEDICAL USERS

This surge of prescription drug abuse has created new dilemmas for cancer pain management, as a heterogeneous group of prescription drug users now exist: pain patients and nonmedical users. Pain patients live with chronic non–cancer- or cancer-related pain and require these medications to improve their quality of life. Nonmedical users consist of people who are not prescribed the medications, but are acquiring them from someone they know or by another illegal means (e.g., stealing, buying). The following sections describe the different subgroups of each type of user and discuss the implications for clinicians in working with this patient population.

CANCER PAIN PATIENTS

Although a vast majority of cancer patients are adherent, clinicians will come in contact with patients who are self-medicating bona fide problems (i.e., "chemical coping pain patients") or who have problems with substance abuse and addiction (Fig. 55-2). When working with cancer pain patients, clinicians must learn how to recognize and manage patients who are not using their medications as prescribed.

Eduardo Bruera and colleagues coined the term "chemical copers" to describe those walking the fine line between adherence and aberrancy,[47] illustrating an archetype of maladaptive coping via substances.[48] This term was first applied to a sample of cancer patients with high rates of historical substance abuse, which was furthered by the distress associated with cancer.[48] Chemical copers tend to be guided by stress and are inclined to increase their drug dose and deviate from the treatment path when stress becomes unbearable. They also tend to be uninterested in nonpharmacologic treatments for pain (e.g., psychotherapy).[47]

Within the construct of chemical coping, four associated features are seen: (1) self-medication,[49] (2) sensation seeking, (3) alexithymia, and (4) somatization. In the self-medication feature, patients misuse substances to relieve feelings of physical or emotional distress and tend to be drawn toward specific pharmacologic substances.[49] Sensation seeking is defined as a proclivity to complicated and powerful experiences. This feature often involves patients going outside the box to attain such feelings and avoid feelings of distress.[50] Alexithymia is characterized as the inability to manage and grasp emotions

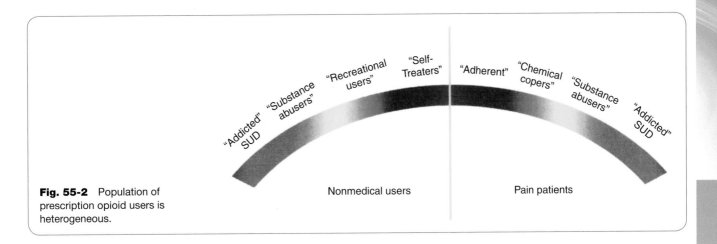

Fig. 55-2 Population of prescription opioid users is heterogeneous.

and feelings. These patients present with somatic complaints and have little to no emotional connection, thereby solely relying on physical feelings.[51] The last associated feature, somatization, is a process whereby mental and emotional stresses are expressed by physical symptoms. With this feature, patients are not always aware that they are misconstruing emotional distress as physical symptoms, but believe these feelings are actual physical pains and discomforts.[52] Overall, these patients are prime candidates for psychiatric intervention coupled with a simplified drug regimen to learn to cope more efficiently and in more adaptive ways.

NONMEDICAL USERS

Nonmedical users run the gamut from experimenters to self-medicators to true addicts. Since the 1980s, pain relievers have become the single most sought after class of nonmedically used substances in our society, and are the top first drug of young users. According to the 2005 National Survey on Drug Use and Health, 2,193,000 people have reported the nonmedical use of prescription pain relievers, and 526,000 of these people are new users of OxyContin.[53]

These nonmedical users are not seen as pain patients, but are self-treating their ailments with medications from nonmedical professionals (e.g., parent, sibling, grandparent, friend). According to the 2005 National Survey on Drug Use and Health, 59.8% of nonmedical users obtain pain relievers from a friend or relative, 16.8% from one doctor, 4.3% from a dealer or stranger, and 0.8% from the Internet.[53]

A fast growing population of nonmedical users of prescription drugs consists of college-aged women.[54] They are often playing "arm chair pharmacist" with one another (e.g., taking someone else's prescription sleeping pill because they cannot sleep, taking someone's methylphenidate because they have to stay up to study).[54] The existence of this phenomenon places new responsibilities on cancer pain clinicians and pain patients. Education about storage and the importance of not sharing medications is essential, even in adherent patients (see Case Study).

ASSESSMENT

The first member of the medical team to suspect drug or alcohol abuse (often a nurse) should alert the team to begin the multidisciplinary assessment and management process. Too

CASE STUDY

Mr. G is in his mid 50s and has advanced bladder cancer. He presented to the pain service via the urgent care center after his first pain crisis. He was seen for "failure to thrive in need of pain control." He was assessed for depression and was reported to have found religion 5 years prior. He is currently in recovery for a lifelong heroin addiction. Notably, Mr. G is living in an unstable social situation. He lives in a rented room in a flop house in a "tough part" of town, where there is a constant flow of younger men and women at all hours. It is important to emphasize that this is the patient's first ever pain crisis. The first line of treatment presented is OxyContin, the most abused medicine on the street, along with hydromorphone rescues. This represents lack of concern at the forefront on the part of most medical oncologists. They are focusing on alleviating the patient's pain, not on the street value of the drug they are prescribing and not on the patient's social situation. This case study represents the need to educate prescribing physicians about the increase in prescription drug abuse and about ways to safely prescribe these medications.

often, the fear of offending or stigmatizing the patient leaves signs of alcohol or drug abuse neglected. A physician must assess the potential for withdrawal and other pressing concerns, and must involve other staff members (e.g., social work, psychiatry) in management strategies.

Recognition of potentially dangerous drug-related behaviors is crucial for successful treatment of ongoing pain. Extensive clinical experience has led to the development of guidelines specifically tailored to monitor chronic pain patients receiving opioid therapy, known as the "4 A's."[55] The "4 A's" incorporate the critical domains of pain management, including (1) analgesia, (2) activities of daily living, (3) adverse side effects, and (4) aberrant drug-taking behaviors. Continuous assessment of these domains during treatment can provide clinicians with a useful framework that informs decision making and fosters compliance with the therapeutic use of controlled substances.[56]

Taking an accurate, detailed history from the patient is essential for proper assessment and treatment of alcohol and drug abuse, as well as for assessment of any comorbid psychiatric disorders. It is also important to ask the patient for information regarding duration, frequency, and desired effect of drug or alcohol use, although alcohol or drug use tends to be underreported because of embarrassment, fear of stigmatization, and/or strong defense mechanisms, primarily denial. With pressure to treat most patients in the ambulatory setting, quick identification of a substance use disorder and needs assessment must begin at initial contact. Empathic and truthful communication is generally the best approach. When time permits, the use of a careful, graduated interview approach can be instrumental in slowly introducing the subject of the patient's drug or alcohol use. The assessment interview should begin with broad questions about the patient's drug or alcohol use (e.g., nicotine, caffeine) in the patient's life, gradually becoming more specific in focus to include more aberrant drug and alcohol use. This type of approach is helpful in reducing denial and resistance from the patient.

Consultations with family members or close friends of the patient may be helpful in verifying the accuracy of the patient's reports and level of denial. However, the presence of co-dependent behavior (i.e., denial or enabling) should also be considered when interviewing family or friends of a drug- or alcohol-abusing cancer patient. In active abusers, time of last drug intake or alcohol consumption should be noted, and prevention of withdrawal should become the first priority. This type of interview will also assist in identifying the presence of coexisting psychiatric disorders that may be present. Assessment and treatment of comorbid psychiatric disorders can enhance management strategies and reduce the risk of relapse. Understanding the patient's desired effects from alcohol or drug use can often point to co-occurring psychiatric disorders (e.g., drinking to relieve panic symptoms).

When prescribing ongoing opioid therapy, particularly outside the context of ongoing cancer treatment (e.g., long-term survivors), it is important to continue to assess the 4 A's (Analgesia, Activities, Adverse effects, and Aberrant behaviors).[57] Documentation is especially helpful if the propriety of ongoing opioid therapy is ever questioned. Predesigned structured chart notes are available[55] in the literature and can be utilized to guide clinicians toward effective note writing and documentation.

Because of the high prevalence of abuse of opioids, clinicians must be aware of associated risk factors and vulnerabilities. The Opioid Risk Tool (ORT) is a screening tool that consists of five self-report items that evaluate risk potential for opioid abuse[58] (Table 55-2). The ORT is designed to be administered to patients whose chronic pain is planned to be treated with opioids at the clinical visit before initiation of treatment. This measure allows for evaluation of patients before the initiation of opioid therapy, thereby allowing clinicians to classify patients into one of three categories: low risk, moderate risk, or high risk. Low risk (scoring 0–3) refers to those unlikely to abuse opioids; moderate risk (scoring 4–7) applies to those just as likely to abuse opioids as they are not to abuse; and high risk (>8) refers to the group with greatest likelihood to abuse.[58] The simplicity of the ORT allows the clinician to begin treatment while monitoring the underlying risk factors presented. Furthermore, the clinician is able to tailor treatment to meet the individual needs of each patient.[58,59]

Table 55-2 Opioid risk tool (ORT)

		Female	Male
Is there a history of substance abuse in your **family**?	Alcohol	1	3
	Illegal drugs	2	3
	Other	4	4
Have **you** had a history of substance abuse?	Alcohol	3	3
	Illegal drugs	4	4
	Prescription drugs	5	5
Is your age between 16 and 45?		1	1
Is there a history of preadolescent (childhood) sexual abuse?		3	0
Do you have a history of any of the following conditions?	ADD, OCD, bipolar, schizophrenia?	2	2
	Depression?	1	1
Low (0–3), moderate (4–7), high (8+)	Total		

ADD, Attention deficit disorder; *OCD*, obsessive-compulsive disorder.

Another risk assessment tool is the CAGE, a four-item instrument used to identify people with a history of alcohol dependency. The acronym CAGE aligns with the four questions: <u>c</u>ut back, <u>a</u>nnoyance by critics, <u>g</u>uilt about drinking, and <u>e</u>ye-opening morning drinking. A positive response to two or more of these items suggests a potential alcohol problem.[60] Using this cutoff value, the sensitivity of CAGE in various populations ranges from 61% to 100%, and its specificity ranges from 77% to 96%.[61,62]

TREATMENT MODALITIES

Substance abuse is often a chronic, progressive disorder that can interfere with the treatment of a medical condition. As a result, the development of clear-cut treatment goals is crucial for treatment. Although abstinence is ideal, it is not necessarily a treatment goal for all patients in the oncology setting. A more realistic approach is a management plan that facilitates the effective implementation and continuation of cancer treatment. The most common approaches to substance abuse can be separated into psychotherapeutic and pharmacologic interventions.[63–65]

PSYCHOTHERAPEUTIC APPROACH

An effective psychotherapeutic treatment approach focuses on the development of effective coping skills, relapse prevention, and, most important, treatment compliance. The substance of choice has been the patient's primary, albeit maladaptive, coping tool. As a result, improvement in coping skills in these individuals is critical. When compounded with the stress associated with having cancer, the cessation can be overwhelming and can contribute to noncompliance and discontinuation of treatment. Teaching specific, illness-related coping methods is essential, and harm reduction with crisis intervention as a central component should be utilized. Support groups and 12-step programs can offer added benefit. Although traditional 12-step groups are based on an abstinence only policy, recent support groups have been tailored to the pain-specific population.

PHARMACOLOGIC APPROACH

Disulfiram (Antabuse) is a pharmacologic agent that has been approved by the U.S. Food and Drug Administration (FDA) since 1951 for the treatment of alcoholism.[66] Antabuse serves as a deterrent by inducing an unpleasant physical state characterized by nausea or vomiting when alcohol is consumed, thus ideally leading to alcohol cessation.[66] The practicality and effectiveness of Antabuse are questionable, because its use has been limited by difficulties with patient adherence for continued use of the drug.[67]

Several studies have suggested that patients often derive the greatest long-term benefit from Antabuse. These individuals tend to (1) be older than 40 years of age, (2) have longer drinking histories, (3) be socially stable, (4) be highly motivated, (5) have a history of prior attendance at Alcoholics Anonymous, (6) be cognitively intact, and (7) be able to maintain and tolerate relationships.[68–70] Further research is needed to ascertain which factors increase the likelihood of successful treatment (Table 55-3).

Table 55-3 Types and characteristics of benzodiazepines for treatment of alcohol withdrawal

Drug	Dose	Duration of action	Half-life, hr
Chlordiazepoxide	25–100 mg every 3 hours IV	Short	5–30
Diazepam	10–20 mg every 1–4 hours IV	Short	20–100
Lorazepam	1–2 mg every 1–4 hours IV	Intermediate	10–20
Midazolam	1–5 mg every 1–2 hours IV	Very short	1–4

CONCLUSION

Managing cancer patients with drug and alcohol abuse/addiction can be labor intensive and difficult; a nonjudgmental, structured approach can lead to satisfying outcomes in even the most difficult patients.

REFERENCES

1. Substance Abuse and Mental Health Services Administration (SAMHSA). *Results from the 2003 National Survey on Drug Use and Health: national findings*. Rockville, MD: SAMHSA, Office of Applied Studies; 2004a. NSDUH Series H-25, DHHS Publication No. SMA 04-3964.

2. Substance Abuse and Mental Health Services Administration (SAMHSA). *Results from the 2004 National Survey on Drug Use and Health: national findings*. Rockville, MD: SAMHSA, Office of Applied Studies; 2005a. NSDUH Series H-28, DHHS Publication No. SMA 05-4062.

3. Passik SD, Olden M, Kirsh KL, Portenoy RK. Substance abuse issues in palliative care. In: Berger A, Portenoy RK, Weissman DE, eds. *Principles and practice of palliative care and supportive oncology*. Philadelphia: Lippincott Williams & Wilkins; 2007:593–603.

4. Burton RW, Lyons JS, Devens M, et al. Psychiatric consultations for psychoactive substance disorders in the general hospital. *Gen Hosp Psychiatry*. 1991;13:83–87.

5. Colliver JD, Kopstein AN. Trends in cocaine abuse reflected in emergency room episodes reported to DAWN. Drug Abuse Warning Network. *Public Health Rep*. 1991;106:59–68.

6. Derogatis LR, Morrow GR, Fetting J, et al. The prevalence of psychiatric disorders among cancer patients. *JAMA*. 1983;249:751–757.

7. Groerer J, Brodsky M. The incidence of illicit drug use in the United States, 1962–1989. *Br J Addict*. 1992;87:1345–1351.

8. Regier DA, Myers JK, Kramer M, et al. The NIMH Epidemiologic Catchment Area program: historical context, major objectives, and study population characteristics. *Arch Gen Psychiatry*. 1984;41:934–941.

9. American Psychiatric Association. *Diagnostic and statistical manual for mental disorders III*. Washington, DC: American Psychiatric Association; 1983.

10. Bruera E, Moyano J, Seifert L, et al. The frequency of alcoholism among patients with pain due to terminal cancer. *J Pain Symptom Manage*. 1995;10:599–603.

11. Reference deleted in proofs.

12. Cloninger CR, Sigvardsson S, Bohman M. Childhood personality predicts alcohol abuse in young adults. *Alcohol Clin Exp Res*. 1988;12:494–505.

13. Kirsh KL, Whitcomb LA, Donaghy K, et al. Abuse and addiction issues in medically ill patients with pain: attempts at clarification of terms and empirical study. *Clin J Pain*. 2002;18:S52–S60.

14. Dole VP. Narcotic addiction, physical dependence and relapse. *N Engl J Med*. 1972;286:988–992.

15. Martin WR, Jasinski DR. Physiological parameters of morphine dependence in man—tolerance, early abstinence, protracted abstinence. *J Psychiatr Res*. 1969;7:9–17.

16. Chapman CR, Hill HF. Prolonged morphine self administration and addiction liability: evaluation of two theories in a bone marrow transplant unit. *Cancer*. 1989;63:1636–1644.

17. Foley KM. Clinical tolerance to opioids. In: Basbaum AU, Besson JM, eds. *Towards a new pharmacotherapy of pain*. Chichester, UK: John Wiley and Sons; 1991:181.

18. France RD, Urban BJ, Keefe FJ. Long-term use of narcotic analgesics in chronic pain. *Soc Sci Med*. 1984;19:1379–1382.

19. Kanner RM, Foley KM. Patterns of narcotic drug use in a pacer pain clinic. *Ann N Y Acad Sci*. 1981;362:161–172.

20. Portenoy RK. Management of common opioid side effects during long-term therapy of cancer pain. *Ann Acad Med Singapore*. 1994;23:160–170.

21. Portenoy RK, Foley KM. Chronic use of opioid analgesics in non-malignant pain: report of 38 cases. *Pain*. 1986;25:171–186.

22. Twycross RG. Clinical experience with dia-morphine in advanced malignant disease. *Int J Clin Pharmacol Ther Toxicol*. 1974;7:187–198.

23. Urban BJ, France RD, Steinberger EK, et al. Long term use of narcotic/antidepressant medication in the management of phantom limb pain. *Pain*. 1986;24:191–196.

24. Zenz M, Strumpf M, Tryba M. Long-term oral opioid therapy in patients with chronic nonmalignant pain. *J Pain Symptom Manage*. 1992;7:69–77.

25. Wikler A. *Opioid dependence: mechanisms and treatment*. New York: Plenum Press; 1980.

26. Ling GS, Paul D, Simantov R, et al. Differential development of acute tolerance to analgesia, respiratory depression, gastrointestinal transit and hormone release in a morphine infusion model. *Life Sci*. 1989;45:1627–1636.

27. Bruera E, Macmillan K, Hanson J, et al. The cognitive effects of the administration of narcotic analgesics in patients with cancer pain. *Pain*. 1989;39:13–16.

28. Redmond Jr DE, Krystal JH. Multiple mechanisms of withdrawal from opioid drugs. *Annu Rev Neurosci*. 1984;7:443–478.

29. American Psychiatric Association. *Diagnostic and statistical manual for mental disorders IV*. Washington, DC: American Psychiatric Association; 1994.

30. World Health Organization. *Youth and drugs*. Technical report no. 516. Geneva, Switzerland: World Health Organization; 1973.

31. Halpern LM, Robinson J. Prescribing practices for pain in drug dependence: a lesson in ignorance. *Adv Alcohol Subst Abuse*. 1985;5:135–162.

32. Dai S, Corrigall WA, Coen KM, et al. Heroin self-administration by rats: influence of dose and

physical dependence. *Pharmacol Biochem Behav.* 1989;32:1009–1015.

33. Passik SD, Kirsh KL, McDonald MV, et al. A pilot survey of aberrant drug-taking attitudes and behaviors in samples of cancer and AIDS patients. *J Pain Symptom Manage.* 2000;19:274–286.

34. Helzer JE, Pryzbeck TM. The co-occurence of alcoholism with other psychiatric disorders in the general population and its impact on treatment. *J Study Alcohol.* 1998;49:219–224.

35. Regier DA, Farmer ME, Rae DS, et al. Comorbidity of mental disorders with alcohol and other drug abuse: results from the Epidemiologic Catchment Area (ECA) study. *JAMA.* 1990;264:2511–2518.

36. Khantzian EJ, Treece C. DSM-III psychiatric diagnosis of narcotic addicts: recent findings. *Arch Gen Psychiatry.* 1985;42:1067–1071.

37. Portenoy RK, Lussier D, Kirsh KL, Passik SD. Pain and addiction. In: Frances RJ, Miller SI, Mack AH, eds. *Clinical textbook of addictive disorders.* New York: Guilford Press; 2005:367–395.

38. Passik SD, Portenoy RK. Substance abuse disorders. In: *Psycho-oncology.* New York, NY: Oxford University Press; 1998:576–586.

39. Passik SD, Kirsh KL, Whitcomb L, et al. Pain clinicians' rankings of aberrant drug-taking behaviors. *J Pain Palliat Care Pharmacother.* 2002;16:39–49.

40. Weissman DE, Haddox JD. Opioid pseudoaddiction—an iatrogenic syndrome. *Pain.* 1989;36:363–366.

41. Passik SD, Portenoy RK, Ricketts PL. Substance abuse issues in cancer patients. Part 1: Prevalence and diagnosis. *Oncology (Williston Park).* 1998;12:517–521 524.

42. Passik SD, Kirsh KL, Donaghy KB, et al. Pain and aberrant drug-related behaviors in medically ill patients with and without histories of substance abuse. *Clin J Pain.* 2006;22:173–181.

43. Brown SA, Inaba RK, Gillin JC, et al. Alcoholism and affective disorder: clinical course of depressive symptoms. *Am J Psychiatry.* 1995;152:45–52.

44. Kushner MG, Sher KJ, Beitman BD. The relation between alcohol problems and the anxiety disorders. *Am J Psychiatry.* 1990;147:685–695.

45. Winokur G, Coryell W, Akiskal HS, et al. Alcoholism in manic-depressive (bipolar) illness: familial illness, course of illness, and the primary-secondary distinction. *Am J Psychiatry.* 1995;152:365–372.

46. Passik SD, Theobald DE. Managing addiction in advanced cancer patients: why bother? *J Pain Symptom Manage.* 2000;19:229–234.

47. Kirsh KL, Bennett JC, Hagen DS, et al. Initial development of a survey tool to detect issues of chemical coping in chronic pain patients. *Palliat Support Care.* 2007;5:219–226.

48. Bruera E, Seifert L, Fainsinger RL, et al. The frequency of alcoholism among patients with pain due to terminal cancer. *J Pain Symptom Manage.* 1995;10:599–603.

49. Khantzian EJ. The self-medication hypothesis revisited: the dually diagnosed patient. *Prim Psychiatry.* 2003;10:47–48 53–54.

50. Kirsh KL, Jass C, Bennett DS, et al. Initial development of a survey tool to detect issues of chemical coping in chronic pain patients. *Palliat Support Care.* 2007;5:219–226.

51. Sifneos PE. Alexithymia: past and present. *Am J Psychiatry.* 1996;153(suppl 7):137–142.

52. Avila LA. Somatization or psychosomatic symptoms? *Psychosomatics.* 2006;47:163–166.

53. Substance Abuse and Mental Health Services Administration (SAMHSA). *National Survey on Drug Use and Health: summary of methodological studies, 1971-2005.* Methodology Series M-6. Rockville, MD: Office of Applied Studies, Department of Health and Human Services, SAMHSA; 2006:140.

54. Boyd CJ, McCabe SE. Coming to terms with the nonmedical use of prescription medications. *Subst Abuse Treat Prev Policy.* 2008;3:22.

55. Passik SD, Kirsh KL, Whitcomb L, et al. A new tool to assess and document pain outcomes in chronic pain patients receiving opioid therapy. *Clin Ther.* 2004;26:552–561.

56. Reference deleted in proofs.

57. Passik SD, Weinreb HJ. Managing chronic nonmalignant pain: overcoming obstacles to the use of opioids. *Adv Ther.* 2000;17:70–83.

58. Webster LR, Webster RM. Predicting aberrant behaviors in opioid-treated patients: preliminary validation of the Opioid Risk Tool. *Pain Med.* 2005;6:432–442.

59. Webster LR. Assessing abuse potential in pain patients. *Medscape Neurol Neurosurg.* 2004;6.

60. Ewing JA. Detecting alcoholism: the CAGE questionnaire. *JAMA.* 1984;252:1905–1907.

61. Cherpitel CJ. Brief screening instruments for alcoholism. *Alcohol Health Res World.* 1997;21:348–351.

62. Cherpitel CJ. *Gender and acculturation differences in performance of screening instruments for alcohol problems among U.S. Hispanic emergency room patients.* Paper presented at: Alcohol Epidemiology Symposium of the Kettil Bruun Society for Social and Epidemiological Research, Reykjavik, Iceland:1997.

63. Maxmen JS, Ward NG. Substance-related disorders. In: *Essential psychopathology and its treatment.* New York, NY: W.W. Norton & Company; 1995:132–172.

64. Erstad BL, Cotugno CL. Management of alcohol withdrawal. *Am J Health Syst Pharm.* 1995;52:697–709.

65. Newman JP, Terris DJ, Moore M. Trends in the management of alcohol withdrawal syndrome. *Laryngoscope.* 1995;105:1–7.

66. Suh JJ, Pettinati HM, Kampman KM, et al. The status of disulfiram: a half of a century later. *J Clin Psychopharmacol.* 2006;26:290–302.

67. Weinrieb RM, O'Brien CP. Diagnosis and treatment of alcoholism. In: Dunner DL, ed. *Current psychiatric therapy.* 2nd ed. Philadelphia: PA; Saunders; 1997.

68. Fuller RK, Gordis E. Does disulfiram have a role in alcoholism treatment today? *Addiction.* 2004;99:21–24.

69. Banys P. The clinical use of disulfiram (Antabuse): a review. *J Psychoactive Drugs.* 1988;20:243–261.

70. Hughes JC, Cook CC. The efficacy of disulfiram: a review of outcome studies. *Addiction.* 1997;92:381–395.

Care of professional caregivers

56

Brenda M. Sabo and Mary L. S. Vachon

The sting of illness and death is the spectre of broken relationships and the loss of the world. Over and against this threat stand the efforts of caregivers and companions to embrace the sufferer and continuously reaffirm his or her capacity for relationship.[1]

Working in supportive and palliative care has been described as both rewarding and stressful for health care professionals.[2–4] This chapter will review the stressors, mediating factors, and sources of satisfaction associated with work in this field. One of the key concepts in the chapter will be the notion that engagement in self-care activities as a fundamental part of care has the potential for transformation and regeneration for patient and professional alike.[5–7] Finally, select strategies supporting self-care will be provided.

OCCUPATIONAL STRESS AMONG ONCOLOGY HEALTH CARE PROFESSIONALS

Research over the past four decades has identified several potential adverse consequences affecting the health and well-being of professionals who provide caring work; consequences cited include stress and problems with physical health,[8] burnout,[9] compassion fatigue,[10,11] moral distress[12] and moral residue,[13] and vicarious traumatization.[14]

Sources of stress and burnout can have their origin in organizational issues (e.g., lack of value, control, poor leadership) as well as "emotion work" (e.g., requirement to display or suppress emotions on the job, requirement to be emotionally empathic). Emotionally laden work has been shown to account for additional variance in burnout scores over and above job stressors.[15] Some nonrelationship factors that may lead health care professionals to experience a sense of ambiguity and/or conflict about their ability to provide the care they think is needed include increased patient complexity, reliance on advancing technology to sustain or prolong life, continued emphasis on medical models supporting "cure" over "care," and perceived "lack of time."[16–20] Ongoing exposure to these factors may lead the professional to experience compassion fatigue, burnout, moral distress, and morale residue and/or vicarious traumatization.

Within oncology, the emotional aspect of working with patients who are in pain, suffering, or at end of life has been recognized repeatedly as potentially stress inducing.[3,7,18,21–30] To a lesser extent, work in palliative care has also been found to be potentially stress inducing.[31–34] Similar to the foundation of nursing practice, which is rooted in the therapeutic relationship and caring,[35–37] researchers have noted that palliative care is given through the medium of a human relationship.[38] Barnard and colleagues[38] found that education for palliative care involves the art of building and sustaining relationships and using the self as a primary instrument for diagnosis and treatment. This involves psychological risk taking that may be unique in the health field. Caregivers in oncology may also use themselves as a major aspect of caring.[7,39] What follows is an overview of the most frequently identified potential consequences of caring work within supportive oncology and palliative care.

BURNOUT

Burnout is rooted in the understanding of the interpersonal context of the job—that is, the relationship between caregiver and recipient of care and the values and beliefs held by the care provider as they pertain to caring work.[15] It is most commonly defined as "a syndrome of emotional exhaustion, depersonalization, and reduced accomplishments that can occur among individuals who do 'people work' of some kind."[40] The emotional exhaustion component (EE) represents the basic individual stress dimension of burnout. It refers to feelings of being overextended and depleted of one's emotional and physical resources. The cynicism (or depersonalization [DP]) component represents the interpersonal context dimension of burnout. It refers to a negative, callous, or excessively detached response to various aspects of the job. The component of reduced efficacy or personal accomplishment (PA) represents the self-evaluation dimension of burnout. It refers to feelings of incompetence and lack of achievement and productivity at work.[15] Initially conceptualized to reflect the effects of people work, burnout has been expanded to include all occupations.[41]

Although a number of theoretical frameworks have been proposed to explain burnout (e.g., individual, interpersonal, organizational, societal), research suggests that the most plausible explanation falls within the category of workplace or organizational environment.[42] Increasingly, research supports the notion that burnout arises out of a mismatch between the person and the job.[9,43] Early conceptualization and research focused on the relationship between the care provider and the care recipient as a necessary element in the development of burnout. In particular, the relationship was seen to contribute to emotional exhaustion, which was thought to be the root cause of burnout. As research shifted from descriptive to inferential study designs, findings strongly suggested that the relationship was not the key driver for experiencing burnout.[44,45] Research now supports six work-life issues involving person-job mismatch as the most likely explanation for cause. They include work overload, lack of control, lack of reward, lack of community, lack of fairness, and value conflict.[9,15,43,46] Burnout is by far the most researched of the models for understanding occupational stress. The following section provides a synthesis of previous reviews of the variables associated with stress and burnout in oncology and palliative care.[30,33,34,47]

Workload

Excessive workload exhausts the individual to the extent that recovery becomes difficult. A review of the literature[47] showed that from the early 1970s, there were perceived difficulties with workload and insufficient staff to do the job at hand in both oncology and palliative care, because the 1970s oncology staff, in particular, reported being overwhelmed with the workload imposed by the increase in cancer and the chronic nature of the illness. In contrast, palliative care physicians in the United Kingdom experienced less of a sense of work overload than did colleagues in clinical and radiation oncology.[29] Depersonalization and high General Health Questionnaire (GHQ) scores were associated with being overloaded.[29] A study of hospice nurses in the United Kingdom found that despite workload being a frequently reported stressor, it was not related to burnout.[31]

More recently, however, a study of 401 specialist registrars in palliative medicine, medical oncology, and clinical oncology[48] found that one in four had GHQ-12 scores above the threshold indicating possible psychiatric morbidity. The occupational stressor with the highest mean score, and ranking as the highest stressor for all three specialties, was "being overstretched at times." However, significant differences were noted between the three groups in mean scores, with medical oncology having the highest mean. As in other studies, the "effect of hours of work on personal/family life" is an important stressor for specialists. Indeed the items with the highest scores appear to relate to the very issue in clinical practice that one might expect these trainees to be concerned about—being competent in the face of conflicting demands on time.

A recent study comparing staff in oncology and palliative care in an oncology center[4] found that 63% reported experiencing "a great deal" of stress at work. The top two variables predicting this stress were greater perceived workload and insufficient time to grieve patients' deaths. A total of 52% felt that their workload negatively affected patient care, and more than 80% felt that it affected their ability to provide emotional support for patients and compassionate end-of-life care. In all, 55% stated that they did not have sufficient time to grieve the death of a patient, and more than 30% felt they did not have enough resources to cope with work-related stress. The actual workplace (palliative care unit vs. oncology unit) did not predict the degree of perceived distress, nor were there any significant associations for age, marital status, or full-time versus part-time status. Stress at home also did not predict work-related stress, indicating that the perceived stress at work was not caused by stress at home. Of interest is previous research conducted at the same oncology center more than 30 years earlier. In that study, nurses reported lack of resource personnel, and physicians reported "a tremendous workload imposed by the prevalence of cancer, the increased life expectancy and chronic nature of the disease."[49]

Control

The issue of control is related to lack of efficacy or reduced personal accomplishment. Mismatches often indicate that individuals have insufficient control over the resources necessary to do their work, or insufficient authority to pursue the work in what they believe is the most effective manner.[9]

Caregivers consistently report having difficulty performing their jobs because of a lack of organizational resources.[4,24,28,29,50]

In addition, they report feeling disenfranchised[25] and having an imbalance between their job and their authority.[51]

Reward

Lack of reward may be financial, when one does not receive a salary or benefits commensurate with achievements, or social, when one's hard work is ignored and is not appreciated by others. The lack of intrinsic rewards (e.g., doing something of importance and doing it well) can also be a critical part of this mismatch. Issues with the financial reward for work were noted by physicians.[50,52,53] Almost half of Italian oncology nurses, compared with one third of oncologists, reported low salaries.[50] Low personal accomplishment and high stress were reported when pay was inequitable,[54] or when resources to do one's work were lacking.[4,52,54]

In a large French study of 574 oncology professionals from 212 centers attached to the Great West Cancerople,[55] the greatest cause of social stress influencing quality of life at work is the need for acknowledgment from peers, the hierarchy, and doctors. Oncology support staff reported feeling a lack of value and recognition. Their lowest satisfaction score was related to job recognition.[56] Reports of communication problems with administration often reflect a lack of social rewards.[23] In the study by Ramirez and colleagues,[29] researchers found that when oncologists derived little satisfaction from their work, they were at greater risk for experiencing burnout.

Community

This mismatch arises when people lose a sense of personal connection with others in the workplace. Social support from people with whom one shares praise, comfort, happiness, and humor affirms membership in a group with a shared sense of values. In the study by Kash et al.,[25] oncologists reported that they received less support from their colleagues than did nurses or fellows. Lack of support from administration was reported by Italian nurses,[50] as well as by support staff at Massachusetts General Hospital.[56] Among Greek staff, a lack of role clarity was associated with burnout.[57] French nurses reported that the absence of a doctor at the time of a patient's death was associated with distress lasting for a week after the patient's death.[23] Gynecologic oncologists had high depersonalization and high job stress if they had difficult relations with colleagues.[54] High EE and high job stress were associated with taking on managerial responsibilities and relationships with colleagues.[54]

Although teamwork has been seen as the best and perhaps the only way of providing palliative care, some of the assumptions of palliative care teamwork have come into question.[58] A group consists of "two or more people who are interacting with one another, who share a set of common goals and norms which direct their activities, and who develop a set of roles and a network of affective relationships."[58] In contrast, a team is a group of people brought together, from within or outside the organization, for a specific purpose or task. In working to achieve the task, it is expected that team members will work interdependently and will take some ownership for the task. The quintessential feature of a small, well-balanced team is leadership that is shared or rotates, depending on the issue involved. Palliative care teams generally function with an identified leader, and there are often prescribed ways of dealing with issues such as standing orders. Within the team, tension may be expressed internally or may be deflected toward others who do not refer to members appropriately, who do not appreciate what members do, or who do not value their work.[34,58]

Research on a new palliative care team in an academic palliative care unit in Germany[59] found that factors crucial to communication in the team members' views were close communication, team philosophy, good interpersonal relationships, high team commitment, autonomy, and the ability to deal with death and dying. Close communication was by far the most frequently mentioned criterion for cooperation. Team performance, good coordination of workflow, and mutual trust underpin the evaluation of efficient teamwork. Inefficient teamwork is associated with the absence of clear goals, tasks, and role delegation, as well as a lack of team commitment. Team members spoke of common understandings; mutual openness, respect, and a positive attitude; a basic trust in one another's contribution to the common goal; reliance on colleagues; and openness and flexibility. Lack of communication and task conflict were the most frequently mentioned factors requiring cooperation. However, at the end of the first year of operation, the three salient outcome criteria for cooperation—team commitment, work satisfaction, and team performance—had evolved positively in the view of the team.

Fairness

This mismatch arises when there is no perceived fairness in the workplace. Fairness communicates respect and confirms people's self-worth. Mutual respect between people is central to a shared sense of community. Recent research in a university setting showed that fairness in the work environment may be the tipping point determining whether people develop job engagement or burnout.[60] Lack of fairness was perceived in unrealistic expectations of the organization.[3] Concerns about funding rivalries between hospices and other settings of care[61] and between different hospices have long been an issue.[3,62]

Barbara Munroe, a social worker with a long history of working in palliative care, and now CEO of St. Christopher's Hospice, suggests there needs to be considerable change in the delivery of palliative care. With the changes being proposed by Munroe,[63] much skill will be required to focus on "first principles," that is, what it is that needs to be done for the highest and best good of the patients and families whom we serve.

Values

People might feel constrained by their job to do something unethical and not in accord with their own values. Alternatively, there may be a mismatch between their personal career goals and the values of the organization. People can also be caught in conflicting values of the organization, as when there is a discrepancy between a lofty mission statement and actual practice, or when the values are in conflict (e.g., high-quality service and cost containment do not always coexist). Staffing problems can lead to not being able to do the job properly, a decrease in quality patient care, and decreased staff morale.[24] Gynecologic oncologists had high EE and high job stress if their expertise was not being put to good use.[54] Burned out oncology surgeons[64] were less satisfied with their career choice. Surgeons in private practice were less likely to say that they would become a physician again, and were less likely to say that they would become a surgical oncologist again. Devoting less than 25% of one's time to research was associated with burnout in that study.[64]

In a national study (n = 3213) exploring the interaction between workload and value congruence (personal and system) among Canadian family physicians, researchers found that both workload and value congruence were strong predictors of emotional exhaustion and cynicism ($P = .01$) for both genders, whereas value congruence was found to be a strong predictor of personal efficacy ($P = .01$).[65] Similarly, an article providing strategies to reduce burnout among oncologists reported that optimization of career fit (balance between personal and professional goals/values) led to increased job satisfaction.[66]

Emotion-work variables

Emotion-work variables require the individual to display or suppress emotions on the job and involve the requirement to be emotionally empathic. Research has found that these emotional factors account for additional variance in burnout scores over and above job stressors.[15] Oncology staff report difficulty in various aspects of communicating with sick, suffering, and dying patients and their family members,[24,50,51] particularly if they are young.[50] Although the literature has been somewhat divided as to whether the care of the dying is a major stressor in hospice palliative care,[3,67] Payne[31] found that the most problematic stressor reported by hospice nurses was "death and dying." In contrast, a survey of 464 palliative care staff from a variety of disciplines in New Zealand[68] did not identify "death and dying" issues as a major contributor to creating a stressful work environment. Participants reported that these issues were manageable as long as there were sufficient and appropriate organizational support practices, such as acknowledgment of the deaths, the use of rituals, and the availability of debriefing, if required. A study of 18 academic oncologists found that some oncologists took a biomedical approach, whereas others incorporated psychosocial elements into their practice in an effort to assist the patient and family to cope with the process of dying.[39] The psychosocial elements integrated into their practice included effective communication, building a therapeutic relationship, and caring for both patient and family.

Boston et al.[69] noted that dying persons experience disruption of the essence of day-to-day living and challenges to their perception of who they are. Through this process, they gain new wisdom and reshape their sense of meaning in life. A different way of knowing the world evolves, characterized by inner know-how and tacit knowledge that defines the self in relation to others. Caregivers and others around them "are perceived to be in another place, or don't seem to be there at all."[69] Patients and caregivers may feel that they just do not connect. Boston and coauthors[69] speak of palliative care as taking caregivers into emotional realms that are neither easy nor comfortable. When patients experience meaning and peacefulness in relation to their approaching death, this enriches the lives of the clinicians involved. This phenomenon appears similar to the "healing connections" identified by Mount, Boston, and Cohen.[70]

COMPASSION FATIGUE

The past 20 years have seen a surge in research linking exposure to pain, suffering, and trauma with the health of professionals providing care.[11,71–74] An offshoot of burnout, the term *compassion fatigue* was first used by a nurse studying burnout among emergency room nurses.[11] Compassion fatigue has been described as the "natural consequent behaviours and emotions resulting from knowing about a traumatizing event experienced by a significant other—the stress resulting from helping, or wanting to help, a traumatized or suffering person."[10] Researchers suggest that the phenomenon is connected to the therapeutic relationship between the health care provider and the patient; the traumatic or suffering experience of the patient triggers a response on multiple levels in the provider. In particular, an individual's capacity for empathy and ability to engage in, or enter into, a therapeutic relationship is considered central to compassion fatigue. Individuals who display high levels of empathy and empathic response to a patient's pain, suffering, or traumatic experience are more vulnerable to experiencing compassion fatigue.[72,75]

The dominant theoretical model postulating the emergence of compassion fatigue draws on a stress process framework.[72,76] Key elements within this model include empathic ability, empathic response, and residual compassion stress. The model is based on the assumption that empathy and emotional energy are the critical elements necessary for forming a therapeutic relationship and a therapeutic response. Although each factor is defined (e.g., empathic ability "is the aptitude of the psychotherapist to notice the pain of others"[76[p. 1436]]), the description of how each factor potentially interacts with another is limited. The model is depicted as a series of cascading events beginning with exposure to a patient's pain, suffering, and/or traumatic event. Empathic concern and empathic ability on the part of the nurse produce an empathic response, which may result in compassion stress (residue of emotional energy). If the nurse feels positive about her/his efforts or distances herself/himself from the story of pain/suffering or trauma, compassion stress may be prevented. If the stress continues to build, compassion fatigue may ensue. This risk is increased if the nurse experiences (1) ongoing exposure to suffering, (2) memories that elicit an emotional response, or (3) unexpected disruptions in her/his life. Limitations of this model include an emphasis on a linear direction and dimension for compassion fatigue (you either have it or you don't). This seems antithetical to human behavior responses in which individuals may express varying degrees of response. For example, an individual may not have compassion fatigue or may be slightly, moderately, or severely affected.

MORAL DISTRESS

Nursing and caring work have often been perceived as synonymous with ethics and ethical practice.[77,78] The goals of nursing, such as (1) protecting the patient from harm, (2) providing safe, effective quality care, and (3) maintain a healing therapeutic environment for patients and families (psychically, psychologically, emotionally, and spiritually), are "demonstrably ethical,"[79] given the inherent vulnerability associated with the patient role. When these goals are compromised, the nurse may experience moral distress. This might occur in situations such as when (1) the nurse feels unable to maintain a safe, healing environment (e.g., working short staffed), or (2) nursing values and beliefs are challenged by the health care system within which she/he works. Indeed these ethical dilemmas are not an uncommon occurrence for nurses working with acutely ill patients such as those on critical care or oncology units.[80]

Nurses are not alone in facing moral dilemmas and experiencing moral distress. Palliative care physicians have written about their personal experiences, along with the ensuing frustrations and thoughts or actions about leaving the profession.[81] Weissman[81] noted that since the beginning of the service, they have "had two nurses and two physicians with an accumulated 30-plus years of palliative care experience, partly or completely hang up their palliative care shingle." The sheer frustration of working within a system that is out of sync with the needs of both patients and care providers, and that impedes their ability to meet the needs of the dying, lingered long after each shift. These thoughts and feelings reflect the concept of moral distress, which occurs when the health care professional knows the correct action to take, but institutional or other constraints impede that action.[80,82,83] This general definition has been broadened to include situations in which one fails to pursue "the right course of action (or failing to do so to one's satisfaction) because of...an error in judgment, some personal failing...or circumstances beyond one's control."[13] Moral distress can have a profound effect on the integrity of the professional leaving, a "moral residue" associated with compromised values and beliefs.[79]

Serious moral compromise can lead to moral residue, the detritus "each of us carries with us from those times in our lives when, in the face of moral distress we have seriously compromised ourselves or allowed ourselves to be compromised."[13] The passage of time may blunt the acute experience of moral distress, but many people who have lived through serious moral compromise may carry the remnants of these experiences for many years, if not for a lifetime. The weight of moral residue over time may lead to fragmentation of one's sense of identity and may erode individuals' sense of meaning and purpose in their lives.[84]

VICARIOUS TRAUMATIZATION

Evidence within trauma research supports the notion that psychological distress affects individuals other than just those who have been personally traumatized.[73,85,86] The psychological distress experienced by health care professionals in their work with patients who are suffering or have been traumatized has been labeled vicarious traumatization.[14] Vicarious traumatization (VT) refers to the "[negative] transformation in the therapist's (or other trauma worker's) inner experience resulting from empathic engagement with clients' trauma material."[86] Researchers suggest that ongoing exposure to graphic accounts of human cruelty, trauma, and suffering, as well as healing work within the therapeutic relationship facilitated through "empathic openness" (as is the case in compassion fatigue), may leave health care providers vulnerable to emotional and spiritual consequences.[87]

In conjunction with empathy, two key sets of factors have been identified as contributing to the development of VT: (1) characteristics of the health care professional (i.e., previous personal history of abuse and/or personal life stressors, personal expectations, need to fulfill all patients' needs, inadequate training/inexperience), and (2) characteristics of the treatment (e.g., invasiveness; life-threatening; long-term side effects) and its context (i.e., type of patient; political, social, and cultural context within which [a] the treatment occurs and [b] the traumatic event took place).[14,88]

Explanatory models for vicarious traumatization are rooted in cognitive theory, which argues that core beliefs influence and filter how the world is viewed and experienced, leading to assimilation or accommodation.[89,90] This process suggests that a health professional's core beliefs may be altered by new information received from the patient, particularly if the information conflicts with her/his existing beliefs. This thinking would appear to be consistent with the transformative process underlying the development of vicarious traumatization.

Building on this, McCann and Pearlman,[91] and later Pearlman and Saakvitne,[86] used constructivist self-development theory (CSDT) to explain the "progressive development of a sense of self and world view in response to life experiences."[88] An individual's unique history (life experience) shapes how she/he will experience, interpret, and adapt to traumatic or highly stressful events. Their interactive model attempts to take into account the variability of life experience, suggesting that vicarious traumatization is unique to the individual.[88,91] For example, if a caregiver grew up in a home environment where one coped by dealing with stressful situations through escape/avoidance behavior (a negative coping strategy), she/he would likely use the same coping strategy in other stressful situations, as when witnessing ongoing patient suffering. If negative coping strategies are coupled with other contributing factors such as inadequate education, lack of emotional support, aggressive invasive treatments, and unrealistic expectations of self in her/his role as care provider, the risk for vicarious traumatization may be increased.[92]

OCCUPATIONAL HEALTH: THE BENEFITS OF CARING FOR ONCOLOGY AND PALLIATIVE PATIENTS

Satisfaction with one's work appears to be a secondary outcome, with the primary objective of studies focused on adverse consequences such as compassion fatigue (secondary trauma), burnout, moral distress, and vicarious traumatization. Few occupational health studies have, as their primary objective, to determine whether or not health care professionals achieve personal satisfaction from their work. This backdoor approach to understanding satisfaction may result in misleading findings. For example, if a researcher assumes that a specific area of oncology practice such as hematopoietic stem cell transplant must be stress inducing and administers an instrument to measure adverse consequences (e.g., burnout without a clear understanding of the nature of the work), it may very well appear that the nature of the work is inherently distressing, emotionally overwhelming, or traumatizing. In fact, the very opposite may be true. The benefits attributed to working with advanced cancer patients or individuals at end of life include compassion satisfaction, job engagement and satisfaction, vitality/hardiness/coherence, exquisite empathy, resilience, and hope.

COMPASSION SATISFACTION

Compassion satisfaction has been defined as "the pleasure you derive from being able to do your work well."[93] It stands in sharp contrast to compassion fatigue, which pertains to the negative effects arising from one's work. A review of occupational health literature highlights the adverse effects of oncology and end-of-life care.[94] In a recent study exploring the predictive factors associated with occupational stress, researchers found that 63% of staff (physicians, nurses, chaplains, and allied health professionals) self-reported work-related stress.[4] Dougherty and colleagues[4] hypothesized that satisfaction would be negatively correlated with work stress. In this descriptive study, researchers administered a 53-question survey to interprofessional oncology staff on two inpatient units (oncology and palliative care). In contrast to high levels of work-related stress, 85% of staff surveyed reported looking forward to work, and 70% reported that they had sufficient resources to offset stress. Although the findings are interesting and support the notion that working with individuals who are suffering, traumatized, or at end of life can be rewarding, further research is needed to clearly demonstrate the benefits of caring work.[94,95]

Additional evidence in support of the concept of work satisfaction may be found in a study by Vachon.[3] In the 1980s, the author conducted a large international study involving interviews with 581 caregivers (71% female and ranging in age from early 20s to early 70s) from a variety of health disciplines working with the critically ill, dying, and bereaved. When asked what kept them going in the face of multiple stressors, the primary reasons for continuing their work included "a sense of competence, control or pleasure in one's work."

Factors that have been identified as supporting compassion satisfaction range from positive affect and optimism to social support networks and work-life balance.[96] These same factors are reminiscent of factors associated with self-care strategies.[97-100] In a study of hospice workers, researchers hypothesized that self-care strategies would enhance compassion satisfaction and lower the likelihood of compassion fatigue.[101] This descriptive exploratory study surveyed health care professionals from two hospice settings. Three data collection instruments were used: demographic questions, self-care assessment worksheet,[102] and Professional Quality-of-Life (ProQOL) assessment.[93] Alkema and colleagues[101] found that compassion satisfaction was negatively correlated with burnout (r = −.612) and compassion fatigue (r = −.300). At the same time, researchers noted that self-care (excluding physical self-care) was negatively correlated with compassion fatigue, suggesting that health care professionals should integrate self-care strategies into their everyday lives. Further, Alkema and colleagues[101] found that emotional and spiritual self-care and personal-professional balance were predictive of higher levels of compassion satisfaction. Limitations of this study include the small sample size, limited sample diversity (hospice professionals were predominantly Caucasian, female, and between 28 and 37 years of age), and inability to infer causation because of the correlational study design. Although the findings are interesting, further research involving multiple methods and cause-effect designs is needed to understand the connection between compassion satisfaction, compassion fatigue, burnout, and self-care.

In an exploratory interpretative phenomenologic study that examined the psychosocial health of hematopoietic stem cell transplant nurses,[94] the author noted that when nurses felt part of a community of practice where they were able to share their experiences, feelings of isolation and emotional distress were perceived as less overwhelming. By sharing their experiences, nurses were able to enhance their current level of knowledge and understanding, both academic and tacit. Researchers

have pointed to the intrinsic value of reflecting and learning from one's clinical practice[103-105] and personal experience.[106] Further, when professionals feel part of a community, they are more likely to experience satisfaction and control, even in work environments that may prove challenging.[60,107]

Perhaps a more helpful approach to understanding the experience of compassion or job satisfaction may be to examine this aspect of quality of life within the context of life satisfaction. Life satisfaction has been defined as one's perception of personal well-being (subjective) when the goal is to optimize positive or pleasant experiences while minimizing the unpleasant.[108] In other words, health care professionals focus on those aspects of their work, such as the patient-family-professional relationship, that give them the most personal and professional benefit or reward.[50,94,95,109,110] Drawing on two theoretical models, top-down[108,111,112] and bottom-up,[113] Swedish researchers sought to understand the connections among life satisfaction, work-life, and personal characteristics in pediatric oncologists.[114] A top-down approach emphasizes the roles of personality, stable life, and cultural diversity in predicting well-being. In contrast, a bottom-up approach highlights the roles of current mood, temporary life circumstances, and context in satisfaction. Stenmarker and colleagues[114] found that "pediatric oncology positively influenced their personal development in spite of the medical, psychosocial and existential challenges."[114] It may be that the work environment (academic treatment facility) supported more positive outcomes for patients, facilitated teamwork, and enhanced access to continuing education. It may also have led to a more positive outlook on life and social nature. What is unique about this study is the focus on life satisfaction informing job satisfaction, rather than the reverse. Limitations of this study include its cross-sectional design, homogeneous sample, and lack of a control group. Further research is needed to understand how personality, general life satisfaction, work-life, and context may influence job satisfaction.

JOB ENGAGEMENT

Job engagement is conceptualized as being the opposite of burnout.[115] It involves energy, involvement, and efficacy. Engagement involves the individual's relationship with work. This includes a sustainable workload, feelings of choice and control, appropriate recognition and reward, a supportive work community, fairness and justice, and meaningful and valued work. Engagement is also characterized by high levels of activation and pleasure.[114,115] Engagement is defined as a persistent, positive-affective-motivational state of fulfillment in employees that is characterized by vigor, dedication, and absorption.[115]

VITALITY, THE TRANSFORMATIVE POWER OF POSITIVE EMOTION, AND RESILIENCE

Vitality has been defined as "the capacity to live and develop or the power to endure."[117] The concept has considerable relevance when considered within the context of supportive oncology and palliative care. Physicians, nurses, and other professionals have identified a "way of living" through personal connections, significant emotional experiences, and meaning as underlying vitality.[61] Further, vitality has been associated with energy, life, animation, and importance.[118]

These very qualities may help to explain why many health care professionals reap immense rewards and personal satisfaction from their work, even in the face of patient/family suffering, trauma, and dying.

Webster and Kristjanson[61] found that the lessons that health care professionals learned from their work added meaning to their personal and professional lives. Described in terms of personal growth, interactions with patients, families, and colleagues added a dimension to palliative care work that shifted their work beyond mere care (technical aspect) to caring. Crucial to the experience of palliative care for the participants were patient and family, holistic care, and the interdisciplinary team.[61] Similarly, in research exploring the meaning of hematopoietic stem cell transplant nursing, Sabo[94] found that when nurses were connected in a compassionate, caring, and fully present manner with patients and families, they were able to transform the experience from one that was emotionally overwhelming to one of privilege, reward, and personal and professional growth.

Relationships continue to remain at the core of supportive and palliative care. Katz[5] has applied the psychiatric concept of counter-transference to end-of-life care. Counter-transference is defined as "…an 'abbreviation' for the totality of our responses to our work—emotional, cognitive, and behavioral—whether prompted by our patients, by the dynamics incumbent to our helping relationships, or by our own inevitable life experiences."[5] End-of-life care professionals of all disciplines and levels of experience, not just therapists, are subject to powerful reactions to their work. These reactions are seen as being far more diverse than "compassion fatigue" or "vicarious traumatization." Drawing on the quantum physics concept that the whole is greater than the sum of its parts, similar to Kearney's *A Place of Healing: Working With Suffering in Living and Dying,*[6] Katz[5] speaks of the alchemical reaction that occurs when two individuals engage together at the most vulnerable time in human existence—the end of life. Alchemy is "that space" that takes its own place in the poignant relationship between helper and patient. Through the experience, both can be transformed.

Vaillant,[119] known for his pioneering work in adult development, has recently written of the transformative power of positive emotion, "All human beings are hardwired for positive emotions, and these positive emotions are a common denominator of all major faiths and of all human beings."[119] He suggests that such positive emotions are essential to the survival of *Homo sapiens* as a species. In contrast, negative emotions such as anger and fear are "all about me" and do little to support growth and change within the individual, in part because of the focus on the present. Vaillant[119] suggests that positive emotions are more expansive and help us to build. They widen our tolerance, expand our moral compass, and enhance our creativity. They help us to survive in time future…while negative emotions narrow attention and miss the forest for the trees; positive emotions, especially joy, make thought patterns more flexible, creative, integrative, and efficient.

Positive emotions have the capacity to undo the physical effects associated with negative emotions, returning the individual to a pre-stressor baseline.[120,121] Positive emotions "serve not only as breathers, providing a psychological break or respite, but also as restorers, replenishing resources."[122] Research has found positive emotions to be associated with resilience. Defined as the ability to bounce back or cope successfully despite considerable adversity,[123] this commonly held trait results "from the operation of basic human adaptational systems."[124] Reinforcing the connection between positive emotions and resilience are the positive attributes of resilience such as "re-integration," sense of purpose or self-determination, positive relationships/social network, flexibility, and self-esteem/self-efficacy.[125] Resilient people may use positive emotions as a mechanism for coping. Although not conclusive, studies suggest that resilient people not only use positive emotions for coping but elicit positive emotions in others, thereby creating a supportive social context that facilitates coping.[122] In their study exploring positive emotions and resilience following a terrorist attack on the World Trade Center, Frederickson et al.[122] found that positive emotions appeared to provide a core buffering effect against depression by broadening postcrisis resources. Further, resilience facilitated the participants' ability to draw on psychological resources such as optimism, life satisfaction, and tranquility (concepts closely related to resilience) and to grow from their crisis experiences.

In a study exploring stress-resilience capacity among pediatric oncologists, researchers found that an optimistic attitude, willingness to discuss existential issues associated with life and death, and high levels of motivation decreased the level of depression and enhanced job satisfaction and resilience.[114] In a similar vein, Ablett and Jones[126] compared palliative care nurses' sense of purpose about their work and commitment with two theoretical concepts underlying resilience: hardiness[127,128] and a sense of coherence.[129,130] Hardiness comprises three closely related aspects of resilience: commitment (sense of meaning and purpose in life), challenge (change as an opportunity for growth), and control (autonomy, self-efficacy).[127,128] Coherence sees one's life as being comprehensible, manageable, and meaningful.[129] Although hardiness and coherence overlap conceptually (e.g., meaning or purpose in life derives from the individual's social context), they also differ. Where hardiness stresses change as the norm, coherence places emphasis on stability and structure. Because some nurses in the study indicated a dislike for change, preferring stability, particularly when faced with mortality and uncertainty, the authors suggested that a sense of coherence might explain resilience for some participants, and hardiness might explain resilience for others, who viewed change as providing a sense of personal satisfaction and achievement.[126] The key factor seems to be the individual's attitude toward change.

In a cross-sectional national survey on predictors of career satisfaction, work-life balance, and burnout, mailed to 2000 physicians (48% response rate), factor analysis confirmed the presence of four domains: work-life balance, career satisfaction, personal accomplishment, and emotional resilience.[131] Measures of burnout strongly predicted career satisfaction. The strongest predictor of work-life balance was having some control over one's schedule. Both women and men reported moderate levels of emotional resilience (51% vs. 53%) and high levels of personal accomplishment (74%). The measures of burnout within personal accomplishment and emotional resilience (the opposite of emotional exhaustion) were both strong and significant predictors of career satisfaction, remaining strong predictors after adjustments were made for both work and demographic variables. Work-life balance, or having some control over schedule and hours worked, was the strongest work characteristic related to emotional resilience.

Being older significantly predicted both personal accomplishment and emotional resilience.[131]

The concept of resilience is important to the delivery of end-of-life care and the significant challenges it poses for those who provide or require care.[132] Resilient people are able to find positive meaning within stressors[133,134] "and have greater access to stored positive information that enables them to avoid being overwhelmed by the negative experiences and emotions that everyone goes through."[132] Monroe and her colleague, David Oliviere, a physician at St. Christopher's Hospice, again present a challenge that palliative care as it is currently being practiced must change, and this will require resilience in caregivers.

Malcolm Payne applies the concept of resilience to palliative care teams. He notes that the idea of resilience comes from attachment theory, which, in turn, comes from psychoanalytic theory. Payne uses ideas about resilience and attachment to enrich ideas about interprofessional teamwork. He notes that achieving resilient interprofessional teams in palliative care "means raising awareness and understanding of how organizations, teams and the individuals within them can respond effectively to adversities."[135] Adversities can come from many sources, both external and internal. A crucial element in adversity is its impact on individuals, the team, and the organization. The emphasis on resilience and attachment theory on emotional responses based in previous relationships draws attention to the importance of dealing with team members' emotional reactions to adversities. This is so because the main purpose of multidisciplinary teamwork is to facilitate more effective and coordinated holistic services to patients and their families."

EMPATHY AND COMPASSION

At the core of both supportive and palliative care is the relationship between the patient-family and the health care professional. It has been postulated that empathy provides the nurse, physician, and others working with patients and families who are suffering, traumatized, or at end of life, the capacity to connect with and understand them.[37,136,137] In essence, empathy conveys the ability of the professional to understand the world of the patient by "walking in their shoes." Empathy has been conceptualized as an innate human trait that can be refined and reinforced,[138] a professional state learned through cognitive and behavioral training,[139–141] a communication process[142]; it has also been conceptualized as caring (an outcome or intervention arising from an understanding the patient)[143,144] and as a reciprocal relationship.[145] Factors that support the development and expression of empathy include familiarity/similarity, self-awareness, experience/knowledge, and socialization.[146]

A recent study exploring protective practices that mitigated the risk of vicarious trauma among mental health therapists found that nine major themes were salient across the six clinicians' narratives of protective practices.[95] Although many of the themes are consistent with other research findings, one theme stood out—"exquisite empathy." Unlike previous studies, the authors found that empathic engagement with traumatized clients appeared to be a protective practice for clinicians working with traumatized clients. Exquisite empathy "required a sophisticated balance on the part of the clinician as s/he simultaneously maintains clear and consistent boundaries, expanded perspective, and highly present, intimate, and heartfelt interpersonal connection in the therapeutic relationship with clients, without fusing or losing sight of the clinician's own perspective."[95]

Qualitative research on peer-nominated, exemplary therapists who were thriving in their work with traumatized clients, including palliative care patients and their families, has identified a variety of protective practices that enhance caregivers' professional satisfaction and help prevent or mitigate compassion fatigue.[7,95] In particular, trauma therapists who engaged in *exquisite empathy* were "invigorated rather than depleted by their intimate professional connections with traumatized clients"[95] and were protected against compassion fatigue and burnout. This idea, which has also been referred to as *bi-directionality*,[95] refutes the commonly held notion that being empathic to dying patients inevitably leads to emotional depletion.[10,86,147,148] The practice of exquisite empathy is facilitated by clinician self-awareness,[95] which was identified in another study as the most important factor in psychologists' healthy functioning in the face of personal and professional stressors.[149]

Dr. Rachel Naomi Remen writes, "basically service is about taking life personally, letting the lives that touch yours touch you."[151] She contends that service is a relationship between equals. When you serve, the work itself keeps you from burnout. Unless you let the patients touch you, you will never last in this work.[151] Protecting ourselves from loss rather than grieving and healing our losses is one of the major causes of burnout[152]: "We burn out not because we don't care but because we don't grieve. We burn out because we have allowed our hearts to become so filled with loss that we have no room left to care."[152] Remen speaks of compassion, which, she says, "begins with the acceptance of what is most human in ourselves, what is most capable of suffering. In attending to our own capacity to suffer, we can uncover a simple and profound connection between our own vulnerability and the vulnerability in all others. Experiencing this allows us to find an instinctive kindness toward life which is the foundation of all compassion and genuine service."[151] Although similar to empathy, compassion is embedded within the context of emotion. It may be thought of as the experience of feeling **with** others, while recognizing that one is not actually feeling what they are feeling.[153] In understanding compassion as emotion, an affective dimension is reflected within feeling, which can be understood as "a mental tone that affects us and which characteristically permeates our perceptions, our desires and actions in ways which we are not aware of."[154] This quality suggests that compassion affects our lives over extended periods of time, not just in the moment, and could exist in the absence of feeling. For example, "the nurse who exhibits compassion will not simply respond with feelings at the time of the patient's suffering but will care for this patient in an ongoing way that may not always be expressed in terms of feeling."[155] Further, displays of compassion include characteristics such as virtue leading to concern for the good of others, awareness of the other's suffering, and a desire to act to relieve suffering.[36,37,155,156]

RELIGION AND SPIRITUALITY

In the early 1990s, academic medical centers, medical and nursing schools, residency programs, and hospitals began to recognize the role of spiritual care as a dimension of palliative care.[157] A recent consensus conference on improving the quality of spiritual care as a dimension of palliative care developed the following definition: "Spirituality is the aspect of humanity that refers to the way individuals seek and express meaning and purpose and the way they experience their connectedness to the moment, to self, to others, to nature, and to the significant or sacred."[(ibid,p.887)] With relationship as the core of spirituality, one might infer that health care, by virtue of its relational quality, is inherently spiritual. As such, Puchalski and colleagues[157] proposed a model of spiritual care reflected in the transformation occurring between professional-patient relationships. For this to occur, health care professionals "must have an awareness of the spiritual dimensions of their own lives and then be supported in the practice of compassionate presence with patients through a reflective process." In developing self-awareness of one's personal values, beliefs, and attitudes, a deeper, more meaningful connection may take place between the professional and the patient-family, as may enhanced coping[7,94,157] (Box 56-1).

The consensus conference proposed that spirituality should be considered a patient vital sign. Institutional policies for spiritual history and screening must be integrated into intake policies and ongoing assessment of care. Consistent with the philosophy of the National Consensus Project (NCP) Guidelines and the National Quality Forum (NQF) Preferred Practices, palliative care is appropriate regardless of disease status and can begin at the time of early diagnosis; in addition, attention to spiritual needs should be integrated across the trajectory of illness. In a study of 155 members of the Israeli Oncology Society, spiritual well-being, extrinsic religiosity, and education demonstrated significant direct relationships in a path analysis of attitudes toward spiritual care. Spiritual well-being of the nurse was the strongest predictor of Israeli oncology nurses' attitudes toward spiritual care.[158]

In a study exploring spirituality within an interdisciplinary palliative care team, researchers found that caregivers struggled to define spirituality.[159] Respondents included concepts related to integrity, wholeness, meaning, and personal journeying. For many, their spirituality was inherently relational,

might involve transcendence, was wrapped up in caring, and often manifested in small daily acts of kindness and of love. For some participants, palliative care was a spiritual calling. A collective spirituality, stemming from common goals, values, and belonging, surfaced. The authors suggest that further research might explore spirituality on a collective level, including a more in-depth study of the relationship between spirituality and tacit skills such as empathy, "being present," and compassion as used by palliative care professionals in caring for the dying. The question arises whether the spiritual belief systems of those in palliative care might serve as protection against burnout and compassion fatigue.

Sinclair's doctoral dissertation[160] involved research on key leaders among palliative hospice care providers (PHCPs), as well as a community of health care professionals within a local hospice who were interviewed regarding spirituality. The spirituality of PHCPs was experiential in nature, embedded within both their souls and the setting, involving an invisible and deeply real connection between the essence of one's self and another, or Other, that affected one's sense of wholeness both within and in relation to an ultimate reality. Spirituality was centered on presence—the outward radiance of soul, or PHCP, underlying discourse (consisting of virtues, vices, beliefs, experiences, and divine immanence). Spiritual care as an involuntary and universal facet of humanity was embedded across all acts of care, residing in the liminal space between PHCPs' own souls and the souls of those in their care, and had a residual effect on both parties' sense of connection and wholeness.[160]

Using Stamm's ProQOL,[161] Peter Huggard[162,163] studied 230 New Zealand physicians. A positive and significant correlation was found between compassion satisfaction[161] and spirituality. This study examined the relationship between compassion fatigue, compassion satisfaction, and burnout versus resilience, spirituality, empathy, emotional competence, and social-support–seeking behaviors. Huggard found a positive correlation between religion and vicarious traumatization.[162,163] Using the Scale of Psychological Well-Being,[164] high scores were noted on the "relationship with a higher power" subscale, which related to high scores on the compassion fatigue subscale. He also demonstrated a negative and significant correlation between spirituality and burnout.

In a study that used in-depth interviews with 10 palliative care physicians regarding their perspectives and experiences in the spiritual domain of care, several key themes emerged.[165] These included the concept of spirituality and the difference between spirituality and religion. The overarching theme involved the concept of how the participants' own spirituality affected their practice and how their practice affected their spirituality. These were inextricably woven together. Addressing spirituality was fundamental to a palliative care physician providing compassionate and holistic care.

BOX 56-1 Selected Recommendations for Staff Providing Palliative Care[157]

1. All members of the palliative care team should be trained in spiritual care. This training should be required as part of continuing education for all clinicians.
2. Team members should have training in self-care, self-reflection, contemplative practice, and spiritual self-care.
3. Health care systems should offer time for professional development of staff with regard to spiritual care and should develop accountability measures in spiritual care for the interprofessional team.
4. Board-certified chaplains can provide spiritual care education and support for interprofessional team members.
5. Clinical sites should offer education for community clergy members and spiritual care providers about end-of-life care procedures in health care facilities.
6. Chaplain certification and training in palliative care are needed.

INTERVENTIONS TO SUPPORT PHYSICAL, PSYCHOSOCIAL, AND EMOTIONAL WELL-BEING IN THE PROFESSIONAL CAREGIVER

Evidence shows that occupational stress may occur as a direct result of caring for cancer patients.[23,110,166] The need for self-care to ensure physical, psychological, and emotional well-being should be integrated into every health care professional's daily personal routine to decrease the risk for adverse effects such as compassion fatigue, burnout, moral distress, and vicarious traumatization.[9,10,88] The notion of self-care would appear to be an intuitive fit, given the relational quality of many of the practices of the health care disciplines.

Shanafelt et al.[66] found greater work satisfaction among oncologists who used wellness strategies in caring for themselves as they care for others. Vachon recently noted that as oncology nurses educate cancer patients about the importance of wellness strategies, they should take their own advice to heart and make wellness changes in their own lives.[167] The reminder that one receives when traveling on airplanes, "First, put on your own seat belt," applies to caregivers. First, make sure you are nurturing yourself. Self-care has even been shown to be associated with mental well-being and increased empathy in internal medicine residents.[168] The importance of a number of personal wellness promotion strategies (aspects of self-care, relationships, work attitudes, religious/spiritual practice, personal philosophies, and strategies related to work-life balance) differed for residents with higher mental well-being on the Short Form (SF)-8. Higher mental well-being was associated with enhanced resident empathy in this cross-sectional survey.

Jayne Huggard[68] inquired into the personal coping mechanisms used by New Zealand hospice staff and found that they fell into four categories: family/Whanau (extended Maori kinship system), religion/spirituality, self-care, and professional. Considerable support was received from family members and friends. Self-care practices included relaxation practices such as massage and meditation, reading, gardening, and time spent with pets. Personal interests such as playing sports, running and jogging, or participating in hobbies were included as part of self-care and therefore were seen as supportive. Other forms of support of a professional nature included educational opportunities taken (courses or conferences), supervision, counseling, coaching, or mentoring, and opportunities for networking; all of these were paid for by the individual, and therefore were seen as support received from outside the organization.[33]

In one of the largest intervention studies, Leblanc and colleagues[169] used a quasi-experimental design to test a team-based burnout intervention in 29 oncology units in the Netherlands. Nine wards were randomly selected to participate in the *Take Care!* intervention. The program consisted of six monthly 3-hour sessions that included education about the mechanisms of stress and feedback about participants' work situation. This feedback was used to help participants structure their subjective feelings by providing them with relevant topics for discussion of their plans to reduce stress on the ward. At the end of the first session, the job stressors that were dealt with during the training session were selected. The remaining sessions consisted of education and action portions. Subjects included unwanted collective behavior, communication and feedback, building a support network, balancing job-related investments and outcomes, personal experiences, and potential problems with change. During the action component, participants formed problem-solving teams. Outcomes from the sessions included the introduction of more efficient reporting procedures (patient, supplies), the appointment of staff as "guardian angels" to monitor staff well-being (support), and the restructuring of weekly staff meetings to give staff a "voice" in decision making. Results of multilevel

analyses showed that staff on the experimental wards experienced significantly less emotional exhaustion at both Time 2 (6 months) and Time 3 (1 year) and less depersonalization at Time 2 compared with control wards. Changes in burnout levels were significantly related to changes in the perception of job characteristics over time.[30]

SELF-AWARENESS AS A MECHANISM FOR ENHANCING SELF-CARE

Self-awareness involves both a "combination of self-knowledge and development of *dual-awareness,* a stance that permits the clinician to simultaneously attend to and monitor the needs of the patient, the work environment, and his or her own subjective experience."[7] When functioning with less self-awareness, clinicians are more likely to lose perspective, experience more stress in interactions with their work environment, experience empathy as a liability, and have a greater likelihood of compassion fatigue and burnout. Self-awareness may both enhance self-care and improve patient care and satisfaction.[149] Additionally, when professionals integrate self-awareness into their practice, this may help them to accept limits (including personal vulnerability, personal influence, responsibility and accountability for change, and limits of the known and unknown) and maintain clarity about self in relation to others, in terms of both interconnections and boundaries.[94,95]

Methods of self-care that do not involve enhanced self-awareness, such as maintaining clear professional boundaries, offer protection from occupational stressors and can make possible renewal outside of work. However, exclusive reliance on such approaches to self-care undermines the health care professional's ability to be emotionally available for patients or to find reward in their work.[6,7] Integrating self-awareness into one's clinical practice supports emotional availability, self-regeneration, and increased personal and professional fulfillment even when faced with difficult and/or emotionally challenging situations.[6,7,95] Several practical ways can be used to enhance self-awareness. These include initiatives such as continuing education,[169,170] peer support (Balint),[171,172] mindfulness meditation,[168,173,174] and reflective writing.[105,175]

Perhaps the most widely recognized means of increasing self-awareness, mindfulness meditation refers to a process of developing careful attention to minute shifts in body, mind, emotions, and environs, while holding a kind, nonjudgmental attitude toward self and others.[176] The practice of mindfulness meditation simultaneously raises the consciousness of one's inner reality (physical, emotional, and cognitive) and of the external reality with which individuals interact.[177] The practice has begun to be utilized and researched in the workplace. Some organizations have used mindfulness meditation as part of a larger intervention, and some have focused on mindfulness meditation. For example, an 8-week mindfulness-based stress reduction (MBSR) program for nurses in a hospital system was introduced and was found to lower burnout and improve well-being.[178] Results from this study showed that the treatment group decreased scores on the Maslach Burnout Inventory, and these changes lasted 3 months. Specifically, significantly decreased emotional exhaustion and depersonalization were noted with a trend toward significance in personal accomplishment.[178] In a matched, randomized controlled trial examining the effect of an 8-week mindfulness-based intervention program for medical students, the authors found that those participating in the intervention experienced less anxiety and depression and greater empathy than those in the control group.[179]

Recently, the concept of compassionate silence has emerged as a component of the patient-clinician encounter in palliative care.[180] This ability may come from contemplative practices such as mindfulness-based meditation. Compassion requires active intention—that is, the health care professional not only gives attention, but maintains focus and clarity of perception. "These compassionate silences arise spontaneously from the clinician who has developed the mental capacities of stable attention, emotional balance, and pro-social mental qualities, such as naturally arising empathy and compassion."[180]

Writing in a reflective and emotionally expressive way is another form of self-care that enhances self-awareness.

Somatic[181-184] and psychological benefits[185,186] of this practice have been demonstrated in patients and have been extended to promote reflection and empathic engagement in physicians.[187,188] Reflective writing has been utilized in a meaning-centered psychoeducational group intervention called *Enhancing Meaning in Palliative Care Nursing*, which was designed to support nurses providing palliative care.[189] This intervention aims to increase job satisfaction and quality of life and to prevent burnout. Based on Breitbart and colleagues' earlier work with palliative patients,[190] (1) characteristics of meaning, (2) sources of meaning, (3) creative values explored in terms of personal historical perspective and a sense of accomplishment at work, (4) suffering as a source of attitudinal change, and (5) affective experiences and humor were explored as experiential avenues to finding meaning. Although the intervention shows promise and has the potential to positively influence quality of life and job satisfaction among other palliative care professionals outside of nursing, more research and evaluation are needed.

PROFESSIONAL AND ORGANIZATIONAL RESPONSIBILITIES

In a study of New Zealand hospice workers, "personal support level, self-care strategies such as spiritual beliefs and reflective pastimes were seen to be a necessary and integral component to the practice of palliative care professionals. However, what was identified was that organizational support strategies appear to be the most important for hospice staff."[191] Huggard[191] identified the following professional responsibilities for staff working in palliative care: collegial support, line manager support, supervision and mentoring, personal debriefing model, being mindful of boundaries, positive team relationships, managing conflict, giving and receiving feedback, reflective practice, professional development, communicating effectively, maintaining motivation, prioritizing workload, managing time, taking meal breaks, maintaining humor, and attending to grief work. Organizational responsibilities included appropriate recruitment and orientation, accurate job descriptions, competencies linked to performance appraisals, human resources policies and procedures, training opportunities and support for study, open communication channels, providing critical incident debriefing, offering regular and timely feedback, healthy rosters, acknowledgment of personal pressures, and staff support.[33]

Mentorship and supervisory programs that facilitate the development of self-awareness skills may be beneficial for health care professionals, given the strong relational component to their practice (e.g., nursing, chaplaincy, social work, psychology). The notion of leading by example, modeled in mentors, has the potential to support change.[192] Mentoring enhances professional development by combining competent clinical practice with increased capacity to enter into, support, and sustain healing relationships with patients and families.[193,194] Further, mentorship and clinical supervisory roles may be beneficial in lowering levels of burnout among nurses by increasing overall job satisfaction, supporting opportunities for discussion of negative experiences with trusted colleagues, and improving practice.[193,194]

EDUCATIONAL INTERVENTIONS

More recently, Chochinov has proposed the A, B, C, and D of dignity-conserving care.[195] Using empirical evidence, he shows that kindness, humanity, and respect, the core values and behaviors of medical professionalism, often relegated to the "niceties" of care, embrace the true essence of medicine. These aspects of care, variably referred to as spiritual care, whole-person care, or dignity-conserving care, involve *attitude, behavior, compassion, and dialogue,*[195] which provide the core framework for dignity-conserving care to guide health care providers to incorporate this important facet of patient care. Hospice and palliative care specialists may feel that they have incorporated these values into their work, but work remains to be done. Box 56-2 identifies some of the challenges to be faced in educating health care professionals.

CONCLUSION

Although adverse consequences of working in oncology and palliative care have received extensive attention in the occupational health research literature, fewer studies have focused specifically on the rewards of working with those who are suffering, in pain, traumatized, or at end of life. Further, research on the integration and evaluation of health-promotional intervention strategies to counter the multiple stressors associated with working in oncology and palliative care is limited. This chapter provides the reader with an overview of current research on occupational stress and strategies to counter stressors; these strategies may in turn enhance psychosocial health and well-being.

BOX 56-2 Challenges of Educating Health Care Professionals[196]

Challenge 1: Develop a philosophy of teaching that promotes relational learning and reflective practice.

Challenge 2: Develop a curriculum that includes goals, learning objectives, and methods of teaching that focus on relationships with the dying, the bereaved, and coworkers.

Challenge 3: Integrate current knowledge into educational programs and supervised clinical applications.

Challenge 4: Evaluate training outcomes as well as the context and process by which learning occurs.

Challenge 5: Integrate formal and informal learning activities into the work context.

REFERENCES

1. Barnard D. The promise of intimacy and fear or our own undoing. *J Palliat Care.* 1995;11:22–26.
2. Vachon M. Motivation and stress experienced by staff working with the terminally ill. *Death Educ.* 1978;2:113–122.
3. Vachon M. *Occupational stress in the care of the critically ill, dying and bereaved.* Washington, DC: Hemisphere; 1987.
4. Dougherty E, Pierce B, Ma C, et al. Factors associated with work stress and professional satisfaction in oncology staff. *Am J Hosp Palliat Med.* 2009;26:105–111.
5. Katz R. When out personal selves influence our professional work: an introduction to emotions and countertransference in end-of-life care. In: Katz R, Johnson T, eds. *When professionals weep: emotional and countertransference responses in end-of-life care.* New York: Routledge; 2006:3–12.
6. Kearney M. *A place of healing: working with suffering in living and dying.* Oxford: Oxford University Press; 2000.
7. Kearney M, Weininger R, Vachon M, et al. Self-care of physicians caring for patients at end-of-life: "Being connected…a key to my survival". *JAMA.* 2009;301:1155–1164.
8. Lyall W, Rogers J, Vachon M. *Report to palliative care unit of Royal Victoria Hospital regarding professional stress in the care of the dying.* Montreal: Royal Victoria Hospital; 1976.
9. Maslach C, Leiter M. *The truth about burnout: how organizations cause personal stress and what to do about it.* San Francisco, CA: Jossey-Boss; 1997.
10. Figley C. *Compassion fatigue: coping with secondary traumatic stress disorder in those who treat the traumatized.* New York, NY: Brunner-Routledge; 1995.
11. Joinson C. Coping with compassion fatigue. *Nursing.* 1992;22:116–122.
12. Austin W. Nursing ethics in an era of globalization. *Adv Nurs Sci.* 2001;24:1–18.
13. Webster C, Baylis F. Moral residue. In: Rubin S, Zoloth I, eds. *The ethics of mistakes in the practice of medicine.* Hagerstown: University Publishing; 2000.
14. Pearlman L, MacIan P. Vicarious traumatization: an empirical study of the effects of trauma work on trauma therapists. *Prof Psychol Res Pract.* 1995;26:558–565.
15. Maslach C, Schaufeli W, Leiter M. Job burnout. *Annu Rev Psychol.* 2001;52:397–422.
16. Blomberg K, Sahlberg-Blom E. Closeness and distance: a way of handling difficult situations in daily care. *J Clin Nurs.* 2007;16:244–254.
17. Edwards D, Burnard P. A systematic review of stress and stress management interventions for mental health nurses. *J Adv Nurs.* 2003;42:169–200.
18. Ekedahl M, Wengstrom Y. Nurses in cancer care—stress when encountering existential issues. *Eur J Oncol Nurs.* 2007;11:228–237.
19. Hertting A. *The healthcare sector: a challenging or draining work environment. Psychosocial work experiences and health among hospital employees during the Swedish 1990's.* Stockholm: Karolinska Institute; 2001.
20. Hertting A, Nilsson K, Theorell T, et al. Downsizing and reorganization: demands, challenges and ambiguity for registered nurses. *J Adv Nurs.* 2004;45:145–154.

21. Bakker D, Fitch M, Green E, et al. Oncology nursing: finding the balance in a changing health care system. *Can Oncol Nurs J.* 2006;16:79–98.
22. Barnard D, Street A, Love A. Relationships between stressors, work supports and burnout among cancer nurses. *Cancer Nurs.* 2006;29:338–344.
23. Escot C, Arteros S, Gandubert C, et al. Stress levels in nursing staff working in oncology. *Stress Health.* 2001;17:273–279.
24. Grunfeld E, Whelan T, Zitzelsberger W, et al. Cancer care workers in Ontario: prevalence of burnout, job stress and job satisfaction. *Can Med Assoc J.* 2000;163:166–169.
25. Kash K, Holland J, Breitbart W, et al. Stress and burnout in oncology. *Oncology (Williston Park).* 2000;14:1621–1633; discussion 1633–1634, 1636–1637.
26. Lyall W, Vachon M. Concerns regarding the professional role in the field of thanatology. In: Schoenberg B, Gerber I, Wiener A, et al., eds. *Bereavement: its psychosocial aspects.* New York: Cambridge University Press; 1975:226–231.
27. McVicar A. Workplace stress in nursing: a literature review. *J Adv Nurs.* 2003;44:633–642.
28. Ramirez A, Graham J, Richards M, et al. Mental health of hospital consultants: the effect of stress and satisfaction at work. *Lancet.* 1996;16:724–728.
29. Ramirez A, Graham J, Richards M, et al. Burnout and psychiatric disorder among cancer clinicians. *Br J Cancer.* 1995;71:1263–1269.
30. Vachon M. Oncology staff stress and related interventions. In: Holland J, Breitbart W, Jacobsen P, et-al, ed. *Psycho-Oncology* 2nd ed. New York: Oxford University Press; in press.
31. Payne N. Occupational stressors and coping as determinants of burnout in female hospice nurses. *J Adv Nurs.* 2001;33:396–405.
32. Vachon M. Staff stress in hospice/palliative care: a review. *Palliat Med.* 1995;9:91–122.
33. Vachon M, Huggard J. The experience of the nurse in end-of-life care in the 21st century: stressors, personal, professional, and organizational responsibilites. In: Ferrell B, Coyle N, ed. *Textbook of palliative care nursing.* 3rd ed. Oxford: Oxford University Press; in press.
34. Vachon M, Mueller M. Burnout and symptoms of stress. In: Breitbart W, Chochinov H, eds *Handbook of psychiatry in palliative medicine.* New York: Oxford University Press; 2009:559–625.
35. Leininger M. *Caring: an essential human need.* Detroit: Wayne State University Press; 1988.
36. Watson J. *Nursing: human science and human care—a theory of nursing.* New York: National League of Nursing Press; 1985.
37. Benner P, Wrubel J. *The primacy of caring: stress and coping in health and illness.* Menlo Park: Addison-Wesley; 1989.
38. Barnard D, Towers A, Boston P, et al. *Crossing over: narratives of palliative care.* New York: Oxford University Press; 2000.
39. Jackson V, Mack J, Matsuyama R, et al. A qualitative study of oncologists' approaches to end-of-life care. *J Palliat Med.* 2008;11:893–906.
40. Maslach C, Jackson S. *Maslach burnout inventory manual.* 2nd ed. Palo Alto, CA: Consulting Psychologists Press; 1986.

41. Leiter M, Schaufeli W. Consistency of the burnout construct across occupations. *Anxiety Stress Coping.* 1996;9:229–243.
42. Schaufeli W, Enzmann D. *The burnout companion to study and practice: a critical analysis.* London: Taylor & Francis; 1998.
43. Leiter M, Laschinger H. Relationships of work and practice environment to professional burnout: testing a causal model. *Nurs Res.* 2006;55:137–146.
44. Lee RT, Ashforth BE. A meta-analytic examination of the correlates of the three dimensions of burnout. *J Appl Psychol.* 1996;81:123–133.
45. Leiter M. Burnout as a developmental process: consideration of models. In: Schaufeli W, Maslach C, Marek T, eds. *Professional burnout: recent developments in theory and research.* London: Taylor & Francis; 1993:237–250.
46. Leiter M, Maslach C. Areas of worklife: a structural approach to organizational predictors of job burnout. In: Perrewe P, Ganster D, eds. *Research in occupational stress and well being, vol 3, Emotional and physiological processes and positive intervention strategies.* Oxford: JAI Press/Elsevier; 2004:91–134.
47. Vachon M, Sherwood C. Staff stress and burnout. In: Berger A, Shuster J, Von Roenn J, eds. *Principles and practice of palliative care and supportive oncology.* 3rd ed.Philadelphia, PA: Lippincott Williams and Wilkins; 2007:667–686.
48. Berman R, Campbell M, Makin W, et al. Occupational stress in palliative medicine, medical oncology and clinical oncology specialist registrars. *Clin Med.* 2007;7:235–242.
49. Vachon M, Lyall W, Freeman S. Measurement and management of stress in health professionals working with advanced cancer patients. *Death Educ.* 1978;1:365–375.
50. Bressi C, Manenti S, Porcellana M, et al. Haemato-oncology and burnout: an Italian study. *Br J Cancer.* 2008;98:1046–1052.
51. Isikhan V, Comez T, Danis M. Job stress and coping strategies in health care professionals working with cancer patients. *Eur J Oncol Nurs.* 2004;8:234–244.
52. Graham J, Ramirez A, Cull A, et al. Job stress and satisfaction among palliative physicians. *Palliat Med.* 1996;10:185–194.
53. Asai M, Morita T, Akechi T, et al. Burnout and psychiatric morbidity among physicians engaged in end-of-life care for cancer patients: a cross-sectional nationwide survey in Japan. *Psychooncology.* 2007;16:421–428.
54. Elit L, Trim K, Mand-Bains I, et al. Job satisfaction, stress, and burnout among Canadian gynecologic oncologists. *Gynecol Oncol.* 2004;94:134–139.
55. Pronost A, Le Gouge A, Leboul D, et al. The effects of various features of haematology-oncology services using the palliative approach and the socio-demographic characteristics of healthcare providers on health indicators: social support, perceived stress, coping strategies, quality of life at work. *Oncology.* 2008;10:125–134.
56. Cashavelly B, Binda K, Mallhot J, et al. The forgotten team member: meeting the needs of oncology support staff. *Oncologist.* 2008;13:530–538.

57. Liakopoulou M, Panaretaki I, Papadakis V, et al. Burnout, staff support, and coping in Pediatric Oncology. *Support Care Cancer.* 2008;16:143–150.

58. Speck P. *Teamwork in palliative care: fulfilling or frustrating?* New York: Oxford University Press; 2006.

59. Jünger S, Pestinger M, Elsner F, et al. Criteria for successful multiprofessional cooperation in palliative care teams. *Palliat Med.* 2007;21:347–354.

60. Maslach C, Leiter M. Early predictors of job burnout and engagement. *J Appl Psychol.* 2008;93:498–512.

61. Webster J, Kristjanson L. "But isn't it depressing?" The vitality of palliative care. *J Palliat Care.* 2002;18:15–24.

62. Vachon M. The experience of the nurse in end-of-life care in the 21st century. In: Ferrell B, Coyle D, eds. *Textbook of palliative nursing.* 2nd ed.Oxford: Oxford University Press; 2006:1011–1029.

63. Munroe B, Speck P. Team effectiveness. In: Speck P, ed. *Teamwork in palliative care: fulfilling or frustrating?* Oxford: Oxford University Press; 2006:201–209.

64. Kuerer H, Eberlein T, Pollock R, et al. Career satisfaction, practice patterns and burnout among surgical oncologists: report on the quality of life of members of the Society of Surgical Oncology. *Ann Surg Oncol.* 2007;14:2043–2053.

65. Leiter M, Frank E, Matheson T. Demands, values and burnout: relevance for physicians. *Can Fam Physician.* 2009;55:1224–1225 e1–6.

66. Shanafelt T, Chung H, White H, et al. Shaping your career to maximize personal satisfaction in the practice of oncology. *J Clin Oncol.* 2006;24:4020–4026.

67. Vachon M. Staff stress in palliative-hospice care: a review. *Palliat Med.* 1995;9:91–122.

68. Huggard J. *A national survey of the support needs of interprofessional hospice staff in Aotearoa.* New Zealand: University of Auckland; 2008.

69. Boston P, Towers A, Barnard A. Embracing vulnerability: risk and empathy in palliative care. *J Palliat Care.* 2001;17:248–253.

70. Mount B, Boston P, Cohen S. Healing connections: on moving from suffering to a sense of well-being. *J Pain Symptom Manage.* 2007;33:372–378.

71. Abendroth M, Flannery J. Predicting the risk of compassion fatigue: a study of hospice nurses. *J Hosp Palliat Nurs.* 2006;8:346–356.

72. Adams R, Boscarino J, Figley C. Compassion fatigue and psychological distress among social workers: a validation study. *Am J Orthopsychiatry.* 2006;76:103–108.

73. Figley C. Compassion fatigue: toward a new understanding of the costs of caring. In: Stamm BH, ed. *Secondary traumatic stress: self care issues for clinicians, researchers and educators.* 2nd ed.Lutherville: Sidran; 1999:3–28.

74. Sabo BM. Compassion fatigue and nursing work: can we accurately capture the consequences of caring work? *Int J Nurs Pract.* 2006;12:136–142.

75. Figley C. *Treating compassion fatigue.* In: Figley CR, ed. New York, NY: Brunner-Routledge; 2002.

76. Figley C. Compassion fatigue: psychotherapists' chronic lack of self care. *Psychother Pract.* 2002;58:1433–1441.

77. Liaschenko J, Peter E. Nursing ethics and conceptualizations of nursing: profession, practice and work. *J Adv Nurs.* 2004;46:488–495.

78. Storch JL, Rodney P, Starzomski R. *Toward a moral horizon: nursing ethics for leadership and practice.* Toronto: Pearson Prentice Hall; 2004.

79. Corley M. Nurse moral distress: a proposed theory and research agenda. *Nurs Ethics.* 2002;9:636–650.

80. Ferrell B. Understanding the moral distress of nurses witnessing medically futile care. *Oncol Nurs Forum.* 2006;33:922–930.

81. Weissman D. Moral distress in palliative care. *J Palliat Med.* 2009;12:865–866.

82. Austin W, Bergum V, Goldberg L. Unable to answer the call of our patients: mental health nurses' experience of moral distress. *Nurs Inq.* 2003;10:177–183.

83. Raines M. Ethical decision making in nurses: relationships among moral reasoning, coping style and ethics stress. *Healthcare Law Ethics Regul.* 2000;2:29–41.

84. Webster G, Vachon M. Personal communication.

85. Collins S, Long A. Too tired to care? The psychological effects of working with trauma. *J Psychiatr Mental Health Nurs.* 2003;10:17–27.

86. Pearlman L, Saakvitne K. *Trauma and the therapist: countertransference and vicarious traumatization in psychotherapy with incest survivors.* London: W.W. Norton; 1995.

87. Dunkley J, Whelan T. Vicarious traumatization: current status and future directions. *Br J Guid Couns.* 2006;34:107–116.

88. Pearlman L, Saakvitne K. Treating therapists with vicarious traumatization and secondary traumatic stress disorders. In: Figley CR, ed. *Compassion fatigue: coping with secondary traumatic stress disorder in those who treat the traumatized.* New York: Brunner-Routledge; 1995.

89. Dalgleish T. Cognitive theories of post-traumatic stress disorder. In: Yule W, ed. *Post-traumatic stress disorders: concepts and therapy.* Wiley: Chichester; 1999:193–220.

90. Brewin CR, Dalgleish T, Joseph S. A dual representation theory of post-traumatic stress disorder. *Psychol Rev.* 1996;103:670–686.

91. McCann L, Pearlman L. Vicarious traumatization: a framework for understanding the psychological effects of working with victims. *J Trauma Stress.* 1990;3:131–149.

92. Saakvitne K, Tennen H, Affleck G. Exploring thriving in the context of clinical trauma theory: constructive self development theory. *J Soc Issues.* 1998;54:279–299.

93. Stamm B. *The concise manual for the Professional Quaity of Life Scale: the ProQOL.* Pocatello, ID: ProQOL.org; 2009.

94. Sabo B. *Nursing from the heart: an exploration of caring work among hematology/blood and marrow transplant nurses in three Canadian tertiary care centres.* Halifax: Dalhousie University; 2009.

95. Harrison R, Westwood M. Preventing vicarious traumatization of mental health therapists: identifying protective practices. *Psychother Theory Res Pract Training.* 2009;46:203–219.

96. Radley M, Figley C. The social psychology of compassion. *Clin Soc Work J.* 2007;35:207–214.

97. Keidel GC. Burnout and compassion fatigue among hospice caregivers. *Am J Hosp Palliat Care.* 2002;19:200–205.

98. Jenaro C, Flores N, Arias B. Burnout and coping in human services practitioners. *Prof Psychol Res Pract.* 2007;38:80–87.

99. Jones S. A self-care plan for hospice workers. *Am J Hosp Palliat Med.* 2005;22:125–128.

100. O'Halloran T, Linton J. Stress on the job: self-care resources for counselors. *J Mental Health Couns.* 2000;22:354–364.

101. Alkema K, Linton J, Davies R. A study of the relationship between self-care, compassion satisfaction, compassion fatigue, and burnout among hospice workers. *J Soc Work End-of-Life Palliat Care.* 2008;4:101–119.

102. Saakvitne K, Pearlman L. *Staff of the Traumatic Stress Institute. Transforming the pain: a workbook on vicarious traumatization.* New York: WW Norton; 1996.

103. Benner P. *From novice to expert: excellence and power in clinical nursing practice.* Menlo Park: Addison-Wesley; 1984.

104. Carper B. Fundamental patterns of knowledge in nursing. *Adv Nurs Sci.* 1978;1:13–23.

105. Johns C. The value of reflective practice for nursing. *J Clin Nurs.* 1995;4:23–30.

106. Quinn B. Exploring nurses' experiences of supporting a cancer patient in their search for meaning. *Eur J Oncol Nurs.* 2003;7:164–171.

107. Arvay MJ. Secondary traumatic stress among trauma counsellors: what does the research say? *Int J Adv Couns.* 2001;23:283–293.

108. Diener E. Subjective well-being. *Psychol Bull.* 1984;95:542–575.

109. Ekedahl M, Wengstrom Y. Coping processes in a multidisciplinary healthcare team—a comparison of nurses in cancer care and hospital chaplains. *Eur J Cancer Care.* 2008;17:42–48.

110. Molassiotis A, van den Akker O. Psychological stress and job satisfaction in marrow transplant nurses. *Cancer Nurs.* 1995;19:449–454.

111. Costa P, McCrae R, Zonderman A. Environmental and dispositional influences on well-being: longitudinal follow-up of an American national sample. *Br J Psychol.* 1987;78:299–306.

112. Diener E, Suh E, Lucas R, et al. Subjective well-being: three decades of progress. *Psychol Bull.* 1999;125:276–302.

113. Strack F, Martin L, Schwarz N. Priming and communication: social determinants of information use in judgments of life satisfaction. *Eur J Soc Psychol.* 1988;18:429–442.

114. Stenmarker M, Palmerus K, Marky I. Life satisfaction of swedish pediatric oncologists: the role of personality, work-related aspects and emotional distress. *Pediatr Blood Cancer.* 2009;53:1308–1314.

115. Maslach C. Job burnout: new directions in research and interventions. *Curr Direct Psychol Sci.* 2003;12:189–192.

116. Reference deleted in proofs.

117. Merriam Webster. *The Merriam-Webster dictionary.* 11th ed. Springfield, MA: Merriam Webster, Inc; 2004.

118. *Compact thesaurus: the ultimate wordfinder.* Glasgow: Harper-Collins Publ Ltd; 1999.

119. Vaillant G. *Spiritual evolution.* New York: Broadway Books; 2008.

120. Fredrickson B, Levenson R. Positive emotions speed the recovery from the cardiovascular sequelae of negative emotions. *Cogn Emot.* 1998;12:191–220.

121. Fredrickson B, Mancuso R, Branigan C, et al. The undoing effect of positive emotions. *Motiv Emot.* 2000;24:237–258.

122. Fredrickson B, Tugade M, Waugh C, et al. What good are positive emotions in crises? A prospective study of resilience and emotions following the terrorist attacks on the United States on September 11th, 2001. *J Person Soc Psychol.* 2003;84:365–376.

123. Walsh F. *Strengthening family resilience.* New York: Guilford Press; 2006.

124. Masten A. Ordinary magic: resilience processes in development. *Am Psychol.* 2001;56:227–238.

125. Earvolino-Ramirez M. Resilience: a concept analysis. *Nurs Forum.* 2007;42:73–82.
126. Ablett J, Jones R. Resilience and well-being in palliative care staff: a qualitative study of hospice nurses' experiences of work. *Psychooncology.* 2007;16:733–740.
127. Kobasa S, Maddi S, Kahn S. Hardiness and health: a prospective study. *J Personal Soc Psychol.* 1982;42:168–177.
128. Maddi S, Kobasa S. *The hardy executive: health under stress.* Chicago: Dorsey Press; 1984.
129. Antonovsky A. *Unraveling the mystery of health: how people manage stress and stay well.* London: Jossey-Bass; 1987.
130. Geyer S. Some conceptual considerations on the sense of coherence. *Soc Sci Med.* 1997;44:1771–1779.
131. Keeton K, Fenner D, Johnson T, et al. Predictors of physician career satisfaction, work-life balance and burnout. *Obstet Gynecol.* 2007;109:949–955.
132. Monroe B, Oliviere D. *Resilience in palliative care: achievment in diversity.* New York: Oxford University Press; 2007.
133. Tugade M, Fredrickson B. Resilient individuals use positive emotions to bounce back from negative emotional experiences. *J Personal Soc Psychol.* 2004;86:320–333.
134. Fredrickson B. The role of positive emotions in positive psychology: the broaden-and-build theory of positive emotions. *Am Psychologist.* 2001;56:218–226.
135. Payne M. Resilient multiprofessional teams. In: Monroe B, Oliviere D, eds. *Resilience in palliative care: achievement in diversity.* New York: Oxford University Press; 2007.
136. Kalisch B. What is empathy? *Am J Nurs.* 1973;73:1548–1552.
137. Peplau H. *Interpersonal relations in nursing: a conceptual frame of reference for psychodynamic nursing.* New York: Putnam; 1952.
138. Alligood MR, May BA. A nursing theory of personal system empathy: interpreting a conceptualization of empathy in King's interacting systems. *Nurs Sci Q.* 2000;13:243–247.
139. Morse J, Anderson G, Botter J, et al. Exploring empathy: a conceptual fit for nursing practice. *Image J Nurs Sch.* 1992;24:273–280.
140. Thompson S. Empathy: towards a clearer meaning for nursing. *Nurs Praxis N Z.* 1996;11:19–26.
141. Alligood M. Empathy: the importance of recognizing two types. *J Psychosoc Nurs.* 1992;30:14–17.
142. La Monica E. Construct validity of an empathy instrument. *Res Nurs Health.* 1981;4:389–400.
143. Hudson G. Empathy and technology in the coronary care unit. *Intens Crit Care Nurs.* 1993;9:55–61.
144. Sutherland J. Historical concept analysis of empathy. *Issues Ment Health Nurs.* 1995;16:555–566.
145. Raudonis B. The meaning and impact of empathic relationships in hospice nursing. *Cancer Nurs.* 1993;19:304–309.
146. Wiseman T. A concept analysis of empathy. *J Adv Nurs.* 1996;23:1162–1167.
147. Salston M, Figley C. Secondary traumatic stress effects of working with survivors of criminal victimization. *J Trauma Stress.* 2003;16:167–174.
148. Pearlman L. Self-care for trauma therapists: ameliorating vicarious traumatization. In: Stamm B, ed. *Secondary traumatic stress: self-care issues for clinicians, researchers, and educators.* Baltimore: The Sidran Press; 1999:51–64.

149. Novak D, Epstein R, Paulsen R. Toward creating physician-healers: fostering medical students' self awareness, personal growth, and well-being. *Acad Med.* 1999;74:516–520.
150. Reference deleted in proofs.
151. Remen R. *My grandfather's blessings.* New York: Riverhead Books; 2000.
152. Remen R. *Kitchen table wisdom.* New York: Riverhead Books; 1996.
153. Blum L. Compassion. In: Rorty AM, ed. *Explaining emotions.* Berkeley, CA: University of California Press; 1980.
154. Oakley J. *Morality and emotions.* London: Routledge; 1992.
155. Pask EJ. Moral agency in nursing: seeing value in the work and believing that I make a difference. *Nurs Ethics.* 2003;10:165–175.
156. Bergum V, Dossetor J. *Relational ethics: the full meaning of respect.* Hagerstown: University Publishing Group; 2005.
157. Puchalski C, Ferrell B, Virani R, et al. Improving the quality of spiritual care as a dimension of palliative care: the report of the Consensus Conference. *J Palliat Med.* 2009;12:885–904.
158. Musgrave C, McFarlane E. Intrinsic and extrinsic religiosity, spiritual well-being and attitudes toward spiritual care: a comparison of Israeli Jewish oncology nurses' scores. *Oncolo Nurs Forum.* 2004;31:1179–1183.
159. Sinclair S, Raffin S, Pereira J, et al. Collective soul: the spirituality of an interdisciplinary palliative care team. *Palliat Support Care.* 2006;4:13–24.
160. Sinclair S. *The spirituality of palliative and hospice care professionals: an ethnographic inquiry.* Calgary: University of Calgary; 2009.
161. Stamm BH. Measuring compassion satsifaction as well as fatigue: developmental hisotry of the compassion satisfaction and fatigue test. In: Figley C, ed. *Treating compassion fatigue.* New York: Brunner-Routledge; 2002:107–122.
162. Huggard P. Taking care of the health professional (presentation at the Idaho conference on health care. In: Vachon M, ed. *Pocatello: Health Care 2005: Emerging issues.* 2005.
163. Huggard P. *Managing compassion fatigue: implications for medical education.* Auckland: University of Auckland; 2008.
164. Ryff C. Beyond Ponce de Leon and life satisfaction: new directions in quest of successful aging. *Int J Behav Dev.* 1989;12:35–55.
165. Seccareccia D, Brown J. Impact of spirituality on palliative care physicians: personally and professionally. *J Palliat Med.* 2009;12:805–809.
166. Barrett L, Yates P. Oncology/hematology nurses: a study of job satisfaction, burnout and intention to leave the specialty. *Aust Health Rev.* 2002;25:109–121.
167. Vachon M. Meaning, spirituality and wellness in cancer survivors. *Semin Oncol Nurs.* 2008;24(Issues on Survivorship):218–225.
168. Shanafelt T, West C, Zhan X, et al. Relationship between increased personal well-being and enhanced empathy among internal medicine residents. *J Gen Intern Med.* 2005;20:559–564.
169. LeBlanc P, Hox J, Schaufeli W, et al. Take care! The evaluation of a team-based burnout intervention program for oncology care providers. *J Appl Psychol.* 2007;92:213–217.
170. Robinson K, Sutton S, von Gunten C, et al. Assessment of the education for physicians on end-of-life care (EPEC) project. *J Palliat Med.* 2004;7:837–845.

171. Kjeldmand D, Holmstrom I, Rosenqvist I. Balint training makes GPs thrive better in their job. *Patient Educ Couns.* 2004;55:230–235.
172. Kjeldmand D, Holmstrom I. Balint groups as a means to increase job satisfaction and prevent burnout among general practitioners. *Ann Fam Med.* 2008;6:138–145.
173. Grossman P, Niemann L, Schmidt S, et al. Mindfulness-based stress reduction and health benefits: a meta-analysis. *J Psychosom Res.* 2004;57:35–43.
174. Davidson R, Kabat-Zinn J, Schumacher J, et al. Alterations in brain and immune function produced by mindfulness meditation. *Psychosom Med.* 2003;65:564–570.
175. Harris A. Does expressive writing reduce health care utilization? A meta-analysis of randomized trials. *J Consult Clin Psychol.* 2006;74:243–252.
176. Shapiro S, Brown K, Biegel G. Teaching self-care to caregivers: effects of mindfulness-based stress reduction on the mental health of therapists in training. *Training Educ Prof Psychol.* 2007;1:105–118.
177. Shapiro S, Astin J, Bishop S, et al. Mindfulness-based stress reduction for health care professionals: results from a randomized trial. *Int J Stress Manage.* 2005;12:164–176.
178. Cohen-Katz J, Wiley S, Capuano T, et al. The effects of mindfulness-based stress reduction on nurse stress and burnout: a quantitative and qualitative study. *J Holistic Nurs.* 2004;18:302–308.
179. Rosenzweig S, Reibel D, Greeson J, et al. Mindfulness-based stress reduction lowers psychological distress in medical students. *Teach Learn Med.* 2003;15:88–92.
180. Back A, Bauer-Wu S, Rushton C, et al. Compassionate silence in the patient–clinician encounter: a contemplative approach. *J Palliat Med.* 2009;J12:1113–1117.
181. Smythe J, Stone A, Hurewitz A, et al. Effects of writing about stressful experiences on symptom reduction in patients with asthma or rheumatoid arthritis. *JAMA.* 1999;281:1304–1309.
182. Petrie K, Fontanilla I, Thomas M, et al. Effect of written emotional expression on immune function in patients with human immunodeficiency virus infection: a randomized trial. *J Psychosom Med.* 2004;66:272–275.
183. O'Cleirigh C, Ironson G, Fletcher M, et al. Written emotional disclosure and processing of trauma are associated with protected health status and immunity in people living with HIV/AIDS. *Br J Health Psychol.* 2008;13(Pt 1):81–84.
184. Cepeda M, Chapman R, Miranda N, et al. Emotional disclosure through patient narrative may improve pain and well-being: results of a randomized controlled trial in patients with cancer pain. *J Pain Symptom Manage.* 2008;35:623–631.
185. Morgan N, Graves K, Poggi E, et al. Implementing an expressive writing study in a cancer clinic. *Oncologist.* 2008;13:196–204.
186. Stanton A, Danoff-Burg S, Sworowski L, et al. Randomized, controlled trial of written emotional expression and benefit finding in breast cancer patients. *J Clin Oncol.* 2002;20:4160–4168.
187. Charon R. Narrative medicine: a model for empathy, reflection, profession, and trust. *JAMA.* 2001;286:1897–1902.
188. Brady D, Corbie-Smith G, Branch W. What's important to you?": the use of narratives to promote self-reflection and to understand the experiences of medical residents. *Ann Intern Med.* 2002;137:220–223.

189. Fillion L, Dupuis R, Tremblay I, et al. Enhancing meaning in palliative care practice: a meaning-centred intervention to promote job satisfaction. *Palliat Support Care*. 2006;4:333–344.

190. Breitbart W. Spirituality and meaning in palliative care: spirituality and meaning-centered group psychotherapy interventions in advanced cancer. *Support Care Cancer*. 2001;10:272–280.

191. Huggard J. *A report of a study of staff support practices in UK and Canadian palliative care units and hospices*. Wellington; 2006.

192. Kotter J, Cohen D. *The heart of change: real life stories of how people change their organization*. Boston: Harvard Business Press; 2002.

193. Edwards D, Burnard P, Hannigan B, et al. Clinical supervision and burnout: the influence of clinical supervision for community mental health nurses. *J Clin Nurs*. 2006;15:1007–1015.

194. Johnson L, Cohen M, Hull M. Cultivating expertise in oncology nursing: methods, mentors and memories. *Oncol Nurs Forum*. 1994;21:27–34.

195. Chochinov H. Dignity and the essence of medicine: the A, B, C & D of dignity-conserving care. *Br Med J*. 2007;334:184–187.

196. Papadatou D. *In the face of death*. New York: Springer; 2009.

57

Sexuality and intimacy after cancer

Jennifer Potter and Katherine T. Johnston

Cancer diagnosis and treatment pose innumerable challenges that affect psychological, interpersonal, physiologic, and spiritual realms. Self-esteem and body image are often profoundly affected, and fear of being rejected or presenting a burden to a partner or prospective partner is a common sentiment. Coupled with the common physical effects of cancer treatment, which can range from general symptoms (e.g., fatigue) to specific effects (e.g., impotence, premature menopause), these reactions can threaten intimacy and hamper sexual satisfaction. Because emotional closeness and sexual gratification provide many benefits—physical comfort, relaxation, stress relief, sleep assistance, pleasure, and relief from pain—that are especially important for people who are coping with trauma, it is crucial for clinicians to assess and address problems in these areas effectively. For many patients and their partners, the specter of infertility, in addition to other losses associated with cancer treatment, compounds the challenge. Therefore, clinicians must learn about fertility preservation and must be able to counsel and refer patients appropriately when questions about childbearing potential arise; the next chapter addresses these issues in greater detail.

Despite an expressed preference to receive information, support, and practical strategies about how to adjust to sexual changes after treatment, most patients in published surveys report receiving little to no counseling about the effects of cancer treatment on sexual function and reproductive health.[1,2] Although research shows that partners of cancer survivors are also significantly affected, even less inquiry has focused on the needs of this group. For example, as of 2002, only 14% of comprehensive cancer centers surveyed by telephone offered specific counseling on the topics of sexuality, intimacy, and fertility.[3] Health professionals frequently presume that once patients are faced with a life-threatening disease, they lose interest in their sexuality and concentrate on fighting their illness; clinicians also make many stereotypical assumptions about patients' sexuality on the basis of age, sex, diagnosis, culture, partnership, and functional status.[4] When sexuality is addressed at all, inordinate emphasis tends to be placed on physiologic parameters such as fertility, contraception, menopause management, or erectile status.[5] Other barriers to open and complete discussion include (1) the idea that patients and their partners cannot possibly digest information about sexual side effects in the midst of taking in a diagnosis of cancer and making major treatment decisions, (2) the reality that clinicians lack training in how to assess and address sexual problems, (3) the fact that they have difficulty finding adequate time for these discussions, and (4) that patients must contend with the fact that many health insurance plans do not provide coverage for sexual difficulties.

To address these needs, we offer this chapter as a practical guide. We acknowledge that the field is still young, particularly with regard to management of female sexual difficulties; however, we believe that there is enough of an evidence base to support making general recommendations about what information should be included in discussions about sexuality and intimacy after cancer, and to outline a rational approach to evaluation and management when patients and their partners express concerns. When possible, we have tried to display this information in tabular fashion to make it easier for clinicians to access efficiently. Because this is an evolving area of study, questions arise frequently to which there are as yet no ready answers. We believe strongly in maintaining an open mind, thinking "outside the box," and being willing to consider new treatment options (as long as they have been shown not to be or are not likely to be harmful). Even when little can be done to change a particular patient's or couple's circumstances, we find repeatedly that people simply value the opportunity to talk, and that mere discussion facilitates acceptance and adaptation, and leads to enhanced relationship satisfaction.

CONCEPTUAL FRAMEWORK FOR UNDERSTANDING SEXUALITY AND INTIMACY AFTER CANCER

It is difficult to address difficulties with sexuality and intimacy without first acquiring a basic understanding of human sexual physiology and an appreciation for the diversity of human sexual experience. Therefore, the first part of this chapter will present a conceptual framework to support our later recommendations regarding evaluation and management. For readers who desire a more comprehensive discussion of normal female and male sexual anatomy and physiology—topics that fall well beyond the scope of this chapter—we suggest two comprehensive background references[6,7]:

1. The neurobiology of human sexual response is complex.

Sexual response requires intact neural, vascular, and muscular circuitry; complex interactions between multiple neurotransmitter systems; and modulating influences from the endocrine system. Although the sexual anatomy of women and men is obviously different, studies done to date have identified a number of neurotransmitters, bioactive substances, and sex steroids that appear to play a role in the sexual physiology of both sexes, including (but not limited to) dopamine, norepinephrine, serotonin, acetylcholine, nitric oxide, vasoactive intestinal peptide, prostaglandin E1, estrogen, testosterone, progesterone, oxytocin, prolactin, melanocortins, endocannabinoids, and opiates.[8] Details regarding key differences between women and men, specific sites of action (central, peripheral, or both), and effects on sexual function (excitatory, inhibitory, or neutral) remain to be fully elucidated. Figure 57-1 is an oversimplified schematic that illustrates purported actions of various substances in central and peripheral loci in women and provides a template to help explain the impact of various anatomic (e.g., removal of key target tissues) and biochemical (e.g.,

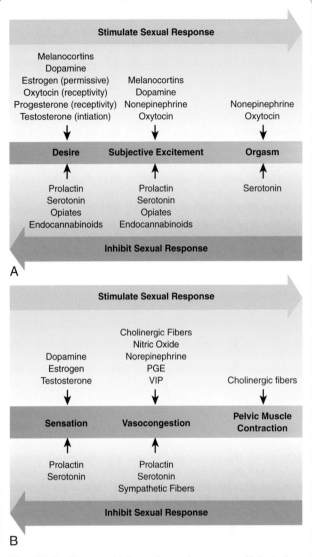

Fig. 57-1 The neurobiology of sexual response. *(Adapted from Potter J. Female sexuality: assessing satisfaction and addressing problems. Posted on ACP Medicine, 2010.)*

changes in neurotransmitter or hormone concentrations) perturbations. The literature is replete with analogous diagrams regarding the impact of various effectors on sexual function in men; readers seeking additional information may refer to Mulcahy's aforementioned text.[7]

2. There are no universally accepted definitions to describe "normal" sexual function; therefore, "dysfunction" is subjectively, rather than objectively, determined.

Definitions of "normal" sexual activity and function vary greatly according to the descriptive criteria one chooses to utilize. Variables to consider include age, gender, choice (sexual orientation) and number (concurrent or lifetime) of partners, frequency of sexual activity, context in which sex occurs (casual or committed relationships), specific sexual acts performed, safety of sexual practices with respect to mutuality/consent and freedom from exposure to unintended pregnancy/sexually transmitted infections, and overall sexual satisfaction. Satisfaction is a complex variable that encompasses general intimacy (feeling close to one's partner), happiness with one's own level of libido and attainment of physically pleasurable sensations (including orgasm), and contentment with the overtures and reactions of one's partner(s).

Because different values are placed on various aspects of sexual function according to a person's age, sexual identity and experience, and culture,[9–11] it is crucial for clinicians to refrain from imposing their own values when talking about sex with patients and their partners, and instead to determine the norm for each individual/couple, to evaluate the extent to which there is distress with the status quo, to encourage open and respectful communication and adherence to safer sex practices and methods to prevent unintended pregnancy, and to set reasonable expectations when embarking on a treatment plan. Because the term "sexual dysfunction" implies the existence of an objectively determined norm, we prefer to use the term "sexual difficulties" instead.

3. Many patients and partners have basic sexual concerns that need to be addressed alongside cancer-related concerns.

Many patients and their partners have significant questions and concerns about their sexuality long before cancer enters their lives; attempts to address sexual difficulties that arise after cancer must therefore include attention to the same basic sexual concerns that many people in the general population experience. These include cultural prohibitions about sex that cause uneasiness about normal sexual anatomy, desires and behaviors, and unrealistic expectations about sexual performance created by media hype. Examples of the former include shame about the appearance of one's genitalia; attraction to people one "should not" be attracted to; and guilt regarding masturbation or sexual activities other than missionary position, penile-vaginal intercourse. Examples of the latter include the idea that normal function includes a proscribed frequency of sexual activity, having an orgasm every time, or experiencing a particular type of orgasm (e.g., simultaneous with one's partner, multiple rather than single, "vaginal" rather than "clitoral").

Provision of accurate information goes a long way toward dispelling myths, helping patients appreciate their bodies and responses as they are, and giving patients the permission to explore their sexuality in ways that did not feel comfortable previously. Permission to consider trying new sexual techniques is especially important after cancer because the physiologic effects of treatment frequently mean that different types of stimulation are needed to produce arousal than were needed in the past. For example, use of erotic materials can be used to stimulate diminished desire, experimentation with different sexual positions may enhance comfort during sexual activity, and openness toward exploring nongenital erogenous zones when genital function has been compromised may reveal new sources of pleasure.

4. Clinically, it is useful to consider three functional domains of sexual response (desire, arousal, orgasm) and their neurobiological correlates.

Desire is a mental state created by external and internal stimuli that generate a wish or a need to participate in sexual activity. Clinical manifestations of increased desire include sexual thoughts or fantasies and the motivation to initiate or the willingness to be receptive to sexual activity. It is helpful

to consider three major components of desire—biological drive (which can be thought of as lust), cognitive motivation, and beliefs/values. As shown in Figure 57-1, sexual desire is physiologically controlled by brain systems involved in sexual excitation and inhibition.[12] Central dopamine pathways that link the hypothalamus and the limbic system appear to form the core of the excitatory system, which also involves the action of melanocortins, oxytocin, and norepinephrine. The excitatory system is balanced by inhibitory actions of opioids (mediate sexual reward), endocannabinoids (induce sedation), and serotonin (induces satiety). Excitatory and inhibitory pathways are modulated hormonally and conditionally by anticipation of a risk (e.g., pain) or reward (e.g., orgasm) associated with initiation of or participation in sexual activity. This schema helps explain the effects of various hormones (e.g., estrogen, testosterone, progesterone, prolactin), medications (e.g., dopaminergic, noradrenergic, serotoninergic agonists or antagonists), and learned or culturally mediated influences that positively or negatively affect the desire to engage in sexual activity.

As shown in Figure 57-2, it is not necessary to have an exuberant libido to enjoy a satisfying sexual life. Diverse cognitive incentives lead patients and their partners to initiate or participate in sexual activity, including physical reasons (attraction, experience seeking, pleasure, stress reduction), goal attainment (conception, social status, revenge), emotional connection or expression, and insecurity factors (boost self-esteem, unable to say no, prevent partner from straying).[13] No matter which factors motivate a person to engage in sexual activity, arousal can often proceed in the presence of appropriate erotic stimulation and intact physiologic pathways and in the absence of inhibiting influences. These truths may be

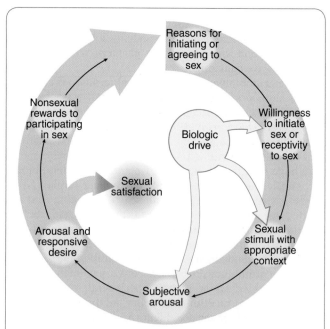

Fig. 57-2 Basson's integrated model of sexual response. *(Redrawn from: Potter J. Female sexuality: assessing satisfaction and addressing problems. Posted on ACP Medicine, 2010.)*

comforting for patients with a reduced biological sex drive, who can be taught by using cognitive restructuring techniques to identify and celebrate intact motivations to participate in sexual activity and to notice and learn to deflect negative thoughts that lead to avoidance of sexual activity or anticipation (and therefore a higher likelihood) of experiencing a negative outcome.

Sexual arousal includes subjective excitement (awareness of, comfort with, and appreciation of erogenous stimulation) and objectively measurable signs of physiologic (both non-genital and genital) arousal,[14] such as cutaneous flushing, vascular engorgement, and penile erection or vaginal lubrication. It is important to distinguish between these two types of arousal because measurable physiologic arousal has been documented in the absence of a subjective sense of excitement or pleasure, particularly in women,[15] and in men and women with neurologic disorders.[16,17] Gender differences appear to be important, as subjective appreciation of sexual arousal seems to be especially dependent on cognitive processing of stimulus meaning and content in women,[18] as opposed to being related predominantly to peripheral vasocongestive and neuromuscular events. These phenomena help to explain why phosphodiesterase inhibitors (PDEIs), which increase genital blood flow fairly consistently in both sexes, do not reliably result in an enhanced subjective appreciation of pleasurable genital sensations in all circumstances. Subjective arousal is a central event that appears to be mediated by neurotransmitter systems analogous to those involved in sexual desire. Genital sexual arousal appears to be mediated by spinal reflexes.

Arousal and orgasm can be viewed on a continuum. Arousal is necessary for buildup of the orgasmic platform; in effect, there can be no orgasm if there is no arousal. The experience of orgasm comprises both central (experience of pleasure) and peripheral (measurable pelvic muscle contraction) events. The central control of orgasm is poorly understood, but it is postulated that norepinephrine has stimulatory effects, and that serotonin (5-HT) and prolactin have inhibitory effects, as they do on the production of subjective excitement. Genital events that take place during orgasm (e.g., the ejaculatory response in men) are controlled by spinal reflexes; similar events are thought to occur in women.[19]

Some authors include a fourth domain of sexual function—pain—to account for the fact that sexual stimulation of genital structures and/or orgasm triggers a painful rather than a pleasurable response in some women.[20] Potential causes of sexual pain in women include vulvovaginal infections (e.g., candidiasis), postmenopausal atrophy, dermatitides (e.g., eczema, psoriasis), dermatoses (e.g., lichen sclerosus), pelvic floor muscle problems (e.g., vaginismus), structural abnormalities of the vagina (e.g., postradiation vaginal stenosis), benign and malignant pelvic processes, and disorders of unknown cause (e.g., vulvodynia-vestibulitis).[21] Sexual pain disorders also occur in men, although they are less well understood and warrant further inquiry.[22] To date, male sexual pain disorders are best described in the context of research on chronic pelvic pain syndrome (CPPS). Men with CPPS report less sexual desire, fewer sexual thoughts, less frequent sexual activity, poor arousal, decreased orgasmic ability, and genital pain with intercourse.[23] Chronic prostatitis is also associated with a high incidence of sexual dysfunction, including pain during sexual activity.[24] Other chronic medical disorders have been associated with impaired male sexual function due to painful

ejaculation, including epididymitis, urethritis, lower urinary tract symptoms (LUTS), posttraumatic urethral strictures, and ureteral tract stones.[25]

5. Cancer treatment is associated with numerous physiologic changes and psychosocial stressors that can negatively affect function in each domain of sexual response.

Cancer treatment causes numerous physical changes that vary according to the location of the primary tumor, the presence or absence of distant (metastatic) disease, and the types of treatment that are rendered. Treatment modalities may include surgery, radiation therapy, chemotherapy, hormonal therapies, and immune-mediated therapies, each of which can cause treatment-specific effects that influence sexual function in multiple response domains. Table 57-1 provides a list of common treatment-associated physical changes and the mechanism(s) by which they are believed to cause sexual difficulties.

Surgery may damage or remove organs, nerves, muscles, and/or blood vessels that are integral to a patient's self-esteem and body image, are key structural elements involved in sexual response, or are important because they produce hormones, neurotransmitters, and other mediators that modulate sexual response. Although there are numerous predictors of sexual health in women after breast cancer treatment, it is clear that younger women in particular often experience body image problems related to breast surgery, with resultant negative impact on sexual function.[26] Radical pelvic surgery, which involves en bloc removal of the uterus, fallopian tubes, and ovaries, along with contiguous pelvic nerves and blood vessels (pelvic exenteration), is also associated with sexual difficulties.[27] Especially when pelvic surgery involves a urostomy or a colostomy, some women express self-consciousness regarding being seen in the nude by their partner.[28] Removal of the uterus can be associated with a shortened vagina, with consequent discomfort during penetration. Removal of the ovaries in formerly premenopausal women results in premature menopause; estrogen deficiency then leads to vasomotor symptoms (with consequent sleep deprivation, fatigue, and decreased libido), as well as vulvovaginal atrophy (with consequent decreased lubrication and dyspareunia). Because ovaries are also an important source of androgens, oophorectomy can cause relative testosterone deficiency, with resultant unfavorable effects on libido. Coincident removal or damage to pelvic nerves and blood vessels can result in reduced sensation and vasocongestion in response to genital stimulation (decreased arousal). Thus, radical pelvic surgery can result in a decremental response in all four functional domains (desire, arousal, orgasm, and pain); this multimodal impact on several domains in combination, rather than on just one discrete domain alone, tends to be the rule rather than the exception, demonstrating the importance of asking patients about problems in each area.

Surgical treatment for prostate, rectal, or penile cancer provides a somewhat analogous example in men. Qualitative studies of men's experiences with surgical treatment reveal worse psychological outcomes such as altered masculinity, self-consciousness, and body image concerns after surgery for prostate and penile cancer[29,30]; male survivors report a need for supportive partners to help them cope with the experience. In addition to psychological challenges, damage to autonomic nerves and arteries during surgery predicts poor physiologic sexual outcomes after surgery for both rectal and prostate cancer,[31,32] with

Table 57-1 Common treatment-associated physical and physiologic changes and mechanisms by which they cause sexual difficulties

Treatment modality	Cause of adverse effects	Clinical examples
Surgery	Reaction to cosmetic changes Damage to critical structures	*Both sexes:* Body image issues associated with head and neck surgery, urostomy, colostomy Lymphedema, pain syndromes *Women:* Body image issues associated with mastectomy Sexual effects of radical cystectomy *Men:* Sexual effects of prostate, testicular, or penile surgery
Radiation therapy	Damage to critical structures	*Both sexes:* Lymphedema, pain syndromes *Women:* Radiation-induced vaginal changes *Men:* Radiation-induced erectile dysfunction
Chemotherapy	Hair loss Weight gain Fatigue Premature menopause Male hypogonadism Peripheral neuropathy	*Both sexes:* Body image issues associated with hair loss Sexual effects of weight gain and decreased physical fitness Reduced sensation associated with neuropathy *Women:* Sexual sequelae of postmenopausal atrophy *Men:* Sexual sequelae of testosterone deficiency
Hormonal therapies	Antiestrogen effects Antiandrogen effects	*Women:* Sexual effects of medical menopause induction (e.g., GnRH agonist) and antiestrogens (e.g., tamoxifen, aromatase inhibitors) *Men:* Sexual effects of androgen deprivation therapies (e.g., GnRH)
Immunotherapies	Graft-versus-host-disease	Sexual effects of genital GVHD

GnRH, Gonadotropin-releasing hormone; *GVHD,* graft-versus-host disease.

a negative impact in each domain of sexual function, including lessened desire, poor arousal, decreased ability to orgasm, and pain with sexual activity. Research indicates that even when male survivors report poor sexual function, their knowledge and use of effective treatments are often limited. Clinicians can play an important role by exploring male survivors' concerns, including perceptions of inadequacy, performance anxiety, depression, unrealistic expectations, partner readiness to resume sexual activity, and openness to experimenting with pharmacologic or mechanical sexual aids.[33]

In both women and men, the specifics of the surgical procedure can make a significant difference. Sometimes, a less drastic procedure results in a better cosmetic outcome, with resultant preservation of self-esteem and body image. For example, a number of studies have shown that body image and sexual satisfaction are superior with breast-conserving surgery compared with mastectomy.[34] Existing data are inconsistent with respect to whether or not reconstructive surgery helps to preserve quality of life when mastectomy is necessary, in part because available assessment tools may not be sufficiently sensitive to detect clinically relevant problems.[35] In some circumstances, care taken to avoid unnecessary damage to critical structures can reduce sexual sequelae. For example, unfavorable effects of radical cystectomy for bladder cancer in women (vaginal dryness, decreased arousal,

and dyspareunia) are less frequent with nerve-sparing surgery than with traditional procedures.[36] Similarly, injury to autonomic nerves during prostate and bladder cancer surgeries can be minimized without compromising oncologic outcomes through nerve sparing and nerve reconstruction procedures.[37] Even when oncologic control requires radical prostatectomy or radical cystectomy (necessitating wide excision and cavernous nerve dissection), erectile dysfunction need not be an automatic outcome. For example, emerging data suggest that nerve reconstruction and replacement of the cavernous nerve with a sural nerve graft result in preserved postoperative sexual function.[38]

Other adverse effects of surgery include lymphedema, which exerts its effect via negative self-esteem and body image issues and/or localized discomfort that detracts from the sexual experience. Fortunately, current emphasis on performance of sentinel lymph node assessment before systematic axillary or pelvic lymphadenectomy results in a lower incidence of lymphedema. Surgical procedures can also result in a multitude of cutaneous pain syndromes that, depending on the anatomic site involved, can cause noxious reactions to sexual stimulation or cognitive inhibition of sexual response by unwelcome distraction of the pain itself. For example, some women experience pain syndromes after breast surgery that manifest as hypersensitivity or neuralgia involving the chest wall and/or axilla. At best, the discomfort serves as a continual reminder that they have lost their breasts as a source of sexual pleasure; at worst, the pain may be so severe that it effectively drowns out any possible pleasure that might be derived by stimulation of other erogenous regions.

Radiation therapy (RT) can also result in damage to critical structures, lymphedema, and pain syndromes. For example, RT to the axilla and groin regions is associated with lymphedema of the upper and lower extremities, respectively; nerve damage, such as brachial plexopathy, can also result. Pelvic irradiation, on the other hand, can be associated with direct effects on genital function. For example, 55% to 70% of women treated with pelvic RT in the form of external beam therapy or intracavitary implants reported sexual impairments in the form of vaginal dryness, pain, bleeding, and stenosis in one study,[39] while in a second study, the rate of vaginal stenosis in women receiving intracavitary treatment was as high as 88%.[40] Erectile dysfunction is also common after radiotherapy for prostate cancer, although the mechanism remains unclear. Predictors of impaired erectile function after radiotherapy include age, pretreatment erectile function, use of androgen deprivation therapy, and the volume of tissue exposed.[41] In men receiving external beam radiation therapy for prostate cancer, postexposure sexual function is most strongly predicted by pre-exposure sexual function. Affected men typically experience a decline in sexual function for approximately 2 years after exposure, after which time sexual function appears to reach a plateau.[42]

Although the harmful effects of chemotherapy are agent and dose dependent, common side effects that can influence sexual function negatively include hair loss and weight gain (via effects on body image), fatigue (via effects on general stamina), premature menopause (via central and peripheral effects of estrogen and testosterone depletion), and peripheral neuropathy (via impairment in genital sensation). Chemotherapy results in irreversible damage to ovarian follicles and stromal function. The incidence and irreversibility of chemotherapy-induced amenorrhea (CIA) vary from approximately 20% to 100%, depending on patient age at the time of administration and the type of chemotherapy given. Alkylating agents typically cause the most significant damage to ovarian reserve. In premenopausal breast cancer patients, younger age (<40) and taxane-based therapy are associated with an increased probability of recovery of menses,[43] with 14% (24% younger than age 40 and 11% age 40 or older) resuming menstruation after an initial period of amenorrhea.[44] Although considerably less information is available about the effects of various leukemia and lymphoma chemotherapy regimens on reproductive function, limited data suggest high overall rates of CIA (>50%) and a similar association of CIA with older age (>30) at the time of administration.[45] It is interesting to note that one small (N = 35) study demonstrated that a substantial proportion—80%—of girls treated for childhood leukemia before the onset of menarche subsequently progressed through puberty normally; however, follow-up was insufficient to allow conclusions about the impact of treatment on later fertility.[46] Other intriguing studies have demonstrated a higher incidence of CIA in women treated during the follicular phase of their menstrual cycle,[47] as well as possible protective effects of coadministration of oral contraceptives[48] or gonadotropin-releasing hormone (GnRH) agonists[49] before and during chemotherapy; these findings warrant further study. In summary, because of the high likelihood of ovarian damage, all women of repro-

ductive age should be informed of the possibility of CIA before beginning treatment, and options for fertility preservation should be discussed (please see the following section on Fertility After Cancer). In addition, because a significant minority of patients will eventually resume menstruation and be fertile after treatment, it is important to provide appropriate contraceptive counseling. Schwarz et al. provide an excellent recent review on this topic.[50]

In men, the most frequent chemotherapeutic culprits are high-dose alkylating agents and cyclophosphamide, which impair sexual function via direct injury to the testes. Cyclophosphamide causes the most sexual dysfunction due to damage to the Leydig cells, with consequent reduced production of testosterone and hypogonadism.[51,52] Alkylating agents are more likely to damage seminiferous tubules and to limit sperm production without affecting testosterone production.

Hormonal cancer therapies can exert unfavorable effects on sexual function in women by precipitating menopause altogether (e.g., lupron, tamoxifen) or by magnifying the effects of preexisting menopause-related hypoestrogenemia (e.g., tamoxifen, aromatase inhibitors).[53] In addition, we have recently observed a very high frequency of vulvar lichen sclerosus in women in our practice who are taking aromatase inhibitors, which is not surprising because vulvar estrogen receptor expression and levels appear to be linked to the etiopathology of this entity[54]: Routine vulvar inspection is therefore a critical aspect of surveillance in patients on these medications.

In men, hormonal cancer therapies cause sexual difficulties via effects on testosterone. Hormonal therapies are most commonly used in advanced prostate cancer for androgen deprivation therapy (ADT); however, ADT is now being increasingly used for short periods of time in men with early-stage disease. The most common form of ADT used in up to 90% of men is medical castration with a GnRH agonist—either leuprolide or goserelin. These agents lower testosterone levels significantly within 1 month, resulting in a decline in libido, erectile dysfunction, decreased size of the penis and/or testes, vasomotor changes, labile mood, fatigue, gynecomastia, and diminished self-image and quality of life.[55] Although these adverse effects can occur after any form of treatment for prostate cancer, symptoms are frequently particularly severe in men using ADT[56] and are exacerbated in men who are obese or of older age.[57] Patients should always be counseled that recovery of sexual function after cessation of therapy is possible but is not guaranteed.[58] Alternative regimens using antiandrogen monotherapy, such as bicalutamide without the addition of a GnRH agonist,[59] or cyclic GnRH agonists with temporary withdrawal periods after an initial induction phase[60] cause significantly less sexual dysfunction and fewer hot flashes, but without clear equality in disease control and survival. Until survival outcomes are more fully understood, these options remain controversial. Estrogens are sometimes used to complement ADT in men with prostate cancer; use of estrogens in men is associated with lethargy, poor libido, and erectile dysfunction.[61]

Immune-mediated cancer therapies can also affect sexual function in several ways. Immunocompromised patients are at increased risk for a number of infections, including candidiasis, which can be associated with vulvovaginal discomfort and pain on penetration. Bone marrow transplantation for hematologic malignancies frequently results in clinically manifest graft-versus-host disease (GVHD), which, in women, can result in a dry, thin, and painful vulvovaginal mucosa that is prone to scarring and stenosis.[62] A recent case series suggests that vulvovaginal GVHD is relatively common, with typical cutaneous and soft tissue changes seen in 17 of 44 (39%) consecutive autologous bone marrow transplant recipients.[63] These numbers suggest that routine perineal inspection should be the standard of care in women following transplantation.

Because of the emphasis that the traditional medical model places on nature over nurture and the human tendency to seek quick pharmacologic fixes for our woes, we find that it is easy to fall into the trap of concentrating mainly on the physical effects of cancer treatment, rather than considering cancer's numerous and equally important psychological and interpersonal effects. To avoid making this mistake, we find it helpful when evaluating patients to refer to a biopsychosocial model of sexual function (Fig. 57-3) that contains all of these features. Specific questions that delve into each of these key areas are presented later, in the section on history taking.

6. If sex was important before cancer, it generally remains important after cancer.

Whether or not their lives are affected by cancer, some individuals and couples choose not to be sexually active and are content with that status. For example, 1% of respondents in a survey of the general population in the United Kingdom indicated that they were asexual (defined as having no sexual attraction to a person of either sex)[64]; approximately 20% to 30% of couples in committed relationships in another general population survey[65] were estimated to be sexually abstinent (defined as engaging in sexual activity fewer than 10 times per year). Abstinence after a cancer diagnosis may not pose a

problem at all for individuals and couples such as these, and it is important to respect their choice. On the other hand, available evidence suggests that sexual activity is a priority for many people whose lives are affected by cancer: Some previously sexually active couples continue to have sex throughout the cancer experience, and most couples recommence or try to recommence sexual activity relatively early during the recovery period, usually in the first few months after treatment ends.[66,67] Accordingly, cancer survivors and their partners typically have many questions about sex that deserve careful consideration (Table 57-2). Accurate information about what practices are safe during treatment (e.g., during chemotherapy and radiation administration in the setting of neutropenia and thrombocytopenia) and about what to expect and how to respond to changes in sexual function after treatment is crucial for these couples.

7. Adjustment and adaptation are heavily influenced by life stage and by both individual and couple coping responses.

Acceptance of and successful adaptation to the physical changes associated with cancer treatment are influenced by each individual's and couple's psychological maturity and coping style, and also by the life phase during which cancer strikes. Significant changes in sexual function occur across the life cycle in association with acute stressors such as illness and the physiologic changes that come with major transitions such as puberty, pregnancy, breastfeeding, menopause, and senescence. Cancer treatment frequently causes an acceleration of the physiologic changes associated with aging. Careful explanation of this reality can help to normalize changes and facilitate adaptation, particularly for older individuals and couples

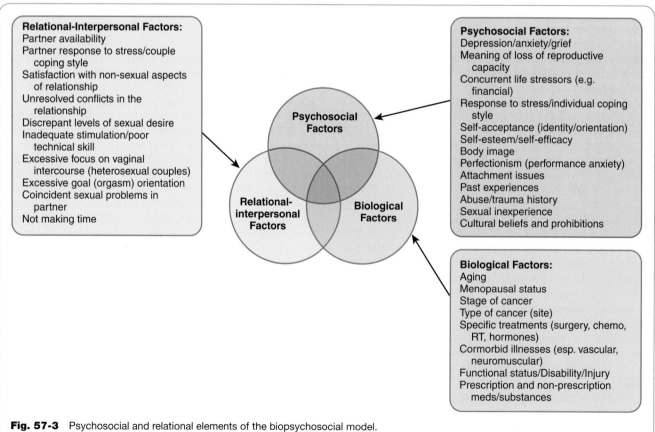

Relational-Interpersonal Factors:
Partner availability
Partner response to stress/couple
   coping style
Satisfaction with non-sexual aspects
   of relationship
Unresolved conflicts in the
   relationship
Discrepant levels of sexual desire
Inadequate stimulation/poor
   technical skill
Excessive focus on vaginal
   intercourse (heterosexual couples)
Excessive goal (orgasm) orientation
Coincident sexual problems in
   partner
Not making time

Psychosocial Factors:
Depression/anxiety/grief
Meaning of loss of reproductive
   capacity
Concurrent life stressors (e.g.,
   financial)
Response to stress/individual coping
   style
Self-acceptance (identity/orientation)
Self-esteem/self-efficacy
Body image
Perfectionism (performance anxiety)
Attachment issues
Past experiences
Abuse/trauma history
Sexual inexperience
Cultural beliefs and prohibitions

Biological Factors:
Aging
Menopausal status
Stage of cancer
Type of cancer (site)
Specific treatments (surgery, chemo,
   RT, hormones)
Cormorbid illnesses (esp. vascular,
   neuromuscular)
Functional status/Disability/Injury
Prescription and non-prescription
   meds/substances

Fig. 57-3 Psychosocial and relational elements of the biopsychosocial model.

Table 57-2 Common questions survivors have about sex

Did sexual activity cause my cancer?

Will sexual activity spread the cancer to my partner?

Will my partner lose hair if we have sex during treatment?

How long should I wait to have sex after (surgery, chemo, radiation)?

What level should my (platelets, absolute neutrophil count) be?

Can I get pregnant while receiving (chemo, radiation)?

How will I know if I can still have children after treatment?

Will sex feel different while I'm having treatment?

If I'm too tired or too sick, how do I let my partner know I still care?

Ever since treatment ended, I just don't seem to be interested anymore, and my vagina feels sore. What can I do?

Adapted from www.stjude.org.

who have weathered the impact of some age-related physical changes already, and in whom the incremental impact of cancer treatment therefore tends to be less severe and abrupt. For example, it can be helpful to explain to a couple that because of treatment-associated changes in genital sensitivity and responsiveness, it is expected that the patient will require more intense and prolonged genital stimulation to achieve orgasm, and that this change is not a manifestation of diminished affection for his or her partner. Younger individuals generally require significant support because it can be extremely daunting to face the challenges of embracing and exploring one's sexuality for the first time in the context of heightened body image concerns and the uncertainty and fear that surround when and how to divulge a history of cancer to prospective partners.

Coping response has an enormous impact on the intensity and duration of sexual difficulties that patients and/or their partners experience after cancer. As shown in Figure 57-4, people tend to develop fairly stereotypical reactions (e.g., the fight-or-flight response) in response to stress, in which exposure to the stressor leads to a cascade of emotions (e.g., fear), automatic thoughts (e.g., I've got to get away), and physical sensations (e.g., elevated heart rate) and/or behaviors (e.g., person runs away). Although the original intent of this type of cascade is generally adaptive (i.e., the goal is to achieve safety and security), the individual is often less well served when automatisms become too deeply ingrained over time. Consider the hypothetical reactions of two different cancer survivors to

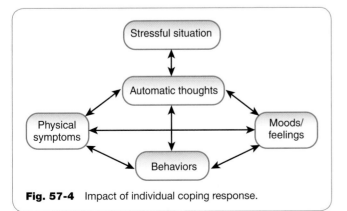

Fig. 57-4 Impact of individual coping response.

the emotional and physical losses associated with cancer treatment. Both women start with a feeling of sadness related to the losses they have experienced ("I miss my old body and sex life"). For one woman, this feeling of sadness immediately triggers a cascade of negative thoughts ("I look really ugly," "No one will ever want me"), which, when coupled with maladaptive physical responses to stress, result in preoccupation or withdrawal and avoidance of intimacy and sexual activity, and ultimately culminate in increased isolation and loneliness. The other woman, who has more highly developed coping skills, is able to transition quickly from a place of sadness into a proactive position with a positive thought ("I need to learn my new body"); this cognitive framing permits her to research and experiment with ways to manage her symptoms and to seek connection and strengthen relationships with others. Although not pictured here, it is easy to imagine how ever more complicated these cascades would become if the reactions of each woman's partner were included. Fortunately, patients and their partners can be taught to recognize and replace negative with positive thoughts, thereby learning how to choose courses of action that facilitate more favorable outcomes. As shown in Figure 57-5, coping in couples can be greatly enhanced when a stressor is perceived as a dyadic stress, and the couple coordinates their efforts to find a shared solution.

8. Although pharmacologic treatments can be helpful, the most successful interventions include attention to psychological and couples issues and lifestyle and behavioral change.

Given the inherent complexity of sexual function and the need to explore all aspects of the biopsychosocial model when evaluating patients who present with sexual difficulties, it should not be surprising that the most effective interventions are also multimodal and include attention to individual and couples counseling and lifestyle and behavioral change, in addition to pharmacologic manipulation. In discussing the need for attention to each of these areas, we find it helpful to review the concept of a "sexual tipping point" when counseling patients (Fig. 57-6). According to this model, the degree of sexual responsiveness that a person experiences at any one point in time is a product of all of the excitatory psychological, interpersonal, cultural, and physiologic factors that act to "turn on" the system at that time balanced against all of the psychological, interpersonal, cultural, and physiologic influences that act to "turn off" the system. An excess of excitatory influences results in faster and/or greater sexual response (e.g., "hot"), whereas a preponderance of inhibitory influences results in slower and/or less intense response (e.g., "not").[68] Optimal results can be achieved only by concentrating on all areas that are amenable to improvement, rather than focusing solely on pharmacologic intervention. For patients and their partners who remain unconvinced, it is helpful to point out that the positive effects of counseling and lifestyle change reach far beyond the realm of sexual function (e.g., improved communication enhances overall relationship satisfaction, weight loss reduces the risks for diabetes and cardiovascular disease). Moreover, in contradistinction to medications, behavioral and counseling techniques are far less likely to be associated with undesirable side effects.

9. Successful intervention has a positive impact on quality of life (QOL) and overall functioning.

Sexual function is an important predictor of QOL. Erectile dysfunction has a significant impact on QOL, for example, in one study of men with erectile dysfunction, the strongest

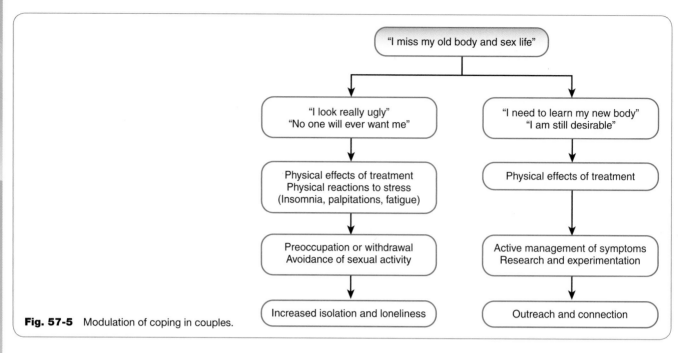

Fig. 57-5 Modulation of coping in couples.

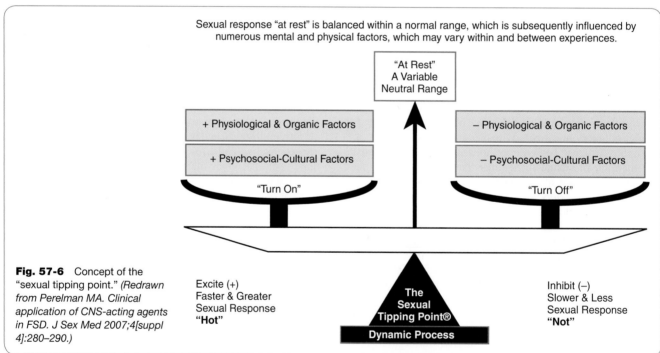

Fig. 57-6 Concept of the "sexual tipping point." *(Redrawn from Perelman MA. Clinical application of CNS-acting agents in FSD. J Sex Med 2007;4[suppl 4]:280–290.)*

predictor of better QOL was better sexual functioning, followed by more positive beliefs about the effects of erectile dysfunction on masculinity.[69] In another study, which evaluated satisfaction with outcome among 1201 men treated for prostate cancer and 625 spouses, sexual difficulties resulting from cancer treatment were significantly associated with reduced satisfaction and reduced QOL in both groups, highlighting the fact that sexual problems after cancer affect not only the survivor, but also the partner.[70] Fortunately, although the field is young, a growing body of literature is beginning to show that interventions that prevent sexual side effects of treatment or that help to restore sexual function after treatment have a positive impact on QOL and overall functioning.[71]

PREVALENCE AND PREDICTORS OF SEXUAL DIFFICULTIES AFTER CANCER

Most of the research on sexual difficulties in female cancer survivors done to date has focused on "reproductive" cancers: An estimated 50% of women with breast cancer and 80% of women with gynecologic cancers experience problems, especially during the first 12 to 18 months after treatment.[72,73] However, many women whose cancers affect geographic sites other than the breasts or genitalia also appear to experience dramatic changes in sexual function after treatment, with one comparative review demonstrating 84% versus 76% prevalence of sexual difficulties in women with "reproductive" versus "nonreproductive" cancer sites.[74] This is likely a result of treatment effects on psychosocial parameters, as well as systemically mediated effects on neurobiological mechanisms of sexual response, as discussed previously. For many women, sexual difficulties can persist for years, despite improvements in mood and overall adjustment; therefore it is important to ascertain the presence of problems and to initiate interventions promptly. Early intervention can be facilitated by identification of various predisposing factors, which include poor perceived health, poor body image, vaginal dryness, urinary incontinence, poor dyadic adjustment, a history of preexisting sexual problems, and having a partner with sexual problems.[75–77] For the aforementioned reasons, younger women are especially vulnerable.[78] Single women in particular experience significant anxiety regarding when to discuss their cancer history with prospective partners and frequently express the fear that they will be found sexually undesirable, will be rejected outright, or perhaps will never find another partner.

Impaired sexual function is also documented in men with a variety of cancers, including prostate, testicular, rectal, bladder, penile, and hematologic malignancies. Difficulties reported include decreased interest in sex and overall dissatisfaction with the frequency and quality of sexual activity.[79] Careful assessment of sexual function before treatment is important to understanding the late and long-term effects of treatment. In one study with rigorous presurgical assessment of sexual function, 50% of men were found to have erectile dysfunction before radical surgery for prostate cancer, which also was associated with depression and fear of the proposed procedure.[80] Surveys demonstrate that treatment for prostate cancer disrupts marital and sexual happiness in 10% to 20% of patients.[81] Disturbances in sexual function and relationships are compounded by cultural norms and perceptions of masculinity, which decrease the likelihood that men will seek help when needed.[82]

Predictors of impaired sexual function in men vary according to cancer diagnosis, strength of the partnered relationship before cancer, and treatments received. However, the greatest predictor of sexual function after cancer therapy is pretherapy sexual function.[80] With controls for type of cancer and pretreatment sexual function level, predictors include (1) patient age, (2) difference in age between the survivor and his partner,[84] (3) preservation of penis size,[85] (4) early use of a vacuum erection device after prostatectomy,[86] (5) poorer psychological function,[87] and (6) lack of a spouse.[87]

In addition to having an impact on the patient, cancer subjects the patient's partner to considerable stress, which may manifest as heightened anxiety, depression, feelings of being unprepared to help, fear of recurrence and eventual death of the spouse, and somatic preoccupations. Limited literature suggests that spouses may keep these fears to themselves, hoping to spare their loved one from additional burden or worry.[89] When queried specifically, many spouses express specific concerns regarding sexual intimacy; although the incidence and origin of diagnosable sexual dysfunction in partners of female cancer survivors are not known, a high proportion—78% of partners in one study—reported adverse effects on their own sexual functioning.[90] These results point to the importance of open communication between partners, particularly given the fact that emotional support provided by either partner to the other plays a critical role in each person's adjustment.[91] Fortunately, coping with cancer tends to strengthen relationships overall. For example, 282 couples affected by breast cancer were surveyed in one study: In 42% of the couples, both partners reported that cancer "brought us closer"; in 14% both partners believed there was "no effect," in 6% one partner reported feeling "distanced," and in 1% both partners reported being "distanced."[92]

HOW TO TAKE A SEXUAL HISTORY FROM PATIENTS AND THEIR PARTNERS

The most important things clinicians can do to make a difference are to take a thorough sexual history and to be prepared to respond proactively when patients and their partners express concerns. Because talking about sex is something many clinicians feel uneasy about, and because it is an area in which most have had limited opportunity to practice their skills, several authors have proposed communication models to ease discussion. These include the P-LI-SS-IT model (Permission, Limited Information, Specific Suggestions, Intensive Therapy)[93]; the ALARM model (Activity, Libido, Arousal, Resolution, Medical)[94]; the BETTER model (Bring up, Explain, Tell, Time, Educate, Record)[95]; and the 5 A's model (Ask, Advise, Assess, Assist, Arrange follow-up).[96] The latter two models were designed specifically for use with cancer survivors. Rather than enumerating the specifics of each of these models, we would like to highlight several key themes: the importance of asking cancer survivors about sex; providing education about basic sexual function and common changes caused by cancer treatment; suggesting strategies to enhance sexual satisfaction in the face of these changes; and facilitating further workup and referral when requested to do so. We would like to emphasize the importance of scrupulously remembering to **involve both patients and partners**; to **initiate discussion before, during, and after treatment**; to **ask questions about multiple dimensions** (e.g., all domains of sexual response, everything in the biopsychosocial model); and to **be mindful of cultural context** (e.g., in some cultures, patients will discuss intimate topics only with a same-gender clinician).

Several brief questionnaires about sexual function have been validated in different populations of cancer survivors, including the UCLA Prostate Cancer Index,[97] the 5-item version of the International Index of Erectile Function,[98] and the Female Sexual Function Index.[99] For clinicians who have the time and are so inclined, use of these instruments may be helpful both during the initial evaluation and subsequently during follow-up, to ascertain benefits achieved using various interventions. However, it is important to note that the questions asked in these measures may not be apropos to all patients, for example, all of the female sexual function measures that have been reviewed to date were developed and tested in heterosexual or presumed heterosexual populations, and therefore may not be applicable to lesbians, who do not participate in vaginal intercourse.[100] Fortunately, ongoing work is being done to develop a more apropos and psychometrically robust measure of sexual function for use in oncology settings, and we are hopeful that an improved assessment tool will be available in the near future.[101] With or without the use of formal assessment tools, we believe strongly that all clinicians can learn to take a thorough sexual history in a sensitive manner, and that increased comfort and skill will inevitably accrue over time and with greater practice. Table 57-3 presents a list of questions that can be used as a starting point.

Table 57-3 Questions to ask when patients and partners present with sexual concerns

Begin With General Opening Questions

- Are you satisfied with your sexual life?
- Are there things about your (or your partner's) sexual function you wish you could change?
- Has cancer treatment affected your sexual function (self-image, comfort showing your body to your partner, interest in sex, responsiveness to sexual stimulation) in any way?
- Did you experience any problems with sexual intimacy before cancer?

Determine Affected Functional Domains

- Desire: Do you notice a change in your interest in sex?
- Arousal: Do you become sufficiently lubricated (women)? Do you have difficulty obtaining or maintaining erections (men)?
- Orgasm: Are you able to reach orgasm?
- Comfort/Pain: Do you experience any discomfort or pain during sex?

Evaluate Distress and Expectations

- How have these changes affected you? Your partner? Your relationship?
- Are you interested in trying to change the current situation?
- Have you tried any interventions already? If so, what were the results?

Evaluate Relationship Quality

- How would you describe the overall quality of your relationship?
- Do you feel comfortable talking with your partner about the kinds of stimulation you enjoy?
- If you do talk about sex with your partner, have you found her/him to be responsive?

Ask Specific Questions About Each Affected Sexual Domain

Questions about Desire

- What was your highest ever level of desire (grade on a 0–10 point scale)? How about now?
- Can you identify any inhibiting feelings or thoughts that interfere with your level of desire?
- Do you participate in sexual activities even though your level of desire has changed? If so, what motivates you?
- Do you experience spontaneous sexual thoughts or fantasies?
- Are you "turned on" by erotic descriptions in books or sex scenes in movies?
- Do you find your partner (or other people) attractive?
- How often do you masturbate?

Questions About Arousal

- (For women): Is dryness a problem? Have you tried using lubricants? Which ones? Are they helpful?
- (For men): Do you experience any difficulty achieving or maintaining an erection? Do you have erections at night, or do you ever wake up with an erection? Is your penis firm enough to go inside your partner?
- Do you experience pleasurable sensations when you masturbate?
- What types of sexual activities do you and your partner engage in? Do you experience pleasurable sensations during these activities?
- Can you identify any distracting feelings or thoughts that seem to inhibit these sensations?
- Have you had any negative experiences that might be interfering with your enjoyment now, such as being sexually abused, raped, or coerced into having sex?

Questions About Orgasm

(For women):

- Have you ever had an orgasm?
- If not…Are you familiar with female genital structures, such as the clitoris? Are you aware that most women need clitoral stimulation to become fully aroused?
- What kinds of sexual activities do you participate in? Do they involve stimulation of the clitoris?
- If so…When did you notice a change? What happens exactly? Are you ever able to achieve orgasm? Does it take longer? Do some kinds of stimulation work better than others?
- Can you identify any distracting feelings or thoughts that seem to interfere with orgasm?
- Do you expect to have an orgasm every time you have sex? Do you ever feel satisfied without reaching climax?

(For men):

- What happens during orgasm?
- Has the character, color, amount, or consistency of your semen changed?

Questions About Pain/Discomfort

- Do you experience any discomfort during sexual activity?

Table 57-3 Questions to ask when patients and partners present with sexual concerns—cont'd

- If so, when did it start? Does it occur every time you have sex or just sometimes? Is it related to how turned on you are feeling or how much foreplay you've had?
- What does the discomfort feel like? Where do you feel it exactly? At what point during sexual activity does it occur?
- (For women): On the outside skin of the vulva as soon as it is touched? At or just inside the vaginal opening at the time of penetration? Deep inside the vagina or in the pelvis? At the time of or following orgasm?
- (For men): Have you been able to identify any triggers? Does anything (e.g., trying different sexual positions, using more lubricant) make it feel better?
- (For women): Have you experienced pain in the past when using tampons or with speculum insertion during pelvic examination? (symptoms of vaginismus)
- (For men): Do you experience penile curvature or pain with erection (symptoms of Peyronie's disease)? Do you have pain during ejaculation?

PHYSICAL EXAMINATION

Few studies have evaluated the reliability and reducibility of the physical examination to diagnose sexual problems; however, abnormal findings may be discovered that suggest specific causes, or that guide treatment (Table 57-4). It is reasonable to palpate the thyroid in all survivors with diminished libido, because hypothyroidism can be a side effect of various cancer treatments and may affect sexual function adversely. Breasts and liver should be examined when hormonal (especially systemic hormonal) treatments are being considered, because of possible toxicities. A careful genital examination should be performed in all patients, especially in those with decreased arousal (erectile dysfunction in men; reduced genital sensation and/or lubrication in women), anorgasmia, or sexual pain. The pelvic examination can be especially challenging in some women, especially those with a past history of abuse, severe postmenopausal atrophy, and/or vaginal stenosis related to pelvic irradiation. Simple measures can help reduce anxiety and discomfort and maximize a woman's sense of control, including the presence of a support person/chaperone; a contract to stop the examination if requested by the patient; the use of a very small and narrow speculum; and adequate lubrication with a water-based gel, which has been shown not to interfere with cytology or culture results.[102,103] In our clinical experience, use of lidocaine jelly as the lubricant may also ease a challenging pelvic examination significantly.

Inspection of male genitalia should begin with assessment of the Tanner staging of hair distribution. Male pubic hair should be dense and in a rhomboid or diamond-shaped pattern at maturity. A level inconsistent with maturity level could indicate a clinically important loss of testosterone. Testicular examination by palpation is an important next step to investigate for atrophy (if testosterone production has been affected by chemotherapy, radiation, or other secondary causes) or masses (signifying concern for additional cancers). Mature male testicular size ranges from 4 to 7 cm in length. Additionally, a complete male examination includes inspection and palpation of the chest for evidence of gynecomastia (glandular breast tissue over the pectoralis muscle), which is caused by a relative imbalance in testosterone. Gynecomastia should be distinguished from pseudogynecomastia (excess adiposity in the chest) and breast cancer, which often manifests as a firm eccentric mass lateral to the nipple. If the tissue type is not obvious after completion of the examination, diagnostic imaging should be performed. The cause of confirmed gynecomastia should be determined to rule out hypogonadism (primary or secondary), hyperthyroidism, hyperprolactinemia, and adrenocortical or germ cell testicular tumors, as well as liver or kidney failure. Gynecomastia is a common side effect of many medications and chemotherapeutic agents.

The integrity of pelvic blood vessels and nerves should be assessed in patients with arousal problems. Blood pressure and peripheral pulses provide an assessment of overall cardiovascular function. Hair distribution on the lower legs can signify arterial insufficiency or peripheral vascular disease, which could be confirmed by the additional assessment of ankle-brachial index. If evidence of peripheral vascular disease is present in the lower extremities, vascular disease is likely to be a factor limiting arterial flow to the genitalia and impairing arousal. The integrity of sacral neurologic outflow can be assessed via digital rectal examination and assessment of anal sphincter tone and bulbocavernosus reflex.

The Q-tip test is useful in determining the location and intensity of pain (graded from 1 to 10) in women with complaints of vulvar pain[104]; sensory testing has not been well published in men with pelvic pain syndromes. More sophisticated tests can provide additional functional information but are not generally necessary in the initial evaluation and usually fall in the province of the specialist. These tests include things such as nocturnal penile tumescence monitoring or duplex Doppler ultrasound of the cavernosal arteries in men, which may reveal arterial blockages amenable to surgical repair.[105] In women, genital sensation can be measured using a device called a biothesiometer, and clitoral blood flow assessed using a vaginal photoplethysmograph. Ultrasound can be done to assess the integrity of pelvic structures in women with deep pelvic pain during sexual activity but is rarely needed.

LABORATORY AND OTHER TESTING

Laboratory testing should be tailored to individual circumstances, with careful consideration given to cost and evidence of clinical usefulness. In noncancer patients with sexual difficulties, measurement of cardiovascular risk factors (lipids, glucose) and hormonal profiles have been recommended by expert consensus[106]; however, few data from randomized controlled trials (RCTs) support this approach. Appropriate laboratory testing is reasonable when hyperprolactinemia,

Table 57-4 Physical examination in patients who report sexual problems

Anatomic feature or examination maneuver	Possible source of sexual difficulty
Nongenital (female and male)	
Blood pressure	Atherosclerosis
Peripheral pulses	
Thyroid examination	Hypothyroidism
Breast examination	Hyperprolactinemia (nipple discharge)
Gynecomastia	
Musculoskeletal examination	Limited comfort and mobility
Neurologic examination	Neurologic impairment
Genital/perineal (female)	
Mons pubis	Low androgens (sparse pubic hair)
Vulvar skin inspection	Changes caused by infection (*Candida,* herpes), dermatitis (allergic, eczema, psoriasis), dermatoses (lichens)
Labia majora and minora	Atrophy, lesions, adhesions, fusion
Clitoris	Phimosis, adhesions, female genital
Circumcision	
Urethra	Infection, prolapse
Vaginal introitus	Atrophy, lesions, scarring, stricture
Vagina	Atrophy, lesions, stenosis, discharge
Valsalva	Cystocele, rectocele, uterine prolapse, urinary incontinence
Bimanual examination	Masses, tenderness
Vaginal and anal muscle contraction	Poor tone
Bulbocavernosus reflex	Pudendal neuropathy
Genital/perineal (male)	
Mons pubis	Low androgens (sparse pubic hair)
Palpate penile shaft for plaque	Peyronie's disease
Testicular size, consistency	Hypogonadism (testosterone deficiency)
Digital rectal examination	Prostate, anal tone
Bulbocavernosus reflex	Pudendal neuropathy

hypothyroidism, or anemia is suspected. Serum androgens are not diagnostically useful in women because there are no precise definitions of androgen deficiency, the "normal" ranges for serum androgens in women of different ages are poorly characterized, and two large population-based studies failed to show a correlation between low serum testosterone level and low sexual desire.[107,108] Androgen testing should always be performed in a man with sexual difficulties. Testosterone is best checked in the morning around 8 AM because of its diurnal variation. Appropriate morning levels should be in the range of 300 to 800 ng/dl. If borderline or lower than the normal range, a repeat testosterone level and follicle-stimulating hormone (FSH) and luteinizing hormone (LH) levels should be checked to confirm the low level and assess for primary or secondary causes. Free testosterone levels are often unreliable and lead to false results but should be considered in obese and older men who may have impaired testosterone binding.[109,110] If desired, a free level can be calculated with total testosterone, albumin, and sex hormone–binding globulin levels through the use of readily available online calculators.

An appropriate evaluation should be performed in the setting of apparent vaginitis/cervicitis or penile discharge, or when male or female genital lesions are discovered, including selected tests for vaginitis and sexually transmitted infections and biopsy of suspicious lesions. Routine screening with clinical breast and prostate examinations, prostate-specific antigen (PSA), mammography, and Pap testing should follow usual age-, gender-, and risk-appropriate guidelines as outlined by the American Society of Clinical Oncology (ASCO)[111] and the National Comprehensive Cancer Network (NCCN).[112]

INTERVENTIONS TO OPTIMIZE EMOTIONAL AND PHYSICAL INTIMACY

Clinicians can do many things to help patients and their partners achieve and maintain optimal emotional and physical intimacy. In discussing potential interventions with patients, we find it helpful to keep several thoughts in mind:

1. Preparation and prevention are worth a pound of cure. Patients and their partners generally do better when they are apprised of potential hurdles that they may encounter before these challenges arise. The most effective ways to prevent emotional distance and problems with sexual function are to explicitly attend to communication and (for couples who want to be sexually active and for whom sexual activity is not clinical inadvisable) to continue regular sexual activity throughout the cancer experience. In women particularly, there is a certain "use it or lose it" aspect of sexual function, that is, ongoing sexual activity in and of itself tends to maintain vaginal lubrication and elasticity, even in the face of untreated postmenopausal estrogen decline.

2. Losses in function need to be acknowledged and grieved before it is possible to embrace the concept of change. It is therefore important for clinicians to listen empathically when patients and their partners express the multitude of emotions (e.g., sadness, anger, guilt) about the ways in which cancer has influenced their lives and their interactions with one another, and to help each partner support the other in dealing with these feelings.

3. There is no such thing as "perfect" sexual function, and there are no "quick fixes." Media hype about sex leads many patients and partners to believe that "good" sex requires rapid, multiple, and simultaneous orgasms, and that magic bullets (e.g., PDEIs) are available that can restore sexual function easily and completely when problems arise. Because this is seldom the case, it is important to help patients and their partners set reasonable expectations, and to point out that restoration and maintenance of emotional and sexual intimacy generally require substantial dedicated time and effort.

4. The complexity of human sexual response, which involves a dance between numerous excitatory and inhibitory influences, may be confusing and even overwhelming to patients and their partners, but it is important to point out that this complexity also means that many different pathways can usually be exploited to enhance pleasure. In our experience, taking the time to review the sexual tipping point diagram (see Fig. 57-6) and enumerating all of the opportunities for positive intervention facilitate better understanding and greater patience with the process of evaluation and treatment, and typically result in both parties becoming more readily engaged as active participants in their care.

EDUCATION, COUNSELING, AND LIFESTYLE CHANGE INTERVENTIONS

Many patients and their partners are surprised by the extent to which their emotional reactions to the whole experience of cancer intrude during intimate moments, and by the degree to which physical changes associated with cancer treatment interfere with sexual functioning. Open discussion about the challenges cancer can pose to intimate relationships, including the need to manage numerous, powerful, conflicting and ever-changing emotions, as well as the need to adjust and adapt to physical changes that affect sexual function, helps prepare patients and their partners, so that these events do not arrive as a shock. Because the challenges cancer brings can be overwhelming, it is crucially important to offer patients and their partners a list of resources that they can use to achieve a greater understanding of and mastery over all of the changes they are experiencing, including books, websites, and referral to appropriate counseling services when additional support and guidance are needed. It is also beneficial to proactively and explicitly discuss various lifestyle strategies that patients and their partners can use to prevent sexual side effects of treatment or to ease adjustment to changes in sexual function when they occur. Table 57-5 lists helpful educational, counseling, and lifestyle interventions. The reader may also find it helpful to refer to Table 57-6 ("A Problem-Oriented Approach to Improving Sexual Function") while reading this section and the following sections on pharmacologic strategies, mechanical devices, and surgical interventions to improve sexual function.

Referral for counseling can help enhance general coping skills; alleviate depression, anxiety, and body image issues; and improve communication between patients and established or prospective partners. Counseling can be beneficial in many forms (e.g., individual, couples, groups), and when in-depth interventions are needed to address sexual communication and technique, dedicated sex therapy may be indicated. It is important to appreciate that body image, self-esteem,

---

Table 57-5 Educational, counseling, and lifestyle interventions

Sexuality education

1. Identify and address any misconceptions about sex.
2. Review sexual anatomy and physiology; expected changes with aging, menopause; and changes associated with specific cancer treatments.
3. Distinguish between lust and other motivations for initiating sexual activity or responding to a partner's advances; identify and celebrate these motivations.
4. Discuss sexual techniques, including identification of both genital (e.g., the clitoris, in women) and nongenital erogenous zones; encourage exploration and experimentation.

Referral for counseling and/or psychopharmacology consultation

1. Individual, couples, or group interventions.
2. Sex therapists have expertise providing counseling that focuses on the sexual aspect of relationships, using various behavioral techniques and homework assignments. AASECT provides a national listing of such therapists.
3. For patients with significant anxiety, depression, PTSD, or compulsive sexual behaviors, a combination of psychotherapy and medications may be appropriate.

Lifestyle changes to enhance sexual satisfaction

1. Create opportunities for intimacy (make "dates," eliminate distractions, create a conducive environment with candles, dimmed lighting, music, etc.).
2. Maximize comfort (encourage use of lubricants, experiment with position changes, strategic analgesic use, etc.).
3. Give permission to explore (masturbation, new positions, new techniques, sex toys, erotica, etc.).
4. Encourage weight loss and exercise.

---

and sexual responsiveness do not occur in isolation. Rather, patients' self views are sculpted by the responses of the people with whom they interact: Positive messages and positive regard that they receive from the significant others in their lives can be profoundly healing.[113] A recent review of couple-based interventions for enhancing women's sexual adjustment and body image after cancer concluded that strategies that produce the strongest effects are couple-focused and include treatment components that (1) educate both partners about the women's diagnosis and treatments, (2) promote couples' mutual coping and support processes, and (3) include specific sexual therapy techniques to address sexual and body image concerns.[114] In men with erectile dysfunction after cancer, both couples-based[115] and group-based[116] therapies have been shown useful in improving male distress and sexual function in both men and their partners; however, these study outcomes are affected by a high concurrent usage rate of pharmacologic therapies for erectile dysfunction. Therefore, whenever possible, we suggest exploiting the power of dyadic interventions with patients who have partners; for un-partnered individuals, group interventions may be particularly beneficial.

Several other strategies may be beneficial in enhancing body image. Chemotherapy-induced hair loss is consistently ranked as one of the most distressing effects of cancer

Table 57-6 A problem-oriented approach to improving sexual function

Affected functional domain	Goal of treatment	Specific interventions
Desire	Address cognitive inhibitors	Stress reduction, work on body image, individual and couples therapy
	Optimize cognitive motivators	Maximize opportunities for closeness, exploit erotica, etc.
	Address biological inhibitors	Treat hypothyroidism, etc.
	Consider biological motivators	Hormone therapy, bupropion, etc.
Arousal	Optimize sensory input	Vibrators
	Optimize blood flow	PDEIs, vacuum therapy devices, penile injections, penile implants
	Optimize lubrication	Lubricants, vaginal estrogen
	Optimize muscle contraction	Pelvic floor exercises
	Optimize positive cognitive feedback	Utilize sexual fantasies
Orgasm/Ejaculation	Reduce premature ejaculation	Desensitizing creams, stop/squeeze techniques, SSRIs, or PDEIs
	Reduce latency to orgasm (frequently caused by SSRI antidepressants)	Switch to a less sex-negative medication, or add an antidote (see text)
	Address concerns about retrograde ejaculation	Reassure (not a harmful condition), remove potentially offending medications, trial of imipramine
Comfort/Pain	Address general comfort	Strategic analgesic dosing, etc.
	Assess specific issues (e.g., vaginal atrophy and stenosis in women)	Lubricants, vaginal estrogen, vaginal dilators

PDEIs, Phosphodiesterase inhibitors; *SSRIs*, selective serotonin reuptake inhibitors.

treatment and has a profoundly negative impact on body image in both women and men.[117,118] Participation in programs such as the American Cancer Society's Look Good… Feel Better program, which provides cosmetic makeovers and hair help, can enhance self-confidence and social comfort for patients whose appearance is altered by cancer treatment.[119] For women who have undergone mastectomy without reconstruction and are bothered by the appearance of their surgical scar, consideration of various interventions, such as temporary or permanent postmastectomy tattooing or delayed surgical reconstruction, may be helpful. Both women and men who are distressed by the presence of a urostomy or colostomy bag may benefit from the use of a wide range of cleverly designed intimate lingerie in the bedroom.

Obesity, weight gain, and physical activity also deserve close attention. Weight gain can be a complication of cancer treatment and is associated with negative effects on body image and sexual functioning among cancer survivors. Obesity after cancer diagnosis is associated with increased recurrence and/or poorer prognosis in breast, prostate, and colon cancer survivors.[120–122] Although evidence to support the beneficial effects of weight reduction in this setting is limited, higher levels of posttreatment physical activity are associated with improved outcomes among breast and colon cancer survivors.[123,124] Moreover, both moderate weight loss and regular physical activity reduce the risk of chronic health conditions other than cancer and are associated with improvements in body image and sexual satisfaction among overweight people in the general population.[125,126] Therefore, cancer survivors should be encouraged to achieve and maintain a healthy weight and to engage in regular physical activity to improve their overall well-being and to enhance health outcomes. The American Cancer Society (ACS) has published a useful set of

guidelines to help direct nutrition and physical activity during and after cancer treatment.[127]

Some cancer patients feel betrayed by their bodies after a cancer diagnosis; others experience their changed bodies as unfamiliar, strange, or alien. It can be difficult to engage in intimate sexual activities with a partner under these circumstances, and it is often helpful for patients to spend some time alone first, getting to know their new bodies and learning what locations and types of touch feel good. It is important to give patients explicit permission to explore masturbation; some may initially be reluctant to do so because of cultural constraints, and for those who are sexually inexperienced, it may be helpful to provide basic information about erogenous zones and sexual technique. Exploration of previously unappreciated nongenital erogenous areas (e.g., ears, breasts, neck, antecubital and popliteal fossae) should be encouraged. Patients can be assured that once they have learned about their own bodies, they can teach their partner what kinds of stimulation they enjoy. A wide variety of books can be recommended to provide guidance (see suggested resources). For patients who feel uncomfortable with erotic self-touch, simple body massage with a pleasantly scented lotion may ease adjustment to a changed body and eventually facilitate acceptance.

For patients who have partners, it may be helpful to deliberately create opportunities for closeness, such as making dates to spend intimate time together, making sure there will be no distractions, and setting a relaxing and/or romantic mood by choosing a conducive setting, music, and/or candles. It is important to stress that physical intimacy encompasses far more than sexual activity: Snuggling, cuddling, and spooning are all to be cherished. Many survivors who experience loss of libido after cancer treatment express great concern that they will never be interested in having sex again. Although it is important to acknowledge their loss, it is most helpful to point out that motivators other than lust (such as the desire to feel close to one's partner) can lead people into participating in sex, and that once engaged in sexual activity, there are many ways to achieve satisfaction (e.g., if sufficient arousal results, orgasm may occur, or one may simply take pleasure in one's partner's enjoyment). This is an example of utilizing cognitive restructuring techniques (e.g., helping patients substitute productive for unproductive thoughts) to effect changes in behavior. For survivors whose instinct is to avoid recommencing genital stimulation because of performance anxiety, discomfort, or fear of discomfort, the use of nondemand, sensual touching exercises ("sensate focus exercises") that focus on the pleasurable sensations associated with nongenital touch can be extremely helpful as a first step. Typically, these exercises begin with the least threatening types of touch, such as back rubs or foot massage, and can progress over time to nude, full-body caressing, including the genitals. As discussed earlier, patients who do not have partners often need help in planning how and when to discuss their cancer history with prospective partners, and may benefit from practicing these conversations using role-play exercises.

Physical comfort during sexual activity may be an issue for many cancer survivors because of hypersensitivity to touch caused by scarring or neuropathy, lymphedema, or reduced mobility. Helpful suggestions include considering a warm bath before sexual activity, optimizing analgesic use, and experimenting with alternative sexual positions. For women with postmenopausal atrophic changes who experience discomfort during penetrative sexual activity, both vaginal moisturizers and sexual lubricants can be recommended. Vaginal moisturizers are used day-to-day to hydrate vulvar and vaginal cells and reduce mucosal fragility; lubricants are used during sexual activity to reduce friction and increase glide. Many different lubricants are available, including water-, oil-, and silicone-based options. Selection should be based on safety (only water-based lubricants should be used with latex safer sex barriers), palatability (some lubricants are designed to taste good—important if partners wish to engage in sequential oral and vaginal sex), and glide (oil- and silicone-based lubricants coat mucosal surfaces more effectively and are more long-lasting). In one small (N = 59) double-blind, randomized, crossover trial of Replens (a moisturizer) versus KY Jelly (a water-based lubricant), both products reduced vaginal dryness; however, a trend toward less dyspareunia was noted in the Replens group (P = .05).[128] In our clinical experience, we find that daily use of a vaginal moisturizer plus use of a lubricant during sexual activity often results in greater comfort during penetration than use of either one alone. A small study (N = 15) in the general population indicated that Replens performs comparably to vaginal estrogen cream (discussed in the next section) in alleviating discomfort associated with vaginal dryness,[129] and is therefore a good option for survivors in whom all estrogen therapies, including low-dose vaginal estrogen, are contraindicated.

Although lifestyle recommendations and risk factor modifications are advised for all men with impaired erectile function,[130,131] no study to date has examined the role of lifestyle changes in improving erectile function in male cancer survivors. It is recommended that all men limit or reduce factors known to exacerbate erectile function, such as obesity, lack of exercise, stress, and tobacco use. One RCT to date has assessed lifestyle modifications and erectile function in men. Esposito et al. examined 110 obese men with sexual dysfunction as determined by International Index of Erectile Function (IIEF) scores <21. The men were randomly assigned to an intervention group, in which they received detailed advice on how to achieve weight loss of 10% through reduced caloric intake and increased physical activity. Men in the control group were given general information about healthy food choices and exercise. After 2 years of follow up, mean IIEF scores improved in the intervention group (from 13.9 to 17; $P < .001$) but remained stable in the control group (from 13.5 to 13.6; $P = .89$). Multivariate analyses revealed that changes in body mass index ($P = .02$), physical activity ($P = .02$), and C-reactive protein ($P = .03$) were independently associated with changes in IIEF score.[132] Criticisms of this study included that improvement in IIEF score was not sufficient to resolve impaired sexual function; however, these data do suggest that recommended dietary and lifestyle changes could lead to improvement in sexual function and could reduce the risks of chronic disease and comorbidities.

Premature ejaculation (PE) can interfere with normal sexual activity in men with and without a history of cancer. PE is defined as an inability to control ejaculation to the degree that allows both partners involved to enjoy the activity to their satisfaction. Men with PE often report less than a minute of duration between achieving a full erection to ejaculation; this is estimated to occur in 20% of all men. It is unknown how many male cancer survivors suffer from PE. Therapies for PE include the pause and squeeze technique, whereby after erection sexual enjoyment is stopped after 5 to 10 seconds, and the man (or his partner) squeezes the glans or head of his penis firmly until the erection loses firmness. Sexual activity then resumes for another 5 to 10 seconds, and the technique is performed again. The process is repeated with gradually increasing durations between squeezes to assist the man in building a tolerance or in conditioning his nervous system to hold back on ejaculation until the desired time.[133] Pharmacologic therapy is also effective for men with PE. For example, the common adverse effects of antidepressants in delaying ejaculation can be useful in this setting. In a prospective double-blind, randomized, crossover study involving 31 men with premature ejaculation, median ejaculation latency time was significantly increased from the pretreatment median of 1 minute up to 3 to 4 minutes, with use of the squeeze technique, clomipramine, sertraline, or paroxetine. Median ejaculation latency time increased from 1 minute to 15 minutes with the use of sildenafil. Each of the drugs was administered 3 to 4 hours before sexual activity. In this study, sildenafil was considered superior to selective serotonin reuptake inhibitor (SSRI) therapy or the pause and squeeze technique.[134] After use of a daily medication for 1 to 3 months, men are usually able to stop use of the medication and have normal ejaculatory latency times. PE is a highly treatable condition and should be assessed in all male survivors.

Retrograde ejaculation appears to be a much more common postoperative problem for male cancer survivors than PE. Retrograde ejaculation occurs when semen is ejaculated into the bladder, rather than outward through the urethra. In normal function, the sphincter of the bladder contracts before ejaculation, which forces semen forward via the urethra. Factors that impair proper sphincter contraction result in differential pressures in the bladder-urethra circuit and permit semen to flow along the path of least resistance—into the bladder. The bladder sphincter is under the control of the autonomic nervous system at the T10-S2 levels of the spinal cord, and this is partially mediated by alpha receptors.[135] Men who have experienced prostate surgery, transurethral or open resection of the prostate, bladder neck surgery, abdomino-perineal rectum excision, or retroperitoneal lymph node dissection for testicular or other pelvic cancers are at risk for damage to these nerve pathways.[136] Certain medications, including antidepressants, antipsychotics, antihypertensives, and alpha blocking agents, can also cause retrograde ejaculation in male cancer survivors.[137] When men present with concerns about retrograde ejaculation, a urinalysis should be obtained after masturbation; the diagnosis is confirmed when an abnormally high sperm count is found in the urine specimen relative to a semen analysis. Reassurance may be all that is needed for some men, in that retrograde ejaculation is not harmful and does not interfere with orgasm; however, many men are disconcerted by its occurrence. Regardless of the cause, 50% of men with or without a history of cancer are effectively treated with medical management.[137] Treatment should begin with cessation of medications known to disturb bladder sphincter function. The second step is to prescribe a medication that increases the sympathetic tone of the bladder or decreases the parasympathetic tone of the bladder; options include alpha agonists, anticholinergics, and antihistamines. The most effective treatments achieve success in a mean of 2 weeks and include chlorpheniramine + phenylpropanolamine 50 mg daily (79% success; n = 14), or imipramine 25 to 75 mg daily (64% success; n = 110).[137] Vibratory stimulation techniques and surgical treatments are also available for men who fail medical therapy, but these approaches often are best managed with the assistance of a urologic specialist.

PHARMACOLOGIC INTERVENTIONS

In addition to utilizing educational, counseling, and lifestyle change strategies, a number of pharmacologic interventions can be considered in selected circumstances. We will discuss these in three categories: hormonal therapies (systemic or vaginal estrogen, testosterone), nonhormonal therapies (PDEIs, prostaglandin E1 agonists), and strategies that can be used to minimize antidepressant-induced sexual dysfunction. Because each of these agents is associated with both benefits and risks, it is always important to have a complete and informed discussion before initiating treatment, and to monitor the patient on treatment to optimize benefits and minimize adverse effects.

Hormonal therapies
FEMALE CANCER SURVIVORS

Systemic estrogen treatment (at doses that raise serum estrogen levels significantly) can be considered for women who experience sexual difficulties after surgical removal of their ovaries or chemotherapy-induced premature ovarian failure, as long as administration of estrogen is not clinically contraindicated on the basis of risk factors (cardiovascular disease, venous thromboembolism [VTE]) or a history of estrogen-sensitive cancer. However, although systemic estrogen treat-

ment reduces vaginal atrophy and improves lubrication and comfort during sexual activity, positive effects on libido have not been as convincingly demonstrated and appear to require doses higher than typically prescribed in this era (conjugated equine estrogen doses greater than 0.625 mg/day).[140] Therefore, when libido is insufficiently enhanced by administration of systemic estrogen, the addition of testosterone (see later) should be considered. Transdermal estrogen formulations are preferable options because they are associated with a lower risk of VTE and, unlike oral estrogens, do not induce hepatic synthesis of sex hormone–binding globulin, high levels of which are associated with reduced desire. In women who still have a uterus, the addition of a progestin is required to prevent the occurrence of endometrial hyperplasia. Use of systemic estrogen with or without progestin is limited by cardiovascular safety considerations,[141,142] and these therapies are not approved by the U.S. Food and Drug Administration (FDA) for sexual indications.

Low-dose vaginal estrogen decreases vaginal dryness and dyspareunia at least as well as systemic estrogen, and with fewer systemic adverse effects. Randomized, controlled trials comparing the effectiveness, safety, and acceptability of various vaginal estrogens in the general population have been reviewed extensively.[143] All forms of vaginal estrogen administration (cream, tablet, silicone ring) are effective, and overall adverse events are infrequent. Both tablets and ring relieve atrophy with minimal systemic absorption, such that the addition of progestin to prevent endometrial hyperplasia is generally not advocated; however, evidence for endometrial safety beyond 1 year of use is lacking, and some authors have suggested periodic progestin withdrawal in longer-term users. Scant literature has addressed the safety of low-dose vaginal estrogen in women with estrogen-sensitive tumors. In one small cohort study, 69 of 1472 breast cancer survivors (36% were estrogen receptor positive [ER+]; 48% were on tamoxifen) received low-dose vaginal estrogen (cream or tablets) for 1 year and were followed for 5.5 years.[144] No increase in breast cancer recurrence was observed among the estrogen users. In a second small study of ER+ breast cancer survivors (N = 7) taking aromatase inhibitors, serum estradiol (E2) levels were monitored during initiation of low-dose vaginal estrogen (tablets).[145] A short-term rise in serum E2 was observed, reversing the estrogen suppression achieved via aromatase inhibition. Therefore, until more definitive information is available, the decision regarding whether or not to use low-dose vaginal estrogen in women with estrogen-sensitive cancers must be individualized and requires careful consideration of recurrence risk and quality of life.

For women who experience vaginal dryness while taking an aromatase inhibitor, and who elect not to use low-dose vaginal estrogens, options include use of vaginal moisturizers and lubricants and/or switching to tamoxifen, which is associated with a lesser severity of atrophic symptoms.[146] Another option that deserves further study is pilocarpine. Systemic pilocarpine is useful for the treatment of xerostomia (a subjective feeling of dryness in the mouth) but is associated with a variety of undesirable side effects, including sweating, bronchoconstriction, transient hemodynamic changes, and visual changes.[147] Anecdotal use suggests that pilocarpine administration also reduces vaginal mucosal dryness; we look forward to learning the results of studies done to determine the potential benefits of topical genital application. We previously mentioned our clinical observation that intensive antiestrogen treatment seems to be associated with an unusually high incidence of vulvar lichen sclerosus. This entity is notable because it can cause severe vulvar pruritus, pain, and scarring, and is associated with an elevated risk of vulvar cancer.[148] Patients who present with typical findings should therefore undergo skin biopsy to confirm the diagnosis, and regular surveillance examinations are highly advisable. Lichen sclerosus is most aptly treated with application of a high-potency topical glucocorticoid steroid ointment, such as clobetasol. A combination of a topical estrogen plus a topical immunosuppressive agent such as a superpotent glucocorticoid, cyclosporine, or tacrolimus is generally effective in treating women who have chronic vulvovaginal GVHD[149]; in those with vaginal scarring, the use of graded vaginal dilators may also be helpful.

Two randomized controlled trials (N = 218, N = 102) showed that the addition of oral methyltestosterone to systemic estrogen increased sexual responsiveness and desire in postmenopausal women in the general population; however, decreased high-density lipoprotein was a consequence of combination oral treatment.[150,151] Four RCTs (combined N = 1619) subsequently demonstrated that the addition of a 300-μg transdermal testosterone patch to systemic estrogen therapy in surgically menopausal women with hypoactive sexual desire disorder (HSDD) resulted in an increase from one to two satisfying sexual episodes per month[152-155]; a subsequent study confirmed that this increase was clinically meaningful.[156] No adverse effects on lipids were observed; nonsignificant increases in acne, alopecia, facial hair, and voice deepening were reported. Administration of estrogen does not appear to be a necessary cofactor, as a fifth RCT (N = 814 postmenopausal women with HSDD) demonstrated an increase from 0.7 to 2.1 satisfying sexual episodes per month with use of the 300-μg testosterone patch alone.[157] In spite of these observed beneficial effects, the FDA has not yet approved the use of testosterone for women for sexual indications because of the short-term duration of all of these studies (24 weeks); clinicians electing to treat do so off-label and must use testosterone products formulated for men. It should be noted that only one study thus far has studied the impact of testosterone treatment on sexual function among postmenopausal cancer survivors specifically. In this phase III crossover trial, 150 breast cancer survivors with HSDD received 2% testosterone versus placebo cream for 4 weeks. Testosterone cream achieved higher serum levels of bioavailable testosterone, but no positive effect on libido was demonstrated.[158] In addition to concerns about effectiveness, questions remain about the safety of testosterone in women with estrogen-sensitive tumors, because testosterone is metabolized to estrogen in vivo. For all of the aforementioned reasons, it is probably best to avoid its use in this population unless patients are concurrently taking an aromatase inhibitor (which blocks conversion of testosterone to estrogen). If prescribing, patients should be carefully informed about potential risks and the limitations of available evidence.

MALE CANCER SURVIVORS

Hormonal therapy (i.e., testosterone replacement) should be considered in hypogonadal men with impaired sexual function. In men with serum testosterone levels below 300 ng/ml

with concurrent LH levels above normal range, testosterone replacement has been shown to improve male sexual function. Although testosterone levels below the lower limit of normal have been linked to adverse effects in men, the level of testosterone that corresponds to the ability to achieve erection has not been defined, and some data suggest that LH level may predict erection ability better than testosterone level.[159,160] Testosterone replacement therapy has been found to be effective in improving sexual function in hypogonadal men and should be considered in all hypogonadal male cancer survivors. A meta-analysis of 16 studies enrolling hypogonadal men without cancer revealed that significant improvement in erectile dysfunction occurred more often in those treated with testosterone than in those who received placebo (57.0% vs. 16.7%),[161] although this effect was more pronounced in men with primary versus secondary hypogonadism. Although some research suggests that testosterone replacement therapy may unmask occult prostate cancers,[162] no study to date has proven that testosterone replacement therapy causes prostate cancer. Emerging data suggest that testosterone therapy can be considered to treat sexual difficulties in selected populations of men with hypogonadism after completion of treatment for prostate cancer. For example, no evidence of cancer recurrence or progression was seen in one study of male prostate cancer survivors treated with brachytherapy who received testosterone to treat symptomatic hypogonadism.[163] Limitations of the data and careful consideration of potential pros and cons should always be reviewed with patients before beginning testosterone supplementation; in addition, monitoring after initiation of therapy is critical to reduce potential adverse effects and to maximize success (Table 57-7).

Men who receive testosterone replacement therapy should be seen and reevaluated 1 to 3 months after initiation of therapy, and then at least annually thereafter. Assessment should begin with a careful history to assess for improvement in symptoms, impact on erectile function, and adverse effects. Testosterone and LH levels should be repeated (at a time appropriate to the type of replacement administered; please see Table 57-7). Testosterone levels should increase to the normal range of 500 to 600 ng/dl after 3 months of therapy, and LH levels should decrease to within normal range. Dosing of testosterone replacement should be adjusted to achieve mid-normal range levels with improvement of symptoms.[164] It is important to note that sexual function may not improve to ideal levels with replacement of testosterone. Additional therapies should be used to complement the effects of testosterone replacement.

Testosterone therapy should begin with use of the lowest effective dose and a delivery mechanism that is conducive to each man's life and situation. Transdermal preparations have been shown to produce the most consistent serum levels, offering steady control of hypogonadal symptoms.[164] Gel preparations, administered daily, are considered the easiest for transdermal use, but they are also the most expensive and contain a box warning for risk of secondary exposure to children. Adverse effects of testosterone therapy include gynecomastia, sleep apnea, development or exacerbation of lower urinary tract symptoms due to benign prostatic hyperplasia, prostate cancer, reduced levels of high-density lipoprotein cholesterol, erythrocytosis, elevations in liver function levels, and impaired fertility.[166] Along with ongoing monitoring of testosterone levels, men on testosterone replacement should

Table 57-7 Options for testosterone replacement in hypogonadal men

Drug	Delivery	Dose	Adverse effects	Monitoring	Cost (drugstore.com)
Testosterone esters (testosterone enanthate and testosterone cypionate)	IM injection (oil)	1. 100 mg weekly 2. 200 mg q2wk 3. 300 mg q3wk	Self- administration Serum levels can fluctuate (increasingly so with increased dose interval), leading to symptom recurrence	Check level midway between injections	100 mg/ml (10 ml vial): $57.99 200 mg/ml (10 ml vial): $88.99
Androderm	Patch (applied to arm or torso) each evening	2.5 or 5 mg per 24 hours	Severe skin rash leading to discontinuation	Check level the following morning after patch application	2.5 mg/24 hr (60 patches): $277.53 5 mg/24 hr (30 patches) $278.56
AndroGel	Gel	2.5 g (25 mg testosterone) and 5.0 g (50 mg testosterone) packets of gel applied daily; metered-dose pump 1.25 g per pump	Minor skin irritation	Check level no sooner than 14 days after starting therapy	25 mg/2.5 g (30 packets): $261.01 50 mg/5 g (30 packets): $274.58 Pump: 1% (150 g total): $290.63
Testim	Gel	5 g tube (50 mg testestosterone) and 10 g (100 mg testosterone)	Reports of odor	No sooner than 14 days of therapy	1% (5 g tube) $302.37
Striant	Buccal tablet	30 mg tablet (applied above the gum line above upper incisors) twice a day		Check level >4 weeks after start of therapy, before AM dose	30 mg (60 tablets): $259.37

receive digital rectal examination and monitoring of complete blood count and PSA.[167]

Nonhormonal therapies

PHOSPHODIESTERASE INHIBITORS (PDEIS)

Male Cancer Survivors

Phosphodiesterase inhibitors (PDEIs) have been shown to improve sexual function in men after treatment of cancer and are often considered first-line therapies. Although the efficacy of PDEIs has been demonstrated most often in prostate cancer survivors, encouraging data suggest that it should be considered for use in any male cancer survivor with erectile dysfunction. Studies have shown that men are often reluctant to present with complaints of impaired sexual function, and that many men who try PDEIs after cancer treatments do not experience improvement or adhere to therapy.[168] Therefore, it is important to identify the ideal preparation for each individual, to time treatment appropriately (e.g., initiate earlier rather than later), and to ensure close follow-up to optimize sexual function after treatment.

Numerous studies have demonstrated the utility of PDEIs in male prostate cancer survivors.[169] Among 11 RCTs examined in a recent Cochrane review, which evaluated a broad spectrum of treatments, the strongest evidence for effective therapy was seen in four studies of oral PDEIs, given after radical prostatectomy or radiation therapy. Combined results from two of the trials showed a significant improvement in erectile function in the therapy groups (odds ratio [OR], 10.09; 95% confidence interval [CI], 6.20%–16.43%). Adverse effects were rare and included symptoms of head-

ache and flushing. Additional studies have examined specific predictors of success; factors that have been shown to decrease the effectiveness of PDEI therapy include poor level of sexual function before cancer treatment,[170] older age, duration of time after cancer therapy before onset of PDEI use, androgen deprivation therapy for longer than 4 months, and radiation dose >85 Gy.[171]

Research demonstrates that simple maintenance of regular sexual activity tends to protect men from developing erectile dysfunction. For example, in one prospective 5-year study of 989 men aged 55 to 79 in the general population who had no impairment in sexual function at baseline (as defined by the IIEF inventory survey), those who reported sexual intercourse less than once per week were twice as likely to develop erectile dysfunction than those who reported sexual intercourse one time or more per week (incidence rate ratio, 2.2; 95% CI, 1.3%–3.8%).[172] Frequent sexual activity is believed to exert its protective effect via maintenance of vascular endothelial function. Accordingly, recent trials have examined prophylactic therapies to maintain erectile function in men after treatment for cancer—a strategy termed "penile rehabilitation." Results from one randomized, double-blind trial (subgroup analysis, N = 54) that examined the effects of nightly sildenafil after bilateral nerve-sparing radical retropubic prostatectomy (BNSRRP) on sexual function are illustrative. Although the placebo group experienced little to no improvement, the men who received prophylactic sildenafil nightly for 36 weeks after surgery demonstrated gradual dose-dependent improvement in erectile function. Up to one third of men receiving sildenafil demonstrated a return of nocturnal erections and erectile function (24% [4/17] of 50-mg sildenafil recipients,

33% [6/18] of 100-mg sildenafil recipients, and 5% [1/19] placebo recipients).[173] Additional randomized, controlled studies of daily prophylactic sildenafil therapy are needed before it can be considered safe and effective for daily use in men undergoing other surgical or radiation therapies for prostate cancer.

Initiation of PDEIs in men with erectile dysfunction after cancer treatment should begin as soon as possible to have the most potent effect. In a study of 110 men found to have impaired sexual function (as measured by the IIEF scale) after radiation therapy for prostate cancer, men who started sildenafil therapy less than 1 year after completing therapy were 60% likely to have normalization sexual function scores, and men who started sildenafil more than 2 to 3 years after completion of radiation were only 26% likely to achieve normal scores.[174] This potential loss of efficacy underscores the importance of talking about sexual function early on and offering effective options for treatment before it is too late to see physiologic improvement.

We recommend following the same dosage guidelines for PDEIs in male noncancer survivors: Start with 50 mg sildenafil, 10 mg of vardenafil, or 10 mg of tadalafil, taken at least 30 minutes before desired activity. Both sildenafil and vardenafil have a mean duration of 4 hours, and tadalafil has a duration up to 36 hours[175]; all are considered equally effective in improving erectile function. Each should be used with caution or avoided in people using CYP3A4 inhibitors, which would prolong their duration of action. PDEIs are contraindicated in men with recent myocardial infarction/stroke, active coronary ischemia/congestive heart failure (CHF), hypotension, or taking nitrates. Men should be questioned about their exercise tolerance before starting therapy. An exercise tolerance level sufficient for sexual activity and orgasm is approximately 4 METS (metabolic equivalent of oxygen consumption)—the equivalent of walking up one flight of stairs, or walking 2 to 4 miles on a level surface without difficulty.[176]

Female Cancer Survivors

PDEIs increase genital perfusion in women in a similar fashion; however, these agents have not been found to be as sexually beneficial as they are in men. One large, multicenter, placebo-controlled trial examined the efficacy of sildenafil, 10 to 100 mg, taken 1 hour before sexual activity in 577 estrogen-replete and 204 estrogen-deficient women with female sexual arousal disorder (FSAD).[177] No increase in sexual arousal was observed in either treatment group at any treatment dose. This study has been criticized because less than half of the women studied had a primary diagnosis of FSAD; many also suffered from diminished sexual desire, which we would not expect to be improved by a medicine that causes vasodilation. Limited data suggest that PDEIs may be useful in treating women in the general population who have isolated FSAD. For example, in a subgroup analysis of women without concomitant HSDD during a randomized controlled trial of sildenafil 50 mg versus placebo in postmenopausal women with FSAD, significant improvements were seen in vaginal lubrication, genital sensation, and ability to achieve orgasm.[178] On the basis of this preliminary information, we believe that PDEIs (off-label use) are worth a try in female cancer survivors in whom genital arousal difficulty predominates, as is sometimes the case among women who have undergone radical pelvic surgery with interruption of genital vascular and nerve supply. As noted later, PDEIs may also be beneficial as antidotes to the sexual side effects of certain antidepressants. To our knowledge, no studies as yet have specifically examined the effects of PDEIs on genital arousal in female cancer survivors. If electing to prescribe PDEIs in this population, we recommend a starting dose of 50 mg sildenafil, or the equivalent, taken 1 hour before sexual activity. As in men, PDEIs are contraindicated in women with recent myocardial infarction/stroke, active coronary ischemia/CHF, or taking nitrates.

PROSTAGLANDIN E1 AGONISTS

In men with insufficient erectile function after use of PDEIs and testosterone (when warranted), alprostadil offers a more effective option for both penile rehabilitation after cancer therapies and maintenance of erectile function throughout survivorship. Alprostadil is a prostaglandin E1 analog that causes vasodilation and smooth muscle relaxation, allowing blood flow and entrapment into the penis for erection to occur. It is administered as an intraurethral pellet suppository (Muse), or as an injection to the dorsolateral aspect of the proximal one third of the penile shaft. Multiple studies have examined the use of intraurethral or intracavernous injection of alprostadil after radical prostatectomy, and significant benefit was found.[179–181] Overall, men who began to use alprostadil within 1 month of their surgery and continued use 3 times per week over a 6-month period were significantly more likely to achieve spontaneous erections at the completion of treatment. All of these studies were limited by no clear preoperative assessment of erectile function, short-term follow-up, and the fact that up to one third of the sample dropped out as the result of penile irritation or lack of initial success. Ongoing studies are needed, but current recommendations include considering alprostadil administration as second-line posttreatment therapy for men who fail to respond adequately to first-line treatment (PDEIs and testosterone in eligible candidates).[182] When alprostadil suppositories are prescribed, the first dose must be given under clinical supervision to monitor for hypotension and severe side effects.

Intracavernous injection therapy is considered the most effective nonsurgical treatment for erectile dysfunction. Injections can be prepared with alprostadil alone, or in combination with papaverine, an arterial vasodilator, and/or phentolamine, an alpha-1-receptor blocker. Although they are sometimes considered more effective, mixtures of these substances require the use of compounding pharmacies. Dosing and mixture should be based on individual effectiveness and side effects for each patient. Limitations include high risk of priapism, invasive approach and technique for the patient to learn, and the requirement that the first dose be administered under clinical supervision. It is also recommended that each patient be given a clear warning to monitor for an erection lasting longer than 4 hours, and a clear plan for how that will be managed with the clinician.[183] To optimize the risks and benefits of therapy, we recommend that intracavernous injection therapies be prescribed in collaboration with a urology specialist.

We are unaware of any studies that have examined the effectiveness of topical alprostadil in improving genital arousal in female cancer survivors specifically. However, in the general population, one RCT (N = 400 women aged 22–62) has shown significant improvement in several arousal parameters after application of a 900-μg alprostadil cream to the clitoris and anterior vaginal wall before intercourse[184]; a previous study showed that the most common adverse effect was a mild, transient genital burning sensation lasting <1 minute.[185] On the basis of these results, we believe that this agent deserves additional, targeted study.

Other nonhormonal pharmacotherapies for erectile dysfunction

Studies continue to examine the potential benefits of other nonhormonal pharmacotherapies for men with erectile dysfunction, but none have yet shown benefit. Use of trazodone, yohimbine, herbal therapies, and topical vasodilators is strongly discouraged at this time because of lack of proven benefit and high risk of adverse effects.[186]

Bupropion and other strategies to minimize antidepressant-induced dysfunction

Sexual dysfunction is extremely common among patients taking antidepressant and/or certain antianxiety medications[187]; this is important for clinicians to realize, because many survivors benefit from using these medications to aid psychosocial adjustment. The SSRIs (citalopram, fluoxetine, paroxetine, and sertraline) do not differ substantially from one another in the prevalence of sexual dysfunction, suggesting a class effect of serotonin reuptake inhibitory medications. Gender differences in sexual side effects have been noted, with men more likely to complain of desire and orgasmic dysfunction, and women more likely to report arousal phase problems. One might expect the serotonin norepinephrine reuptake inhibitors (SNRIs) to have fewer sexual side effects than the SSRIs because of the central excitatory effect of norepinephrine; however, this appears to be the case only for duloxetine and not for venlafaxine. Compared with other antidepressants, bupropion (a norepinephrine and dopamine reuptake inhibitor) and nefazodone (a $5-HT_2$ antagonist used infrequently because of the risk of hepatotoxicity) have the lowest rates of sexual dysfunction. Based on its mechanism of action (antagonist at alpha-2, $5-HT_{2A}$ and $5-HT_3$ receptors), mirtazapine might be expected to spare sexual function as well. Finally, transdermal application of the monoamine oxidase inhibitor (MAOI) selegiline does not seem to be associated with greater sexual dysfunction than placebo. With respect to treatment of anxiety, buspirone (a $5-HT_{1A}$ partial agonist) tends to improve rather than cause sexual problems in patients with generalized anxiety disorder.[188] Few data address the effects of benzodiazepines, although anecdotal experience suggests potential utility in managing sexual difficulties related to performance anxiety. Although choosing the medication that is most likely to be effective in treating a patient's depression or anxiety generally trumps concerns about potential sexual side effects, the differential impact of various antidepressant and antianxiety medications on sexual function should be kept in mind when making a selection and should always be discussed with the recipient.

Several strategies have been described to treat sexual dysfunction associated with psychotropic medications; most have not been rigorously studied in randomized, placebo-controlled trials. Proposed methods include waiting for tolerance to develop (low success rate), lowering the dose of the culprit medication (associated with the possibility of relapse), taking a drug holiday (relapse also a concern), substituting a medication with a lower likelihood of sexual side effects (associated with fear of therapeutic failure), and adding another medication as an antidote (associated with risk of drug interactions and additional side effects, as well as increased cost).[189] Antidotes with a reasonable success rate include bupropion,[190] sildenafil,[191,192] and buspirone (a $5-HT_{1A}$ partial agonist approved for the treatment of generalized anxiety disorder).[193] Although not yet demonstrated in controlled trials, the addition of mirtazapine may be helpful.[194] According to a review conducted by Taylor, best evidence supports the use of PDEIs for antidepressant-induced erectile dysfunction and bupropion for antidepressant-associated low libido.[195]

The optimal dose of bupropion and the breadth of its effects have not yet been definitively delineated. In two small RCTs (N = 31, N = 41) that studied the effects of bupropion SR 150 mg per day as an antidote to sexual side effects in euthymic patients taking SSRIs, no change in sexual function was observed after 3 and 6 weeks, respectively.[196,197] In a third trial (N = 42) in which a higher dose of bupropion SR (300 mg/day) was used, sexual *desire* and *frequency* of sexual activity increased in treated patients at 4 weeks.[198] Bupropion SR 300 mg per day has also been studied as a general sexual stimulant in a nondepressed population of premenopausal women (N = 75); in the active treatment group, significant increases were seen in sexual *arousal, orgasm* completion, and sexual *satisfaction* but not desire at 112 days.[199] We are not aware of any randomized trials that have studied the use of bupropion in cancer survivors. However, results from one small (N = 20 breast cancer survivors), open-label study in which subjects were treated with bupropion 150 mg per day show that ASEX scores (an assessment tool that evaluates *libido, excitability,* and ability to reach *orgasm*) were significantly better at 4 weeks.[200] If no contraindications to its use (e.g., a history of seizures) are known, we therefore consider a trial of bupropion in a dose of at least 150 mg per day for male and female cancer survivors with diminished desire, and for female cancer survivors with sexual difficulties in the arousal or orgasm domain.

Investigational medications that show additional promise

Two additional compounds with novel mechanisms of action may eventually prove useful in treating male and female cancer survivors who have sexual difficulties. The first of these, bremelanotide, is a synthetic melanocortin analog of melanocyte-stimulating hormone (an agonist at melanocortin receptors MC3R and MC4R) that is administered intranasally. Preliminary studies demonstrate improvements in erection response in men with mild to moderate erectile dysfunction[201] and in men with erectile dysfunction unresponsive to sildenafil,[202] as well as improvement in both arousal and subjective excitement in premenopausal women with FSAD.[203] The second compound, flibanserin, initially developed as an antidepressant, is a postsynaptic $5-HT_{1A}$ agonist, a very weak partial D4 agonist, and a $5-HT_{2A}$ antagonist. In preliminary studies in premenopausal women with HSDD, 24 weeks' treatment with flibanserin 100 mg at every bedtime was associated with significant improvement in various measures of sexual desire and an increase from 1.0 to 1.7 satisfying sexual episodes per month.[204] We await with great interest results from additional studies of these two agents.

MECHANICAL DEVICES

Use of mechanical devices (e.g., vibrators) may be helpful for women and men who have experienced vascular or neurologic injury to genital structures and therefore require more intense stimulation for longer periods of time to achieve arousal.[205] The prevalence of vibrator use during solo or partnered sexual activity was 52.5% and 44.8% in nationally representative, Internet-based surveys of 3800 women and 1047 men aged 18 to 60, respectively.[206,207] Recent vibrator users demonstrated higher scores in a wide variety of sexual function domains; adverse effects associated with vibrator use were infrequent. Vibrators are now available in a wide variety of shapes and sizes and can be bought discreetly from online sex boutiques. Other mechanical devices may be useful in selected circumstances. For example, a clitoral vacuum pump—the Eros clitoral therapy device (Eros Therapy, San Francisco, CA)—significantly improved genital sensation, vaginal lubrication, ability to orgasm, and overall sexual satisfaction in a small (N = 19) sample of women in the general population with and without arousal difficulties.[208] Use of this device to increase clitoral blood flow during 15 to 30 minutes of intermittent vacuum therapy, 4 times per week for 3 months, was also found to significantly increase desire, arousal, lubrication, orgasm, and satisfaction, and to reduce pain in a similarly small (N = 15) group of irradiated cervical cancer patients with sexual dysfunction 2 years post treatment.[209]

In men seeking mechanical therapies to augment erectile function, vacuum constriction devices are considered effective and are widely available at low cost through online drugstores and websites, with no prescription required. However, they often require much patience and dexterity, and therefore tend to have lower patient acceptability compared with other interventions. The vacuum pressure encourages arterial influx of blood into the shaft of the penis, with an occlusive ring applied at the base to prevent egress of venous blood until after intercourse is completed. Research on the effectiveness of the vacuum erection device (VED) after radical prostatectomy shows preservation of penile length and sexual function. A small trial by Köhler et al. (N = 28) examined the use of a VED daily for 10 minutes without a constricting ring, over 5 months of follow-up. Subjects were divided into two groups, one starting therapy at 1 month and the other at 6 months after nerve-sparing radical retropubic prostatectomy. IIEF scores were measured at baseline, 3 months, and 6 months; scores were significantly higher in the early treatment group than in the group starting 6 months postoperatively at 3 months (11.5 [9.4] vs. 1.8 [1.4], P = .008) and at 6 months (12.4 [8.7] vs. 3.0 [1.9], P = .012).[210] Vacuum constriction devices are generally considered safe for use, with monitoring to enhance penile rehabilitation strategies after radical prostatectomy.[211] It is strongly recommended that patients seeking to purchase vacuum devices be warned to use only those with a vacuum limiter to prevent excessively high negative pressures from harming penile tissue.[212]

VAGINAL DILATORS AND PELVIC FLOOR PHYSICAL THERAPY

Additional interventions may be useful for female cancer survivors who, as a result of radical pelvic surgery and/or irradiation, experience vaginal stenosis and/or other pelvic floor problems. According to a 2003 Cochrane review, the strongest evidence for benefit consists of grade IC data on the use of topical estrogen and benzydamine in the prevention and treatment of acute radiation-induced vaginal changes.[213] The use of vaginal dilators to prevent the development of vaginal stenosis is supported by grade IIC evidence. However, little consensus has been reached on when to begin dilatation, how often it should be performed, and for how long.[214] The value of hyperbaric oxygen therapy and surgical reconstruction is supported by much weaker grade IIIC evidence in the form of case reports.[215] Studies are urgently needed to investigate this topic further, and discussion of various options that may prevent and/or ameliorate the complications of pelvic irradiation must become much more consistent and routine.

Urinary and fecal incontinence must also be addressed, if present, because either of these can have a profoundly negative impact on the sexual function of affected women and men and their partners. The potential role of pelvic floor physical therapy in restoring continence in postoperative cancer survivors has not yet been fully evaluated. A systematic literature review concluded that pelvic floor muscle training hastens the return of continence in male prostate cancer survivors who experience urinary incontinence after radical prostatectomy[216]; it may therefore be of value in this circumstance. We are not aware of any studies that have addressed the effectiveness of similar interventions in female cancer survivors who develop urinary incontinence after pelvic surgery. Evidence to support the utility of anal sphincter exercises to reduce the severity of fecal incontinence in noncancer patients is mixed. One small, nonrandomized trial demonstrated equivalent improvements in the modified Cleveland Incontinence Score among both irradiated and nonirradiated postoperative colon cancer survivors who received anal sphincter muscle training[217]; this modality may therefore be worth a try in affected patients, as it does not appear to be associated with any significant morbidities. The impact of pelvic floor physical therapy is only just beginning to be studied in noncancer patients with sexual dysfunction related to chronic pelvic pain[218]; we hope that studies that examine the effectiveness of this modality in populations of cancer survivors with chronic pelvic pain will soon be forthcoming.

GENITAL SURGERIES TO IMPROVE SEXUAL FUNCTION

Surgical therapies to improve male erectile function include vascular surgeries to improve arterial and venous blood flow and penile prosthesis implantation. Vascular surgeries, such as arterial reconstructive surgery with anastomosis of the inferior epigastric artery to the dorsal penile artery or vein, are currently recommended in selected patients only. Men who benefit from vascular surgery have recent onset of erectile dysfunction with evidence of focal arterial occlusive disease. The procedure has not been shown to be helpful in men with diffuse vascular disease or cavernous myopathy from chronic ischemia[219]; therefore, it is unlikely that cancer survivors would benefit. No study to date has proven that vascular surgery in male cancer survivors improves erectile function significantly; however, studies are ongoing, and future research or new techniques may prove beneficial.

Penile prosthesis implantation provides male cancer survivors with a surgical alternative to improve erectile function.

Prosthesis implantation offers men two options: (1) malleable, noninflatable, semirigid rod-type prostheses, associated with lower cost, better mechanical reliability, and ease of use, or (2) inflatable prostheses, associated with flaccidity and erections considered closer to normal for men, but also with the risk of pump displacement and autoinflation.[220] Implantation of any device carries the risk of infection, erosion, penile shortening, and mechanical failure (estimated as 6%–16% at 5 years), as well as the need for repeat operations and reduced effectiveness for any subsequent therapy attempt in the future.[221] Men who undergo penile prosthesis placement in conjunction with radical prostatectomy (RP) have been shown to have higher quality-of-life (QOL) and sexual health scores than men who undergo radical prostatectomy without prosthesis implantation. Ramsawh et al. mailed questionnaires to men who had undergone both RP and penile prosthesis placement (n = 51) and compared their results against those of a group of men who underwent RP without prosthesis placement (n = 47). Men who chose simultaneous placement of a penile prosthesis with RP reported greater overall QOL and erectile function and more frequent sexual contact than men who underwent RP alone. The benefit seemed to be greatest for men who were not candidates for a nerve-sparing RP.[222] Given the limited efficacy of other treatments for erectile dysfunction after prosthesis implantation, we recommend this procedure in selected candidates who may not be eligible for other first- and second-line therapies for erectile dysfunction.

Researchers are just beginning to recognize the need for studies that examine the impact of various genital reconstructive procedures on postoperative sexual function in female cancer survivors. Reconstructive surgery at the time of radical pelvic surgery can facilitate wound healing, minimize acute and chronic morbidity, and restore anatomic form and function. A wide range of reconstruction techniques can be implemented to address the various vulvar, vaginal, and pelvic floor defects that commonly occur, including but not limited to skin grafting, simple tissue transposition flaps, fasciocutaneous flaps, and myocutaneous flaps. Optimal cosmetic and anatomic outcomes are achieved when the reconstruction is planned and effected at the time of the primary surgical procedure.[223] It is not surprising to note that attempted reconstruction in previously irradiated tissue is particularly challenging. To date, few studies have assessed the impact of vulvar and vaginal reconstruction on functional outcomes (e.g., libido, arousal, orgasm, overall sexual satisfaction). These endpoints are critical to address because mere restoration of a vaginal vault that permits a woman to engage in vaginal intercourse may not be associated with enhanced subjective enjoyment in the absence of sensate tissue. One small prospective study demonstrated higher female sexual function index (FSFI) scores in a subgroup of sexually active cancer survivors after sigmoid loop vaginal reconstruction. However, these scores were lower than those achieved in noncancer patients after equivalent vaginoplasty, and 85% of the women developed subsequent vaginal stenosis requiring operative recanalization.[224] Additional prospective, randomized studies are clearly needed to examine functional outcomes.

WHEN AND TO WHOM TO REFER

In summary, this chapter provides a practical guide to the assessment and management of patients (and their partners) who present with intimacy and/or sexuality problems after cancer. We believe that most of what we have outlined falls within the purview of the general medical oncologist or primary care provider; however, we also recognize that lack of familiarity with these topics and competing demands on a provider's time may make it difficult, if not impossible, to substantively address these issues. At a minimum, we therefore urge all clinicians who come into contact with cancer survivors to raise the importance of these issues, ascertain the need for support and/or evaluation, and provide resources and referrals (please see Table 57-7) to individuals/couples who wish to pursue targeted intervention.

REFERENCES

1. Hordern A, Street A. Issues of intimacy and sexuality in the face of cancer: the patient perspective. *Cancer Nurs.* 2007;30:E11–E18.
2. Huber C, Ramnarace T, McCaffrey R. Sexuality and intimacy issues facing women with breast cancer. *Oncol Nurs Forum.* 2006;33:1163–1167.
3. Tesauro GM, Rowland JH, Lustig C. Survivorship resources for post-treatment cancer survivors. *Cancer Pract.* 2002;10:277–283.
4. Hordern A. Intimacy and sexuality after cancer: a critical review of the literature. *Cancer Nurs.* 2008;31:E9–E17.
5. Hordern AJ, Street AF. Communicating about patient sexuality and intimacy after cancer: mismatched expectations and unmet needs. *Med J Aust.* 2007;186:224–227.
6. Potter J. *Female sexuality: assessing satisfaction and addressing problems.* Posted on ACP medicine, 2010
7. Mulcahy JJ, ed. *Male sexual function: a guide to clinical management.* Totowa, NJ: Humana Press Inc; 2006.
8. Pfaus JG. Pathways of sexual desire. *J Sex Med.* 2009;6:1506–1533.
9. Avis NE, Zhao X, Johannes CB. Correlates of sexual function among multi-ethnic, middle-aged women: results from the Study of Women's health Across the Nation (SWAN). *Menopause.* 2005;12:385–397.
10. Sand MS, Fisher W, Rosen R, et al. Erectile dysfunction and constructs of masculinity and quality of life in the multinational Men's Attitudes to Life Events and Sexuality (MALES) study. *J Sex Med.* 2008;5:583–594.
11. Tolman DL, Diamond LM. Desegregating sexuality research: cultural and biological perspectives on gender and desire. *Annu Rev Sex Res.* 2001;12:33–74.
12. Pfaus JG. Pathways of sexual desire. *J Sex Med.* 2009;6:1506–1533.
13. Meston CM, Buss DM. Why humans have sex. *Arch Sex Behav.* 2007;36:477–507.
14. Clayton AH. Sexual function and dysfunction in women. *Psychiatr Clin North Am.* 2003;26:673–682.
15. Basson R, Leiblum S, Brotto L, et al. Definitions of women's sexual dysfunction reconsidered: advocating expansion and revision. *J Psychosom Obstet Gynecol.* 2003;24:221–229.
16. Rees PM, Fowler CJ, Mass CP. Sexual function in men and women with neurological disorders. *Lancet.* 2007;369:512–525.
17. Alexander M, Rosen RC. Spinal cord injuries and orgasm: a review. *J Sex Marital Ther.* 2008;34:308–324.
18. Graziottin A. The challenge of sexual medicine for women: overcoming cultural and educational limits and gender biases. *J Endocrinol Invest.* 2003;26(suppl 3):139–142.
19. McKenna KE. The neurophysiology of female sexual function. *World J Urol.* 2002;20:93–100.
20. Hatzimouratidis K, Hatzichristou D. Sexual dysfunctions: classifications and definitions. *J Sex Med.* 2007;4:241–250.
21. Stewart EG. Treatment options for vulvar vestibulitis. *Contemp Obstet Gynecol.* 2003;48:47–61.
22. Davis SN, Binik YM, Carrier S. Sexual dysfunction and pelvic pain in men: a male sexual pain disorder? *J Sex Marital Ther.* 2009;35:182–205.
23. Aubin S, Berger RE, Heiman JR, et al. The association between sexual function, pain, and psychological adaptation of men diagnosed with chronic pelvic pain syndrome type III. *J Sex Med.* 2008;5:657–667.
24. Lee SW, Liong ML, Yuen KH, et al. Adverse impact of sexual dysfunction in chronic prostatitis/chronic pelvic pain syndrome. *Urology.* 2008;71:79–84.

25. Basson R, Schultz WW. Sexual sequelae of general medical disorders. *Lancet*. 2007;369:409–424.

26. Ganz P, Desmond KA, Belin TR, et al. Predictors of sexual health in women after a breast cancer diagnosis. *J Cin Oncol*. 1999;17:2371–2380.

27. Pieterse QD, Maas CP, ter Kuile MM, et al. An observational longitudinal study to evaluation micturition, defecation, and sexual function after radical hysterectomy with pelvic lymphadenectomy for early-stage cervical cancer. *Int J Gynecol Cancer*. 2006;16:1119–1129.

28. Ratliff CR, Gershenson DM, Morris M, et al. Sexual adjustment of patients undergoing gracilis myocutaneous flap vaginal reconstruction in conjunction with pelvic exenteration. *Cancer*. 1996;78:2229–2235.

29. Bullen K, Edwards S, Marke V, et al. Looking past the obvious: experiences of altered masculinity in penile cancer. *Psychooncology*. 2010;19:933–940.

30. Wittman D, Northouse L, Foley S, et al. The psychosocial aspects of sexual recovery after prostate cancer treatment. *Int J Impot Res*. 2009;21:99–106.

31. Lange MM, Marijnen CA, Maas CP, et al. Cooperative clinical investigators of the Dutch: risk factors for sexual dysfunction after rectal cancer treatment. *Eur J Cancer*. 2009;45:1578–1588.

32. Wittmann D, Northouse L, Foley S, et al. The psychosocial aspects of sexual recovery after prostate cancer treatment. *Int J Impot Res*. 2009;21:99–106.

33. Matthew AG, Goldman A, Trachtenberg J, et al. Sexual dysfunction after radical prostatectomy: prevalence, treatments, restricted use of treatments and distress. *J Urol*. 2005;174:2105–2110.

34. Montazeri A. Health-related quality of life in breast cancer patients: a bibliographic review of the literature from 1974 to 2007. *J Exp Clin Cancer Res*. 2008;27:32.

35. Potter S, Thomson HJ, Greenwood RJ, et al. Health-related quality of life assessment after breast reconstruction. *Br J Surg*. 2009;96:613–620.

36. Zippe C, Nandipati K, Agarwal A, et al. Sexual function after pelvic surgery. *Int J Impot Res*. 2006;18:1–18.

37. Rodriguez E, Melamud O, Ahlering TE. Nerve-sparing techniques in open and laparoscopic prostatectomy. *Expert Rev Anticancer Ther*. 2008;8:475–479.

38. Anastasiadis AG, Benson MC, Rosenwasser MP, et al. Cavernous nerve graft reconstruction during radical prostatectomy or radical cystectomy: safe and technically feasible. *Prostate Cancer Prostatic Dis*. 2003;6:56–60.

39. Bergmark K, Avall-Lundquist E, Dickman PW, et al. Vaginal changes and sexuality in women with a history of cervical cancer. *N Engl J Med*. 1999;340:1383–1389.

40. Bruner DW, Lanciano R, Keegan M, et al. Vaginal stenosis and sexual function following intracavitary radiation for the treatment of cervical and endometrial carcinoma. *Int J Radiat Oncol*. 1993;27:825–830.

41. Mendenhall WM, Henderson RH, Indelicato DJ, et al. Erectile dysfunction after radiotherapy for prostate cancer. *Am J Clin Oncol*. 2009;32:443–447.

42. Siglin J, Kubicek GJ, Leiby B, et al. Time of decline in sexual function after external beam radiotherapy for prostate cancer. *Int J Radiat Oncol Biol Phys*. 2010;76:31–35.

43. Minisini AM, Menis J, Valent F, et al. Determinants of recovery from amenorrhea in premenopausal breast cancer patients receiving adjuvant chemotherapy in the taxane era. *Anticancer Drugs*. 2009;20:503–507.

44. Lee S, Kil WJ, Chun M, et al. Chemotherapy-related amenorrhea in premenopausal women with breast cancer. *Menopause*. 2009;16:98–103.

45. Behringer K, Breuer K, Reineke T, et al. Secondary amenorrhea after Hodgkin's lymphoma is influenced by age at treatment, stage of disease, chemotherapy regimen, and the use of oral contraceptives during therapy: a report from the German Hodgkin's Lymphoma Study Group. *J Clin Oncol*. 2005;23:7555–7564.

46. Siris ES, Leventhal BG, Vaitukaitis JL. Effects of childhood leukemia and chemotherapy on puberty and reproductive function in girls. *N Engl J Med*. 1976;294:1143–1146.

47. DiCosimo S, Alimonti A, Ferretti G, et al. Incidence of chemotherapy-induced amenorrhea depending on the timing of treatment by menstrual cycle phase in women with early breast cancer. *Ann Oncol*. 2004;15:1065–1071.

48. Behringer K, Breuer K, Reineke T, et al. Secondary amenorrhea after Hodgkin's lymphoma is influenced by age at treatment, stage of disease, chemotherapy regimen, and the use of oral contraceptives during therapy: a report from the German Hodgkin's Lymphoma Study Group. *J Clin Oncol*. 2005;23:7555–7564.

49. Badawy A, Elnashar A, El-Ashry M, et al. Gonadotropin-releasing hormone agonists for prevention of chemotherapy-induced ovarian damage: prospective randomized study. *Fertil Steril*. 2009;91:694–697.

50. Schwarz EB, Hess R, Trussell J. Contraception for cancer survivors. *J Gen Intern Med*. 2009;24(suppl 2):S401–S406.

51. Kulkarni SS, Sastry PS, Saikia TK, et al. Gonadal function following ABVD therapy for Hodgkin's disease. *Am J Clin Oncol*. 1997;20:354–357.

52. Kenney LB, Laufer MR, Grant FD, et al. High risk of infertility and long term gonadal damage in males treated with high dose cyclophosphamide for sarcoma during childhood. *Cancer*. 2001;91:613–621.

53. Kwan KW, Chlembowski RT. Sexual dysfunction and aromatase inhibitor use in survivors of breast cancer. *Clin Breast Cancer*. 2009;9:219–224.

54. Taylor AH, Guzail M, Al-Azzawi F. Differential expression of oestrogen receptor isoforms and androgen receptor in the normal vulva and vagina compared with vulval lichen sclerosus and chronic vaginitis. *Br J Dermatol*. 2008;158:319–328.

55. Loblaw DA, Mendelson DS, Talcott JA, et al. American Society of Clinical Oncology recommendations for the initial hormonal management of androgen-sensitive metastatic, recurrent, or progressive prostate cancer. *J Clin Oncol*. 2004;22:2927–2941.

56. Smith DP, King MT, Egger S, et al. Quality of life three years after diagnosis of localised prostate cancer: population based cohort study. *BMJ*. 2009;339:b4817.

57. Sanda MG, Dunn RL, Michalski J, et al. Quality of life and satisfaction with outcome among prostate-cancer survivors. *N Engl J Med*. 2008;358:1250–1261.

58. Wilke DR, Parker C, Andonowski A, et al. Testosterone and erectile function recovery after radiotherapy and long-term androgen deprivation with luteinizing hormone-releasing hormone agonists. *BJU Int*. 2006;97:963–968.

59. Smith MR, Goode M, Zietman AL, et al. Bicalutamide monotherapy versus leuprolide monotherapy for prostate cancer: effects on bone mineral density and body composition. *J Clin Oncol*. 2004;22:2546–2553.

60. de Leval J, Boca P, Yousef E, et al. Intermittent versus continuous total androgen blockade in the treatment of patients with advanced hormone-naive prostate cancer: results of a prospective randomized multicenter trial. *Clin Prostate Cancer*. 2002;1:163–171.

61. Oh WK. The evolving role of estrogen therapy in prostate cancer. *Clin Prostate Cancer*. 2002;1:81–89.

62. Stratton P, Turner ML, Childs R, et al. Vulvovaginal chronic graft-versus-host disease with allogeneic hematopoietic stem cell transplantation. *Obstet Gynecol*. 2007;110:1041–1049.

63. Smith Knutsson E, Broman AK, Bjork Y, et al. *Sexual life in women after bone marrow transplantation*. Presented at: 19th WAS World Congress for Sexual Health, Goteborg, Sweden; June 2009 Abstract # OP1.5–5.

64. Bogaert AF. Asexuality: prevalence and associated factors in a national probability sample. *J Sex Res*. 2004;41:279–287.

65. Michael R, Gagnon J, Laumann E, et al. *Sex in America*. Boston: Little, Brown; 1994.

66. Fobair P, Stewart SL, Chang S, et al. Body image and sexual problems in young women with breast cancer. *Psychooncology*. 2006;15:579–594.

67. Wimberly SR, Carver CS, Laurenceau JP, et al. Perceived partner reactions to diagnosis and treatment of breast cancer: impact on psychosocial and psychosexual adjustment. *J Consult Clin Psychol*. 2005;73:300–311.

68. Perelman MA. The sexual tipping point: a mind/body model for sexual medicine. *J Sex Med*. 2009;6:629–632.

69. Stamogiannou I, Grunfeld EA, Denison K, et al. Beliefs about illness and quality of life among men with erectile dysfunction. *Int J Impot Res*. 2005;17:142–147.

70. Sanda MG, Dunn RL, Michalski J, et al. Quality of life and satisfaction with outcome among prostate-cancer survivors. *N Engl J Med*. 2008;358:1250–1261.

71. Weber BA, Roberts BL, Yarandi H, et al. Dyadic support and quality-of-life after radical prostatectomy. *J Mens Health Gen*. 2007;4:156–164.

72. Schover LR. The impact of breast cancer on sexuality, body image and intimate relationships. *CA Cancer J Clin*. 1991;41:112–120.

73. Anderson BL, van Der Does J. Surviving gynecologic cancer and coping with sexual morbidity: an international problem. *Int J Gynecol Cancer*. 1994;4:225–240.

74. Hawkins Y, Ussher J, Gilbert E, et al. Changes in sexuality and intimacy after the diagnosis and treatment of cancer: the experience of partners in a sexual relationship with a person with cancer. *Cancer Nurs*. 2009;32:271–280.

75. Greendale GA, Petersen L, Zibecchi L, et al. Factors related to sexual function in postmenopausal women with a history of breast cancer. *Menopause*. 2001;8:111–119.

76. Carmack Taylor CL, Basen-Engquist K, Shinn EH, et al. Predictors of sexual functioning in ovarian cancer patients. *J Clin Oncol*. 2004;22:881–889.

77. Ganz PA, Desmond KA, Belin TR, et al. Predictors of sexual health in women after a breast cancer diagnosis. *J Clin Oncol*. 1999;17:2371–2380.

78. Schover LR. Sexuality and body image in younger women with breast cancer. *J Natl Cancer Inst Monogr*. 1994;16:177–182.

79. Incrocci L. Changes in sexual function after treatment of male cancer. *J Men's Health Gender*. 2005;2:236–243.

80. Trinchieri A, Nicola M, Masini F, et al. Prospective comprehensive assessment of sexual function after retropubic non nerve sparing radical prostatectomy

for localized prostate cancer. *Arch Ital Urol Androl.* 2005;77:219–223.

81. Schover LR, Eschenbach AC. Sexual and marital relationships after treatment for nonseminomatous testicular cancer. *Urology.* 1985;25:251–255.

82. Addis ME, Mahalik JR. Men, masculinity, and the context of help-seeking. *Am Psychol.* 2003;58:5–14.

83. Reference deleted in proofs.

84. Descazeaud A, Debre B, Flam TA. Age difference between patient and partner is a predictive factor of potency rate following radical prostatectomy. *J Urol.* 2006;176(6 Pt 1):2594–2598.

85. Briganti A, Fabbri F, Salonia A, et al. Preserved postoperative penile size correlates well with maintained erectile function after bilateral nerve-sparing radical retropubic prostatectomy. *Eur Urol.* 2007;52:702–707.

86. Kohler TS, Pedro R, Hendlin K, et al. A pilot study on the early use of the vacuum erection device after radical retropubic prostatectomy. *BJU Int.* 2007;100:858–862.

87. Syrjala KL, Roth-Roemer SL, Abrams JR, et al. Prevalence and predictors of sexual dysfunction in long-term survivors of marrow transplantation. *J Clin Oncol.* 1998;16:3148–3157.

88. Reference deleted in proofs.

89. Germino BB, Fife BL, Funk SG. Cancer and the partner relationship: what is its meaning? *Semin Oncol Nurs.* 1995;11:43–50.

90. Hawkins Y, Ussher J, Gilbert E, et al. Changes in sexuality and intimacy after the diagnosis and treatment of cancer: the experience of partners in a sexual relationship with a person with cancer. *Cancer Nurs.* 2009;32:271–280.

91. Hoskins CN, Baker S, Budin W, et al. Adjustment among husbands of women with breast cancer. *J Psychosoc Oncol.* 1996;14:41–69.

92. Dorval M, Guay S, Mondor M, et al. Couples who get closer after breast cancer: frequency and predictors in a prospective investigation. *J Clin Oncol.* 2005;23:3588–3596.

93. Annon JS. The PLISSIT model: a proposed conceptual scheme for the behavioral treatment of sexual problems. *J Sex Educ Ther.* 1976;2:1–15.

94. Shell JA. Evidence based practice for symptom management in adults with cancer: sexual dysfunction. *Oncol Nurs Forum.* 2002;29:53–66.

95. Mick J, Hughes M, Cohen MZ. Using the BETTER model to assess sexuality. *Clin J Oncol Nurs.* 2004;8:84–86.

96. Park ER, Norris RL, Bober SL. Sexual health communication during cancer care: barriers and recommendations. *Cancer J.* 2009;15:74–77.

97. Litwin MS, Hays RD, Fink A, et al. The UCLA Prostate Cancer Index: development, reliability, and validity of a health-related quality of life measure. *Med Care.* 1998;36:1002–1012.

98. Rosen R, Brown C, Heiman J, et al. The Female Sexual Function Index (FSFI): a multidimensional self-report instrument for the assessment of female sexual function. *J Sex Marital Ther.* 2000;26:191–208.

99. Rosen RC, Cappelleri JC, Smith MD, et al. Development and evaluation of an abridged, 5-item version of the International Index of Erectile Function (IIEF-5) as a diagnostic tool for erectile dysfunction. *Int J Impot Res.* 1999;11:319–326.

100. Boehmer U, Potter J, Bowen DJ. Sexual functioning after cancer in sexual minority women. *Cancer J.* 2009;15:65–69.

101. Jeffery DD, Tzeng JP, Kefe FJ, et al. Initial report of the cancer Patient-Reported Outcomes Measurement Information System (PROMIS) Sexual Function Committee. *Cancer.* 2009;115:1142–1153.

102. Amies AM, Miller L, Lee SK, et al. The effect of vaginal speculum lubrication on the rate of unsatisfactory cervical cytology diagnosis. *Obstet Gynecol.* 2002;100(5 Pt 1):889–892.

103. Griffith WF, Stuart GS, Gluck KL, et al. Vaginal speculum lubrication and its effects on cervical cytology and microbiology. *Contraception.* 2005;72:60–64.

104. Stewart EG. Treatment options for vulvar vestibulitis. *Contemp Obstet Gynecol.* 2003;48:47–61.

105. Lewis RW. Venous surgery for impotence. *Urol Clin North Am.* 1988;15:115–121.

106. Hatzichristou D, Rosen RC, Broderick G, et al. Clinical evaluation and management strategy for sexual dysfunction in men and women. *J Sex Med.* 2004;1:49–57.

107. Davis SR, Davison SL, Donath A, et al. Circulating androgen levels and self-reported sexual function in women. *JAMA.* 2005;294:91–96.

108. Santoro N, Torrens J, Crawford S, et al. Correlates of circulating androgens in midlife women: the Study of Women's Health Across the Nation. *J Clin Endocrinol Metab.* 2005;90:4836–4845.

109. Glass AR, Swerdloff RS, Bray GA, et al. Low serum testosterone and sex hormone binding globulin in massively obese men. *J Clin Endocrinol Metab.* 1977;45:1211.

110. Purifoy FE, Koopmans LH, Mayes DM. Age differences in serum androgen levels in normal adult males. *Hum Biol.* 1981;53:499.

111. Khatcheressian JL, Wolff AC, Smith TJ, et al. American Society of Clinical Oncology 2006 update of the breast cancer follow-up and management guidelines in the adjuvant setting. *J Clin Oncol.* 2006;24:5091–5097.

112. National Comprehensive Cancer Network. *Practice guidelines in oncology, version 1.* 2010. Available at: www.nccn.org.

113. Kayser K, Scott J. *Helping couples cope with cancer: an evidence-based approach for practitioners.* New York: Springer Science + Business Media; 2008.

114. Scott JL, Kayser K. A review of couple-based interventions for enhancing women's sexual adjustment and body image after cancer. *Cancer J.* 2009;15:48–56.

115. Canada AL, Neese LE, Sui D, et al. Pilot intervention to enhance sexual rehabilitation for couples after treatment for localized prostate carcinoma. *Cancer.* 2005;104:2689–2700.

116. Melnik T, Soares BG, Nasselo AG. Psychosocial interventions for erectile dysfunction. *Cochrane Database Syst Rev.* 2007;(3):CD004825.

117. Lemieux J, Maunsell E, Provencher L. Chemotherapy-induced alopecia and effects on quality of life among women with breast cancer: a literature review. *Psychooncology.* 2008;4:317–328.

118. Hilton S, Hunt K, Emslie C, et al. Have men been overlooked? A comparison of young men and women's experiences of chemotherapy-induced alopecia. *Psychooncology.* 2008;6:577–583.

119. American Cancer Society. *Look good feel better program.* Information available at: http://www. lookgoodfeelbetter.org/index.htm.

120. Carmichael AR. Obesity and prognosis of breast cancer. *Obes Rev.* 2006;4:333–340.

121. Amling CL. Relationship between obesity and prostate cancer. *Curr Opin Urol.* 2005;15:167–171.

122. Siegel EM, Ulrich CM, Poole EM, et al. The effects of obesity and obesity-related conditions on colorectal cancer prognosis. *Cancer Control.* 2010;17:52–57.

123. Holmes MD, Chen WY, Feskanich D, et al. Physical activity and survival after breast cancer diagnosis. *JAMA.* 2005;293:2479–2486.

124. Meyerhardt JA, Giovannucci EL, Holmes MD, et al. Physical activity and survival after colorectal cancer diagnosis. *J Clin Oncol.* 2006;24:3527–3534.

125. Kolotkin RL, Binks M, Crosby RD, et al. Improvements in sexual quality of life after moderate weight loss. *Int J Impot Res.* 2008;20:487–492.

126. Berber JR, Johnson JV, Bunn JY, et al. A longitudinal study of the effects of free testosterone and other psychosocial variables on sexual function during the natural traverse of menopause. *Fertil Steril.* 2005;83:643–648.

127. Doyle C, Kushi LH, Byers T, et al. Nutrition and physical activity during and after cancer treatment: an American Cancer Society Guide for informed choices. *CA Cancer J Clin.* 2006;56:323–353.

128. Loprinzi CL, Abu-Ghazaleh S, Sloan JA, et al. Phase III randomized double-blind study to evaluate the efficacy of a polycarbophil-based vaginal moisturizer in women with breast cancer. *J Clin Oncol.* 1997;15:969–973.

129. Nachtigall LE. Comparative study: Replens versus local estrogen in menopausal women. *Fertil Steril.* 1994;61:178–180.

130. Montague DK, Jarow JP, Broderick GA, et al. Erectile Dysfunction Guideline Update Panel. Chapter 1: The management of erectile dysfunction: an AUA update. *J Urol.* 2005;174:230–239.

131. Peltier A, van Velthoven R, Roumeguère T. Current management of erectile dysfunction after cancer treatment. *Curr Opin Oncol.* 2009;21:303–309.

132. Esposito K, Giugliano F, Di Palo C, et al. Effect of lifestyle changes on erectile dysfunction in obese men: a randomized controlled trial. *JAMA.* 2004;291:2978–2984.

133. Gregore A. ABC of sexual health: assessing and managing male sexual problems. *BMJ.* 1999;318:315.

134. Abdel-Hamid IA, El Naggar EA, El Gilany AH. Assessment of as needed use of pharmacotherapy and the pause-squeeze technique in premature ejaculation. *Int J Impot Res.* 2001;13:41–45.

135. Ohl DA, Quallich SA, Sønksen J, et al. Anejaculation and retrograde ejaculation. *Urol Clin North Am.* 2008;35:211–220 viii.

136. Kamischke A, Nieschlag E. Treatment of retrograde ejaculation and anejaculation. *Hum Reprod Update.* 1999;5:448–474.

137. Kamischke A, Nieschlag E. Treatment of retrograde ejaculation and anejaculation. *Hum Reprod Update.* 1999;5:448–474.

138. Reference deleted in proofs

139. Reference deleted in proofs.

140. Potter J. A 60-year old woman with sexual difficulties. *JAMA.* 2007;297:620–633.

141. Anderson GL, Limacher M, Assaf AR, et al. Effects of conjugated equine estrogen in postmenopausal women with hysterectomy: the Women's Health Initiative randomized controlled trial. *JAMA.* 2004;291:1701–1712.

142. Rossouw JE, Anderson GL, Prentice RL, et al. Risks and benefits of estrogen in healthy postmenopausal women: principal results from the Women's Health Initiative randomized controlled trial. *JAMA.* 2002;288:321–333.

143. Suckling J, Lethaby A, Kennedy R. Local oestrogen for vaginal atrophy in postmenopausal women. *Cochrane Database Syst Rev.* 2003;(4): CD001500.

144. Dew JE, Wren BG, Eden JA. A cohort study of topical vaginal estrogen therapy in women previously treated for breast cancer. *Climacteric.* 2003;6:45–52.

145. Kendall A, Dowsett M, Folkerd E, et al. Caution: vaginal estradiol appears to be contraindicated in postmenopausal women on adjuvant aromatase inhibitors. *Ann Oncol.* 2006;17:584–587.

146. Kwan KW, Chlebowski RT. Sexual dysfunction and aromatase inhibitor use in survivors of breast cancer. *Clin Breast Cancer.* 2009;9:219–224.

147. Berk L. Systemic pilocarpine for treatment of xerostomia. *Drug Metab Toxicol.* 2008;4:1333–1340.

148. van de Nieuwenhof HP, van der Avoort IAM, de Hullu JA. Review of squamous premalignant vulvar lesions. *Crit Rev Oncol Hematol.* 2008;68:131–156.

149. Spiryda LB, Laufer MR, Soiffer RJ, et al. Graft-versus-host-disease of the vulva and/or vagina: diagnosis and treatment. *Biol Blood Marrow Transplant.* 2003;9:60–66.

150. Lobo RA, Rosen RC, Yang HM, et al. Comparative effects of oral esterified estrogens with and without methyltestosterone on endocrine profiles and dimensions of sexual function in postmenopausal women with hypoactive desire disorder. *Fertil Steril.* 2003;79:1341–1352.

151. Warnock JK, Swanson SG, Borel RW, et al. Combined esterified estrogens and methyltestosterone versus esterified estrogens alone in the treatment of loss of sexual interest in surgically menopausal women. *Menopause.* 2005;12:374–384.

152. Shifren JL, Braunstein G, Simon J, et al. Transdermal testosterone treatment in women with impaired sexual function after oophorectomy. *N Engl J Med.* 2000;343:682–688.

153. Braunstein G, Sundwall DA, Katz M, et al. Safety and efficacy of a testosterone patch for the treatment of hypoactive sexual desire disorder in surgically menopausal women: a randomized, placebo-controlled trial. *Arch Intern Med.* 2005;165:1582–1589.

154. Buster JE, Kingsberg SA, Aguirre O, et al. Testosterone patch for low sexual desire in surgically menopausal women: a randomized trial. *Obstet Gynecol.* 2005;105:944–952.

155. Simon J, Braunstein G, Nachtigall L, et al. Testosterone patch increases sexual activity and desire in surgically menopausal women with hypoactive sexual desire disorder. *J Clin Endocrinol Metab.* 2005;90:5226–5233.

156. DeRogatis LR, Graziottin A, Bitzer J, et al. Clinically relevant changes in sexual desire, satisfying sexual activity and personal distress as measured by the profile of female sexual function, sexual activity log, and personal distress scale in postmenopausal women with hypoactive sexual desire disorder. *J Sex Med.* 2009;6:175–183.

157. Davis SR, Moreau M, Kroll R, et al. Testosterone for low libido in postmenopausal women not taking estrogen. *N Engl J Med.* 2008;359:2005–2017.

158. Barton DL, Wender DB, Sloan JA, et al. Randomized controlled trial to evaluate transdermal testosterone in female cancer survivors with decreased libido: North Central Cancer Treatment Group protocol N02C3. *J Natl Cancer Inst.* 2007;99:672–679.

159. Bhasin S, Cunningham GR, Hayes FJ, et al. Testosterone therapy in adult men with androgen deficiency syndromes: an Endocrine Society clinical practice guideline. *J Clin Endocrinol Metab.* 2006;91:1995–2010.

160. Guay AT, Spark RF, Bansal S, et al. American Association of Clinical Endocrinologists medical guidelines for clinical practice for the evaluation and treatment of male sexual dysfunction: a couple's problem—2003 update. *Endocr Pract.* 2003;9:77–95.

161. Jain P, Rademaker AW, McVary KT. Testosterone supplementation for erectile dysfunction: results of a meta-analysis. *J Urol.* 2000;164:371–375.

162. Rhoden EL, Morgentaler A. Risks of testosterone-replacement therapy and recommendations for monitoring. *N Engl J Med.* 2004;350:482–492.

163. Sarosdy MF. Testosterone replacement for hypogonadism after treatment of early prostate cancer with brachytherapy. *Cancer.* 2007;109:536–541.

164. Bhasin S, Cunningham GR, Hayes FJ, et al. Testosterone therapy in adult men with androgen deficiency syndromes: an Endocrine Society clinical practice guideline. *J Clin Endocrinol Metab.* 2006;91:1995–2010.

165. Reference deleted in proofs.

166. Guay AT, Spark RF, Bansal S, et al. American Association of Clinical Endocrinologists medical guidelines for clinical practice for the evaluation and treatment of male sexual dysfunction: a couple's problem—2003 update. *Endocr Pract.* 2003;9:77–95.

167. Rhoden EL, Morgentaler A. Risks of testosterone-replacement therapy and recommendations for monitoring. *N Engl J Med.* 2004;350:482–492.

168. Stephenson RA, Mori M, Hsieh YC, et al. Treatment of erectile dysfunction following therapy for clinically localized prostate cancer: patient reported use and outcomes from the Surveillance, Epidemiology, and End Results Prostate Cancer Outcomes Study. *J Urol.* 2005;174:646–650.

169. Miles CL, Candy B, Jones L, et al. Interventions for sexual dysfunction following treatments for cancer. *Cochrane Database Syst Rev.* 2007;(4):CD005540.

170. Lee IH, Sadetsky N, Carroll PR, et al. The impact of treatment choice for localized prostate cancer on response to phosphodiesterase inhibitors. *J Urol.* 2008;179:1072–1076.

171. Teloken PE, Parker M, Mohideen N, et al. Predictors of response to sildenafil citrate following radiation therapy for prostate cancer. *J Sex Med.* 2009;6:1135–1140.

172. Koskimäki J, Shiri R, Tammela T, et al. Regular intercourse protects against erectile dysfunction: Tampere Aging Male Urologic Study. *Am J Med.* 2008;121:592–596.

173. McCullough AR, Levine LA, Padma-Nathan H. Return of nocturnal erections and erectile function after bilateral nerve-sparing radical prostatectomy in men treated nightly with sildenafil citrate: subanalysis of a longitudinal randomized double-blind placebo-controlled trial. *J Sex Med.* 2008;5:476–484.

174. Ohebshalom M, Parker M, Guhring P, et al. The efficacy of sildenafil citrate following radiation therapy for prostate cancer: temporal considerations. *J Urol.* 2005;174:258–262.

175. Tadalafil (cialis) for erectile dysfunction. *Med Lett Drugs Ther.* 2003;45:101–102.

176. Cheitlin MD, Hutter AM, Brindis RG, et al. ACC/AHA expert consensus document: use of sildenafil (Viagra) in patients with cardiovascular disease. American College of Cardiology/American Heart Association. *J Am Coll Cardiol.* 1999;33:273–282.

177. Basson R, McInnes R, Smith MD, et al. Efficacy and safety of sildenafil citrate in women with sexual dysfunction associated with female sexual arousal disorder. *J Womens Health Gend Based Med.* 2002;11:367–377.

178. Berman JR, Berman LA, Toler SM, et al. Safety and efficacy of sildenafil citrate for the treatment of female sexual arousal disorder: a double-blind, placebo controlled study. *J Urol.* 2003;170(6 Pt 1):2333–2338.

179. Raina R, Pahlajani G, Agarwal A, et al. The early use of transurethral alprostadil after radical prostatectomy potentially facilitates an earlier return of erectile function and successful sexual activity. *BJU Int.* 2007;100:1317–1321.

180. Montorsi F, Luigi GG, Strambi LF, et al. Recovery of spontaneous erectile function after nerve-sparing radical retropubic prostatectomy with and without early intracavernous injections of alprostadil: results of a prospective, randomized trial. *J Urol.* 1997;158:1408–1410.

181. Gontero P, Fontana F, Bagnasacco A, et al. Is there an optimal time for intracavernous prostaglandin E1 rehabilitation following non nerve sparing radical prostatectomy? Results from a hemodynamic prospective study. *J Urol.* 2003;169:2166–2169.

182. Peltier A, van Velthoven R, Roumeguère T. Current management of erectile dysfunction after cancer treatment. *Curr Opin Oncol.* 2009;21:303–309.

183. Montague DK, Jarow JP, Broderick GA, et al. Erectile Dysfunction Guideline Update Panel. Chapter 1: The management of erectile dysfunction: an AUA update. *J Urol.* 2005;174:230–239.

184. Liao Q, Zhang M, Geng L, et al. Efficacy and safety of alprostadil cream for the treatment of female sexual arousal disorder: a double-blind, placebo-controlled study in a Chinese population. *J Sex Med.* 2008;5:1923–1931.

185. Heiman JR, Gittelman M, Costabile R, et al. Topical alprostadil (PGE1) for the treatment of female sexual arousal disorder: in-clinic evaluation of safety and efficacy. *J Psychosom Obstet.* 2006;27:31–41.

186. Montague DK, Jarow JP, Broderick GA, et al. Erectile dysfunction guideline update panel. Chapter 1: The management of erectile dysfunction: an AUA update. *J Urol.* 2005;174:230–239.

187. Clayton AH, Pradko JF, Croft HA, et al. Prevalence of sexual dysfunction among newer antidepressants. *J Clin Psychiatry.* 2002;63:357–366.

188. Othmer E, Othmer SC. Effect of buspirone on sexual dysfunction in patients with generalized anxiety disorder. *J Clin Psychiatry.* 1987;48:201–203.

189. Clayton AH, Balon R. The impact of mental illness and psychotropic mediations on sexual functioning: the evidence and management. *J Sex Med.* 2009;6:1200–1211.

190. Clayton AH, Waarnock JK, Kornstein SG, et al. A placebo-controlled trial of bupropion SR as an antidote for selective serotonin reuptake inhibitor-induced sexual dysfunction. *J Clin Psychiatry.* 2004;65:62–67.

191. Fava M, Nurnberg HG, Seidman SN, et al. Efficacy and safety of sildenafil in men with serotonergic antidepressant-associated erectile dysfunction: results from a randomized, double-blind, placebo-controlled trial. *J Clin Psychiatry.* 2006;67:240–246.

192. Nurnberg HG, Hensley PL, Heiman JR, et al. Sildenafil treatment of women with antidepressant-associated sexual dysfunction: a randomized controlled trial. *JAMA.* 2008;300:395–404.

193. Landon M, Eriksson E, Agren H, et al. Effect of buspirone on sexual dysfunction in depressed patients

treated with selective serotonin reuptake inhibitors. *J Clin Psychopharmacol.* 1999;19:268–271.

194. Ozmenler NK, Karlidere T, Bozhurt A, et al. Mirtazapine augmentation in depressed patients with sexual dysfunction due to selective serotonin reuptake inhibitors. *Hum Psychopharmacol Clin Exp.* 2008;23:321–326.

195. Taylor MJ. Strategies for managing antidepressant-induced sexual dysfunction: a review. *Curr Psychiatry Rep.* 2006;8:431–436.

196. Masand PS, Ashton AK, Gupta S, et al. Sustained-release bupropion for selective serotonin reuptake inhibitor-induced sexual dysfunction: a randomized, double-blind, placebo-controlled, parallel-group study. *Am J Psychiatry.* 2001;158:805–807.

197. DeBattista C, Solvason B, Poirier J, et al. A placebo-controlled, randomized, double-blind study of adjunctive bupropion sustained release in the treatment of SSRI-induced sexual dysfunction. *J Clin Psychiatry.* 2005;66:844–848.

198. Clayton AH, Warnock JK, Kornstein SG, et al. A placebo-controlled trial of bupropion SR as an antidote for selective serotonin reuptake inhibitor-induced sexual dysfunction. *Clin Psychiatry.* 2004;65:62–67.

199. Segraves RT, Clayton A, Croft H, et al. Bupropion sustained release for the treatment of hypoactive sexual desire disorder in premenopausal women. *J Clin Psychopharmacol.* 2004;24:339–342.

200. Mathias C, Cardeal Mendes CM, Ponde de Sena E, et al. An open-label, fixed-dose study of bupropion effect on sexual function scores in women treated for breast cancer. *Ann Oncol.* 2006;17:1792–1796.

201. Diamond LE, Earle DC, Rosen RC, et al. Double-blind, placebo-controlled evaluation of the safety, pharmacokinetic properties and pharmacodynamic effects of intranasal PT-141, a melanocortin receptor agonist, in healthy males and patients with mild-to-moderate erectile dysfunction. *Int J Impot Res.* 2004;16:51–59.

202. Safarinejad MR, Hosseini SY. Salvage of sildenafil failures with bremelanotide: a randomized, double-blind, placebo controlled study. *J Urol.* 2008;179:1066–1071.

203. Safarinejad MR. Evaluation of the safety and efficacy of premelanotide, a melanocortin receptor agonist, in female subjects with arousal disorder: a double-blind placebo-controlled, fixed dose, randomized study. *J Sex Med.* 2008;5:887–897.

204. Jolly E, Clayton A, Thorp J, et al. Efficacy of flibanserin 100 mg qhs as a potential treatment for hypoactive sexual desire disorder in premenopausal women. *J Sex Med.* 2009;6(suppl 5):465 Abstract #PO-11–004.

205. Billups KL. The role of mechanical devices in treating female sexual dysfunction and enhancing the female sexual response. *World J Urol.* 2002;20:137–141.

206. Herenick D, Reece M, Sanders S, et al. Prevalence and characteristics of vibrator use by women in the United States: results from a nationally representative study. *J Sex Med.* 2009;6:1857–1866.

207. Herenick D, Reece M, Sanders S, et al. Prevalence and characteristics of vibrator use by men in the United States: results from a nationally representative study. *J Sex Med.* 2009;6:1867–1874.

208. Wilson SK, Delk JR, Billups KL. Treating symptoms of female sexual arousal disorder with the Eros-Clitoral Therapy Device. *J Gend Specif Med.* 2001;4:54–58.

209. Schroder MA, Mell LK, Hurteau JA, et al. Clitoral therapy device for treatment of sexual dysfunction in irradiated cervical cancer patients. *Int J Radiat Oncol Biol Phys.* 2005;61:1078–1086.

210. Köhler TS, Pedro R, Hendlin K, et al. A pilot study on early use of the vacuum erection device after radical retropubic prostatectomy. *BJU Int.* 2007;100:858–862.

211. Mulhall JP, Morgentaler A. Penile rehabilitation should become the norm for radical prostatectomy patients. *J Sex Med.* 2007;4:538–543.

212. Montague DK, Jarow JP, Broderick GA, et al. Erectile Dysfunction Guideline Update Panel. Chapter 1: The management of erectile dysfunction: an AUA update. *J Urol.* 2005;174:230–239.

213. Denton AS, Maher EJ. Interventions for the physical aspects of sexual dysfunction in women following pelvic radiotherapy. *Cochrane Database Syst Rev.* 2003;(1):CD003750.

214. Lancaster L. Preventing vaginal stenosis after brachytherapy for gynaecological cancer: an overview of Australian practices. *Eur J Oncol Nurs.* 2004;8:30–39.

215. Denton AS, Maher EJ. Interventions for the physical aspects of sexual dysfunction in women following pelvic radiotherapy. *Cochrane Database Syst Rev.* 2003;(1:CD003750).

216. MacDonald R, Fink HA, Huckaby C, et al. Pelvic floor muscle training to improve urinary incontinence after radical prostatectomy: a systematic review of effectiveness. *BJU Int.* 2007;100:76–81.

217. Allgayer H, Dietrich CF, Rohde W, et al. Prospective comparison of short- and long-term effects of pelvic floor exercise/biofeedback training in patients with fecal incontinence after surgery plus irradiation versus surgery alone for colorectal cancer: clinical, functional and endoscopic/endosonographic findings. *Scand J Gastroenterol.* 2005;40:1168–1175.

218. Rosenbaum TY, Owens A. The role of pelvic floor physical therapy in the treatment of pelvic and genital pain-related sexual dysfunction. *J Sex Med.* 2008;5:513–523.

219. Montague DK, Jarow JP, Broderick GA, et al. Erectile Dysfunction Guideline Update Panel. Chapter 1: The management of erectile dysfunction: an AUA update. *J Urol.* 2005;174:230–239.

220. Montague DK, Jarow JP, Broderick GA, et al. Erectile Dysfunction Guideline Update Panel. Chapter 1: The management of erectile dysfunction: an AUA update. *J Urol.* 2005;174:230–239.

221. Montague DK, Jarow JP, Broderick GA, et al. Erectile Dysfunction Guideline Update Panel. Chapter 1: The management of erectile dysfunction: an AUA update. *J Urol.* 2005;174:230–239.

222. Ramsawh HJ, Morgentaler A, Covino N, et al. Quality of life following simultaneous placement of penile prosthesis with radical prostatectomy. *J Urol.* 2005;174(4 Pt 1):1395–1398.

223. Fowler JM. Incorporating pelvic/vaginal reconstruction into radical pelvic surgery. *Gynecol Oncol.* 2009;115:154–163.

224. Fotopoulou C, Neumann U, Klapp C, et al. Long-term effects of neovaginal reconstruction with sigmoid loop technique on sexual function and self image in patients with gynecologic malignancies: results of a prospective study. *Gynecol Oncol.* 2008;111:400–406.

SUGGESTED RESOURCES

Internet Websites
General Sexuality
www.siecus.org Sexuality Information and Education Council of the United States.Sexuality After Cancer
www.LAF.org The Lance Armstrong Foundation.
www.lbbc.org Living Beyond Breast Cancer.
www.mautnerproject.org The Mautner Project for Lesbians With Cancer.
www.oncolink.org Comprehensive, Web-based cancer resource.

Books and Other Resources
Body Image
"Look Good…Feel Good" program offered by the American Cancer Society, 1-800-395-LOOK.
Cash TF. *The body image workbook: an 8 step program for learning to like your looks.* New York: Harbinger Publications; 1997.

General Sexuality
Heiman JR, LoPiccolo L, LoPiccolo J. *Becoming orgasmic: a sexual and personal growth program for women.* New York: Fireside; 1988.
Renshaw D. *Seven weeks to better sex.* Redondo Beach, CA: Westcom Press; 2004.

Sexuality After Cancer
Harpham WS. *After cancer: a guide to your new life.* New York: Harper Perennial; 1995.
Hill Schnipper H. *After breast cancer: a common-sense guide to life after treatment.* New York: Bantam Dell; 2006.
Kydd S, Rowett D. *Intimacy after cancer: a woman's guide.* Big Think Media: Seattle; 2006.
Laken V, Laken K. *Making love again: hope for couples facing loss of sexual intimacy.* Kansas City, MO: Ant Hill Press; 2002.

Mulhall JP. *Saving your sex life: a guide for men with prostate cancer.* Munster, IN: Hilton Publishing; 2008.
NCI/PDQ. *Sexuality and reproductive issues.* 2009. Available at: http://www.oncolink.org/coping/article.cfm?c=4&s=46&ss=95&id=801.
Schover LR. *Sexuality and cancer: for the man who has cancer and his partner.* New York: American Cancer Society; 1997.
Schover LR. *Sexuality and cancer: for the woman who has cancer and her partner.* New York: American Cancer Society; 2001.

For Referral to a Certified Sex Therapist
The American Association of Sex Educators, Counselors, and Therapists (AASECT). http://www.aasect.org (804) 644 3288.

Fertility assessment and preservation

58

Katherine T. Johnston and Jennifer Potter

SCOPE OF THE PROBLEM

The number of reproductive-age cancer survivors has increased over the past 20 years. This group comprises people who are affected by cancers of the pelvic organs, as well as those with cancers whose treatments are known to be damaging to reproductive organs. It is estimated that approximately 78,500 new cancers are diagnosed each year in people younger than 39 years, 58,000 of which occur in persons aged 25 to 39 years—the most common years for childbearing.[1] Cancer and its treatments can permanently alter the reproductive potential of young people and are more likely to do so if not addressed and managed as an integral aspect of treatment planning, as well as later on, during the survivorship time period. Concerns for future fertility are present in all young survivors at different stages throughout the cancer care process. However, when patients and their partners present to clinicians, they may not always voice their reproductive concerns; therefore, it is crucial to ask questions proactively. Clinicians can offer support, guidance, and appropriate planning and referral for reproductive-age women and men whose lives are affected by cancer, at the time of diagnosis, during treatment, and after treatment.

The most common types of cancers that affect men of reproductive age are testicular cancer, prostate cancer, lymphomas, and leukemias; breast cancer, cervical cancer, lymphomas, and leukemias cause reproductive challenges most frequently in women.[2] Currently, breast cancer is the most common cancer that affects women, with 1 in 200 women younger than age 40 diagnosed with the disease each year. Unfortunately, the percentage of young women diagnosed with breast cancer is increasing; this trend coincides with the fact that many women choose to defer the start of their families until their later 30s and early 40s.[3] Overall, 25% of women with breast cancer are premenopausal at the time of diagnosis.[4]

The opportunity to biologically parent a child after cancer is most strongly dependent on the survivors' gender and the age at which they received cancer treatment. The critical window during which cancer treatment affects fertility most adversely differs for men versus women. Men are significantly less likely to father a child if treated for cancer before age 14, whereas women are most strongly affected when cancer treatment is administered between ages 20 and 34.[5] As assessed in multiple observational studies, rates of postcancer parenthood are estimated to be reduced by 30% to 50% for female survivors and by 20% to 30% for male survivors, compared with their healthy siblings.[6] This variation reveals a clear gender difference in the degree of effect of cancer treatments on later fertility.

CONCERNS OF SURVIVORS

It is important for clinicians caring for cancer survivors to understand the common concerns that survivors have about parenting. Surveys show that the experience of cancer commonly increases the perceived significance of fertility[7] because of an increase in the value that survivors place on family ties. Additionally, a patient attitude survey revealed that many survivors want to have biological children, feel they will be better parents as survivors,[8] and consider fertility to be an issue vital to their quality of life.[9] Women report both distress about delaying childbearing after cancer[10] and unmet information needs about fertility and late or long-term effects of adjuvant treatment.[11] Qualitative studies show that young women perceive childbearing after cancer to reflect a return to normalcy and consider loss of fertility to represent as great a threat as cancer itself poses to their survival.[7] Similarly, qualitative studies in young men reveal considerable distress about the potential for infertility after cancer, most notably in men who were childless at the time of diagnosis.[7] Addressing these concerns and assisting survivors in achieving parenthood are important roles for clinicians who care for cancer survivors.

Cancer often challenges people's values and focus in life. Individuals who did not wish to parent previously may change their minds after experiencing cancer themselves, or by sharing the cancer experience of their partner. Clinicians therefore should ask about parenting desires and should not make assumptions based on their previous knowledge of the person. Research indicates that survivors' fertility information needs and concerns are rarely addressed by health care providers.[12] Useful opening questions include the following: "Have you considered parenting a child?" "Would you like the option of having children in the future?" "What are your concerns?" Based on the patient's and/or partner's responses, clinicians can provide appropriate information and resources to facilitate informed decision making. Information on both biological and nonbiological parenting options should be included; however, it should be noted that a history of cancer often precludes some forms of adoption.

Clinicians also have a key role in helping patients estimate the risk for infertility, both before and after cancer treatment, as well as the risk of complications for themselves or for biological children conceived after cancer treatment. Many survivors worry that cancer treatments will have an adverse effect on future pregnancies, or will predispose future offspring to birth defects and genetic abnormalities. Fortunately, no study to date has shown an increased rate of birth defects in cancer survivors. Pregnancy outcomes have not been shown to be altered by previous chemotherapy exposure, although women who undergo therapeutic pelvic or uterine radiation have an increased miscarriage rate and are more likely to have low-birthweight infants.[7] Many women have a disproportionate fear that pregnancy will increase the chance of cancer recurrence[7]; thus far, no evidence indicates that pregnancy reduces survival rates when cancer stage and histology are controlled.[4,13,14] Moreover, many cancer chemotherapies can be safely administered during pregnancy,[15] reducing concern regarding potential treatment delay. Caring for cancer survivors mandates a focus on quality of life, which includes helping patients and their partners manage the fear of recurrence by providing information and support, while balancing the desire to optimize fertility or to pursue parenting a nonbiological child.

ATTITUDES OF CANCER HEALTH CARE PROVIDERS

Research on the knowledge and attitudes of primary care and oncology clinicians is limited; a preponderance of existing information is based on surveys with low response rates. Most surveys focus on the self-reported knowledge of oncology providers regarding fertility preservation and frequency of referral for preservation procedures. It is generally recommended that all male patients of reproductive age should be referred for sperm cryopreservation before cancer treatment is initiated. Despite this general recommendation and the fact that 91% of respondents stated that sperm cryopreservation should be discussed with all eligible men, one survey revealed that 48% of oncologists never broached the topic.[16] Additional surveys demonstrate that oncology providers may be unaware of many options to preserve fertility, or may overestimate the perceived cost burden, and thus do not consistently refer all eligible patients for appropriate procedures.[17] Research on primary care providers, who provide the majority of care for long-term cancer survivors, indicates that that they lack adequate training and do not know how to access even general resources for survivorship care.[18] Discussion points that should be addressed during fertility assessment are outlined in Table 58-1.

General guidelines on fertility preservation for cancer survivors are available through the American Society of Clinical Oncology (ASCO),[19,20] as well as a number of other organizations and websites (Table 58-2). Clinicians should review all late and long-term side effects of treatments with patients, including the risk of infertility and options to reduce this risk.[20,21] Discussion should take place before treatment is begun, and the topic may be continually readdressed over time after exposure to injurious agents has occurred.[20] Finding adequate time for these discussions is challenging: A visit dedicated to this purpose would be ideal but frequently is not possible. The process may be aided by enlisting the cooperation of clinicians across the multiple disciplines involved in cancer care. For example, starting the conversation can be the role of the primary care provider or the clinician making the cancer diagnosis. General information and resources about fertility assessment and preservation and nonbiological parenting options can be provided; a detailed review of fertility options can be deferred to a specialist to preserve time. Although fertility preservation is most successful when elected before treatment, discussion of parenting options

---

Table 58-1 ASCO guidelines for fertility preservation in cancer survivors

- Address the possibility of infertility in all people undergoing cancer treatment during reproductive years.
- Counsel patients about the effects of treatments on their fertility, including individual factors such as disease, age, treatment type, dosages, and pretreatment fertility.
- Consider fertility preservation approaches as early as possible, before treatment is preferred.
- At this time, there appears to be no detectable increased risk of cancer recurrence after use of fertility sparing procedures.
- Treatment-related infertility is associated with psychosocial distress; early referral for counseling support may be beneficial.

Table 58-2 Additional resources for clinicians and survivors

Resource	Website	Options
American Society for Clinical Oncology (ASCO)	www.asco.org/ guidelines/fertility	Guidelines for fertility preservation and survivorship care
Lance Armstrong Foundation (LAF)	www.livestrong.org (note—not livestrong.com)	Resources for cancer survivors and providers
Fertile Hope	www.fertilehope. org	Fertility options, risk calculators, nonbiological parenting information, financial support options, and specialist referral guide
American Society for Reproductive Medicine (ASRM)	www.asrm.org	Patient information booklets and factsheets about adoption, reproductive procedures, and infertility, including cancer survivors
		This site also lists a directory of mental health professionals for persons needing increased support options.
Resolve	www.resolve.org	Online community for women and men with infertility
Hope for Two	www. pregnantwithcancer. org	Online support for women diagnosed with cancer while pregnant

should continue after treatment, as many patients who did not initially express interest may change their minds and become interested in pursuing parenting after treatment is completed.

IMPACT OF CANCER AND ITS TREATMENTS ON FERTILITY

CANCER TYPE

In men, testicular cancer and Hodgkin's lymphoma are known to affect fertility directly, with many men having impaired sperm quality or seminal vesicle abnormalities when assessed before treatment.[20] The cause of the impaired sperm quality is unknown in this situation but is postulated to be related to tumor infiltration, cytokine-induced abnormalities, or underlying genetic causes. In women, fertility can be directly affected by ovarian, fallopian, uterine, and later-stage cervical cancer.

SURGERY

Operative removal of cancer often necessitates removal of affected reproductive organs, or potential damage to nerves and vessels proximal to reproductive organs. To date, no prospective studies have quantified the risks of impaired

fertility related to anatomic, neurologic, or vascular changes. The cancer type, location, and regional spread often determine the degree to which fertility is compromised in testicular, prostate, ovarian, uterine, and cervical cancer. Research on fertility-sparing surgical procedures is limited to case reports, series, and retrospective reviews, a few of which will be discussed later in this chapter.

Retrograde ejaculation and anejaculation are specific adverse effects of cancer surgery that affect 10% of men after prostate surgery and 30% to 60% of men after retroperitoneal lymph node dissection for testicular cancer.[22] These conditions occur when nerve damage hinders closure and contraction of the bladder sphincter during orgasm, leading to little or no anterograde flow of semen through the urethra. The more severe form—anejaculation—is a common consequence of bilateral retroperitoneal lymph node dissection, caused by profound nerve damage. Both conditions can occur in men without cancer histories and are diagnosed in the presence of a typical history, associated medications (such as antidepressants, antihypertensives, antipsychotics, or alpha blockers), and medical disorders or surgeries known to affect nerve function adversely. Diagnosis is confirmed by post-masturbation urine testing with sperm count evaluation.[22] Either condition can cause male factor infertility as the result of low or no ejaculate produced at the time of orgasm.

RADIATION THERAPIES

Similar to surgical treatment, therapeutic radiation directed toward cancers affecting pelvic organs leads to anatomic and neurovascular changes that impair fertility in most recipients. Fertility sparing techniques, which limit radiation dose and beam direction, are under investigation and are often used but have not been shown to guarantee later fertility. For men, the most common cause of radiation-induced azoospermia is receipt of >2.5 Gy to the testis, whereas in women, external beam radiation to any field that involves the ovaries has a >80% risk of causing amenorrhea. Women who have experienced total-body irradiation or uterine radiation are thought to be at increased risk for miscarriage, prematurity, and low-birthweight delivery.[20]

CHEMOTHERAPIES

The most common cause of impaired fertility after cancer is exposure to chemotherapeutic agents. Any effect is dependent on dose, cycle number, and the age and pretreatment fertility function of the recipient. In women and men, the chemotherapeutic agents most likely to cause prolonged azoospermia or amenorrhea are alkylating agents, including cyclophosphamide, ifosfamide, nitrosoureas, chlorambucil, procarbazine, melphalan, and busulfan. Data on the degree to which fertility is impaired by specific chemotherapeutic regimens and dosages are outside the scope of this chapter but are nicely stratified in the ASCO guidelines.[20] It is impossible to estimate the precise impact of various chemotherapeutic agents on gonadal function, as many studies report proxy outcomes, such as azoospermia or amenorrhea, rather than actual conception rates or positive pregnancy outcomes. For example, many studies report on the likelihood of return to normal menstruation in women after receipt of chemotherapy, but resumption of cyclic menstruation does not indicate the degree of remaining

Table 58-3 Fertility preservation methods

Technique	Optimal timing with cancer therapies	Advantages	Considerations
Males			
Sperm cryopreservation after masturbation	Before treatment (but may be performed after)	The most established technique Lowest cost No partner required at time of decision Ease of use at any age Fewer ethical concerns	• Outpatient procedure • ≈$1500 for three samples stored over 3 years
Sperm cryopreservation after electroejaculation	Before treatment (but may be performed after)	Effective when nerve impairment is present	• Outpatient surgical procedure • Requires some testicular function
Sperm cryopreservation after testicular sperm extraction	Before treatment (but may be performed after)	Effective in males with azoospermia	• Outpatient surgical procedure • Requires some testicular function
Females			
Embryo cryopreservation	Before treatment in women (but may be performed after)	Effective and well-established procedure	• Outpatient surgical procedure • Requires 10–14 days of ovarian stimulation from the beginning of the menstrual cycle • ≈$8000 per cycle; $350 per year storage fees • Partner or donor required at time of decision
Oocyte cryopreservation	Before treatment (but may be performed after)	No partner or donor needed at time of decision	• Experimental/Investigational • Outpatient surgical procedure • Live birth rate 3–4× lower than standard IVF
Ovarian tissue extraction ± transplantation	Before treatment	No partner or donor needed at time of decision	• Experimental/Investigational • Outpatient surgical procedure • Not suitable if ovarian cancer involvement possible

IVF, In vitro fertilization.

ovarian reserve or the risk for early menopause. It is clearly important to review with patients limitations in our ability to predict fertility when attempting to select an optimal chemotherapeutic regimen.

OPTIONS FOR FERTILITY PRESERVATION BEFORE OR AFTER CANCER TREATMENT

As previously noted, the best time to assess interest in fertility preservation is at the time of diagnosis or before initiation of treatment. For example, in women with breast cancer, an optimal 6-week window of opportunity exists after breast surgery and before chemotherapy administration, during which fertility preservation can be pursued without delaying cancer treatment. This time period can perhaps be extended further, as delays of up to 12 weeks between surgery and chemotherapy have not been shown to affect disease outcome.[23] Multiple methods of preservation are available to both women

and men (Table 58-3), but the optimal methods by which to preserve ovarian and testicular tissue have not yet been delineated. Current studies are limited in size, lack randomization or adequate controls, use surrogate endpoints, and likely carry inherent bias caused by lack of referral or concern of physicians for recurrence potential. According to ASCO guidelines, anything other than sperm cryopreservation and embryo cryopreservation should be considered experimental.[20] The availability and effectiveness of other preservation techniques remain in question, but this should not deter clinicians from referring patients to discuss all potential options with fertility preservation specialists.

FERTILITY OPTIONS FOR MEN WITH CANCER
Sperm cryopreservation

The ideal preservation technique for men is sperm cryopreservation. As stated previously, it should be offered to all men,[24,25] has been proven effective,[26] and has been shown to help men cope emotionally with the effects of treatment.[27] The procedure involves extraction of sperm, through various methods, and exposure to cryopreservatives. The sperm retains much function and can be saved for thawing and future use with any fertilization procedure.

METHODS OF SPERM EXTRACTION

Options for sperm extraction depend on the timing of the extraction and previous treatment for cancer. Whether sperm is extracted for immediate use with assisted reproductive technologies or cryopreservation, pregnancy success rates are similar.[28] Before cancer treatment, a baseline functional appraisal can be obtained by collecting a semen sample via masturbation, with assessment of sperm count and motility. After treatment, remaining gonadal structure and function should be assessed. For men with at least one remaining testicle and with impairment of the nervous system (due to radiation, surgery, or chemotherapies), electroejaculation may be used. Electroejaculation is an operative procedure performed under anesthesia through direct electrical stimulation of the sympathetic nerves responsible for ejaculation.[29] When successful, intraoperative ejaculation permits sperm collection for use with other reproductive technologies. For men with at least one testicle, testicular sperm extraction (TESE), the direct retrieval of sperm from the testes, is also effective. TESE involves a surgical procedure in which microdissection of the testes allows extraction of sperm from tubules most likely to be actively engaged in spermatogenesis.[30] For later fertilization, any technique of sperm extraction can be combined with intracytoplasmic sperm injection (ICSI), or injection of a single live sperm into the center of an oocyte. Even in cases in which men have a preexisting diagnosis of azoospermia on assessment of ejaculate, TESE has been used successfully to extract sperm directly from the testicles before surgery or after chemotherapy. TESE plus ICSI is effective in producing live offspring in men with azoospermia, before or after chemotherapy.[31,32]

Treatment of retrograde ejaculation or anejaculation

Retrograde ejaculation is considered highly treatable with removal of offending medications or, when due to nerve damage, through the use of medications such as imipramine 25 to 75 mg daily.[33] For prompt restoration of fertility, referral to a specialist is often indicated. Sperm can be recovered from post-masturbation urine samples for use during assisted reproductive procedures. For men who are unable to achieve anterograde ejaculation with medications, electrovibration stimulation (EVS) can be used. EVS is performed by the affected patient by applying a specialized vibrator to the base of the penile surface. The vibrations initiate a reflex in the spinal cord that leads to anterograde ejaculation. The vibrator is applied for cycles of 3 minutes duration with 2 minutes of rest until anterograde ejaculation is achieved. EVS can be performed in a clinical setting, or within the privacy of one's home, through the guidance of a clinician. Surgical options for management of retrograde ejaculation are also available but are rarely advised. For men with anejaculation, medical treatment can be attempted but is rarely successful because of the degree of nerve impairment. Most men with anejaculation seeking fertility require EVS for fertility assistance.[33]

FERTILITY OPTIONS FOR WOMEN WITH CANCER

Embryo cryopreservation

Embryo cryopreservation is the most effective technique for fertility preservation in women. Because of its relatively high cost and the high rate of success of sperm cryopreservation options for men, embryo cryopreservation is reserved for use in preserving fertility in women before or after cancer. Embryo cryopreservation requires the presence of an available and willing partner or use of donor semen. The process involves oocyte retrieval from the woman and subsequent in vitro fertilization with her partner's or donor sperm. The embryos are then exposed to cryoprotectants and are stored at subzero temperatures until desired for use. Upon making the decision to use the embryo, thawing takes place and arrangements are made for implantation. Survival rates per thawed embryo are estimated to be around 70% but vary considerably, depending on the conditions and the procedures performed.[34,35] Rates of successful transfer and implantation can be as low as 10%.[34,35] Despite these low numbers, cumulative pregnancy rates as high as 60% have been reported.[35] Currently, few data inform the effectiveness of embryo cryopreservation with implantation and subsequent successful pregnancy outcome in cancer survivors specifically. Advantages of embryo cryopreservation include its relatively high success rate in the general population and the existence of well-tested protocols. Disadvantages include the need for a partner or donor gametes, as well as the potential exposure risk of ovarian stimulants needed for oocyte retrieval.

Oocyte retrieval options for women with cancer who are considering embryo cryopreservation must be considered in the context of whether the tumor is estrogen sensitive. Conventional protocols of ovarian stimulants, such as clomiphene, interfere with the negative feedback mechanism of endogenous estrogens on the pituitary gland and hypothalamus.[36] This cessation of feedback leads the pituitary gland to secrete follicle-stimulating hormone (FSH), which leads to ovarian follicle development and increased production of estrogen. Use of ovarian stimulants, such as clomiphene, or daily injections of FSH during the first 2 to 3 weeks of a menstrual cycle have been shown to increase serum estradiol levels in women up to 10-fold higher than normal cyclic levels. These high estradiol levels limit the safety of ovarian stimulation in women with estrogen-sensitive cancers.[35] Newer regimens involve the use of selective estrogen receptor modulators (SERMs) such as tamoxifen, or aromatase inhibitors such as letrozole, as ovarian stimulants are also effective and are believed to be safer.[37,38] Both tamoxifen and aromatase inhibitors are thought to work similarly to clomiphene, by interfering with negative feedback of endogenous estrogen on the pituitary gland and hypothalamus. Tamoxifen-based ovarian stimulation protocols result in lower serum estradiol levels than clomiphene or FSH stimulation (with a concomitant protective effect of blocking estrogen receptors on breast tissue), yet tamoxifen results in higher serum estradiol levels compared with aromatase inhibitors, such as letrozole. Despite the differences in serum estradiol levels produced by the use of tamoxifen or letrozole for ovarian stimulation, no study has documented a difference in cancer recurrence rates.[39] For any female survivor considering embryo cryopreservation, an individualized approach is needed and will depend on whether she is awaiting or has already completed treatment, as well as the specific characteristics of her tumor type.[40] As stated previously, when retrieval is planned during the time between surgical excision and initiation of chemotherapy, it is desirable to complete the retrieval process within 12 weeks to prevent potential adverse effects on cancer treatment.[23] Clinicians referring patients for fertility preservation can provide introductory information about these options, while noting that the optimal approach will require a team approach in collaboration with oncology providers and a reproductive specialist.

Experimental techniques for fertility preservation

For female cancer survivors who are not eligible for the fertility preservation procedures mentioned previously, a number of experimental procedures with limited efficacy are currently available. These techniques are not widely available and are most often applied in women who have not yet undergone exposure to cancer therapies. Experimental techniques include oocyte cryopreservation and ovarian tissue extraction. Oocyte cryopreservation is a technique in which no partner or donor sperm is needed. Oocytes are extracted via the same hormonal stimulation procedures described earlier in this chapter.[35] Unfortunately, cryopreservation techniques have not progressed to the point where oocytes consistently retain an effective level of function; consequently, reproductive outcomes thus far are poor. Another option is cryopreservation of ovarian tissue with later transplantation. Through this procedure, ovarian tissue is extracted from a woman's body and is cryopreserved and/or later transplanted to another part of her body.[41] This technique is currently used in women who need radiation therapy for cervical cancer or lymphomas.[42,43] Transplantation of a woman's ovarian tissue into an area outside the radiation field, such as into her arm, permits the tissue to remain reproductively active and capable of producing oocytes for extraction at a later date.[44,45] Currently, long-term data for ovarian tissue transplant are promising, and this procedure may become more effective with future research.[46]

ADDITIONAL FERTILITY SPARING TECHNIQUES

Gonadal shielding is an option for women and men who need to have radiation therapy directed at pelvic organs. The shielding is used to decrease the dose of radiation delivered to reproductive organs. Research on the effectiveness of gonadal shielding is limited to case series for both women and men. Limitations include the need for expertise to ensure that shielding does not magnify the doses delivered, and the fact that shielding techniques are feasible only with specific radiation fields and anatomy.[19,20]

For women with early-stage cervical cancer, hysterectomy is not necessarily required. Trachelectomy is useful for preserving fertility in women who are appropriate candidates. This procedure involves removal of the cervix with preservation of the uterus.[19] In a retrospective review of 32 consecutive women with early-stage cervical cancer who opted for trachelectomy, after a median of 31 months' follow-up, 24 women regained normal menstruation, six women attempted conception, three conceived, and one had cancer recurrence and death from recurrence.[47] Trachelectomy is considered by ASCO to be a standard therapeutic option for appropriate candidates with early-stage cervical cancer.

Finally, the use of gonadotropin-releasing hormone (GnRH) agonists to "protect" ovarian or testicular tissue during administration of chemotherapy or radiation therapy is widely studied but is still considered investigational.[19] The medication is administered before the start of therapy and is continued through to completion. No studies to date have shown consistent effectiveness for fertility preservation in humans.[48] Side effects of therapy include moderate to severe hot flashes estimated to occur in the majority of recipients and a transient rise in serum estrogen and testosterone levels, in women and men respectively, which may have a detrimental effect on hormonally sensitive cancers.

SUMMARY

Studies show that patients and their partners frequently have many questions and fears about their reproductive capacity after cancer. They rarely spontaneously ask their clinicians about these concerns. A growing number of interventions are available to help interested survivors realize their parenting goals. Therefore, regardless of cancer type or the duration of time since treatment was received, clinicians need to ask all survivors of reproductive age about their desires regarding future childbearing. As noted in this chapter, clinicians can impart valuable information and offer resources to help survivors cope with the many difficult decisions that cancer and the possibility of childbearing present. This information and support are desired and highly valued by patients and their partners and may help them cope well throughout their cancer experience.

REFERENCES

1. Bleyer A, Viny A, Barr RD. *Cancer epidemiology in older adolescents and young adults 15 to 29 years: SEER incidence and survival, 1975–2000.* Bethesda: National Cancer Institute; 2006.
2. Jemal A, Murray T, Ward E, et al. Cancer statistics, 2005. *CA Cancer J Clin.* 2005;55:10–30.
3. Jones AL. Fertility and pregnancy after breast cancer. *Breast.* 2006;15(suppl 2):S41–S46.
4. Calhoun K, Hansen N. The effect of pregnancy on survival in women with a history of breast cancer. *Breast Dis.* 2005;23:81–86.
5. Madanat LM, Malila N, Dyba T, et al. Probability of parenthood after early onset cancer: a population-based study. *Int J Cancer.* 2008;123:2891–2898.
6. Schover LR. Rates of postcancer parenthood. *J Clin Oncol.* 2009;27:321–322.
7. Schover LR. Motivation for parenthood after cancer: a review. *J Natl Cancer Inst Monogr.* 2005;34:2–5.
8. Schover LR, Rybicki LA, Martin BA, et al. Having children after cancer: a pilot survey of survivors' attitudes and experiences. *Cancer.* 1999;86:697–709.
9. Partridge AH. Fertility preservation: a vital survivorship issue for young women with breast cancer. *J Clin Oncol.* 2008;26:2612–2613.
10. Schover LR. Premature ovarian failure and its consequences: vasomotor symptoms, sexuality, and fertility. *J Clin Oncol.* 2008;26:753–758.
11. Thewes B, Meiser B, Taylor A, et al. Fertility- and menopause-related information needs of younger women with a diagnosis of early breast cancer. *J Clin Oncol.* 2005;23:5155–5165.
12. Peate M, Meiser B, Hickey M, et al. The fertility-related concerns, needs and preferences of younger women with breast cancer: a systematic review. *Breast Cancer Res Treat.* 2009;116:215–223.
13. Surbone A, Petrek JA. Childbearing issues in breast carcinoma survivors. *Cancer.* 1997;79:1271–1278.

14. Sutton R, Buzdar AU, Hortobagyi GN. Pregnancy and offspring after adjuvant chemotherapy in breast cancer patients. *Cancer*. 1990;65:847–850.

15. Berry DL, Theriault RL, Holmes FA, et al. Management of breast cancer during pregnancy using a standardized protocol. *J Clin Oncol*. 1999;17:855–861.

16. Schover LR, Brey K, Lictin A, et al. Oncologists' attitudes and practices regarding banking sperm before cancer treatment. *J Clin Oncol*. 2002;20:1890–1897.

17. Zapzalka DM, Redmon JB, Pryor JL. A survey of oncologists regarding sperm cryopreservation and assisted reproductive techniques for male cancer patients. *Cancer*. 1999;86:1812–1817.

18. Bober SL, Recklitis CJ, Campbell EG, et al. Caring for cancer survivors: a survey of primary care physicians. *Cancer*. 2009;115(18 suppl):4409–4418.

19. ASCO. Recommendations on fertility preservation in cancer patients: guideline summary. *J Oncol Pract*. 2006;2:143–146.

20. Lee SJ, Schover LR, Partridge AH, et al. American Society of Clinical Oncology recommendations on fertility preservation in cancer patients. *J Clin Oncol*. 2006;24:2917–2931.

21. Fertility guidelines address often-ignored treatment side effect. *CA Cancer J Clin*. 2006;56:251–253.

22. Ohl DA, Quallich SA, Sønksen J, et al. Anejaculation and retrograde ejaculation. *Urol Clin North Am*. 2008;35:211–220, viii.

23. Lohrisch C, Paltiel C, Gelmon K, et al. Impact on survival of time from definitive surgery to initiation of adjuvant chemotherapy for early-stage breast cancer. *J Clin Oncol*. 2006;24:4888–4894.

24. Foley SJ, De Winter P, McFarlane JP, et al. Storage of sperm and embryos: cryopreservation of sperm should be offered to men with testicular cancer. *BMJ*. 1996;313:1078.

25. Lass A, Abusheikha N, Akagbosu F, et al. Cancer patients should be offered semen cryopreservation. *BMJ*. 1999;318:1556.

26. Neal MS, Nagel K, Duckworth J, et al. Effectiveness of sperm banking in adolescents and young adults with cancer: a regional experience. *Cancer*. 2007;110:1125–1129.

27. Saito K, Suzuki K, Iwasaki A, et al. Sperm cryopreservation before cancer chemotherapy helps in the emotional battle against cancer. *Cancer*. 2005;104:521–524.

28. Schmidt KL, Larsen E, Bangsbøll S, et al. Assisted reproduction in male cancer survivors: fertility treatment and outcome in 67 couples. *Hum Reprod*. 2004;19:2806–2810.

29. Electroejaculation (EEJ). *Fertil Steril*. 2004;82(suppl 1):S204.

30. Tsujimura A. Microdissection testicular sperm extraction: prediction, outcome, and complications. *Int J Urol*. 2007;14:883–889.

31. Chan PT, Palermo GD, Veeck LL, et al. Testicular sperm extraction combined with intracytoplasmic sperm injection in the treatment of men with persistent azoospermia postchemotherapy. *Cancer*. 2001;92:1632–1637.

32. Descombe L, Chauleur C, Gentil-Perret A, et al. Testicular sperm extraction in a single cancerous testicle in patients with azoospermia: a case report. *Fertil Steril*. 2008;90:443, e1–4.

33. Kamischke A, Nieschlag E. Treatment of retrograde ejaculation and anejaculation. *Hum Reprod Update*. 1999;5:448–474.

34. Wang JX, Yap YY, Matthews CD. Frozen-thawed embryo transfer: influence of clinical factors on implantation rate and risk of multiple conception. *Hum Reprod*. 2001;16:2316–2319.

35. Sonmezer M, Oktay K. Fertility preservation in female patients. *Hum Reprod Update*. 2004;10:251–266.

36. Brown J, Farquhar C, Beck J, et al. Clomiphene and anti-oestrogens for ovulation induction in PCOS. *Cochrane Database Syst Rev*. 2009;(4):CD002249.

37. Azim AA, Costantini-Ferrando M, Oktay K. Safety of fertility preservation by ovarian stimulation with letrozole and gonadotropins in patients with breast cancer: a prospective controlled study. *J Clin Oncol*. 2008;26:2630–2635.

38. Oktay K. Further evidence on the safety and success of ovarian stimulation with letrozole and tamoxifen in breast cancer patients undergoing in vitro fertilization to cryopreserve their embryos for fertility preservation. *J Clin Oncol*. 2005;23:3858–3859.

39. Oktay K, Buyuk E, Libertella N, et al. Fertility preservation in breast cancer patients: a prospective controlled comparison of ovarian stimulation with tamoxifen and letrozole for embryo cryopreservation. *J Clin Oncol*. 2005;23:4347–4353.

40. Oktay K. An individualized approach to fertility preservation in women with cancer. *J Support Oncol*. 2006;4:181–182, 184.

41. Dobson R. Ovarian transplant raises hope for women facing cancer treatment. *BMJ*. 1999;319:871.

42. Clough KB, Goffinet F, Labib A, et al. Laparoscopic unilateral ovarian transposition prior to irradiation: prospective study of 20 cases. *Cancer*. 1996;77:2638–2645.

43. Pahisa J, Martínez-Román S, Martínez-Zamora MA, et al. Laparoscopic ovarian transposition in patients with early cervical cancer. *Int J Gynecol Cancer*. 2008;18:584–589.

44. Hilders CG, Baranski AG, Peters L, et al. Successful human ovarian autotransplantation to the upper arm. *Cancer*. 2004;101:2771–2778.

45. Oktay K. Successful human ovarian autotransplantation to the upper arm. *Cancer*. 2005;103:1982–1983 author reply 1983.

46. Kim SS, Lee WS, Chung MK, et al. Long-term ovarian function and fertility after heterotopic autotransplantation of cryobanked human ovarian tissue: 8-year experience in cancer patients. *Fertil Steril*. 2009;91:2349–2354.

47. Kim JH, Park JY, Kim DY, et al. Fertility-sparing laparoscopic radical trachelectomy for young women with early stage cervical cancer. *BJOG*. 2010;117:340–347.

48. Meistrich ML, Shetty G. Hormonal suppression for fertility preservation in males and females. *Reproduction*. 2008;136:691–701.

59 Bereavement care

Wendy G. Lichtenthal, David W. Kissane,
Maureen E. Clark, and Holly G. Prigerson

The practice of supportive oncology extends beyond the course of the patient's illness to support family, significant others, and even professional providers of care. All witness grief in many forms, beginning with the multiple losses that cancer patients suffer before their death. The patient and family members may grieve the patient's loss of physical capacity, important personal roles and activities, significant relationships, and even future plans as the patient's health declines. Health care providers help optimize coping with these losses as the disease progresses. Through the development of trusting relationships with the patient and family over the course of the illness, practitioners are in a unique position to provide continuity of care from pre-bereavement to post-bereavement.

By taking a family-centered approach during palliative care, clinicians can more readily facilitate bereavement care[1] by helping the family to understand the dying process. This may provide surviving family members with a sense of predictability and comfort. Providers should be aware of risk factors for morbid bereavement outcomes, recognize the multiple presentations of grief, and be able to manage such expressions or make appropriate referrals when risk factors are apparent or clinical intervention seems necessary.

Reactions to loss are described by many terms, which are often used interchangeably by clinicians, patients, and their families. The following are definitions that grief theorists maintain in the literature:

- *Bereavement* is the **state of having experienced a** loss resulting from death.[2,3]
- *Grief* is the distressing **emotional response** to any loss, including related feelings, cognitions, and behaviors.[2]
- *Mourning* is the **process of adaptation to a loss,** which includes expression of grief and behaviors influenced by culture, religion, and social events, such as grieving rituals.[4]
- *Anticipatory grief* is the distress and related emotions, cognitions, and behaviors that occur **before an expected loss.**[4]
- *Pathologic grief* is a severely distressing and disabling **abnormal emotional response** to loss that involves mental and/or physical dysfunction.[5–8]
- *Disenfranchised grief* occurs with losses that are not recognized by society, resulting in **less social permission to express one's grief.**[9]

This chapter begins with a brief overview of theoretical models of bereavement that have influenced our understanding of the clinical presentation of grief. We then provide descriptions of various clinical presentations that may occur over the course of the palliative care and bereavement trajectory. We consider the reactions of specific populations, including parents who lose a child to cancer and children who lose a parent. Pathologic reactions to bereavement, such as prolonged grief disorder (PGD), and related risk factors are also discussed. Finally, we present a summary of grief interventions, including broad descriptions, indications, and, when available, efficacy data.

THEORIES OF GRIEF AND BEREAVEMENT

By gaining an understanding of general bereavement theories, staff may be better able to comprehend and contextualize observed behaviors and make appropriate referrals when necessary. Theoretical models suggest adaptive tasks as well as potential preventive strategies and interventions (see references 2 and 10 for summaries).

One of the most influential frameworks for understanding separation and loss is attachment theory. This model, advanced largely by Bowlby,[11] focuses on the attachment that naturally occurs between social animals. It posits that children have an instinctual drive to bond with their caregivers, who provide safety and security, to survive. Reactions such as crying and searching when separated from an attachment figure serve the function of reuniting individuals. Studies of infants have distinguished secure from insecure attachment styles, which may be anxious, avoidant, or disorganized/hostile.[12] Theorists believe that individuals internalize working models of these early attachments,[11] and that having a more insecure attachment style increases one's risk for separation distress and prolonged grief reactions.[7,13] Adaptive grief reactions may involve continuing bonds to the deceased (i.e., maintaining connection to and the influence of the deceased in the survivor's present-day life) as a healthy by-product of attachment and the grief process.[10,14]

Early relationships are also a focal point of psychodynamic theories. Freud argued that "grief work" is necessary for adaptation to bereavement.[15] This process involves working through one's emotions to loosen the bond to, and detach libido invested in, the deceased.[2,10] Pathologic grief occurs when grief work is not accomplished.[15] Although there has not been substantial empirical support of Freud's hypotheses, some have argued that aspects of his contributions have validity and should not be completely dismissed.[2,10] Object relations theory, rooted in psychodynamics, considers the influence of the initial separation between infant and mother, which is thought to serve as a template for reactions to subsequent separations.[16] Yearning for the lost object and preserving rather than relinquishing ties are considered adaptive responses to these separations, including bereavement.[10]

Interpersonal theories of bereavement focus on the way interaction patterns and roles shape identity and self schemata, influencing how individuals grieve.[17] Past experiences are believed to influence relationship patterns, including current interpersonal choices and behaviors. Interactions and relationship roles shape the individual's identity and associated self schemata. Person schemata may be related to a lost relationship, such as an "ambivalent" schema rooted in mixed feelings about the deceased.[18] Horowitz described a treatment for stress responses to events such as bereavement that viewed these person schemata as modifiable once they are identified in current relationships.[18]

Several theories focus on the cognitive processes that are involved in adaptation to bereavement.[3,19] Parkes proposed that death forces individuals to alter their assumptions about the world being safe and predictable so they can cope with life's challenges.[3] The psychosocial transitions necessary for adaptation to a loss involve accommodating the inevitability of death into one's assumptive world.[3,20] With a constructivist perspective, Neimeyer focused on a related adaptive task, "meaning reconstruction."[21] This process involves individuals making sense of and finding meaning in the loss by developing a coherent narrative about how the loss fits into their lives. According to cognitive stress theory, cognitive appraisals of a situation determine the extent to which the event is perceived as stressful, the manner in which an individual copes with the event, and its related physiologic impact.[22] In addition to decreasing distress, making meaning of adverse life events such as bereavement can yield positive reactions, which can improve or maintain physical health. The social-functional perspective highlights the interpersonal benefits that these positive emotions can foster.[2,10,23]

Sociologic models of bereavement consider the impact of society on the individual's grief and mourning process, including culture-specific rituals such as self-mutilation. Some cultural rituals support continuing, not severing, bonds with the deceased, for instance by revering and seeking spiritual guidance from deceased ancestors.[10] The social constructionist perspective posits that the expression of grief, including the sanctioning of public and private grieving practices, is largely shaped by culture and social norms.[24] Social support also plays a large role in facilitating the grieving process, providing an outlet for emotional expression, buffering against negative consequences of other stressful events, and reducing isolation of bereaved individuals. Family systems theorists propose that individual members of a bereaved family have reciprocal influences on the grief reactions of one another.[25] Grief responses are affected by the role that the deceased individual played in the family system, as well as the family's level of functioning before the loss.[1] Poor communication, low cohesion, and increased conflict in the family have been associated with negative psychosocial outcomes during bereavement.[1,26]

The focus of cognitive-behavioral theory is on the interplay between grief-related emotions, thoughts, and behaviors, particularly those that are maladaptive and play a role in prolonged or severe grief responses.[10,27,28] Distorted cognitions (e.g., unrealistic thoughts that one should have done more to care for the deceased) and associated feelings (e.g., guilt) can result in unhelpful ruminations about the deceased. Cognitive-behavioral theory also considers the role of avoidance of triggers of painful emotions, such as reminders of the deceased, in prolonging the course of grief. Avoidance can become negatively reinforcing and may reduce opportunities to process the loss and to engage in pleasurable, corrective experiences.[28]

One of the most widely accepted contemporary theories is Stroebe and Schut's[29] dual process model of coping. This theory proposes that engagement in both loss-oriented and restoration-oriented tasks is necessary for adaptive coping, highlighting the value of both approaching and avoiding the loss.[10,29] Loss-oriented thoughts, emotions, and behaviors focus on the deceased, confronting the reality of the loss and processing positive and negative memories about the deceased, the relationship, and the future without him/her. Restoration-oriented thoughts, emotions, and behaviors are those that involve restoring functioning through assimilation in the world without the deceased. Normal functioning is reestablished as the bereaved gradually resumes and develops valued activities and relationships. Oscillation between loss-oriented and restoration-oriented phases allows bereaved individuals to actively confront their grief for a time and then find respite from their pain as they attempt to reengage in life.[2,10] Grief interventions have incorporated the dual process model into their theoretical rationales as a means of facilitating adaptive coping.[26,27,30]

All of the theories described previously may be considered within a biopsychosocial framework. In fact, initiatives to develop a neurobiopsychosocial model of grief have been advanced through the use of technology such as functional magnetic resonance imaging (fMRI).[31] For example, a recent fMRI study gave participants a grief arousal task and found increased activity in the posterior cingulate cortex, a brain region believed to be involved in retrieval of emotion-laden episodic memories.[32] The sheer number of theoretical models of bereavement developed suggests that grief is a complex process with numerous influences. Integration of biological, psychological, social, and behavioral viewpoints is critical to a comprehensive understanding of observed bereavement phenomena.[2]

CLINICAL PRESENTATIONS OF GRIEF

Supportive care clinicians may witness grieving in numerous contexts, including the emergence of anticipatory grief as illness progresses, acute grief at the time of death, and, in some cases, prolonged grieving that does not dissipate over time.

ANTICIPATORY GRIEF

The grief of cancer patients and their families may begin well before the patient's death. In fact, both patients and family members may perceive the illness as fatal at the initial moment of diagnosis.[4] Cognitive and emotional acceptance of a terminal prognosis is a dynamic process, waxing and waning as acknowledgment of the prognosis competes with a desire to maintain hope for a cure. Loved ones may present with unrealistic optimism, protest, anger, or heightened protectiveness of the patient. The challenge of accepting that the patient is going to die involves a complex interplay between one's basic personality, the availability of social support, and one's spiritual and existential views on life. A psychological process of adaptation evolves throughout the course of an illness.[33,34] Achieving cognitive and emotional acceptance is important to bereavement care because of the role it can play in facilitating adjustment post loss.[35] Without the ability or opportunity to come to terms with a patient's prognosis, survivors are more at risk for a complicated course of bereavement and developing PGD after the patient dies.[35]

Anticipatory grieving may intensify when bad news or serious disease progression is communicated to the patient and family. By using sensitive communication approaches, providers can assist the family in processing clinical information and revising their expectations if necessary. This may allow loved ones the chance to mentally prepare for the loss. As additional losses associated with advanced illness occur, there may be opportunities for family members to express their attachment through acts of caregiving. Through these acts and through efforts to resolve any relationship issues, families may grow closer and more cohesive. However, families with greater dysfunction may experience more tension and conflict as some members react with denial, hostility, avoidance, or other maladaptive behaviors.[26]

Although some theorists have suggested that the presence of anticipatory grief diminishes the intensity of post-loss grief, studies in this area have yielded inconsistent findings. Intense anticipatory grief is a risk factor for clinical depression.[36] These discrepancies may be due to variations in how anticipatory grief is operationally defined. The experience of grieving before the death should be distinguished from being prepared for the loss, which has been associated with the presence of PGD.[37] Even when the course of illness is lengthy, survivors may perceive the death as sudden. Providers can help patients and families psychologically prepare for the patient's death and foster positive emotions during stressful times by encouraging open communication and opportunities to say goodbye, allowing them to address unfinished business and express appreciation for one another.[1]

GRIEF AROUND THE TIME OF DEATH

Family members at the patient's bedside are often emotional and exceptionally attentive to details associated with the patient's well-being. The final moments of the patient's life often remain as vivid memories in the survivors' minds long after the patient's death. Even though many sources of distress may not be readily visible or easily articulated by patients, their influence on the end-of-life experience can be profound.[38] Clinicians must exhibit the utmost respect and sensitivity at this time. Practitioners working at the patient's bedside frequently have the opportunity to provide important consoling information, including reassurance about the patient's comfort and clear explanations in layperson's terms about the dying process, including the meaning of sounds, secretions, changes in breathing, and alterations in levels of consciousness. Providing family members with information about what to expect can be extremely helpful in preparing them for the death and reducing distress as they witness end-of-life symptoms.

When death appears imminent, providers should contact family members who are not present. Relatives who cannot visit before the death occurs should be offered an opportunity to view the patient's body and be given information about the sequence of events leading up to the death. Clinicians should take time to provide support and answer questions thoroughly. Culture may play a significant role in expressions of acute grief. Staff ought to respect and honor cultural and religious practices, including those related to autopsy and time alone with the patient. Providers may facilitate pastoral counseling and may wish to consult with a cultural intermediary to assist with sensitive and appropriate responses to a family's practices and needs. Clinicians should make efforts to prevent disenfranchised grief,[9] encouraging expression of sorrow for relationships that may not have been accepted and making efforts not to minimize expected deaths. Families are often deeply appreciative when providers communicate their sympathy through a phone call or other personal channels. A letter of condolence can provide a grieving family with concrete expression of the provider's care that may be reviewed in the future, while also providing a sense of closure for the professional.[39] Support may also be offered through provision of prescriptions for anxiolytics or sleep aids, referrals for psychosocial services, and guidance about making funeral arrangements.

ACUTE GRIEF FOLLOWING THE DEATH

The first empirical investigation of acute grief phenomena was conducted by Lindemann, who examined the reactions of bereaved relatives of individuals who perished in a 1942 Boston nightclub fire.[40] Lindemann described acute grief as a characteristic syndrome of affective and somatic symptoms, such as sadness, anger, guilt, shortness of breath, and physical identification symptoms that the deceased experienced.[40] Because these distressing symptoms may be intense and variable, even within a given family system, it is often difficult to distinguish between "normal" and pathologic responses during the first months of bereavement. Adaptive acute grief has characteristic emotions, cognitions, behaviors, and physical symptoms that come and go in waves. Emotional reactions include sadness, guilt, anger, distress, and anxiety.[3,10] Initially, a profound sense of yearning occurs for the lost individual. When patients are significantly suffering as they approach death, surviving family members may, in parallel to their sadness, experience a sense of relief. They may also experience numbness or disbelief if the death was not expected to occur so soon, particularly if the death was sudden and due to disease-related complications. Grief-related thoughts range from purposeful reminiscing about the deceased to intrusive images and memories. The bereaved may anticipate the absence of the deceased in expected future life events (e.g., graduations, weddings). Behaviors include searching for the deceased, particularly when confronted with personal reminders of their loved one, and social withdrawal. Individuals may also seek support and comfort. Physical symptoms include difficulty sleeping, fatigue, anorexia, mild weight loss, numbness, restlessness, tension, tremors, and sometimes pain.

Acute grief and its associated features may reflect difficulty in informational and emotional processing of the reality of the loss. Research has demonstrated that as grief decreases over time, acceptance increases.[41] Grief at its height might reflect the emotional consequences of the inability to accept the loss and to continue wanting what one cannot have.[41] Acceptance of the loss, by contrast, may represent emotional equanimity, that is, a sense of inner peace and tranquility that comes with relinquishing the struggle to regain what is lost or is being taken away as one rebuilds his/her life.[42] Greater acceptance has been associated with less suffering, implying that benefits may be derived from promoting acceptance.[42] Clinicians may be uniquely positioned to facilitate this process.

For many years, the stage theory of grief resolution was widely accepted in the bereavement field. This theory proposed that "normal" or adaptive grief required consecutive passing through the stages of shock—yearning or angry protest to sad or depressed mood to, finally, acceptance of the loss.[43,44] The top panel of Figure 59-1 illustrates this sequence.

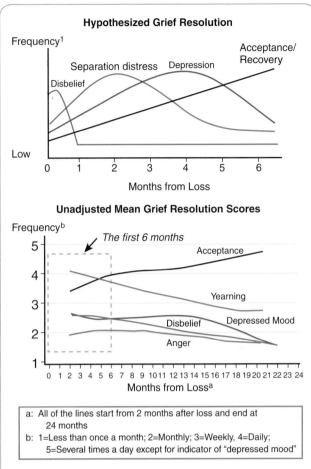

Fig. 59-1 Proposed grief resolution model and observed grief symptoms over time. (*Redrawn from Pathologic grief: maladaptation to loss [Copyright 1993, American Psychiatric Publishing, Inc.].*[1])

To examine its validity, an empirical study of the stage theory was conducted with bereaved participants in the community-based Yale Bereavement Study.[45] Results showed that, rather than shock and disbelief, the most common initial grief symptom was yearning,[45] as presented in the bottom panel of Figure 59-1. Participants were assessed between 2 and 24 months post loss, and it is possible that shock or other symptoms were elevated during the first 2 months, but were not captured in this investigation.[45] A trajectory of gradual reductions in levels of shock, yearning, and sad mood represents the pattern of normal mourning. Anger levels remained low and relatively stable, and acceptance increased over time. When these grief indicators were rescaled and compared, their respective peak frequencies in the first 6 months post loss occurred in a sequence similar to the order of stages proposed by past bereavement theorists[3,44] (see Fig. 59-1).

The common contemporary perspective is that stages of grief overlap and intense emotions may wax and wane in the early phases of bereavement. Bereaved individuals may continue their bond to the deceased and reexperience grief symptoms intermittently throughout their lives.[10] Bereavement theorists widely believe that adaptive coping involves the dynamic oscillation between confrontation of the loss and related emotions and reengagement in life without the deceased, as proposed by the dual process model of coping.[29] Cultural sanctions may influence expressions of grief, including its duration. However, no absolute timeline exists for the adaptation process, as the duration and intensity of symptoms are often proportionate to the strength of the attachment to the deceased. The absence of grief symptoms may reflect, therefore, either a weak attachment to the deceased or coping with strong emotions through denial or dissociation.

Although grief often does not completely "resolve," studies suggest that 80% to 90% of bereaved individuals have largely begun to accept the death of their loved one and to adapt by 6 months after the loss.[7] This adaptation is characterized by individuals' ability to acknowledge the death and to begin to transform their relationship to the deceased. It also involves restoring functioning through reengagement in work, leisure, and creative activities and the development of new and existing personal relationships. As time passes, bereaved individuals are able to find meaning and purpose in their lives and to consider the future as fulfilling and satisfying.[42] Although they may continue to grieve throughout their lives, particularly when reminders of the deceased or anniversaries present, the intensity and duration of their reactions will gradually diminish. In fact, resilience following bereavement is common.[2,10,46]

PATHOLOGIC RESPONSES TO BEREAVEMENT

Intense distress and periods of sadness and anxiety are typical in the acute phase of grief. When bereavement-related psychological symptoms interact with an individual's existing vulnerabilities, however, symptoms of depressive and anxiety disorders may emerge. In a longitudinal study of bereaved widows, Zisook and Schucter[47] found that 24% of their sample met criteria for major depression 2 months after their loss, with rates decreasing to 16% by 13 months post loss. Given that sadness is common during the early months of bereavement, the diagnosis of clinical depression becomes warranted when more pathologic features, such as profound loss of interest, pervasive sadness, psychomotor retardation, deep guilt, worthlessness, hopelessness, helplessness, loss of meaning, and/or suicidal ideation, are present.[48] Neurovegetative depressive symptoms are less discriminatory. Anxiety disorders are also prevalent, and bereaved individuals may present with separation anxiety, generalized anxiety, phobic, and somatic symptoms. When family members witness circumstances that they perceive as traumatic, such as gross disfigurement, bedsores, foul odor, agitated confusion, or even an insufficient goodbye, symptoms of posttraumatic stress disorder (PTSD) may manifest. Individuals with a history of alcohol or other substance use, psychosis, or bipolar disorder are at increased risk of relapsing following bereavement. According to the *Diagnostic and Statistical Manual of Mental Disorders, Fourth Edition, Text Revision (DSM-IV-TR)*[49] guidelines, clinicians should not make a diagnosis of an adjustment disorder if the clinical symptoms are due to the stress of bereavement.

PROLONGED GRIEF DISORDER

Normatively, as bereaved individuals move toward acceptance of their loss and adaptation to life without the deceased, the intensity and severity of grief symptoms dissipate over time. However, approximately 10% to 20% exhibit a more prolonged and severe grief response.[7,8] These individuals often seem "stuck" in their grief, with the acute, intense grief symptoms that are frequently observed immediately after a loss persisting over time. To assist clinicians in identifying these individuals, researchers have empirically derived diagnostic criteria of PGD, which is characterized by a cluster of symptoms that is distinct from symptoms of bereavement-related depression and anxiety.[7,8] Although PGD may be comorbid with depression or anxiety, discriminating symptoms include intense yearning and longing for the deceased, preoccupying ruminations, intrusive painful thoughts, disbelief and trouble accepting the reality of the loss, and difficulty finding meaning and moving forward in their lives without their loved one. These are clinically distinct from symptoms of depression, such as depressed mood, psychomotor retardation, and changes in appetite or weight.[50] Diagnoses of PGD and PTSD may co-occur, but PGD may manifest following traumatic or nontraumatic losses. In a study of bereaved individuals assessed for major depressive disorder, PTSD, and PGD, Barry et al.[37] found that PGD was the most common disorder 4 and 9 months post loss, and that overlap between these diagnoses was modest. Silverman et al.[51] similarly examined the prevalence of these mental disorders in a different cohort and found that PGD was most prevalent and had the lowest comorbidity rate. PGD has been associated with increased risk of negative mental and physical health outcomes, including cancer, hypertension, cardiac events, adverse health behaviors, hospitalization, depressive symptoms, functional impairment, and suicidal ideation.[52-54]

Bereavement experts have proposed that PGD, formerly referred to in the literature as complicated grief and traumatic grief, should be established as a distinct mental disorder in the next edition of the *Diagnostic and Statistical Manual of Mental Disorders*[36] (i.e., *DSM-V*).[8,50] The proposed diagnostic criteria[8] are presented in Box 59-1. Note that a diagnosis of PGD should not be made until at least 6 months has elapsed since the death. This criterion is sensitive enough to identify individuals who might benefit from intervention because their grief is persisting, while attempting to avoid pathologizing the reactions of those individuals whose grief will resolve naturally with time.[8] Typically, onset of symptoms occurs at the time of death, but delayed and chronic grief can also meet the 6-month timing criterion.

Bereavement experts have described pathologic grief responses for decades. Many subtypes have been used to characterize grief pathology in the literature, including *chronic grief, inhibited grief,* and *delayed grief*.[3,10] Despite a consensus that pathologic responses to bereavement exist, debates about whether symptoms of PGD should be established as a distinct mental disorder remain, as "normal" and abnormal grief responses are believed to fall on the same continuum. Pathologic symptoms consist of intensified and prolonged manifestations of acute grief symptoms. Advocates of establishing PGD as a mental disorder argue that doing so will allow consistent identification of individuals in need by researchers, clinicians, and even insurance companies, to facilitate the development and delivery of appropriate interventions.[7,8,50] Detractors worry that PGD will result in stigmatization and potential medicalization of normal reactions to loss and will inhibit family members' willingness to intervene.[55]

BOX 59-1 Proposed Diagnostic Criteria for Prolonged Grief Disorder (PGD)

A. Event Criterion: Bereavement (loss of a significant other).

B. Separation Distress: The bereaved person experiences yearning (e.g., craving, pining, longing for the deceased; physical or emotional suffering as a result of the desired, but unfulfilled, reunion with the deceased) daily or to a disabling degree.

C. Cognitive, Emotional, and Behavioral Symptoms: The bereaved person must have five (or more) of the following symptoms experienced daily or to a disabling degree:
(1) Confusion about one's role in life or diminished sense of self (i.e., feeling that a part of oneself has died)
(2) Difficulty accepting the loss
(3) Avoidance of reminders of the reality of the loss
(4) Inability to trust others since the loss
(5) Bitterness or anger related to the loss
(6) Difficulty moving on with life (e.g., making new friends, pursuing interests)
(7) Numbness (absence of emotion) since the loss
(8) Feeling that life is unfulfilling, empty, and meaningless since the loss
(9) Feeling stunned, dazed, or shocked by the loss

D. Timing: Diagnosis should not be made until at least 6 months has elapsed since the death.

E. Impairment: The disturbance causes clinically significant impairment in social, occupational, or other important areas of functioning (e.g., domestic responsibilities).

F. Relation to Other Mental Disorders: The disturbance is not better accounted for by Major Depressive Disorder, Generalized Anxiety Disorder, or Posttraumatic Stress Disorder.

Note: Proposed diagnostic criteria for PGD outlined by Prigerson HG, Horowitz MJ, Jacobs SC, et al.[8]

Table 59-1 Risk factors for pathologic grief outcomes

Category	Description
Circumstances of death	• Perceived lack of preparedness for loss • Untimely within the life cycle (e.g., death of child) • Sudden and unexpected (e.g., death from septic neutropenia during chemotherapy) • Traumatic (e.g., shocking cachexia and debility) • Stigmatized (e.g., AIDS, suicide)
Personal vulnerability	• History of psychiatric disorder (e.g., clinical depression, separation anxiety) • Childhood adversity (e.g., abuse, neglect, controlling parenting) • Personality and coping style (e.g., intense worrier, low self-esteem) • Attachment style (e.g., insecure) • Cumulative experience of losses
Nature of the relationship to the deceased	• Overly dependent (e.g., security-enhancing relationship) • Ambivalent (e.g., angry and insecure with alcohol abuse, infidelity, gambling)
Family and social support	• Family dysfunction (e.g., poor cohesion and communication, high conflict) • Isolated (e.g., new migrant, new residential move) • Alienated (e.g., perception of low social support)

AIDS, Acquired immunodeficiency syndrome.

RISK FACTORS

A majority of bereaved individuals will adapt over time to the death of a loved one from cancer without requiring intervention. When support resources are limited, it is particularly important to triage those at heightened risk for poor outcomes to psychosocial support services. Staff should hold a regular multidisciplinary death review to identify family members at risk for psychopathology.[1,10] Table 59-1 presents common risk factors for negative bereavement outcomes. Individuals at risk for psychiatric disorders in general are vulnerable to the onset or recurrence of disturbances during bereavement. Studies of the causes of PGD have demonstrated the key role of early disturbances in secure attachment. Empirically identified risk factors include insecure attachment styles[56,57]; high marital dependency and close, security-enhancing relationships[57,58]; close kinship relationships to the deceased[57,59]; childhood separation anxiety[13]; childhood adversity[51] (e.g., abuse, serious neglect, parent death); and controlling parents.[60] PGD has also been associated with being African American,[42] having lower perceived preparedness for the loss,[37] and having lower levels of social support.[61] Although peaceful acceptance of dying may reduce survivors' risk for poor outcomes, clearly not all dying patients or bereaved family members will be able to confront loss with peace and equanimity.[35] However, clinicians may be ble to foster death acceptance and to provide support or referrals to those individuals who appear to be at greater risk for psychological distress and prolonged suffering.

SPECIFIC CIRCUMSTANCES

SUDDEN DEATH

Sudden death in oncology occurs in one quarter of patients, when infection, clots, or cardiac events interrupt the predicted cancer trajectory.[62] Perceptions that a death was sudden are often due to the family member's expectations about the amount of time they had left with the patient. These expectations might be based on the prognosis given or on the number of times the patient had near-fatal experiences but eventually recovered. Such experiences can reduce the family's preparedness for the death actually occurring following an acute secondary condition, such as sepsis, pulmonary emboli, cardiac events, or hemorrhage.

Although families may have an intellectual understanding that the illness is terminal, they might still be unable to process this information on an emotional level. Emotional acceptance of a terminal prognosis is associated with feeling less terrified and more supported.[63] Family members with greater acceptance that the patient is dying are more likely to feel prepared for the loss and less likely to experience negative bereavement outcomes.[37] Improved quality of life among bereaved family members has also been associated with patients' peaceful awareness of their prognosis, which is predictive of advance care planning, and greater mental and physical health in the last week of life.[35] Conversely, those who experience the death as sudden or themselves as psychologically unprepared for the loss are at greater risk for PGD and depression, particularly when the death is perceived as violent.[7,37] Clinicians should assess family members' understanding of the circumstances surrounding the death and help the bereaved make sense of any aspects that were perplexing.

GRIEF DURING CHILDHOOD

The grief reaction of a child who loses a parent or other attachment figure is dependent on his/her developmental stage.[4,10] Children may not understand the irreversibility of death until they have developed the capacity for abstract thinking, which usually occurs around ages 8 to 10. Mourning can be facilitated and supported through open discussion of the death by the surviving parent and family. Clinicians can provide guidance to surviving parents by encouraging the child's attendance at and participation in bereavement rituals and fostering emotional expression through family activities and creation of a memory book, to continue the child's connection to the deceased.[4,10]

LOSS OF A CHILD

The loss of a child to cancer is one of the most intense and prolonged types of bereavement.[64] It often occurs after a lengthy battle with the illness and deep investment in providing care for the child. When caregiving for the child has long been the priority, parents may become disconnected from other relationships and roles that were meaningful. The intense pain of acute grief often deepens their sense of isolation. Parents may find solace in connecting with other bereaved parents through support groups. They may need additional assistance coping with guilt related to concerns that they could have done more to prevent the death. Finding ways to honor and memorialize their child's life may help parents to move forward, and so staff should facilitate this when possible.

Many aspects of parental grief that have been viewed as pathologic in other settings of bereavement (e.g., prolonged yearning) may, in fact, be typical of the experience of losing a child.[64] Researchers have found heightened anxiety and depression among parents bereaved by cancer that persists 4 to 6 years after the loss.[65] Among those parents with unresolved grief, poorer mental and physical health, increased health service use, and increased sick leave from work have been reported.[66] The course of parental bereavement is highly individual, and many factors can influence it.[67] Parents who appear to be at greater risk for poor adjustment are those who, before their loss, have difficulty accepting the possibility of death and have weak emotional bonds with others, and following their loss, have difficulties relating to others and redefining their identity and purpose in life.[67]

Clinicians can play an influential role in parents' adjustment to bereavement before the child's death. Parents often do not recognize their dying child's poor prognosis, resulting in aggressive care at the end of life. Research suggests that parents who report the highest quality of care are those who feel most prepared for the end-of-life care period. Although providers may be reluctant to discuss the child's prognosis because it is painful and difficult to predict, sensitive, open, clear, and supportive communication about how the end of the child's life may unfold can be very helpful.[68] Following the child's death, providers should use the child's name when speaking of him or her to the family and should offer to be available to answer questions if any arise over the course of the parents' bereavement. Clinicians should recognize that they, themselves, often have strong emotional reactions to the death of a child and can benefit from outlets to express their own feelings.

INTERVENTIONS

Research on grief interventions has yielded inconclusive findings, which, in large part, may be due to the inconsistent methodologic rigor of treatment outcome studies. Many studies have lacked adequate control groups, random assignment, treatment adherence monitoring, and standardized and blinded outcome assessments, and have had unexplained dropouts. A number of systematic reviews and meta-analyses of grief interventions have been conducted to determine which bereaved populations might benefit from psychotherapy and counseling.[69–72] Table 59-2 presents a summary of these studies. With small to moderate effects for grief interventions, the research suggests that psychosocial treatment generally is not efficacious. Researchers have debated the meaning of these results. Some have argued that the effects are small because, for the majority of individuals, grief and related symptoms diminish naturally over time.[72,73] Others have advocated cautious optimism about the utility of grief counseling.[74] Although the results of grief intervention trials in general have been variable, interventions that target bereaved individuals at high risk for or exhibiting poorer adjustment have consistently demonstrated stronger effects.[72]

STAFF SUPPORT

Families generally appreciate when oncology staff members connect with them following the patient's death, particularly when close relationships have developed over the course of the patient's care. Condolences may be offered over the telephone, through a sympathy card or personal visits, or by attending the funeral. Staff may also choose to hold an annual commemoration service for the deceased and include bereaved families in this ritual.

INDIVIDUAL PSYCHOTHERAPY
Supportive counseling

Support is a key component of many therapeutic approaches. Interventions that focus on support create a safe forum for emotional expression and time to focus on the loss, which can facilitate the natural adaptive grieving process.[19] Providing validation and encouragement, supportive counselors also promote adaptation and restoration through discussion of future personal goals related to moving forward with life in the absence of the deceased.

Table 59-2 Systematic reviews and meta-analyses of bereavement interventions

Authors	Number of studies included	Study characteristics	Effect size	Possible conclusions
Currier, Neimeyer, and Berman[72]	61	Randomized and nonrandomized studies No-intervention control group Participants did not choose study condition 48 peer-reviewed articles and 16 dissertations	0.16*	Generally, all participants (intervention and control) improved over time Clinical and self-referrals associated with better outcomes, although differences diminished at follow-up Age/sex of participants and timing of intervention did not appear to influence effects
Currier, Holland, and Neimeyer[71]	13	Controlled studies of interventions for children	0.14	Lack of support for efficacy of interventions Earlier intervention yielded stronger effects Targeting distressed associated with better outcomes
Allumbaugh and Hoyt[69]	35	Controlled and noncontrolled	0.43	Effects stronger for self-identified participants Low statistical power Moderating variables influence effects
Kato and Mann[70]	13	Randomized controlled trials Treatment and control groups recruited similarly Post-loss interventions	0.11	Interventions may be ineffective Control groups also improve May need stronger dose of interventions Methodologic problems common
Fortner and Neimeyer[84†]	23	Randomized controlled trials	0.13	Greater effects with high-risk populations
Schut, Stroebe, van den Bout, and Terheggen[85]	16 primary; 7 secondary; 7 tertiary‡	Organized help Focused on treating grief Methodologically sound	Low to Modest effects	Strongest effects with individuals exhibiting psychopathology/pathologic grief Greater effects with self-referred
Jordan and Neimeyer[73]	4	Reviews and meta-analyses	N/A	Generally low efficacy of interventions Intervention may not be necessary for most bereaved Need to develop new approaches Need to improve study methods

*The effect size of $d = 0.16$ was for randomized studies at posttreatment; for nonrandomized studies (n = 12), the effect size was $d = 0.51$ at posttreatment. Tests of both effect size estimates were statistically significant.
†From unpublished work of Fortner and Neimeyer (1999) as described by Neimeyer.[84]
‡Primary preventive interventions were open to all bereaved individuals. Secondary preventive interventions were open to high-risk individuals. Tertiary preventive interventions were open to individuals with complicated grief or other psychopathology.

Psychodynamic and interpersonal psychotherapies

Psychodynamic approaches consider the influence that childhood experiences and internalized object relations may be playing in the patient's unconscious conflicts and current related grief response. Psychotherapy is typically a longer-term process. There is a limited but growing evidence base for psychodynamic therapies, with the majority of trials focusing on supportive-expressive approaches.[75] Individuals who struggle with unresolved issues influenced by early relationships and conflicts, including those related to attachment security, might benefit from a psychodynamic approach.

Another treatment based on psychodynamic theory is interpersonal psychotherapy (IPT), a short-term (12 to 16 weeks) manualized approach that focuses on relationship problems that are believed to maintain symptoms. It was originally designed to treat depression but has been applied to treat a variety of disorders in several populations.[76] IPT therapists choose a target area to focus on, which may include role disputes, role transitions, interpersonal deficits, or complicated grief. When unresolved grief is targeted, patients work on reengaging in or developing relationships using strategies such as communication skill building. IPT is indicated for bereaved individuals exhibiting current interpersonal functioning issues.

Cognitive-behavioral therapy

Cognitive-behavioral therapy (CBT) focuses on identifying and restructuring maladaptive thoughts and behaviors. For bereaved individuals, CBT approaches involve modification of dysfunctional thinking that prevents adaptive processing of the loss. Behavioral strategies include exposure to avoided thoughts and situations, as well as engagement in restoration-oriented, pleasurable activities.[28] CBT is indicated when individuals are struggling with excessive guilt and anger that may be fueled by cognitive distortions about, for example, the relationship to the deceased or circumstances surrounding the death. CBT also may be helpful for those avoiding reminders of the loss or avoiding resuming functional activities. For individuals suffering from severe depression following bereavement, research suggests that CBT is more effective than IPT.[76]

GROUP PSYCHOTHERAPY

Bereavement groups permit mutual support among individuals who have experienced similar types of losses. Members can provide validation to one another, while reducing the isolation that may occur during bereavement. Groups additionally facilitate emotional expression and processing and share effective coping strategies. In studies of short-term group psychotherapy for individuals with complicated grief (i.e., PGD), Piper and colleagues[77–79] found that bereaved individuals were more likely to benefit from the treatment group if they had more social support; a history of mature relationships; and higher levels of extraversion, openness, and conscientiousness.

FAMILY THERAPY

Using a family-centered approach throughout the course of cancer treatment and palliative care permits providers to identify those who might be at risk for poor psychological outcomes after death. Kissane et al.[1,26] developed family-focused grief therapy (FFGT), a 6- to 10-session preventive intervention designed to facilitate continuity of care. Families are screened to identify those with high conflict, low cohesion, and/or communication deficits while the patient is receiving palliative care. Therapy begins at this time and continues through bereavement, targeting dysfunctional families and "intermediate" families, who exhibit moderate challenges in their ability to relate effectively. Commencing therapy while the patient is still alive allows clinicians to understand the impact of the illness on the family and how it may affect their adjustment post loss. The goals of FFGT are to facilitate mutual support and the sharing of grief. A randomized controlled trial (RCT) of FFGT demonstrated significant reductions in distress among family members 13 months after the patient's death.[26,80] An ongoing RCT is comparing the dose intensity of 6 or 10 sessions of FFGT for high-risk families at Memorial Sloan-Kettering Cancer Center and other local institutions. By implementing routine screening of family functioning and interventions such as FFGT in oncology settings, more dysfunctional families can be identified, and morbid grief outcomes may be prevented.

INTERNET INTERVENTIONS

Internet-based mental health interventions provide a promising vehicle to promote mental health and overcome barriers to accessing care by offering mental health information and home-based, self-help treatments to underserved populations.[81] Self-disclosure may be facilitated by the anonymity of the computer.[82] It may also provide much needed assistance to grieving individuals who find it too painful to return to the institution where their loved one was treated. Internet delivery of more directive intervention approaches (e.g., CBT) may help reduce symptoms of psychiatric disorders such as PGD, depression, and PTSD.[81]

Combined psychopharmacologic approaches

Bereavement-related mental disorders are wisely treated using appropriate combinations of standard psychopharmacologic and psychotherapeutic approaches.[2,10] Anxiolytics and sleep aids may be particularly useful during the acute phase of bereavement. Selective serotonin and noradrenergic reuptake inhibitors may be used to reduce depressive symptoms.

Treatments for PGD

Symptoms of PGD can be resistant to traditional treatments for bereavement-related depression (e.g., IPT, antidepressants).[7,50] Specific interventions designed to treat PGD have been developed. Shear et al.[27] developed Complicated Grief Treatment (CGT), a 16-session manualized treatment that incorporates psychoeducation about the dual process model of bereavement coping with CBT approaches such as exposure to avoided loss-related thoughts, retelling the story of the death, imaginal conversations with the deceased, and development of personal goals to assist with restorative behaviors. An RCT comparing CGT to IPT found that a larger percentage of patients responded to CBT (51%) than to IPT (28%), and that the time to response for patients receiving CGT was more rapid.[27]

Boelen et al.[83] compared a 12-session CBT intervention designed to treat PGD versus supportive counseling. They found that CBT was more efficacious in reducing PGD and other psychopathologic symptoms than the comparison arm. Greater benefits were found with exposure than with cognitive restructuring techniques, and when treatment began with exposure followed by cognitive restructuring, as opposed to when the order of these techniques was reversed.[83]

CONCLUSIONS

Several theoretical models of bereavement have been proposed, each offering a unique perspective on the grieving experience of individuals who survive the loss of a loved one to cancer. These models are not mutually exclusive and can be integrated within a biopsychosocial framework to provide a comprehensive understanding of observed reactions and to develop effective interventions. Given the variety of disciplines and theoretical perspectives of grief, it is not surprising that a significant divide between clinical practice and research often exists in this field.[2] Grief intervention research has been hindered by this and the challenges of recruiting and designing methodologically rigorous treatment outcome studies with vulnerable bereaved populations. Despite these issues, clinicians should make efforts to provide support to bereaved individuals through the application of, or referral for, empirically supported treatments.

Controversial issues in the field of bereavement include whether it is appropriate to distinguish normal, or typical, grief from more pathologic reactions such as PGD. Efforts are being made to establish PGD as a mental disorder in *DSM-V*. Psychotherapy for grief should target those individuals who are at greatest risk and would likely benefit the most. Lower effect sizes observed in past grief intervention clinical trials were likely related to the inclusion of well-adjusted bereaved individuals whose grief dissipated naturally over time.[72,85] By studying bereaved individuals who exhibit resilience after their loss,[10,46] we can learn more about adaptive pathways that can be promoted through support and intervention.

The importance of continuity of care for families from end of life through bereavement is gaining increasing recognition in palliative care. Oncology clinicians are uniquely positioned to facilitate this continuity, but there remains a great need to establish infrastructures that support these efforts within cancer treatment settings. Bereavement care begins before the patient's death by screening for risk factors to identify family members who may be in need of continued support post loss, and by applying evidence-based interventions to reduce the suffering of those in greatest need.

REFERENCES

1. Kissane DW, Bloch S. *Family focused grief therapy: a model of family-centered care during palliative care and bereavement*. Buckingham: Open University Press; 2002.

2. Genevro J, Marshall T, Miller T. Report on bereavement and grief research. *Death Stud*. 2004;28:491–575.

3. Parkes C. *Bereavement studies of grief in adult life*. 3rd ed. Madison, CT: International Universities Press; 1998.

4. Raphael B. *The anatomy of bereavement*. London: Hutchinson; 1983.

5. Klass D, Walter T. Processes of grieving: how bonds are continued. In: Stroebe MS, Hansson RO, et al., eds. *Handbook of bereavement research: consequences, coping, and care*. Washington, DC: American Psychological Association; 2001:431–448.

6. Jacobs S. *Pathologic grief: maladaptation to loss*. Washington, DC: American Psychiatric Press; 1993.

7. Prigerson HG, Vanderwerker LC, Maciejewski PK. A case for inclusion of prolonged grief disorder in DSM-V. In: Stroebe M, Hansson R, et al., eds. *Handbook of bereavement research and practice: advances in theory and intervention*. Washington, DC: American Psychological Association; 2008:165–186.

8. Prigerson HG, Horowitz MJ, Jacobs SC, et al. Prolonged grief disorder: psychometric validation of criteria proposed for DSM-V and ICD-11. *PLoS Med*. 2009;6:e100–e121.

9. Doka K. Disenfranchised grief. In: Doka K, ed. *Disenfranchised grief: recognizing hidden sorrow*. Lexington, MA: Lexington Books; 1989:3–11.

10. Stroebe M, Hansson R, Stroebe W, et al., eds. *Handbook of bereavement research: consequences, coping, and care*. Washington, DC: American Psychological Association; 2001.

11. Bowlby J. The making and breaking of affectional bonds I & II. *Br J Psychiatry*. 1977;130:201–210 421–431.

12. Ainsworth M, Blehar M, Waters E, et al. *Patterns of attachment: a psychological study of the strange situation*. Hillsdale, NJ: Erlbaum; 1978.

13. Vanderwerker LC, Jacobs SC, Parkes CM, et al. An exploration of associations between separation anxiety in childhood and complicated grief in later life. *J Nerv Mental Dis*. 2006;194:121–123.

14. Field NP, Gao B, Paderna L. Continuing bonds in bereavement: an attachment theory based perspective. *Death Stud*. 2005;29:277–299.

15. Freud S. *Mourning and melancholia*. vol 14. London: Hogarth; 1917.

16. Field NP, Sturgeon SE, Puryear R, et al. Object relations as a predictor of adjustment in conjugal bereavement. *Dev Psychopathol*. 2001;13:399–412.

17. Shapiro ER. Grief in interpersonal perspective: theories and their implications. In: Stroebe M, Hansson R, et al., eds. *Handbook of bereavement research: consequences, coping, and care*. Washington, DC: American Psychological Association; 2001:301–327.

18. Horowitz MJ. A model of mourning: change in schemas of self and other. *J Am Psychoanal Assoc*. 1990;38:297–324.

19. Worden JW. *Grief counseling and grief therapy: a handbook for the mental health practitioner*. 4th ed. New York: Springer Publishers; 2008.

20. Janoff-Bulman R. *Shattered assumptions: towards a new psychology of trauma*. New York: Free Press; 1992.

21. Neimeyer R. *Meaning reconstruction and the experience of loss*. Washington, DC: American Psychological Association; 2001.

22. Stroebe MS, Folkman S, Hansson RO, et al. The prediction of bereavement outcome: development of an integrative risk factor framework. *Soc Sci Med*. 2006;63:2440–2451.

23. Bonanno GA, Kaltman S. Toward an integrative perspective on bereavement. *Psychol Bull*. 1999;125:760–776.

24. Rosenblatt PC. A social constructionist perspective on cultural differences in grief. In: Stroebe MS, Hansson RO, et al., eds. *Handbook of bereavement research: consequences, coping, and care*. Washington, DC: American Psychological Association; 2001:298–300.

25. Walsh F, McGoldrick M. Loss and the family: a systemic perspective. In: Walsh F, McGoldrick M, eds. *Living beyond loss: death in the family*. New York: Norton; 1991:1–29.

26. Kissane D, Bloch S, McKenzie M, et al. Family focused grief therapy: a randomized controlled trial in palliative care and bereavement. *Am J Psychiatry*. 2006;163:1208–1218.

27. Shear K, Frank E, Houck PR, et al. Treatment of complicated grief: a randomized controlled trial. *JAMA*. 2005;293:2601–2608.

28. Boelen PA, van den Hout MA, van den Bout J. A cognitive-behavioral conceptualization of complicated grief. *Clin Psychol Sci Pract*. 2006;13:109–128.

29. Stroebe M, Schut H. The dual process model of coping with bereavement: rationale and description. *Death Stud*. 1999;23:197–224.

30. Stroebe M, Stroebe W, Schut H, et al. Does disclosure of emotions facilitate recovery from bereavement? Evidence from two prospective studies. *J Consult Clin Psychol*. 2002;70:169–178.

31. Freed PJ, Mann JJ. Sadness and loss: toward a neurobiopsychosocial model. *Am J Psychiatry*. 2007;164:28–34.

32. O'Connor MF, Gundel H, McRae K, et al. Baseline vagal tone predicts BOLD response during elicitation of grief. *Neuropsychopharmacology*. 2007;32:2184–2189.

33. Pollock SE, Sands D. Adaptation to suffering: meaning and implications for nursing. *Clin Nurs Res*. 1997;6:171–185.

34. Thompson GN, Chochinov HM, Wilson KG, et al. Prognostic acceptance and the well-being of patients receiving palliative care for cancer. *J Clin Oncol*. 2009;27:5757–5762.

35. Ray A, Block SD, Friedlander RJ, et al. Peaceful awareness in patients with advanced cancer. *J Palliat Med*. 2006;9:1359–1368.

36. Levy LH. Anticipatory grief: its measurement and proposed reconceptualization. *Hosp J*. 1991;7:1–28.

37. Barry LC, Kasl SV, Prigerson HG. Psychiatric disorders among bereaved persons: the role of perceived circumstances of death and preparedness for death. *Am J Geriatr Psychiatry*. 2002;10:447–457.

38. Chochinov HM, Hassard T, McClement S, et al. The landscape of distress in the terminally ill. *J Pain Symptom Manage*. 2009;38:641–649.

39. Bedell SE, Cadenhead K, Graboys TB. The doctor's letter of condolence. *N Engl J Med*. 2001;344:1162–1164.

40. Lindemann E. Symptomatology and management of acute grief. *Am J Psychiatry*. 1944;101:141–148.

41. Prigerson HG, Maciejewski PK. Grief and acceptance as opposite sides of the same coin: setting a research agenda to study peaceful acceptance of loss. *Br J Psychiatry*. 2008;193:435–437.

42. Goldsmith B, Morrison R, Vanderwerker L, et al. Elevated rates of prolonged grief disorder in African Americans. *Death Stud*. 2008;32:352–365.

43. Kübler-Ross E. *On death and dying*. New York: Macmillan; 1969.

44. Bowlby J. Processes of mourning. *Int J Psychoanal*. 1961;42:317–340.

45. Maciejewski PK, Zhang B, Block SD, et al. An empirical examination of the stage theory of grief. *JAMA*. 2007;297:716–723.

46. Bonanno GA. Loss, trauma, and human resilience: have we underestimated the human capacity to thrive after extremely aversive events? *Am Psychol*. 2004;59:20–28.

47. Zisook S, Shuchter SR. Depression through the first year after the death of a spouse. *Am J Psychiatry*. 1991;148:1346–1352.

48. Kendler KS, Myers J, Zisook S. Does bereavement-related major depression differ from major depression associated with other stressful life events? *Am J Psychiatry*. 2008;165:1449–1455.

49. American Psychiatric Association. *Diagnostic and statistical manual of mental disorders*. 4th ed. Washington, DC: American Psychiatric Association; 2000 text revision (DSM-IV-TR).

50. Lichtenthal WG, Cruess DG, Prigerson HG. A case for establishing complicated grief as a distinct mental disorder in DSM-V. *Clin Psychol Rev*. 2004;24:637–662.

51. Silverman GK, Johnson JG, Prigerson HG. Preliminary explorations of the effects of prior trauma and loss on risk for psychiatric disorders in recently widowed people. *Israel J Psychiatry Rel Sci*. 2001;38:202–215.

52. Latham AE, Prigerson HG. Suicidality and bereavement: complicated grief as psychiatric disorder presenting greatest risk for suicidality. *Suicide Life Threat Behav*. 2004;34:350–362.

53. Prigerson HG, Bierhals AJ, Kasl SV, et al. Traumatic grief as a risk factor for mental and physical morbidity. *Am J Psychiatry*. 1997;154:616–623.

54. Ott CH. The impact of complicated grief on mental and physical health at various points in the bereavement process. *Death Stud*. 2003;27:249–272.

55. Stroebe M, Schut H, Finkenauer C. The traumatization of grief? A conceptual framework for understanding the trauma-bereavement interface. *Israel J Psychiatry Rel Sci*. 2001;38:185–201.

56. Wijngaards-de Meij L, Stroebe M, Schut H, et al. Patterns of attachment and parents' adjustment to the death of their child. *Person Soc Psychol Bull*. 2007;33:537–548.

57. van Doorn C, Kasl SV, Beery LC, et al. The influence of marital quality and attachment styles on traumatic grief and depressive symptoms. *J Nerv Mental Dis*. 1998;186:566–573.

58. Carr D, House JS, Kessler RC, et al. Marital quality and psychological adjustment to widowhood among older adults: a longitudinal analysis. *J Gerontol B Psychol Sci Soc Sci*. 2000;55:S197–S207.

59. Cleiren M, Diekstra RFW, Kerkhof AJ, et al. Mode of death and kinship in bereavement: focusing on "who" rather than "how.". *Crisis*. 1994;15:22–36.

60. Johnson JG, Zhang B, Greer JA, et al. Parental control, partner dependency, and complicated grief among widowed adults in the community. *J Nerv Mental Dis*. 2007;195:26–30.

61. Vanderwerker LC, Prigerson HG. Social support and technological connectedness as protective factors in bereavement. *J Loss Trauma.* 2004;9:45–57.

62. Costantini-Ferrando MF, Foley KM, Rapkin BD. Communicating with patients about advanced cancer. *JAMA.* 1998;280:1403.

63. Mack JW, Nilsson M, Balboni T, et al. Peace, Equanimity, and Acceptance in the Cancer Experience (PEACE): validation of a scale to assess acceptance and struggle with terminal illness. *Cancer.* 2008;112:2509–2517.

64. Rando TA. *Parental loss of a child.* Champaign, IL: Research Press Co; 1986.

65. Kreicbergs U, Valdimarsdottir U, Onelov E, et al. Anxiety and depression in parents 4–9 years after the loss of a child owing to a malignancy: a population-based follow-up. *Psychol Med.* 2004;34:1431–1441.

66. Lannen PK, Wolfe J, Prigerson HG, et al. Unresolved grief in a national sample of bereaved parents: impaired mental and physical health 4 to 9 years later. *J Clin Oncol.* 2008;26:5870–5876.

67. Barrera M, O'Connor K, D'Agostino NM, et al. Early parental adjustment and bereavement after childhood cancer death. *Death Stud.* 2009;33:497–520.

68. Mack JW, Hilden JM, Watterson J, et al. Parent and physician perspectives on quality of care at the end of life in children with cancer. *J Clin Oncol.* 2005;23:9155–9161.

69. Allumbaugh D, Hoyt W. Effectiveness of grief therapy: a meta-analysis. *J Couns Psychol.* 1999;46:370–380.

70. Kato PM, Mann T. A synthesis of psychological interventions for the bereaved. *Clin Psychol Rev.* 1999;19:275–296.

71. Currier JM, Holland JM, Neimeyer RA. The effectiveness of bereavement interventions with children: a meta-analytic review of controlled outcome research. *J Clin Child Adolesc Psychol.* 2007;36:253–259.

72. Currier JM, Neimeyer RA, Berman JS. The effectiveness of psychotherapeutic interventions for the bereaved: a comprehensive quantitative review. *Psychol Bull.* 2008;134:648–661.

73. Jordan JR, Neimeyer RA. Does grief counseling work? *Death Stud.* 2003;27:765–786.

74. Larson DG, Hoyt WT. What has become of grief counseling? An evaluation of the empirical foundations of the new pessimism. *Prof Psychol Res Pract.* 2007;38:347–355.

75. Crits-Christoph P, Connolly MB. Empirical basis of supportive-expressive psychodynamic psychotherapy. In: Bornstein RF, Masling JM, eds. *Empirical studies of the therapeutic hour.* Washington, DC: American Psychological Association; 1998:109–151.

76. Luty SE, Carter JD, McKenzie JM, et al. Randomised controlled trial of interpersonal psychotherapy and cognitive-behavioural therapy for depression. *Br J Psychiatry.* 2007;190:496–502.

77. Piper WE, Ogrodniczuk JS, Joyce AS, et al. Group composition and group therapy for complicated grief. *J Consult Clin Psychol.* 2007;75:116–125.

78. Ogrodniczuk JS, Piper WE, Joyce AS, et al. Social support as a predictor of response to group therapy for complicated grief. *Psychiatry.* 2002;65:346–357.

79. Ogrodniczuk JS, Piper WE, Joyce AS, et al. NEO-five factor personality traits as predictors of response to two forms of group psychotherapy. *Int J Group Psychother.* 2003;53:417–442.

80. Kissane D, Lichtenthal WG, Zaider T. Family care before and after bereavement. *Omega (Westport).* 2007;56:21–32.

81. Lange A, Schrieken B, van de Ven J-P, et al. Interapy": the effects of a short protocolled treatment of posttraumatic stress and pathological grief through the Internet. *Behav Cogn Psychother.* 2000;28:175–192.

82. Joinson AN. Self-esteem, interpersonal risk, and preference for e-mail to face-to-face communication. *CyberPsycholog Behav.* 2004;7:472–478.

83. Boelen PA, de Keijser J, van den Hout MA, et al. Treatment of complicated grief: a comparison between cognitive-behavioral therapy and supportive counseling. *J Consult Clin Psychol.* 2007;75:277–284.

84. Fortner B, Neimeyer RA. *The effectiveness of grief counseling and therapy: a quantitative review.* San Antonio, TX: Annual Meeting of the Association for Death Education and Counseling, 1999.

85. Schut H, Stroebe M, van den Bout J, et al. The efficacy of bereavement interventions: determining who benefits. In: Stroebe M, Hansson R, et al., eds. *Handbook of bereavement research: consequences, coping, and care.* Washington, DC: American Psychological Association; 2001:705–738.

Index

Page numbers followed by b indicate boxes; f, indicate figures; t, indicate tables.